Red Book

D0356472

2015 REPORT OF THE COMMITTEE ON INFECTIOUS DISEASES
30TH EDITION

Author: Committee on Infectious Diseases,
American Academy of Pediatrics

David W. Kimberlin, MD, FAAP, Editor

Michael T. Brady, MD, FAAP, Associate Editor
Mary Anne Jackson, MD, FAAP, Associate Editor
Sarah S. Long, MD, FAAP, Associate Editor

American Academy of Pediatrics
141 Northwest Point Blvd
Elk Grove Village, IL 60007-1019

Suggested citation: American Academy of Pediatrics. [Chapter title.] In: Kimberlin DW, Brady MT, Jackson MA, Long SS, eds. *Red Book: 2015 Report of the Committee on Infectious Diseases.* 30th ed. Elk Grove Village, IL: American Academy of Pediatrics; 2015:[chapter page numbers]

30th Edition
1st Edition – 1938
2nd Edition – 1939
3rd Edition – 1940
4th Edition – 1942
5th Edition – 1943
6th Edition – 1944
7th Edition – 1945
8th Edition – 1947
9th Edition – 1951
10th Edition – 1952
11th Edition – 1955
12th Edition – 1957
13th Edition – 1961
14th Edition – 1964
15th Edition – 1966
16th Edition – 1970
16th Edition Revised – 1971
17th Edition – 1974
18th Edition – 1977
19th Edition – 1982
20th Edition – 1986
21st Edition – 1988
22nd Edition – 1991
23rd Edition – 1994
24th Edition – 1997
25th Edition – 2000
26th Edition – 2003
27th Edition – 2006
28th Edition – 2009
29th Edition – 2012

ISSN No. 1080-0131
ISBN No. 978-1-58110-926-9
MA0749

Quantity prices on request. Address all inquiries to:
American Academy of Pediatrics
141 Northwest Point Blvd
Elk Grove Village, IL 60007-1019

or Phone:
1-888-227-1770 Publications

The recommendations in this publication do not indicate an exclusive course of treatment or serve as a standard of medical care. Variations, taking into account individual circumstances, may be appropriate.

Publications from the American Academy of Pediatrics benefit from expertise and resources of liaisons and internal (AAP) and external reviewers. However, publications from the American Academy of Pediatrics may not reflect the views of the liaisons or the organizations or government agencies that they represent.

The American Academy of Pediatrics has neither solicited nor accepted any commercial involvement in the development of the content of this publication.

3-334/0415   1 2 3 4 5 6 7 8 9 10

Committee on Infectious Diseases, 2012-2015

Collaborators

Mark J. Abzug, MD, Children's Hospital Colorado and University of Colorado School of Medicine, Aurora, CO

Edward P. Acosta, PharmD, University of Alabama at Birmingham, Birmingham, AL

Paula Ehrlich Agger, MD, MPH, Food and Drug Administration, Silver Spring, MD

Iyabode Akinsanya-Beysolow, MD, MPH, Centers for Disease Control and Prevention, Atlanta, GA

Andrés Esteban Alarcón, MD, Food and Drug Administration, Silver Spring, MD

John J. Alexander, MD, MPH, Food and Drug Administration, Silver Spring, MD

Upton D. Allen, MBBS, MSc, FRCPC, The Hospital for Sick Children, University of Toronto, Toronto, Ontario, Canada

Maria C. Allende, MD, Food and Drug Administration, Silver Spring, MD

Jon R. Almquist, MD, University of Washington, Burien, WA

Alicia D. Anderson, DVM, MPH, Centers for Disease Control and Prevention, Atlanta, GA

Margot Anderson, MD, University of Malawi College of Medicine, Lilongwe, Malawi

Marsha Anderson, MD, University of Colorado School of Medicine, Aurora, CO

Jon Kim Andrus, MD, Pan American Health Organization, Washington, DC

Kristie E. Appelgren, MD, MSCR, Centers for Disease Control and Prevention, Atlanta, GA

Grace D. Appiah, MD, MS, Food and Drug Administration, Silver Spring, MD

Jorge Arana, MD, MPH, Centers for Disease Control and Prevention, Atlanta, GA

Paul M. Arguin, MD, Centers for Disease Control and Prevention, Atlanta, GA

Stephen S. Arnon, MD, California Department of Public Health, Richmond, CA

Negar Ashouri, MD, Children's Hospital of Orange County, Orange, CA

John W. Baddley, MD, MSPH, University of Alabama at Birmingham, Birmingham, AL

Carol J. Baker, MD, Baylor College of Medicine, Texas Children's Hospital, Houston, TX

M. Douglas Baker, MD, Johns Hopkins University, School of Medicine, Owings Mills, MD

Robert S. Baltimore, MD, Yale University School of Medicine, New Haven, CT

Elizabeth D. Barnett, MD, Maxwell Finland Laboratory for Infectious Diseases, Boston, MA

Allison H. Bartlett, MD, MS, The University of Chicago Medicine, Chicago, IL

Casey Barton Behravesh, MS, DVM, DrPH, Centers for Disease Control and Prevention, Atlanta, GA

Daniel G. Bausch, MD, MPH & TM, Tulane University Health Sciences Center, New Orleans, LA

Melisse S. Baylor, MD, Food and Drug Administration, Silver Spring, MD

Michael J. Beach, PhD, Centers for Disease Control and Prevention, Atlanta, GA

Judy A. Beeler, MD, Food and Drug Administration, Bethesda, MD

Ermias Belay, MD, Centers for Disease Control and Prevention, Atlanta, GA

Ozlem Belen, MD, MPH, Food and Drug Administration, Silver Spring, MD

David M. Bell, MD, Centers for Disease Control and Prevention, Atlanta, GA

Melissa Bell, BS, Centers for Disease Control and Prevention, Atlanta, GA

Kaitlin M. Benedict, MPH, Centers for Disease Control and Prevention, Atlanta, GA

Daniel K. Benjamin, Jr, MD, Duke University, Durham, NC

Sarah D. Bennett, MD, MPH, Centers for Disease Control and Prevention, Atlanta, GA

Tina J. Benoit, MPH, Centers for Disease Control and Prevention, Atlanta, GA

Henry H. Bernstein, DO, MHCM, Cohen Children's Medical Center of New York, New Hyde Park, NY

Niranjan Bhat, MD, Food and Drug Administration, Silver Spring, MD

Stephanie Bialek, MD, MPH, Centers for Disease Control and Prevention, Atlanta, GA

David D. Blaney, MD, MPH, Centers for Disease Control and Prevention, Atlanta, GA

Karen C. Bloch, MD, MPH, Vanderbilt University School of Medicine, Nashville, TN

Joseph A. Bocchini, Jr, MD, Louisiana State University Health Sciences Center-Shreveport, Shreveport, LA

Cheryl A. Bopp, MS, Centers for Disease Control and Prevention, Atlanta, GA

Suresh Babu Boppana, MD, University of Alabama at Birmingham, Birmingham, AL

Elizabeth A. Bosserman, MPH, Centers for Disease Control and Prevention, Atlanta, GA

Anna Bowen, MD, MPH, Centers for Disease Control and Prevention, Atlanta, GA

William Bower, MD, Centers for Disease Control and Prevention, Atlanta, GA

Heather Bradley, PhD, Centers for Disease Control and Prevention, Atlanta, GA

John S. Bradley, MD, Rady Children's Hospital San Diego, San Diego, CA

Michael T. Brady, MD, Nationwide Children's Hospital, Columbus, OH

Mary E. Brandt, PhD, Centers for Disease Control and Prevention, Atlanta, GA

Bernard M. Branson, MD, Centers for Disease Control and Prevention, Atlanta, GA

Joseph Bresee, MD, Centers for Disease Control and Prevention, Atlanta, GA

Elizabeth C. Briere, MD, MPH, Centers for Disease Control and Prevention, Atlanta, GA

William J. Britt, MD, University of Alabama at Birmingham Medical Center, Birmingham, AL

Karen R. Broder, MD, Centers for Disease Control and Prevention, Atlanta, GA

Kevin Brown, MD, Virus Reference Department, Public Health England, Colindale, London, United Kingdom

June M. Brown, BS, Centers for Disease Control and Prevention, Atlanta, GA

Patricia C. Brown, MD, Food and Drug Administration, Silver Spring, MD

Gary Brunette, MD, MS, Centers for Disease Control and Prevention, Alpharetta, GA

Heather M. Burke, MA, MPH, Centers for Disease Control and Prevention, Atlanta, GA

Barbara Burleigh, PhD, Harvard School of Public Health, Boston, MA

Jane L. Burns, MD, University of Washington School of Medicine, Seattle, WA

Jane C. Burns, MD, Rady Children's Hospital San Diego, La Jolla, CA

Gale R. Burstein, MD, MPH, Erie County Department of Health, Buffalo, NY

Carrie L. Byington, MD, University of Utah Health Science Center, Salt Lake City, UT

Carlos C. Campbell, MD, MPH, Program for Appropriate Technology in Health (PATH), Seattle, WA

Doug Campos-Outcalt, MD, MPA, American Academy of Family Physicians, Phoenix, AZ

Maria Cano, MD, MPH, Centers for Disease Control and Prevention, Atlanta, GA

Paul T. Cantey, MD, MPH, Centers for Disease Control and Prevention, Atlanta, GA

Michael Cappello, MD, Yale School of Medicine, New Haven, CT

Mary T. Caserta, MD, University of Rochester Medical Center, Rochester, NY

Corey Casper, MD, MPH, University of Washington, Seattle, WA

Larisa Cervenakova, MD, American Red Cross, Rockville, MD

Ellen G. Chadwick, MD, Ann & Robert H. Lurie Children's Hospital of Chicago, Chicago, IL

Rana Chakraborty, MD, MSc, FRCPCH, DPhil, Emory University, Atlanta, GA

Archana Chatterjee, MD, PhD, University of South Dakota, Sanford School of Medicine, Sioux Falls, SD

Rana Chattopadhyay, PhD, Food and Drug Administration, Silver Spring, MD

John C. Christenson, MD, Indiana University School of Medicine, Indianapolis, IN

Paul R. Cieslak, MD, Oregon Health Authority, Portland, OR

Angela Ahlquist Cleveland, MPH, Centers for Disease Control and Prevention, Atlanta, GA

Susan E. Coffin, MD, MPH, The Children's Hospital of Philadelphia, Philadelphia, PA

Amanda C. Cohn, MD, Centers for Disease Control and Prevention, Atlanta, GA

Melissa G. Collier, MD, MPH, Centers for Disease Control and Prevention, Atlanta, GA

Wayne Conlan, PhD, National Research Council Canada, Ottawa, Ontario, Canada

Jennifer R. Cope, MD, MPH, Centers for Disease Control and Prevention, Atlanta, GA

Judith U. Cope, MD, MPH, Food and Drug Administration, Silver Spring, MD

Margaret M. Cortese, MD, Centers for Disease Control and Prevention, Atlanta, GA

C. Buddy Creech, MD, MPH, Vanderbilt University School of Medicine and Monroe Carell, Jr. Children's Hospital, Nashville, TN

James E. Crowe, Jr, MD, Vanderbilt University Medical Center, Nashville, TN

Lee (Toni) A. Darville, MD, University of Pittsburgh, Children's Hospital of Pittsburgh of UPMC, Pittsburgh, PA

Gregory A. Dasch, PhD, Centers for Disease Control and Prevention, Atlanta, GA

Alma C. Davidson, MD, Food and Drug Administration, Silver Spring, MD

H. Dele Davies, MD, University of Nebraska Medical Center, Omaha, NE

Roberta L. DeBiasi, MD, Children's National Medical Center, George Washington University School of Medicine, Washington, DC

Walter N. Dehority, MD, MSc, University of New Mexico, Albuquerque, NM

Michael S. Deming, MD, MPH, Centers for Disease Control and Prevention, Atlanta, GA

Alicia Demirjian, MD, MMSc, Centers for Disease Control and Prevention, Atlanta, GA

Penelope H. Dennehy, MD, Alpert Medical School of Brown University and Hasbro Children's Hospital, Providence, RI

Dickson Despommier, PhD, Columbia University, New York, NY

Frank DeStefano, MD, MPH, Centers for Disease Control and Prevention, Atlanta, GA

Sahera Dirajlal-Fargo, MS, DO, Food and Drug Administration, Cleveland, OH

Thomas J. Doker, DVM, MPH, Centers for Disease Control and Prevention, Atlanta, GA

Sheila C. Dollard, PhD, Centers for Disease Control and Prevention, Atlanta, GA

Ken L. Dominguez, MD, MPH, Centers for Disease Control and Prevention, Atlanta, GA

Samuel R. Dominguez, MD, University of Colorado School of Medicine, Denver, CO

Jonathan Duffy, MD, MPH, Centers for Disease Control and Prevention, Atlanta, GA

Eileen F. Dunne, MD, MPH, Centers for Disease Control and Prevention Atlanta GA

Mark L. Eberhard, PhD, Centers for Disease Control and Prevention, Atlanta, GA

Kathryn M. Edwards, MD, Vanderbilt University, Nashville, TN

Morven S. Edwards, MD, Baylor College of Medicine, Houston, TX

Sean P. Elliott, MD, University of Arizona Health Network, Tucson, AZ

Dean D. Erdman, DrPH, Centers for Disease Control and Prevention, Atlanta, GA

Geoffrey Evans, MD, Former Director, Division of Vaccine Injury Compensation, HHS, Winchester, MA

Karen M. Farizo, MD, Food and Drug Administration, Silver Spring, MD

Meghan Ferris, MD, MPH, Food and Drug Administration, Silver Spring, MD

Amy Parker Fiebelkorn, MSN, MPH, Centers for Disease Control and Prevention, Atlanta, GA

Doran L. Fink, MD, PhD, Food and Drug Administration, Silver Spring, MD

Theresa M. Finn, PhD, Food and Drug Administration, Silver Spring, MD

Marc Fischer, MD, MPH, Centers for Disease Control and Prevention, Fort Collins, CO

Margaret C. Fisher, MD, The Unterberg Children's Hospital at Monmouth Medical Center, Long Branch, NJ

Collette Fitzgerald, PhD, Centers for Disease Control and Prevention, Atlanta, GA

Patricia M. Flynn, MD, St Jude Children's Research Hospital, Memphis, TN

LeAnne M. Fox, MD, MPH, DTM&H, Centers for Disease Control and Prevention, Atlanta, GA

Anne B. Francis, MD, University of Rochester Medical Center, Rochester, NY

Richard Franka, DVM, PhD, Centers for Disease Control and Prevention, Atlanta, GA

Robert W. Frenck, Jr, MD, Cincinnati Children's Hospital Medical Center, Cincinnati, OH

Sheila Friedlander, MD, University of California San Diego School of Medicine, San Diego, CA

Renee Galloway, MPH, Centers for Disease Control and Prevention, Atlanta, GA

Hayley A. Gans, MD, Stanford University Medical Center, Stanford, CA

Julianne Gee, MPH, Centers for Disease Control and Prevention, Atlanta, GA

Bruce Gellin, MD, MPH, National Vaccine Program Office, Washington, DC

Jon R. Gentsch, MSc, PhD, Centers for Disease Control and Prevention, Atlanta, GA

Susan I. Gerber, MD, Centers for Disease Control and Prevention, Atlanta, GA

Anne A. Gershon, MD, Columbia University Medical Center, New York, NY

Mayurika Ghosh, MD, Food and Drug Administration, Silver Spring, MD

Francis Gigliotti, MD, University of Rochester School of Medicine and Dentistry, Rochester, NY

Janet R. Gilsdorf, MD, University of Michigan Medical Center, Ann Arbor, MI

Lori M. Gladney, BS, Centers for Disease Control and Prevention, Atlanta, GA

Carol Ann Glaser, DVM, MPVM, MD, California Department of Public Health, Richmond, CA

Mary P. Glode, MD, University of Colorado School of Medicine, Children's Hospital Colorado, Golden, CO

Brittany Goldberg, MD, Food and Drug Administration, Silver Spring, MD

Richard L. Gorman, MD, National Institutes of Health, Bethesda, MD

Rachel Gorwitz, MD, MPH, Centers for Disease Control and Prevention, Atlanta, GA

L. Hannah Gould, MS, PhD, Centers for Disease Control and Prevention, Atlanta, GA

Sara H. Goza, MD, Fayetteville, GA

Kim Y. Green, PhD, National Institutes of Health, Bethesda, MD

Patricia M. Griffin, MD, Centers for Disease Control and Prevention, Atlanta, GA

Lisa A. Grohskopf, MD, MPH, Centers for Disease Control and Prevention, Atlanta, GA

Charles F. Grose, MD, University of Iowa, Iowa City, IA

Marta A. Guerra, DVM, MPH, PhD, Centers for Disease Control and Prevention, Atlanta, GA

Penina Haber, MPH, Centers for Disease Control and Prevention, Atlanta, GA

Caroline B. Hall, MD, University of Rochester School of Medicine & Dentistry, Rochester, NY

Aron J. Hall, DVM, MSPH, Centers for Disease Control and Prevention, Atlanta, GA

Scott A. Halperin, MD, Dalhousie University, Canadian Center for Vaccinology, Halifax, Nova Scotia, Canada

Theresa Harrington, MD, MPH&TM, Centers for Disease Control and Prevention, Atlanta, GA

Aaron Harris, MD, MPH, Centers for Disease Control and Prevention, Atlanta, GA

Jason B. Harris, MD, Massachusetts General Hospital, Boston, MA

Christopher J. Harrison, MD, Children's Mercy Hospital, Kansas City, MO

Joshua D. Hartzell, MD, Walter Reed National Military Medical Center, Potomac, MD

Amber K. Haynes, MPH, Centers for Disease Control and Prevention, Atlanta, GA

C. Mary Healy, MD, Baylor College of Medicine, Houston, TX

J. Owen Hendley, MD, University of Virginia School of Medicine, Charlottesville, VA

Katherine Hendricks Walters, MD, MPH&TM, Centers for Disease Control and Prevention, Atlanta, GA

Thomas W. Hennessy, MD, MPH, Centers for Disease Control and Prevention, Anchorage, AK

Adam L. Hersh, MD, PhD, University of Utah, Salt Lake City, UT

Barbara L. Herwaldt, MD, MPH, Centers for Disease Control and Prevention, Atlanta, GA

Beth Hibbs, RN, MPH, Centers for Disease Control and Prevention, Atlanta, GA

Sheila M. Hickey, MD, University of New Mexico, Albuquerque, NM

Carole J. Hickman, PhD, Centers for Disease Control and Prevention, Atlanta, GA

Lauri A. Hicks, DO, Centers for Disease Control and Prevention, Atlanta, GA

Alison Hinckley, PhD, Centers for Disease Control and Prevention, Fort Collins, CO

William P. Hitchcock, MD, Rady Children's Hospital, San Diego, CA

Michele C. Hlavsa, RN, MPH, Centers for Disease Control and Prevention, Atlanta, GA

Cynthia M. Holland-Hall, MD, MPH, Nationwide Children's Hospital, The Ohio State University College of Medicine, Columbus, OH

Scott Holmberg, MD, MPH, Centers for Disease Control and Prevention, Atlanta, GA

Karen W. Hoover, MD, MPH, Centers for Disease Control and Prevention, Atlanta, GA

Peter J. Hotez, MD, PhD, Baylor College of Medicine, Houston, TX

Christine Hughes, MPH, Centers for Disease Control and Prevention. Atlanta, GA

Dmitri Iarikov, MD, PhD, Food and Drug Administration, Silver Spring, MD

Joseph Icenogle, PhD, Centers for Disease Control and Prevention, Atlanta, GA

Shahed Iqbal, PhD, MBBS, MPH, Centers for Disease Control and Prevention, Atlanta, GA

Martha Iwamoto, MD, MPH, Centers for Disease Control and Prevention, Atlanta, GA

Marika K.Iwane, PhD, MPH, Centers for Disease Control and Prevention, Atlanta, GA

Mary Anne Jackson, MD, Children's Mercy Hospital, Kansas City, MO

Richard F. Jacobs, MD, Arkansas Children's Hospital, Little Rock, AR

Ruth A. Jajosky, DMD, MPH, Centers for Disease Control and Prevention, Atlanta, GA

John A. Jereb, MD, Centers for Disease Control and Prevention, Atlanta, GA

James F. Jones, MD, Centers for Disease Control and Prevention, Atlanta, GA

Jeffrey L. Jones, MD, MPH, Centers for Disease Control and Prevention, Atlanta, GA

Tim Jones, MD, Tennessee Department of Health, Nashville, TN
Sheldon L. Kaplan, MD, Baylor College of Medicine, Houston, TX
Cecilia Y. Kato, PhD, Centers for Disease Control and Prevention, Atlanta, GA
Carol A. Kauffman, MD, University of Michigan, Ann Arbor, MI
Gilbert J. Kersh, PhD, Centers for Disease Control and Prevention, Atlanta, GA
David L. Kettl, MD, Food and Drug Administration, Silver Spring, MD
Harry L. Keyserling, MD, Emory University School of Medicine, Atlanta, GA
Sarah Kidd, MD, MPH, Centers for Disease Control and Prevention, Atlanta, GA
Peter W. Kim, MD, MS, Food and Drug Administration, Silver Spring, MD
David W. Kimberlin, MD, University of Alabama at Birmingham, Birmingham, AL
Charles H. King, MD, Case Western Reserve University, Cleveland, OH
Robert D. Kirkcaldy, MD, MPH, Centers for Disease Control and Prevention, Atlanta, GA
Martin B. Kleiman, MD, Indiana University School of Medicine, Indianapolis, IN
Nicola Klein, MD, PhD, Kaiser Permanente Vaccine Study Center, Oakland, CA
R. Monina Klevens, DDS, Centers for Disease Control and Prevention, Atlanta, GA
Mark W. Kline, MD, Texas Children's Hospital, Houston, TX
Keith P. Klugman, MD, PhD, Bill and Melinda Gates Foundation, Seattle, WA
Athena P. Kourtis, MD, PhD, MPH, Centers for Disease Control and Prevention,
   Atlanta, GA
Philip R. Krause, MD, Food and Drug Administration, Silver Spring, MD
Andrew T. Kroger, MD, MPH, Centers for Disease Control and Prevention, Atlanta, GA
Matthew J. Kuehnert, MD, Centers for Disease Control and Prevention, Atlanta, GA
Preeta K. Kutty, MD, MPH, Centers for Disease Control and Prevention, Atlanta, GA
Paul M. Lantos, MD, Duke University, Greensboro, NC
Tatiana M. Lanzieri, MD, MPH, Centers for Disease Control and Prevention, Atlanta, GA
Lucia Lee, MD, Food and Drug Administration, Silver Spring, MD
Grace M. Lee, MD, MPH, Children's Hospital Boston, Boston, MA
Zanie C. Leroy, MD, MPH, Centers for Disease Control and Prevention, Chamblee, GA
Myron M. Levine, MD, DTPH, University of Maryland School of Medicine,
   Baltimore, MD
Linda L. Lewis, MD, Food and Drug Administration, Bethesda, MD
Jennifer L. Liang, DVM, MPVM, Centers for Disease Control and Prevention,
   Atlanta, GA
Allan S. Lieberthal, MD, Kaiser Permanente, Agoura Hills, CA
Jane E. Liedtka, MD, Food and Drug Administration, Silver Spring, MD
Jill A. Lindstrom, MD, Food and Drug Administration, Silver Spring, MD
Eloisa Llata, MD, MPH, Centers for Disease Control and Prevention, Atlanta, Ga
Mark N. Lobato, MD, Centers for Disease Control and Prevention, Atlanta, GA
Cortland Lohff, MD, MPH, Chicago Department of Public Health, Chicago, IL
Sarah S. Long, MD, St. Christopher's Hospital for Children, Philadelphia, PA
Benjamin A. Lopman, PhD, Centers for Disease Control and Prevention, Atlanta, GA
Bennett Lorber, MD, MACP, Temple University School of Medicine, Philadelphia, PA
Benjamin D. Lorenz, MD, Food and Drug Administration, Silver Spring, MD
Jessica R. MacNeil, MPH, Centers for Disease Control and Prevention, Atlanta, GA
Ryan A. Maddox, PhD, Centers for Disease Control and Prevention, Atlanta, GA
Barbara E. Mahon, MD, MPH, Centers for Disease Control and Prevention, Atlanta, GA
Yvonne A. Maldonado, MD, Stanford University School of Medicine, Stanford, CA

Mario J. Marcon, PhD, Ohio State University College of Medicine, Mt. Carmel Health System, Westerville, OH

S. Michael Marcy, MD, University of California Los Angeles, Los Angeles, CA

Harold Margolis, MD, Centers for Disease Control and Prevention, San Juan, PR

Mona Marin, MD, Centers for Disease Control and Prevention, Atlanta, GA

Lauri E. Markowitz, MD, Centers for Disease Control and Prevention, Atlanta, GA

Diana L. Martin, PhD, Centers for Disease Control and Prevention, Atlanta, GA

Kimberly C. Martin, DO, MPH, Food and Drug Administration, Silver Spring, MD

Daniel W. Martin, MSPH, Centers for Disease Control and Prevention, Atlanta, GA

Robert F. Massung, PhD, Centers for Disease Control and Prevention, Atlanta, GA

Anita McElroy, MD, PhD, Centers for Disease Control and Prevention, Atlanta, GA

Michael M. McNeil, MD, MPH, Centers for Disease Control and Prevention, Atlanta, GA

Jennifer H. McQuiston, DVM, MS, Centers for Disease Control and Prevention, Atlanta, GA

John R. McQuiston, PhD, Centers for Disease Control and Prevention, Atlanta, GA

Paul S. Mead, MD, MPH, Centers for Disease Control and Prevention, Fort Collins, CO

Felicita M. Medalla, MD, MS, Centers for Disease Control and Prevention, Atlanta, GA

H. Cody Meissner, MD, Tufts Medical Center, Boston, MA

Elissa Meites, MD, MPH, Centers for Disease Control and Prevention, Atlanta, GA

Joette M. Meyer, PharmD, Food and Drug Administration, Silver Spring, MD

Marian G. Michaels, MD, MPH, University of Pittsburgh School of Medicine, Pittsburgh, PA

Ian C. Michelow, MD, DTM&H, Warren Alpert Medical School of Brown University, Providence, RI

Elaine R. Miller, RN, MPH, Centers for Disease Control and Prevention, Atlanta, GA

Nancy B. Miller, MD, Food and Drug Administration, Silver Spring, MD

John F. Modlin, MD, Dartmouth Medical School, Lebanon, NH

Rajal K. Mody, MD, MPH, Centers for Disease Control and Prevention, Atlanta, GA

Tina Khoie Mongeau, MD, MPH, Food and Drug Administration, Silver Spring, MD

Susan P. Montgomery, DVM, MPH, Centers for Disease Control and Prevention, Atlanta, GA

Jose G. Montoya, MD, Stanford University School of Medicine, Palo Alto, CA

Matthew Moore, MD, MPH, Centers for Disease Control and Prevention, Atlanta, GA

Pedro L. Moro, MD, MPH, Centers for Disease Control and Prevention, Atlanta, GA

Dean S. Morrell, MD, University of North Carolina Department of Dermatology, Chapel Hill, NC

Samuel M. Moskowitz, MD, Massachusetts General Hospital for Children, Boston, MA

Trudy V. Murphy, MD, Centers for Disease Control and Prevention, Atlanta, GA

Dennis L. Murray, MD, Georgia Regents University Children's Hospital of Georgia, Augusta, GA

Henry W. Murray, MD, Weill Cornell Medical College, New York, NY

Oidda Ikumboka Museru, MSN, MPH, Centers for Disease Control and Prevention, Atlanta, GA

Angela L. Myers, MD, MPH, Children's Mercy Hospitals & Clinics, University of Missouri, Kansas City School of Medicine, Kansas City, MO

Martin G. Myers, MD, University of Texas Medical Branch, Annapolis, MD

Sumathi Nambiar, MD, MPH, Food and Drug Administration, Germantown, MD

Roger S. Nasci, PhD, Centers for Disease Control and Prevention, Fort Collins, CO

James P. Nataro, MD, PhD, MBA, University of Virginia Charlottesville, Charlottesville, VA

Eileen E. Navarro Almario, MD, Food and Drug Administration, Silver Spring, MD

Robyn Neblett Fanfair, MD, MPH, Centers for Disease Control and Prevention, Atlanta, GA

Karen P. Neil, MD, MSPH, Centers for Disease Control and Prevention, Atlanta, GA

Christina Nelson, MD, MPH, Centers for Disease Control and Prevention, Fort Collins, CO

Noele P. Nelson, MD, PhD, MPH, Centers for Disease Control and Prevention, Atlanta, GA

Steven R. Nesheim, MD, Centers for Disease Control and Prevention, Atlanta, GA

Jason G. Newland, MD, MEd, Children's Mercy Hospitals & Clinics, Kansas City, MO

William L. Nicholson, MS, PhD, Centers for Disease Control and Prevention, Atlanta, GA

Thomas B. Nutman, MD, National Institutes of Health, Bethesda, MD

Ann-Christine Nyquist, MD, MSPH, Children's Hospital Colorado, Aurora, CO

Richard A. Oberhelman, MD, Tulane University School of Medicine, New Orleans, LA

M. Steven Oberste, PhD, Centers for Disease Control and Prevention, Atlanta, GA

Paul A. Offit, MD, The Children's Hospital of Philadelphia, Philadelphia, PA

Ciara E. O'Reilly, PhD, Centers for Disease Control and Prevention, Atlanta, GA

Walter A. Orenstein, MD, Emory University, Atlanta, GA

Elizabeth O'Shaughnessy, MB, BCh, Food and Drug Administration, Silver Spring, MD

Gary D. Overturf, MD, University of New Mexico School of Medicine, Los Ranchos, NM

Laura Pabst, MPH, Centers for Disease Control and Prevention, Atlanta, GA

Mark A. Pallansch, PhD, Centers for Disease Control and Prevention, Atlanta, GA

Monica E. Parise, MD, Centers for Disease Control and Prevention, Atlanta, GA

Benjamin J. Park, MD, Centers for Disease Control and Prevention, Atlanta, GA

Manish Patel, MD, Centers for Disease Control and Prevention, Atlanta, GA

Andrew T. Pavia, MD, University of Utah, Salt Lake City, UT

Georgina Peacock, MD, MPH, Centers for Disease Control and Prevention, Atlanta, GA

Stephen Ira Pelton, MD, Boston University School of Medicine, Boston, MA

Carol Pertowski, MD, Centers for Disease Control and Prevention, Atlanta, GA

Thomas A. Peterman, MD, MSc, Centers for Disease Control and Prevention, Atlanta, GA

Clarence J. Peters, MD, University of Texas Medical Branch, Galveston, TX

Brett W. Petersen, MD, MPH, Centers for Disease Control and Prevention, Atlanta, GA

Larry K. Pickering, MD, Centers for Disease Control and Prevention, Atlanta, GA

Andreas Pikis, MD, Food and Drug Administration, Silver Spring, MD

Tamara Pilishvili, MPH, Centers for Disease Control and Prevention, Atlanta, GA

Ariel R. Porcalla, MD, MPH, Food and Drug Administration, Silver Spring, MD

Drew L. Posey, MD, MPH, Centers for Disease Control and Prevention, Atlanta, GA

Susan M. Poutanen, MD, MPH, FRCPC, Mount Sinai Hospital, Toronto, ON

R. Douglas Pratt, MD, Food and Drug Administration, Silver Spring, MD

Gary Procop, MD, MS, Cleveland Clinic, Cleveland, OH

Anne E. Purfield, PhD, Centers for Disease Control and Prevention, Atlanta, GA

Conrad P. Quinn, PhD, Centers for Disease Control and Prevention, Atlanta, GA

Roshan Ramanathan, MD, MPH, Food and Drug Administration, Silver Spring, MD

Octavio Ramilo, MD, Nationwide Children's Hospital & Ohio State University, Columbus, OH

Agam K. Rao, MD, Centers for Disease Control and Prevention, Atlanta, GA

Anuja Rastogi, MD, MHS, Food and Drug Administration, Silver Spring, MD

Mobeen H. Rathore, MD, University of Florida Center for HIV/AIDS Research, Jacksonville, FL

Jennifer S. Read, MD, MS, MPH, DTM&H, Food and Drug Administration, Rockville, MD

Sergio Recuenco, MD, MPH, DrPH, Centers for Disease Control and Prevention, Atlanta, GA

Joanna J. Regan, MD, MPH, Centers for Disease Control and Prevention, Atlanta, GA

Mary G. Reynolds, PhD, Centers for Disease Control and Prevention, Atlanta, GA

Frank O. Richards, Jr, MD, The Carter Center, Atlanta, GA

Jeffrey N. Roberts, MD, Food and Drug Administration, Silver Spring, MD

Joan Robinson, MD, University of Alberta, Edmonton Alberta, Canada

Pierre E. Rollin, MD, Centers for Disease Control and Prevention, Atlanta, GA

José R. Romero, MD, University of Arkansas for Medical Sciences, Arkansas Children's Hospital, Little Rock, AR

Sandra W. Roush, MT, MPH, Centers for Disease Control and Prevention, Atlanta, GA

Janell A. Routh, MD, MHS, Centers for Disease Control and Prevention, Atlanta, GA

Sharon L. Roy, MD, MPH, Centers for Disease Control and Prevention, Atlanta, GA

Lorry G. Rubin, MD, Hofstra North Shore-Long Island Jewish School of Medicine, New Hyde Park, NY

Francis E. Rushton, Jr, MD, University of South Carolina, Birmingham, AL

Marco Aurelio Palazzi Safadi, MD, Santa Casa de Sao Paulo School of Medicine, Sao Paulo, Brazil

Hugh A. Sampson, MD, Icahn School of Medicine at Mount Sinai, New York, NY

Pablo J. Sanchez, MD, Nationwide Children's Hospital, Columbus, OH

Mathuram Santosham, MD, MPH, Johns Hopkins University, Baltimore, MD

Jason B. Sauberan, PharmD, University of California San Diego Medical Center, San Diego, CA

Mark H. Sawyer, MD, University of California San Diego School of Medicine, Rady Children's Hospital San Diego, San Diego, CA

Sarah Schillie, MD, MPH, MBA, Centers for Disease Control and Prevention, Atlanta, GA

D. Scott Schmid, MS, PhD, Centers for Disease Control and Prevention, Atlanta, GA

Eileen Schneider, MD, MPH, Centers for Disease Control and Prevention, Atlanta, GA

Lawrence B. Schonberger, MD, MPH, Centers for Disease Control and Prevention, Atlanta, GA

Gordon E. Schutze, MD, Baylor College of Medicine, Houston, TX

Robert A. Schwartz, MD, MPH, University of Medicine & Dentistry of New Jersey, Newark, NJ

Ann Talbot Schwartz, MD, Food and Drug Administration, Gaithersburg, MD

Kathleen B. Schwarz, MD, The Johns Hopkins Hospital, Baltimore, MD

Ranee Seither, MPH, Centers for Disease Control and Prevention, Atlanta, GA

James J. Sejvar, MD, Centers for Disease Control and Prevention, Atlanta, GA

Rangaraj Selvarangan, BVSc, PhD, D(ABMM), Children's Mercy Hospital, Kansas City, MO

Deborah Sesok-Pizzini, MD, MBA, The Children's Hospital of Philadelphia, Philadelphia, PA

Jane F. Seward, MBBS, MPH, Centers for Disease Control and Prevention, Atlanta, GA

Sean V. Shadomy, DVM, MPH, Centers for Disease Control and Prevention, Atlanta, GA

Samir Suresh Shah, MD, Cincinnati Children's Hospital Medical Center, Cincinnati, OH

Hala Shamsuddin, MD, Food and Drug Administration, Silver Spring, MD

Andi L. Shane, MD, MPH, MSc, Emory Children's Center, Atlanta, GA

Eugene D. Shapiro, MD, Yale University, New Haven, CT

Alan M. Shapiro, MD PhD, Food and Drug Administration, Silver Spring, MD

Devindra Sharma, MSN, MPH, Centers for Disease Control and Prevention, Atlanta, GA

Tom T. Shimabukuro, MD, MPH, MBA, Centers for Disease Control and Prevention, Atlanta, GA

Stanford T. Shulman, MD, Ann & Robert H. Lurie Children's Hospital of Chicago, Chicago, IL

Benjamin J. Silk, PhD, MPH, Centers for Disease Control and Prevention, Atlanta, GA

Geoffrey R. Simon, MD, Nemours duPont Pediatrics, Wilmington, DE

Rosalyn J. Singleton, MD, MPH, Alaska Native Tribal Health Consortium, Anchorage, AK

Anders Sjöstedt, MD, PhD, Umeå University, Sweden

Bryce D. Smith, PhD, Centers for Disease Control and Prevention, Atlanta, GA

Rachel M. Smith, MD, MPH, Centers for Disease Control and Prevention, Atlanta, GA

Kirk Smith, DVM, MS, PhD, Minnesota Department of Health, St Paul, MN

Thomas D. Smith, MD, Food and Drug Administration, Silver Spring, MD

Sunil K. Sood, MD, Cohen Children's Medical Center of New York, Bay Shore, NY

Paul W. Spearman, MD, Emory University and Children's Healthcare of Atlanta, Atlanta, GA

Stanley M. Spinola, MD, Indiana University School of Medicine, Indianapolis, IN

Arjun Srinivasan, MD, Centers for Disease Control and Prevention, Atlanta, GA

Joseph W. St. Geme III, MD, The Children's Hospital of Philadelphia, Philadelphia, PA

Mary Allen Staat, MD, MPH, Cincinnati Children's Hospital Medical Center, Cincinnati, OH

J. Erin Staples, MD, PhD, Centers for Disease Control and Prevention, Fort Collins, CO

Jeffrey R. Starke, MD, Baylor College of Medicine, Houston, TX

William J. Steinbach, MD, Duke University, Durham, NC

Shannon Stokley, MPH, Centers for Disease Control and Prevention, Atlanta, GA

Raymond A. Strikas, MD, MPH, Centers for Disease Control and Prevention, Atlanta, GA

John R. Su, MD, PhD, MPH, Centers for Disease Control and Prevention, Atlanta, GA

John L. Sullivan, MD, University of Massachusetts Medical School, Worcester, MA

Wellington Sun, MD, Food and Drug Administration, Silver Spring, MD

Anil G. Suryaprasad, MD, Centers for Disease Control and Prevention, Atlanta, GA

Deborah F. Talkington, PhD, Centers for Disease Control and Prevention, Atlanta, GA

Jonathan L. Temte, MD, PhD, University of Wisconsin School of Medicine and Public Health, Madison, WI

Tina Q. Tan, MD, Northwestern University Feinberg School of Medicine, Chicago, IL

Eyasu H. Teshale, MD, Centers for Disease Control and Prevention, Atlanta, GA
Tejpratap S. P. Tiwari, MD, Centers for Disease Control and Prevention, Atlanta, GA
Melissa Tobin-D'Angelo, MD, MPH, Georgia Department of Public Health, Atlanta, GA
Suzanne R. Todd, DVM, Centers for Disease Control and Prevention, Atlanta, GA
Robert W. Tolan, Jr, MD, The Children's Hospital at Saint Peter's University Hospital,
    New Brunswick, NJ
Kay M. Tomashek, MD, MPH, DTM, Centers for Disease Control and Prevention,
    San Juan, PR
Elizabeth A. Torrone, MPSH, PhD, Centers for Disease Control and Prevention,
    Atlanta, GA
Rita M. Traxler, MHS, Centers for Disease Control and Prevention, Atlanta, GA
James R. Treat, MD, The Children's Hospital of Philadelphia, Philadelphia, PA
Richard W. Truman, PhD, Louisiana State University School of Veterinary Medicine,
    Baton Rouge, LA
Elizabeth R. Unger, PhD, MD, Centers for Disease Control and Prevention, Atlanta, GA
Tim Uyeki, MD, MPH, MPP, Centers for Disease Control and Prevention, Atlanta, GA
Chris Van Beneden, MD, MPH, Centers for Disease Control and Prevention, Atlanta, GA
John A. Vanchiere, MD, PhD, Louisiana State University, Health Sciences Center,
    Shreveport, LA
Tafadzwa S. Vargas-Kasambira, MD, MPH, Food and Drug Administration,
    Silver Spring, MD
Claudia Vellozzi, MD, MPH, Centers for Disease Control and Prevention, Atlanta, GA
Jennifer Rabke Verani, MD, MPH, Centers for Disease Control and Prevention,
    Atlanta, GA
Joseph M. Vinetz, MD, University of California San Diego School of Medicine,
    LaJolla, CA
Jan Vinje, PhD, Centers for Disease Control and Prevention, Atlanta, GA
Prabha Viswanathan, MD, Food and Drug Administration, Silver Spring, MD
Neil M. Vora, MD, Centers for Disease Control and Prevention, Atlanta, GA
Duc J. Vugia, MD, MPH, California Department of Public Health, Richmond, CA
Ken B. Waites, MD, University of Alabama at Birmingham, Birmingham, AL
Henry T. Walke, MD, MPH, Centers for Disease Control and Prevention, Atlanta, GA
Gregory S. Wallace, MD, MS, MPH, Centers for Disease Control and Prevention,
    Tucker, GA
Richard J. Wallace, Jr, MD, University of Texas Health Science Center at Tyler, Tyler, TX
Richard L. Wasserman, MD, PhD, Dallas Allergy, Dallas, TX
Donna L. Weaver, RN, MN, Centers for Disease Control and Prevention, Atlanta, GA
Cindy M. Weinbaum, MD, MPH, Centers for Disease Control and Prevention,
    Atlanta, GA
Michelle S. Weinberg, MD, MPH, Centers for Disease Control and Prevention,
    Atlanta, GA
Eric S. Weintraub, MPH, Centers for Disease Control and Prevention, Atlanta, GA
Richard J. Whitley, MD, Children's Hospital of Alabama, Birmingham, AL
Patricia P. Wilkins, PhD, Centers for Disease Control and Prevention, Atlanta, GA
Warren Williams, MPH, Centers for Disease Control and Prevention, Atlanta, GA
Rodney E. Willoughby, Jr, MD, Medical College of Wisconsin, Milwaukee, WI
JoEllen Wolicki, BSN, RN, Centers for Disease Control and Prevention, Atlanta, GA

Emily Jane Woo, MD, MPH, Food and Drug Administration, Silver Spring, MD
Dana Woodhall, MD, Centers for Disease Control and Prevention, Atlanta, GA
Kimberly A. Workowski, MD, Centers for Disease Control and Prevention, Atlanta, GA
Jonathan Wortham, MD, Centers for Disease Control and Prevention, Atlanta, GA
Mary A. Worthington, PharmD, BCPS, McWhorter School of Pharmacy, Stamford
    University, Birmingham, AL
Peter F. Wright, MD, Geisel School of Medicine at Dartmouth, Lebanon, NH
Albert C. Yan, MD, FAAD, The Children's Hospital of Philadelphia, University of
    Pennsylvania School of Medicine, Philadelphia, PA
Sixun Yang, MD, PhD, Food and Drug Administration, Silver Spring, MD
Yuliya Yasinskaya, MD, Food and Drug Administration, Silver Spring, MD
Zhiping Ye, MD, PhD, Food and Drug Administration, Silver Spring, MD
Jonathan S. Yoder, MPH, Centers for Disease Control and Prevention, Atlanta, GA
Theoklis E. Zaoutis, MD, MSCE, The Children's Hospital of Philadelphia,
    Philadelphia, PA
Jon E. Zibbell, PhD, Centers for Disease Control and Prevention, Atlanta, GA

AAP Bright Futures Steering Committee
AAP Committee on Child Abuse and Neglect
AAP Committee on Foster Care, Adoption, and Kinship Care
AAP Committee on Medical Liability and Risk Management
AAP Committee on Native American Child Health
AAP Committee on Nutrition
AAP Committee on Pediatric AIDS
AAP Committee on Practice and Ambulatory Medicine
AAP Council on Early Childhood
AAP Council on Environmental Health
AAP Council on Injury, Violence, and Poison Prevention
AAP Council on School Health
AAP Section on Allergy and Immunology
AAP Section on Bioethics
AAP Section on Breastfeeding
AAP Section on Child Abuse and Neglect
AAP Section on Epidemiology, Public Health, and Evidence
AAP Section on Gastroenterology, Hepatology, and Nutrition
AAP Section on Hematology/Oncology
AAP Section on Infectious Diseases
AAP Section on Nephrology
AAP Section on Ophthalmology
AAP Section on Pediatric Pulmonology and Sleep Medicine
AAP Section on Perinatal Pediatrics
AAP Section on Rheumatology
AAP Section on Tobacco Control

Committee on Infectious Diseases, 2012–2015

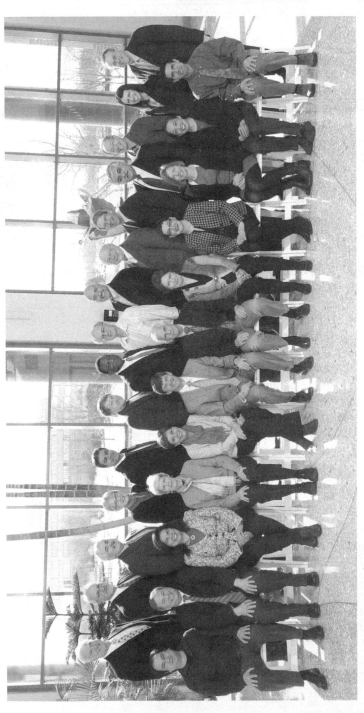

SEATED, LEFT TO RIGHT: Geoffrey R. Simon, Henry H. Bernstein, Yvonne A. Maldonado, Jane F. Seward, Mary Anne Jackson, David W. Kimberlin, Michael T. Brady, Sarah S. Long, Carrie L. Byington, Joan L. Robinson, Tina Q. Tan, Marc Fischer

STANDING, LEFT TO RIGHT: Rodney E. Willoughby, Jr, Gordon E. Schutze, Richard L. Gorman, Kathryn M. Edwards, Marco Aurelio Palazzi Safadi, Dennis L. Murray, H. Dele Davies, Jeffrey R. Starke, Theoklis E. Zaoutis, Joseph A. Bocchini, Jr, Mark H. Sawyer, Mobeen H. Rathore, Walter A. Orenstein, Jennifer M. Frantz, H. Cody Meissner

NOT PICTURED: Elizabeth D. Barnett, Doug Campos-Outcalt, Karen M. Farizo, Bruce Gellin, Mary P. Glode, Harry L. Keyserling, Lucia H. Lee, Ann-Christine Nyquist, R. Douglas Pratt, Jennifer S. Read

2015 *Red Book* Dedication For Stanley A. Plotkin, MD, FAAP

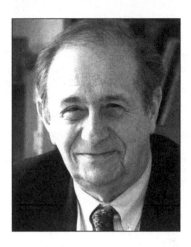

This edition of the *Red Book* is dedicated to Stanley A. Plotkin, MD, FAAP, who served on the AAP Committee on Infectious Diseases for 8 years, was chairman of this committee from 1987 to1990, and was *Red Book* Associate Editor for the 1982 and 1986 editions.

Stanley earned his Bachelor of Arts degree from New York University and then his Doctor of Medicine degree from the State University of New York Medical School in Brooklyn. Following an internship at Cleveland Metropolitan General Hospital and pediatric residency at the Children's Hospital of Philadelphia (CHOP) and the Hospital for Sick Children in London, Stanley served in the Epidemic Intelligence Service of the US Centers for Disease Control and Prevention (CDC). Stanley then joined the faculty at the University of Pennsylvania and at the Wistar Institute, where he rose to be the Director of Infectious Diseases and Senior Physician at the Children's Hospital of Philadelphia. While at the Wistar Institute, Stanley performed the pivotal trial showing that an anthrax vaccine prevents inhalational disease, collaborated with his lifelong mentor and friend, Hillary Koprowski, on an oral polio and rabies vaccine, and was the inventor of the RA27/3 strain of rubella vaccine, which has virtually eliminated congenital rubella syndrome from many countries throughout the world. While at CHOP, Stanley was the coinventor of the pentavalent rotavirus vaccine, now estimated to save hundreds of lives in the developing world, and conducted seminal studies on cytomegalovirus and varicella vaccines. In 1991, Stanley left the university setting to join Pasteur-Mérieux-Connaught, where he was Medical and Scientific Director. He now has emeritus appointments at Wistar and the University of Pennsylvania.

Stanley is a giant in the field of pediatric infectious diseases. He is the founding father of the Pediatric Infectious Diseases Society (PIDS), has published nearly 700 articles, and has edited several books, including *Vaccines*, the most complete work on vaccinology that now is in its 6th edition. Stanley was elected to the Institute of Medicine in 2005 and to the French Academy of Medicine in 2007. He has received scores of awards from around the world, including the French Legion of Honor Medal, the Sabin Foundation Medal, the Fleming Award of the Infectious Diseases Society of America, the Finland Award of the National Foundation for Infectious Disease, the Hilleman Award of the American Society for Microbiology, the Marshall Award of the European Society for Pediatric Infectious Diseases, and the Distinguished Physician Award of the Pediatric Infectious Diseases Society.

To this day, Stanley regularly attends international academic meetings such as IDWeek and the Pediatric Academic Societies annual meeting, and virtually every meeting of the Advisory Committee on Immunization Practices (ACIP) of the CDC. When Stanley approaches the microphone at ACIP meetings, all heads turn to hear his sage observations and comments, and the direction of the debate following such interjections frequently reflects his guidance. Stanley and his wife Susan's support of the next generation of physician scientists includes an endowment that they established in 2009 with PIDS that already has supported the career development of 3 pediatric infectious disease fellows as they begin promising academic careers.

A measure of one's life can be seen in the lives that are touched during our travels on this earth. Few men or women have touched more lives than Stanley Plotkin. Because of his passion and his genius, countless lives across scores of years have been kept whole. At the 2010 PIDS St. Jude's meeting for pediatric infectious diseases fellows, Stanley reflected back on the road that he has traveled, and guided those in attendance to "be patient… follow your dream." The world is a better place because of Stanley and his dreams. This edition of the *Red Book* is dedicated to Stanley as a small thank you on behalf of all the children and pediatricians whose lives are better through his contributions.

PREVIOUS RED BOOK DEDICATION RECIPIENTS:
2012 Samuel L. Katz, MD, FAAP
2009 Ralph Feigin, MD, FAAP
2006 Caroline Breese Hall, MD, FAAP
2003 Georges Peter, MD, FAAP
2000 Edgar O. Ledbetter, MD, FAAP
1997 Georges Peter, MD, FAAP

Preface

The *Red Book* is a unique and valuable source of information on infectious diseases and immunizations for practitioners who care for children. The practice of pediatric infectious diseases is changing rapidly. With the limited time available to the practitioner, the ability to quickly obtain current, accurate, and easily accessible information about new vaccines and vaccine recommendations, emerging infectious diseases, new diagnostic modalities, and treatment recommendations is essential. The Committee on Infectious Diseases of the American Academy of Pediatrics (AAP), the editors of the *Red Book*, and the 500 *Red Book* contributors are dedicated to providing the most current and accurate information available in the concise, practical format for which the *Red Book* is known.

Publishing is rapidly evolving, so the value of the *Red Book* is continuously enhanced by the *Red Book* Online (**www.aapredbook.org**). AAP policy statements, clinical reports, and technical reports and recommendations endorsed by the AAP are posted online as they become available during the 3 years between editions of *Red Book*. *Red Book* users are encouraged to sign up for e-mail alerts on **www.aapredbook.org** to receive new information and policy updates between editions. Another important resource is the visual library of *Red Book* Online, which has been updated and expanded to include more images of infectious diseases, examples of classic radiologic and other findings, and recent information on epidemiology of infectious diseases.

The Committee on Infectious Diseases relies on information and advice from many experts, as evidenced by the lengthy list of contributors to *Red Book*. We especially are indebted to the many contributors from other AAP committees, the American Thoracic Society, the Canadian Paediatric Society, the Centers for Disease Control and Prevention, the Food and Drug Administration, the National Institutes of Health, the National Vaccine Program Office, la Sociedad Latinoamericana de Infectología Pediátrica, the Pediatric Infectious Diseases Society, the World Health Organization, and many other organizations and individuals who have made this edition possible. In addition, suggestions made by individual AAP members to improve the presentation of information on specific issues and on topic selection have been incorporated into this edition.

Most important to the success of this edition is the dedication and work of the editors, whose commitment to excellence is unparalleled. Under the able leadership of David W. Kimberlin, MD, editor, with associate editors Michael T. Brady, MD, Mary Anne Jackson, MD, and Sarah S. Long, MD, this new edition was made possible. We also are indebted to H. Cody Meissner, MD, for his invaluable and untiring efforts to gather and organize the slide materials that make up the visual library of *Red Book* Online and are part of the electronic versions of the *Red Book*, and to Henry H. Bernstein, DO, MHCM, for his continuous efforts to maintain up-to-date content as editor of *Red Book* Online.

As noted in previous editions of the *Red Book*, some omissions and errors are inevitable in a book of this type. We ask that AAP members continue to assist the committee actively by suggesting specific ways to improve the quality of future editions.

Carrie L. Byington, MD, FAAP
Chair, Committee on Infectious Diseases

Introduction

The Committee on Infectious Diseases (COID) of the American Academy of Pediatrics (AAP) is responsible for developing and revising guidance for the AAP for control of infectious diseases in infants, children, and adolescents. Every 3 years, the committee issues the *Red Book: Report of the Committee on Infectious Diseases,* which contains a composite summary of current AAP recommendations representing the policy of the AAP on various aspects of infectious diseases, including updated vaccine recommendations for the most recent US Food and Drug Administration (FDA)-licensed vaccines for infants, children, and adolescents. These recommendations represent a consensus of opinions based on consideration of the best available evidence by members of the COID, in conjunction with liaison representatives from the Centers for Disease Control and Prevention (CDC), the FDA, the National Institutes of Health, the National Vaccine Program Office, the Canadian Paediatric Society, the American Thoracic Society, the Pediatric Infectious Diseases Society, *Red Book* consultants, and numerous collaborators. This edition of the *Red Book* is based on information available as of February 2015. The *Red Book* is formatted as hard copy, mobile app, and online Web version, with the electronic versions containing links to supplemental information, including visual images, graphs, maps, and tables. Policy updates between editions are posted on *Red Book* Online (**www.aapredbook.org**).

Preparation of the *Red Book* is a team effort in the truest sense of the term. Soon after publication of each *Red Book* edition, all *Red Book* chapters are sent for updates to primary reviewers who are leading national and international experts in their specific areas. For the 2015 *Red Book*, 62% of primary reviewers were new to this process, ensuring that the most up-to-date information has been included in this new edition. Following review by the primary reviewer, each chapter is returned to the assigned Associate Editor for incorporation of the reviewer's edits. The chapter then is disseminated to content experts at the CDC and FDA and to members of all AAP Sections that agree to review specific chapters for their additional edits as needed, following which it again is returned to the assigned Associate Editor for harmonization and incorporation of edits as appropriate. Two designated COID reviewers then complete their final review of the chapter, and it is returned to the assigned Associate Editor for inclusion of any needed additional modifications. Finally, each chapter is discussed and debated by the full committee at the COID "Marathon Meeting" held at the AAP during the spring of the year prior to publication, where it is finalized. Copyediting by the Editor and senior medical copy editor follows, and the book then is reviewed by the *Red Book* reviewers appointed by the AAP Board of Directors. In all, more than 1000 hands have touched the 2015 *Red Book* prior to its publication! That so many contributors dedicate so much time and expertise to this product is a testament to the role the *Red Book* plays in the care of children.

Through this deliberative and inclusive process, the COID endeavors to provide current, relevant, evidence-based recommendations for prevention and management of infectious diseases in infants, children, and adolescents. Seemingly unanswerable scientific questions, the complexity of medical practice, ongoing innovative technology, continuous new information, and inevitable differences of opinion among experts all are addressed during production of the *Red Book*. In some cases, other committees and experts may differ in their interpretation of data and resulting recommendations. In certain instances, no single recommendation can be made because several options for management are equally acceptable.

In making recommendations in the *Red Book*, the committee acknowledges differences in viewpoints by use of the phrases "most experts recommend..." and "some experts recommend..." Both phrases indicate valid recommendations, but the first phrase signifies more agreement and support among the experts. Inevitably in clinical practice, questions arise that cannot be answered easily on the basis of currently available data. When this happens, the COID still provides guidance and information that, coupled with clinical judgment, will facilitate well-reasoned, clinically relevant decisions. For many conditions, an expert in the field of infectious diseases should be consulted. The COID appreciates receiving questions, different perspectives, and alternative recommendations that will improve future editions of the *Red Book*. Through this process of lifelong learning, the committee seeks to provide a practical guide for physicians and other health care professionals in their care of infants, children, and adolescents.

To aid physicians and other health care professionals in assimilating current changes in recommendations in the *Red Book*, a list of major changes has been compiled (see Summary of Major Changes, p xxxiii). However, this list only begins to cover the many in-depth changes that have occurred in each chapter and section. Therefore, health care professionals should consult individual chapters and sections of the book for current guidance. Throughout the *Red Book*, Web site addresses enable rapid access to new information. In order to ensure widespread dissemination between editions, the AAP publishes new recommendations from the COID in *Pediatrics* and in *AAP News*. In addition, all AAP policies concerning infectious diseases published between editions of the *Red Book* will be posted on *Red Book* Online (**www.aapredbook.org**). Use of *Red Book* Online enables AAP members to enroll to receive e-mail alerts automatically when new information becomes available.

Information on use of antimicrobial agents is included in the package inserts (product labels) prepared by manufacturers, including contraindications and adverse events. The *Red Book* does not attempt to provide this information comprehensively, because it is available readily in the *Physicians' Desk Reference* (**www.pdr.net**) and in package inserts. As in previous editions of the *Red Book*, recommended dosage schedules for antimicrobial agents are provided (see Section 4, Antimicrobial Agents and Related Therapy) and may differ from those of the manufacturer as provided in the package insert. Physicians also can reference additional information in the package inserts of vaccines licensed by the FDA (which also may differ from COID and ACIP/CDC recommendations for use) and of immune globulins, as well as recommendations of other committees (see Sources of Vaccine Information, p 3), many of which are included in the *Red Book*.

This book could not have been prepared without the dedicated professional competence of many people. Joseph A. Bocchini, MD, Sara H. Goza, MD, H. Cody Meissner, MD, and Francis E. Rushton Jr, MD, served as *Red Book* reviewers appointed by the AAP Board of Directors.

The commitment of the AAP to the production of the *Red Book* starts at the very top, with the leadership of Errol R. Alden, MD. During his nearly 10-year tenure as Executive Director/CEO of the AAP, Dr. Alden has supported the production of 4 editions of the *Red Book*, including this one. As he retires from the AAP around the time of publication of the 2015 edition, we all express our gratitude for his unfailing commitment to the *Red Book* and the pediatricians and children that benefit from it.

The AAP staff has been outstanding in its committed work and contributions, particularly Jennifer Frantz, manager, who served as the administrative director for the COID and coordinated preparation of the *Red Book;* Jennifer Shaw, senior medical copy editor, who has improved every aspect of the *Red Book;* Linda Rutt, division assistant; Theresa Wiener, manager of publishing and production services; Jeff Mahony, Mark Grimes, and Mark Ruthman for their adaptation of the *Red Book* content to the online and app electronic versions; and the staff of the Department of Marketing, all of whom make the full *Red Book* product line possible.

Marc Fischer, MD, of the CDC, and R. Douglas Pratt, MD, and Lucia H. Lee, MD, of the FDA, devoted time and effort in providing significant input from their organizations. Special thanks is also due to Rangaraj Selvarangan, BVSc, PhD, D(ABMM), for his careful review of all diagnostic tests portions of the chapters in section 3. I am especially indebted to the associate editors Michael T. Brady, MD, Mary Anne Jackson, MD, and Sarah S. Long, MD, for their expertise, tireless work, good humor, and immense contributions in their editorial and committee work. Members of the COID contributed countless hours and deserve appropriate recognition for their patience, dedication, revisions, and reviews. The COID appreciates the guidance and dedication of the past and current COID chairpersons, Michael T. Brady, MD, and Carrie L. Byington, MD, respectively, whose knowledge, dedication, insight, and leadership are reflected in the quality and productivity of the committee's work. I thank my wife, Kim, for always being there and for her patience, understanding, and never-ending support as this edition of the *Red Book* came to fruition.

There are many other contributors whose professional work and commitment have been essential in the committee's preparation of the *Red Book.* Of special note is the person to whom this edition of the *Red Book* is dedicated, Stanley A. Plotkin, MD, truly a giant in the field of pediatric infectious diseases whose lifetime of work has improved the lives and health of literally millions of people worldwide.

David W. Kimberlin, MD, FAAP
Editor

Table of Contents

SECTION 2
RECOMMENDATIONS FOR CARE OF CHILDREN
IN SPECIAL CIRCUMSTANCES

SECTION 3
SUMMARIES OF INFECTIOUS DISEASES

SECTION 4
ANTIMICROBIAL AGENTS AND RELATED THERAPY

SECTION 5
ANTIMICROBIAL PROPHYLAXIS

APPENDICES

Summary of Major Changes in the 2015 *Red Book*

MAJOR CHANGES: GENERAL

1. To ensure that the information presented in the *Red Book* is based on the most accurate and up-to-date scientific data, the primary reviewers of each *Red Book* chapter were selected for their specific academic expertise in each particular area. In this edition of the *Red Book*, 62% of the primary reviewers were new for their assigned chapters. This ensures that the *Red Book* content is viewed with fresh eyes with each publication cycle.

2. Every chapter of the *Red Book* has been modified since the 2012 edition. The listing below outlines the more major changes throughout the 2015 edition.

3. All Diagnostic Tests portions of the pathogen-specific chapters in Section 3 were reviewed by a single microbiology laboratory director to ensure that they include the state-of-the-art diagnostic modalities.

4. Throughout the *Red Book*, the number of Web sites where additional current and future information can be obtained has been updated. All Web sites are in bold type for ease of reference, and all have been verified for accuracy and accessibility.

5. Reference to evidence-based policy recommendations from the American Academy of Pediatrics (AAP), the Advisory Committee on Immunization Practices (ACIP) of the Centers for Disease Control and Prevention (CDC), and other select professional organizations have been updated throughout the *Red Book*.

6. Standardized approaches to disease prevention through immunizations, antimicrobial prophylaxis, and infection-control practices have been updated throughout the *Red Book*.

7. Wording regarding doxycycline has been harmonized throughout the *Red Book*. Tetracycline-based antimicrobial agents, including doxycycline, may cause permanent tooth discoloration for children younger than 8 years if used for repeated treatment courses. However, doxycycline binds less readily to calcium compared with older tetracyclines, and in some studies, doxycycline was not associated with visible teeth staining in younger children (see Tetracyclines, p 873).

8. Policy updates released after publication of this edition of the *Red Book* will be posted on *Red Book* Online.

9. Appropriate chapters throughout the *Red Book* have been updated to be consistent with AAP and CDC 2015 vaccine recommendations, CDC sexually transmitted disease guidelines, CDC recommendations for immunization of health care personnel, and drug recommendations from *2015 Nelson's Pediatric Antimicrobial Therapy*. (Bradley JS, Nelson JD, Cantey JB, Kimberlin DW, Leake JAD, Palumbo PE, Sauberan J, Steinbach WJ, eds. 21st ed. Elk Grove Village, IL: American Academy of Pediatrics; 2015), as well as recommendations for treatment and prevention of opportunistic infections among children infected with or exposed to human immunodeficiency virus (HIV) from the CDC, National Institutes of Health, and Infectious Diseases Society of America.

10. Several tables and figures have been added for ease of information retrieval.
11. The appendices have been consolidated where appropriate, decreasing the number from 13 to 8 and increasing the ease of data retrieval.

SECTION 1. ACTIVE AND PASSIVE IMMUNIZATION

1. An expanded presentation of discussing the benefits of immunization and addressing parental questions about vaccines has been consolidated in **Informing Patients and Parents** about vaccination rather than in multiple areas of Section 1.
2. Discussion of vaccine ingredients, conjugating agents, preservatives, stabilizers, and adjuvants has been greatly expanded under **Vaccine Ingredients**.
3. Also under **Vaccine Ingredients**, the AAP extends its strongest support to the recent Strategic Advisory Group of Experts (SAGE) on immunization recommendations to retain the use of thimerosal in the global vaccine supply. **(www.who. int/wer/2012/wer8721.pdf).** As advocates for the health of all children, the AAP strongly supports global immunization efforts and recognizes that these programs rely on multidose vials, which require a preservative to ensure vaccine safety. A recent World Health Organization (WHO) assessment supported the continued use of thimerosal-containing vaccines and noted that immunization prevents approximately 2.5 million deaths a year globally **(www.who.int/biologicals/ Report_THIMEROSAL_WHO_Mtg_3-4_April_2012.pdf).** The preponderance of available evidence has failed to demonstrate harm associated with thimerosal in vaccines.
4. **Vaccine Handling and Storage** has been enhanced, consistent with the renewed emphasis on equipment and procedures as outlined in the June 2012 Office of the Inspector General report.
5. **Managing Injection Pain** has been significantly expanded on the basis of recent evidence-based recommendations.
6. **Inactivated influenza vaccine (IIV) and 13-valent pneumococcal conjugate vaccine (PCV13) can be administered simultaneously**, as outlined under the Simultaneous Administration of Multiple Vaccines.
7. **Tuberculosis (TB) testing** relative to administration of live–virus vaccines has been harmonized with advances in recommendations on TB testing in general, as outlined in the **Tuberculosis** chapter and the recent AAP Technical Report published in December 2014.
8. The difference between coincidental and causal relationships of a suspected adverse event following vaccination have been expanded upon in the **Vaccine Safety** chapter. Discussion of the **Brighton Collaborative** has been incorporated in this chapter as well.
9. Information regarding the FDA's **Postlicensure Rapid Immunization Safety Monitoring (PRISM) system** has been added to discussion of active surveillance of vaccine safety.
10. Explanation of the services and benefits provided by the CDC's **Clinical Immunization Safety Network (CISA)** has been expanded.
11. The distinction between **vaccine contraindications and precautions** is clarified and expanded in the **Vaccine Safety** portion of Section 1.
12. **Table 1.12, Managing Immune Globulin Intravenous (IGIV) Reactions,** has been added.

13. Because in the United States animal serum immune globulins are available only from the CDC, information on **desensitization to animal serum products** has been removed from the *Red Book*.

14. Recommendations on **tetanus toxoid, reduced diphtheria toxoid, and acellular pertussis vaccine (Tdap) administration with each pregnancy** have been updated in the **Immunization in Special Clinical Circumstances** and the **Pertussis** chapters.

15. **Immunization in Immunocompromised Children** has been completely restructured to provide general principles of vaccination in this population as well as to deal in specifics with examples a practitioner is likely to encounter. The new section is harmonized with the 2013 Infectious Diseases of America (IDSA) Clinical Practice Guideline for Vaccination of the Immunocompromised Host, with references to this document being provided for additional specific examples and unusual circumstances.

16. The discussion of **biologic response modifiers** has been expanded to include preventive strategies that should be employed prior to use of these agents, as well as specific vaccine recommendations.

17. **Central nervous system anatomic barrier defects** have been added to the consideration of vaccination of immunocompromised children.

18. **Active Immunization After Exposure to Disease** has been deleted as a chapter in Section 1, and all of the information incorporated into the disease-specific chapters in Section 3.

19. **Children in Residential Institutions** has been deleted as a chapter in Section 1, and all of the information has been incorporated into the disease-specific chapters in Section 3.

20. Discussion of an **accelerated schedule of routine vaccination** has been added to the presentation of immunization in US children living outside of the United States.

21. Use of a **meningococcal serogroup B vaccine in college settings** has been added to the discussion of immunization in college populations.

22. Presentations of **immunizations received outside of the United States** and **unknown or uncertain immunization status of vaccines received in the United States** have been consolidated into 1 chapter and expanded in scope.

SECTION 2. RECOMMENDATIONS FOR CARE OF CHILDREN IN SPECIAL CLINICAL CIRCUMSTANCES

1. The list of **potential bioterrorism agents** that US public health system and primary health care providers must be prepared to address has been updated and is consistent with guidance from the CDC.

2. A preference for **hand washing** over alcohol-based hand sanitizers for prevention of *Clostridium difficile* and **norovirus** infections has been emphasized.

3. **Human papillomavirus (HPV) vaccination** is recommended **following sexual victimization**; in such circumstances, the HPV vaccine series should be started as early as 9 years of age.

4. **Diagnosis and Treatment of Sexually Transmitted Infections in Adolescents and Children** have been updated to harmonize with new AAP and CDC guidelines.

5. Screening for sexually transmitted infections in **children who are victims of sexual abuse** has been updated to harmonize with new AAP and CDC guidelines.
6. The chapters on **evaluation of internationally adopted children, refugees, and immigrant children** have been consolidated and completely revised.
7. **Tuberculosis testing modalities** have been updated by age.
8. Recommendations have been added for **repeating HIV serologic testing in children who acquire hepatitic C virus** following a needlestick from a discarded needle.

SECTION 3. SUMMARIES OF INFECTIOUS DISEASES

1. **Actinomycosis.** Exclusively oral therapy for cases of cervicofacial actinomycosis has been included.
2. **Amebiasis.** Identification of the trophozoites or cysts of *Entamoeba histolytica* provides definitive (rather than presumptive) diagnosis for intestinal tract amebiasis. Clarification has been added that the majority of infected individuals are asymptomatic. The recent association of *Entamoeba dispar* and *E moshkovskii* with intestinal and extraintestinal pathology, raising questions about whether they are always nonpathogenic, has been added to the chapter.
3. **Amebic Meningoencephalitis.** Miltefosine, available through the CDC (770-488-7100), has been added to the chapter as a treatment that has been used successfully *Naegleria fowleri*.
4. **Anthrax.** The chapter has been harmonized with the 2014 anthrax preparedness publications of the CDC and AAP.
5. **Arboviruses.** Licensure of the inactivated Vero cell culture-derived Japanese encephalitis vaccine (IXIARO [JE-VC]) in children has been added to the chapter. The expansion of **chikungunya virus** into the Caribbean, South America, and North America (local transmission in Florida) has been added to the chapter.
6. **Aspergillosis.** The epidemiology portion of the chapter has been expanded to include additional modes of transmission and specific times in which acquisition is more likely. Dosing of voriconazole and prioritization of second-line agents has been added to the chapter.
7. ***Bacillus cereus* Infections.** For intraocular *Bacillus cereus* infections, a recommendation has been added that an ophthalmologist should be consulted regarding use of intravitreal vancomycin therapy in addition to systemic therapy.
8. **Bacterial Vaginosis.** The diagnostic portion of the chapter has been updated and expanded, including use of rapid tests and molecular diagnostics.
9. **Infections With *Blastocystis hominis* and Other Subtypes.** The chapter has been broadened to include discussion of subtypes other than *Blastocystis hominis*.
10. **Blastomycosis.** The treatment portion of the chapter has been harmonized with recommendations from the Infectious Diseases Society of America (IDSA).
11. **Candidiasis.** Treatment recommendations have been harmonized with those of the IDSA.
12. ***Chlamydia trachomatis*.** Diagnostic evaluations for *Chlamydia trachomatis* were updated to harmonize with the 2014 AAP policy statement on screening for nonviral sexually transmitted infections in adolescents and young adults.
13. ***Clostridium difficile*.** The Treatment portion of the chapter has been expanded to more prominently include nitazoxanide and fecal transplant (intestinal microbiota transplantation).

14. **Coccidioidomycosis.** The increasing incidence in coccidioidomycosis over the past 15 years has been added to the chapter.

15. **Coronaviruses, Including SARS and MERS.** MERS-CoV, the human coronavirus that causes Middle Eastern respiratory syndrome, has been added to the chapter. Advancements in the diagnostics for the other human coronaviruses also have been updated.

16. **Cryptosporidiosis.** The occurrence of cryptosporidiosis in solid organ transplant patients has been emphasized.

17. **Cytomegalovirus Infection.** Diagnosis and treatment of congenital cytomegalovirus (CMV) infection and disease has been updated, including a recommendation to treat patients with symptomatic congenital CMV disease with or without central nervous system involvement for 6 months with oral valganciclovir.

18. **Dengue.** The clinical manifestations of dengue have been updated.

19. *Ehrlichia, Anaplasma,* **and Related Infections.** The diagnostic portion of the chapter has been updated, including enhanced presentation of molecular diagnostics. The list of human ehrlichiosis and anaplasmosis that occur worldwide has been expanded. Heartland virus also has been added to the differential diagnosis.

20. **Enterovirus (Nonpoliovirus).** The **enterovirus D68** outbreak during the summer and fall of 2014 has been incorporated into the chapter, including respiratory manifestations and the potential relationship with acute flaccid myelitis. Antiviral options for the management of enteroviral infections have been expanded. Parechoviruses have been separated out as their own specific chapter.

21. **Epstein-Barr Virus Infections.** The pathogenesis of Epstein-Barr virus has been expanded, and management of primary Epstein-Barr virus infections relating to return to sport activities has been updated.

22. *Escherichia coli* **and Other Gram-Negative Bacilli.** The diagnostic portion of the chapter has been updated, including enhanced presentation of molecular diagnostics. Recommendations for treatment of infections caused by carbapenemase-producing gram-negative organisms have been added.

23. *Escherichia coli* **Diarrhea.** New molecular diagnostic tests are discussed.

24. *Giardia intestinalis* **(formerly *Giardia lamblia* and *Giardia duodenalis*) Infections.** Treatment of *Giardia intestinalis* infections in HIV-infected people has been harmonized with recommendations from the IDSA.

25. **Gonococcal Infections.** Information on diagnosis and treatment of gonococcal infections has been updated extensively to harmonize with the 2014 AAP policy statement and CDC guidelines. This includes expanded recommendations for use of molecular diagnostic testing, and thorough presentation of treatment recommendations that have been modified in response to emerging antibiotic resistance and treatment failure data.

26. *Haemophilus influenzae* **Infections.** The HibMenCY vaccine has been added to the chapter. Vaccine recommendations have been updated for immunocompromised people and those with other underlying conditions.

27. *Helicobacter pylori* **Infections.** The treatment portion of the chapter has been harmonized with recent childhood guidelines from the European Society for Pediatric Gastroenterology, Hepatology and Nutrition and North American Society for Pediatric Gastroenterology, Hepatology and Nutrition.

28. **Hemorrhagic Fevers Caused by Arenaviruses.** Access to intravenous ribavirin in the management of Lassa fever has been added to the chapter.

29. **Hemorrhagic Fevers Caused by Bunyaviruses.** Discussion of Heartland virus has been added to the chapter.

30. **Hemorrhagic Fevers Caused by Filoviruses: Ebola and Marburg.** A new chapter on Hemorrhagic Fevers Caused by Filoviruses, including Ebola and Marburg, has been added to the *Red Book*. The chapter was released in advance of publication in November 2014 to aid in pediatric management of Ebola, marking the first time in its 77-year history that a *Red Book* chapter was released before publication.

31. **Hepatitis C.** Treatment advances, including protease inhibitors, polymerase inhibitors, and inhibitors of the nonstructural NS5A enzyme replication complex of hepatitis C virus, have been incorporated into the chapter.

32. **Herpes Simplex Virus.** The AAP management algorithm for infants born to women with active herpetic lesions has been added to the chapter. Diagnostic and management updates have been added to the portion of the chapter addressing neonatal herpes simplex virus infections.

33. **Human Herpesvirus 6.** Human herpesvirus 6 now is separated into 2 species: HHV-6A and HHV-6B. Previously, these were classified as 2 distinct subgroups known as variants A and B. With the designation as separate species, the number of known human herpesviruses has increased to 9.

34. **Human Immunodeficiency Virus.** The chapter has been updated with the new recommendations for treatment and prevention of opportunistic infections among children infected with or exposed to HIV from the CDC, National Institutes of Health, and Infectious Diseases Society of America. The natural history of the disease in the antiretroviral era also has been updated.

35. **Influenza.** The chapter has been updated to reflect the most recent seasons' epidemiology, including circulating strains. The discussion of molecular diagnostics has been expanded. Use of oseltamivir down to 2 weeks of age has been added, following the expansion of the ages for which the drug is licensed by the US Food and Drug Administration (FDA). Data on febrile seizures following concomitant use of IIV and PCV13 has been updated.

36. **Kawasaki Disease.** The identification of a respiratory virus by molecular testing does not necessarily exclude the diagnosis of Kawasaki disease in infants and children who otherwise meet diagnostic criteria. Wording also has been added that hemolysis requiring transfusion has occurred after IGIV treatment in children with Kawasaki disease because of isoagglutinins in the products; hemoglobin concentrations should be monitored after high/repeated-dose IGIV infusions in at-risk children.

37. **Leishmaniasis.** Clinical manifestations of leishmaniasis have been expanded. Treatment of cutaneous, mucosal, and visceral leishmaniasis has been updated with the oral agent miltefosine, now approved as treatment for infection caused by particular *Leishmania* species in patients who are at least 12 years of age, weigh at least 30 kg (66 pounds), and are not pregnant or breastfeeding.

38. **Leprosy.** The clinical manifestations of leprosy have been expanded, and the recommendation for routine household screening has been removed.

39. ***Listeria monocytogenes* Infections.** Options for the treatment of *Listeria monocytogenes* infections have been expanded, although penicillin and gentamicin remain the standards.

40. **Lyme Disease.** Treatment duration has been clarified, and antimicrobial agents of choice have been specified for select disease manifestations (eg, facial nerve palsy). Discussion of "chronic Lyme disease" and post-Lyme disease symptoms has been added.

41. **Measles.** Evidence of immunity for measles has been revised since the last publication of the *Red Book*. Use of Immune Globulin products for measles prevention, vaccination for people with HIV infection, and vaccination of health care personnel born before 1957 also have been updated. Management of exposed susceptible patients also has been expanded.

42. **Meningococcal Infections.** Vaccination ages and recommendations have been updated to account for recently licensed products and age indications. Ciprofloxicin has been added to rifampin as a drug of choice for most children in whom chemoprophylaxis is indicated.

43. **Microsporidia Infections.** Microsporidia infections in people who have received organ transplantation are emphasized to a greater extent than in previous editions. Treatment options for keratoconjunctival infections caused by microsporidia have been added.

44. *Mycoplasma pneumoniae* **Infections.** Presentation on the use of molecular diagnostics has been expanded. Recommendations limiting use of macrolide therapies in the outpatient setting, and especially among preschool-aged children, have been updated.

45. **Nocardiosis.** The diagnostic tests portion of the chapter has been expanded.

46. **Human Papillomavirus.** Human papillomavirus vaccine is recommended beginning at 9 years of age in children with suspected child sexual abuse. Additionally, information has been added on the 9-valent human papillomavirus vaccine that was licensed for use in the United States in December 2014.

47. **Human Parechovirus Infections.** A new chapter on human parechovirus infections has been incorporated into the *Red Book*. Previously, parechoviruses were included in the Enterovirus chapter.

48. **Pediculosis Capitis.** Language regarding use of lindane shampoo for the treatment of head lice has been strengthened from "no longer is recommended" in the 2012 *Red Book* to "should not be used in the treatment of pediculosis capitis" in the 2015 *Red Book*. A table has been added comparing the costs of the different over-the-counter and prescription treatment options.

49. **Pertussis (Whopping Cough).** The correlation of lack of natural booster events plus waning immunity since the most recent immunization, particularly when acellular pertussis vaccine is used for the entire immunization series, with the increased cases of pertussis reported in school-aged children, adolescents, and adults is addressed. The definition of "close contact" for purposes of postexposure prophylaxis has been added. Administration of Tdap to pregnant women with every pregnancy irrespective of previous Tdap history has been added. Contraindications and precautions language for Tdap has been streamlined.

50. **Pneumococcal Infections.** Vaccination recommendations using PCV13 and 23-valent pneumococcal polysaccharide vaccine (PPSV23) for the prevention of pneumococcal infections in high-risk patients 6 to 18 years of age have been updated.

51. **Poliovirus.** The status of the worldwide poliovirus eradication program has been added to the chapter. Clinical presentation and history also have been expanded, and new recommendations have been included for poliovirus vaccination among travelers who are residing for 4 or more consecutive weeks in countries with ongoing poliovirus transmission and are leaving those countries to go to polio-free countries.

52. **Polyomaviruses.** Additional treatments under evaluation have been added to the chapter.

53. **Prion Diseases: Transmissible Spongiform Encephalopathies.** New diagnostic tests in development have been added to the chapter.

54. **Q fever (*Coxiella burnetii* Infection).** Diagnosis and management have been updated in accordance with 2013 guidance from the CDC.

55. **Respiratory Syncytial Virus.** The chapter has undergone substantial modification. Management of bronchiolitis has been updated to include recommendations in the 2014 AAP bronchiolitis clinical practice guideline, including limitations on use of alpha- and beta-adrenergic agents and corticosteroids. Recommendations for use of palivizumab have been updated to reflect the 2014 AAP policy statement on palivizumab immunoprophylaxis. The most substantial change from previous guidance is the recommendation limiting use of palivizumab in preterm infants without chronic lung disease or congenital heart disease to those born at less than 29 weeks' gestational age.

56. **Rocky Mountain Spotted Fever.** Polymerase chain reaction detection of *R rickettsii* DNA in acute whole blood and serum specimens now is the diagnostic modality of choice for Rocky Mountain spotted fever, although a fourfold or greater rise in antigen-specific immunoglobulin G between acute and convalescent sera obtained 2 to 6 weeks apart also remains an acceptable way to confirm the diagnosis.

57. **Rotavirus Infections.** The chapter has been updated with current data on the small risk of intussusception from the currently licensed rotavirus vaccines in the United States.

58. ***Salmonella* Infections.** The recent recognition of invasive disease in sub-Saharan Africa caused by certain serovars of nontyphoidal *Salmonella* that are highly lethal and distinct genetically from their serovar counterparts causing pediatric disease in industrialized countries has been added to the chapter.

59. ***Shigella* Infections.** Antibiotic treatment options, including emerging resistance to azithromycin, have been added to the chapter.

60. **Staphylococcal Infections.** New data on methods of reducing skin and soft tissue infection recurrences attributable to *Staphylococcus aureus* have been added to the chapter.

61. **Group A Streptococcal Infections.** A more definitive recommendation has been added to the chapter stating that a throat swab specimen with a negative rapid antigen test result from children be submitted to laboratory for isolation of group A streptococci. Additionally, the recommended dosages for several antibiotics for the treatment of group A streptococcal pharyngitis have been updated.

62. **Group B Streptococcal Infections.** Recently defined long-term neurologic sequelae among survivors of neonatal group B streptococcal infections have been added to the chapter. A smart phone app has been developed to guide management of pregnant women and their infants regarding testing for group B streptococcal infection.

63. **Syphilis.** The chapter has been updated with recent epidemiologic data. Treponemal specific tests have been revised to include new assays that have been recently released or are in development.

64. **Tetanus.** Antibody kinetics following administration of tetanus toxoid and Tetanus Immune Globulin (TIG) have been added to the chapter.

65. **Tinea capitis.** A treatment table has been added to the chapter, detailing recommended treatment options.

66. ***Toxoplasma gondii* Infections.** The seasonality and the transmission within families of *Toxoplasma gondii* infections have been updated.

67. ***Trichomonas vaginalis* Infections.** The molecular diagnostic modalities and screening recommendations for diagnosis of *Trichomonas vaginalis* infections have been updated to harmonize with the 2014 AAP policy statement on screening for nonviral sexually transmitted infections in adolescents and young adults.

68. **Trichuriasis.** The treatment of choice for trichuriasis now is albendazole, because mebendazole no longer is available in the United States.

69. **Tuberculosis.** Tuberculosis testing modalities have been updated by age, including a flow diagram guiding the use of tuberculin skin test (TST) and interferon-g release assay (IGRA) by age and bacille Calmette-Guérin (BCG) immunization status that is consistent with the AAP technical report published in November 2014. Dosing of commonly used drugs for treatment of tuberculosis in infants, children, and adolescents has been harmonized with WHO dosing recommendations. Several treatment options are provided for management of latent tuberculosis infection, with prioritization provided by regimen to manage likelihood of satisfactory completion of therapy and, therefore, risk of development of resistance. Discussion of populations at risk of tuberculosis has been expanded.

70. **Diseases Caused by Nontuberculous Mycobacteria.** Cutaneous infections following cosmetic surgery increasingly are recognized among the diseases caused by nontuberculous mycobacteria. Recognition that biologic response modifiers increase the risk of nontuberculous mycobacterial disease has been added.

71. **Tularemia.** Gentamicin has been designated the treatment of choice for tularemia because of the limited availability of streptomycin.

72. **Varicella-Zoster Infections.** A flow diagram outlining management of exposures to people with varicella-zoster infections has been added.

73. ***Vibrio cholerae* Infections.** Antibiotic treatment recommendations for *Vibrio cholerae* infections are provided in a new table.

SECTION 4. ANTIMICROBIAL AGENTS AND RELATED THERAPY

1. The fluoroquinolone portion of the **Antimicrobial Agents and Related Therapy** chapter has been updated to include data recently incorporated into package inserts for this class of drug.

2. The **Antimicrobial Resistance and Antimicrobial Stewardship: Appropriate and Judicious Use of Antimicrobial Agents** chapter has been broadened and updated with the principles of antimicrobial stewardship, judicious use of antibiotics for respiratory tract infections, and antimicrobial resistance. Chapter content has been harmonized with AAP and CDC publications.

3. Information has been added on whether generic formulations are available for each of the antimicrobial agents in **Table 4.3: Antibacterial Drugs for Pediatric Patients Beyond the Newborn Period.**

4. The table on treatment of **Sexually Transmitted Infections** has been updated extensively to harmonize with the 2014 CDC sexually transmitted infection guidelines.

5. A table with the relative susceptibilities of different fungal species has been added to the **Antifungal Drugs for Systemic Fungal Infections** chapter.

6. Target concentrations for therapeutic drug monitoring for itraconazole and voriconazole have been added to the **Recommended Doses of Parenteral and Oral Antifungal Drugs** table.

7. The rapidly expanding repertoire of antiviral agents to treat hepatitis C virus infection has been added to the **Non-HIV Antiviral Drugs** table.

8. The **Drugs for Parasitic Infections** table has been completely revised to reflect up-to-date treatment guidance from the CDC Web site for each parasitic pathogen, rather than the periodically published *Medical Letter* that had been reproduced previously.

SECTION 5. ANTIMICROBIAL PROPHYLAXIS

1. The **Antimicrobial Prophylaxis** chapter has been updated to reflect results from the Randomized Intervention for Children with VesicoUreteral Reflux (RIVUR) study, sponsored by the National Institute of Diabetes and Digestive and Kidney Diseases, of chemoprophylaxis of recurrent febrile or symptomatic urinary tract infections.

2. The 2013 clinical practice guidelines on antimicrobial prophylaxis prior to and during surgery from the American Society of Health-System Pharmacists (ASHP), the IDSA, the Surgical Infection Society (SIS), and the Society for Healthcare Epidemiology of America (SHEA) have been incorporated into the **Antimicrobial Prophylaxis in Pediatric Surgical Patients** chapter. This includes use of preoperative nasal mupirocin and chlorhexidine baths for *Staphylococcus aureus* carriers to reduce the risk of deep surgical site infections as an adjunct to intravenous prophylaxis in adult cardiac and orthopedic surgery patients.

APPENDICES

1. The **Directory of Resources (Appendix I)** has been updated with current Web links and telephone numbers. Several additional vaccine safety Web sites have been added.

2. The **Codes for Commonly Administered Pediatric Vaccines/Toxoids and Immune Globulins (Appendix II)** has been updated with the *International Statistical Classification of Diseases and Related Health Problems, 10th Revision* (ICD-10) codes that are scheduled to be released on October 1, 2015.

3. The table of **Nationally Notifiable Infectious Diseases in the United States (Appendix IV)** has been updated to match those infectious agents listed at the time of publication of the 2015 *Red Book.*

4. Norovirus has been added as the most common cause of foodborne illness in **Prevention of Infectious Disease From Contaminated Food Products (Appendix VI).**

Active and Passive Immunization

⋯⋯⋯⋯⋯⋯⋯⋯⋯
PROLOGUE

The ultimate goal of immunization is control of infection transmission, elimination of disease, and eventually eradication of the pathogen that causes the infection and disease; the immediate goal is prevention of disease in people or groups. To accomplish these goals, physicians must make timely immunization a high priority in the care of infants, children, adolescents, and adults. The global eradication of smallpox in 1977, elimination of polio-myelitis disease from the Americas in 1991, elimination of year-round ongoing measles transmission in the United States in 2000 and in the Americas in 2002, and elimination of rubella and congenital rubella syndrome from the United States in 2004 serve as models for fulfilling the promise of disease control through immunization. These accomplishments were achieved by combining a comprehensive immunization program providing consistent, high levels of vaccine coverage with intensive surveillance and effective public health disease-control measures. The resurgence of pertussis and measles in the United States, however, illustrates how precarious the substantial gains to date can be without vigilant commitment by physicians, public health officials, and members of the public themselves. Worldwide eradication of polio, measles, and rubella remains possible through implementation of proven prevention strategies, but diligence must prevail until eradication is achieved, or success itself is imperiled.

High immunization rates, in general, have reduced dramatically the incidence of all vaccine-preventable diseases (see Tables 1.1 and 1.2, p 2) in the United States. Yet, because organisms that cause vaccine-preventable diseases persist in the United States and elsewhere around the world, continued immunization efforts must be maintained and strengthened. Discoveries in immunology, molecular biology, and medical genetics have resulted in burgeoning vaccine research. Licensing of new, improved, and safer vaccines; establishment of an adolescent immunization platform; development of vaccines against cancer (eg, human papillomavirus and hepatitis B vaccines); and application of novel vaccine-delivery systems promise to continue the advances in preventive medicine achieved during the course of the 20th century. The advent of population-based postlicensure studies of new vaccines facilitates detection of rare adverse events temporally associated with immunization that were undetected during large prelicensure clinical trials.

Each edition of the *Red Book* provides recommendations for immunization of infants, children, and adolescents. These recommendations, which are harmonized among the American Academy of Pediatrics (AAP), the Advisory Committee on Immunization Practices (ACIP) of the Centers for Disease Control and Prevention (CDC), and the American Academy of Family Physicians, are based on careful analysis of disease epidemiology, benefits, and risks of immunization; feasibility of implementation; and cost-benefit analysis. ACIP recommendations utilize Grading of Recommendations Assessment, Development and Evaluation (GRADE) in evaluating the evidence of benefits and risks for a given vaccine, further ensuring that the recommendations are evidence-based and objectively assessed. Use of trade names

Table 1.1. Comparison of 20th Century Annual Morbidity and Current Morbidity: Vaccine-Preventable Diseases[a]

Disease	20th Century Annual Morbidity[b]	2013 Reported Cases[c]	Percent Decrease
Smallpox	29 005	0	100
Diphtheria	21 053	0	100
Measles	530 217	184	>99
Mumps	162 344	438	>99
Pertussis	200 752	24 231	88
Polio (paralytic)	16 316	0	100
Rubella	47 745	9	>99
Congenital rubella syndrome	152	0	100
Tetanus	580	19	97
Haemophilus influenzae	20 000	18[d]	>99

[a]National Center for Immunization and Respiratory Diseases. Historical Comparisons of Vaccine-Preventable Disease Morbidity in the U.S. Atlanta, GA: Centers for Disease Control and Prevention.
[b]Roush SW, Murphy TV, Vaccine-Preventable Disease Table Working Group. Historical comparisons of morbidity and mortality for vaccine-preventable diseases in the United States. *JAMA.* 2007;298(18):2155-2163.
[c]Centers for Disease Control and Prevention. Notifiable diseases and mortality tables. *MMWR Morb Mortal Wkly Rep.* 2014;62(52):ND-719-ND-732. Available at: **www.cdc.gov/mmwr/mmwr_wk/wk_cvol.html.**
[d]*Haemophilus influenzae* type b (Hib) in children younger than 5 years. An additional 13 cases of Hib are estimated to have occurred among the 212 reports of *Haemophilus influenzae* (younger than 5 years) with unknown serotypes.

Table 1.2. Comparison of Prevaccine Era Estimated Annual Morbidity With Current Estimates: Vaccine-Preventable Diseases[a]

Disease	Prevaccine Era Annual Estimate	2012 Estimate	Percent Decrease
Hepatitis A	117 333[b]	2890[c]	98
Hepatitis B (acute)	66 232[b]	18 800[c]	72
Pneumococcus (invasive)			
All ages	63 067[b]	31 600[d]	50
<5 y	16 069[b]	1800[e]	89
Rotavirus (hospitalizations, <3 y)	62 500[f]	1250[g]	98
Varicella	4 085 120[b]	216 511[h]	95

[a]National Center for Immunization and Respiratory Diseases. Historical Comparisons of Vaccine-Preventable Disease Morbidity in the U.S. Atlanta, GA: Centers for Disease Control and Prevention
[b]Roush SW, Murphy TV, Vaccine-Preventable Disease Table Working Group. Historical comparisons of morbidity and mortality for vaccine-preventable diseases in the United States. *JAMA.* 2007;298(18):2155-2163
[c]Centers for Disease Control and Prevention. Viral Hepatitis Surveillance – United States, 2011. Available at: **www.cdc.gov/hepatitis/Statistics/2011Surveillance/.**
[d]Centers for Disease Control and Prevention. Active Bacterial Core Surveillance Provisional Report; *S. pneumoniae* 2012. Available at: **www.cdc.gov/abcs/reports-findings/survreports/spneu12.html.**
[e]Centers for Disease Control and Prevention. Active Bacterial Core Surveillance (unpublished data).
[f]Centers for Disease Control and Prevention. Prevention of rotavirus gastroenteritis among infants and children: recommendations of the Advisory Committee on Immunization Practices (ACIP). *MMWR Recomm Rep.* 2009;58(RR-02):1-25
[g]New Vaccine Surveillance Network 2012 data (unpublished); U.S. rotavirus disease now has biennial pattern.
[h]Centers for Disease Control and Prevention. Varicella Program 2012 data (unpublished).

and commercial sources in the *Red Book* is for identification purposes only and does not imply endorsement by the AAP. Internet sites referenced in the *Red Book* are provided as a service to readers and may change without notice; citation of Web sites does not constitute AAP endorsement.

SOURCES OF VACCINE INFORMATION

In addition to the *Red Book*, which is published every 3 years, physicians have evidence-based literature and other sources available to answer specific vaccine questions encountered in practice. Such sources include the following:

- *Pediatrics.* Policy statements developed by the Committee on Infectious Diseases (COID) providing updated recommendations are published in *Pediatrics* between editions of the *Red Book*. Policy statements also may be accessed via the American Academy of Pediatrics (AAP) Web site (**pediatrics.aappublications.org/site/ aappolicy/index.xhtml**). Recommendations of the COID become official when approved by the Board of Directors of the AAP and published in *Pediatrics*.

- The Recommended Immunization Schedule for Persons Age 0 Through 18 Years for the United States is published annually in February (**http://redbook. solutions.aap.org/SS/Immunization_Schedules.aspx**). This is a harmonized schedule developed by the AAP, Centers for Disease Control and Prevention (CDC), and American Academy of Family Physicians.

- *AAP News.* Policy statements (or statement summaries) from the COID often are published initially in *AAP News*, the monthly newsmagazine of the AAP (**http:// aapnews.aappublications.org**), to inform the membership promptly of new recommendations.

- *Red Book* **Online.** The AAP has vaccine status table link on Red Book Online (**http://aapredbook.aappublications.org/news/vaccstatus.xhtml**) to provide current information about the vaccine licensure process and AAP recommendations about vaccines listed in the table. This table is updated as changes occur.

- *Morbidity and Mortality Weekly Report (MMWR).* Published weekly by the CDC, the *MMWR* contains current vaccine recommendations, reports of specific disease activity, alerts concerning vaccine availability, changes in vaccine formulations, vaccine safety issues, policy statements, and other infectious disease and vaccine information. New and updated vaccine recommendations made by the ACIP are published as policy notes or as recommendation and reports in the *MMWR* and are posted on the CDC Web site (**www.cdc.gov/mmwr**). Recommendations of the ACIP are not official until endorsed by the CDC director and published in the *MMWR*.

- **Manufacturers' prescribing information (package inserts/product information).** Manufacturers provide product-specific information with each vaccine product. The product label must be in full compliance with US Food and Drug Administration (FDA) regulations pertaining to labeling for vaccines, including indications and usage, dosage and administration, contraindications, warnings and precautions, adverse reactions, use in specific populations, and clinical studies. Each product insert lists contents of the vaccine, including preservatives, stabilizers, antimicrobial agents, adjuvants, and suspending fluids. Vaccine prescribing information is accessible through the FDA Web site (**www.fda.gov/cber/vaccines.htm**). Most manufacturers maintain Web sites with current information concerning new vaccine releases and changes in labeling. Additionally, 24-hour contact telephone numbers for medical questions are available in the *Physicians' Desk Reference* (**www.pdr.net**). Indications contained in a product insert reflect data from clinical trials conducted by the sponsor and submitted to the FDA for drug licensure. The FDA does not issue guidelines or recommendations for vaccine use. In some instances, AAP recommendations for use of a vaccine differ from what is stated in the product insert.

- ***Health Information for International Travel (The Yellow Book).*** This useful monograph is published approximately every 2 years by the CDC as a guide to requirements of various countries for specific immunizations. The monograph also provides information about other vaccines recommended for travel in specific areas and additional information for travelers. This document can be purchased from Oxford University Press. This information also is available on the CDC Web site (**www.cdc. gov/travel**), which is updated frequently as circumstances change, including regarding travel watches, alerts, and warnings. For additional sources of information on international travel, see International Travel (p 101).

- **CDC materials.** The National Center for Immunization and Respiratory Diseases (NCIRD) of the CDC maintains a comprehensive Web site (**www.cdc.gov/ vaccines**) that includes a section for health care professionals to facilitate immunization delivery. The CDC has partnered with the AAP and American Academy of Family Physicians to develop "Provider Resources for Vaccine Conversations with Parents" (**www.cdc.gov/vaccines/hcp/patient-ed/conversations/index.html**). All current and past ACIP/CDC vaccine recommendations are available online (**www. cdc.gov/vaccines/acip/index.html**). A CDC textbook, *Epidemiology and Prevention of Vaccine-Preventable Diseases,* also referred to as the Pink Book, is available online (**www. cdc.gov/vaccines/pubs/pinkbook/index.html**) and provides comprehensive information on use and administration of childhood vaccines, as well as selected ACIP recommendations and other vaccine-related information (for purchase of the Pink Book, contact the Public Health Foundation at 877-252-1200 or visit **www.cdc. gov/vaccines/pubs/#text**). A CDC publication titled *Manual for Surveillance of Vaccine-Preventable Diseases* provides current guidance for surveillance for vaccine preventable diseases including laboratory confirmation and principles used to investigate and control cases and outbreaks of disease. The NCIRD publishes a series of brochures on immunization topics and produces a CD-ROM that contains a wide range of resources, including vaccine information statements (VISs) and the complete text of the Pink Book. To obtain CDC materials, contact the CDC information center (**www. cdc.gov/info**) or visit the NCIRD publication Web site (**www.cdc.gov/vaccines/ pubs/default.htm**).

- **Satellite broadcasts and Web-based training courses.** The NCIRD conducts several immunization-related "train the trainer" courses that are available on DVD, live via satellite and through the Internet via Webcast, Web-on-demand, or self-study sessions each year. Annual course offerings include the Immunization Update, Vaccines for International Travel, Influenza, and an 11-module introductory course on the Epidemiology and Prevention of Vaccine-Preventable Diseases. The course schedule, slide sets, and written materials can be accessed online (**www.cdc.gov/vaccines/ ed/default.htm**). In addition, each meeting of the ACIP in February, June, and

October is Webcast for viewing. See the CDC Web site (**www.cdc.gov/vaccines/ acip/index.html**) for details and specific dates.
- **CDC immunization information e-mail–based inquiry system.** This system responds to immunization-related questions submitted from health care professionals and members of the public. Individualized responses to inquiries typically are sent within 24 hours. Inquiries can be submitted online (**www.cdc.gov/vaccines/ about/contact/nipinfo_contact_form.htm**).
- **Independent sources of reliable immunization information.** Appendix I (p 975) provides a list of reliable immunization information resources, including facts concerning vaccine efficacy, clinical applications, schedules, and unbiased information about safety. Two resources comprehensively address concerns of practicing physicians: the National Network for Immunization Information (**www.immunizationinfo.org**), and the Immunization Action Coalition (**www.immunize.org**), which also provides state-specific requirements for immunizations.
- **Vaccine price list.** Information about pediatric and adolescent vaccines, types of packaging, and CDC and private-sector costs are available online (**www.cdc.gov/vaccines/ programs/vfc/awardees/vaccine-management/price-list/index.html**).
- **Other resources**[1] include the FDA and the Institute of Medicine; infectious disease and vaccine experts at university-affiliated hospitals, at medical schools and children's hospitals, and in private practice; and state immunization programs and local public health departments. Information can be obtained from state and local health departments about current epidemiology of diseases; immunization recommendations; legal requirements; public health policies; and nursery school, child care, and school health concerns or requirements. Information regarding global health matters can be obtained from the World Health Organization (**www.who.int/**).
- **Immunization schedulers.** Online on-time and catch-up immunization schedulers are available for use by parents, other care providers, and health care professionals. The schedulers are based on the recommended immunization schedules for children, adolescents, and adults. The schedulers, which can be downloaded, allow the user to determine vaccines needed by age and are useful for viewing missed or skipped vaccines quickly according to the recommended childhood and adult immunization schedules. The interactive vaccine schedules are available at the following sites:
  - Childhood scheduler (0 through 6 years of age): **www2a.cdc.gov/nip/kidstuff/ newscheduler_le/**
  - catch-up scheduler: **www.vacscheduler.org**
  - adolescent scheduler: **www.cdc.gov/vaccines/schedules/Schedulers/ adolescent-scheduler.html**
  - adult scheduler: **www.cdc.gov/vaccines/schedules/Schedulers/ adult-scheduler.html**

Several health care professional associations, nonprofit groups, universities, and government organizations provide Internet resources containing accurate immunization information.

---

[1]Appendix I, Directory of Resources, p 975.

HEALTH PROFESSIONAL ASSOCIATIONS

American Academy of Family Physicians (AAFP)
www.familydoctor.org
American Academy of Pediatrics (AAP)
www.aap.org/immunization
American Medical Association (AMA)
www.ama-assn.org
American Nurses Association (ANA)
www.nursingworld.org
Association of State and Territorial Health Officials (ASTHO)
www.astho.org
Association for Prevention Teaching and Research
www.aptmweb.org
National Medical Association (NMA)
www.nmanet.org

NONPROFIT GROUPS AND UNIVERSITIES

Allied Vaccine Group (AVG)
www.vaccine.org
Every Child By Two (ECBT)
www.ecbt.org
www.vaccinateyourbaby.org
GAVI Alliance
www.gavialliance.org
Health on the Net Foundation (HON)
www.hon.ch
History of Vaccines, The College of Physicians of Philadelphia
www.historyofvaccines.org
National Healthy Mothers, Healthy Babies Coalition (HMHB)
www.hmhb.org
Immunization Action Coalition (IAC)
www.immunize.org
Institute for Vaccine Safety (IVS), Johns Hopkins University
www.vaccinesafety.edu
Institute of Medicine (IOM)
www.iom.edu/?ID=4705
National Alliance for Hispanic Health
www.hispanichealth.org
National Network for Immunization Information (NNii)
www.immunizationinfo.org
Parents of Kids with Infectious Diseases (PKIDS)
www.pkids.org
Sabin Vaccine Institute
www.sabin.org

Texas Children's Hospital Vaccine Center
   www.texaschildrens.org/Locate/Departments-and-Services/Vaccine/
University of Pennsylvania
   www.vaccineethics.org
Vaccine Education Center at the Children's Hospital of Philadelphia
   www.vaccine.chop.edu
Vaccine Page
   www.vaccines.com
World Health Organization
   www.who.int/topics/immunization/en/

GOVERNMENT ORGANIZATIONS

Centers for Disease Control and Prevention (CDC)
   www.cdc.gov/vaccines
   www.cdc.gov/vaccinesafety
Food and Drug Administration (FDA)
   www.fda.gov/BiologicsBloodVaccines/Vaccines/
   ApprovedProducts/ucm093830.htm
National Vaccine Program Office (NVPO)
   www.hhs.gov/nvpo/
National Institute of Allergy and Infectious Diseases (NIAID)
   www3.niaid.nih.gov/topics/vaccines/default.htm

······································

DISCUSSING VACCINES WITH PATIENTS AND PARENTS

Patients and their parents and/or legal guardians should be informed about the benefits of vaccines in preventing diseases in immunized people and in their community and about possible risks of disease-preventive and therapeutic procedures, including immunizations. Questions should be encouraged, and adequate time should be allowed so that information is understood (**www.cdc.gov/vaccines/hcp/patient-ed/conversations/index.html**).

The National Childhood Vaccine Injury Act (NCVIA) of 1986 included requirements for notifying *all* patients and parents about vaccine benefits and risks. Whether vaccines are purchased with private or public funds, this legislation mandates that a vaccine information statement (VIS) be provided *each* time a vaccine covered under the National Vaccine Injury Compensation Program (VICP), established by the NCVIA, is administered (see Table 1.3, p 8). This applies in all settings, including clinics, offices, hospitals (eg, for the birth dose of hepatitis B vaccine), and pharmacies. The VIS must be provided at the time of the immunization and for take-away, if desired. For vaccines not yet included in the VICP, VISs are available but are not mandated unless the vaccine is purchased through a contract with the Centers for Disease Control and Prevention (CDC [ie, the

Vaccines for Children Program, state immunization grants, or state purchases through the CDC]). Physicians can verify that the VIS provided is the current version by noting the date of publication. Copies of current official VISs in English and Spanish are available online from the CDC (**www.cdc.gov/vaccines/pubs/vis/default.htm**). In addition, the Immunization Action Coalition (**www.immunize.org**) has both the official VIS documents as well as translations of many of the VIS into more than 40 other languages. Copies also can be obtained from the American Academy of Pediatrics (AAP), state and local health departments, and vaccine manufacturers or by sending a request through the CDC Internet hotline service (**www.cdc.gov/info**). Every attempt should be made to provide a VIS in the patient or caregivers' native language. If the translated VIS version is older than the current official VIS, it is acceptable to give the translated VIS even though it is not the most current.

The NCVIA requires that personnel administering VICP-covered vaccines, whether purchased with private or public funds, record in the patient's health record the information shown in Table 1.4, as well as confirmation that the relevant VIS was provided at the time of each immunization (see Record Keeping and Immunization Information Systems, p 40). For vaccines purchased through CDC contract, physicians are required to record the VIS date of publication as well as the date on which the VIS was provided to the patient or parent/legal guardian. Although VIS distribution and vaccine record-keeping requirements do not apply to privately purchased vaccines not covered by the VICP, the AAP recommends following the same record-keeping practices for all vaccines. The AAP also recommends recording the site and route of administration and vaccine expiration date when administering any vaccine.

Parents' or patients' signatures are not required by federal NCVIA but may be required by state law to indicate that they have read and understood material in the VIS. Health care professionals should be familiar with requirements of the state in which they practice; the health care professional always has the option to request a signature. Whether or not a signature is obtained, health care professionals should document in the chart that the VIS has been provided and discussed with the patient or parent/legal guardian.

Table 1.3. Guidance in Using Vaccine Information Statements (VISs)[a]

Distribution
Must be provided each time a VICP-covered vaccine is administered[b]
Must be given to patient (nonminor), parent, and/or legal representative[b,c]
Must be the current version[d]
Can provide (not substitute) other written materials or audiovisual aids in addition to VISs[e]

VICP indicates Vaccine Injury Compensation Program.
[a] VISs are available on the Centers for Disease Control and Prevention (CDC) Web site (**www.cdc.gov/vaccines/pubs/vis/default.htm**).
[b] Required under the National Childhood Vaccine Injury Act.
[c] Consenting adolescent may vary by state.
[d] Required by CDC regulations for vaccines purchased through CDC contract. See the VIS Web site for current versions.
[e] An electronic version of the VIS can be transmitted to the patient's electronic device.

Table 1.4. Documentation Requirements Under the National Childhood Vaccine Injury Act

Documentation in the patient's health record

Vaccine manufacturer, lot number, and date of administration[a]

Name and business address of the health care professional administering the vaccine[a]

Date that VIS is provided (and VIS publication date[b])

Site (eg, deltoid area) and route (eg, intramuscular) of administration and expiration date of the vaccine[c]

[a] Required under the National Childhood Vaccine Injury Act.
[b] Required by Centers for Disease Control and Prevention (CDC) regulations for vaccines purchased through CDC contract. See the VIS Web site for current versions.
[c] Recommended by the American Academy of Pediatrics.

Addressing Parents' Questions About Vaccine Safety and Effectiveness

People understand and react to information regarding vaccines on the basis of many factors, including past experience, education, perception of the risk of disease and the vaccine offered, ability to control risk, and personal values. Although parents receive information from multiple sources, they consider health care professionals their most trusted source of health information. Acknowledging parents' concerns, listening respectfully, and providing accurate information about both benefits and risks of vaccines helps forge a meaningful relationship. Several factors contribute to parental vaccine concerns, hesitancy, or lack of confidence in the benefits of vaccines, including: (1) lack of information about the vaccine being given and about immunizations in general; (2) lack of understanding of the severity of and communicability of vaccine-preventable diseases; (3) opposing information and misinformation from other sources (eg, alternative medicine practitioners, anti-vaccination organizations and Web sites, and some religious groups); (4) perceived risk of serious vaccine adverse effects; (5) mistrust of the source of information regarding vaccines (eg, vaccine manufacturer, the government); (6) concern regarding number of injections to be administered simultaneously; (7) delivery of information in a culturally insensitive manner or that is not tailored to individual concern; and (8) delivery of information at an inconvenient time or in a hurried manner. Some people view the risk of immunization as disproportionately greater than the risk of disease, in part because of the relative infrequency of vaccine-preventable diseases in the United States because of the success of the immunization program. Others may dwell on sociopolitical issues, such as mandatory immunization, informed consent, and the primacy of individual rights over that of societal benefit.

Health care professionals should determine, in general terms, what parents understand about vaccines their children will be receiving, the nature of their concerns, and what information should be provided to address their concerns.

Common Misconceptions About Immunizations and the Institute of Medicine Findings

Misconceptions and misinformation regarding vaccines must be addressed clearly. Table 1.5 includes facts that refute common misconceptions/myths about immunizations. Misconceptions that are contrary to the science-based evidence about vaccine safety and effectiveness are associated with delayed immunization and underimmunization. The Institute of Medicine (IOM) has performed a number of reviews of the scientific evidence of vaccine safety. In 2004, the IOM developed and published several conclusions after scientific expert review of the now-debunked hypotheses that either measles-mumps-rubella (MMR) vaccine or thimerosal-containing vaccines are associated with autism. Conclusions of the IOM were: (1) scientific evidence rejects a causal relationship between MMR vaccine and autism; (2) available funding for autism research should be channeled to more promising areas of inquiry; and (3) risk-benefit communication requires attention to the needs of both the scientific community and the public.

Table 1.5. Common Misconceptions/ Myths About Immunizations[a,b]

Claims	Facts
Natural methods of enhancing immunity are better than vaccinations.	The only "natural way" to be immune is to have the disease. Immunity from a preventive vaccine provides protection against disease when a person is exposed to it in the future. That immunity is usually similar to what is acquired from natural infection, although several doses of a vaccine may have to be given for a child to develop an adequate immune response.
Epidemiology—often used to establish vaccine safety—is not science but number crunching.	Epidemiology is a well-established scientific discipline that, among other things, identifies the cause of diseases and factors that increase a person's risk of acquiring a disease. It is also part of the science base that can distinguish a causal association from a temporal association (coincident in time).
Giving multiple vaccines at the same time causes an "overload" of the immune system.	Vaccination does not overburden a child's immune system; the recommended vaccines use only a small portion of the immune system's "memory." The Institute of Medicine (IOM) has concluded that there is no evidence that the immunization schedule is unsafe (see text).
Vaccines are ineffective.	Vaccines have spared millions of people the effects of devastating diseases.
Prior to the use of vaccinations, these diseases had begun to decline because of improved nutrition and hygiene.	In the 19th and 20th centuries, some infectious diseases began to be better controlled because of improvements in sanitation, clean water, pasteurized milk, and pest control. However, vaccine-preventable diseases decreased dramatically after the vaccines for those diseases were licensed and were given to large numbers of children.

Table 1.5. Common Misconceptions/Myths About Immunizations,[a,b] continued

Claims	Facts
Vaccines cause poorly understood illnesses or disorders, such as autism, sudden infant death syndrome (SIDS), immune dysfunction, diabetes, neurologic disorders, allergic rhinitis, eczema, and asthma.	Scientific evidence does not support these claims. See IOM reports.
Vaccines weaken the immune system.	Vaccinated children are not at greater risk of infection, regardless of cause. Importantly, natural infections like influenza, measles, and chickenpox do weaken the immune system, increasing the risk of other infections.
Giving many vaccines at the same time is untested.	Concomitant use studies require all new vaccines to be tested with existing vaccines. These studies are performed to ensure that new vaccines do not affect the safety or effectiveness of existing vaccines given at the same time and that existing vaccines administered at the same time do not affect the safety or effectiveness of new vaccines.
Vaccines can be delayed, separated, and spaced out without consequences.	Many vaccine-preventable diseases occur in early infancy. Optimal vaccine-induced immunity may require a series of vaccines over time. Any delay in receiving age-appropriate immunization increases the risk of diseases that vaccines are administered to prevent.

Adapted from: Myers MG, Pineda D. *Do Vaccines Cause That? A Guide for Evaluating Vaccine Safety Concerns.* Galveston, TX: Immunizations for Public Health; 2008:79.
[a] Institute of Medicine Reviews of Adverse Events After Immunization (p 44).
[b] Other common misconceptions are detailed online (**www.cdc.gov/vaccines/vac-gen/6mishome.htm**).

In 2011, the IOM reviewed evidence on the safety of 8 individual vaccines (**www.iom.edu/Reports/2011/Adverse-Effects-of-Vaccines-Evidence-and-Causality.aspx**) and, in 2013, the immunization schedule (**iom.edu/Reports/2013/The-Childhood-Immunization-Schedule-and-Safety.aspx**). Conclusions were: (1) few health problems are caused by or clearly associated with individual vaccines; and (2) there is no evidence that the immunization schedule is unsafe. The IOM specifically found no links between the immunization schedule and autoimmune diseases, asthma, hypersensitivity, seizures, child developmental disorders, learning or developmental disorders, or attention deficit or disruptive disorders. Additionally, use of nonstandard schedules is harmful, because it increases the period of risk of acquiring vaccine-preventable diseases and increases the risk of incomplete immunization.

Parents may be aware through the media, social media, or information from alternative Web sites about issues that may be portrayed as controversial regarding scheduled vaccines. Many issues about childhood vaccines communicated by these means are presented incompletely, inaccurately, and in an inflammatory way. When a parent initiates discussion about an alleged vaccine controversy, the health care professional should listen carefully and then nonjudgmentally but confidently and definitively discuss specific concerns using factual information and language appropriate for parents and other care providers.

Resources for Optimizing Communications With Parents About Vaccines

Vaccine information is available that can help health care professionals respond to questions and misconceptions about immunizations and vaccine-preventable diseases (see list of Internet resources for accurate immunization information, p 6). Helpful credible information sources that can be provided to parents or to which parents can be directed include the "Parent's Guide to Childhood Immunization" (**www.cdc.gov/vaccines**), the Centers for Disease Control and Prevention (CDC) Internet hotline service (**www. cdc.gov/info**), the American Academy of Pediatrics (AAP) Immunization Initiative Web site (**www2.aap.org/immunization/**), and the Vaccine Education Center at Children's Hospital of Philadelphia (**www.vaccine.chop.edu**).

The CDC, the AAP, and the American Academy of Family Physicians developed **"Provider Resources for Vaccine Conversations with Parents"** (**www.cdc. gov/vaccines/hcp/patient-ed/conversations/**). These educational materials build on the latest research in vaccine and communication science and are designed to help health care professionals remain current on vaccine topics; strengthen communication and trust between health care professionals and parents; and share with parents up-to-date, easy-to-use information about vaccines and vaccine-preventable diseases. People can download these materials and enroll for e-mail updates when new resources are posted (**www.cdc.gov/vaccines/hcp/patient-ed/conversations/**). The materials include the following:

- Strategies on Talking with Parents about Vaccines for Infants.
- Current vaccine safety topics, such as Understanding MMR and Vaccine Safety; Understanding Thimerosal, Mercury, and Vaccine Safety; Ensuring the Safety of US Vaccines; The Childhood Immunization Schedule; and more.
- Basic and in-depth fact sheets on 14 vaccine-preventable diseases for parents. Fact sheets are available in English and Spanish for a variety of reading levels, and many include stories of families whose children have experienced a vaccine-preventable disease.
- If You Choose Not to Vaccinate Your Child, Understand the Risks and Responsibilities shares the risks for parents who choose to delay or decline a vaccine and offers steps for parents to take to protect their child, family, and others.
- Interactive, online childhood immunization scheduler and waiting room videos, such as Get the Picture: Childhood Immunization Video.

Parental Refusal of Immunizations

Many parents have concerns related to 1 or 2 specific vaccines. Pediatricians and other health care providers should discuss benefits and risks of each vaccine, because a parent who is reluctant to accept administration of 1 vaccine may be willing to accept others. Parents who have concerns about administering multiple vaccines to a child in a single visit may have their concerns addressed by using methods to reduce the pain of injection (see Managing Injection Pain, p 30) or by using combination vaccines. Any schedule should adhere to age ranges of vaccine administration provided in the Recommended Immunization Schedule for Persons Age 0 Through 18 Years (**http://redbook. solutions.aap.org/SS/Immunization_Schedules.aspx**). Physicians also should explore the possibility that cost is a reason for refusing immunization and assist parents by helping them obtain recommended immunizations for their children.

Parents who refuse vaccines for their child should be advised that all states have laws prohibiting unimmunized children from attending school during outbreaks of vaccine-preventable diseases. Parents should be encouraged to read the applicable law(s) in their state. Information on state-specific religious, philosophical, and nonmedical exemptions for immunization is available online (**http://vaccinesafety.edu/cc-exem.htm**). Discussions about vaccine delay and refusal should be documented in the patient's health record and may decrease any potential liability should a vaccine-preventable disease occur in an unimmunized patient with resulting harm to them or to other children, including immunocompromised children or those too young to receive the vaccine, to whom they might spread the infection. This *informed refusal* documentation should note that the parent was informed about why the immunization was recommended, the risks and benefits of immunization, and the possible consequences of not being immunized. Parents also should be encouraged to inform health care providers when children who are not immunized are seeking care for an acute illness, because they could be a risk to other vulnerable children who might also be in the health care facility. A sample Refusal to Vaccinate form can be found on the AAP Web site (**www2.aap.org/immunization/ pediatricians/pdf/RefusaltoVaccinate.pdf**).

For all cases in which parents refuse vaccine administration for their child, pediatricians should make the most of their ongoing relationship with the family and revisit the immunization discussion on subsequent visits. Such repeated discussions should be documented in the health record. Continued refusal after adequate discussion should be acknowledged and no further action taken unless the child is put at additional risk of serious harm (eg, during an epidemic). Only then should state agencies be involved to override parental discretion on the basis of medical neglect. When significant differences in philosophy of care and concerns about practice of care (eg, recalling that a child is underimmunized at each sick visit and urgent call) emerge or poor quality of communication persists, a substantial level of distrust may develop. The pediatrician may choose to encourage the family to find another physician or practice after providing sufficient advance notice in writing to the patient or parent/legal guardian. The physician must provide medical care for a reasonable period until a new physician can be secured and in accordance with local and state regulations.

ACTIVE IMMUNIZATION

Active immunization involves administration of all or part of a microorganism or a modified product of a microorganism (eg, a toxoid, a purified antigen, or an antigen produced by genetic engineering) to evoke an immunologic response and clinical protection that mimics that of natural infection but usually presents little or no risk to the recipient. Immunization can result in antitoxin, antiadherence, anti-invasive, or neutralizing activity or other types of protective humoral or cellular responses in the recipient. Some vaccines provide nearly complete and lifelong protection against disease, some provide protection against the more severe manifestations and/or consequences of the infection if exposed, and some must be readministered periodically to maintain protection. The immunologic response to vaccination is dependent on the type and dose of antigen, the effect of adjuvants, and host factors related to age, preexisting antibody, nutrition, concurrent disease, or drug effect and genetics of the host. The effectiveness of a vaccine is assessed by evidence of protection against the natural disease. Induction of antibodies is an indirect measure of protection (eg, antitoxin against *Clostridium tetani* or neutralizing antibody against measles virus), but for some infectious diseases, an immunologic response that correlates with protection is understood poorly, and serum antibody concentration does not always predict protection.

Vaccines are categorized as live (viral or bacterial, which almost always are attenuated) or inactivated ("nonlive"). The term "inactivated vaccines," for simplicity, includes antigens that are toxoids or other purified proteins, purified polysaccharides, protein-polysaccharide or oligosaccharide conjugates, inactivated whole or partially purified viruses, and proteins assembled into virus-like participles. Vaccines recommended routinely for immunocompetent individuals are updated annually in the harmonized schedule developed by the AAP, Centers for Disease Control and Prevention (CDC), and American Academy of Family Physicians (**http://redbook.solutions.aap.org/SS/Immunization_Schedules.aspx**) and for simplicity are referred to as "on the annual immunization schedule." Vaccines licensed for use in the United States are listed in Table 1.6 (p 15). The US Food and Drug Administration (FDA) maintains and updates a Web site listing vaccines and all components licensed for immunization and distribution in the United States with supporting documents (**www.fda.gov/BiologicsBloodVaccines/vaccines/ApprovedProducts/ucm093830.htm**). Appendix II provides the *Current Procedural Terminology* (CPT) and *International Classification of Diseases* (ICD-9 and ICD-10) codes used for vaccine administration.

Among currently licensed vaccines in the United States, there are 2 live-attenuated bacterial vaccines (oral typhoid and bacille-Calmette Guérin vaccines) and several live-attenuated viral vaccines. Although active bacterial or viral replication ensues after administration of these vaccines, because the pathogen has been attenuated, infection is modified greatly and little or no illness or other effect occurs. Vaccines for some viruses (eg, hepatitis A, hepatitis B, human papillomavirus) and most bacteria are inactivated, component, subunit (purified components) preparations or inactivated toxins. Some vaccines contain purified bacterial polysaccharides conjugated chemically to immunobiologically active proteins (eg, tetanus toxoid, nontoxic variant of mutant diphtheria toxin, meningococcal outer membrane protein complex). Viruses and bacteria in inactivated, subunit, and conjugate vaccine preparations are not capable of replicating in the host; therefore, these vaccines must contain a sufficient antigen content and possibly include an adjuvant to stimulate a desired response. In the case of conjugate polysaccharide vaccines, the linkage between the polysaccharide and the carrier protein enhances vaccine immunogenicity. Maintenance of long-lasting immunity with inactivated viral or bacterial vaccines and toxoid vaccines may require periodic administration of booster doses. Although inactivated vaccines may not elicit the range of immunologic response provided by live-attenuated agents, efficacy of licensed inactivated vaccines in children is high. For example, an injected inactivated viral vaccine may evoke sufficient serum antibody or cell-mediated immunity but evoke only minimal mucosal antibody in the form of secretory immunoglobulin (Ig) A. Mucosal protection after administration of inactivated vaccines generally is inferior to mucosal immunity induced by live-attenuated vaccines. Nonetheless, the demonstrated efficacy for such vaccines against invasive infection is high. Bacterial polysaccharide conjugate vaccines (eg, *Haemophilus influenzae* type b and pneumococcal conjugate vaccines) reduce nasopharyngeal colonization through exudated IgG. Viruses and bacteria in inactivated vaccines cannot replicate in or be excreted by the vaccine recipient as infectious agents and, thus, do not present the same safety concerns for

Table 1.6. Vaccines Licensed for Immunization and Distributed in the United States and Their Routes of Administration[a]

Vaccine	Type	Route of Administration
Adenovirus	Live viruses	Oral
BCG	Live bacteria	ID (preferred) or SC
Diphtheria-tetanus (DT, Td)	Toxoids	IM
DTaP	Toxoids and inactivated bacterial components	IM
DTaP, hepatitis B, and IPV	Toxoids and inactivated bacterial components, recombinant viral antigen, inactivated virus	IM
DTaP-IPV	Toxoids and inactivated bacterial components, inactivated virus	IM
DTaP-IPV/Hib (PRP-T reconstituted with DTaP-IPV)	Toxoids and inactivated bacterial components, polysaccharide-protein conjugate, inactivated virus	IM
Hepatitis A	Inactivated virus	IM
Hepatitis B	Recombinant viral antigen	IM
Hepatitis A-hepatitis B	Inactivated virus and recombinant viral antigens	IM
Hib conjugate	Bacterial polysaccharide-protein conjugate	IM
Hib conjugate (meningococcal protein conjugate)	Bacterial polysaccharide-protein conjugate	IM
Hib conjugate (PRP-T) meningococcal conjugate CY	Bacterial polysaccharide-protein conjugate combined with bacterial polysaccharide	IM
Human papillomavirus (HPV2, HPV4, and HPV9)	Recombinant viral antigens	IM
Influenza	Inactivated viral components	IM
Influenza	Live-attenuated viruses	Intranasal
Japanese encephalitis	Inactivated virus	IM
Meningococcal polysaccharide (MPSV4)	Bacterial polysaccharide	SC
Meningococcal conjugate (MCV4)	Bacterial polysaccharide-protein conjugate	IM
Meningococcal serogroup B	Bacterial lipoprotein	IM

Table 1.6. Vaccines Licensed for Immunization and Distributed in the United States and Their Routes of Administration,[a] continued

Vaccine	Type	Route of Administration
MMR	Live-attenuated viruses	SC
MMRV	Live-attenuated viruses	SC
Pneumococcal polysaccharide (PPSV23)	Bacterial polysaccharide	IM or SC
Pneumococcal conjugate (PCV13)	Bacterial polysaccharide-protein conjugate	IM
Poliovirus (IPV)	Inactivated viruses	SC or IM
Rabies	Inactivated virus	IM
Rotavirus (RV1 and RV5)	Live-attenuated virus	Oral
Tdap	Toxoids and inactivated bacterial components	IM
Tetanus	Toxoid	IM
Typhoid	Bacterial capsular polysaccharide	IM
Typhoid	Live-attenuated bacteria	Oral
Varicella	Live-attenuated virus	SC
Zoster	Live-attenuated virus	SC
Yellow fever	Live-attenuated virus	SC

BCG indicates bacille Calmette-Guérin; ID, intradermal; SC, subcutaneous; DT, diphtheria and tetanus toxoids (for children 7 years of age or older and adults); IM, intramuscular; DTaP, diphtheria and tetanus toxoids and acellular pertussis, adsorbed; IPV, inactivated poliovirus; Hib, *Haemophilus influenzae* type b; PRP-T, polyribosylribitol phosphate-tetanus toxoid; HPV, human papillomavirus; MMR, live measles-mumps-rubella; MMRV, live measles-mumps-rubella-varicella (monovalent measles, mumps, and rubella components are not being produced in the United States); Tdap, tetanus toxoid, reduced diphtheria toxoid, and acellular pertussis.

[a] Other vaccines licensed in the United States but not distributed include anthrax, smallpox, H5N1 influenza vaccines, influenza A (H1N1) monovalent 2009 vaccine, JE-virus vaccine (JE-VAX), pneumococcal conjugate vaccine (PCV7), and tetanus toxoid. The FDA maintains a Web site listing currently licensed vaccines in the United States (**www.fda.gov/BiologicsBloodVaccines/ Vaccines/ApprovedProducts/ucm093830.htm**). The AAP maintains a Web site (**http://aapredbook.aappublications.org/news/vaccstatus.dtl**) showing status of licensure and recommendations for newer vaccines.

[b] See Table 3.11, p 374.

immunosuppressed vaccinees or contacts of vaccinees as might live-attenuated vaccines. However, only the oral poliovirus vaccine (OPV), which no longer is licensed or recommended for use in the United States, is contraindicated for administration to someone living in the home of an immunosuppressed person.

Recommendations for dose, vaccine storage and handling (see Vaccine Handling and Storage, p 20), route and technique of administration (see Vaccine Administration, p 26), and immunization schedules should be followed for predictable, effective immunization (also see disease-specific chapters in Section 3). Adherence to recommended guidance is critical to the success of immunization practices at both the individual and the societal levels.

Vaccine Ingredients

A vaccine's principal constituents are listed in its package insert. As part of the licensure process, the FDA considers all of a vaccine's ingredients—the antigen/immunogen as well as vaccine additives that have specific purposes (eg, stabilizers that protect the vaccine's integrity, preservatives that prevent the growth of bacteria or fungi, and residual components from the manufacturing process) (**www.cdc.gov/vaccines/vac-gen/ additives.htm** and **www.cdc.gov/vaccines/pubs/pinkbook/downloads/ appendices/B/excipient-table-2.pdf**).

ACTIVE IMMUNIZING ANTIGENS/IMMUNOGENS

Some vaccines consist of a single antigen that is a highly defined constituent (eg, tetanus or diphtheria toxoid). Other vaccines consist of multiple antigens, which vary substantially in chemical composition, structure, and number (eg, acellular pertussis components, pneumococcal and meningococcal protein conjugate vaccines, and human papillomavirus [HPV] vaccines). Other vaccines contain live-attenuated viruses (eg, measles-mumps-rubella [MMR], measles-mumps-rubella-varicella [MMRV], varicella, OPV, live-attenuated influenza vaccine [LAIV], oral rotavirus vaccine), killed viruses or portions of virus (eg, enhanced inactivated poliovirus [IPV], hepatitis A, and inactivated influenza vaccines), or recombinant viral proteins (eg, hepatitis B vaccine, HPV vaccine, and 1 influenza vaccine, FluBlok [Protein Sciences Corp, Meriden, CT]).

CONJUGATING AGENTS

Vaccines based on bacterial polysaccharides (*Haemophilus influenzae* type b [Hib], pneumococcal, and meningococcal vaccines) have limited immunogenicity in children younger than 18 months and fail to induce immunologic memory. To overcome these limitations and to facilitate polysaccharide processing by antigen-presenting cells, vaccine antigens are chemically conjugated to a protein carrier with proven immunologic potential (eg, tetanus toxoid, nontoxic variant of diphtheria toxin, meningococcal outer membrane protein complex) to improve the immune response.

VACCINE ADDITIVES

Vaccine additives are substances added to a vaccine for a specific purpose: adjuvants, preservatives, and stabilizers. Allergic reactions may occur if the recipient is sensitive to one or more of these additives. Whenever feasible, these reactions should be anticipated by a careful screening for known allergy to specific vaccine components. Porcine gelatin, a stabilizing agent used in several vaccines, is the additive most likely to induce an allergic reaction. Standardized forms are available to assist clinicians in screening for allergies and other potential contraindications to immunization (**www.immunize.org/catg.d/ p4060.pdf**).

ADJUVANTS. From the Latin word for "to help," adjuvants are materials that are added to a vaccine to improve the immune response to the antigen. Aluminum salts, the most commonly used adjuvants, have been used in vaccines for more than 80 years and often are used in vaccines containing inactivated microorganisms or toxoids (eg, hepatitis B vaccine and diphtheria and tetanus toxoids). Despite their well-known clinical effect, their mechanism of action of stimulating an immune response via cytokine release was demonstrated only recently. New adjuvants include molecules that stimulate innate immune responses to enhance immunogenicity of vaccine antigens (eg, deacylated monophosphoryl lipid A plus aluminum hydroxide [ASO4], as used in HPV2 vaccine) or oil-in-water emulsions (MF59 and ASO3, neither licensed for use in the United States), which, by improving the immune response to influenza antigens, also have the benefit of antigen sparing, thereby allowing more vaccine doses to be available to more people when vast numbers of doses are needed (eg, pandemic influenza).

PRESERVATIVES. Preservatives are added to multidose vials to prevent the growth of bacteria or fungi that may be introduced into the vaccine during its use. In some cases, preservatives are used during the vaccine manufacturing process to inhibit microbial growth, which can leave trace amounts in the final product.

Thimerosal has been the most commonly used preservative in vaccines. In use since the 1930s, thimerosal is added to multidose vaccine vials specifically to kill or inhibit growth of microorganisms that might inadvertently contaminate the vial with repeated penetrations to withdraw a dose. However, in shifting to single-dose formulations, all routinely recommended vaccines for infants and children in the United States are available only as preservative-free (eg, thimerosal-free) formulations or contain only trace amounts of thimerosal. The single exception is inactivated influenza vaccines in multidose vials, which contain thimerosal for its antimicrobial, preservative properties. This multidose preparation is produced to meet the needs of practitioners who often prefer this formulation, because it requires less refrigerator space and is believed to be more efficient in the clinical setting given the number of influenza vaccines that are administered in the early fall, between the time when vaccines become available and the onset of the influenza season. Inactivated influenza vaccines for pediatric use are available as thimerosal-free formulation, trace thimerosal-containing formulation, and thimerosal preservative-containing formulation. Information about the thimerosal content of vaccines is available from the FDA (**www.fda.gov/cber/vaccine/thimerosal.htm**). Thimerosal has been studied extensively and is associated with only rare, mild allergic reactions or other adverse events. Independent safety reviews by the Institute of Medicine regarding thimerosal-containing vaccines as well as vaccines and autism are available (**www.iom.edu/Reports/2004/Immunization-Safety-Review-Vaccines-and-Autism.aspx**). The only nonvaccine biologic agents that contain thimerosal in production and distributed in the United States are certain antivenins. Immune Globulin Intravenous (IGIV) does not contain thimerosal or other preservatives, and none of the Rho (D) Immune Globulin (human) products contain thimerosal (**www.fda.gov/ BiologicsBloodVaccines/SafetyAvailability/BloodSafety/ucm095529.htm**).

In circumstances in which preservatives are required and thimerosal has been shown to affect vaccine potency, alternative preservatives (eg, 2-phenoxyethanol in IPV and phenol in 23-valent pneumococcal vaccine) have been used. A recent review of vaccine preservatives by the World Health Organization highlighted that alternative preservatives, such as 2-phenoxyethanol, have variable antimicrobial effectiveness in some formulations. In addition, as for many ingredients, 2-phenoxyethanol has different compatibilities with different antigens and may affect a vaccine's immunogenicity, stability, and safety profile, which underscores the requirement to study each formulation for safety and immuno-genicity (**www.who.int/biologicals/Report_THIOMERSAL_WHO_Mtg_3-4_April_2012.pdf**). The effort to remove thimerosal (ethyl mercury) from vaccines was driven in large part by initial concerns about toxicity of methyl mercury, a mercury-containing compound not related to thimerosal, and a number of subsequent studies have not supported a link between thimerosal exposure and neurodevelopmental disorders, including autism. It is very clear that the use of thimerosal in vaccines does not put vaccine recipients at increased risk of neurodevelopmental problems. Overwhelmingly, the evidence collected over the past 15 years has failed to yield any evidence of harm from thimerosal-containing vaccines: dozens of studies from countries around the world have examined the safety of thimerosal containing vaccines and failed to find harm. Even in the United States, having the option for including thimerosal could be critical for dealing with emergencies and the need to increase vaccine supply and delivery rapidly, such as during a serious pandemic of influenza.

However, thimerosal as a preservative remains an important component of many vaccines used in resource-limited countries, particularly because of extensive use of multidose vials in global immunization programs. Multidose vials provide a number of efficiencies in resource-limited settings, among them cost, storage, cold-chain requirements, and waste disposal. Multiple re-entries into multidose vials, however, increase the risk of microbial contamination, which is the impetus for thimerosal use in multidose vials in resource-limited settings. In advocating for the health of all children, the AAP strongly supports global immunization efforts and recognizes that these programs rely on multidose vials, which require a preservative to ensure vaccine safety. A recent WHO assessment supported the continued use of thimerosal-containing vaccines and noted that immunization prevents approximately 2.5 million deaths a year globally (**www.who.int/biologicals/Report_THIMEROSAL_WHO_Mtg_3-4_April_2012.pdf**). The preponderance of available evidence has failed to demonstrate harm associated with thimerosal in vaccines. As such, the AAP extends its strongest support for the recent recommendations of the Strategic Advisory Group of Experts on immunization to retain the use of thimerosal in the global vaccine supply (**www.who.int/wer/2012/wer8721.pdf**).

More information on thimerosal in vaccines is available (**www.fda.gov/BiologicsBloodVaccines/Vaccines/QuestionsaboutVaccines/ucm070430.htm** and **www.cdc.gov/vaccinesafety/Concerns/thimerosal/index.html**).

STABILIZERS. Stabilizers are added to vaccines to ensure that their potency is not affected by adverse conditions during the manufacturing process (eg, freeze drying) or during transport and storage (eg, mild temperature excursion). Stabilizers commonly added to vaccines for this purpose include sugars (sucrose or lactose), amino acids (eg, glycine), or proteins (eg, gelatin).

OTHER INGREDIENTS

Although steps in the manufacturing process are designed to remove nonessential constituents (formaldehyde, glutaraldehyde, antibiotics, and bacterial or cell culture components), small residual amounts may remain in the final product. Such ingredients are noted in the package label.

SUSPENDING FLUID

Sterile water for injection or saline solution are used commonly as a vaccine vehicle or suspending fluid. Some vaccine products use more complex suspending fluids, such as tissue-culture fluid, which may contain proteins or other constituents derived from the growth medium or from the biological system in which the vaccine was produced (eg, egg antigens, gelatin, or cell culture-derived antigens). These are also considered in the licensing process.

ANTIMICROBIAL AGENTS

Certain vaccines contain trace amounts of neomycin, polymyxin B, or streptomycin. Penicillins, cephalosporins, or fluoroquinolones are not present in vaccines.

Vaccine Handling and Storage

For vaccines to be optimally effective, they must be stored properly from the time of manufacturing until they are administered. Immunization providers are responsible for proper storage and handling from the time the vaccine arrives at their facility until the vaccine is given. All staff should be knowledgeable about the importance of proper storage and handling of vaccines.

A written vaccine-specific storage and handling plan should be available for reference by all staff members and kept on or near the unit used for storing vaccines. This plan should be updated annually. It should detail both routine management of vaccines and emergency measures for vaccine retrieval and storage.

Most vaccines are designated for optimal storage between 2°C and 8°C (35°F and 46°F), and such vaccines are referred to as "refrigerated vaccines." Of vaccines routinely used in pediatric offices, only those containing varicella virus are required to be stored frozen between −50°C and −15C° (−58°F and +5°F). These are referred to as "freezer vaccines." There is only 1 vaccine, MMR, that can be stored in either location with a safe temperature range between −50°C and 8C° (−58°F and +46°F).

It is imperative that great care be taken to avoid exposing "refrigerated vaccines" to freezing temperatures, even for brief periods. Such exposure can compromise the integrity of refrigerated vaccine even without generating ice crystals or other changes in physical appearance of the vaccine. Visual inspection cannot reliably detect a vaccine that has been destroyed by freeze exposure; thus, only careful monitoring of the temperatures used to store these vaccines will allow identification of potentially altered vaccines. It is recommended that refrigerators be set to maintain 5°C (40°F) for storage of these vaccines.

"Refrigerated vaccines" may tolerate limited exposure to elevated temperatures, but care should be taken to maintain storage temperatures within the licensed safe storage temperature ranges.

Vaccines exposed to temperatures outside their licensed safe storage ranges should be segregated in a bag or container that is kept in an environment safe for storing these vaccines. They should not be used until specifics of the temperature excursion are reviewed. Protocols after the event vary depending on individual state or agency policies. Providers should contact their immunization program, vaccine manufacturer(s), or both for guidance. Advice regarding disposition of vaccines should be documented.

Some vaccines, including HPV and MMR, must be protected from light exposure of more than 30 minutes. This can be accomplished by keeping each vial or syringe in its original carton while in recommended storage and until immediate use. Some products may show physical evidence of altered integrity, and others may retain their normal appearance despite a loss of potency. All personnel responsible for handling vaccines in an office or clinic setting should be familiar with standard procedures designed to minimize risk of vaccine failure. A protocol should be in place for personnel to know under what situations they should contact the immunization program, vaccine manufacturers, or both. Brief "warm" temperature excursions that may occur with vaccine stock management (eg, inventory, stock rotation, identifying expired vaccines), as well as those noted during freezer defrost cycling, should not require contact with the manufacturer because they are accounted for in the "cold chain modeling" used by manufacturers to license their products. Contact phone numbers of the manufacturers are available online (**www. cdc.gov/vaccines/recs/storage/manufact-dist-contact.pdf**) as well as in the package inserts and the annual *Physicians' Desk Reference*.

Recommendations for handling and storage of selected biologics are summarized in the package insert for each product (**www.immunize.org/packageinserts/**). The most accurate information about recommended vaccine storage conditions, handling instructions, and survivability for specific temperature excursions must be obtained directly from manufacturers. The following guidance is suggested as part of a quality-control system for safe handling and storage of vaccines in an office or clinic setting.

PERSONNEL

A primary staff vaccine coordinator and an alternate vaccine coordinator should be trained and responsible for vaccine storage and handling. In addition, a physician or manager with understanding of the value and importance of appropriate vaccine storage should be engaged with the responsible vaccine coordinating staff.

The vaccine coordinator should be responsible for:

- Ordering vaccines.
- Overseeing proper receipt and storage of shipments.
- Creating and maintaining a vaccine log book.
- Organizing vaccines in storage units.
- Temperature monitoring of storage units at least twice daily and monitoring of minimum and maximum temperatures daily, preferably in the morning.
- Recording temperature readings on a log.
- Daily physical inspection of the storage unit.
- Rotating stock so that vaccines closest to expiration date are used first.
- Contacting state Vaccines for Children (VFC) program vaccine coordinator if it appears VFC vaccines will expire before they will be used in the practice.
- Monitoring expiration dates and ensuring expired vaccines are removed from the refrigerator/freezer.

- Responding to potential storage temperature excursions and calling the manufacturer, VFC program, or both to obtain guidance for temperature excursion events.
- Overseeing proper vaccine transport, either routine or in an emergency. Routine off-site transport generally is not recommended by vaccine manufacturers. If possible, have vaccines delivered directly to an off-site facility.
- Maintaining all appropriate vaccine storage and handling documentation, including temperature excursion responses.
- Maintaining storage equipment and records, including VFC program documentation.
- Informing all people who will be handling vaccines about specific storage requirements and stability limitations of the products they will encounter. The details of proper storage conditions should be posted on or near each refrigerator or freezer used for vaccine storage or should be readily available to staff. Receptionists, mail clerks, and other staff members who also may receive shipments should be educated.

EQUIPMENT

- Ensure that refrigerators and freezers in which vaccines are to be stored are working properly and are capable of meeting storage requirements.
- Do not connect refrigerators or freezers to a computer uninterrupted power supply or an outlet controlled by a ground fault circuit interrupter or one activated by a wall switch. Use plug guards and warning signs to prevent accidental dislodging of the wall plug. Post **"Do Not Unplug"** warning signs on circuit breakers.
- Store vaccines in refrigerator and freezer units that can maintain the appropriate temperature range and are large enough to maintain the largest anticipated inventory without crowding, along with temperature-buffering water bottles. Stand-alone units are recommended; these are self-contained units that only refrigerate or only freeze and are suitable for vaccine storage. For refrigerated vaccine storage, medical-grade units with an electronic thermostat and digital display are preferred. Household combination refrigerator/freezer units with separate exterior doors and separate thermostats are considered acceptable by the Centers for Disease Control and Prevention (CDC) at this time to store refrigerated vaccines only, with careful monitoring and certain cautionary notes. The risk of freeze damage to refrigerated vaccines is increased greatly in combination refrigerator/freezer units. By design, super cold air from the freezer is circulated in the refrigerator to cool that space. This subfreezing air can freeze temperature-sensitive vaccines. In addition, the freezer portion of many combination units is insufficiently cold to store frozen vaccines and, thus, is not permitted for storage of VFC vaccines. A separate stand-alone freezer should be used to store frozen vaccines. Use of dormitory or bar-style refrigerator/freezer units with 1 exterior door is not recommended for any vaccine storage and not allowed for vaccine storage of VFC program products.
- Use refrigerators with wire—not glass—shelving to improve air circulation in the unit. Do not use the top shelf of domestic combination refrigerator-freezer units for vaccine storage. Do not use the refrigerator door for vaccine storage. To improve air circulation, place vaccine storage trays used to separate different vaccines away from the walls and rear of the refrigerator. Each vaccine storage compartment should be monitored by a digital thermometer with accuracy of +/− 0.5°C (1°F). The thermometer should be capable of continuous frequent measurements (with a detachable probe in a temperature buffer [eg, biosafe glycol or similar]), should display daily maximum and minimum temperatures, and should be readable without opening the unit door. The buffered

probes should be located near the vaccines, away from the walls, vents, and floor of the vaccine storage unit. The temperature data should be displayed graphically and should be able to be stored for 3 years. The graphic data should be reviewed and corrective efforts documented if daily maximum and minimum values are found to be outside of acceptable ranges.

- Use a certified calibrated thermometer with a Certificate of Traceability and Calibration Testing (also known as Report of Calibration). Such thermometers have been individually tested for accuracy against a recognized reference standard by a laboratory with accreditation from an International Laboratory Accreditation Cooperation (ILAC) Mutual Recognition Arrangement (MRA) signatory body or by a laboratory or manufacturer with documentation that calibration testing performed meets ISO/IEC 17025 international standards for calibration testing and traceability. These thermometers are sold with an individually numbered certificate documenting this testing. Old certified glass thermometers should be replaced by calibrated data-logging thermometers with a detachable probe that is kept in a glycol-filled bottle. This type of probe can provide a more accurate reading of actual vaccine temperature than one that measures air temperature. Providers who receive VFC vaccines or other vaccines purchased with public funds should consult their immunization program regarding the required methods and timeframe for thermometer calibration testing. The National Institute of Standards and Technology maintains a Web site devoted to vaccine storage education (**www.nist.gov/pml/div685/grp01/vaccines.cfm**). Calibration testing and traceability must be performed every 1 to 2 years from the last calibration testing date (date certificate issued) or using suggested calibration timelines from the manufacturer of the device. Temperature accuracy of thermometers can be checked using an ice melting point test (**www.nist.gov/pml/div685/grp01/upload/Ice-Melting-Point-Validation-Method-for-Data-Loggers.pdf**).

PROCEDURES

- A vaccine log should be maintained and should include vaccine name, number of doses, arrival condition of the vaccine, manufacturer and lot numbers, and expiration date.
- Formally accept vaccine on receipt of shipment:
  - Ensure that the expiration date of the delivered product has not passed.
  - Examine the merchandise and its shipping container for any evidence of damage during transport.
  - Consider whether the interval between shipment from the supplier and arrival of the product at its destination is excessive (more than 48 hours) and whether the product has been exposed to excessive heat or cold that might alter its integrity. Review vaccine time and temperature indicators, both chemical and electronic, if included in the vaccine shipment.
  - Do not accept the shipment if reasonable suspicion exists that the delivered product may have been damaged by environmental insult or improper handling during transport. Find and inspect any temperature excursion devices (electronic or temperature-tape) found in the shipment for evidence of temperature excursions.
  - Contact the vaccine supplier or manufacturer when unusual circumstances raise questions about the stability of a delivered vaccine. Store suspect vaccine under proper conditions and label it **"Do Not Use"** until the viability has been determined.

- Refrigerator and freezer inspection:
  - If using a combination refrigerator-freezer, determine the placement of the cold air vents and do not put vaccines on the top shelf or near the vents. Measure the temperature of the central part of the storage compartment twice a day, and record this temperature on a temperature log. A minimum-maximum thermometer in a thermal buffer is preferred to record extremes in temperature fluctuation and reset to baseline daily. Consider use of an alarm system capable of phone/text message/e-mail notification if there is equipment failure, power outage, or temperature excursion. The refrigerator temperature should be maintained between 2°C and 8°C (35°F and 46°F), with a target temperature of 5°C (40°F), and the freezer temperature should be −15°C (5°F) or colder. A **"Do Not Unplug"** sign should be affixed directly next to the refrigerator electrical outlet and to the circuit breaker controlling that circuit.
- Train and designate staff to respond immediately to temperature recordings outside the recommended range and to document response and outcome.
  - Inspect the unit weekly for outdated vaccine and either dispose of or return expired products appropriately.
- Establish routine procedures:
  - Store vaccines according to temperatures recommended in the package insert.
  - Rotate vaccine supplies so that the shortest-dated vaccines are in front to reduce wastage because of expiration.
  - Promptly remove expired (outdated) vaccines from the refrigerator or freezer and dispose of them appropriately or return to manufacturer to avoid accidental use.
  - Store both opened and unopened vials in the original packaging, which facilitates temperature stability, inventory management, and rotation of vaccine by expiration date and avoids light exposure. Mark the outside of boxes of opened vaccines with a large "X" to indicate that it has been opened.
  - Keep opened vials of vaccine in a tray so that they are readily identifiable.
  - Indicate on the label of each vaccine vial the date and time the vaccine was reconstituted or first opened.
  - Unless immediate use is planned, avoid reconstituting multiple doses of vaccine or drawing up multiple doses of vaccine in multiple syringes. Predrawing vaccine increases the possibility of medication errors and causes uncertainty of vaccine stability.
  - Because different vaccines can share similar components/names (eg, diphtheria and tetanus and acellular pertussis vaccines [DTaP and Tdap] or meningococcal polysaccharide vaccine [MPSV4] and meningococcal conjugate vaccine [MCV4]), care should be taken during storage to ensure that the different products are stored separately in a manner to avoid confusion and possible medication errors.
  - Each vaccine and diluent vial should be inspected carefully for damage or contamination prior to use. The expiration date printed on the vial or box should be checked. Vaccine can be used through the last day of the month indicated by the expiration date unless otherwise stated on the package labeling. The expiration date or time for some vaccines changes once the vaccine vial is opened or the vaccine is reconstituted. This information is available in the manufacturer's package insert. Regardless of expiration date, vaccine and diluent should only be used as long as they are normal in appearance and have been stored and handled properly. Expired vaccine or diluent should never be used.

- When feasible, use prefilled unit-dose syringes supplied by the vaccine manufacturer to prevent contamination of multidose vials and errors in labeling syringes or dosing.
- Discard reconstituted live-virus and other vaccines if not used within the time interval specified in the package insert. Examples of discard times following reconstitution include varicella vaccine after 30 minutes and MMR vaccine after 8 hours. All reconstituted vaccines should be refrigerated during the interval in which they may be used.
- Always store vaccines in the refrigerator or freezer as indicated until immediately prior to delivery. Do not open more than 1 vial of a specific vaccine at a time.
- Store vaccine where temperature remains constant.
- Do not keep food or drink in refrigerators in which vaccine is stored; this will limit frequent opening of the unit that leads to thermal instability.
- Do not store radioactive materials in the same refrigerator in which vaccines are stored.
- Discuss with all clinic or office personnel any violation of protocol for handling vaccines or any accidental temperature excursion. Segregate the affected vaccine to avoid use until the vaccine manufacturers can be contacted to determine the disposition of the affected vaccine.

SUMMARY

To summarize best equipment and practices for storage of refrigerated vaccines:
1. Medical refrigerator with electronic thermostat and an external digital display, set to 4°C or 5°C.
2. Wire shelving and an interior circulating fan.
3. One or more data-logging certified thermometers with a detachable or wireless probe in a thermal buffer collocated with vaccine.
4. Displays with current temperature and resettable maximum and minimum temperatures visible on the outside of the unit.
5. Audible temperature alarm with capability for rapid user notification via phone/text message/e-mail should temperature excursion be detected.
6. Extra space in the unit should be filled with water bottles to serve as a cold mass and to prolong safe storage in the event of refrigerator failure.

EMERGENCY VACCINE RETRIEVAL AND STORAGE

Develop a written plan for emergency storage of vaccine in the event of a catastrophic event. Refrigerators can maintain their 2°C to 8°C temperature for only 2 to 3 hours without power. Office personnel should have a written and easily accessible procedure that outlines vaccine packing and transport. Vaccines that have been exposed to temperatures outside the recommended storage range may be ineffective. Vaccines should be packed using a qualified container and pack-out or portable refrigerator/freezer and moved to a location where the appropriate storage temperatures can be maintained. Alternatively, because transportation of a large amount of vaccine in itself carries the risk of inadequacy, sheltering in place can be undertaken if an adequate supply of conditioned frozen water bottles and coolers sufficient to hold the vaccine are available. Frozen vaccine should be packed in a smaller cooler with frozen gel packs and taken quickly to another facility with a freezer capable of −15°C to −50°C temperature. Office personnel need to be aware of alternate storage sites and trained in the correct techniques to shelter and/or store and transport vaccines safely. Special care must be taken to avoid freezing refrigerated vaccine either by transport coolant or by environment (as in the winter). If a certified wireless thermometer is not available to be placed in the cooler with the vaccine, several simple home wireless indoor/outdoor thermometers can be helpful staples in the evacuation kit.

After a power outage or mechanical failure, do not assume that vaccine exposed to temperature outside the recommended range is unusable; contact the vaccine manufacturer for guidance before discarding vaccine.

Additional materials are available from the CDC National Center for Immunization and Respiratory Diseases (**www.cdc.gov/vaccines/recs/storage/default.htm**) and the American Academy of Pediatrics (AAP) (**www.aap.org/immunization/ pediatricians/storagehandling.html**).

Vaccine Administration

GENERAL CONSIDERATIONS FOR VACCINE ADMINISTRATION

Personnel administering vaccines should take appropriate precautions to minimize risk of spread of disease to or from patients. Hand hygiene should be used before and after each new patient contact. Gloves are not required when administering vaccines unless the health care professional has open hand lesions or will come into contact with potentially infectious body fluids. Syringes and needles must be sterile and disposable. To prevent inadvertent needlesticks or reuse, a needle should **not** be recapped after use, and disposable needles and syringes should be discarded promptly in puncture-proof, labeled containers placed in the room where the vaccine is administered.

Vaccines should be prepared just prior to administration. A separate needle and syringe should be used for each injection. If the vaccine requires reconstitution, the diluent supplied by the manufacturer should be used. Each vaccine and diluent vial should be inspected carefully for damage or contamination prior to use. The expiration date printed on the vial or box should be checked. Expired vaccine or diluent should not be administered. Different vaccines should not be mixed in the same syringe unless specifically licensed and labeled for such use. Changing needles between drawing a vaccine into a syringe and injecting the child is not necessary.

A patient should be restrained adequately, if indicated, before any injection (see Managing Injection Pain, p 30). Information about atraumatic care, positioning, comfort restraint, and comfort care is available (**www.immunize.org/catg.d/p3085.pdf; www.cdc.gov/vaccines/pubs/pinkbook/downloads/appendices/D/vacc_ admin.pdf,** and **http://eziz.org/assets/docs/IMM-898**).

Because of the rare possibility of a severe allergic reaction to a vaccine component, people administering vaccines or other biologic products should be prepared to recognize and treat allergic reactions, including anaphylaxis (see Hypersensitivity Reactions After Immunization, p 54). Facilities and personnel should be available for treating immediate allergic reactions. This recommendation does not preclude administration of vaccines in school-based or other nonclinic settings.

Syncope can occur following any immunization, particularly in adolescents and young adults. Personnel should be aware of presyncopal manifestations and take appropriate measures to prevent injuries if weakness, dizziness, or loss of consciousness occurs. However, syncope can occur without any presyncopal symptoms. The relatively rapid onset of syncope in most cases suggests that health care professionals should consider observing adolescents for 15 minutes after they are immunized. Adolescents should be seated or lying down during vaccination, and having vaccine recipients *sit or lie down for at least 15 minutes* after immunization could avert many syncopal episodes and secondary injuries. If syncope develops, patients should be observed until symptoms resolve.[1] Syncope following receipt of a vaccine is not a contraindication to subsequent doses.

SITE AND ROUTE OF IMMUNIZATION (ACTIVE AND PASSIVE)

ORAL VACCINES. Rotavirus vaccines (RV1 [Rotarix], RV5 [RotaTeq], both liquid formulations) and oral typhoid vaccine (TY21a [Vivotif], a capsule formulation) are the only US-licensed vaccines for children that are administered by the oral route. Oral vaccines generally should be administered prior to administering injections or performing other procedures that might cause discomfort. The liquid RV1 and RV5 vaccines should be administered slowly down 1 side of the inside of the cheek (between the cheek and gum) toward the back of the infant's mouth. Care should be taken not to go far enough back to initiate the gag reflex. Never administer or spray (squirt) the vaccine directly into the throat. Detailed information on oral delivery of these vaccines is included in each manufacturer's product information guide. Breastfeeding does not interfere with successful immunization with rotavirus vaccines or with oral poliovirus (OPV) vaccine (no longer licensed or available for use in the United States). Vomiting within 10 minutes of receiving an oral dose is an indication for repeating the dose of OPV, but not rotavirus vaccine. If the repeated dose of OPV vaccine also is not retained, neither dose should be counted, and the vaccine should be readministered.

INTRANASAL VACCINE. Live-attenuated influenza vaccine (LAIV) is the only vaccine currently licensed for intranasal administration. This vaccine is licensed for healthy, nonpregnant people 2 through 49 years of age. With the recipient in the upright position, approximately 0.1 mL (ie, half of the total sprayer contents) is sprayed into 1 nostril. An attached dose-divider clip is removed from the sprayer to administer the second half of the dose into the other nostril. If the recipient sneezes after administration, the dose should not be repeated. The vaccine can be administered during minor illnesses. However, if clinical judgment indicates that nasal congestion might impede delivery of the vaccine to the nasopharyngeal mucosa, vaccine deferral should be considered until resolution of the illness.

PARENTERAL VACCINES.[2] Injectable vaccines should be administered using aseptic technique at a site as free as possible from risk of local neural, vascular, or tissue injury. Recommended routes of administration are included in package inserts of vaccines and are listed in Table 1.6 (p 15). The recommended route is based on studies designed to demonstrate maximum safety and immunogenicity. To minimize untoward local or systemic effects and to ensure optimal efficacy of the immunizing procedure, vaccines should be administered by the recommended route. Preferred sites for vaccines administered via the subcutaneous (SC) or intramuscular (IM) route include the anterolateral aspect of the

---

[1]Centers for Disease Control and Prevention. Syncope after vaccination—United States, January 2005–July 2007. *MMWR Morb Mortal Wkly Rep.* 2008;57(17):457–460

[2]For a review on intramuscular injections, see Centers for Disease Control and Prevention. *Epidemiology and Prevention of Vaccine-Preventable Diseases (Pink Book).* Atlanta, GA: Centers for Disease Control and Prevention; 2012 (**www.cdc.gov/vaccines/pubs/pinkbook/index.html**). For hard copies, contact the Public Health Foundation at 877-252-1200.

upper thigh (SC or IM); upper, outer triceps area of the upper arm (SC); and the deltoid area of the upper arm (IM).

For IM injections, the choice of site, thigh or arm, depends on the age of the individual and the degree of muscle development. In children younger than 1 year, the anterolateral aspect of the thigh provides the largest muscle and is the preferred site. In older children, the deltoid muscle usually is large enough for IM injection. A 22- to 25-gauge needle is recommended for IM injections. Decisions on needle length must be made for each person on the basis of the size of the muscle and the thickness of adipose tissue at the injection site. Suggested needle lengths are shown in Table 1.7 (p 28). Needles should be long enough to reach the muscle mass and prevent vaccine from seeping into subcutaneous tissue and causing local reactions, yet not so long as to involve underlying nerves, blood vessels, or bone.

Ordinarily, the upper, outer aspect of the buttocks should not be used for active immunization, because the gluteal region is covered by a significant layer of subcutaneous fat. Because of diminished immunogenicity, hepatitis B and rabies vaccines should not be given in the buttocks at any age.

When the upper, outer quadrant of the buttocks is used for large-volume passive immunization, such as IM administration of large volumes of Immune Globulin (IG), care must be taken to avoid injury to the sciatic nerve. The site selected should be well into the upper, outer quadrant of the gluteus maximus, away from the central region of the buttocks, and the needle should be directed anteriorly—that is, if the patient is lying prone, the needle is directed perpendicular to the table's surface, not perpendicular to the skin plane. The ventrogluteal site may be less hazardous for IM injection, because it is free

Table 1.7. Site and Needle Length by Age for Intramuscular Immunization

Age Group	Needle Length, inches (mm)[a]	Suggested Injection Site
Newborns (preterm and term) and infants <1 mo of age	⅝ (16)[b]	Anterolateral thigh muscle
Term infants, 1–12 mo of age	1 (25)	Anterolateral thigh muscle
Toddlers and children	⅝–1 (16–25)[b]	Deltoid muscle of the arm
	1–1¼ (25–32)	Anterolateral thigh muscle
Adults		
Female and male, weight <60 kg	1 (25)[c]	Deltoid muscle of the arm
Female and male, weight 60–70 kg	1 (25)	Deltoid muscle of the arm
Female, weight 70–90 kg	1 (25)–1½ (38)	Deltoid muscle of the arm
Male, weight 70–118 kg	1 (25) 1½ (38)	Deltoid muscle of the arm
Female, weight >90 kg	1½ (38)	Deltoid muscle of the arm
Male, weight >118 kg	1½ (38)	Deltoid muscle of the arm

[a] Assumes that needle is inserted fully.
[b] If the skin is stretched tightly and subcutaneous tissues are not bunched.
[c] Some experts recommend a 5/8-inch needle for men and women who weigh less than 60 kg.

of major nerves and vessels. This site is the center of a triangle for which the boundaries are the anterior superior iliac spine, the tubercle of the iliac crest, and the upper border of the greater trochanter. Rabies Immune Globulin (RIG), Hepatitis B Immune Globulin (HBIG), palivizumab, and other similar products administered for passive immunoprophylaxis also are injected intramuscularly, except that as much of the RIG as possible should be infiltrated around the site of a bite wound.

Vaccines containing adjuvants (eg, aluminum present in certain vaccines recommended for IM injection) must be injected deep into the muscle mass. These vaccines should not be administered subcutaneously or intracutaneously, because they can cause local irritation, inflammation, granuloma formation, and tissue necrosis.

Serious complications resulting from IM injections are rare. Reported adverse events include broken needles, muscle contracture, nerve injury, bacterial (eg, staphylococcal, streptococcal, or clostridial) abscesses, sterile abscesses, skin pigmentation changes, hemorrhage, cellulitis, tissue necrosis, gangrene, local atrophy, periostitis, cyst or scar formation, and inadvertent injection into a joint space. For patients with a known bleeding disorder or people receiving anticoagulant therapy, bleeding complications following IM immunization can occur. Such events can be minimized by administration immediately after the patient's receipt of replacement factor if appropriate, by utilization of a finer needle (23-gauge or less and of appropriate length), and by applying firm pressure at the immunization site for at least 2 minutes. Scheduling immunizations after factor replacement therapy, if feasible, may be considered.

SC injections can be administered at a 45° angle into the anterolateral aspect of the thigh or the upper outer triceps area by inserting the needle in a pinched-up fold of skin and tissue. A 23- to 25-gauge needle of 5/8 inch length is recommended. Immune responses after SC administration of hepatitis B or recombinant rabies vaccine are decreased compared with those after IM administration of either of these vaccines; therefore, these vaccines should not be given subcutaneously. Quadrivalent meningococcal polysaccharide vaccine (MPSV4) is administered subcutaneously, whereas quadrivalent meningococcal conjugate vaccine (MCV4) is administered intramuscularly (see Table 1.6).

No intradermal vaccines are licensed for use in pediatric patients, because people younger than 18 (or older than 64) years may not have sufficient skin thickness for intradermal administration. Intradermal influenza vaccine is the only vaccine licensed currently for intradermal administration, but it is for people 18 through 64 years of age. The site of administration is the deltoid region of the upper arm. A manufacturer-prefilled microinjection syringe is used to administer a 0.1-mL dose into the dermal layer of the skin. The syringe contains a 30-gauge, 1.5 mL microneedle. This formulation is not the same as IM formulations of inactivated influenza vaccine. Because of the decreased antigenic mass administered with intradermal injections, attention to technique is essential to ensure that material is not injected subcutaneously. Other influenza vaccine formulations should not be administered by the intradermal route.

When multiple vaccines are administered, separate sites should be used. When necessary, 2 or more vaccines can be given in the same limb at a single visit. The anterolateral aspect of the thigh is the preferred site for multiple simultaneous IM injections because of its greater muscle mass. The distance separating the injections is arbitrary but should be at least 1 inch, if possible, so that local reactions are unlikely to overlap. Multiple vaccines should not be mixed in a single syringe unless specifically licensed and labeled for administration in 1 syringe. A different needle and syringe should be used for each injection.

Aspiration before injection of vaccines or toxoids (ie, pulling back on the syringe plunger after needle insertion, before injection) is not recommended, because no large blood vessels are located at the preferred injection sites, and the process of aspiration has been demonstrated to increase pain (see Managing Injection Pain).

A brief period of bleeding at the injection site is common and usually can be controlled by applying gentle pressure.

Additional information on vaccine administration and safe injection practices is available on the Centers for Disease Control and Prevention (CDC) Web site (**www.cdc.gov/vaccines/recs/vac-admin/default.htm** and **www.cdc.gov/injectionsafety/**).

Managing Injection Pain

A planned approach to decreasing the child's anxiety before, during, and after immunization and to decreasing pain from the injection is helpful for children of any age.[1] The Canadian Medical Association recently conducted a systematic review of the literature on injection site pain and published a clinical practice guideline for Canadian physicians and families.[2] Parents should be educated about techniques for reducing injection pain or distress. Truthful and empathetic preparation for injections is beneficial, using words that are explanatory without evoking anxiety—for example, "pressure," "squeezing," and "poking" rather than "pain," "hurt," and "shot." Parents and medical care providers should not tell children that "it won't hurt" because this type of statement has been shown to be ineffective in reducing pain at the time of injection. Parents also should be advised not to threaten children with injections or use them as a punishment for inappropriate behavior. Techniques for minimizing pain can be divided into physical, psychological, and pharmacologic. Combinations of these techniques are useful. Routine preemptive administration of acetaminophen is not recommended because of concern for potential detrimental effect on the immune response to the vaccine(s) being administered.

PHYSICAL TECHNIQUES FOR MINIMIZING INJECTION PAIN

Breastfeeding has demonstrable analgesic effects attributable to skin-to-skin contact, the child being held, the act of sucking, and the sweet taste of human milk, and should be encouraged during vaccination. For infants younger than 12 months who cannot breastfeed, a sweet-tasting solution such as 2 mL of 25% sucrose can be provided during vaccine administration. Children should not be placed in a supine position during vaccination but should be held on the lap of a parent or other caregiver. Older children may be more comfortable sitting on the examination table edge and hugging their parent chest to chest while an immunization is administered. The limb should be positioned to facilitate relaxation of the muscle to be injected. For the deltoid, some flexion of the elbow may be required. For the anterolateral thigh, some degree of internal rotation may be helpful. A rapid plunge of the needle through the skin without aspirating and rapid injection may decrease discomfort. Rubbing or stroking the skin near the

---

[1]Schechter NL, Zempsky WT, Cohen LL, McGrath PJ, McMurtry CM, Bright NS. Pain reduction during pediatric immunizations: evidence-based review and recommendations. *Pediatrics.* 2007;119(5):e1184-e1198

[2]Taddio A, Appleton M, Bortolussi R, et al. Reducing the pain of childhood vaccination: an evidence-based clinical practice guideline. *CMAJ.* 2010;182(18):E843-E855

injection site with moderate intensity before and during vaccination also may reduce the sensation of pain.

PSYCHOLOGICAL TECHNIQUES FOR MINIMIZING INJECTION PAIN

Parent-led or physician-led age-appropriate distraction can reduce pain-related distress at the time of injection. Parental behaviors such as nonprocedural conversation in a calm voice and humor to distract the child are beneficial, whereas reassurance and apologies may increase distress and pain. Physician-led distraction, including encouragement of slow, deep breathing or blowing performed by the child, also can decrease injection pain and distress.

PHARMACOLOGIC TECHNIQUES FOR MINIMIZING INJECTION PAIN

Topically applied agents may reduce the pain of injection. Because currently available topical anesthetics require 30 to 60 minutes to provide adequate anesthesia, planning ahead is necessary so that cream is applied en route to the office visit or immediately on arrival. Lidocaine 4% is approved by the US Food and Drug Administration (FDA) for children older than 2 years, is available over the counter, and takes effect 30 minutes after application. EMLA (lidocaine 2.5%/prilocaine 2.5%), available by prescription, is approved by the FDA for patients >37 weeks' estimated gestational age and takes effect 60 minutes after application. Topical application of ethyl chloride, sprayed onto a cotton ball that is then placed over the injection site for 15 seconds prior to administering the injection, also has been shown to decrease injection pain in school-aged children.

Scheduling Immunizations

A vaccine is intended to be administered to a person capable of an appropriate immunologic response and likely to benefit from the protection given. However, the optimal immunologic response for a person must be balanced against the need to achieve timely protection against disease. For example, pertussis-containing vaccines may be less immunogenic in early infancy than in later infancy, but the benefit of conferring protection in young infants—who experience the highest morbidity and mortality from pertussis—mandates that immunization occur early, despite a lessened serum antibody response. For this reason, in some developing countries, oral polio-virus vaccine is given at birth, in accordance with recommendations of the World Health Organization.

With parenterally administered live-virus vaccines, the inhibitory effect of residual specific maternal antibody determines the optimal age of administration. For example, live-virus measles-containing vaccine in use in the United States provides suboptimal rates of seroconversion during the first year of life, mainly because of interference by trans-placentally acquired maternal antibody. If a measles-containing vaccine is administered before 12 months of age (eg, because of travel or increased risk of exposure), the child should receive 2 additional doses of measles-containing vaccine at the recommended ages and interval (see Measles, p 535).

An additional factor in selecting an immunization schedule is the need to achieve a uniform and regular response. With some products, an immune response is achieved after 1 dose. For example, live-virus rubella vaccine evokes a predictable response at high rates after a single dose. With many inactivated or component vaccines, a primary series of several doses is necessary to achieve an optimal initial response in recipients. Some people require multiple doses to respond to all included antigens. For example, some people respond only to 1 or 2 types of poliovirus after a single dose of oral poliovirus vaccine, but several doses are needed to stimulate antibody against all 3 types, thereby ensuring complete protection for the person and maximum response rates for the population. For some vaccines, periodic booster doses (eg, with tetanus and diphtheria toxoids and acellular pertussis antigen) are required to maintain protection.

Vaccines are safe and effective when administered simultaneously. This information is particularly important for scheduling immunizations for children with lapsed or missed immunizations and for people preparing for international travel (see Simultaneous Administration of Multiple Vaccines, p 35). Data indicate possible impaired immune responses when 2 or more parenterally administered live-virus vaccines are not given simultaneously but rather within 28 days of each other; therefore, live-virus vaccines not administered on the same day should be given at least 28 days (4 weeks) apart whenever possible (Table 1.8). No minimum interval is required between administration of different inactivated vaccines, with a few exceptions. In people with functional or anatomic asplenia, quadrivalent meningococcal conjugate vaccine (MCV4-D; Menactra [Sanofi Pasteur, Swiftwater, PA]) should not be given until at least 4 weeks after all doses of 13-valent pneumococcal conjugate vaccine (PCV13) have been administered because of interference with the immune response to the PCV13 series since both vaccines are conjugated to diphtheria toxin carrier protein. PCV13 and 23-valent pneumococcal polysaccharide vaccine (PPSV23) should not be administered simultaneously and should be spaced at least 8 weeks apart; when both vaccines are indicated, PCV13 should be administered first, if possible.

The Recommended Immunization Schedule for Persons Age 0 Through 18 Years for the United States represents a consensus of the American Academy of Pediatrics (AAP), the Advisory Committee on Immunization Practices (ACIP) of the Centers for Disease Control and Prevention (CDC), and the American Academy of Family Physicians (AAFP). The schedule is reviewed regularly, and the updated schedule is issued annually in February. Schedules are available at **www.cdc.gov/vaccines/schedules/index. html** and are posted at *Red Book* Online (**http://redbook.solutions.aap.org/SS/ Immunization_Schedules.aspx**). Interim recommendations occasionally may be made when issues such as a shortage of a product or a safety concern arise, or a new

Table 1.8. Guidelines for Spacing of Live and Inactivated Antigens

Antigen Combination	Recommended Minimum Interval Between Doses
2 or more inactivated[a]	None; can be administered simultaneously or at any interval between doses
Inactivated plus live	None; can be administered simultaneously or at any interval between doses
2 or more live[b]	28-day minimum interval if not administered simultaneously

[a]See text for exceptions.
[b]An exception is made for some live oral vaccines (ie, Ty21a typhoid vaccine, oral poliovirus vaccine, oral rotavirus vaccine) that can be administered simultaneously or at any interval before or after inactivated or live parenteral vaccines.

recommendation may be added to incorporate a new vaccine or vaccine indication. Special attention should be given to footnotes on the schedule, which summarize major recommendations for routine childhood immunizations.

Combination vaccine products may be given whenever any component of the combination is indicated and its other components are not contraindicated, provided they are licensed by the FDA for that dose in the schedule for each component and for the child's age. The use of a combination vaccine generally is preferred over separate injections of its equivalent component vaccines. Considerations for separate administration include provider assessment and patient preference. The provider assessment should include the number of injections, vaccine availability, the likelihood of improved coverage, the likelihood of patient return, and storage and cost considerations.

Web-based childhood immunization schedulers using the current vaccine recommendations are available for parents, caregivers, and health care professionals to facilitate making schedules for children, adolescents, and adults in the immunization setting (see Immunization Schedulers, p 5, or **www.cdc.gov/vaccines**). Most state and regional immunization information systems (also known as immunization registries) also will forecast immunizations that are due based on the consensus AAP/ACIP/AAFP schedule.

For children in whom early or rapid immunization is required or for children not immunized on schedule, simultaneous immunization with multiple products allows for more rapid protection. In some circumstances, immunization can be initiated earlier than at the usually recommended time or schedule, or doses can be given at shorter intervals than are recommended routinely (for guidance, see the disease-specific chapters in Section 3).

Physicians or localities using such a compressed schedule should be certain to observe the 6-month minimum interval between doses 3 and 4 of DTaP vaccine as well as other minimal interval recommendations. The final dose of the hepatitis B vaccine series should be administered at least 16 weeks after the first dose and no earlier than 24 weeks of age. Influenza vaccine should be administered before the start of influenza season but provides benefit if administered at any time during the influenza season (see Influenza, Timing of Vaccine Administration, p 489).

The immunization schedule issued by the AAP, ACIP, and AAFP primarily is intended for children and adolescents in the United States. In many instances, the guidance will be applicable to children in other countries, but individual pediatricians and recommending committees in each country are responsible for determining the appropriateness of the recommendations for their settings. The schedule recommended by the Expanded Programme on Immunization of the World Health Organization (**www. who.int**) can serve as a resource, with modifications made by the ministries of health in individual countries on the basis of local considerations. Recommendations for vaccine schedules in Europe are available from the European Center for Disease Prevention and Control (**www.ecdc.europa.eu**).

Minimum Ages and Minimum Intervals Between Vaccine Doses

Immunizations generally are recommended for members of the youngest age group at risk of experiencing the disease for whom efficacy, effectiveness, immunogenicity, and safety of the vaccine have been demonstrated. Most vaccines in the childhood and adolescent immunization schedule require 2 or more doses for stimulation of an adequate and persisting immune response. Studies have demonstrated that the recommended age and interval between doses of the same antigen(s) (**www.cdc.gov/vaccines/schedules/index.html**) provide optimal protection.

Vaccines generally should not be administered at intervals less than the recommended minimum or at an earlier age than the recommended minimum (ie, accelerated schedules). Administering doses of a multidose vaccine at intervals shorter than those recommended in the childhood and adolescent immunization schedule might be necessary in circumstances in which an infant or child is behind schedule and needs to be brought up to date quickly or when international travel is anticipated. During a measles outbreak or for international travel, measles vaccine may be given as early as 6 months of age. However, if a measles-containing vaccine is administered before 12 months of age, the dose is not counted toward the 2-dose measles vaccine series. The child should be reimmunized at 12 through 15 months of age with a measles-containing vaccine. A third dose of a measles-containing vaccine is indicated at 4 through 6 years of age but can be administered as early as 4 weeks after the second dose (see Measles, p 535). Another possibility when an "accelerated" schedule could be considered involves administering a vaccine dose a few days earlier than the minimum interval or age, which is unlikely to have a substantially negative effect on the immune response to that dose. Although immunizations should not be scheduled at an interval or age less than those recommended in the childhood and adolescent immunization schedule, a child may be in the office early for a routine visit or for an appointment not specifically scheduled for immunization (eg, recheck of otitis media). In this situation, the clinician can consider administering the vaccine before the minimum interval or age. If the child is known to the clinician and follow-up can be ensured, rescheduling the child for immunization closer to the recommended interval is preferred. If the parent or child is not known to the clinician or follow-up cannot be ensured (eg, habitually misses appointments), administration of the vaccine at that visit rather than rescheduling the child for a later visit is preferable. Vaccine doses administered 4 days or fewer before the minimum interval or age can be counted as valid. Doses administered 5 days or more before the minimum interval or age should not be counted as valid doses and should be repeated as age appropriate. The repeat dose should be spaced after the invalid dose by the recommended minimum interval. Health care professionals need to be aware of local or state requirements to be certain that doses of selected vaccines (eg, MMR) administered within 4 days of the minimal interval will be accepted as valid. This 4-day recommendation does not apply to rabies vaccine because of the unique schedule for this vaccine. The latest recommendations can be found in the annual immunization schedule (**http://redbook.solutions.aap.org/SS/Immunization_Schedules.aspx**).

Interchangeability of Vaccine Products

Similar vaccines made by different manufacturers can differ in the number and amount of their specific antigenic components and formulation of adjuvants and conjugating agents, thereby eliciting different immune responses. When possible, effort should be made to complete a series with vaccine made by the same manufacturer. Although data documenting the effects of interchangeability are limited, most experts have considered vaccines interchangeable when administered according to their recommended indications. Licensed vaccines that may be used interchangeably during a vaccine series from different manufacturers, according to recommendations from the AAP or ACIP, include diphtheria and tetanus toxoids vaccines, hepatitis A vaccines, hepatitis B vaccines, and rabies vaccines (see Rabies, p 658). An example of similar vaccines used in different schedules that are not recommended as interchangeable is the 2-dose schedule of the adult formulation of Recombivax HB that is licensed for adolescents 11 through 15 years of age; adolescent patients begun on a 3-dose hepatitis B vaccine schedule are not candidates to complete their series with the adult formulation of Recombivax HB, and the 2-dose schedule is applicable only to Recombivax HB (Merck and Co Inc, Whitehouse Station, NJ; see Hepatitis B, p 400).

Licensed rotavirus (RV) vaccines (RV5, RotaTeq [Merck and Co Inc]; RV1, Rotarix [GlaxoSmithKline]) are considered interchangeable as long as recommendations concerning conversion from a 2-dose regimen (RV-1) to a 3-dose regimen (RV-5) are followed (see Rotavirus, p 684). Similarly, licensed *Haemophilus influenzae* type b (Hib) conjugate vaccines are considered interchangeable as long as recommendations for a total of 3 doses in the first year of life are followed (ie, if 2 doses of Hib-OMP are not given, 3 doses of a Hib-containing vaccine are required).

Minimal data on safety and immunogenicity and no data on efficacy are available for interchangeability of DTaP vaccines from different manufacturers. When feasible, DTaP from the same manufacturer should be used for the primary series (see Pertussis, p 608). However, in circumstances in which the DTaP product received previously is not known or the previously administered product is not readily available, any of the DTaP vaccines may be used according to licensure for dose and age. Matching of booster doses of DTaP and adolescent Tdap by manufacturer is not necessary. Whenever possible, the same HPV vaccine product should be used for the 3-dose series, particularly because the 3 vaccines differ in serotype content (see Human Papillomaviruses, p 576). However, if the product previously received is not known or is not readily available, either HPV vaccine (HPV4, Gardasil [Merck and Co Inc]; HPV2, Cervarix [GlaxoSmithKline]) can be used to continue the series in females and should provide protection for HPV types 16 and 18. HPV2 vaccine is not licensed or recommended for use in males. Single-component vaccines from the same manufacturer of combination vaccines, including DTaP-HepB-IPV and DTaP-IPV/Hib are interchangeable (see Combination Vaccines, p 36).[1] If any products that require 3 doses are used, then 3 doses are required to complete the series.

Simultaneous Administration of Multiple Vaccines

Simultaneous administration of most vaccines is safe, effective, and recommended. Infants and children have sufficient immunologic capacity to respond to multiple vaccines. There is no contraindication to simultaneous administration of multiple vaccines routinely recommended for infants and children, with 2 exceptions: (1) in people with functional or anatomic asplenia, MCV4-D (Menactra [Sanofi Pasteur, Swiftwater, PA]) should not be given until at least 4 weeks after all doses of PCV13 have been administered because of interference with the immune response to the PCV13 series since both vaccines are conjugated to diphtheria toxin carrier protein; and (2) PCV13 and PPSV23 should not be administered simultaneously and should be spaced at least 8 weeks apart; when both vaccines are indicated, PCV13 should be administered first, if possible.

---

[1]Centers for Disease Control and Prevention. General Recommendations on Immunization—recommendations of the Advisory Committee on Immunization Practices (ACIP). *MMWR Recomm Rep.* 2011;60(RR-02):1-64

Immune response to 1 vaccine generally does not interfere with responses to other vaccines. Simultaneous administration of IPV, MMR, varicella, or DTaP vaccines results in rates of seroconversion and of adverse events similar to those observed when the vaccines are administered at separate visits. A slightly increased risk of febrile seizures is associated with the higher likelihood of fever following the first dose of MMRV compared with MMR and monovalent varicella among children 12 through 23 months of age; after dose 1 of MMRV vaccine, 1 additional febrile seizure is expected to occur per approximately 2300 to 2600 young children immunized, compared with MMR and monovalent varicella. During the 2 influenza seasons between 2010–2012, there were increased reports of febrile seizures in the United States in young children who received inactivated influenza vaccine (IIV) and PCV13 concomitantly. This has not persisted in subsequent seasons. Simultaneous administration of IIV and PCV13 continues to be recommended when both vaccines are indicated.

Because simultaneous administration of routinely recommended vaccines is not known to alter the effectiveness or safety of any of the recommended childhood vaccines, simultaneous administration of all vaccines that are appropriate for the age and immunization status of the recipient is recommended.[1] When vaccines are administered simultaneously, separate syringes and separate sites should be used, and injections into the same extremity should be separated by at least 1 inch so that any local reactions can be differentiated. Simultaneous administration of multiple vaccines can increase immunization rates significantly. Individual vaccines should never be mixed in the same syringe unless they are specifically licensed and labeled for administration in 1 syringe. If an inactivated vaccine and an Immune Globulin product are indicated concurrently (eg, hepatitis B vaccine and Hepatitis B Immune Globulin, rabies vaccine and Rabies Immune Globulin, tetanus-containing vaccine and Tetanus Immune Globulin), they should be administered at separate anatomic sites.

Combination Vaccines

Combination vaccines represent one solution to the issue of increased numbers of injections during single clinic visits and generally are preferred over separate injections of equivalent component vaccines. Combination vaccines can be administered instead of separately administered vaccines if licensed and indicated for the patient's age. Table 1.9 lists combination vaccines licensed for use in the United States. Combination vaccines should not be used outside the age groups for which they are licensed. These vaccine components also are available for separate administration (eg, MMRV also is available as MMR and varicella vaccine, although single-component measles, mumps, or rubella vaccines are not available in the United States). All available types or brand-name products do not need to be stocked by each health care professional, and it is recognized that the decision of health care professionals to implement use of new combination vaccines involve complex economic and logistical considerations. Factors that should be considered by the provider, in consultation with the parent, include the potential for improved vaccine coverage, the number of injections needed, vaccine safety, vaccine availability, interchangeability, storage and cost issues, and whether the patient is likely to return for follow-up.

---

[1]Centers for Disease Control and Prevention. General Recommendations on Immunization—recommendations of the Advisory Committee on Immunization Practices (ACIP). *MMWR Recomm Rep.* 2011;60(RR-02):1-64

Table 1.9. Combination Vaccines Licensed by the US Food and Drug Administration (FDA)[a]

| Vaccine[b] | FDA Licensure | | Use in Immunization Schedule |
	Trade Name (Year Licensed)	Age Group	
HepA-HepB	Twinrix (2001)	≥18 y	Three doses on a 0-, 1-, and 6-mo schedule
DTaP-HepB-IPV	Pediarix (2002)	6 wk through 6 y	Three-dose series at 2, 4, and 6 mo of age
MMRV	ProQuad (2005)	12 mo through 12 y	Two doses (see Varicella-Zoster Infections, p 846)
DTaP-IPV	Kinrix (2008)	4 y through 6 y	Booster for fifth dose of DTaP and fourth dose of IPV
DTaP-IPV/Hib	Pentacel (2008)	6 wk through 4 y	Four-dose series administered at 2, 4, 6, and 15 through 18 mo of age
Hib-MenCY	MenHibrix (2013)	6 wk through 18 mo	Four-dose series administered at 2, 4, 6, and 12 through 15 mo of age

HepA indicates hepatitis A vaccine; HepB, hepatitis B vaccine; DTaP, diphtheria and tetanus toxoids and acellular pertussis vaccine; IPV, inactivated poliovirus vaccine; MMRV, measles-mumps-rubella-varicella vaccine; Hib, *Haemophilus influenzae* type b; MenCY meningococcal conjugate vaccine serogroups C and Y.
[a] Excludes measles-mumps-rubella (MMR), DTaP, Tdap, Td, and IPV vaccines, for which individual components are not available. DTaP/Hib (TriHIBit) no longer is manufactured.
[b] Dash (-) indicates products in which the active components are supplied in their final (combined) form by the manufacturer; slash (/) indicates products in which active components must be mixed by the user.

When patients have received the recommended immunizations for some of the components in a combination vaccine, administering the extra antigen(s) in the combination vaccine is permissible if they are not contraindicated (**www.cdc.gov/mmwr/preview/mmwrhtml/rr6002a1.htm?s_cid=rr6002a1_e**) and doing so will reduce the number of injections required. Excessive doses of toxoid vaccines (diphtheria and tetanus) may result in extensive local reactions. To overcome the potential for recording errors and ambiguities in the names of vaccine combinations, systems that eliminate error are needed to enhance the convenience and accuracy of transferring vaccine-identifying information into health records and immunization information systems.

Lapsed Immunizations

A lapse in the immunization schedule does not require reinitiating the entire series or addition of doses to the series for any vaccine in the recommended schedule. If a dose of vaccine is missed, subsequent immunizations should be given at the next visit as if the usual interval had elapsed. For RV vaccine, the doses to be administered are age limited, so catch-up may not be possible (see Rotavirus Infections, p 684). See specific influenza vaccine recommendations in the Influenza chapter (p 476) and annual influenza policy statement for children younger than 9 years whose first 2 doses were not administered in the same season, because recommendations will vary depending on the formulation of each season's vaccine. The health records of children for whom immunizations have been missed or postponed should be flagged to remind health care professionals to resume the child's immunization regimen at the next available opportunity. Minimum age and interval recommendations should be followed for administration of all doses. A computer-based tool is available for downloading and can be used to determine which vaccines a child 6 years or younger needs according to the childhood immunization schedule, including timing of missed or skipped vaccines (**www.vacscheduler.org**).

Unknown or Uncertain Immunization Status

Many children, adolescents, and young adults do not have adequate documentation of their immunizations. Parent or guardian recollection of a child's immunization history may not be accurate. Only written, dated records should be accepted as evidence of immunization. In general, when in doubt, a person with unknown or uncertain immunization status should be considered disease susceptible, and recommended immunizations should be initiated without delay on a schedule commensurate with the person's current age. Serologic testing is an alternative to vaccination for certain antigens (eg, measles, rubella, hepatitis A, and tetanus). No evidence suggests that administration of vaccines to already immune recipients is harmful. In general, initiation of revaccination with an age-appropriate schedule of pertussis, diphtheria, and tetanus toxoid-containing vaccine is appropriate, with performance of serologic testing for specific IgG antibody needed only if a severe local reaction occurs.[1]

Vaccine Dose

Reducing or exceeding a recommended dose volume is never recommended. Reducing or dividing doses of DTaP or any other vaccine, including vaccines given to preterm or low birth weight infants, can result in inadequate immune response. A previous immunization with a dose that was less than the standard dose or one administered by a nonstandard route should not be counted as valid, and the person should be reimmunized as recommended for age.

Active Immunization of People Who Recently Received Immune Globulin and Other Blood Products

Live-virus vaccines may have diminished immunogenicity when given within 2 weeks before or up to 11 months following receipt of IG (either standard or hyperimmune globulins following intramuscular, intravenous, or subcutaneous administration). In particular, IG administration inhibits the response to measles vaccine for up to 11 months. Inhibition of immune response to rubella vaccine also has been demonstrated, but the effect on response to mumps or varicella vaccines is not known. The appropriate interval between IG administration and measles immunization varies with the dose of IG and the specific product. Suggested intervals are provided in Table 1.10 but may be shortened if exposure to measles is likely (see Measles, p 535). Because of potential interference with the immune response, varicella, mumps, or rubella vaccine administration should be delayed as recommended for measles vaccine (see Table 1.10). If IG must be given within 14 days

---

[1]Centers for Disease Control and Prevention. General recommendations on immunization: recommendations of the Advisory Committee on Immunization Practices (ACIP). *MMWR Recomm Rep.* 2011;60(RR-02):1-64

Table 1.10. Suggested Intervals Between Immune Globulin Administration and Measles Immunization (MMR or MMRV)

Indications or Product	Route	Dose U or mL	Dose mg IgG/kg	Interval, mo[a]
RSV prophylaxis (palivizumab monoclonal antibody)[b]	IM	...	15 (monoclonal)	None
Tetanus prophylaxis (as TIG)	IM	250 U	10	3
Hepatitis A prophylaxis (as IG)				
Contact prophylaxis	IM	0.02 mL/kg	3.3	3
International travel	IM	0.06 mL/kg	10	3
Hepatitis B prophylaxis (as HBIG)	IM	0.06 mL/kg	10	3
Rabies prophylaxis (as RIG)	IM	20 IU/kg	22	4
Varicella prophylaxis (as VariZIG)	IM	125 U/10 kg (maximum 625 U)	20–40	5
Measles prophylaxis (as IG)				
Standard	IM	0.25 mL/kg	40	5
Immunocompromised host	IM	0.50 mL/kg	80	6
Botulinum Immune Globulin Intravenous (Human [as BabyBIG])	IV	1.5 mL/kg	75	6
Blood transfusion				
Washed RBCs	IV	10 mL/kg	Negligible	0
RBCs, adenine-saline added	IV	10 mL/kg	10	3
Packed RBCs	IV	10 mL/kg	20–60	5
Whole blood	IV	10 mL/kg	80–100	6
Plasma or platelet products	IV	10 mL/kg	160	7
Replacement (or therapy) of immune deficiencies (as IGIV)	IV	...	300–400	8
Therapy for ITP (as IGIV)	IV	...	400	8
Varicella prophylaxis (as IGIV)	IV		400	8
Therapy for ITP (as IGIV)	IV	...	1000	10
Therapy for ITP or Kawasaki disease (as IGIV)	IV	...	1600–2000	11

MMR indicates measles-mumps-rubella; MMRV, measles-mumps-rubella-varicella; RSV, respiratory syncytial virus; IM, intramuscular; TIG, Tetanus Immune Globulin; IG, Immune Globulin; HBIG, Hepatitis B Immune Globulin; RIG, Rabies Immune Globulin; VariZIG, Varicella-Zoster Immune Globulin; IV, intravenous; RBCs, Red Blood Cells; IGIV, Immune Globulin Intravenous; ITP, immune (formerly termed "idiopathic") thrombocytopenic purpura.

[a] These intervals should provide sufficient time for decreases in passive antibodies in all children to allow for an adequate response to measles vaccine. Physicians should not assume that children are protected fully against measles during these intervals. Additional doses of IG or measles vaccine may be indicated after exposure to measles (see text).

[b] RSV monoclonal antibody (palivizumab) does not interfere with the immune response to vaccines.

after administration of measles- or varicella-containing vaccines, these vaccines should be administered again after the interval specified in Table 1.10. One exception to this rule is when serologic testing at an appropriate interval after IG administration documents seroconversion.

Administration of IG preparations does not interfere with antibody responses to yellow fever, oral poliovirus (OPV), or oral rotavirus vaccines and is not expected to affect response to live-attenuated influenza vaccine. Hence, these live vaccines can be administered simultaneously with or at any time before or after administration of IG.

In contrast to the effect on some live-virus vaccines, administration of an IG preparation does not significantly inhibit the immune responses to inactivated vaccines or toxoids. Concurrent administration of recommended doses of Hepatitis B Immune Globulin (HBIG), Tetanus Immune Globulin, or Rabies Immune Globulin (RIG) and standard doses of the corresponding inactivated vaccine or toxoid for postexposure prophylaxis provides immediate protection and long-term immunity and does not impair the efficacy of the vaccine. Vaccines should be administered at a separate anatomic site from that of intramuscularly administered IG. For additional information, see chapters on specific diseases in Section 3.

Respiratory syncytial virus monoclonal antibody (palivizumab) does not interfere with the response to any vaccines.

Testing for *Mycobacterium tuberculosis* Infection

Testing for *Mycobacterium tuberculosis* infection at any age is not a prerequisite for administering live-virus vaccines. A tuberculin skin test (TST) or interferon-gamma release assay (IGRA [see Tuberculosis, p 804]) can be performed at the same visit during which any vaccines are administered, but the testing should not be performed for at least 6 weeks after the administration of measles-containing vaccine (including MMR and MMRV) or smallpox vaccine, because the vaccine temporarily could suppress tuberculin sensitivity for at least 4 to 6 weeks. The effect of live-virus varicella, mumps, rubella, yellow fever, and live-attenuated influenza vaccines on the TST or IGRA result is not known. Infection with wild varicella-zoster virus suppresses TST response, and although the effect of live-virus vaccines on IGRA results has not yet been studied, in theory it could be similar to the effect on the TST. In the absence of data, the same spacing recommendation for TST and IGRA should be applied to these live-virus vaccines as is described for measles, which means waiting at least 6 weeks after administration of vaccine before testing, if the test is not performed at the same time as vaccination (see Tuberculosis portion of Medical Evaluation for Infectious Diseases for Internationally Adopted, Refugee, and Immigrant Children, p 198, and Tuberculosis, p 804). However, if a child is being evaluated for tuberculosis disease, tests for tuberculosis infection should be performed regardless of time after vaccination; a positive test result is valid. Inactivated vaccines, polysaccharide vaccines, and recombinant or subunit vaccines and toxoids do not interfere with clinical interpretation of the TST or IGRA.

Record Keeping and Immunization Information Systems

The National Vaccine Advisory Committee in 1993 recommended a set of standards to improve immunization practices for health care professionals serving children, and revised the standards in 2002. More recently, the ACIP has reviewed and updated these standards for immunization practices.[1] The standards include the recommendation that immunizations of patients be documented through use of immunization records that are accurate, complete, and easily accessible. In addition, the standards also recommend use of tracking systems to provide reminder/recall notices to nonminor patients, parents or legal guardians, and physicians when immunizations are due or overdue. Immunization information systems address record-keeping needs and tracking functions and have additional capacities, such as vaccine inventory management; generation of reports on vaccine usage, including those required for vaccines provided through the Vaccines for Children program; vaccine forecasting; adverse event reporting; interoperability with electronic health records; emergency preparedness functions; and linkage with other public health programs. Additional information about immunization information systems can be found online (**www.cdc.gov/vaccines/programs/iis/index.html**).

Almost all states, territories, and large metropolitan areas have computerized immunization information systems (IISs) to collect and consolidate immunization data for all children residing in the geopolitical area, regardless of where the immunization services are provided. IISs help facilitate children's full immunization by identifying unimmunized and underimmunized children. Children typically enter IISs at birth through linkages with vital records and/or birth hospitals; children also may enter IISs at the time of first clinical encounter for immunizations. Most IISs can consolidate records from physicians' offices, help remind parents and health care professionals when immunizations are due or overdue, help health care professionals determine the immunization needs of their patients at each visit, and generate official immunization records to meet child care or school requirements. IISs also can provide summaries of immunization coverage by age, immunization series, and physician or clinic practice. The AAP urges physicians and all other immunization providers to cooperate with state and local health officials in providing immunization data for state or local IISs.

IMMUNIZATION DOCUMENTATION

Every physician should document and maintain the immunization history of each patient in a confidential record that can be reviewed easily and updated when subsequent immunizations are administered. The health record maintained by the primary health care professional and by the state or regional IIS (see previous discussion) should document all vaccines received, including vaccines received in another health care setting. The format of the record should facilitate identification and recall of patients in need of immunization and, if maintained in a hard-copy health record, should be kept as a single summary sheet of all immunizations administered.

Records of children whose immunizations have been delayed or missed should be flagged to indicate the need to complete immunizations. For data that are required by the National Childhood Vaccine Injury Act of 1986 as well as data recommended by the AAP to be recorded in each patient's medical record for each immunization, see Discussing Vaccines With Patients and Parents (p 7).

Congress passed the Health Information Technology for Economic and Clinical Health (HITECH) Act in 2009 to support adoption and use of electronic health records (EHRs). The purpose of the HITECH Act is to achieve significant improvements in care through meaningful use of EHRs by health care professionals. The HITECH Act

---

[1]www.cdc.gov/mmwr/preview/mmwrhtml/rr6002a1.htm

established incentive payments to eligible professionals and hospitals to promote adoption and meaningful use of interoperable health information technology systems and qualified EHRs. The HITECH Act contains 2 regulations: the first defines the "meaningful use" objectives that providers must meet to qualify for Medicare and Medicaid incentive payments, and the other identifies the technical capabilities required for certified EHR technology. Among the meaningful use objectives is submission to IISs by eligible providers who administer immunizations.

The meaningful use program is to be implemented in at least 3 stages. In stage 1, eligible providers are required to test the capacity of their EHR to submit immunization data to an IIS and to continue to submit if successful. In stage 2, providers must demonstrate ongoing submission to an IIS. In stage 3 (not yet finalized), EHR systems will likely be required to query an IIS for patient records.

Approval by the FDA for use of 2-dimensional bar codes on individual vaccines should facilitate improved efficacy and safety in entering vaccine data, including product type, manufacturer, vaccine lot number, and expiration dates, into electronic systems. Interest in use of EHRs prompted the AAP to issue a revised statement in 2007 outlining functions that would need to be performed in a pediatric practice for EHR systems to be useful.[1]

PERSONAL IMMUNIZATION RECORDS HELD BY PARENTS/PATIENTS

The AAP and state health departments have developed an official written immunization record. This record should be given to parents of every newborn infant, and parents should be encouraged to safeguard the record for subsequent referral and updates. Physicians should cooperate with this endeavor by recording immunization data in this record and by encouraging parents/patients not only to preserve the record but also to present it at each visit to a health care professional. An alternative to written records is the use of patient portals that interface with EHRs and allow patients and caregivers access to immunization records electronically.

Vaccine Shortages

When vaccine shortages occur, temporary changes in childhood or adolescent immunization recommendations by the AAP and CDC may be necessary, including temporary deferral of certain vaccines or specific doses in the schedule for those vaccines, establishment of vaccine priorities for high-risk children, and suspension of school and child care entry immunization requirements in some states.

When vaccines are in short supply, physicians and other health care professionals should maintain lists of children and adolescents who do not receive vaccines at the recommended time or age so they can be recalled when the vaccine supply becomes adequate. For current information about vaccine shortages and resulting recommendations, see the Web sites of the CDC (**www.cdc.gov/vaccines/vac-gen/shortages/default.htm**), FDA (**www.fda.gov/BiologicsBloodVaccines/SafetyAvailability/Shortages/default.htm**), or *Red Book* Online (**http://aapredbook.aappublications.org**). The FDA Web site also provides information on other biologic products in short supply (eg, Immune

---

[1]American Academy of Pediatrics, Council on Clinical Information Technology. Special requirements of electronic health record systems in pediatrics. *Pediatrics.* 2007;119(3):631–637. Reaffirmed May 2012

Globulin products) as well as products permanently discontinued. For analyses of vaccine shortages and recommended solutions, see the published recommendations from the National Vaccine Advisory Committee.[1]

Vaccine Safety

RISKS AND ADVERSE EVENTS

Prior to licensure, all vaccines in the United States undergo rigorous safety and efficacy/immunogenicity testing. However, adverse events after vaccination occasionally occur. Furthermore, some individuals still may acquire a vaccine-preventable disease despite receiving the corresponding vaccine. Adverse events following vaccination may be true causally associated vaccine adverse events or reactions, such as local pain and tenderness at the injection site. However, many adverse events may be coincidental events that occur in temporal association after vaccination but are unrelated to vaccination. Highly effective vaccines have dramatically reduced the threat of infectious diseases, and because of this success some people now worry more about potential vaccine adverse effects than the illnesses vaccines prevent. As vaccinations successfully control their target diseases, providers need to communicate benefits and risks of vaccination to a population whose first-hand experience with vaccine-preventable diseases increasingly is rare.

As with all aspects of medicine, the benefits and risks from vaccines must be weighed against each other, and vaccine recommendations are based on this assessment. Recommendations are made to maximize protection and minimize risk by providing specific advice on dose, route, and timing and by identifying precautions or contraindications to vaccination.

Common vaccine adverse reactions usually are mild to moderate in severity (eg, fever or injection site reactions, such as swelling, redness, and pain) and have no permanent sequelae. Examples include local inflammation after administration of DTaP, Td, or Tdap vaccines, and fever and rash 1 to 2 weeks after administration of MMR or MMRV vaccines.

The occurrence of an adverse event following vaccination does not mean the vaccine caused the symptoms or signs. The Brighton Collaboration is a nonprofit international voluntary consortium formed to develop globally accepted and standardized case definitions for adverse events following immunization to be used in vaccine safety surveillance and research. The project began in 2000 with formation of a steering committee and creation of work groups composed of international experts in vaccine safety, patient care, pharmacology, regulatory affairs, public health, and vaccine delivery. It is the world's largest network of vaccine safety science experts. The Brighton Collaboration provides guidelines for collecting, analyzing, and presenting vaccine safety data, which facilitates sharing and comparison of vaccine data among professionals working in the area of vaccine safety worldwide. Additional information, including current definitions and updates of progress, can be found online (**https://brightoncollaboration.org/public/resources.html**). As of January 2015, a total of 28 case definitions have been developed and completed, and all definitions can be accessed online.

---

[1]Santoli JM, Peter G, Arvin AM, et al. Strengthening the supply of routinely recommended vaccines in the United States: recommendations from the National Vaccine Advisory Committee. *JAMA.* 2003;290(23):3122–3128

Because many suspected adverse events are merely coincidental with administration of a vaccine, a true causal association usually requires that the event occur at a significantly higher rate in vaccine recipients than in nonvaccinated groups of similar age and residence, or that the event has previously been determined to be associated with vaccination through prelicensure clinical trials or postlicensure epidemiologic studies. Although rare, a causal link with a live-virus vaccine may be established if the vaccine-type virus can be identified in biologic specimens from an ill child with compatible symptoms (eg, rotavirus vaccine-associated diarrhea in a patient with severe combined immunodeficiency). Clustering in time of unusual adverse events following vaccination may suggest a possible causal relationship that requires further evaluation. Because many adverse events following immunization include clinical syndromes that also occur in the absence of vaccination, definitive assessment of causality often requires careful epidemiologic studies comparing the incidence of the event in vaccinees to nonvaccinees or the incidence of the adverse event in a specific time frame following immunization (the postulated risk interval) with the incidence in other timeframes.

Health care professionals are mandated by law to report specific adverse events found on the Vaccine Adverse Event Reporting System (VAERS) Table of Reportable Events Following Vaccination (Appendix III, p 987) (**http://vaers.hhs.gov/resources/ VAERS_Table_of_Reportable_Events_Following_Vaccination.pdf**). Reporting of any clinically significant adverse event following vaccination to VAERS (see p 46) is important because, when analyzed in conjunction with other VAERS reports, this information can provide evidence of safety signals for unanticipated potentially causally related vaccine adverse events (Appendix III, p 987). It is important to understand that VAERS is not designed to assess whether a vaccine caused an adverse event, but rather as a system to generate hypotheses (to detect signals) to be tested subsequently through well-designed epidemiologic studies. Other vaccine safety monitoring systems, such as the Vaccine Safety Datalink (VSD), which uses large-linked databases (**www.cdc.gov/ vaccinesafety/Activities/vsd.html**) or the Clinical Immunization Safety Assessment (CISA) project (**www.cdc.gov/vaccinesafety/Activities/cisa.html**) provide mechanisms to implement such studies. A nationally notifiable vaccine-preventable disease that occurs in a child or adolescent at any time, including after vaccination (vaccine failure), should be reported to the local or state health department (see Appendix IV, p 992). An Institute of Medicine report published in January 2013[1] reviewed and affirmed existing data sources and systems involved in vaccine safety surveillance and research (also see Addressing Parents' Questions About Vaccine Safety and Effectiveness [p 9] and Institute of Medicine [IOM] Reviews of Adverse Events After Immunization [p 44]).

INSTITUTE OF MEDICINE REVIEWS OF ADVERSE EVENTS AFTER IMMUNIZATION

In a series of comprehensive reviews, the IOM of the National Academy of Sciences determined that the childhood immunization schedule is safe and that following the complete childhood immunization schedule is associated strongly with a reduction in vaccine-preventable diseases.

---

[1]Institute of Medicine. *The Childhood Immunization Schedule and Safety: Stakeholder Concerns, Scientific Evidence, and Future Studies*. Washington, DC: National Academies Press; 2013

The Health Resources and Services Administration (HRSA) of the US Department of Health and Human Services, with support provided by the CDC and the National Vaccine Program Office, had commissioned the IOM to convene a committee of experts on several occasions to review the epidemiologic, clinical, and biological evidence regarding adverse health events associated with specific vaccines covered by the Vaccine Injury Compensation Program (VICP) and to assess the adequacy of the current childhood and adolescent immunization schedule and its safety (**http://www.iom.edu/Activities/ PublicHealth/ImmunizationSafety.aspx**). These committees included members with expertise in pediatrics, internal medicine, neurology, immunology, immunotoxicology, neurobiology, rheumatology, epidemiology, biostatistics, and law. The initial reviews were expected to provide the scientific basis for review and adjudication of claims of vaccine injury by the VICP.[1] The most recent review assessed the adequacy and safety of the current immunization schedules.[2]

In the initial IOM report on vaccine safety, 8 different vaccines covered by the VICP were reviewed: varicella-zoster vaccines, influenza vaccines, HepB vaccines, HPV vaccines; tetanus toxoid-containing vaccines other than those containing whole-cell pertussis component; hepatitis A vaccines; meningococcal vaccines; and MMR vaccine. HRSA provided a list of specific adverse events for the committee to review, and the committee had the flexibility to add additional adverse events as the review progressed. Two lines of evidence supported the committee's causality conclusions: epidemiologic evidence and mechanistic evidence. The benefit and effectiveness of vaccines were not assessed during this review. On the basis of scientific evidence, the IOM committee developed 158 causality conclusions and assigned each to 1 of 4 relationships between vaccines and adverse events. A summary of the IOM committee causality conclusions regarding evidence for a causal relationship between the specified vaccine and adverse event follows[3]:

Category 1: Evidence convincingly supports a causal relationship between vaccines and some adverse events:

- Varicella vaccines and 5 specific adverse events:
    - disseminated vaccine-strain varicella-zoster virus (VZV) infection without other organ involvement
    - disseminated vaccine-strain VZV infection with other organ involvement, including pneumonia, meningitis, or hepatitis, in immunodeficient individuals
    - vaccine-strain viral reactivation without other organ involvement
    - vaccine-strain viral reactivation with subsequent infection resulting in meningitis or encephalitis
    - anaphylaxis

[1]Institute of Medicine. *Adverse Effects of Vaccines: Evidence and Causality*. Washington, DC: National Academies Press; 2011

[2]Institute of Medicine. *The Childhood Immunization Schedule and Safety: Stakeholder Concerns, Scientific Evidence and Future Studies*. Washington, DC: National Academies Press; 2013. Available at: **www.iom.edu/Reports/2013/ The-Childhood-Immunization-Schedule-and-Safety.aspx**

[3]Institute of Medicine. *The Childhood Immunization Schedule and Safety: Stakeholder Concerns, Scientific Evidence and Future Studies*. Washington, DC: National Academies Press; 2013. Available at: **www.iom.edu/Reports/2013/ The-Childhood-Immunization-Schedule-and-Safety.aspx**

- MMR vaccine and 3 specific adverse events:
  - measles inclusion body encephalitis in immunodeficient individuals
  - febrile seizures
  - anaphylaxis
- Influenza vaccines and anaphylaxis
- Hepatitis B vaccines and anaphylaxis
- Tetanus toxoid vaccines and anaphylaxis
- Meningococcal vaccines and anaphylaxis
- Injection-related events and deltoid bursitis
- Injection-related events and syncope

Category 2: Evidence favors acceptance of a causal relationship (evidence is strong and generally suggestive but not firm enough to be described as convincing):
- Certain inactivated influenza vaccines previously used in Canada and oculorespiratory syndrome
- HPV vaccines and anaphylaxis
- MMR vaccine and transient arthralgia in women and in children

Category 3: Evidence favors rejection of a causal relationship:
- MMR vaccine and autism
- MMR vaccine and type 1 diabetes mellitus
- DT, TT, or acellular pertussis-containing vaccines and type 1 diabetes mellitus
- Inactivated influenza vaccines and Bell palsy
- Inactivated influenza vaccines and exacerbation of asthma or reactive airways disease in children and adults

Category 4: Evidence is inadequate to accept or reject a causal relationship for the vast majority (135 vaccine-adverse event pairs).

During the years 2001-2004, the Immunization Safety Review Committee evaluated 8 existing and emerging vaccine safety concerns. One of these reports examined hypotheses about associations between vaccines and autism. The committee concluded that the evidence favors rejection of a causal relationship between the MMR vaccine and autism and between thimerosal-containing vaccines and autism.

In the 2013 report, the IOM expert committee further reviewed scientific findings and stakeholder concerns related to the overall safety of the childhood immunization schedule. This review determined that the childhood immunization schedule is safe and that following the complete childhood immunization schedule is strongly associated with reducing vaccine-preventable diseases.[1,2]

VACCINE ADVERSE EVENT REPORTING SYSTEM

The Vaccine Adverse Event Reporting System (VAERS) is a national passive surveillance system that monitors the safety of vaccines licensed for use in the United States. Jointly administered by the CDC and the FDA, VAERS accepts reports of suspected

[1]Institute of Medicine. *The Childhood Immunization Schedule and Safety: Stakeholder Concerns, Scientific Evidence and Future Studies*. Washington, DC: National Academies Press; 2013. Available at: **www.iom.edu/Reports/2013/ The-Childhood-Immunization-Schedule-and-Safety.aspx**

[2]Institute of Medicine. *Immunization Safety Review*. Available at: **www.iom.edu/Activities/PublicHealth/ ImmunizationSafety.aspx**

adverse events after administration of any vaccine. The strengths of VAERS are that it is national in scope, can rapidly detect safety signals, and can detect rare and unexpected adverse events. VAERS is also useful for monitoring vaccine safety trends and for evaluating lot-specific frequencies of adverse events. Like all passive surveillance systems, VAERS is subject to limitations, including reporting biases such as underreporting, inconsistent data quality and completeness, lack of denominator data, and absence of an unvaccinated comparison group. Because of these limitations, determining causal associations between vaccines and adverse events from VAERS reports usually is not possible.

The National Childhood Vaccine Injury Act of 1986 requires physicians and other health care professionals who administer vaccines covered under the National Vaccine Injury Compensation Program to maintain permanent vaccination records and to report to VAERS any condition listed on the VAERS Table of Reportable Events Following Vaccination (see Appendix III, p 987) or listed in the manufacturer's package insert as a contraindication to further doses. Vaccines covered under this act include those that are recommended by the CDC for routine administration to children. The vaccines to which these requirements apply are measles, mumps, rubella, varicella, poliovirus, hepatitis A, hepatitis B, pertussis, diphtheria, tetanus, rotavirus, *Haemophilus influenzae* type b, pneumococcal conjugate, meningococcal (conjugate and polysaccharide), human papillomavirus, and influenza (inactivated and live intranasal [see Record Keeping and Immunization Information Systems, p 40]). Health care professionals who suspect that any clinically significant adverse event occurred after any vaccination are strongly encouraged to report the event, regardless of whether or not it is listed on the VAERS Table of Reportable Events Following Vaccination. People other than health care professionals also may submit a report of a suspected adverse event to VAERS. In addition to adverse events, vaccine product problems and vaccine administration errors may be reported.

The Health Insurance Portability and Accountability Act (HIPAA) Privacy Rule permits reporting of protected health information to public health authorities. Submission of a VAERS report does not necessarily indicate that the vaccine or vaccination procedure caused or contributed to the event. All patient-identifying information is kept confidential. Written notification that the report has been received is provided to the person submitting the report. VAERS forms (see Fig 1.1, p 48) are available for download (**http://vaers.hhs.gov**), by e-mailing VAERS (info@vaers.org), or by calling 1-800-822-7967.

Reports can be submitted through a secure online system (**https://vaers.hhs.gov/esub/index**) or by mail or facsimile. Online reporting is preferred. VAERS data, excluding personal identifiers, are made available to the public and can be accessed on the VAERS Web site. These deindentified data are also available by search engine on the CDC Wide-ranging Online Data for Epidemiologic Research (WONDER) Web site (**http://wonder.cdc.gov/vaers.html**).

Information in VAERS reports is evaluated and analyzed by CDC and FDA staff to determine whether there are unusual patterns of adverse events associated with vaccines or concerns about specific vaccine lots. Reports are coded as serious when at least 1 of the following outcomes is reported: death, life-threatening illness, hospitalization, prolongation of an existing hospitalization, permanent disability, or an intervention was required to prevent any of the aforementioned outcomes. Medical records are obtained,

FIG 1.1 VAERS FORM

FOR DIRECTIONS FOR COMPLETING FORM AND FOR A NEW ELECTRONIC
REPORTING FORM, SEE HTTP://VAERS.HHS.GOV/ESUB/INDEX

WEBSITE: www.vaers.hhs.gov   E-MAIL: info@vaers.org   FAX: 1-877-721-0366

VACCINE ADVERSE EVENT REPORTING SYSTEM
24 Hour Toll-Free Information 1-800-822-7967
P.O. Box 1100, Rockville, MD 20849-1100
PATIENT IDENTITY KEPT CONFIDENTIAL

VAERS

For CDC/FDA Use Only

VAERS Number _____

Date Received _____

Patient Name:

Last   First   M.I.

Address

City   State   Zip

Telephone no. (___) _____

Vaccine administered by (Name):

Responsible
Physician _____
Facility Name/Address

City   State   Zip

Telephone no. (___) _____

Form completed by (Name):

Relation   ☐ Vaccine Provider ☐ Patient/Parent
to Patient ☐ Manufacturer   ☐ Other
Address (if different from patient or provider)

City   State   Zip

Telephone no. (___) _____

1. State	2. County where administered	3. Date of birth mm / dd / yy	4. Patient age	5. Sex ☐ M ☐ F	6. Date form completed mm / dd / yy

7. Describe adverse events(s) (symptoms, signs, time course) and treatment, if any

8. Check all appropriate:
☐ Patient died   (date ___ / ___ / ___)
                           mm   dd   yy
☐ Life threatening illness
☐ Required emergency room/doctor visit
☐ Required hospitalization (_____days)
☐ Resulted in prolongation of hospitalization
☐ Resulted in permanent disability
☐ None of the above

9. Patient recovered   ☐ YES ☐ NO ☐ UNKNOWN

12. Relevant diagnostic tests/laboratory data

10. Date of vaccination mm / dd / yy Time _____ AM PM	11. Adverse event onset mm / dd / yy Time _____ AM PM

13. Enter all vaccines given on date listed in no. 10

	Vaccine (type)	Manufacturer	Lot number	Route/Site	No. Previous Doses
a.					
b.					
c.					
d.					

14. Any other vaccinations within 4 weeks prior to the date listed in no. 10

	Vaccine (type)	Manufacturer	Lot number	Route/Site	No. Previous doses	Date given
a.						
b.						

15. Vaccinated at:
☐ Private doctor's office/hospital   ☐ Military clinic/hospital
☐ Public health clinic/hospital   ☐ Other/unknown

16. Vaccine purchased with:
☐ Private funds   ☐ Military funds
☐ Public funds   ☐ Other/unknown

17. Other medications

18. Illness at time of vaccination (specify)

19. Pre-existing physician-diagnosed allergies, birth defects, medical conditions (specify)

20. Have you reported this adverse event previously?	☐ No ☐ To doctor	☐ To health department ☐ To manufacturer

Only for children 5 and under

22. Birth weight _____ lb. _____ oz.

23. No. of brothers and sisters

21. Adverse event following prior vaccination (check all applicable, specify)

	Adverse Event	Onset Age	Type Vaccine	Dose no. in series
☐ In patient				
☐ In brother or sister				

Only for reports submitted by manufacturer/immunization project

24. Mfr./imm. proj. report no.

25. Date received by mfr./imm.proj.

26. 15 day report?   ☐ Yes ☐ No

27. Report type   ☐ Initial ☐ Follow-Up

Health care providers and manufacturers are required by law (42 USC 300aa-25) to report reactions to vaccines listed in the Table of Reportable Events Following Immunization. Reports for reactions to other vaccines are voluntary except when required as a condition of immunization grant awards.

Form VAERS-1(FDA)

when available, by VAERS staff for serious reports and other reports of special interest and then are reviewed by FDA and CDC physicians. FDA physicians perform postmarketing safety evaluations 18 months after approval (or approval for expanded indication) of a vaccine or after its use in 10 000 individuals, whichever is later. The FDA also presents a safety summary to an independent pediatric advisory committee after the first 12 months of safety data after licensure of a vaccine for use in children. Periodically, reviews of vaccine and adverse event-specific surveillance summaries from VAERS data are published by CDC and FDA staff. These summary reports may provide reassurance of the safety of a vaccine, or they may describe findings ("signals") of associations that require further evaluation. Vaccine safety concerns identified through VAERS nearly always require further studies for confirmation using established systems, such as the Vaccine Safety Datalink (VSD) or other controlled epidemiologic methods. At a minimum, determination of causality requires the demonstration that the incidence of an adverse event following immunization is significantly higher than would be expected in an unvaccinated population or that the incidence in a specific time frame following vaccination is higher than would be expected in an unvaccinated population within that time frame and not attributed to other factors.

VACCINE SAFETY DATALINK PROJECT

To supplement the VAERS program, which is a passive surveillance system, the CDC formed partnerships with several large managed-care organizations to establish the Vaccine Safety Datalink (VSD) project in 1990, an active surveillance system designed to monitor and evaluate vaccine safety. The VSD project includes comprehensive medical and immunization histories on more than 9 million people. The VSD project allows for both retrospective and prospective observational vaccine safety studies as well as for timely investigations of newly licensed vaccines or emerging vaccine safety concerns. Rates of potential adverse events following immunization can be compared with rates in control windows, rates in a historical cohort, or other unexposed populations in the VSD cohort, as feasible. The VSD has been a critical part of the public health immunization system in the United States. Information about the VSD can be found on the CDC Web site (**www.cdc.gov/vaccinesafety/Activities/vsd.html**).

POSTLICENSURE RAPID IMMUNIZATION SAFETY MONITORING (PRISM)

The VSD is complemented by the vaccine safety portion of the FDA's Mini-Sentinel project (**www.fda.gov/safety/FDAsSentinelInitiative/ucm2007250.htm**), called the Postlicensure Rapid Immunization Safety Monitoring (PRISM) system. PRISM includes medical and drug coverage for more than 50 million individuals in partnership with 4 large, national data partners in the United States. In addition, linkages have been established between health plans and state immunization information systems to enhance data on vaccine exposure. PRISM currently is conducting retrospective vaccine safety evaluations and preparing for prospective, active surveillance of FDA-licensed vaccines and biologics in the United States.

CLINICAL IMMUNIZATION SAFETY ASSESSMENT (CISA) PROJECT

Serious and other uncommon clinically important adverse events (AEs) following immunization rarely occur in prelicensure clinical trials, and health care professionals may see them too infrequently to be able to provide standardized evaluation. In addition, high-quality studies are needed to identify risk factors for AEs following immunization, especially in special populations, and to develop strategies to prevent or reduce the severity of AEs following immunization. The CDC supports the CISA Project to improve the understanding of AEs following immunization at the individual patient level. The CISA Project's goals are: (1) to serve as a vaccine safety resource for consultation on clinical vaccine safety issues, including individual case reviews, and to assist with immunization decision making; (2) to assist the CDC in developing strategies to assess individuals who may be at increased risk of AEs following immunization; and (3) to conduct studies to identify risk factors and preventive strategies for AEs following immunization, particularly in special populations. The CISA Project consists of 7 academic centers with expertise in vaccines and vaccine safety, epidemiology, biostatistics, and a wide range of specialty areas, such as allergy, immunology, neurology, infectious diseases, immunology, and obstetrics and gynecology.

The CISA Project advises US clinicians who have vaccine safety questions about specific patients who have received US-licensed vaccines. For example, CISA may provide an opinion on whether a patient who had an AE following immunization after 1 dose of a vaccine should receive a future dose of the same vaccine. In a CISA evaluation, vaccine safety experts from the CDC's Immunization Safety Office and the CISA academic medical centers meet via scheduled teleconferences to review complex vaccine safety cases from US health care providers. The experts discuss the findings and form a general assessment and plan. These conclusions are then shared with the health care provider. Advice from the CDC and CISA is meant to assist in decision making rather than provide direct patient management, because patient-management decisions are the responsibility of the treating health care provider. The CISA Project also conducts clinical research to advance knowledge of vaccine safety after licensure. National strategic plans and public health needs guide the research priorities of the CISA Project. Current priority areas for CISA research studies are: influenza vaccine safety, safety in people with autoimmune diseases, and safety in pregnant women. The CISA complements vaccine safety surveillance systems and usually studies clinical vaccine safety questions that can be addressed by prospectively enrolling up to hundreds of subjects. Whereas large linked database systems like the VSD are best used to assess risk for rare, medically attended events in vaccinated populations, CISA is well suited to study more common, nonmedically attended events (eg, fever) and to collect biological specimens after vaccination. CISA investigators also have access to special populations (eg, people with autoimmune diseases) and specialists who care for these patients.

US health care providers who need expert opinion or with a vaccine safety question about a specific patient residing in the United States can contact the CDC (**CISAeval@cdc.gov**) to request a CISA evaluation. Current information about the CISA Project is available online (**www.cdc.gov/vaccinesafety/Activities/CISA.html**).

VACCINE INJURY COMPENSATION

The Vaccine Injury Compensation Program (VICP) was established in 1988 as a means to stabilize the nation's vaccine supply by reducing excess liability that could lead vaccine manufacturers to exit the US market. It was developed as an alternative to civil litigation to simplify the process of settling vaccine injury claims. VICP is a no-fault system in which compensation may be sought if people are thought to have suffered death or other injury as a result of administration of a covered vaccine. A "covered vaccine" is any vaccine that is recommended by the CDC for routine use in children and has an excise tax placed on it by Congress. Claims must be filed within 36 months after the first symptom appeared following immunization, and death claims must be filed within 3 years after the first symptom of the vaccine injury or within 2 years of a death and 4 years after the start of the first symptom of the vaccine injury that resulted in the death (**www.hrsa.gov/vaccinecompensation/fileclaim.html**). People seeking compensation for alleged injuries from covered vaccines must first file claims with the VICP before pursuing civil litigation against manufacturers or vaccine providers. For a death or other injury, reasonable lawyers' fees and other legal costs may be paid if the claim was filed on a reasonable basis and in good faith. To ensure that legal expenses are not a barrier to entry into the program, assuming that certain minimal requirements are met, the VICP may pay lawyer's fees and other legal costs related to a claim, regardless of whether the claimant is paid for a vaccine injury or death. If the claimant accepts the judgment of the VICP, neither vaccine providers nor manufacturers can be sued in civil litigation. If the claimant rejects the VICP judgment, he or she has the option of filing a claim against the health care professional on such grounds as failure to adequately warn, negligent vaccine administration, or negligent postvaccination care. Experience to date has demonstrated that the program has had the effect that was intended—that is, it has simplified the process, decreased the number of lawsuits against health care professionals and vaccine manufacturers, and assisted in establishing a stable vaccine supply while ensuring access to compensation for vaccine-associated injury and death.

The program is based on the Vaccine Injury Table (VIT [see Appendix III, p 987] or **www.hrsa.gov/vaccinecompensation/vaccinetable.html**), which lists the vaccines covered by the program as well as injuries, disabilities, illnesses, and conditions (including death) for which compensation may be awarded. The VIT defines the time during which the first symptoms or significant aggravation of an injury must appear after immunization. If an injury listed in the VIT is proven, claimants receive a "legal presumption of causation," thus avoiding the need to prove causation in an individual case. If the claim pertains to conditions not listed in the VIT, claimants may prevail if they prove causation. Contact information for the VICP and the VIT follow:

Parklawn Building
5600 Fishers Lane
Room 11C-26
Rockville, MD 20857
Telephone: 800-338-2382
Web site: **www.hrsa.gov/vaccinecompensation**

People wishing to file a claim for a vaccine injury should telephone or write to the following:

United States Court of Federal Claims
717 Madison Place, NW
Washington, DC 20005-1011
Telephone: 202-357-6400

Information on the VICP is available to parents or guardians through Vaccine Information Statements (**www.cdc.gov/vaccines/pubs/vis/default.htm**), which are required to given prior to administering each dose of vaccines covered through the program.

VACCINE CONTRAINDICATIONS AND PRECAUTIONS

A **contraindication** to vaccination is a condition in a patient that increases the risk of a serious adverse reaction and for whom this increased risk of an adverse reaction outweighs the benefit of the vaccine. A vaccine should **not** be administered when a contraindication is present. The only contraindication applicable to all vaccines is a history of anaphylaxis to a previous dose or to a vaccine component, unless the patient has undergone desensitization. A **precaution** is a condition in a recipient that might increase the risk or seriousness of an adverse reaction or complicate making another diagnosis because of a possible vaccine-related reaction. A precaution also may exist for conditions that might compromise the ability of the vaccine to produce immunity (eg, administering measles vaccine to a person with passive immunity to measles from a blood transfusion).

Vaccinations may be deferred when a precaution is present until the health condition resulting in the precaution improves or resolves. However, vaccination may be recommended in the presence of a precaution if the benefit of protection from the vaccine outweighs the risk. Most precautions are the result of temporary conditions (eg, moderate or severe illness), and a vaccine can be administered when the illness abates.

Failure to understand true contraindications and precautions can result in administration of a vaccine when it should be withheld (see Immunization in Immunocompromised Children, p 74). National standards for pediatric vaccination practices have been established. Screening for contraindications and precautions is important to prevent potential serious adverse reactions following vaccination. Everyone should be screened before every vaccine dose, even if screened during a prior visit.

Vaccine manufacturers may be required to update vaccine package inserts with new information on vaccine contraindications and precautions as additional safety data become available. A change in a patient's condition may also place him or her in a category for a contraindication or precaution, which can be identified with screening before vaccination. A standardized screening form may be helpful. A current screening form for children and adults, available in several languages, can be obtained from each state immunization program or the Immunization Action Coalition (**www. immunize.org**).

The only contraindication applicable to all vaccines is a history of a severe allergic reaction (ie, anaphylaxis) after a previous dose of that vaccine or a component of that vaccine. Severely immunocompromised people generally should not receive live vaccines. Children who experienced encephalopathy within 7 days after administration of a previous dose of diphtheria and tetanus toxoids and pertussis vaccine (DTwP, DTaP, or Tdap), not attributable to another identifiable cause, should not receive additional doses of a vaccine that contains pertussis. Pregnant women should not receive live-virus vaccines because of a theoretical risk to the fetus. In contrast, a personal or family history of seizures is a precaution, rather than a contraindication, for MMRV vaccination in a child.

The presence of a moderate or severe acute illness with or without a fever is a precaution to administration of all vaccines. The decision to administer or delay vaccination because of a current or recent acute illness depends on the severity of symptoms and etiology of the condition. Delaying avoids causing diagnostic confusion between manifestations of the underlying illness and possible adverse effects of vaccination or superimposing adverse effects of the vaccine on the underlying illness. People who have had vaccine administration delayed because of moderate or severe acute illness should be vaccinated as soon as the acute illness has improved.

Vaccination should not be delayed because of the presence of mild respiratory tract illness or other acute mild illnesses with or without fever. The safety and immunogenicity of vaccinating people with mild illnesses have been documented. Routine physical examinations and procedures (eg, measuring temperatures) are not prerequisites for vaccinating people who appear to be healthy, but the provider should ask the parent or guardian whether the child is ill.

Contraindications, precautions, and reasons for deferral of immunizations are addressed in disease-specific chapters in Section 3 and are listed in Appendix V (p 994). For more detailed information, physicians should consult vaccine manufacturer package inserts and published recommendations of the ACIP and AAP. Health care providers, including school physicians, should adhere strictly to contraindications to each vaccine as listed in Appendix V when granting medical exemption from vaccination.

Clinicians might misperceive certain conditions or circumstances as valid contraindications or precautions to vaccination when they do not preclude vaccination. Common conditions that should not delay vaccination but often are considered mistakenly to be contraindications include:

- Diarrhea
- Minor upper respiratory tract illnesses (including otitis media) with or without fever
- Mild to moderate local reactions to a previous dose of vaccine
- Exposure to an infectious disease
- Current antimicrobial therapy (see Appendix V)
- Being in the convalescent phase of an acute illness
- Allergy to duck meat or duck feathers
- Allergy to an antibiotic (except anaphylactic reaction to neomycin, gentamicin, or streptomycin, if any of these are in the vaccine to be administered)
- History of nonanaphylactic allergy to egg
- Personal or family history of seizures
- Family history of sudden unexpected death
- Family history of an adverse event following immunization
- Breastfeeding or pregnancy in a household contact

Misconceptions about vaccine contraindications can result in missed opportunities to provide vaccines and can leave people susceptible to serious diseases.

HYPERSENSITIVITY REACTIONS AFTER IMMUNIZATION

Hypersensitivity reactions to constituents of vaccines are rare; however, facilities and health care professionals should be available for treating anaphylaxis in all settings in which vaccines are administered. This recommendation includes administration of vaccines in school-based, pharmacy, or other complementary or nontraditional settings. Health care professionals should consider observing adolescents for 15 minutes after they are immunized to be able to intervene if a hypersensitivity reaction or nonhypersensitivity reaction event, such as syncope, occurs.

Children who have experienced an apparent allergic reaction to a vaccine or vaccine constituent should be evaluated by an allergist before receiving subsequent doses of the suspect vaccine or other vaccines containing one or more of the same ingredients. This evaluation and appropriate allergy testing may determine whether the child currently is allergic, which vaccines pose a risk, and whether alternative vaccines (without the allergen) are available. Even when the child truly is allergic and no alternative vaccines are available, in almost all cases, the risk of remaining unimmunized exceeds the risk of careful vaccine administration under observation in a facility with personnel and equipment prepared to recognize and treat anaphylaxis, should it occur.

Hypersensitivity reactions related to vaccine constituents can be immediate or delayed and often are attributable to an excipient rather than the immunizing agent itself.

IMMEDIATE-TYPE ALLERGIC REACTIONS

As with most IgE-mediated, immediate-type allergic reactions, the allergens usually are proteins. The proteins most often implicated in vaccine reactions are ovalbumin or other egg white proteins and gelatin, with perhaps rare reactions to yeast or latex. On rare occasions, nonprotein antimicrobial agents present in some vaccines can be the cause of an allergic reaction.

ALLERGIC REACTIONS TO EGG PROTEIN (OVALBUMIN). Current measles and mumps vaccines (and some rabies vaccines) are derived from chicken embryo fibroblast tissue cultures and do not contain significant amounts of egg proteins. Studies indicate that children with egg allergy, even children with severe hypersensitivity, are at low risk of anaphylactic reactions to these vaccines, singly or in combination (eg, MMR or MMRV), and skin testing with the vaccine may not be predictive of an allergic reaction to immunization. Most immediate hypersensitivity reactions after measles or mumps immunization appear to be reactions to other vaccine components, such as gelatin. Therefore, children with egg allergy may be given MMR or MMRV vaccines without special precautions.

The approach to a patient who may be allergic to eggs and requires influenza vaccine should be distinguished from the approach to a patient who has had an apparent allergic reaction to influenza vaccination described previously under "Hypersensitivity Reactions After Immunization." Although both inactivated influenza vaccine (IIV) and live-attenuated influenza vaccine (LAIV) are produced in eggs, data have shown that IIV administration in a single, age-appropriate dose is well tolerated by nearly all recipients who have an egg allergy. No data have been published on the safety of administering LAIV to egg-allergic recipients. More conservative approaches, such as skin testing or a 2-step graded challenge, no longer are recommended.[1] For recommendations regarding administration of influenza vaccine to people with egg allergy, see Influenza (p 476).

Yellow fever vaccine may contain a larger amount of egg protein than influenza vaccines, and there are fewer reports on administering the vaccine to egg-allergic patients. The vaccine package insert describes a protocol involving skin testing the patient with the vaccine and if positive, giving the vaccine in graded doses. Such a procedure would best be performed by an allergist.

ALLERGIC REACTIONS TO GELATIN. Some vaccines, such as MMR, MMRV, varicella, yellow fever, zoster, and some influenza and rabies vaccines, contain gelatin as a stabilizer. The Vero cell culture-derived Japanese encephalitis (JE-VC) vaccine available in the United States does not contain gelatin stabilizers. People with a history of food allergy to gelatin may develop anaphylaxis after receipt of gelatin-containing vaccines. Additionally, people who experience an immediate hypersensitivity reaction following receipt of a vaccine containing gelatin may, in fact, be allergic to gelatin, despite not having a known gelatin food allergy. In either case, such a patient should be evaluated by an allergist before receiving gelatin-containing vaccines to confirm the gelatin allergy and to administer the vaccine under observation and in accordance with established protocols.

ALLERGIC REACTIONS TO YEAST. Hepatitis B and quadrivalent human papillomavirus (HPV4 and HPV9) vaccines are manufactured using recombinant technology in yeast cells. In theory, vaccine recipients with hypersensitivity to yeast could experience an allergic reaction to these vaccines. Allergy to yeast is rare; however, patients claiming such an allergy should be evaluated by an allergist prior to receiving yeast-containing vaccines to confirm the yeast allergy and to administer the vaccine under observation and in accordance with established protocols.

ALLERGIC REACTIONS TO LATEX. Dry natural rubber latex contains naturally occurring proteins that may be responsible for allergic reactions. Some vaccine vial stoppers and syringe plungers contain latex. Other vaccine vials and syringes contain synthetic rubber that poses no risk to the latex-allergic child. Information about latex used in vaccine packaging is available in the manufacturer's package inserts or on the CDC Web site (**www.cdc.gov/vaccines/pubs/pinkbook/downloads/appendices/B/ latex-table.pdf**). Hypersensitivity reactions to latex after immunizations are rare; however, latex-allergic patients should be evaluated by an allergist before receiving vaccines with natural rubber latex in the packaging to confirm the latex allergy and to administer the vaccine under observation and in accordance with established protocols.

DELAYED-TYPE ALLERGIC REACTIONS

As with most cell-mediated, delayed-type allergic reactions, the allergens usually are small molecules. The small molecules present in vaccines include thimerosal, aluminum, and antimicrobial agents.

ALLERGIC REACTIONS TO THIMEROSAL. Most patients with localized or delayed-type hypersensitivity reactions to thimerosal tolerate injection of vaccines containing thimerosal uneventfully or with only temporary swelling at the injection site. This is not a contraindication to receive a vaccine that contains thimerosal.

---

[1]American Academy of Pediatrics, Committee on Infectious Diseases. Recommendations for prevention and control of influenza in children, 2014-2015. *Pediatrics.* 2014;134(5):e1–e17

ALLERGIC REACTIONS TO ALUMINUM. Sterile abscesses or persistent nodules have occurred at the site of injection of certain inactivated vaccines. These abscesses may result from a delayed-type hypersensitivity response to the vaccine adjuvant, aluminum (alum). In some instances, these reactions may be caused by inadvertent subcutaneous inoculation of a vaccine intended for intramuscular use (Table 1.6). Alum-related abscesses recur frequently with subsequent dose(s) of vaccines containing alum. Only if such reactions were severe would they constitute a contraindication to further vaccination with aluminum-containing vaccines.

ALLERGIC REACTIONS TO ANTIMICROBIAL AGENTS. Many vaccines contain trace amounts of streptomycin, neomycin, and/or polymyxin B. Some people have delayed-type allergic reactions to these agents and may develop an injection site papule 48 to 96 hours after vaccine administration. This minor reaction is not a contraindication to future doses of vaccines containing these agents. People with a history of an anaphylactic reaction to one of these antimicrobial agents should be evaluated by an allergist prior to receiving vaccines containing them. No vaccine currently licensed for use in the United States contains penicillin or its derivatives, cephalosporins, or fluoroquinolones.

OTHER VACCINE REACTIONS

People who have high serum concentrations of tetanus IgG antibody, usually as the result of frequent booster immunizations, may have an increased incidence of large injection site swelling after vaccine administration, presumed to be immune complex mediated (Arthus reaction). These reactions are self-limited and do not contraindicate future doses of vaccines at appropriate intervals. Such reactions had been thought to be common with tetanus-containing vaccines, but studies suggest that the reactions are uncommon, even with short intervals between immunizations. Therefore, when indicated, Tdap should be administered regardless of interval since the last tetanus-containing vaccine.

Reactions resembling serum sickness have been reported in approximately 6% of patients after a booster dose of human diploid rabies vaccine, probably resulting from sensitization to human albumin that had been altered chemically by the virus-inactivating agent. Such patients should be evaluated by an allergist but likely will be able to receive additional vaccine doses.

Reporting of Vaccine-Preventable Diseases

Most vaccine-preventable diseases are reportable throughout the United States (see Appendix IV, p 992) as a legal obligation of health care providers. Public health officials depend on health care professionals to report promptly to state or local health departments all suspected cases of vaccine-preventable disease. These reports are transmitted weekly to the CDC and are used to detect outbreaks, monitor disease-control strategies, and evaluate national immunization practices and policies. Reports provide useful information about vaccine effectiveness, changing or current epidemiology of vaccine-preventable diseases, and possible epidemics that could threaten public health. Additionally, reporting allows public health departments to take action, when appropriate, to immunize contacts or to perform other control measures to prevent additional cases. See Appendix IV (p 992) for the list of nationally notifiable diseases. Practitioners should be aware of the reporting requirements, including timeframes, of their state public health departments.

••

PASSIVE IMMUNIZATION

Passive immunization entails administration of preformed antibody to a recipient and, unlike active immunization, confers immediate protection but for only a short period of time. Passive immunization is indicated in the following general circumstances for prevention or amelioration of infectious diseases:

- As replacement, when people are deficient in synthesis of antibody as a result of congenital or acquired antibody production defects, alone or in combination with other immunodeficiencies (eg, severe combined immunodeficiency or human immunodeficiency virus [HIV] infection).
- Prophylactically, when a person susceptible to a disease is exposed to or has a high likelihood of exposure to a specific infectious agent, especially when that person has a high risk of complications from the disease or when time does not permit adequate protection by active immunization alone (eg, rabies immune globulin).
- Therapeutically, when a disease already is present, administration of preformed antibodies (ie, passive immunization) may ameliorate or aid in suppressing the effects of a toxin (eg, foodborne, wound, or infant botulism; diphtheria; or tetanus) or suppress the inflammatory response (eg, Kawasaki disease).

Passive immunization can be accomplished with several types of products. The choice is dictated by the types of products available, the type of antibody desired, the route of administration, timing, and other considerations. These products include standard Immune Globulin (IG) for intramuscular (IM) use; standard Immune Globulin Intravenous (IGIV); hyperimmune globulins, some of which are for intramuscular use (eg, hepatitis B, rabies, tetanus, varicella) and some of which are for intravenous use (eg, botulism, cytomegalovirus [CMV], hepatitis B, vaccinia); antibodies of animal origin (foodborne botulism, black widow spider, rattlesnake, and scorpion antitoxins); and monoclonal antibodies (respiratory syncytial virus [RSV]). Immune Globulin Subcutaneous (Human [IGSC]) is licensed for treatment of patients 2 years or older with primary humoral immunodeficiency.

Indications for administration of IG preparations other than those relevant to infectious diseases or Kawasaki disease are not reviewed in the *Red Book*.

Human plasma used by US-licensed establishments to manufacture derivatives, such as IGIV, IGSC, IGIM, and specific immune globulins, similar to whole blood and blood components for transfusion from US registered blood banks, are released only after appropriate donor screening and testing for presence of bloodborne pathogens, including syphilis, hepatitis B virus, hepatitis C virus, HIV-1 and HIV-2, human T-lymphotropic virus (HTLV)-1 and HTLV-2, *Trypanosoma cruzi* (Chagas disease), and West Nile virus. Selected donations are screened for CMV. Some products are screened for parvovirus B19. Whole blood and blood components also are batch tested for West Nile virus; during an outbreak in a particular geographic area, individual units may be screened by nucleic acid amplification testing (see Blood Safety, p 112; and West Nile Virus, p 865). Blood products are not routinely screened for human parvovirus B19, *Anaplasma* or *Ehrlichia* species, or *Babesia microti*. Since 1993, The US Food and Drug Administration (FDA) requires that IGIV and other IG preparations for intravenous (IV) or IM administration undergo additional manufacturing procedures that inactivate or remove viruses. Most products are subject to at least 2 viral removal/inactivation steps, and some products are nanofiltered to remove prions.

Immune Globulin Intramuscular (IGIM)

IGIM is derived from pooled plasma of adults by a cold ethanol fractionation procedure (Cohn fraction II). IGIM consists primarily of the immunoglobulin (Ig) fraction (at least 90% IgG and trace amounts of IgA and IgM), is treated with solvent/detergent to inactivate lipid-enveloped viruses, is sterile, and is not known to transmit any virus or other infectious agent. IGIM is a concentrated protein solution (approximately 16.5% or 165 mg/mL) containing specific antibodies that reflect the infectious and immunization experience of the population from whose plasma the IGIM was prepared. Many donors (1000 to 60 000 donors per lot of final product) are used to include a broad spectrum of antibodies. Products sold in the United States are derived from plasma collected exclusively in the United States.

IGIM is licensed and recommended for IM administration. Therefore, IGIM should be administered deep into a large muscle mass (see Site and Route of Immunization, p 27). Ordinarily, no more than 5 mL should be administered at one site in an adult, adolescent, or large child; a lesser volume per site (1–3 mL) should be given to small children and infants. Health care professionals should refer to the package insert for total maximal dose at one time. Peak serum concentrations usually are obtained 2 to 3 days after IM administration.

Standard human IGIM should not be administered intravenously. Intradermal use of IG is not recommended. Specific preparations of subcutaneous IG have been shown to be safe and effective in children and adults with primary immune deficiencies (see Immune Globulin Subcutaneous, p 64).

INDICATIONS FOR THE USE OF IGIM

REPLACEMENT THERAPY IN ANTIBODY DEFICIENCY DISORDERS. Most experts no longer consider IGIM appropriate for replacement therapy in immunodeficiency because of the extreme pain of administration and the inability to achieve therapeutic blood concentrations of IgG. If IGIM is used for this indication, the usual dose (limited by muscle mass and the volume that should be administered) is 100 mg/kg (equivalent to 0.66 mL/kg) every 3 weeks. Customary practice is to administer twice this dose initially and to adjust the interval between administration of the doses (2–4 weeks) on the basis of trough IgG concentrations and clinical response (absence of or decrease in infections).

HEPATITIS A PROPHYLAXIS. In people 12 months through 40 years of age, hepatitis A immunization is preferred over IGIM for postexposure prophylaxis against hepatitis A virus infection for people not previously vaccinated against hepatitis A. Hepatitis A vaccination any time before departure is recommended for protection of travelers going to areas with high or intermediate hepatitis A endemicity. For people younger than 12 months or older than 40 years, immunocompromised people of all ages, and people who have chronic liver disease, IGIM is preferred (see Hepatitis A, p 391). IGIM is not indicated for people with clinical manifestations of hepatitis A infection or for people exposed more than 14 days earlier.

MEASLES PROPHYLAXIS. IGIM administered to exposed, measles-susceptible people will prevent or attenuate infection if administered within 6 days of exposure (see Measles, p 535). Measles vaccine and IGIM should not be administered at the same time. The appropriate interval between IGIM administration and measles immunization varies with the dose of IGIM and the specific product (see Table 1.10, p 39).

RUBELLA PROPHYLAXIS. IGIM administered to rubella-susceptible pregnant women after rubella exposure may decrease the risk of fetal infection but should only be offered to women who decline a therapeutic abortion (see Rubella, p 688). Infants with congenital rubella syndrome have been born to women who received IG shortly after exposure.

ADVERSE REACTIONS TO IGIM

- Almost all recipients experience local discomfort, and some experience pain at the site of IGIM administration that is related to the volume administered per injection site. Discomfort is lessened if the preparation is at room temperature at the time of injection. Less common reactions include flushing, headache, chills, and nausea.
- Serious reactions are uncommon; these reactions may involve anaphylaxis manifest as chest pain or constriction, dyspnea, or hypotension and shock. An increased risk of systemic reaction results from inadvertent intravenous administration. Standard IGIM should not be administered intravenously. People requiring repeated doses of IGIM have been reported to experience systemic reactions, such as fever, chills, sweating, and shock.
- IGIM should not be administered to people with selective IgA deficiency (serum IgA concentration <7 mg/dL; IgG and IgM concentrations normal). Because IGIM contains trace amounts of IgA, people who have selective IgA deficiency may develop anti-IgA antibodies on rare occasions and on a subsequent dose of IGIM may experience an anaphylactic reaction with systemic symptoms such as chills, fever, and shock. In rare cases in which reactions related to anti-IgA antibodies have occurred, subsequent use of a licensed IGIV preparation with the lowest IgA concentration may decrease the likelihood of further reactions. Because these reactions are rare, routine screening for IgA deficiency is not recommended.

PRECAUTIONS FOR THE USE OF IGIM

- Caution should be used when administering IGIM to a patient with a history of adverse reactions to IGIM. In this circumstance, some experts recommend administering a test dose (1%–10% of the intended dose) before the full dose.
- Although systemic reactions to IGIM are rare (see Adverse Reactions to IGIM, p 62), epinephrine and other means of treating serious acute reactions (eg, saline for intravenous administration) should be available immediately. Health care professionals administering IGIM should have training to manage emergencies (particularly anaphylactic shock).
- Unless the benefit will outweigh the risk, IGIM should not be used in patients with severe thrombocytopenia or any coagulation disorder that would preclude IM injection. In such cases, use of IGIV is recommended.

Immune Globulin Intravenous (IGIV)

IGIV is a highly purified preparation of IgG antibodies prepared from pooled plasma of qualified adult donors. Different manufacturers use various methods to prepare products for intravenous use. The FDA recommends that the number of donors contributing to a pool used for IGIV be greater than 1000 but no more than 60 000. IGIV consists of more than 95% IgG and trace amounts of IgA and IgM. IGIV is available as a lyophilized powder or as a formulated liquid solution, with final concentrations of IgG ranging from 3% to 12%, depending on the product. IGIV does not contain thimerosal or any other preservative. IGIV products vary in their sodium content, type of stabilizing excipients (sugars, amino acids), osmolarity/osmolality, pH, IgA content, and recommended infusion rate. Each of these factors may contribute to tolerability and the risk of serious adverse events. The FDA specifies that all IGIV preparations must have a minimum concentration of antibodies to measles virus, *Corynebacterium diphtheriae*, poliovirus, and hepatitis B virus. Antibody concentrations against other pathogens, such as *Streptococcus pneumoniae*, cytomegalovirus, and respiratory syncytial virus, vary widely among products and even among lots from the same manufacturer.

INDICATIONS FOR THE USE OF IGIV

Initially, IGIV was developed as an infusion product that allowed patients with primary immunodeficiencies to receive enough IgG at monthly intervals to protect them from infection until their next infusion. IGIV preparations available in the United States currently are licensed by the FDA for use in 6 conditions (Table 1.11). IGIV products may be useful for other conditions, although demonstrated efficacy from controlled trials is not available for many of them. If needed for diagnostic serologic tests for infectious diseases or to evaluate for immunologic disorders, blood sample(s) must be obtained before IGIV administration.

FDA licensure of specific indications for a manufacturer's IGIV product is based on availability of data from one or more clinical trials demonstrating that the product is safe and effective for that indication. All IGIV products are licensed to prevent serious infections in primary immunodeficiency, and many are licensed to treat immune-mediated thrombocytopenia, but not all licensed products are approved for the other indications listed in Table 1.11. In some cases, only a single product has certain indications. Therapeutic differences among IGIV products from different manufacturers may exist, but only 1 comparative clinical trial has been performed. Most experts believe that licensed IGIV and IGSC products are therapeutically equivalent. Among the licensed IGIV products, but not necessarily for each product individually, indications for prevention or treatment of infectious diseases in children and adolescents include the following:

- **Replacement therapy in antibody-deficiency disorders.** The typical dose of IGIV in primary immune deficiency is 400 to 600 mg/kg, administered by infusion approximately every 21 to 28 days. Dose and frequency of infusions should be based

Table 1.11. Uses of Immune Globulin Intravenous (IGIV) for Which There is Approval by the US Food and Drug Administration[a]

Primary immunodeficiency disorders

Kawasaki disease, for prevention of coronary aneurysms

Immune-mediated thrombocytopenia, to increase platelet count

Secondary immunodeficiency in B-cell chronic lymphocytic leukemia

Chronic inflammatory demyelinating polyneuropathy

Multifocal motor neuron neuropathy

[a] Not all IGIV products are approved by the FDA for all indications.

on clinical effectiveness in an individual patient and in conjunction with an expert on primary immune deficiency disorders. When possible, the same brand of IGIV should be administered longitudinally, because changing products is associated with excessive allergic reactions.

- **Kawasaki disease.** Administration of IGIV at a dose of 2 g/kg as a single dose within the first 10 days of onset of fever, when combined with salicylate therapy, decreases the frequency of coronary artery abnormalities and shortens the duration of symptoms. IGIV treatment for children with symptoms of Kawasaki disease for more than 10 days is recommended, although data on efficacy are not available (see Kawasaki Disease, p 494).
- **Pediatric HIV infection.** In children with HIV infection and hypogammaglobulinemia, IGIV may be used to prevent serious bacterial infection.[1] IGIV also might be considered for HIV-infected children who have recurrent serious bacterial infection but is recommended only in unusual circumstances (see Human Immunodeficiency Virus Infection, p 453).
- **Hypogammaglobulinemia in chronic B-cell lymphocytic leukemia.** Administration of IGIV to adults with this disease has been demonstrated to decrease the incidence of serious bacterial infections.
- **Varicella postexposure prophylaxis.** If VariZIG is not available, IGIV can be considered for use in certain people up to 10 days after exposure to a person with varicella or zoster (see Varicella-Zoster Infections, p 846). For maximum benefit, it should be administered as soon as possible after exposure.

IGIV has been used for many other conditions, some of which are listed below.

- **Low birth weight infants.** Results of most clinical trials have indicated that IGIV does not decrease the incidence or mortality rate of late-onset infections in infants who weigh less than 1500 g at birth. Trials have varied in IGIV dose, time of administration, and other aspects of study design. IGIV is not recommended for routine use in preterm infants to prevent late-onset infection.
- **Guillain-Barré syndrome and chronic inflammatory demyelinating polyneuropathy.** In Guillain-Barré syndrome and chronic inflammatory demyelinating polyneuropathy, IGIV treatment has been demonstrated to have efficacy equivalent to that of plasmapheresis and is easier to manage.
- **Toxic shock syndrome.** IGIV has been administered to patients with severe staphylococcal or streptococcal toxic shock syndrome and necrotizing fasciitis. Therapy appears most likely to be beneficial when used early in the course of illness.
- **Other potential uses.** IGIV may be useful for severe anemia caused by parvovirus B19 infection and for neonatal autoimmune thrombocytopenia that is unresponsive to other treatments, immune-mediated neutropenia, decompensation in myasthenia gravis, dermatomyositis, polymyositis, and severe thrombocytopenia that is unresponsive to other treatments.

---

[1]Panel on Opportunistic Infections in HIV-Exposed and HIV-Infected Children. *Guidelines for the Prevention and Treatment of Opportunistic Infections in HIV-Exposed and HIV-Infected Children.* Washington, DC: Department of Health and Human Services; 2013. Available at: **http://aidsinfo.nih.gov/contentfiles/lvguidelines/oi_guidelines_pediatrics.pdf**

SHORTAGES AND SAFETY OF IGIV

Periodic shortages of IGIV have occurred in the United States for various reasons, including manufacturing compliance issues, product withdrawals for theoretical or actual safety concerns, plasma availability, increased use, or decreased production. Physicians should review their IGIV use to ensure consistency with current recommendations. Off-label use of IGIV should be limited until there is adequate scientific evidence of effectiveness. The FDA monitors supply issues and can take actions to ameliorate shortages partially. Supply shortages can be reported to the FDA online (**www.fda.gov/Drugs/DrugSafety/DrugShortages/ucm142398.htm**).

An outbreak of hepatitis C virus infection occurred in the United States in 1993 among recipients of IGIV lots from a single domestic manufacturer. Changes in the preparation of IGIV, including additional viral inactivation steps (such as solvent/detergent exposure, pH 4 incubation, trace enzyme exposure, nanofiltration, and heat treatment) subsequent to this episode have been instituted to prevent transmission of hepatitis C virus and other enveloped viruses, nonenveloped viruses, and prions via IG preparations. Most manufacturers use 3 different pathogen removal/inactivation procedures. All products currently available in the United States are believed to be free of known pathogens. HIV infection never has been transmitted by any IGIV product licensed in the United States.

ADVERSE REACTIONS TO IGIV

Reactions such as fever, headache, myalgia, chills, nausea, and vomiting often are related to the rate of IGIV infusion and usually are mild to moderate and self-limited (Table 1.12). These reactions may result from formation of IgG aggregates during manufacture or storage, or from the presence of trace contamination with vasoactive mediators. Product-to-product variations in adverse effects occur among individual patients, but it is not possible at this time to predict the reactogenicity of one product relative to others. Isoimmune hemolytic reactions can occur, especially if large doses of IGIV (≥ 2 g/kg) are infused. Less common but severe reactions include hypersensitivity and anaphylactoid reactions marked by flushing, changes in blood pressure, and tachycardia; thrombotic events; aseptic meningitis; noncardiogenic pulmonary edema; transfusion-related acute lung injury, and renal insufficiency and failure. Renal failure occurs mainly in patients with preexisting renal dysfunction, diabetes mellitus, and advanced age receiving sucrose-containing products and, in such cases, likely is attributable to sucrose-mediated acute tubular necrosis. Many thrombotic adverse events could be linked to presence of trace amounts of clotting factors that copurify with IgG and occur more commonly (but not exclusively) in patients with risk factors for thrombosis, including advanced age and history of previous thrombotic events. Determining the precise cause and how to prevent thrombotic complications is an area of active investigation. Aseptic meningitis syndrome beginning several hours to 2 days following IGIV treatment may be associated with severe headache, nuchal rigidity, fever, nausea, and vomiting. Pleocytosis frequently is present in the cerebrospinal fluid.

Anaphylactic reactions induced by anti-IgA can occur rarely in patients with primary IgA deficiency (ie, total absence of circulating IgA, IgA <7 mg/dL) who develop IgE antibodies to IgA. These rare reactions have been reported only in patients with selective IgA deficiency. Infusion of licensed IGIV products with a low concentration of IgA may reduce the likelihood of further reactions. Because of the extreme rarity of these

Table 1.12. Managing IGIV Reactions[a]

Timing	Symptoms	Management
During infusion	Anaphylactic/anaphylactoid	Stop the infusion. Administer epinephrine and fluid support, diphenhydramine, and glucocorticoid.
	Headache, fever, chills, sinus tenderness, cough, mild hypotension	Slow the infusion until symptoms resolve. Administer diphenhydramine, NSAID; consider glucocorticoid. When symptoms resolve, the infusion rate may be increased. Pretreatment with NSAID, diphenhydramine, or glucocorticoid or a combination may lesson or prevent a reaction.
After infusion	Headache	Administer NSAID, tryptan, glucocorticoid. Consider an alternative product if there are repeated reactions.
	Myalgia/malaise	Administer NSAID, glucocorticoid. Consider an alternative product if there are repeated reactions.

NSAID indicates nonsteroidal anti-inflammatory drug.
[a] There are no studies of the management of IGIV adverse effects, only expert opinion.

reactions, however, screening for IgA deficiency is not recommended. An assay for anti-IgA antibodies is not available. Similar non-IgE mediated reactions may occur in any IgG recipient, but the etiology of such reactions is uncertain.

PRECAUTIONS FOR THE USE OF IGIV

- Caution should be used when giving IGIV to a patient with a history of adverse reactions to IG.
- Because anaphylactic or anaphylactoid reactions to IGIV can occur (see Adverse Reactions to IGIV, p 62), epinephrine, saline for intravenous administration, and other means of treating acute reactions should be immediately available. If an anaphylactic or anaphylactoid reaction occurs, the risk versus benefit of further infusions should be evaluated; if further IGIV therapy is given, the product eliciting the reaction should not be used.
- Reducing either the rate of infusion or the IGIV dose often can alleviate infusion-related nonallergic adverse reactions (excluding renal failure, thrombosis, and aseptic meningitis). Patients sensitive to one product often tolerate alternative products. Although there are no studies to support the practice, most experts pretreat patients who have experienced significant reactions with a nonsteroidal anti-inflammatory agent such as ibuprofen or aspirin, acetaminophen, diphenhydramine, or a glucocorticoid (prednisone, 1 mg/kg; solucortef, 5–6 mg/kg in children or 100–150 mg in adults; or solumedrol, 1–2 mg/kg) to modify or relieve symptoms. Significant adverse effects of IGIV administration should prompt consultation with an immunologist or other specialist experienced in managing this problem.

- Seriously ill patients with compromised cardiac function who are receiving large volumes of IGIV may be at increased risk of vasomotor or cardiac complications manifested as elevated blood pressure, cardiac failure, or both. In this setting, a low-sodium, high-IgG concentration product should be used if available.
- Screening for selective IgA deficiency is not recommended routinely for potential recipients of IGIV (see Adverse Reactions to IGIV, p 62).

Immune Globulin Subcutaneous (IGSC)

Subcutaneous (SC) administration of IG using mechanical or battery-driven pumps has been shown to be safe and effective in adults and children with primary immunodeficiencies. Many experts prefer IGSC, particularly in small children, because SC administration obviates the need for intravenous access and avoids implanted venous access devices. Smaller doses, administered more frequently (ie, weekly), result in markedly less fluctuation of serum IgG concentrations between infusions. The efficacy of IGSC in preventing infection is at least comparable with that of IGIV. Both mild and severe systemic reactions are less frequent than with IGIV therapy, and most parents or patients can be taught to infuse at home. Infusion reactions should be treated as discussed for IGIV (p 62). The most common adverse effects of IGSC are infusion-site reactions, including local swelling, redness, itching, soreness, induration, and local heat. The most common systemic reaction is headaches. Some experts recommend IGSC infusions daily or up to every 2 weeks to minimize adverse effects and enhance adherence to the treatment regimen. Three products are licensed in the United States for SC use (Hizentra [CSL Behring, Kankakee, IL], Gammagard 10% [Baxter Health care Corp, Westlake Village, CA], and Gamunex-C [Grifols Therapeutics, Research Triangle Park, NC]). There are no data on administration of IGSC for conditions requiring high-dose IG, such as Kawasaki disease and immune-mediated thrombocytopenic purpura. Only IGIV should be used for the treatment of Kawasaki disease.

Specific Immune Globulins

Specific immune globulins differ from other preparations in selection of donors and may differ in number of donors whose plasma is included in the pool from which the product is prepared. These include preparations for which random plasma donations are selected for high titers against certain pathogens (such as CMV), or for which donors are vaccinated to produce high titers ("hyperimmune" globulins). Specific human plasma-derived immune globulins are prepared by the same procedures as other immune globulin preparations. Specific immune globulin preparations for use in infectious diseases include Hepatitis B Immune Globulin, Rabies Immune Globulin, Tetanus Immune Globulin, Varicella-Zoster Immune Globulin (VariZIG), Cytomegalovirus Immune Globulin (CMV-IGIV), Vaccinia IGIV, and Botulism IGIV (BabyBIG to treat infant botulism). Recommendations for use of these immune globulins are provided in the discussions of specific diseases in Section 3. The precautions and adverse reactions for IGIM and IGIV are applicable to specific immune globulins. An intramuscularly administered humanized mouse monoclonal antibody preparation (palivizumab) that helps to reduce the risk of hospitalization attributable to respiratory syncytial virus is available.

Antibodies of Animal Origin (Animal Antisera)

Products of animal origin used to neutralize toxins or for prophylaxis of infectious diseases are derived from serum of horses or sheep immunized with the agent/toxoid of interest. These animal-derived immunoglobulin products are referred to here as "serum" for convenience. Experimental products prepared in other species also may be available. These products are derived by isolating the serum globulin fraction. Some, but not all, products are subjected to an enzyme digestion process to decrease clinical reactions to administered foreign proteins.

Antibody-containing products prepared from animal sera pose a special risk to the recipient, and the use of such products should be limited strictly to certain indications for which specific IG preparations of human origin are not available. Before any animal immune globulin is injected, the patient must be questioned about his or her history of asthma, allergic rhinitis, or urticaria after previous exposure to animals or injections of animal sera. Patients with a history of asthma or allergic symptoms, especially from exposure to horses, can be dangerously sensitive to equine sera and should be given these products with the utmost caution. People who previously have received animal sera are at increased risk of developing acute allergic reactions and serum sickness after administration of sera from the same animal species.

In the United States, animal serum immune globulins are available only from the CDC. Emergency access to experts in diagnostics, decision making, serum procurement, testing for preexisting sensitivity, desensitization, and serum administration are available as noted in relevant pathogen-specific chapters (eg, Clostridial Infections [p 294], Botulism and Infant Botulism [p 294], Diphtheria [p 325]).

TYPES OF REACTIONS TO ANIMAL SERA

The following reactions can occur as the result of administration of animal sera. Of these, only anaphylaxis is mediated by IgE antibodies, and thus, occurrence may be predicted by skin testing results.

ANAPHYLAXIS. The rapidity of onset and overall severity of anaphylaxis may vary considerably. Anaphylaxis usually begins within minutes of exposure to the causative agent, and in general, the more rapid the onset, the more severe the overall course. Major symptomatic manifestations include (1) cutaneous: pruritus, flushing, urticaria, and angioedema; (2) respiratory: hoarse voice and stridor, cough, wheeze, dyspnea, and cyanosis; (3) cardiovascular: rapid weak pulse, hypotension, and arrhythmias; and (4) gastrointestinal: cramps, vomiting, diarrhea, and dry mouth. Anaphylaxis is a medical emergency. Any symptom of an IgE-mediated reaction is reason to terminate administration of the serum and to reassess the need for and the method of administration of the animal antibody. If the antibody is needed, desensitization may be initiated once the patient has been stabilized.

ACUTE FEBRILE REACTIONS. These reactions usually are mild and can be treated with antipyretic agents. Severe febrile reactions should be treated with antipyretic agents or other safe, available methods to physically decrease temperature.

SERUM SICKNESS. Manifestations, which usually begin 7 to 10 days (occasionally as late as 3 weeks) after primary exposure to the foreign protein, consist of fever, urticaria, or a maculopapular rash (90% of cases); arthritis or arthralgia; and lymphadenopathy.

Local edema can occur at the serum injection site a few days before systemic signs and symptoms appear. Angioedema, glomerulonephritis, Guillain-Barré syndrome, peripheral neuritis, and myocarditis also can occur. However, serum sickness may be mild and may resolve spontaneously within a few days to 2 weeks. People who previously have received serum injections are at increased risk after readministration; manifestations in these patients usually occur shortly (from hours to 3 days) after administration of serum. Antihistamines can be helpful for management of serum sickness for alleviation of pruritus, edema, and urticaria. Fever, malaise, arthralgia, and arthritis can be controlled in most patients by administration of aspirin or other nonsteroidal anti-inflammatory agents. Corticosteroids may be helpful for controlling serious manifestations that are inadequately controlled by other agents; prednisone or prednisolone in therapeutic dosages (1.5–2 mg/kg per day; maximum 60 mg/day) for 5 to 7 days are appropriate regimens.

Treatment of Anaphylactic Reactions

Health care professionals administering biologic products or serum must be able to recognize and be prepared to treat systemic anaphylaxis. Medications, equipment, and competent staff necessary to maintain the patency of the airway and to manage cardiovascular collapse must be available.[1]

The emergency treatment of systemic anaphylactic reactions is based on the type of reaction. **In all instances, epinephrine is the primary drug.** Mild manifestations, such as skin reactions alone (eg, pruritus, erythema, urticaria, or angioedema), may be the first signs of an anaphylactic reaction, but intrinsically and in isolation are not dangerous and can be treated with antihistamines (Table 1.13, p 67). However, using clinical judgment, an injection of epinephrine may be given depending on the clinical situation (Table 1.14, p 67). Epinephrine should be injected promptly (eg, goal of <4 minutes) for anaphylaxis, which is likely (although not exclusively) occurring if the patient has 2 or more organ systems involved: (1) skin and mucosal involvement (generalized hives, flush, swollen lips/tongue/uvula); (2) respiratory compromise (dyspnea, wheeze, bronchospasm, stridor, or hypoxemia); (3) low blood pressure; or (4) gastrointestinal tract involvement (eg, persistent crampy abdominal pain or vomiting). If a patient is known to have had a previous severe allergic reaction to the biologic product/serum, onset of skin, cardiovascular, or respiratory symptoms alone may warrant treatment with epinephrine.[2] Because concentrations of epinephrine are higher and are achieved more rapidly after IM administration, SC administration no longer is recommended. Use of readily available commercial epinephrine autoinjectors (available in 2 dosages by weight) and epinephrine prefilled syringes are preferred and have been shown to reduce time to drug administration. Aqueous epinephrine 1:1000 dilution, 0.01 mg/kg (maximum dose, 0.5 mg), usually is administered intramuscularly every 5 to 15 minutes, as necessary, to control symptoms and maintain blood pressure. Injections can be given at shorter than 5-minute intervals if deemed necessary. When the patient's condition improves and remains stable, oral

---

[1] Hegenbarth MA; American Academy of Pediatrics, Committee on Drugs. Preparing for pediatric emergencies: drugs to consider. *Pediatrics.* 2008;121(2):433–443 (Reaffirmed September 2011)

[2] Sampson HA, Munoz-Furlong A, Campbell RL, et al. Second Symposium on the Definition and Management of Anaphylaxis: Summary Report-Second National Institute of Allergy and Infectious Disease/Food Allergy and Anaphylaxis Network Symposium. *J Allergy Clin Immunol.* 2006;117(2):391–397

Table 1.13. Dosages of Commonly Used Secondary Drugs in the Treatment of Anaphylaxis

Drug	Dose
H₁ receptor-blocking agents (antihistamines)	
Diphenhydramine	Oral, IM, IV: 1–2 mg/kg, every 4–6 h (50 mg, maximum single dose <12 y; 100 mg, maximum single dose for 12 y and older)
Hydroxyzine	Oral, IM: 0.5–1 mg/kg, every 4–6 h (100 mg, maximum single dose)
Cetirizine	Oral: 2.5 mg, 6–23 mo; 2.5–5 mg, 2–5 y; 5–10 mg, >5 y (single dose daily)
H₂ receptor-blocking agents (also antihistamines)	
Cimetidine	IV: 5 mg/kg, slowly over a 15-min period, every 6–8 h (300 mg, maximum single dose)
Ranitidine	IV: 1 mg/kg, slowly over a 15-min period, every 6–8 h (50 mg, maximum single dose)
Corticosteroids	
Methylprednisolone	IV: 1.5–2 mg/kg, every 4–6 h (60 mg, maximum single dose)
Prednisone	Oral: 1.5–2 mg/kg, single morning dose (60 mg, maximum single dose); use corticosteroids as long as needed
B₂-agonist	
Albuterol	Nebulizer solution: 0.5% (5 mg/mL), 0.05–0.15 mg/kg per dose in 2–3 mL isotonic sodium chloride solution, maximum 5 mg/dose every 20 min over a 1-h to 2-h period, or 0.5 mg/kg/h by continuous nebulization (15 mg/h, maximum dose)

IM indicates intramuscular; IV, intravenous.

Table 1.14. Epinephrine in the Treatment of Anaphylaxis[a]

Intramuscular (IM) administration
Epinephrine 1:1000 (aqueous): IM (anterolateral thigh), 0.01 mL/kg per dose, up to 0.5 mL, repeated every 5–15 min, up to 3 doses.[b]

Intravenous (IV) administration
An initial bolus of IV epinephrine is given to patients not responding to IM epinephrine using a dilution of 1:10 000 rather than a dilution of 1:1000. This dilution can be made using 1 mL of the 1:1000 dilution in 9 mL of physiologic saline solution. The dose is 0.01 mg/kg or 0.1 mL/kg of the 1:10 000 dilution. A continuous infusion should be started if repeated doses are required. One milligram (1 mL) of 1:1000 dilution of epinephrine added to 250 mL of 5% dextrose in water, resulting in a concentration of 4 µg/mL, is infused initially at a rate of 0.1 µg/kg per minute and increased gradually to 1.5 µg/kg per minute to maintain blood pressure.

[a] In addition to epinephrine, maintenance of the airway and administration of oxygen are critical.
[b] If agent causing anaphylactic reaction was given by injection, epinephrine can be injected into the same site to slow absorption.

antihistamines and possibly oral corticosteroids (1.5–2.0 mg/kg per day of prednisone; maximum 60 mg/day) can be given for an additional 24 to 48 hours.

Maintenance of the airway and administration of oxygen should be instituted promptly. Severe or potentially life-threatening systemic anaphylaxis involving severe bronchospasm, laryngeal edema, other airway compromise, shock, and cardiovascular collapse necessitates additional therapy. Rapid IV infusion of physiologic saline solution, lactated Ringer solution, or other isotonic solution adequate to maintain blood pressure must be instituted to compensate for the loss of circulating intravascular volume.

Epinephrine is administered intramuscularly immediately while IV access is being established. IV epinephrine (note further dilution: 1:10 000 dilution) may be indicated for bolus infusion and is provided in most emergency carts (see Table 1.14, p 67). Administration of epinephrine intravenously can lead to lethal arrhythmia; cardiac monitoring is recommended. A slow, continuous, low-dose infusion is preferable to repeated bolus administration, because the dose can be titrated to the desired effect, and accidental administration of large boluses of epinephrine can be avoided. Nebulized albuterol is indicated for bronchospasm (see Table 1.13, p 67). In some cases, the use of inotropic agents, such as dopamine (see Table 1.13, p 67), may be necessary for blood pressure support. The combination of histamine H_1 and H_2 receptor-blocking agents (see Table 1.13, p 67) may be synergistic in effect and could be used as adjunctive therapy. Corticosteroids should be used in all cases of anaphylaxis except cases that are mild and have responded promptly to initial therapy (see Table 1.13, p 67). However, no data support the usefulness of corticosteroids alone in treating anaphylaxis, and therefore they should not be administered in lieu of treatment with epinephrine and should be considered as adjunctive therapy.

All patients showing signs and symptoms of systemic anaphylaxis, regardless of severity, should be observed for several hours in an appropriate facility, even after remission of immediate symptoms. Anaphylactic reactions can be uniphasic, biphasic, or protracted over 24 to 36 hours despite early and aggressive management. Although a specific period of observation has not been established, a reasonable period of observation would be 4 hours for a mild episode and as long as 24 hours for a severe episode.

Anaphylaxis occurring in people who already are taking beta-adrenergic–blocking agents can be more profound and significantly less responsive to epinephrine and other beta-adrenergic agonist drugs. More aggressive therapy with epinephrine may override receptor blockade in some patients. Some experts recommend use of IV glucagon for epinephrine-refractory anaphylaxis and inhaled atropine for management of bradycardia or bronchospasm in these patients.

··

IMMUNIZATION IN SPECIAL CLINICAL CIRCUMSTANCES

Immunization in Preterm and Low Birth Weight Infants

Infants born preterm (at less than 37 weeks of gestation) or of low birth weight (less than 2500 g) should, with few exceptions, receive all routinely recommended childhood vaccines at the same chronologic age as term and normal birth weight infants. Gestational age and birth weight are not limiting factors when deciding whether a clinically stable preterm infant is to be immunized on schedule. Although studies have shown decreased immune responses to several vaccines given to neonates with very low birth weight (less than 1500 g) and neonates of very early gestational age (less than 29 weeks of gestation), most preterm infants, including infants who receive dexamethasone for chronic lung disease, produce sufficient vaccine-induced immunity to prevent disease. Vaccine dosages given to term infants should not be reduced or divided when given to preterm or low birth weight infants.

Preterm and low birth weight infants tolerate most childhood vaccines as well as do term infants. Apnea with or without bradycardia was reported in some extremely low birth weight (less than 1000 g) infants after use of diphtheria and tetanus toxoids and whole-cell pertussis vaccine (DTwP). More recent reports demonstrate that apnea episodes were neither more frequent nor more severe in extremely low birth weight infants immunized with acellular pertussis-containing vaccines (diphtheria and tetanus toxoids and acellular pertussis [DTaP]) compared with matched controls. However, cardiorespiratory events, including apnea and bradycardia with oxygen desaturation, frequently increase in very low birth weight infants given the combination DTaP, inactivated poliovirus, hepatitis B, and *Haemophilus influenzae* b (Hib) conjugate vaccines. Apnea within 24 hours prior to immunization, younger age, or weight less than 2000 g at the time of immunization and 12-hour Score for Neonatal Acute Physiology II[1] less than 10 have been associated with development of postimmunization apnea, and it may be prudent to monitor infants with these characteristics for 48 hours after immunization if they are still in the hospital. However, these postimmunization cardiorespiratory events do not appear to have a detrimental effect on the clinical course of immunized infants.

Medically stable preterm infants who remain in the hospital at 2 months of chronologic age should be given all inactivated vaccines recommended at that age (see Recommended Immunization Schedule for Persons Aged 0 Through 18 Years **[http://redbook. solutions.aap.org/SS/Immunization_Schedules.aspx]**). A medically stable infant is defined as one who does not require ongoing management for serious infection; metabolic disease; or acute renal, cardiovascular, neurologic, or respiratory tract illness and who demonstrates a clinical course of sustained recovery and a pattern of steady growth. All immunizations required at 2 months of age can be administered simultaneously to preterm or low birth weight infants, except for oral rotavirus vaccine, which should be deferred until the infant is being discharged from the hospital (see Rotavirus, p 684) to prevent the potential nosocomial spread of this live vaccine virus. The same volume of vaccine used for term infants is appropriate for medically stable preterm infants. The number of injections of other vaccines at 2 months of age can be minimized by using combination vaccines. When it is difficult to administer 3 or 4 injections simultaneously to hospitalized preterm infants because of limited injection sites, the vaccines recommended at 2 months of age can be administered at different times. Because recommended parenteral vaccines are inactivated, any interval between doses of individual vaccines is acceptable. However, to avoid superimposing local reactions, 2-week intervals may be reasonable. The choice of needle lengths used for intramuscular vaccine administration is determined by available muscle mass of the preterm or low birth weight infant (see Table 1.7, p 28).

---

[1]Zupancic JAF, Richardson DK, Horbar JD, Carpenter JH, Lee SK, Escobar GJ. Vermont Oxford Network SNAP Pilot Project Participants. Revalidation of the Score for Neonatal Acute Physiology in the Vermont Oxford Network. *Pediatrics*. 2007;119(1):e156-e163

Hepatitis B vaccine given to preterm or low birth weight infants weighing more than 2000 g at birth produces an immune response comparable to that in term infants. Medically stable and thriving infants weighing less than 2000 g demonstrate a lower but sufficient hepatitis B antibody response. Hepatitis B vaccine schedules for infants weighing <2000 g and infants weighing ≥2000 g born to mothers with positive, negative, and unknown hepatitis B surface antigen (HBsAg) status are provided in Hepatitis B, Special Considerations, including Tables 3.22 (p 416) and 3.23 (p 418). Only monovalent hepatitis B vaccine should be used for preterm or term infants younger than 6 weeks. Administration of a total of 4 doses of hepatitis B vaccine is permitted when a combination vaccine containing hepatitis B vaccine is administered after the birth dose.

Because all preterm infants are considered at increased risk of complications of influenza, 2 doses of inactivated influenza vaccine, administered 1 month apart, should be offered for all preterm infants beginning at 6 months of chronologic age as soon as influenza vaccine is available (see Influenza, p 476). Because preterm infants younger than 6 months and infants of any age with chronic complications of preterm birth are extremely vulnerable to influenza virus infection, household contacts, child care providers, and hospital nursery personnel caring for preterm infants should receive influenza vaccine annually (see Influenza, p 476).

Preterm infants younger than 6 months, who are too young to have completed the primary immunization series, are at increased risk of pertussis infection and pertussis-related complications. Tetanus toxoid, reduced diphtheria toxoid, and acellular pertussis (Tdap) vaccine should be administered to all pregnant women (optimally between weeks 27 and 36 of gestation to yield high antibody levels in the infant) during every pregnancy. Tdap should be administered immediately postpartum for women who never have received a previous dose of Tdap. Health care personnel caring for pregnant women and infants and household contacts and child care providers of all infants who have not previously received Tdap should be targeted for vaccination. A single dose of Tdap is recommended for all nonpregnant adolescents as well as nonpregnant adults of any age (see Pertussis, p 608).

Preterm infants born before 29 weeks, 0 days of gestation, infants born with certain congenital heart defects, and certain infants with chronic lung disease of prematurity may benefit from monthly immunoprophylaxis with palivizumab (respiratory syncytial virus monoclonal antibody) during respiratory syncytial virus season (see Respiratory Syncytial Virus, p 667). Palivizumab use does not interfere with the immune response to routine childhood immunizations.

Preterm infants can receive rotavirus vaccine under the following circumstances: the infant is between 6 and 15 weeks, 0 days of chronologic age; the infant is medically stable; and the first dose is given at the time of or after hospital discharge.

Immunization in Pregnancy[1]

Immunization during pregnancy poses only theoretical risks to the developing fetus. Although no evidence indicates that vaccines currently in use have detrimental effects on the fetus, the traditional approach to use of vaccines during pregnancy has been that pregnant women should receive a vaccine only when the vaccine is unlikely to cause harm, the risk of disease exposure is high, and the infection would pose a significant risk

---

[1]See adult immunization schedule available at **www.cdc.gov/vaccines/schedules/hcp/adult.html**

to the pregnant woman, fetus, or newborn infant. Increased recognition of the severity of some vaccine-preventable diseases during pregnancy and of the potential benefit of selected vaccines to the pregnant woman as well as to her newborn infant through either reducing exposure to the vaccine-preventable disease and/or providing protection through maternally acquired antibodies has led to policy recommendations and promotion of selected vaccines during pregnancy.[1]

Two vaccines now are recommended for routine administration during pregnancy in the United States: Tdap and inactivated influenza vaccines. Diphtheria and tetanus toxoids (for children 7 years or older and adults) (Td) vaccine may be indicated in some circumstances.

- **Tdap Vaccine With Each Pregnancy.** The Centers for Disease Control and Prevention (CDC) and the American Academy of Pediatrics (AAP) recommend administration of Tdap during the third trimester of every pregnancy, preferably between 27 and 36 weeks' gestation, to optimize placental transfer of antibodies, although Tdap may be given at any time during pregnancy.[2] For women never previously vaccinated with Tdap, if Tdap is not administered during the current pregnancy, Tdap should be administered immediately postpartum. For women who have been immunized with Tdap, if Tdap is not administered during pregnancy, Tdap is not required postpartum. Pregnant women who are unimmunized or only partially immunized against tetanus should complete the primary series, using Tdap for only 1 of the doses. If a Td booster is indicated for wound management during pregnancy, Tdap should be given if the woman has not already received Tdap during the current pregnancy (see Pertussis, p 608). In resource-limited countries with a high incidence of neonatal tetanus, Td vaccine routinely is administered during pregnancy without evidence of adverse effects and with striking decreases in the occurrence of neonatal tetanus.
- **Inactivated Influenza Vaccine Each Influenza Season.** Studies indicate that women who are pregnant and have no other underlying medical conditions are at increased risk of complications and hospitalization from influenza. Therefore, inactivated influenza vaccine (IIV), using any of the licensed vaccines, should be administered to all women who are or will be pregnant during each influenza season, regardless of trimester (see Influenza, p 476). IIV immunization of pregnant women can help reduce preterm birth and low birth weight and also protects infants younger than 6 months who cannot be immunized actively and in whom antiviral prophylaxis and treatment options are limited. The immunogenicity of IIV has been demonstrated in human immunodeficiency virus (HIV)-infected pregnant women. Live-attenuated influenza vaccine should not be given to pregnant women.

LIVE-VIRUS VACCINES

Pregnancy is a contraindication to administration of all live-virus vaccines, except when susceptibility and exposure are highly probable and the disease to be prevented poses a greater threat to the pregnant woman or fetus than does the vaccine. Although only a theoretical risk to the fetus exists with a live-virus vaccine administered to the pregnant

---

[1]**www.cdc.gov/vaccines/pubs/downloads/b_preg_guide.pdf**

[2]Centers for Disease Control and Prevention. Updated recommendations for use of tetanus toxoid, reduced diphtheria toxoid, and acellular pertussis vaccine (Tdap) in pregnant women—Advisory Committee on Immunization Practices (ACIP), 2012. *MMWR Morb Mortal Wkly Rep.* 2013;62(7):131-135

woman, the background rate of anomalies in uncomplicated pregnancies may result in a defect that could be attributed inappropriately to a vaccine. Therefore, in general, live-virus vaccines should be avoided during pregnancy.

- **Measles, Mumps, Rubella Vaccine.** Because measles, mumps, rubella, and vari-cella vaccines are contraindicated for pregnant women, efforts should be made to immunize women without evidence of immunity against these illnesses before they become pregnant or in the immediate postpartum period. Although of theoretical concern, no case of embryopathy caused by live rubella vaccine has been reported. However, a rare theoretical risk of embryopathy from inadvertent rubella vaccine administration cannot be excluded. Because pregnant women might be at higher risk for severe measles and complications, IGIV should be administered to pregnant women without evidence of measles immunity who have been exposed to measles. The IGIV dose should be high enough to achieve estimated protective levels of measles antibody titers (see Measles, p 535).

- **Varicella Vaccine.** The effect of varicella vaccine on the fetus, if any, is unknown. The manufacturer, in collaboration with the Centers for Disease Control and Prevention (CDC), established the VARIVAX Pregnancy Registry to monitor the fetal outcomes of women who inadvertently were given varicella vaccine during the 3 months before or at any time during pregnancy. Through March 2012, more than 850 women (more than 170 of whom were known to be seronegative before vaccina-tion) were enrolled prospectively in the Pregnancy Registry and had known pregnancy outcomes. More than 550 received varicella vaccine within 30 days prior to their last menstrual period or within the first trimester of pregnancy. No case of congenital vari-cella syndrome and no increased risk of other birth defects after exposure to varicella vaccine were detected. However, the registry data cannot rule out a maximal theoreti-cal risk for congenital varicella syndrome lower than 4% among susceptible women exposed during the high-risk period (the first 2 trimesters of pregnancy) compared with a risk of 1% documented after infection with wild-type varicella-zoster virus. The registry was discontinued for new enrollments in October 2013, because statistically more robust data on the risk of congenital varicella syndrome would likely not accrue given the diminishing seronegative population (because of implementation of universal vaccination) and diminished inadvertent immunization during pregnancy (because of completion of vaccination at a younger age). All exposures to varicella-containing vac-cines (VARIVAX, ProQuad, and ZOSTAVAX) continue to be monitored by the manufacturer (Merck and Co Inc, Whitehouse Station, NJ), and reporting of instances of inadvertent immunization with one of these vaccines during pregnancy or within 3 months prior to conception is encouraged (telephone: 1-877-888-4231). Reports of aggregate data are available by request on the registry's Web site (**www.merckpregnancyregistries.com/varivax.html**).

A pregnant woman in the household is not a contraindication for varicella immu-nization of a child or other household member. Transmission of vaccine virus from an immunocompetent vaccine recipient to a susceptible person has been reported only rarely, and only when a vaccine-associated rash develops in the vaccine recipi-ent (see Varicella-Zoster Infections, p 846). Breastfeeding is not a contraindication for immunization of varicella-susceptible women after pregnancy. In a small study of breastfeeding mothers who were administered varicella vaccine, varicella-zoster virus was not detected by polymerase chain reaction assay in human milk specimens after immunization, and their breastfed infants did not seroconvert to varicella. Varicella-Zoster Immune Globulin (VariZIG) is recommended for pregnant women without evidence of immunity who have been exposed to natural varicella infection (see Varicella-Zoster Virus Infections, p 846). If VariZIG is not available, some experts suggest use of Immune Globulin Intravenous; use of acyclovir in this circumstance has not been evaluated. Zoster vaccine is a live-virus vaccine recommended for people 60 years and older. It should not be administered to pregnant women, and pregnancy should be avoided for 1 month following a dose.

- **Yellow Fever Vaccine.** Yellow fever vaccine is a live-attenuated virus vaccine. Pregnant women and nursing mothers should avoid or postpone travel to an area where there is risk of yellow fever. If travel of a pregnant woman cannot be postponed and mosquito exposure cannot be avoided, immunization should be considered.
- **Smallpox Vaccine.** Vaccinia virus vaccine is a live-virus vaccine and should be given only when there is a definite exposure to smallpox virus. Because smallpox causes more severe disease in pregnant than nonpregnant women, the risks to the mother and fetus from experiencing the disease may substantially outweigh the risks of immunization. Immunized household contacts should avoid contact with pregnant women until the vaccination site is healed.
- **Typhoid Vaccine.** Both live and inactivated typhoid vaccines are available. No information is available on the safety of any of the typhoid vaccines in pregnancy; it therefore is prudent on theoretical grounds to avoid vaccinating pregnant women.[1]

INACTIVATED VACCINES

- **Pneumococcal and Meningococcal Vaccines.** Pneumococcal and meningococcal vaccines can be given to a pregnant woman at high risk of serious or complicated illness from infection with *Streptococcus pneumoniae* or *Neisseria meningitidis*. Meningococcal conjugate vaccine can be given to a pregnant woman when there is increased risk of disease, such as during epidemics or before travel to an area with hyperendemic infection.
- **Hepatitis A and Hepatitis B Vaccines.** Infection with hepatitis A or hepatitis B can result in severe disease in a pregnant woman and, in the case of hepatitis B, chronic infection in the newborn infant. Hepatitis A or hepatitis B immunizations, if indicated, can be given to pregnant women.
- **Inactivated Poliovirus Vaccine.** Although data on safety of inactivated poliovirus (IPV) vaccine for a pregnant woman or developing fetus are limited, no adverse effect has been found, and no risk would be expected. IPV vaccine can be given to pregnant women who never have received poliovirus vaccine, are immunized partially, or are immunized completely but require a booster dose (see Poliovirus Infections, p 644). Oral poliovirus (OPV) vaccine should not be administered to pregnant women.
- **Human Papillomavirus Vaccine.** Human papillomavirus (HPV) vaccine contains no live virus, but data on immunization during pregnancy are limited. Initiation of the vaccine series should be delayed until after completion of the pregnancy. If a woman is determined to be pregnant after initiating the immunization series, the remainder of the 3-dose regimen should be delayed until after completion of the pregnancy. If a vaccine dose has been administered during pregnancy, no intervention is needed.

---

[1]wwwnc.cdc.gov/travel/yellowbook/2014/chapter-3-infectious-diseases-related-to-travel/typhoid-and-paratyphoid-fever

- **Rabies Virus Vaccine.** Rabies vaccine should be given to pregnant women after exposure to rabies under the same circumstances as nonpregnant women. No association between rabies immunization and adverse fetal outcomes has been reported. If the risk of exposure to rabies is substantial, preexposure prophylaxis also may be indicated.
- **Anthrax Vaccine.** Anthrax vaccine is inactivated and has no theoretical risk to the fetus, but the vaccine has not been evaluated for safety in pregnant women, so it should be avoided unless in a postevent situation with a high risk of exposure (see Anthrax, p 234).
- **Japanese Encephalitis Virus Vaccine.** No specific information is available on the safety of Japanese encephalitis virus vaccine for pregnant women. Women should be immunized before conception, if possible, but Japanese encephalitis virus vaccine should be considered if travel to regions with endemic infection and mosquito exposure is unavoidable and the risk of disease outweighs the theoretical risk of adverse events in the pregnant woman and fetus (see Arboviruses, p 240).[1]

Immunization in Immunocompromised Children

The safety and effectiveness of vaccines in people with immune deficiency depend on the nature and degree of immunosuppression. Immunocompromised people vary in their degree of immunosuppression and susceptibility to infection and, therefore, represent a heterogeneous population with regard to immunization. Immunodeficiency conditions can be grouped into primary and secondary disorders. Primary disorders of the immune system generally are inherited, usually as single-gene disorders; can involve any part of the immune defenses, including B-lymphocyte (humoral) immunity, T-lymphocyte (cell)-mediated immunity, complement and phagocytic function, and innate immunity; and share the common feature of increased susceptibility to infection.[2] Secondary disorders of the immune system are acquired and occur in people with HIV infection/acquired immunodeficiency syndrome (AIDS), malignant neoplasm, stem cell or solid organ transplantation, functional asplenia (such as in sickle cell disease or anatomic absence); people receiving immunosuppressive, antimetabolic, or radiation therapy; and people with severe malnutrition, protein loss, chronic inflammatory conditions, and uremia (see Table 1.15, p 75). The Infectious Diseases Society of America, in conjunction with the American Academy of Pediatrics (AAP), CDC, and other professional societies and organizations, has developed immunization guidelines for children and adults with primary and secondary immune deficiencies[3] (**www.idsociety.org/Templates/Content.aspx?id=32212256011**). This document should be consulted for specific conditions, unusual circumstances (eg, international travel), and vaccinations for adults and recommendations for organ donors. The following include general principles and specific recommendations when the primary physician is more likely to deliver care without the patient's continuous management by a subspecialist. Subspecialists who care

---

[1] Centers for Diseases Control and Prevention. Japanese encephalitis virus vaccines—recommendations of the Advisory Committee on Immunization Practices (ACIP). *MMWR Recomm Rep.* 2010;59 (RR-01):1–27

[2] Centers for Disease Control and Prevention. Applying public health strategies to primary immunodeficiency diseases: a potential approach to genetic disorders. *MMWR Recomm Rep.* 2004;53(RR-1):1–29

[3] Rubin LG, Levin MJ, Ljungman P, et al. 2013 IDSA clinical practice guideline for vaccination of the immunocompromised host. *Clin Infect Dis.* 2014;58(3):309-318. Available at: **www.idsociety.org/Templates/Content.aspx?id=32212256011**

Table 1.15. Immunization of Children and Adolescents With Primary and Secondary Immune Deficiencies

Category	Example of Specific Immunodeficiency	Vaccine Contraindications	Effectiveness and Comments, Including Risk-Specific Vaccines[a]
Primary[b]			
B lymphocyte (humoral)	Severe antibody deficiencies (eg, X-linked agammaglobulinemia and common variable immunodeficiency)	OPV,[c] BCG, smallpox, LAIV, yellow fever (YF), and live-bacteria vaccines[d]; no data for rotavirus vaccines	Effectiveness of any vaccine is uncertain if dependent only on humoral response (eg, PPSV23 or MPSV4); IGIV therapy interferes with response to all vaccines, therefore, annual IIV is the only vaccine given to patients receiving IGIV therapy; routine inactivated vaccines can be given if not receiving IGIV.
	Less severe antibody deficiencies (eg, selective IgA deficiency and IgG subclass deficiencies)	OPV,[c] BCG, YF vaccines; other live-vaccines[e] appear to be safe	All vaccines probably are effective; immune response may be attenuated; vaccines should be given as on the annual immunization schedule for immunocompetent people.
T lymphocyte (cell-mediated and humoral)	Complete defects (eg, severe combined immunodeficiency, complete Di-George syndrome)	All live vaccines[d,e,f]	All inactivated vaccines probably are ineffective. The only vaccine that should be given if the patient is receiving IGIV is annual IIV if there is some residual antibody production.
	Partial defects (eg, most patients with DiGeorge syndrome, hyperIgM syndrome, Wiskott-Aldrich syndrome, ataxia telangiectasia)	All live vaccines[d,e]	Effectiveness of any inactivated vaccine depends on degree of immune suppression. Routine inactivated vaccines should be given. Those with ≥500 CD3+ T lymphocytes/mm³, ≥200 CD8+ T lymphocytes/mm³, and normal mitogen response should receive MMR and VAR vaccine (but not MMRV). PPSV23 in addition to PCV13 is indicated in ataxia telangiectasia.

Table 1.15. Immunization of Children and Adolescents With Primary and Secondary Immune Deficiencies, continued

Category	Example of Specific Immunodeficiency	Vaccine Contraindications	Effectiveness and Comments, Including Risk-Specific Vaccines[a]
Complement	Persistent complement component, properdin, or mannan-binding lectin (MBL) deficiency	None	All inactivated and live-virus vaccines on the annual immunization schedule are safe and probably are effective; PPSV23 at 2 years or older and an MCV4 vaccine are recommended in addition to standard vaccines.
Phagocytic function	Chronic granulomatous disease, leukocyte adhesion defects, myeloperoxidase deficiency	Live-bacteria vaccines[d] OPV;[e] smallpox, BCG, combined MMRV, LAIV[e]; withhold MMR and varicella in highly immunocompromised children; YF vaccine may have a contraindication or precaution depending on indicators of immune function[h]	All inactivated vaccines are safe and probably are effective[g]; live-virus vaccines probably are safe and effective.
Secondary[a]	HIV/AIDS		Rotavirus vaccine is recommended on standard schedule; MMR and VAR are recommended for HIV-infected children who are asymptomatic and are not highly immunocompromised[i,j]; all inactivated vaccines, including IIV, may be effective; PPSV23 is recommended in addition to the standard PCV13 vaccine; consider Hib vaccine if not administered during infancy and MCV4 at 2 through 10 years of age.

Table 1.15. Immunization of Children and Adolescents With Primary and Secondary Immune Deficiencies, continued

Category	Example of Specific Immunodeficiency	Vaccine Contraindications	Effectiveness and Comments, Including Risk-Specific Vaccines[a]
	Malignant neoplasm, transplantation, autoimmune disease, immunosuppressive or radiation therapy	Live-virus and live-bacteria vaccines, depending on immune status[d,e]	Effectiveness of any vaccine depends on degree of immune suppression; annual IIV is recommended unless receiving intensive chemotherapy or on anti-B cell antibodies; inactivated standard; PPSV23 is recommended at least 8 weeks after last dose of PCV13. Vaccines are indicated if not highly immunosuppressed, but doses should be repeated after chemotherapy ends.
	Asplenia (functional, congenital anatomic, surgical)	None	All standard vaccines are safe and likely effective; PPSV23 at 24 months or older; MCV4-D (Menactra [Sanofi Pasteur, Swiftwater, PA]) should not be used before 4 weeks after completion of the 4-dose series of PCV13 (eg, 22 months of age or older) because of interference with antibody response to PCV13 when vaccines are administered concurrently; other MCV4 vaccines are used in infants and toddlers as licensed by age without concern for interference with PCV13. In addition to standard vaccines, consider Hib vaccine if not administered during infancy.
	Chronic renal disease	LAIV	All standard vaccines are indicated; PPSV23 is recommended at 24 months or older in addition to standard PCV13.

Table 1.15. Immunization of Children and Adolescents With Primary and Secondary Immune Deficiencies, continued

Category	Example of Specific Immunodeficiency	Vaccine Contraindications	Effectiveness and Comments, Including Risk-Specific Vaccines[a]
	CNS anatomic barrier defect (cochlear implant, congenital dysplasia of the inner ear, persistent CSF communication with naso-/oropharynx)	None	All standard vaccines are indicated; PCV13 if not received as standard; PPSV23 at 2 years or older (≥8 weeks after receipt of PCV13).

OPV indicates oral poliovirus; BCG, bacille Calmette-Guérin; LAIV, live-attenuated influenza vaccine; PPSV23, 23-valent pneumococcal polysaccharide vaccine; MPSV4, quadrivalent meningococcal polysaccharide vaccine; IGIV, Immune Globulin Intravenous; Ig, immunoglobulin; IIV, inactivated influenza vaccine; IgA, immunoglobulin A; IgG, immunoglobulin G; MMR, measles-mumps-rubella; VAR, varicella vaccine; MMRV, measles-mumps-rubella-varicella; PCV13, 13-valent pneumococcal conjugate vaccine; MCV4, quadrivalent meningococcal conjugate vaccine; HIV, human immunodeficiency virus; AIDS, acquired immune deficiency syndrome; Hib, *Haemophilus influenzae* type b; CNS, central nervous system; CSF, cerebrospinal fluid.

[a] Other vaccines that are recommended universally or routinely should be given if not contraindicated.

[b] All children and adolescents should receive an annual age-appropriate inactivated influenza vaccine. LAIV is indicated only for healthy people 2 through 49 years of age.

[c] OPV vaccine no longer is available in the United States.

[d] Live-bacteria vaccines: BCG and Ty21a *Salmonella typhi* vaccine.

[e] Live virus vaccines: LAIV, MMR, VAR, MMRV, herpes zoster (HZV), OPV, YF, vaccinia (smallpox), and rotavirus.

[f] Regarding T-lymphocyte immunodeficiency as a contraindication to rotavirus vaccine, data only exist for severe combined immunodeficiency syndrome.

[g] Additional pneumococcal vaccine is not indicated for children with chronic granulomatous disease beyond age-based standard recommendations for PCV13, because these children are not at increased risk for pneumococcal disease.

[h] YF vaccine is contraindicated in HIV-infected children younger than 6 years who are highly immunosuppressed (see text). There is precaution for use of YF vaccine in asymptomatic HIV-infected children younger than 6 years with total lymphocyte percentage of 15% to 24%, and older than 6 years with CD4+ T-lymphocyte counts of 200–499 cells/mm^3 (Centers for Disease Control and Prevention. Yellow fever vaccine: recommendations of the Advisory Committee on Immunization Practices [ACIP]. *MMWR Recomm Rep.* 2010;59[RR-07];1-27).

[i] HIV-infected children should receive Immune Globulin after exposure to measles (see Measles, p 535) and may receive varicella vaccine if CD4+ T-lymphocyte count ≥15% of expected for age for those younger than 5 years, or CD4+ T-lymphocyte count ≥200 cells/mm^3 for those 5 years or older (see Varicella-Zoster Infections, p 846).

[j] People with perinatal HIV infection who were vaccinated with a measles, rubella, or mumps-containing vaccine prior to the establishment of cART should be considered unvaccinated and should receive 2 appropriately spaced doses of MMR vaccine once effective combination antiretroviral therapy (cART) has been established (at least 6 months with CD4+ T-lymphocyte percentage ≥15% for children younger than 5 years or CD4+ T-lymphocyte count ≥200 cells/mm^3 for children 5 years or older).

for immunocompromised patients share responsibility with the primary care physician for ensuring appropriate vaccinations for immunocompromised patients, and they share responsibility for recommending appropriate vaccinations for members of the patients' household.

GENERAL PRINCIPLES

Certain generalizations regarding degree of immune impairment in patients with primary or secondary immunodeficiency are useful for the practitioner and were adopted in the Infectious Diseases Society of America guideline.[1]

High-level immunosuppression includes patients:

- with combined B- and T-lymphocyte primary immunodeficiency (eg, severe combined immunodeficiency [SCID]);
- receiving cancer chemotherapy;
- with HIV infection and a CD4+ T-lymphocyte count <200 cells/mm^3 for people 5 years or older or a CD4+ T-lymphocyte percentage <15% for infants and children younger than 5 years;
- receiving daily corticosteroid therapy at a dose ≥20 mg (or >2 mg/kg/day for patients weighing <10 kg) of prednisone or equivalent for ≥14 days;
- receiving certain biologic immune modulators, for example, tumor necrosis factor-alpha (TNF-α) antagonists (eg, adalimumab, certolizumab, infliximab, etanercept, and golimumab) or anti–B-lymphocyte monoclonal antibodies (eg, rituximab);
- within 2 months after solid organ transplantation (SOT); and
- within 2 months after hematopoietic stem cell transplant (HSCT) and frequently for a much longer period; HSCT recipients can have prolonged high degrees of immunosuppression, depending on type of transplant (longer for allogeneic than for autologous), type of donor and stem cell source, and post-transplant complications such as graft versus host disease (GVHD) and their treatments.

Low-level immunosuppression includes patients:

- with HIV infection without symptoms and with CD4+ T-lymphocyte counts of 200 to 499 cells/mm^3 for children 5 years or older or CD4+ T-lymphocyte percentages 15% to 24% for those younger than 5 years;
- receiving a lower daily dose of systemic corticosteroid than for high-level immunosuppression for ≥14 days, or receiving alternate-day corticosteroid therapy; and
- receiving methotrexate at a dosage of ≤0.4 mg/kg/week, azathioprine at a dosage of ≤3 mg/kg/day, or 6-mercaptopurine at a dosage of ≤1.5 mg/kg/day.

TIMING OF VACCINES. For patients in whom initiation of immunosuppressive medication is planned, vaccinations should be administered prior to immunosuppression when feasible. Live vaccines should be administered ≥4 weeks prior to initiation of immunosuppression and should not be given within 2 weeks before initiation. Inactivated vaccines should be administered ≥2 weeks prior to immunosuppression.

Certain vaccines may be administered to children while they are modestly immunosuppressed, especially when the state is likely to be lengthy or lifelong. Examples include inactivated and live vaccines in some HIV-infected children and inactivated vaccines during maintenance chemotherapy for acute leukemia or 2 to 6 months after SOT.

[1]Rubin LG, Levin MJ, Ljungman P, et al. 2013 IDSA clinical practice guideline for vaccination of the immunocompromised host. *Clin Infect Dis.* 2014;58(3):309–318. Available at: **www.idsociety.org/Templates/Content.aspx?id=32212256011**

The interval until immune reconstitution varies with the intensity and type of immunosuppressive therapy, radiation therapy, underlying disease, and other factors. Therefore, often it is not possible to make a definitive recommendation for an interval after cessation of immunosuppressive therapy when inactivated vaccines can be administered effectively or when live-virus vaccines can be administered safely and effectively. Immunodeficiency that follows use of recombinant human proteins with anti-inflammatory properties, including TNF-α antagonists (eg, adalimumab, certolizumab, infliximab, etanercept, and golimumab) or anti–B-lymphocyte monoclonal antibodies (eg, rituximab), appears to be prolonged (ie, patients are unlikely to respond to inactivated vaccine within 6 months [see Biologic Response Modifiers, p 83]).

Resumption of vaccinations after reduction or cessation of immunosuppression following transplantation varies by the vaccine, underlying disorder, specific immunosuppressive therapy, and presence of GVHD.[1] Timing for inactivated and live-virus vaccines could vary from as early as 3 months after cessation of chemotherapy for acute leukemia to as long as 24 months for measles-mumps-rubella (MMR) or varicella vaccine after HSCT and only in a patient without ongoing immunosuppression or GVHD.

SAFETY OF VACCINES IN PEOPLE WITH CHRONIC INFLAMMATORY DISORDERS. The Institute of Medicine (IOM) assessed relationships between vaccines (MMR, acellular pertussis-containing diphtheria and tetanus, tetanus toxoid, influenza, hepatitis A, hepatitis B, and HPV vaccines) as potential triggers for a flare or the onset of chronic inflammatory diseases. Evidence was inadequate to establish or refute a causal relationship between each vaccine and onset or exacerbation of multiple sclerosis, systemic lupus erythematosus, vasculitis, rheumatoid arthritis, or juvenile idiopathic arthritis.[2] The IOM concluded that overall, the preponderance of clinical evidence indicates that vaccines are not important triggers of disease or flares and should not be withheld because of this concern.

LIVE VACCINES. In general, people who are severely immunocompromised or in whom immune function is uncertain should not receive live vaccines, either viral or bacterial, because of the risk of disease caused by the vaccine strains. There are particular immune deficiency disorders for which some live vaccines are safe, and for certain immunocompromised children and adolescents the benefits may outweigh risks for use of particular live vaccines (see Table 1.15).

INACTIVATED VACCINES AND PASSIVE IMMUNIZATION. Inactivated vaccines and Immune Globulin (IG) preparations should be used when indicated by age or circumstance. The immune response to inactivated vaccines generally is not affected by circulating antibody. Safety is not a concern, nor is risk of graft rejection or exacerbation of immune-mediated disorders. Annual influenza vaccination with IIV is recommended for immunocompromised patients 6 months and older with primary and secondary immunodeficiencies, except if they are very unlikely to respond (although also unlikely to be harmed), such as those receiving intensive chemotherapy and those who have received anti-B-lymphocyte antibody therapy within 6 months. Immune responses of immunocompromised children to inactivated vaccines, including IIV, may be inadequate. Inactivated vaccines other than IIV are not routinely given to patients receiving immunoglobulin therapy for major antibody deficiency

[1]Rubin LG, Levin MJ, Ljungman P, et al. 2013 IDSA clinical practice guideline for vaccination of the immunocompromised host. *Clin Infect Dis.* 2014;58(3):309–318. Available at: **www.idsociety.org/Templates/Content.aspx?id=32212256011**

[2]Stratton K, Andrew F, Rusch E, Clayton E. *Adverse Effects of Vaccines: Evidence and Causality.* Washington, DC: National Academies Press; 2012

disorders or severe combined immunodeficiencies. Inactivated vaccines administered during immunosuppressive therapy generally are not counted as valid in the recommended annual immunization schedule.

PRIMARY IMMUNODEFICIENCIES (SEE TABLE 1.15)

Vaccine recommendations for primary immunodeficiency disorders depend on the specific immunologic abnormality. All live-virus and inactivated vaccines can be given to children with isolated *immunoglobulin A deficiency*. Inactivated vaccines other than IIV are not routinely given to patients with *major antibody deficiencies or SCID* during IG therapy. For these 2 groups, inactivated vaccines can be administered as part of immunologic assessment prior to Immune Globulin Intravenous (IGIV) therapy without safety concerns.

Table 1.15 contains a list used internationally for exclusions for use of certain live vaccines. Live-virus vaccines should not be given to patients with any of the following conditions: *major antibody deficiencies, severe-combined immunodeficiencies, DiGeorge syndrome with CD3+ T-lymphocyte count <500 cells/mm³,* other *combined immunodeficiencies with similar CD3+ T-lymphocyte counts, Wiskott-Aldrich syndrome,* or *X-linked lymphoproliferative disease* or *familial disorders that predispose to hemophagocytic lymphohistiocytosis.*

Patients with *primary complement deficiencies* (ie, of early classic pathway, alternate pathway, or severe mannose-binding lectin deficiency) should receive all routine inactivated and live vaccines on the annual immunization schedule; none is contraindicated.

Patients with *phagocytic cell deficiencies* (ie, chronic granulomatous disease [CGD], leukocyte adhesion deficiency [LAD], Chediak-Higashi syndrome, cyclic neutropenia) and patients with *innate immune defects* that result in defects of cytokine generation/response or cellular activation (eg, defects of interferon-gamma/interleukin-12 axis) should receive all inactivated vaccines on the annual immunization schedule. Live-virus vaccines should be administered to patients with CGD and cyclic neutropenia. Live-bacterial and live-virus vaccines should not be given to patients with LAD, Chediak-Higashi syndrome, or defects of interferon production.

Additional vaccines not given universally are indicated for children with certain conditions. Patients with primary *complement deficiencies* should be given vaccines in addition to the annual immunization schedule to protect against meningococcal disease, starting early in infancy, and those with *complement deficiencies* and *phagocytic cell deficiencies other than CGD* should be given pneumococcal conjugate vaccine (PCV) doses at the earliest appropriate time on the annual immunization schedule and then 23-valent pneumococcal polysaccharide vaccine (PPSV23) at 2 years of age or older and at least 8 weeks after PCV, followed by a second dose 5 years later (see Special Situations/Hosts, p 82).

SECONDARY (ACQUIRED) IMMUNODEFICIENCIES

Several factors should be considered in immunization of children with secondary immunodeficiencies, including the underlying disease, the specific immunosuppressive regimen (dose and schedule), and the patient's infectious disease and immunization history. Live-virus vaccines generally are contraindicated because of a proven or theoretical increased risk of prolonged shedding of vaccine virus and vaccine virus disease. Exceptions include administration of MMR and varicella vaccine (but not combined measles-mumps-rubella-varicella [MMRV]) in children with HIV infection who are not severely immunosuppressed. Many experts also advise use of rotavirus vaccine in infants exposed to or infected with HIV. Although varicella vaccine has been studied in children with acute lymphoblastic leukemia in remission, varicella vaccine should not be given to children with acute lymphocytic leukemia or another malignancy because (a) many children will have received varicella vaccine prior to immune suppression and may retain protective immunity; (b) the risk of acquiring varicella has diminished in countries with universal immunization programs; (c) most deaths from varicella, although rare, occur within the first year of diagnosis and thus would not be prevented by immunization; (d) hyperimmune globulin is available for postexposure prophylaxis; (e) antiviral agents are available for treatment; and (f) chemotherapy regimens change frequently and often are more immunosuppressive than regimens under which the safety and efficacy of varicella vaccine was studied (see Varicella-Zoster Infections, p 846).

Because patients with congenital or acquired immunodeficiencies may not have an adequate response to vaccines, they may remain susceptible despite having been immunized. If there is an available test for a known antibody correlate of protection, specific postimmunization serum antibody titers can be determined 4 to 6 weeks after immunization (unless the patient has received passive immunoglobulin therapy in recent months) to assess immune response and guide further immunization and management of future exposures. If chemotherapy is ongoing or other immunosuppressive therapy is escalated, protective antibody titer should be verified again at the time of an exposure (eg, to varicella) to guide management.

HOUSEHOLD MEMBERS OF IMMUNOCOMPROMISED PATIENTS

Immunocompetent individuals who live in a household with immunocompromised patients should receive inactivated vaccines on the annual immunization schedule or for travel. Household members who are 6 months or older should receive influenza vaccine annually. Household members should receive IIV or live-attenuated influenza vaccine (LAIV), as recommended routinely. Exceptions to the latter are that LAIV should not be used in a household member (or contact should be avoided for 7 days if LAIV is given) when the immunocompromised household contact has severe SCID or received an HSCT within 2 months or has GVHD requiring therapy.

Healthy immunocompetent members who live in a household with immunocompromised patients of all degrees of severity can and should receive the following live vaccines, as indicated on the annual immunization schedule: MMR, varicella-containing vaccines (Varivax, MMRV, and zoster), rotavirus vaccine for infants 2 through 7 months of age, and yellow fever and oral typhoid vaccines for travel. OPV, which is still available in countries outside the United States, should *not* be administered to individuals who live in a household with immunocompromised patients. Immunocompromised patients should avoid contact with people who develop skin lesions after receipt of varicella or zoster vaccines until lesions clear. If contact occurs inadvertently, risk of transmission is low. When transmission of vaccine strain varicella virus has occurred, the virus has maintained its attenuated characteristics. Therefore, administration of VariZIG or IGIV is not indicated.

SPECIAL SITUATIONS/HOSTS
CORTICOSTEROIDS

Inactivated vaccines, including IIV, and live-virus vaccines should be administered to patients prior to commencement of corticosteroid therapy for inflammatory or autoimmune diseases, when feasible, as for immunocompetent people and indicated on the annual immunization schedule. Inactivated vaccines should be completed ≥ 2 weeks prior and live virus vaccines ≥ 4 weeks prior to commencement of corticosteroid therapy.

Guidance for Administration of Inactivated Vaccines

Inactivated vaccines, if not given prior to commencement, should be given to patients while receiving corticosteroid therapy chronically. Inactivated vaccine administration can be deferred temporarily until corticosteroids are discontinued if the hiatus is expected to be brief and adherence to return appointment is likely. Inactivated vaccines (or live vaccines, when recommended as follows) should not be avoided because of concern for exacerbation of an inflammatory or immune-mediated condition.

Guidance for Administration of Live-Virus Vaccines to Recipients of Corticosteroids

Recommendations are as follows:

- **Topical therapy, local injections, or aerosol use of corticosteroids.** Application of low-potency topical corticosteroids to localized areas on the skin; administration by aerosolization; application on conjunctiva; or intraarticular, bursal, or tendon injections of corticosteroids usually do not result in immunosuppression that would contraindicate administration of live-virus vaccines.
- **Physiologic maintenance doses of corticosteroids.** Children who are receiving only maintenance physiologic doses of corticosteroids can receive live-virus vaccines.
- **Low or moderate doses of systemic corticosteroids given daily or on alternate days.** Children receiving <2 mg/kg per day of prednisone or its equivalent, or <20 mg/day if they weigh more than 10 kg, can receive live-virus vaccines during corticosteroid treatment.
- **High doses of systemic corticosteroids given daily or on alternate days for fewer than 14 days.** Children receiving ≥ 2 mg/kg per day of prednisone or its equivalent, or ≥ 20 mg/day if they weigh more than 10 kg, can receive live-virus vaccines immediately after discontinuation of treatment. Some experts, however, would delay immunization with live-virus vaccines until 2 weeks after discontinuation.
- **High doses of systemic corticosteroids given daily for 14 days or more.** Children receiving ≥ 2 mg/kg per day of prednisone or its equivalent, or ≥ 20 mg/day if they weigh more than 10 kg, for 14 days or more should not receive live-virus vaccines until 4 weeks after discontinuation.
- **Children who have a disease (eg, systemic lupus erythematosus) that, in itself, is considered to suppress the immune response and/or are receiving immunosuppressant medication other than corticosteroids and who are receiving systemic or locally administered corticosteroids.** These children should not be given live-virus vaccines, except in special circumstances.

BIOLOGIC RESPONSE MODIFIERS USED TO DECREASE INFLAMMATION

Biologic response modifiers, also known as cytokine inhibitors, are drugs used to treat immune-mediated conditions, including juvenile idiopathic arthritis, rheumatoid arthritis, and inflammatory bowel disease. These drugs are antibodies to proinflammatory cytokines or proteins that target cytokine receptors. Their purpose is to block the action of cytokines involved in inflammation. Their immune-modulating effects can last for weeks to months after discontinuation. TNF-α inhibitors (adalimumab, certolizumab, etanercept, golimumab, infliximab) are the prototype agents, but newer biologic response modifiers in this class target other cytokines, such as interleukin-1 (anakinra), -6 (tocilizumab), -12, and -23, or the proteins that target cytokine receptors on lymphocytes. These agents often are used in combination with other immunosuppressive drugs, such as methotrexate or corticosteroids.

Patients treated with biologic response modifiers are at increased risk of infections caused by *Mycobacterium tuberculosis*, nontuberculous mycobacterium, molds and endemic fungi (eg, *Pneumocystis jirovecii*), *Legionella* species, *Listeria* species, and other intracellular pathogens, as well as lymphomas and other cancers. Inhibition of this inflammatory immune response potentially permits reactivation of infections that have been controlled previously and/or leads to an inadequate immune response to new pathogens requiring cell-mediated immunity for control. Adverse events related to use of biologic response modifying drugs should be reported to the US Food and Drug Administration (FDA) MedWatch Program (**www.fda.gov/Safety/MedWatch/HowToReport/ ucm053087.htm**). Table 1.16 shows preventive strategies that should be considered in patients who will be or are taking immune-modifying agents (Table 1.16, p 85). Vaccination status should be assessed pretreatment, and recommended vaccines should be administered with timing as for planned corticosteroid use (see Timing of Vaccines). Recommended vaccines include PPSV23 for patients 2 years or older (after PCV13 doses on the routine schedule are completed, or PCV13 for patients 6 years or older who previously did not receive PCV13).

Biologic response modifiers are considered highly immunosuppressive. Live-virus vaccines are contraindicated during therapy and for weeks to months following discontinuation. Inactivated vaccines, including IIV, are recommended during therapy as recommended for age or catch-up on the annual immunization schedule and should not be withheld because of concern for an exaggerated inflammatory response.

HEMATOPOIETIC STEM CELL TRANSPLANTATION

Patients for whom HSCT is planned should receive all routinely recommended inactivated vaccines (including IIV) when the interval to the start of the conditioning period is ≥2 weeks. Routinely recommended live-virus vaccines should be administered if the patient is not already immunosuppressed and the interval to the start of the conditioning period is ≥4 weeks. The HSCT donor also should be current with routinely recommended vaccines, but if he or she is not then vaccination of the donor for benefit of the recipient is not recommended. Administration of MMR, MMRV, varicella, and zoster vaccines should be avoided within 4 weeks of stem cell harvest.

Household members should be counseled regarding risks of infection and should be fully immunized, with certain restriction for use of LAIV (see Household Members of Immunocompromised Patients). Timing of immune reconstitution of HSCT recipients varies greatly depending on type of transplantation, interval since transplantation, receipt of immunosuppressive medications, and presence of GVHD and other complications. Vaccinations (both routine and additional) are an important part of management and are considered according to specific guidelines and in collaboration with the patient's oncologist/hematologist.

Table 1.16. Recommendations for Evaluation Prior to Initiation of Biologic Response Modifying Drugs

- Perform tuberculin skin test (TST) or interferon gamma release assay (IGRA) (see Tuberculosis, p 804)
- Consider chest radiograph on the basis of clinical and epidemiologic findings
- Document vaccination status and, if required, administer:
  - inactivated vaccines (including annual IIV) a minimum of 2 weeks before initiation of biologic response modifying drug
  - live-virus vaccines a minimum 4 weeks before initiation of biologic response modifier therapy, unless contraindicated by condition or other therapies.
- Counsel household members regarding risk of infection and ensure vaccination (see Household Members of Immunosuppressed Patients, p 82)
- Consider serologic testing for *Histoplasma* species, *Toxoplasma* species, and other intracellular pathogens depending on risk of past exposure
- Perform serologic testing for hepatitis B virus
- Consider testing for varicella-zoster virus and Epstein-Barr virus
- Counsel regarding:
  - food safety (**www.cdc.gov/foodsafety**)
  - maintenance of dental hygiene
  - risks of exposure to garden soil, pets, and other animals
  - avoiding high-risk activities (eg, excavation sites or spelunking because of risk of *Histoplasma capsulatum*)
  - avoiding travel to areas with endemic pathogenic fungi (eg, southwestern United States for risk of *Coccidioides* species) or to areas where tuberculosis is endemic

Modified from Le Saux N; Canadian Paediatric Society, Infectious Diseases and Immunization Committee. *Paediatric and Child Health.* Ottawa, Ontario: Canadian Paediatric Society; 2012;17(3):147-150

SOLID ORGAN TRANSPLANTATION

Children and adolescents with chronic or end-stage kidney, liver, heart, or lung disease or intestinal failure, including SOT candidates, should receive all vaccinations as appropriate for age, exposure history, and immune status based on the annual immunization schedule for immunocompetent people. Patients 2 years or older with the these conditions also should have received, or should be given as a candidate for SOT, a dose of PPSV23, if not previously given. (Patients with end-stage kidney disease should receive PPSV23 if they have not received a dose within 5 years and have not received 2 lifetime doses.) PCV13 is administered if not previously received, even for those 6 years or older. When PCV13 and PPSV23 both are indicated, PPSV23 should be given at least 8 weeks after the last PCV13 dose. SOT candidates who are hepatitis B surface antibody (anti-HBs) negative should receive the hepatitis B vaccine (HepB) series, followed by serologic testing and further doses if serologic test results are negative (as indicated for an immunocompetent vaccinee who remains seronegative). Patients 12 months or older who have not received hepatitis A vaccine (HepA), did not complete the vaccination series, or who are seronegative should receive the HepA vaccine series. MMR vaccine can be given to infants 6 through 11 months of age who are SOT candidates and who are not immunocompromised, repeating the dose at ≥12 months if still awaiting a transplant that will not occur within 4 weeks of vaccination. Living SOT donors should have up-to-date vaccination status, with considerations for required vaccines the same as for HSCT donors (see Hematopoietic Stem Cell Transplantation). Household members of these patients should be counseled about risks of infection and should have vaccination status made current.

HIV INFECTION (ALSO SEE HUMAN IMMUNODEFICIENCY VIRUS INFECTION, P 454)

HIV-infected children and adolescents should receive all inactivated vaccines, including annual IIV, as indicated on the annual immunization schedule. PPSV23 should be administered to people 2 years or older, at least 8 weeks after the last required PCV13 dose. HIV-exposed or -infected infants should receive rotavirus vaccine according to the schedule for uninfected infants. MMR and varicella vaccines should be administered to children 12 months or older who are stable clinically and who have low level of immunosuppression (see General Principles, p 79).

For HIV-infected people with low-level immunosuppression (ie, CD4+ count >200 cells/mm^3 for people 5 years and older, or a CD4+ T-lymphocyte percentage ≥15% for children younger than 5 years), a first dose of varicella vaccine is indicated for children 12 months or older. For those receiving varicella vaccine between 1 and 8 years of age, the second dose (usually given at 4–6 years of age) can be administered to HIV-infected children 3 months after the first. A varicella vaccine 2-dose series is indicated for previously unimmunized nonimmune people 9 years or older. HIV-infected children should not be given MMRV or LAIV vaccines.

In the United States, bacille Calmette-Guérin (BCG) vaccine is contraindicated for HIV-infected patients. In areas of the world with a high incidence of tuberculosis, the World Health Organization (WHO) recommends giving BCG vaccine to HIV-infected children who are asymptomatic.

ASPLENIA AND FUNCTIONAL ASPLENIA

The asplenic state results from the following: (1) surgical removal of the spleen (eg, after trauma, for treatment of hemolytic conditions); (2) functional asplenia (eg, from sickle cell disease or thalassemia); or (3) congenital asplenia or polysplenia. Special recommendations for patients with asplenia apply to all 3 categories. All infants, children, adolescents, and adults with asplenia, regardless of the reason for the asplenic state, have an increased risk of fulminant septicemia, especially associated with encapsulated bacteria, which is associated with a high mortality rate. In comparison with immunocompetent children who have not undergone splenectomy, the incidence of and mortality rate from septicemia are increased in children who have had splenectomy after trauma and in children with sickle cell disease by as much as 350-fold, and the rate may be even higher in children who have had splenectomy for thalassemia. The risk of invasive bacterial infection is higher in younger children than in older children, and the risk may be greater during the years immediately after surgical splenectomy. Fulminant septicemia, however, has been reported in adults as long as 25 years after splenectomy.

Streptococcus pneumoniae is the most common pathogen causing septicemia in children with asplenia. Less common causes include *Haemophilus influenzae* type b, *Neisseria meningitidis*, other streptococci, *Escherichia coli*, *Staphylococcus aureus*, and gram-negative bacilli, such as *Salmonella* species, *Klebsiella* species, and *Pseudomonas aeruginosa*. Those with functional or anatomic asplenia also are at increased risk of fatal malaria and severe babesiosis.

Immunization

Pneumococcal conjugate and polysaccharide vaccines are vital for all children with asplenia (see Pneumococcal Infections, p 626). Following administration of an appropriate number of doses of PCV13, PPSV23 should be administered a minimum of 8 weeks later, but only at the age of 24 months or older. A second dose should be administered 5 years later (see Pneumococcal Infections, p 626). For children 2 through 18 years of age who have not received PCV13, even if they completed a PCV7 series, a supplemental dose of PCV13 should be administered. When splenectomy is planned for a patient 2 years or older who is PPSV23 naïve, PPSV23 should be administered ≥2 weeks prior to surgery (and following indicated dose[s] of PCV13 by ≥8 weeks).

H influenzae type b (Hib) immunization should be initiated at 2 months of age, as recommended for otherwise healthy young children on the annual immunization schedule. Previously unimmunized children with asplenia younger than 5 years should receive Hib vaccine according to the catch-up schedule. Unimmunized children 5 years or older should receive a single dose of Hib vaccine.

Quadrivalent meningococcal conjugate vaccine (MCV4) should be administered to all children with asplenia 2 months or older, as recommended for those with primary complement deficiencies (see Primary Immunodeficiencies, p 81), with one important restriction to type/brand of MCV4. MCV4-D (Menactra [Sanofi Pasteur, Swiftwater, PA]) should not be used before 4 weeks after completion of the 4-dose series of PCV13 (eg, 22 months of age or older) because of interference with antibody response to PCV13 when vaccines are administered concurrently. Other MCV4 vaccines are used in infants and toddlers as licensed by age without concern for interference with PCV13. Revaccination with any MCV4 vaccine is recommended 3 years after the primary series and then every 5 years for patients with asplenia who are younger than 7 years; for asplenic patients who are 7 years and older, the initial booster dose following the primary series should be at 5 years (instead of 3 years) and then every 5 years thereafter.

When surgical splenectomy is planned, immunization status for Hib, pneumococcus, and meningococcus should be ascertained, and all indicated vaccines should be administered at least 2 weeks before surgery. If splenectomy is emergent, or vaccination was not performed before splenectomy, indicated vaccines should be initiated as soon as possible 2 weeks or more after surgery. Whenever possible, alternatives to splenectomy should be considered. Management options include postponement of splenectomy for as long as possible in people with congenital hemolytic anemia, preservation of accessory spleens, performance of partial splenectomy for benign tumors of the spleen, conservative (non-operative) management of splenic trauma, or when feasible, repair rather than removal. Splenectomy should be avoided if possible, especially when immunodeficiency is present (eg, Wiskott-Aldrich syndrome).

Antimicrobial Agents

Daily antimicrobial prophylaxis against pneumococcal infections is recommended for many children with asplenia, regardless of immunization status. For infants with sickle cell anemia, oral penicillin prophylaxis against invasive pneumococcal disease should be initiated as soon as the diagnosis is established and preferably by 2 months of age. Although the efficacy of antimicrobial prophylaxis has been proven only in patients with sickle cell anemia, other children with asplenia at particularly high risk, such as children with malignant neoplasms or thalassemia, also should receive daily chemoprophylaxis. Less agreement exists about the need for prophylaxis for children who have had splenectomy after trauma. In general, antimicrobial prophylaxis (in addition to immunization) should be considered for all children with asplenia younger than 5 years of age and for at least 1 year after splenectomy at any age.

The age at which chemoprophylaxis is discontinued often is an empiric decision. On the basis of a multicenter study, prophylactic penicillin can be discontinued at 5 years of age in children with sickle cell disease who are receiving regular medical attention, are fully immunized, and have not had a severe pneumococcal infection or surgical splenectomy. The appropriate duration of prophylaxis for children with asplenia attributable to other causes is unknown. Some experts continue prophylaxis throughout childhood and into adulthood for particularly high-risk patients with asplenia.

For antimicrobial prophylaxis, oral penicillin V (125 mg, twice a day, for children younger than 3 years; and 250 mg, twice a day, for children 3 years or older) is recommended. Some experts recommend amoxicillin (20 mg/kg per day). For children with anaphylactic allergy to penicillin, erythromycin can be given (250 mg, twice daily). A substantial percentage of pneumococcal isolates have intermediate- or high-level resistance to penicillin, resistance to macrolides and azalides, or both. When antimicrobial prophylaxis is used, these limitations must be stressed to parents and patients, who should be made aware that all febrile illnesses potentially are serious in children with asplenia and that immediate medical attention should be sought because the initial signs and symptoms of fulminant septicemia can be subtle. Likewise, medical attention should be sought for asplenic patients who suffer animal bites. When bacteremia or septicemia is a possibility, health care professionals should obtain specimens for blood and other cultures as indicated and begin treatment immediately with an antimicrobial regimen effective against *S pneumoniae, H influenzae* type b, and *N meningitidis* and should consider hospitalizing the child. In some clinical situations, other antimicrobial agents, such as aminoglycosides, may be indicated. If a child with asplenia travels to or resides in an area where medical care is not accessible, an appropriate antimicrobial agent should be readily available and the child's caregiver should be instructed in appropriate use.

CENTRAL NERVOUS SYSTEM ANATOMIC BARRIER DEFECTS

Patients of all ages with profound deafness scheduled to receive a cochlear implant; congenital dysplasias of the inner ear; or persistent cerebrospinal fluid (CSF) communication with the nasopharynx or oropharynx should receive all vaccines recommended routinely on the annual immunization schedule for immunocompetent people. No vaccine is contraindicated. Patients with a cochlear implant, those scheduled to receive a cochlear implant, and those with persistent communication between the CSF and nasopharynx/oropharynx should receive PCV13 as in the standard schedule and as recommended for children with asplenia. At 24 months or older, these patients should receive PPSV23 (≥8 weeks after receipt of PCV13 if indicated). PCV13 and PPSV23 should be administered ≥2 weeks prior to cochlear implant surgery when feasible.

There is no well-established evidence for use of antimicrobial prophylaxis for patients with CSF communication with the nasopharynx, oropharynx, or middle ear. Risk of bacterial meningitis is highest in the first 7 to 10 days following acute traumatic breach. Some physicians recommend empiric parenteral antimicrobial therapy in the immediate post-traumatic period. Parenteral antimicrobial therapy also is given in the perioperative period for cochlear implantation and reparative neurosurgical procedures. Chronic antimicrobial prophylaxis is not indicated for persistent CSF communications or following cochlear implantation.

Immunization in Children With a Personal or Family History of Seizures

Studies have demonstrated a short-term increase in the risk of a febrile seizure (ie, generalized, brief self-limited seizure) following receipt of several vaccines: DTwP, MMR, MMRV, and PCV13. Infants and children with a personal or family history of seizures of any etiology might be at greater risk of having a febrile seizure after receipt of one of these vaccines compared with children without such histories. No evidence indicates that febrile seizures cause permanent brain damage or epilepsy, aggravate neurologic disorders, or affect the prognosis for children with underlying disorders. An increased incidence of seizures has not been found with the currently recommended DTaP vaccines that have replaced the whole-cell DTwP vaccines in the United States.

In the case of pertussis immunization during infancy, vaccine administration could coincide with or hasten the recognition of a disorder associated with seizures, such as infantile spasms or severe myoclonic epilepsy of infancy, which could cause confusion about the role of pertussis immunization. Hence, pertussis immunization in infants with a history of recent seizures generally should be deferred until a progressive neurologic disorder is excluded or the cause of the earlier seizure has been determined. DTaP should be administered to infants and children with a stable neurologic condition, including well-controlled seizures. The nature of seizures and related neurologic status are more likely to have been established in children by the age of 12 months. This difference by age is the basis for the recommendation that measles (MMR) and varicella vaccines should not be deferred for children with a history of seizures.

A family history of a seizure disorder is not a contraindication to pertussis, PCV13, influenza, MMR, or varicella vaccine or a reason to defer immunization. Children with a personal or family history of seizures generally should be given MMR and varicella vaccine as separate immunizations rather than MMRV for the first dose at 12 through 47 months of age. Postimmunization seizures in these children are uncommon, and if they occur usually are febrile in origin, have a benign outcome, and are not likely to be confused with manifestations of a previously unrecognized neurologic disorder.

Immunization in Children With Chronic Diseases

Chronic disease in children can be defined as requiring 3 components: (1) diagnosis on the basis of medical knowledge; (2) not curable currently; and (3) either has been present for at least 3 months, will likely last longer than 3 months, or has occurred at least 3 times in the past year and will likely recur. Chronic diseases may make children more susceptible to the severe manifestations and complications of common infections. Unless specifically contraindicated, immunizations recommended for healthy children should be given to children with chronic diseases. However, live-virus vaccines are contraindicated in children with severe immunologic disorders, including children receiving chronic immunosuppressive therapy (see Immunocompromised Children, p 74). Children with HIV infection who are not severely immunocompromised may receive MMR, varicclla, and rotavirus vaccines. For children with conditions that may require organ transplantation or immunosuppression, administering recommended immunizations before the start of immunosuppressive therapy is important. Children with certain chronic diseases (eg, allergic, cardiorespiratory, hematologic, metabolic, and renal disorders; cystic fibrosis; and diabetes mellitus) are at increased risk of complications of influenza, varicella, and pneumococcal infection and should be targeted to receive IIV, varicella vaccine, and PCV13 or pneumococcal polysaccharide vaccine or both, as recommended for age and immunization status and condition (see Influenza, p 476, Varicella-Zoster Infections, p 846, and Pneumococcal Infections, p 626). All children with chronic liver disease are at risk of severe clinical manifestations of acute infection with hepatitis viruses and should receive hepatitis A (HepA) and hepatitis B (HepB) vaccines on a catch-up schedule if they have not received vaccines routinely (see Hepatitis A, p 391, and Hepatitis B, p 400). MCV4 is recommended for children as young as 2 months with certain immune deficiencies or those who will travel to or reside in areas with high risk of exposure (see Meningococcal Infections, p 547). Siblings of children with chronic diseases and children in households of adults with chronic diseases should receive recommended vaccines, including both live and inactivated vaccines (**www.cdc.gov/vaccines/schedules/index.html**).

The Institute of Medicine assessed relationships between vaccines (MMR, acellular pertussis-containing DT, tetanus toxoid, influenza, HepA, HepB, and HPV vaccines) as potential triggers for a flare or the onset of chronic inflammatory diseases. Evidence was inadequate to establish or refute a causal relationship between each vaccine and onset or exacerbation of multiple sclerosis, systemic lupus erythematosus, vasculitis, rheumatoid arthritis, or juvenile idiopathic arthritis.[1] Overall, the preponderance of clinical evidence indicates that vaccines are not important triggers of disease or flares and should not be withheld because of this concern.

Immunization in American Indian/Alaska Native Children

Although indigenous populations worldwide have high morbidity and mortality from infectious diseases, including vaccine-preventable infections, all indigenous populations are not the same (**wwwnc.cdc.gov/eid/article/7/7/pdfs/01-7732.pdf**).

This chapter focuses on US populations, American Indian and Alaska Native (AI/AN) people, and uses of vaccine and biologic products that are special to these populations. Geographic isolation, cultural barriers, economic factors, and inadequate sewage disposal are some of the reasons why health among AI/AN populations is poorer than other groups. Although the Indian Health Service (IHS) is charged with serving the health needs of these populations, more than half of AI/AN people do not reside permanently on a reservation and, therefore, have limited access to IHS care. Little information is known about relative risks of vaccine-preventable and other infectious diseases in individuals not living on reservations.

---

[1]Rubin LG, Levin MJ, Ljungman P, et al. 2013 IDSA clinical practice guideline for vaccination of the immunocompromised host. *Clin Infect Dis.* 2014;58(3):309–318. Available at: **www.idsociety.org/Templates/Content.aspx?id=32212256011**

Historically, compared with children from other racial groups, AI/AN children living in certain communities (reservations and villages in Alaska) have been documented to have greater risk of acquiring certain vaccine-preventable diseases, such as hepatitis A, hepatitis B, *Haemophilus influenzae* type b, *Streptococcus pneumoniae,* and HPV infections. Mortality from pneumonia and influenza among AI/AN infants is 5 times higher than the rate reported for white infants in the United States. The rate of diarrhea-associated hospitalizations has been significantly higher in AI/AN infants than in other US infants but has declined since introduction of rotavirus vaccine. HIV infection affects the AI/AN community in ways that may not always be apparent because of the small population size. Compared with other races/ethnicities, AI/AN people have poorer survival rates after an HIV diagnosis. They face special challenges to HIV prevention, including poverty and culturally based stigma (**wwwnc.cdc.gov/eid/article/7/7/pdfs/01-7732.pdf**).

During the past 2 decades, childhood immunizations for hepatitis B and targeted immunization for hepatitis A in the United States have eliminated disease disparities for these pathogens in most populations of AI/AN children, and significant decreases in invasive disease have been demonstrated for *H influenzae* type b and *S pneumoniae,* and in varicella hospitalizations. Continued immunization is critical to maintaining this success. Disparities for some vaccine-preventable diseases persist, however, likely related in part to adverse living conditions, such as poverty, household crowding, poor indoor air quality, and absence of indoor plumbing. The historically high rates of infection and ongoing disparities highlight the importance of ensuring that recommendations for universal childhood immunization be optimally implemented in AI/AN children. This is especially relevant to HPV vaccine implementation. Children in AI/AN communities should receive immunizations on time and should receive the full schedule of immunizations, even in times of vaccine shortages. Specific vulnerabilities are noted as follows.

- *Haemophilus influenzae* **type b (Hib).** There are important differences among the currently available Hib vaccines that should be considered by physicians caring for AI/AN children. Before availability and routine use of conjugated Hib vaccines, the incidence of invasive Hib disease was approximately 10 times higher among young AI/AN children compared with non-AI/AN children. Because of the high risk of invasive Hib disease within the first 6 months of life in many AI/AN infant populations, the IHS and AAP recommend that the first dose of Hib conjugate vaccine contain polyribosylribitol phosphate-meningococcal outer membrane protein (PRP-OMP; PedvaxHIB; Merck and Co Inc, Whitehouse Station, NJ). The administration of a PRP-OMP–containing vaccine leads to more rapid development of protective concentrations of antibody compared with other Hib vaccines, and failure to use vaccine containing PRP-OMP has been associated with excess cases of Hib disease in Alaska Native infants. For subsequent doses, any of the Hib conjugate vaccines can be used with apparently equal efficacy (see *Haemophilus influenzae* Infections, p 368), but if the second dose is a vaccine other than PRP-OMP, a third dose of Hib vaccine should be given approximately 2 months later. Availability of more than one Hib vaccine product in a clinic has been shown to lead to errors in vaccine administration. To avoid confusion for health care professionals who serve AI/AN children predominantly, it may be prudent to use only PRP-OMP–containing Hib vaccines.
- *Haemophilus influenzae* **type a (Hia).** Among some indigenous populations, Hia is now the most common *H influenzae* serotype. Hia can cause clinical illness similar to Hib: meningitis, bacteremic pneumonia, septic arthritis, and cellulitis. Elevated rates

of invasive disease attributable to Hia have been reported among Alaska Native (18 per 100 000 in children younger than 5 years), White Mountain Apache/Navajo (20 per 100 000), and Canadian indigenous children (102 per 100 000 in children younger than 2 years), compared with other US children (0.8 per 100 000 in children younger than 5 years). In Alaska, rates of Hia have increased since 2008, raising concerns about the emergence of this pathogen in other AI/AN populations. It is unclear whether an apparent increase in Hia disease is attributable to improved surveillance, higher attention since the dramatic decrease in Hib disease, or replacement.

- ***Streptococcus pneumoniae* (pneumococcus).** Recommendations for PCV13 for AI/AN children are the same as for other US children. Prior to introduction of PCV7, the incidence of invasive pneumococcal disease (IPD) in certain AI/AN children was 5 to 24 times higher than the incidence among other US children. Use of PCV7 in AI/AN infants resulted in near-elimination of disease from vaccine serotypes and decreased incidence of overall IPD. However, AI/AN children continue to have a two- to fourfold increased risk of developing IPD compared with non-AI/AN children. PCV13 has been evaluated among both AI/AN and other children in postmarketing studies and gives promise of further reducing IPD rates. In special situations, public health authorities also may recommend use of PPSV23 after the PCV13 series for AI/AN children who are living in areas where the risk of IPD is documented to be increased (**www.cdc.gov/mmwr/preview/mmwrhtml/rr5911a1.htm**).
- **Hepatitis viruses.** Before the introduction of hepatitis vaccines, rates of hepatitis A and hepatitis B in the AI/AN population greatly exceeded those of the general US population. Universal immunization reduced the incidence of hepatitis A and hepatitis B to that of the general US population (**http://minorityhealth.hhs.gov/templates/content.aspx?lvl=3&lvlid=541&ID=6494**). To maintain these low rates, special efforts should be made to ensure catch-up hepatitis B immunization of previously unimmunized adolescents.
- **Influenza virus.** The disparity in influenza-related mortality rates in the AI/AN population compared with the general US population was confirmed during the 2009 H1N1 epidemic; the H1N1 death rate among AI/AN in 12 states (representing 50% of the AI/AN population in the United States) was 4 times higher than the H1N1 death rate of all other racial and ethnic populations combined. For this reason, the AI/AN population is listed among the groups at risk of severe complications from influenza; therefore, when vaccine or antiviral medication supplies are limited, AI/AN people are considered a high-risk priority group. The 2009 pandemic highlighted the value of maternal immunization to protect both the mother and the neonate. Given the elevated risk of influenza in the AI/AN population, maternal influenza immunization is especially important.
- **Respiratory syncytial virus.** The rates of hospitalization for respiratory syncytial virus (RSV) are much higher for AI/AN infants in rural Alaska and southwest IHS regions (113 and 91 RSV hospitalizations per 1000 births, respectively) than for other US infants (27 per 1000 births). Hospitalization rates for AI/AN infants in these areas are similar to rates among preterm infants in the overall US population. Use of RSV-specific monoclonal antibody prophylaxis (palivizumab), as recommended by the AAP, should be optimized among high-risk AI/AN infants (see Respiratory Syncytial Virus, p 667). RSV season length may be prolonged in northern latitudes, including Alaska, and RSV prophylaxis should reflect local seasonality and risk factors in this population.

Immunization in US Children Living Outside the United States

In general, US children living outside the United States should receive the same immunizations as children living in the United States, but they may require additional vaccines related to the prevalence of regional pathogens. Influenza vaccine appropriate to the hemisphere may be needed; unless the influenza formulation is the same for the southern hemisphere as for the northern hemisphere, there will not be a vaccine licensed by the FDA. The risk of exposure to vaccine-preventable infections may be increased, and additional immunizations against infections not given routinely in the United States, such as typhoid disease, yellow fever, and Japanese encephalitis, may be indicated. To provide the best protection prior to departure, accelerated schedules for routine immunizations can be used, and country-specific risks should be examined to determine the need for additional immunizations. Vaccines received outside the United States should be documented carefully. The CDC *Yellow Book* and disease-specific chapters of the *Red Book* should be reviewed for specific diseases, and tables for accelerated immunization should be consulted. Considerations for tuberculosis and BCG vaccine are provided in the Tuberculosis chapter (p 804).

ACCELERATED SCHEDULE FOR ROUTINE IMMUNIZATIONS FOR US CHILDREN RESIDING OUTSIDE OF THE UNITED STATES

For infants, the schedule for DTaP, IPV, Hib, and PCV13 can be accelerated by giving the primary series at 4-week intervals. For infants between 6 and 12 months of age who are traveling outside the United States, MMR should be administered at 6 months of age to provide early protection. In this case, 2 additional doses of MMR will be needed after 12 months of age. For children older than 12 months who have received the first MMR dose already, the second dose of MMR can be given 1 month after the first dose instead of at 4 to 6 years of age. Similarly, for varicella vaccine, the second dose can be given 3 months after the first dose. Hepatitis A vaccine should be given to children and adolescents who were too young to have received the vaccine as an infant and who do not have a history of receiving hepatitis A vaccine for other reasons. Children younger than 1 year may receive Immune Globulin Intramuscular (IGIM) for hepatitis A protection (see Active Immunization of People Who Recently Received Immune Globulin and Other Blood Products, p 38). For children traveling to areas with hyperendemic or epidemic meningococcal disease, MCV4 can be given to children as young as 2 months. Three meningococcal conjugate vaccines (MCVs) are licensed for use in children (see Meningococcal Infections p 547). The conjugate vaccines are preferred, but the polysaccharide vaccine can be administered in children 2 years or older if MCVs are not available.

Annual immunization with influenza vaccine is recommended for all children 6 months and older and should be given prior to departure, if available. Influenza may not have a typical seasonal pattern in tropical regions and may be present year-round in some areas.

TRAVEL VACCINES FOR US CHILDREN RESIDING OUTSIDE OF THE UNITED STATES

The parenteral typhoid vaccine can be given to children as young as 2 years, and the oral typhoid vaccine can be given to children 6 years and older. Yellow fever vaccine should be given to children 9 months or older who will reside in areas where yellow fever is endemic in South America and Africa. The vaccine is absolutely contraindicated in children younger than 6 months; arrangements will need to be made to receive this vaccine in the destination country when age is appropriate. Other vaccines such as BCG vaccine, rabies vaccine, and Japanese encephalitis virus vaccine may be indicated for some destinations (see International Travel, p 101).

For children (especially children younger than 5 years) who will reside for several months or longer in countries with high rates of tuberculosis and who cannot get access to the tuberculosis-prevention services as are available in most of the United States, some experts recommend BCG immunization. Other methods of preventing tuberculosis exposure and disease often are not practical or available. In many cases, it may be desirable for the child to receive the BCG vaccine as soon as possible after entering the foreign country.

Advice regarding Japanese encephalitis virus vaccine is available in International Travel (p 103).

Families should be educated about the risk of rabies in resource-limited countries. Children should be educated to avoid contact with animals and to report any bites or scratches from animals while abroad. For some children, preexposure rabies vaccine may be indicated.

For information on the risk of specific diseases by country and recommended preventive measures, see International Travel (p 101) or consult the CDC Web site (**wwwn.cdc. gov/travel/default.aspx**) or the WHO Web site (**www.who.int/ith/en/**).

Immunization in Adolescent and College Populations

Immunization recommendations for adolescents and college students have expanded significantly as vaccines have been developed to protect against pertussis, meningococcal disease, and human papillomavirus infections, and this age group was included in the recommendation for yearly influenza vaccination. The adolescent immunization schedule is published annually (**www.cdc.gov/vaccines/schedules/index.html**).

The adolescent population presents many challenges with regard to immunization, including infrequent visits with health care providers and, for some, lack of payer coverage for annual visits. As a result, many adolescents do not receive routine preventive care that provides opportunities for immunization.

To ensure age-appropriate immunization, all youth should have a routine appointment at 11 through 12 years of age for administration of appropriate vaccines and to provide comprehensive preventive health care.[1] Tdap, MCV4 (A, C, Y, W135), and HPV vaccines should be given at the 11- through 12-year-old visit. Arrangements for follow-up visits for subsequent doses of HPV vaccine at 2 and 6 months following the first dose should be made to enhance completion of the 3-dose series on schedule. The 11- through 12-year age platform for administration of these 3 vaccines was chosen to offer the best protection against these potentially serious and life-threating infections. As with all immunizations, the health care provider should give a confident message on the merits of routine HPV vaccine and the importance of providing immune protection well in advance of the potential exposure. If there is reluctance to receive HPV vaccine, the provider should discuss the risks of HPV infection and the risk for cancer in both females and males. Adolescents who do not receive these vaccines on schedule should be immunized at the next available visit. Influenza vaccine should be given annually.

[1]American Academy of Pediatrics, Committee on Practice and Ambulatory Medicine and Bright Futures Periodicity Schedule Workgroup. 2014 recommendations for pediatric preventive health care. *Pediatrics.* 2014;133(3):568-570

During all adolescent visits, immunization status should be reviewed, and deficiencies should be corrected according to the recommended vaccine schedule. Lapses in the immunization schedule are common among adolescents and do not necessitate reinitiation of the entire series or extra doses of any individual dose that was valid.

A history should be obtained to assess for risk factors that would require consideration for administration of hepatitis A and pneumococcal vaccines. These vaccines should be given as soon as the risk condition is identified. Specific indications for each of these vaccines are provided in the respective disease-specific chapters in Section 3.

School immunization laws encourage "catch-up" programs for older adolescents. Accordingly, school and college health services should establish a system to ensure that all students are protected against vaccine-preventable diseases. Because outbreaks of vaccine-preventable diseases, including measles, mumps, and meningococcal disease, have occurred at colleges and universities, the American College Health Association encourages a comprehensive institutional prematriculation immunization policy consistent with recommendations from the CDC Advisory Committee on Immunization Practices (**www.acha.org/topics/vaccine.cfm**). Many colleges and universities are mandated by state law to require vaccination against meningococcal disease and/or hepatitis B, either for all matriculating students or only those living in campus housing. Information regarding state laws requiring prematriculation immunization is available (**www.immunize.org/laws**). A meningococcal serogroup B mixed peptide vaccine that was not licensed for use in the United States at the time was made available through a CDC-sponsored investigational new drug application in response to recent outbreaks of *Neisseria meningitidis* serogroup B in several college settings.

Because adolescents and young adults commonly travel internationally, their immunization status and travel plans should be reviewed 2 or more months before departure to allow time to administer any needed vaccines (see International Travel, p 101). Pediatricians should assist in providing information on benefits and risks of immunization to ensure that adolescents are immunized appropriately. In addition, pediatricians should help facilitate transfer of immunization information to schools and colleges when applicable. This may include completion of necessary forms, giving copies of vaccine records to patients, and participating in electronic immunization registries through which information can be shared in a secure manner. Should vaccines be refused after emphasis of the importance of immunization, this should be documented.

The possible occurrence of illness attributable to a vaccine-preventable disease in a school or college should be reported promptly to local health officials for aid in management, for consideration of public health considerations, and according to individual state law (see Appendix IV, p 992).

Immunization in Health Care Personnel[1]

Adults whose occupations place them in contact with patients with contagious diseases are at increased risk of contracting vaccine-preventable diseases and, if infected, transmitting them to their coworkers and patients. For the purposes of this section, health care personnel (HCP) are defined as those who have face-to-face contact with patients or

---

[1]Centers for Disease Control and Prevention. Immunization of health-care providers: recommendations of the Advisory Committee on Immunization Practices (ACIP) and the Hospital Infection Control Practices Advisory Committee (HICPAC). *MMWR Recomm Rep.* 2011;60(RR-7):1-45

to anyone who works in a building where patient care is delivered or some other group of people employed by a health care facility (eg, laboratory workers). The definition of HCP includes trainees and volunteers. All HCP should protect themselves and susceptible patients by receiving appropriate immunizations. Physicians, health care facilities, and schools for health care professionals should play an active role in implementing policies to maximize immunization of HCP. Vaccine-preventable diseases of special concern to people involved in the health care of children are as follows (see the disease-specific chapters in Section 3 for further recommendations).

- **Pertussis.** Pertussis outbreaks involving adults occur in the community and the workplace. HCP frequently are exposed to *Bordetella pertussis,* have substantial risk of illness, and can be sources for spread of infection to their patients, colleagues, families, and the community. HCP of all ages who work in hospitals or ambulatory-care settings should receive a single dose of tetanus toxoid, reduced diphtheria toxoid, and acellular pertussis (Tdap) vaccine as soon as is feasible if they previously have not received Tdap. Hospitals and ambulatory-care facilities should provide Tdap for HCP using approaches that maximize immunization rates.[1]

- **Hepatitis B.** Hepatitis B vaccine (HepB) is recommended for all HCP whose work- and training-related activities involve reasonably anticipated risk for exposure to blood or other infectious body fluids. The Occupational Safety and Health Administration of the US Department of Labor issued a regulation requiring employers of personnel at risk of occupational exposure to hepatitis B to offer HepB immunization to personnel at the employer's expense. The employer shall ensure that employees who decline to accept HepB immunization offered by the employer sign the declination statement. To determine the need for revaccination and to guide postexposure prophylaxis, postvaccination serologic testing should be performed for all HCP at high risk of occupational percutaneous or mucosal exposure to blood or body fluids. Postvaccination serologic testing is performed 1 to 2 months after administration of the last dose of the vaccine series using a method that allows detection of the protective concentration of anti-HBs ($\geq$10 mIU/mL). People determined to have anti-HBs concentrations of $\geq$10 mIU/mL after receipt of the primary vaccine series are considered immune, and the result should be documented.

  In some cases, susceptible HCP immunized appropriately with HepB vaccines fail to develop serologic evidence of immunity. People who do not respond to the primary immunization series (remain anti-HBs negative) should complete a second 3-dose vaccine series with reevaluation of anti-HBs titers 1 to 2 months after the series is completed. People who do not respond to the second series and remain hepatitis B surface antigen (HBsAg) negative should be considered susceptible to hepatitis B virus infection and will need to receive Hepatitis B Immune Globulin (HBIG) prophylaxis after any known or probable exposure to blood or body fluids infected with hepatitis B virus.[2]

- **Influenza.** Because HCP can transmit influenza to patients and because health care-associated outbreaks do occur, annual influenza immunization should be considered a patient safety responsibility and a requirement for employment in a health care facility

---

[1] Centers for Disease Control and Prevention. Immunization of health-care personnel: recommendations of the Advisory Committee on Immunization Practices (ACIP) and the Hospital Infection Control Practices Advisory Committee (HICPAC). *MMWR Recomm Rep.* 2011;60(RR-7):1-45

[2] Centers for Disease Control and Prevention. CDC guidance for evaluating health-care personnel for hepatitis B virus protection and for administering post-exposure management. *MMWR Recomm Rep.* 2013;62(RR-10):1-19

unless an individual has a recognized medical contraindication to immunization.[1] HCP should be educated about the benefits of influenza immunization and the potential health consequences of influenza illness for themselves and their patients. Influenza vaccine should be offered at no cost annually to all eligible people, and efforts should be made to ensure that vaccine is readily available to personnel on all shifts, such as through use of mobile immunization carts. A signed declination form should be obtained from personnel who decline for reasons other than medical contraindications in any facility that does not have a formal mandatory vaccine policy. Mandatory education about the benefits of vaccination should be required for all people who decline influenza immunization. The utility of mandatory masking for unimmunized HCP is not clear.[2] Either inactivated vaccine or live-attenuated vaccine (according to age and health status limitations) is appropriate. Live-attenuated vaccine should not be used for personnel who will have direct contact with hematopoietic stem cell transplant recipients prior to immune reconstitution in the 7 days following vaccine administration.

- **Measles.** Because measles in HCP has contributed to spread of this disease during outbreaks, evidence of immunity to measles should be required for HCP. Proof of immunity is established by laboratory confirmation of infection, positive serologic test result for measles antibody, or documented receipt of 2 appropriately spaced doses of live virus-containing measles vaccine, the first of which was given on or after the first birthday. HCP born before 1957 generally have been considered immune to measles. However, because measles cases have occurred in HCP in this age group, health care facilities should consider offering 2 doses of measles-containing vaccine to health care personnel who lack proof of immunity to measles. In communities with documented measles outbreaks, 2 doses of MMR vaccine are recommended for unvaccinated health care professionals born before 1957 unless evidence of serologic immunity is demonstrated.

- **Mumps.** Transmission of mumps in health care facilities can be disruptive and costly. All people who work in health care facilities should be immune to mumps. Proof of immunity is established by written documentation of adequate immunization (2 doses of MMR or live mumps vaccine administered ≥28 days apart), laboratory evidence of immunity or laboratory confirmation of disease, or birth before 1957.[3] During an outbreak, a second dose of MMR vaccine should be offered to health care personnel born during or after 1957 who have only received 1 dose of MMR vaccine. HCP born before 1957 without a history of MMR immunization should obtain a mumps antibody titer to document their immune status and, if negative, should receive 2 appropriately spaced doses of MMR vaccine.

- **Rubella.** Transmission of rubella from HCP to pregnant women has been reported. Although the disease is mild in adults, the risk to a fetus necessitates documentation of rubella immunity in HCP of both genders. People should be considered immune on the basis of a positive serologic test result for rubella antibody or documented proof of 1 dose of rubella-containing vaccine. A history of rubella disease is unreliable and

[1]American Academy of Pediatrics, Committee on Infectious Diseases. Recommendation for mandatory influenza immunization of all health care personnel. *Pediatrics.* 2010;126(4):809-815 (Reaffirmed February 2014)

[2]See **www.cdc.gov/flu/professionals/vaccination/index.htm#ACIP**

[3]Centers for Disease Control and Prevention. Immunization of health-care personnel: recommendations of the Advisory Committee on Immunization Practices (ACIP) and the Hospital Infection Control Practices Advisory Committee (HICPAC). *MMWR Recomm Rep.* 2011;60(RR-7):1-45

should not be used in determining immune status. All susceptible HCP who may be exposed to patients with rubella or who take care of pregnant women, as well as people who work in educational institutions or provide child care, should be immunized with 1 dose of MMR to prevent infection for themselves and to prevent transmission of rubella to pregnant patients.

- **Varicella.** Proof of varicella immunity is recommended for all HCP. In health care institutions, serologic screening of personnel who lack evidence of immunity to varicella before immunization is likely to be cost-effective but need not be performed. All health care personnel without evidence of immunity to varicella should receive 2 doses of varicella vaccine. Evidence of immunity to varicella in health care professionals includes any of the following: (1) documentation of 2 doses of varicella vaccine at least 4 weeks apart; (2) history of varicella diagnosed or verified by a health care professional (for a patient reporting a history of or presenting with an atypical case, a mild case, or both, health care professionals should seek either an epidemiologic link with a typical varicella case or evidence of laboratory confirmation, if it was performed at the time of acute disease); (3) history of herpes zoster diagnosed by a health care professional; or (4) laboratory evidence of immunity or laboratory confirmation of disease. The CDC Advisory Committee on Immunization Practices and Health Infection Control Practices Advisory Committee (HICPAC) do not recommend serologic testing of HCP for immunity to varicella after receiving varicella-zoster virus vaccine. Commercially available serologic assays may not be sufficiently sensitive to detect immunization-induced antibody.

Vaccination During Hospitalization, Including Anesthesia and Surgery

Most studies that have explored the effect of surgery or anesthesia on the immune system have been observational, have included only infants and children, and were small and indirect in that they did not evaluate the immune effect on the response to vaccination specifically. They do not provide convincing evidence that recent anesthesia or surgery significantly affect the response to vaccines. Current, recent, or upcoming anesthesia/surgery/hospitalization is not a contraindication to vaccination. Efforts should be made to ensure vaccine administration during the hospitalization or at discharge. For patients who are deemed moderately or severely ill throughout the hospitalization, vaccination should occur at the earliest opportunity (ie, during immediate posthospitalization follow-up care, including home or office visits) when patients' clinical symptoms have improved.

Children Who Received Immunizations Outside the United States or Whose Immunization Status is Unknown or Uncertain

IMMUNIZATIONS RECEIVED OUTSIDE THE UNITED STATES

People immunized in other countries, including exchange students, internationally adopted children, refugees, and other immigrants, should be immunized according to recommended schedules (including minimal ages and intervals) in the United States for healthy infants, children, and adolescents (**http://redbook.solutions.aap.org/SS/ Immunization_Schedules.aspx**). The Immigration and Nationality Act (INA) of 1996 requires all people immigrating to the United States as legal permanent residents (ie, green card holders) to provide "proof of vaccination" with vaccines recommended by the CDC Advisory Committee on Immunization Practices (ACIP) before entry into the United States (**www.cdc.gov/immigrantrefugeehealth/exams/ti/panel/ vaccination-panel-technical-instructions.html**). Specific vaccines required for immigration must fulfill the following criteria: (1) must be an age-appropriate vaccine as recommended by the ACIP for the general US population; and (2) either must protect against a disease that has the potential to cause an outbreak or protects against a disease that has been eliminated or is in the process of being eliminated in the United States. For example, hepatitis B vaccine is not required. Information about immunization requirements for immigrants is available on the CDC Web site (**www.cdc.gov/ immigrantrefugeehealth/**). Internationally adopted children who are 10 years of age and younger may obtain a waiver of exemption from the INA regulations pertaining to immunization of immigrants before arrival in the United States. Children adopted from countries that are not part of the Hague Convention can receive waivers to have their immunizations delayed until arrival in the United States (**www.adoption.state. gov**). When an exemption is granted, adoptive parents are required to sign a waiver indicating their intention to comply with ACIP-recommended immunizations within 30 days after the child arrives in the United States.

Refugees are not required to meet immunization requirements of the INA at the time of initial entry into the United States but must show proof of immunization when they apply for permanent residency, typically 1 year after arrival. However, selected refugees bound for the United States are immunized in their country of origin before arrival in the United States. Clinicians should review the CDC Refugee Health Web site (**www.cdc. gov/ncidod/dq/refugee/index.htm**) for information about which refugee populations currently are receiving immunization outside the United States. Refugee children, however, almost universally are immunized incompletely and often have no immunization records.

In general, only written documentation should be accepted as evidence of previous immunization. BCG, DTwP or DTaP, poliovirus, measles, and hepatitis B vaccines are given routinely and may be documented in an immunization record. However, immunizations to prevent infection caused by agents such as *H influenzae* type b, *S pneumoniae*, mumps, rubella, hepatitis A, and varicella often are given less frequently or are not part of the routine immunization schedule in other countries, and therefore there may not be written documentation for these vaccines. Increasingly, more of these vaccines are being incorporated into the immunization schedules in countries outside the United States. In general, written documentation of immunizations can be accepted as evidence of adequacy of previous immunization if the vaccines, dates of administration, number of doses, intervals between doses, and age of the child at the time of immunization are consistent internally and are comparable to current US or World Health Organization schedules. (**http://apps.who.int/immunization_monitoring/en/globalsummary/ countryprofileselect.cfm**). Inaccuracies, fraudulent data, or other problems, such as recording MMR vaccine but giving a product that did not contain one or more of the components (eg, mumps and/or rubella) should be considered during review of records. Any vaccination documented on the official Department of State health immigration form (DS 3025) should be accepted. Studies performed in internationally adopted children have demonstrated that the majority of children with documentation of immunizations have antibodies consistent with those immunizations. Limited country-specific data are available regarding serologic verification of immunization records for other categories of immigrant children. Evaluation of concentrations of antibody to vaccine-preventable diseases sometimes is useful to ensure that vaccines were given and were immunogenic, as well as to document immunity from past infection (see Serologic Testing to Document Immunization Status). If serologic testing is not available or is too costly, or if a positive result would not mitigate need for further immunization, the prudent course is to repeat administration of the immunizations in question.

UNKNOWN OR UNCERTAIN IMMUNIZATION STATUS IN US CHILDREN

There are circumstances in which the immunization status for a child born in the United States is uncertain or unknown because of lack of paper or electronic documentation of immunizations, an incomplete or inaccurate record, or a recording inconsistent with a recommended product or schedule. For US-born children, serologic testing can be performed to determine whether antibody concentrations are present for some of the vaccine-preventable diseases (see Serologic Testing to Document Immunization Status). A combined strategy of serologic testing for antibodies for some vaccine antigens and immunization for others may be used. If serologic testing is not available or is too costly, or if a positive result would not mitigate need for further immunization, the prudent course is to repeat administration of the immunizations in question.

SEROLOGIC TESTING TO DOCUMENT IMMUNIZATION STATUS

The usefulness, validity, and interpretation of serologic testing to guide management of vaccinations can be complex and varies by age. The cost of testing versus the cost of administering a given immunization series, as well as the likelihood of adherence for completing the immunization series, also should be considered in these decisions. In most situations, a record verifying the administration of a complete vaccine series would be more reliable than serologic testing. In children older than 6 months with or without written documentation of immunization, serologic testing to document antibodies to diphtheria and tetanus toxoids (ie, $\geq$0.1 IU/mL), or H influenzae type b for a child younger than 60 months (ie, $\geq$0.15 U/mL), may be considered to determine whether the child likely has received and responded to dose(s) of the vaccine in question. If the child has "protective" antibodies, the immunization series should be completed as appropriate for that child's age. If a child does not have "protective" antibodies, the series should be restarted, with the understanding that for some vaccine-preventable diseases, fewer doses of vaccine are needed to complete the series as a child ages. The immunization record, plus presence of antibody to diphtheria and tetanus toxoids, can be used as proxy for receipt of pertussis-containing vaccine dose(s). No serologic test is available to assess immunity to pertussis or rotavirus. In children older than 12 months, hepatitis A, measles, mumps, rubella, and varicella antibody concentrations could be measured to determine whether the child is immune; these antibody tests should not be performed in children younger than 12 months because of the potential presence of maternal antibody. Usefulness of measuring measles antibody is limited, because the majority of foreign-born children will need mumps and rubella vaccines, available in the United States only as MMR vaccine, because mumps and rubella vaccines are administered infrequently in resource-limited countries. Two doses of MMR vaccine should be administered for mumps coverage, even if measles antibodies are present. Rubella coverage is achieved following 1 dose of a rubella-containing vaccine. The documented receipt of 2 doses of varicella vaccine is the best indication of immunity to varicella, because commercially available varicella antibody tests are insensitive. Neutralizing antibody tests for poliovirus are not available generally, and only presence of antibody to all 3 serotypes would preclude need for poliovirus vaccine. For immunocompetent children 5 years or older, Hib vaccine is not indicated even if none was given previously; serologic testing should not be performed, because children in this age group frequently have antibody levels <0.15 U/mL yet are not susceptible to *H influenzae* type b infection. Age-appropriate pneumococcal vaccine dose(s) should be administered if a completed series is not documented; serologic testing should not be performed for validation or evidence of immunity.

For immigrants, serologic testing for HBsAg should be performed for all children to identify chronic hepatitis B virus infection. When the HBsAg test result is negative, the results of the anti-HBs and core antibody (anti-HBc) tests will determine whether the child is immune (from immunization or disease, respectively). Some immigrant or refugee children may have had previous hepatitis A infection; presence of immunoglobulin (Ig) G-specific antibody to hepatitis A virus would preclude need for hepatitis A vaccine.

International Travel

Up to 60% of children will become ill during international travel, and up to 19% will require medical care. At particular risk are children of immigrants visiting friends and relatives abroad. Medical planning for travel requires 6 to 8 weeks at minimum. Parents should be made aware that there is increased risk for their children of exposure to vaccine-preventable diseases overseas, even in many countries in Europe. Routinely recommended immunizations should be up-to-date before international travel; some routinely recommended immunizations should be given early or on an accelerated schedule. Additional vaccines to prevent yellow fever, meningococcal disease, typhoid fever, rabies, and Japanese encephalitis may be indicated depending on the destination and type of international travel (see specific disease chapters). Yellow fever vaccine is only available at certified centers in the United States. Japanese encephalitis virus immunization requires 28 days to complete, and catch-up immunization for routine pediatric vaccines may take longer. Travelers to tropical and subtropical areas often risk exposure to malaria, dengue, diarrhea, and skin diseases for which vaccines are not available. For travelers to areas with endemic malaria, antimalarial chemoprophylaxis and insect precautions are vitally important (see Malaria, p 528). Attention to hand hygiene, safer foods, insect vectors, and contaminated sand, soil, and water reduce travelers' risk of acquiring other communicable diseases.

Up-to-date information, including alerts about current disease outbreaks that may affect international travelers, is available on the CDC Travelers' Health Web site (**wwwnc. cdc.gov/travel/**) or the WHO Web site (**www.who.int/ith/**). *Health Information for International Travel* (the "Yellow Book") is revised every 2 years by the CDC and is an excellent reference for travelers and for practitioners who advise international travelers of health risks. Travel information and recommendations can be obtained from the CDC (800-CDC-INFO). Local and state health departments and travel clinics also can provide updated information. Information about cruise ship sanitation inspection scores and reports can be found on the CDC Web site (**www.cdc.gov/nceh/vsp/default.htm**). In June 2007, federal agencies developed a public health Do Not Board (DNB) list, enabling domestic and international public health officials to request that people with communicable diseases who meet specific criteria and pose a serious threat to the public be restricted from boarding commercial aircraft from or arriving in the United States.[1]

RECOMMENDED IMMUNIZATIONS

Transmission of pathogens prevented by the US childhood and adolescent immunization schedule continues in other areas of the world, including some industrialized nations. Infants and children embarking on international travel should be up-to-date on receipt of immunizations recommended for their age. To optimize immunity before departure, vaccines may need to be given on an accelerated schedule.

HEPATITIS A. Hepatitis A vaccine (HepA) is recommended routinely in a 2-dose series ≥6 months apart for all children at 12 through 23 months of age in the United States. HepA should be considered for all people who were born before universal recommendations or who are unimmunized or underimmunized and traveling to areas with intermediate or high rates of hepatitis A infection. These include *all areas of the world except* Australia, Canada, Japan, New Zealand, and Western Europe. Inactivated HepA is used for immunoprophylaxis for people 1 year of age and older. A combination HepA-HepB vaccine is available for people 18 years of age and older. For children younger than 1 year, Immune Globulin Intramuscular (IGIM) may be indicated, because HepA is not licensed in the United States for use in this age group. The dose of IGIM administered for preexposure prophylaxis of hepatitis A infection may interfere with the immune response to varicella and MMR vaccines for up to 3 months (Table 1.10, p 39).

HEPATITIS B. Hepatitis B vaccine (HepB) is recommended routinely for all children in the United States and should be considered for susceptible travelers of all ages (ie, those born before universal recommendations) visiting areas where hepatitis B infection is endemic, such as countries in Asia, Africa, and some parts of South America (see Hepatitis B, p 400). An accelerated dosing schedule is licensed for 1 hepatitis B vaccine (Engerix-B [GlaxoSmithKline Biologicals, Research Triangle Park, NC), during which the first 3 doses are given at 0, 1, and 2 months. In another accelerated schedule, doses are given on days 0, 7, and 14. This schedule may benefit travelers who have insufficient time to complete a standard schedule before departure. If the accelerated schedule is used, a fourth dose should be given at least 6 months after the third dose (see Hepatitis B, p 400). A combination HepA-HepB vaccine is available for people 18 years of age and older.

MEASLES. People traveling abroad should be immune to measles to provide personal protection and minimize importation of the infection. Importation of measles remains an important source for measles cases in the United States.[2] People should be considered susceptible to measles unless they have documentation of appropriate immunization, physician-diagnosed measles, laboratory evidence of immunity to measles, or were born in the United States before 1957. For people born in the United States in 1957 or after, 2 doses of measles vaccine, the first administered at or after 12 months of age, are required to ensure immunity (see Measles, p 535). Children who travel or live abroad should be vaccinated at an earlier age than recommended for children remaining in the United States. Before their departure from the United States, children 12 months and

[1]Centers for Disease Control and Prevention. Federal air travel restrictions for public health purposes—United States, June 2007–May 2008. *MMWR Morb Mortal Wkly Rep.* 2008;57(37):1009–1012

[2]Centers for Disease Control and Prevention. Measles—United States, January–May 20, 2011. *MMWR Morb Mortal Wkly Rep.* 2011;60(20):666-668

older should have received 2 doses of MMR vaccine separated by at least 28 days, with the first dose administered on or after the first birthday. Children 6 through 11 months of age should receive 1 dose of MMR vaccine before departure; 2 doses of MMR vaccine separated by at least 28 days will be required at 12 months or older to complete the required schedule.

POLIOVIRUS. Polio remains endemic in a few countries in Africa and Asia (an up-to-date listing of polio cases can be found at **www.polioeradication.org**). The Western Hemisphere was declared free of wild-type poliovirus in 1994, and the Western Pacific Region was declared free in 2000. The finding of vaccine-derived poliovirus in stool samples from several asymptomatic unimmunized people in a United States community raises concerns about the risk of transmission of polio within other communities with a low level of immunization.[1] To ensure protection, all children should be immunized fully against poliovirus. The ACIP recommends the following[2] (see Poliovirus Infections, p 644):

- The 4-dose IPV series should be administered at 2 months, 4 months, 6 through 18 months, and 4 through 6 years of age.
- The final dose in the IPV series should be administered at 4 through 6 years of age, regardless of the number of previous doses.
- The minimum interval from dose 3 to dose 4 is 6 months.
- The minimum interval from dose 1 to dose 2, and from dose 2 to dose 3, is 4 weeks.
- The minimum age for dose 1 remains 6 weeks of age.

Travelers 18 years or older visiting regions identified on the CDC travel Web site as polio vulnerable should receive a booster dose of IPV.

REQUIRED OR RECOMMENDED TRAVEL-RELATED IMMUNIZATIONS

Depending on the destination, planned activity, and length of stay, other immunizations may be required or recommended (see **wwwnc.cdc.gov/travel/** and disease-specific chapters in Section 3).

CHOLERA. The whole-cell inactivated cholera vaccine no longer is produced in the United States. According to WHO regulations, no country may require cholera immunization as a condition for entry. However, despite WHO recommendations, some local authorities may require documentation of immunization. In such cases, a notation of vaccine contraindication should be sufficient to satisfy local requirements.

JAPANESE ENCEPHALITIS.[3] Japanese encephalitis (JE) virus, a mosquitoborne flavivirus, is the most common cause of encephalitis in Asia. The overall incidence of JE reported among people from countries without endemic infection traveling to Asia is less than 1 case per million travelers. Short-term travelers whose visits are restricted to major urban areas are at minimal risk of JE, but risk varies on the basis of season, destination, duration, and activities. JE virus transmission occurs principally in rural agricultural areas,

---

[1]Centers for Disease Control and Prevention. Poliovirus infections in four unvaccinated children—Minnesota, August–October 2005. *MMWR Morb Mortal Wkly Rep.* 2005;54(41):1053–1055

[2]Centers for Disease Control and Prevention. Updated recommendations of the Advisory Committee on Immunization Practices (ACIP) regarding routine poliovirus vaccination. *MMWR Morb Mortal Wkly Rep.* 2009;58(30):829-830

[3]Centers for Disease Control and Prevention. Japanese encephalitis vaccines: recommendations of the Advisory Committee on Immunization Practices (ACIP). *MMWR Recomm Rep.* 2010;59(RR-01):1-26

often associated with rice production. In temperate areas of Asia, JE cases usually peak in summer and fall. In the tropics, transmission varies with monsoon rains and irrigation practices, and cases may occur year-round. Short-term travelers should be encouraged to avoid high-risk areas or not to take their children to these high-risk areas. Expatriates and travelers staying for prolonged periods in rural areas with active JE virus transmission likely are at similar risk as the susceptible resident population (0.1 to 2 cases per 100 000 people per week). Only one JE vaccine is available commercially for use in the United States. An inactivated Vero cell culture-derived vaccine (IXIARO [JE-VC], distributed in the US by Novartis Vaccines and Diagnostics Inc, Cambridge, MA) is licensed for people 2 months of age or older in a 2-dose primary series. Because of low risk of acquiring disease and high cost of vaccine, JE-VC should be targeted to travelers who are at increased risk for disease on the basis of their planned itinerary. Vaccine is recommended for travelers (including long-term travelers, recurrent travelers, and expatriates) who plan to spend 1 month or longer who are likely to visit rural or agricultural areas with endemic disease during a high-risk period of JE virus transmission. JE vaccine also should be considered for short-term (<1 month) travelers to endemic areas during the JE virus transmission season if they plan to travel outside of an urban area and have an increased risk for JE virus exposure (eg, spending substantial time outdoors in rural or agricultural areas; participating in extensive outdoor activities; staying in accommodations without air conditioning, screens, or bed nets). JE-VC also should be considered for travelers to an area with an ongoing JE outbreak and travelers to endemic areas who are uncertain of specific destinations, activities, or duration of travel. JE-VC is not recommended for short-term travelers whose visit will be restricted to urban areas or to times outside of a well-defined JE virus transmission season (see Arboviruses, p 240).

INFLUENZA. In addition to recommended annual influenza immunization, influenza vaccine may be warranted at other times for international travelers depending on the destination, duration of travel, risk of acquisition of disease (in part on the basis of the season of the year), and the travelers' underlying health status. Because the influenza season is different in the northern and southern hemispheres and epidemic strains may differ, the antigenic composition of influenza vaccines used in North America may be different from those used in the southern hemisphere, and timing of administration may vary (see Influenza, p 476).

MENINGOCOCCUS. Three meningococcal conjugate vaccines (MCVs) can be considered for use in infants traveling to areas where meningococcal disease is hyperendemic, such as serogroups A and W in sub-Saharan Africa or another area with current meningococcal epidemics. Saudi Arabia requires a certificate of immunization for pilgrims to Mecca or Medina during the Hajj. MCVs vary in serogroups covered, conjugating protein, ages of licensed use, and dosing schedules. The following MCVs are licensed for traveling infants and older people for protection against serogroups contained in the vaccines: MenACWY-CRM (Menveo, Novartis Vaccines and Diagnostics Inc, Cambridge, MA; for people 2 months to 55 years of age), MenACWY-D (Menactra, Sanofi Pasteur, Swiftwater, PA; for people 9 months to 55 years of age), and HibMenCY-TT (MenHibrix, GlaxoSmithKline, Research Triangle Park, NC; for people 6 weeks to 18 months of age). The last is not appropriate for people traveling to sub-Saharan Africa or another area where serogroup A or W disease is prevalent. Completion of the entire series is preferred prior to travel. The schedule follows for those receiving MCV4-CRM and MCV4-D: (1) children younger than 9 months—2, 4, and 6 months (with booster at 12-18 months of age) (MCV4-CRM); (2) children 9 months through 23 months of age—2 doses separated by at least 8 weeks (MCV4-D), or 2 doses with the second dose at ≥12 months and ≥3 months following the first dose (MCV4-CRM); and (3) children 24 months or older—a single dose (MCV4-CRM or MCV4-D). Revaccination with a conjugate vaccine is recommended for people who are at continuous or repeated increased risk of meningococcal infection (see Meningococcal Infections, p 547).

RABIES.[1] Rabies immunization should be considered for children who will be traveling to areas with endemic rabies where they may encounter wild or domestic animals (particularly dogs). The 3-dose preexposure series is administered by intramuscular injection (see Rabies, p 658). In the event of a bite by a potentially rabid animal, all travelers (whether they have received preexposure rabies vaccine or not) should be counseled to clean the wound thoroughly with soap and water and then promptly receive postexposure prophylaxis (PEP; see Rabies, p 658). Prior receipt of preexposure vaccination avoids the need for Rabies Immune Globulin, which is critical to the success of PEP but often is not available or of equine origin in developing countries. Travelers who have completed a 3-dose pre-exposure series or have received the full PEP series do not require routine boosters, except after a likely rabies exposure. Periodic serum testing for rabies virus neutralizing antibody is not necessary for routine international travelers.

TUBERCULOSIS. The risk of being infected with *Mycobacterium tuberculosis* during international travel depends on the activities of the traveler and the epidemiology of tuberculosis in the areas in which travel occurs. In general, the risk of acquiring infection during usual tourism activities appears to be low, and no pre- or post-travel testing is recommended routinely. When travelers live or work among the general population of a country with a high prevalence of tuberculosis, the risk may be appreciably higher. In most high-prevalence countries, contact investigation of tuberculosis cases is not performed, and diagnosis and treatment of latent tuberculosis infection (LTBI) is uncommon or is restricted to high-risk people. Children returning to the United States who have signs or symptoms compatible with tuberculosis should be evaluated immediately for tuberculosis disease. It is advisable to perform a tuberculin skin test or interferon-gamma release assay 8 to 10 weeks after return for children who spent 1 month or longer in a country with high prevalence of tuberculosis and for children who had a known tuberculosis exposure, regardless of time abroad or the countries that were visited. Pretravel administration of BCG vaccine generally is not recommended. However, some countries may require BCG vaccine for issuance of work and residency permits for expatriate workers and their families. Physicians can obtain BCG from the US distributor, Organon USA Inc, 56 Livingston Ave, Roseland, NJ (telephone: 973-992-1652).

TYPHOID. Typhoid vaccine is recommended for travelers who may be exposed to contaminated food or water. Two typhoid vaccines are available in the United States: an oral vaccine containing live-attenuated *Salmonella typhi* (Ty21a strain) licensed for ≥6 year olds, and a parenteral Vi capsular polysaccharide (ViCPS) vaccine licensed for ≥2 year olds. Travelers should be reminded that typhoid immunization is not 100% effective, and typhoid fever still can occur; both vaccines protect 50% to 80% of recipients. Revaccination is required after 5 years for oral and 2 years for inactivated vaccine. For

---

[1]Centers for Disease Control and Prevention. Human rabies prevention—United States, 2008: recommendations of the Advisory Committee on Immunization Practices. *MMWR Recomm Rep.* 2008;57(RR-3):1–28

specific recommendations, see *Salmonella* Infections (p 695). Mefloquine or chloroquine can be administered simultaneously with oral Ty21a vaccine. The oral vaccine capsules should be refrigerated. Because the vaccine is not completely efficacious, typhoid immunization is not a substitute for careful selection of food and beverages.

YELLOW FEVER. Yellow fever vaccine, a live-attenuated virus vaccine, is required by some countries as a condition of entry, including travelers arriving from regions with endemic infection.[1] The vaccine is available in the United States only in centers designated by state health departments. Current requirements and recommendations for yellow fever immunization on the basis of travel destination can be obtained from the CDC Travelers' Health Web site (**wwwnc.cdc.gov/travel/**). Yellow fever occurs year-round, predominantly in rural areas of sub-Saharan Africa and South America; in recent years, outbreaks have been reported, including in some urban areas. Although rare, yellow fever continues to be reported among unimmunized travelers and may be fatal. Prevention measures against yellow fever should include protection against mosquito bites (see Prevention of Mosquitoborne Infections, p 213) and immunization. Yellow fever (YF) vaccine rarely has been found to be associated with a risk of viscerotropic disease (multiple-organ system failure) and neurotropic disease (postvaccinal encephalitis). There is increased risk of adverse events in people of any age with thymic dysfunction and people older than 60 years of age. YF vaccine, like all live-virus vaccines, should be avoided during pregnancy. Meningoencephalitis has been reported in neonates (8 days and 38 days old) exposed to vaccine virus through breastfeeding. Administration of YF vaccine should be delayed in breastfeeding women until infants are at least 6 months of age unless exposure to YF is unavoidable. Administration of YF vaccine is recommended for people 9 months and older who are traveling to or living in areas of South America and Africa in which risk exists for yellow fever transmission. Because serious adverse events can follow YF vaccine administration, only people at risk of exposure to yellow fever or who require proof of vaccination for country entry should be immunized. The contraindications and precautions should be followed (Table 1.17). Consultation with a travel medicine expert or the CDC Division of Vector-Borne Infectious Diseases (970-221-6400) or the Division of Global Migration and Quarantine (404-498-1600) to weigh risks and benefits is advised. YF vaccine is contraindicated before 6 months of age, and whenever possible, immunization should be delayed until 9 months of age to minimize the risk of vaccine-associated encephalitis. People who cannot receive YF vaccine because of contraindications should consider alternative itineraries or destinations.

OTHER CONSIDERATIONS. In addition to vaccine-preventable diseases, travelers to the tropics will be exposed to other diseases, such as malaria, which can be life threatening. Prevention strategies for malaria are twofold: prevention of mosquito bites and use of antimalarial chemoprophylaxis. For recommendations on appropriate use of chemoprophylaxis, including recommendations for pregnant women, infants, and breastfeeding mothers, see Malaria (p 528). Prevention of mosquito bites will decrease the risk of malaria, dengue, chikungunya, and other mosquito-transmitted diseases (see Prevention of Mosquitoborne Infections, p 213).

---

[1]Centers for Disease Control and Prevention. Yellow fever vaccine. Recommendations of the Advisory Committee on Immunization Practices. *MMWR Recomm Rep.* 2010;59(RR-07):1–27

Table 1.17. Contraindications and Precautions to Yellow Fever Vaccine Administration

Contraindications	Precautions
Allergy to vaccine component	Age 6 through 8 mo
Age less than 6 mo	Age ≥60 y
Symptomatic HIV infection or CD4+ T-lymphocyte count <200/mm³ (or <15% of total in children younger than 6 y)[a]	Asymptomatic HIV infection and CD4+ T-lymphocyte count 200–499/mm³ (or 15%–24% of total in children younger than 6 y)
Thymus disorder associated with abnormal immune function	Pregnancy
Primary immunodeficiencies	Breastfeeding
Malignant neoplasms	
Transplantation	
Immunosuppressive and immunomodulatory therapies	

[a] Symptoms of HIV have been classified (Panel on Antiretroviral Guidelines for Adults and Adolescents. Guidelines for the use of antiretroviral agents in HIV-1-infected adults and adolescents; US Department of Health and Human Services; 2008. Available at: **http://aidsinfo.nih.gov/Guidelines/html/1/adult-and-adolescent-treatment-guidelines/0/** and Working Group on Antiretroviral Therapy and Medical Management of HIV-Infected Children. Guidelines for the Use of Antiretroviral Agents in Pediatric HIV Infection; 2009. Available at: **http://aidsinfo.nih.gov/ContentFiles/PediatricGuidelines.pdf**).

Traveler's diarrhea affects up to 60% of travelers but may be mitigated by attention to foods and beverages ingested (including ice). Chemoprophylaxis is generally not recommended. Educating families about self-treatment, particularly oral rehydration, is critical. Packets of oral rehydration salts can be obtained before travel and are available in most pharmacies throughout the world, including in developing countries where diarrheal diseases are most common. During international travel, families may want to carry an antimicrobial agent (eg, fluoroquinolone for people 16 years and older and azithromycin for younger children) for treatment of significant diarrheal symptoms. The choice of agent will be influenced by the resistance pattern within the particular region to be visited. Antimotility agents may be considered for older children and adolescents (see *Escherichia coli* Diarrhea, p 343) but should not be used if diarrhea is bloody or for patients with diarrhea attributable to Shiga toxin-producing *Escherichia coli*, *Clostridium difficile*, or *Shigella* species.

Travelers should be aware of potential acquisition of respiratory tract viruses, including novel strains of influenza. They should be counseled on hand hygiene and avoidance of close contact with animals (dead or live). Swimming, water sports, and ecotourism around freshwater carry risks of acquisition of infections from environmental contamination (notably schistosomiasis). Pyogenic skin infections and cutaneous larva migrans are common. Travelers should avoid direct skin contact with sand, soil, and animals.

Recommendations for Care of Children in Special Circumstances

....
BIOLOGICAL TERRORISM

Some infectious agents have the potential to be used in acts of bioterrorism. The Centers for Disease Control and Prevention (CDC) designates biological agents of concern for bioterrorism based on the potential impact and risk to civilians and in order to guide national public health bioterrorism preparedness and response (Table 2.1).[1] The highest-priority agents for preparedness have a moderate to high potential for large-scale dissemination, cause high rates of mortality with potential for major public health effects, could cause public panic and social disruption, and require special action for public health preparedness. These include organisms such as anthrax, smallpox, plague, tularemia, botulism, and viral hemorrhagic fevers, including Ebola, Marburg, Lassa, Junin, and other related viruses. **Moderate risk agents** are fairly easy to disseminate, cause moderate morbidity and low mortality rates, but still require enhanced diagnostic capacity and disease surveillance to respond effectively and mitigate health effects. Some examples of moderate risk agents include *Coxiella burnetii* (Q fever), *Brucella* species (brucellosis), *Burkholderia mallei* (glanders), *Burkholderia pseudomallei* (melioidosis), alphaviruses (Venezuelan equine, eastern equine, and western equine encephalitis), *Rickettsia prowazekii* (typhus), and toxins such as ricin toxin from *Ricinus communis* (castor beans) and *Staphylococcus* enterotoxin B. Additional organisms that could create foodborne or waterborne safety threats include, but are not limited to, *Salmonella* species, *Shigella dysenteriae*, *Escherichia coli* O157:H7, and *Vibrio cholerae*. Finally, emerging pathogens that could present a potential bioterrorism threat as scientific knowledge about these organisms increases include Nipah virus, hantavirus, tickborne hemorrhagic fever viruses, and tickborne encephalitis viruses. The US Department of Homeland Security conducts bioterrorism risk assessments for evaluation and prioritization of potential bioterrorism threats, as mandated by the Homeland Security Presidential Directive 10 (**www.fas.org/irp/offdocs/nspd/hspd-10.html**).

Children may be particularly vulnerable to a bioterrorist attack because they have a more rapid respiratory rate, frequent hand-to-mouth behavior, increased skin permeability, a higher ratio of skin surface area to body mass, and less fluid reserve compared with adults. Accurate and rapid diagnosis may be more difficult in children because of their inability to describe symptoms. In addition, children depend on others for their health and safety, and those individuals may become ill or require quarantine during a bioterrorism event. Many preventive and therapeutic agents recommended for adults exposed or potentially exposed to agents of bioterrorism have not been studied in infants and children. The lack of approval by the US Food and Drug Administration (FDA) means that many medications must be administered through emergency use authorizations (EUAs) or

---

[1]Rotz LD, Khan AS, Ostroff S, Hughes J, Lillibridge SR. Public health assessment and prioritization of potential biological terrorism agents. *Emerg Infect Dis.* 2002;8(2):225-230

Table 2.1. Potential Bioterrorism Agents

Agents

The US public health system and primary health care providers must be prepared to address various biological agents, including pathogens that are rarely seen in the United States. These pathogens might require specific diagnostic testing and require special action for public health preparedness.

- Anthrax (*Bacillus anthracis*)
- Botulism (*Clostridium botulinum* toxin)
- Brucellosis (*Brucella* species)
- Epsilon toxin of *Clostridium perfringens*
- Food safety threats (eg, *Salmonella* species, *Escherichia coli* O157:H7, *Shigella* species)
- Glanders (*Burkholderia mallei*)
- Melioidosis (*Burkholderia pseudomallei*)
- Plague (*Yersinia pestis*)
- Psittacosis (*Chlamydia psittaci*)
- Q fever (*Coxiella burnetii*)
- Ricin toxin from *Ricinus communis* (castor beans)
- Smallpox (variola major)
- Staphylococcal enterotoxin B
- Tularemia (*Francisella tularensis*)
- Typhus fever (*Rickettsia prowazekii*)
- Viral encephalitis (alphaviruses [eg, Venezuelan equine encephalitis, eastern equine encephalitis, western equine encephalitis])
- Viral hemorrhagic fevers (filoviruses [eg, Ebola, Marburg] and arenaviruses [eg, Lassa, Machupo])
- Water safety threats (eg, *Vibrio cholerae, Cryptosporidium parvum*)

Emerging Pathogens

Pediatricians also should be aware of emerging pathogens that could potentially be engineered for mass dissemination in the future and present a potential bioterrorism threat because of availability, ease of production and dissemination, and potential for high morbidity and mortality rates and major health impact. Examples include Nipah virus, hantavirus, tickborne hemorrhagic fever viruses, and tickborne encephalitis viruses. Risk assessments for evaluation and prioritization of potential bioterrorism threats are conducted by the Department of Homeland Security.

investigational new drug (IND) protocols for use in children.[1] Children also may be at risk of unique adverse effects from preventive and therapeutic agents that are recommended for treating exposure to agents of bioterrorism. Parents, pediatricians, and other adults should be cognizant of the psychological responses of children to a disaster or terrorist incident to reduce the possibility of long-term psychological morbidity.[2]

---

[1] American Academy of Pediatrics, Committee on Environmental Health and Committee on Infectious Diseases. Chemical-biological terrorism and its impact on children. *Pediatrics*. 2006;118(3):1267-1278 (Reaffirmed January 2011)

[2] Hagan JF Jr; American Academy of Pediatrics, Committee on Psychosocial Aspects of Child and Family Health. Psychosocial implications of disaster or terrorism on children: a guide for the pediatrician. *Pediatrics*. 2005;116(3):787-795 (Reaffirmed October 2014)

Table 2.2. Emergency Contacts and Educational Resources

Health Department Information
- State Health Department Web sites: **www.cdc.gov/mmwr/international/relres.html**

Emergency Contacts
- Centers for Disease Control and Prevention (CDC) 24-Hour Emergency Operations Center:
- **770-488-7100 (www.bt.cdc.gov/emcontact/)**
- US Army Medical Research Institute of Infectious Disease (USAMRIID) Emergency Response Line: **888-872-7443**

Selected Web Information Resources
- American Academy of Pediatrics bioterrorism information: **www.aap.org/en-us/advocacy-and-policy/aap-health-initiatives/Children-and-Disasters/Pages/default.aspx**
- CDC Emergency Preparedness and Response: **http://emergency.cdc.gov**
- Infectious Diseases Society of America: **www.idsociety.org/Bioterrorism_Agents/**
- American Society for Microbiology Sentinel level clinical laboratory protocols for suspected biological threat agents and emerging infectious diseases: **www.asm.org/index.php/issues/sentinel-laboratory-guidelines**
- US Department of Health and Human Services Public Health Emergency: **www.phe.gov/emergency/pages/default.aspx**
- University of Pittsburgh Medical Center, Center for Biosecurity: **www.upmc-biosecurity.org**
- USAMRIID: **www.usamriid.army.mil/**
- US Food and Drug Administration (FDA) Drug Preparedness: **www.fda.gov/Drugs/EmergencyPreparedness/BioterrorismandDrugPreparedness/default.htm**
- Federal Bureau of Investigation, Web site to report concern about bioterror event: **https://tips.fbi.gov/**
- MedlinePlus from the National Institutes of Health **www.nlm.nih.gov/medlineplus/biodefenseandbioterrorism.html**
- Department of Labor, Occupational Safety and Health Administration: **www.osha.gov/SLTC/bioterrorism/**

Fever, malaise, headache, vomiting, and diarrhea are common early manifestations of illness caused by many bioterrorism agents and other infectious diseases. Some bioterrorism agents can cause typical distinctive signs and symptoms and have specific incubation periods. Each of the bioterrorism agents require unique diagnostic tests, isolation precautions, and recommended treatment and prophylaxis. Agents are discussed in Section 3 under specific pathogens, and extensive information and advice are available elsewhere. Table 2.2 lists resources, including telephone numbers and Internet sites, where updated information can be found concerning clinical recognition, prevention, diagnosis, and treatment of illness caused by potential agents of bioterrorism.

Clinicians should be familiar with reporting requirements within their public health jurisdiction for these conditions. When clinicians suspect that illness is caused by a reportable condition or an act of bioterrorism, they should contact their local public health authority immediately so that appropriate infection-control measures and outbreak investigations can begin. In addition, local public health professionals will determine whether and when to notify local law enforcement. In the event of a bioterrorist attack, clinicians should review the CDC Emergency Preparedness and Response Web site (**http://emergency.cdc.gov**) for current information and specific prophylaxis and treatment guidelines. Public health authorities should be contacted before obtaining and submitting patient specimens for identification of suspected agents of bioterrorism. During a large-scale bioterrorism event, prophylactic medications will be distributed by public health officials through supplemental approaches, including at points of dispensing sites (PODS). Practicing pediatricians would be expected to help support these activities through maintaining the medical home for patients and assisting with questions and concerns about side effects.

Pediatricians play an important role in response and recovery. It is prudent that every pediatrician have both personal and professional preparedness plans. Pediatricians should be aware of preparedness and response plans at institutions in which they provide care, and should have a plan for their own office and staff. They should be aware of sources of information, including training before an event, and methods for receipt of alerts during an event. In addition, pediatricians are in a good position to advise patients and their families on personal preparedness and to provide information during an event. The AAP Web site (**www.aap.org/disasters**) is a source of information on preparedness, including training for pediatricians.

··

BLOOD SAFETY: REDUCING THE RISK OF TRANSFUSION-TRANSMITTED INFECTIONS

In the United States, the risk of transmission of screened infectious agents through transfusion of blood components (Red Blood Cells, Platelets, and Plasma) and plasma derivatives (clotting factor concentrates, immune globulins, and protein-containing plasma volume expanders) is extremely low. Continued vigilance is crucial, however, because of risk from newly identified or emerging infections as well as lack of a mandatory nationwide system for transfusion reaction surveillance. This chapter reviews blood and plasma collection procedures in the United States, factors that have contributed to enhancing the safety of the blood supply, some of the known and emerging infectious agents transmitted by transfusions, and approaches to decreasing the risk of transfusion-transmitted infections.

Blood Components and Plasma Derivatives

Blood collection, preparation, and testing are regulated by the Food and Drug Administration (FDA). In the United States, Whole Blood is collected from volunteer donors and separated into **components,** including Red Blood Cells, Platelets, Plasma, and Cryoprecipitate. Granulocytes and other white blood cells, although sometimes transfused, are not FDA-licensed products (but they generally are collected using apheresis in FDA-registered facilities). Platelets, Red Blood Cells, and Plasma also can be collected through apheresis, in which blood passes through a machine that separates blood components and returns uncollected components to the donor. Plasma for transfusion or further manufacturing into plasma protein derivatives, such as Albumin (Human), clotting factor concentrates, and Immune Globulin Intravenous (IGIV), can be prepared from Whole

Blood or collected by apheresis. Plasma proteins are derived from plasma collected specifically for the purposes of manufacturing these derivatives or from plasma recovered from whole blood. **Plasma protein derivatives** are prepared by pooling plasma from many donors and subjecting the plasma to a fractionation process that separates the desired proteins, including immune globulins and clotting factors.

From an infectious disease standpoint, plasma derivatives differ from blood components in several ways. For economic and therapeutic reasons, plasma from thousands of donors is pooled, and therefore, recipients of plasma derivatives have a vastly greater donor exposure than do blood component recipients. However, plasma derivatives are able to withstand vigorous viral inactivation processes that would destroy Red Blood Cells and Platelets. Most recognized infectious organisms, with the notable exception of non–lipid-enveloped viruses (eg, hepatitis A virus [HAV], parvovirus B19) and prions, are inactivated easily by plasma processing methods. Development and evaluation of various novel strategies for inactivation of infectious agents are ongoing for cellular components.

Current Blood Safety Measures

The safety of the blood supply relies on multiple steps, including donor interview and selection, donor screening by serologic testing and use of nucleic acid amplification tests (NAATs) for markers of infection, deferral registries to avoid collection and use of unsuitable units, inventory quarantines and controls to prevent release of unsuitable or untested blood, investigation of errors and accidents followed by corrective action, inactivation procedures for plasma-derived products, and leukodepletion of certain blood components (see Tables 2.3, p 114, and 2.4, p 115). Blood donors are interviewed to exclude individuals with a history of exposures or behaviors that increase the risk that their blood contains an infectious agent. All blood donations are tested routinely for syphilis, hepatitis B virus (HBV), hepatitis C virus (HCV), human T-lymphotropic virus (HTLV) types I and II, human immunodeficiency virus (HIV) types 1 and 2, and West Nile Virus (WNV) and *Treponema pallidum*. Selected donations also are tested for cytomegalovirus (CMV) antibodies. Because of changing demographics in the United States, the risk of transfusion-transmitted Chagas disease appears to be increasing. Since January 2007, most donations have been tested for antibodies to *Trypanosoma cruzi*, the etiologic agent of Chagas disease. In December 2010, the FDA recommended steps to reduce the risk of transfusion-transmitted Chagas disease, including one-time testing of all donors of allogeneic units of blood using a licensed test for antibodies to *T cruzi*. Other emerging pathogens for which laboratory screening is being performed in selective geographic settings include Dengue virus and *Babesia microti*. Both of these pathogens are detailed in the following sections and currently are under investigation for donor screening in select areas in the United States and its territories. Blood is not routinely screened for parvovirus B19, *Anaplasma* species, or *Ehrlichia* species that infrequently may be transmitted by donated blood.

Transfusion-Transmitted Agents: Known Threats and Potential Pathogens

Any infectious agent that has an infectious blood phase potentially can be transmitted by transfusion. Factors that influence the risk of transmission and development of clinical disease include the prevalence and incidence of the agent in donors, the duration of its hematogenous phase (particularly when asymptomatic), tolerance of the agent to

Table 2.3. Blood Donor Screening Measures[a]

Measure	Targeted Infectious Agents
General interview and screening	
Previous donor history (ie, no deferral in effect)	Bloodborne phase of multiple agents
General health, current illness, temperature at time of donation	
Donor confidential unit exclusion option[b]	
Remember to notify blood collector of illness (eg, fever, diarrhea after donation, or any other pertinent information recalled)	
Specific risk factor history	
High-risk sexual behaviors or injection drug use in donor or donor's partner(s)	HIV, HCV, HBV, HTLV
Geographic risks (travel and residence)	Malaria, vCJD, leishmaniasis, Chagas disease, babesiosis (within the United States)
History of specific infections	HIV, HBV, HCV, other hepatitis agents, parasites (those causing malaria, Chagas disease, babesiosis, and leishmaniasis)
Previous parenteral exposure to blood via transfusion or occupational exposure; not lifetime deferral	HIV, HCV, HBV
Laboratory screening	HIV-1 (antibody and NAAT); HIV-2 (antibody); HCV (antibody and NAAT); HBV (HBsAg and anti-HBc; ALT sometimes is performed but not recommended by the FDA); HTLV-I and HTLV-II (antibodies); syphilis (antibodies); WNV (NAAT); screens for bacteria; *Trypanosoma cruzi* (antibody)

HIV indicates human immunodeficiency virus; HCV, hepatitis C virus; HBV, hepatitis B virus; HTLV, human T-lymphotropic virus; vCJD, variant Creutzfeldt-Jakob disease; NAAT, nucleic acid amplification test; HBsAg, hepatitis B surface antigen; anti-HBc, hepatitis B core antibody; ALT alanine transaminase; FDA, US Food and Drug Administration; WNV, West Nile virus.

[a]Screening of source Plasma (paid) donors is similar but not identical. For example, because HTLV-I and HTLV-II are cell-associated agents, Plasma donations are not tested for anti-HTLV-I and anti-HTLV-II. Donors are tested for syphilis at least every 4 months.

[b]Donor is given the opportunity during the screening process to exclude himself or herself without disclosing the reason.

processing and storage, the infectivity and pathogenicity of the agent, and the recipient's health status. Table 2.4 (p 115) lists major known transfusion-transmitted infections and some of the emerging agents under investigation.

VIRUSES

HIV (P 453), HCV (P 423), HBV (P 400). The probability of infection in recipients who are exposed to HIV, HCV, or HBV in transfused blood products is more than 90%. Although blood donations are screened for these viruses, there is a very small residual risk of infection resulting almost exclusively from donations collected during the "window period" of

Table 2.4. Selected Known and Potential Transfusion-Transmitted Agents[a]

Agents and Products	Transfusion Transmitted	Pathogenic	Estimated per-Unit Risk of Contamination (US Studies, Except as Noted)[b]
Viruses for which all blood donors tested			
HIV	Yes	Yes	1 in 1 467 000
HCV	Yes	Yes	1 in 1 149 000
HBV	Yes	Yes	1 in 357 000 to 280 000
HTLV-I and HTLV-II	Yes	Yes	1 in 4 364 000
WNV	Yes	Yes	1 per 4 570 000, seasonal and geographic variation
Other viruses not routinely tested			
CMV	Yes	Yes	1%–4% with leukoreduced blood
Parvovirus B19	Yes	Yes	1 in 10 000
HAV	Yes	Yes	Less than 1 in 1 million contaminated per units transfused
TT virus	Yes	No	1 in 10 (Japan), 1 in 50 (Scotland)
SEN virus	Yes	No	Unknown
Murine leukemia virus	Probable	No	Unknown
HHV-8	Probable	Yes	Unknown
Bacteria associated with transfusion			
Red Blood Cells: *Yersinia enterocolitica* and other gram-negative bacteria	Yes	Yes	1 in 5 million units
Platelets: *Staphylococcus epidermidis, Bacillus* species, *Staphylococcus aureus, Salmonella* species, *Serratia* species	Yes	Yes	1 in 2000–3000 units
Parasites[c]			
Malaria *(Plasmodium falciparum)*	Yes	Yes	<0.1 per 10^6
Chagas disease *(Trypanosoma cruzi)*	Yes	Yes	<1 per 15 million
Prion diseases (TSEs)			
CJD/vCJD	Yes	Yes	4 cases worldwide vCJD

Table 2.4. Selected Known and Potential Transfusion-Transmitted Agents,[a] continued

Agents and Products	Transfusion Transmitted	Pathogenic	Estimated per-Unit Risk of Contamination (US Studies, Except as Noted)[b]
Tickborne agents infrequently transmitted by transfusion			
Babesia species	Yes	Yes	1 per 10^6 units
Rickettsia rickettsii	Yes	Yes	Unknown
Colorado tick fever virus	Yes	Yes	Unknown
Borrelia burgdorferi	Unknown	Yes	Unknown
Ehrlichia species	Unknown	Yes	Unknown

HIV indicates human immunodeficiency virus; HCV, hepatitis C virus; HBV, hepatitis B virus; HTLV, human T-lymphotropic virus; WNV, West Nile virus; CMV, cytomegalovirus; HAV, hepatitis A virus; HHV, human herpes virus; TSE, transmissible spongiform encephalopathy; CJD, Creutzfeldt-Jakob disease; and vCJD, variant CJD. (TT and SEN viruses were named for the initials of patients from whom the viruses first were isolated.)

[a]Adapted from: A Compendium of Transfusion Practice Guideline, 2010 American Red Cross.

[b]Not all studies are performed by all blood centers.

[c]Other parasites that can be transmitted by transfusion include *Toxoplasma gondii* and leishmanial species.

infection—the period soon after infection during which a blood donor is infectious but screening results are negative.

To decrease the time period when donor HIV and HCV infection may be undetected, routine use of NAATs for blood and plasma donations in the United States was implemented in 1999. At present, the NAAT for HBV is an optional donor screening test. Various estimates suggest that performing NAATs on pooled units can decrease the preantibody seroconversion window period from 22 days to 7 to 15 days for HIV and from 70 days to 7 to 29 days for HCV. Mathematical models have been developed to estimate the low risks of transfusion transmission of HIV, HCV, and HBV using currently accepted screening policies (Table 2.4, p 115).

HTLV-I AND HTLV-II. Infections with HTLV are relatively common in certain geographic areas of the world and in specific populations. For example, HTLV-I is more common in Japan, the Caribbean, and the southern United States, and HTLV-II is more common in indigenous people of North America, Central America, and South America and among injection drug users in the United States and Europe. HTLV-I and HTLV-II are transmitted by transfusion of cellular components of blood but not by Plasma or plasma derivatives. The risk of HTLV transmission from screened blood donated during the window period has been estimated at 1 per 641 000 units screened. However, transmission of HTLV from an infected unit is less likely to lead to infection than transmission of HIV, HBV, or HCV, with an approximate 27% seroconversion rate in people in the United States who receive non–leukocyte-reduced cellular blood components from infected donors.

CYTOMEGALOVIRUS (P 317). Immunocompromised people, including preterm infants and stem cell and solid organ transplant recipients, are at risk of severe, life-threatening illness from transfusion-transmitted CMV. The seroprevalence of CMV in the United States is estimated at 20% to 80%. Consequently, it is difficult to find donors who are negative for CMV antibodies. In some centers, only blood from donors who lack CMV antibodies is given to people in these categories. In contrast, other centers use blood with white blood cells removed or leukoreduced as a means to reduce CMV transmission and improve blood utilization. Red Blood Cells or Platelets that are leukoreduced are labeled as "CMV safe," because CMV resides in a latent phase within white blood cells. CMV-seronegative or leukoreduced blood reduces the risk of CMV transmission to 1% to 4%.

PARVOVIRUS B19 (P 593). Blood donations cannot be effectively screened serologically for parvovirus B19, because previous infection with this virus is common in adults. Seroprevalence rates in adult blood donors range from 29% to 79%, with estimates of parvovirus B19 viremia in blood donors ranging from 0 to 2.6 per 10 000 donors. Parvovirus, like CMV, usually does not cause severe disease in immunocompetent hosts but may be a serious health threat to fetuses of pregnant women lacking immunity; people with hemoglobinopathies, such as sickle cell disease and thalassemia; and immunocompromised patients. Although not precisely known, the risk of transmission of parvovirus B19 from Whole Blood donations is thought to be low. However, treated pooled plasma derivatives commonly test positive for parvovirus B19 DNA, because plasma is pooled from many donors and the virus survives despite treatment. Because parvovirus B19 lacks a lipid envelope, it is resistant to solvent/detergent. To increase safety, manufacturers of plasma derivatives test plasma mini-pools for parvovirus DNA and exclude those containing parvovirus above a threshold concentration.

HEPATITIS A VIRUS (P 391). Like parvovirus, HAV lacks a lipid envelope and survives solvent/detergent treatment. Infection with HAV leads to a relatively short period of viremia, and a chronic carrier state does not occur. Cases of transfusion-transmitted HAV infection have been reported but are rare. However, clusters of HAV infections transmitted from clotting factor concentrates have occurred among people with hemophilia in Europe, South Africa, and the United States.

HUMAN HERPESVIRUS 8 (P 452). Human herpesvirus 8 (HHV-8) is associated with Kaposi sarcoma, particularly in people with HIV infection and certain rare malignant neoplasms. The predominant modes of transmission are male-to-male sexual contact in the United States and close, nonsexual contact in Africa and Mediterranean Europe. Because HHV-8 DNA has been detected in peripheral blood mononuclear cells and serum, there is concern that HHV-8 could be transmitted through blood and blood products. Serologic evidence from several US-based studies suggests that HHV-8 infection may result from receipt of nonleukoreduced blood components as well as from injection drug use. More direct evidence for HHV-8 transmission by blood transfusion was provided by a case-controlled transfusion study in Uganda, where HHV-8 is endemic. However, HHV-8 seroprevalence rates are far lower in the general population in the United States than in areas with endemic infection (2%–5% versus 40%–60%, respectively). In the United States, seroprevalence for HHV-8 is higher in intravenous drug users and men who have sex with men (MSM). Transmission has not been shown in US studies with small numbers of recipients of blood from known HHV-8–seropositive donors. Among people with exposure to blood and blood products (eg, people with hemophilia), HHV-8 seroprevalence generally is comparable with that seen in healthy, HIV-seronegative people. Studies on larger populations of recipients of blood or blood products from HHV-8–positive people are needed.

WEST NILE VIRUS (P 865). WNV can be transmitted through blood transfusions. To reduce transfusion-associated transmission, blood collection agencies have implemented the use of NAATs for WNV. They primarily use an algorithm starting with mini-pools of donation samples. Donations constituting positive mini-pools are retested individually, and if results are positive, the reactive units are removed from the blood supply. If there is evidence of local epidemic WNV transmission, local blood collection agencies switch to individual donation testing to improve the sensitivity of finding WNV. Along with an overall decline in WNV incidence in recent years, these steps have reduced substantially but not eliminated the risk of WNV transmission via blood products. Unlike most other transfusion-transmitted infections, the risk of WNV transmission is highly dependent on season and geography. Cases of WNV disease in patients who have received blood transfusions within 28 days before illness onset should be reported promptly to the appropriate blood center and the Centers for Disease Control and Prevention (CDC) through state and local public health authorities. In addition, cases of WNV disease diagnosed in people who have donated blood within 2 weeks before onset of illness should be reported promptly.

DENGUE VIRUSES (P 322). A case of transfusion-transmitted dengue hemorrhagic fever was recognized during a recent outbreak of dengue fever in Puerto Rico, and other transfusion-transmitted dengue cases have been reported in East Asia. Small outbreaks of dengue fever in Florida, Texas, and Hawaii have not resulted in recognized transfusion transmissions. In 2009, the Transfusion Transmitted Diseases Committee of the AABB (formerly known as the American Association of Blood Banks) identified dengue viruses as among the emerging pathogens that pose a risk of transmission by transfusion. Currently, healthy blood donors recently returning to the continental United States from areas with endemic or epidemic dengue are not deferred, and no licensed tests to screen donors for dengue infection are available, although some blood donor establishments have implemented investigational donor screening and deferral programs; similar programs are under consideration nationally.

OTHER VIRUSES FOUND IN DONOR BLOOD. Murine leukemia virus, marseilleviruses (nucleocytoplasmic large DNA viruses), hepatitis G virus/GB virus type C, TT virus (torque teno virus, anellovirus), and SEN virus can result in persistent infection and may be identified in blood donors. These viruses may be transmitted by transfusion, but they generally are not considered to be pathogenic or clinically significant.

BACTERIA

Although major advances in blood safety have been made, bacterial contamination of blood products remains an important cause of transfusion reactions and can occur during collection, processing, or transfusion of blood components.

Platelets are stored at room temperature, which can facilitate the growth of contaminating bacteria. The predominant bacterium that contaminates Platelets is *Staphylococcus epidermidis. Bacillus* species, *Staphylococcus aureus,* and various gram-negative bacteria, including *Salmonella* species and *Serratia* species, also have been reported to have contaminated blood products. Transfusion reactions attributable to contaminated Platelets are likely underappreciated, because bacteremia with skin organisms is common in patients requiring Platelets, and the link to the transfusion may not be suspected.

Although there is no FDA requirement for testing of platelet products for bacterial contamination, on March 1, 2004, the AABB adopted a new standard that requires member blood banks and transfusion services to implement measures to detect and limit bacterial contamination of Platelet components. As a result, most apheresis and whole blood derived Platelets are tested by FDA-cleared culture methods and/or rapid bacterial detection methods. In 2007, the FDA cleared a rapid test to screen for bacterial contamination of Platelets before transfusion, the Verax PGD Assay. Another rapid test, BacTX Bacterial Detection System, now also is FDA cleared for whole-blood derived Platelets that are pooled within 4 hours. Alternatively, Acrodose Platelets are available through blood centers and are a pooled whole-blood-derived platelet product that allows for bacterial culture testing with the eBDS Bacteria Detection System. The most recent AABB standard, implemented in 2011, requires that only FDA-cleared test methods or methods validated to provide equivalent sensitivity be used for bacterial detection. Data show that after these newer standards were implemented, septic transfusion reactions decreased by approximately 70%, with a similar decrease in septic fatalities (**www.aabb. org/advocacy/regulatorygovernment/bloodcomponents/platelets/Pages/ default.aspx**). Less sensitive testing methods, such as pH testing, no longer are recommended. However, all widely used detection methods have been associated with failures. The residual risk of transfusion-associated bacterial infection is approximately 1 in 2000 to 1 in 3000 transfusions of Platelets. Hospitals should ensure that protocols are in place to communicate results of bacterial contamination tests, both for quarantine of components from individual donors and for prompt treatment of any transfused recipients. Posttransfusion notification of appropriate personnel is required if cultures identify bacteria after product release or transfusion. If bacterial contamination of a component is suspected, the transfusion should be stopped immediately, the unit should be saved for Gram stain and culture testing, and blood should be obtained from the recipient for culture. The blood center should be notified immediately to quarantine other products from the same donor and to complete their investigation of culture results at the time of issuance.

Red Blood Cell units are much less likely than Platelets to contain bacteria at the time of transfusion, because refrigeration kills or inhibits growth of many bacteria. However, certain bacteria, most notably gram-negative organisms such as *Yersinia enterocolitica*, may contaminate Red Blood Cells because they survive and grow in cold storage. Cases of septic shock and death attributable to transfusion-transmitted *Y enterocolitica* and other gram-negative organisms have been documented.

Reported rates of transfusion-associated bacterial sepsis have varied widely depending on study methodology and microbial detection methods used. A prospective, voluntary multisite study (the Assessment of the Frequency of Blood Component Bacterial Contamination Associated with Transfusion Reaction [BaCon] Study) estimated the rate of transfusion-transmitted sepsis to be 1 in 100 000 units for single-donor and pooled Platelets and 1 in 5 million units for Red Blood Cells. Other studies that did not require matching bacterial cultures and/or molecular typing of both the component and the recipient's blood, as in the BaCon Study, or that included less severe recipient reactions in addition to sepsis, have found higher rates of bacterial transmission.

PARASITES

Several parasitic agents have been reported to cause transfusion-transmitted infections, including malaria, Chagas disease, babesiosis, toxoplasmosis, and leishmaniasis. Increasing travel to and immigration from areas with endemic infection have led to a need for increased vigilance in the United States. Babesiosis and toxoplasmosis are endemic in the United States.

MALARIA (SEE P 528). The incidence of transfusion-associated malaria has decreased over the last 30 years in the United States. During the last decade, the rate has declined to 0 to 0.18 cases per million units transfused—that is, no more than 1 to 2 cases per year. Most cases are attributed to infected donors who have immigrated to the United States rather than to people who have traveled to areas with endemic infection. *Plasmodium falciparum* is the species most commonly transmitted. Prevention of transfusion-transmitted malaria relies on interviewing donors for risk factors related to residence in or travel to areas with endemic infection or to previous treatment for malaria. Donation should be delayed until 3 years after either completing treatment for malaria or living in a country where malaria is endemic and until 12 months after returning from a trip to an area where malaria is endemic. There is no licensed laboratory test to screen donated blood for malaria, and donor history is used as the primary screening tool for possible infection.

CHAGAS DISEASE (SEE AMERICAN TRYPANOSOMIASIS, P 803). The immigration of millions of people from areas with endemic *T cruzi* infection (parts of Central America, South America, and Mexico) and increased international travel have raised concern about the potential for transfusion-transmitted Chagas disease. To date, fewer than 10 cases of transfusion-transmitted Chagas disease have been reported in North America. However, studies of blood donors likely to have been born in or to have traveled to areas with endemic infection have found antibodies to *T cruzi* in as many as 0.5% of people tested. Although recognized transfusion transmissions of *T cruzi* in the United States have been rare, detection of antibodies appears to have increased in recent years. In the absence of treatment, seropositive people can remain potential sources of infection by transfusion for decades after immigration from a region of the world with endemic disease. Screening for Chagas disease by donor history is not adequately sensitive or specific to identify infected donors. In December 2006, the FDA approved the first test to screen for antibodies to *T cruzi* (**www. fda.gov/NewsEvents/Newsroom/PressAnnouncements/2006/ucm108802. htm**); a second manufacturer's test was approved in 2010 (**www.fda.gov/NewsEvents/ Newsroom/PressAnnouncements/2010/ucm210429.htm**). The American Red Cross and Blood Systems Inc began screening all blood donations for *T cruzi* in January 2008, and currently most of the US blood supply is screened. In the first 16 months of screening, more than 14 million donations were tested, yielding a seroprevalence of 1:27 500; the highest seroprevalence rates were in Florida (1:3800) and California (1:8300). In December 2010, the FDA issued guidance for appropriate use of screening tests (**www. fda.gov/biologicsbloodvaccines/guidancecomplianceregulatoryinformation/ guidances/blood/ucm235855.htm**). In its guidance, the FDA recommended one-time testing of donors. Donors who have negative (nonreactive) test results can donate again, and those subsequent donations will not be tested for antibodies to *T cruzi*.

BABESIOSIS (P 253). Babesiosis is the most commonly reported transfusion-associated tickborne infection in the United States. More than 150 transfusion-associated cases have been documented, with most attributed to *Babesia microti*, but *Babesia duncani* (formerly the WA1-type *Babesia* parasite) also has been implicated. *Babesia* organisms are intracellular parasites that infect red blood cells. However, at least 4 cases have been associated with the receipt of whole-blood-derived platelets, which often contain a small number of red blood cells. Although most infections are asymptomatic, *Babesia* infection can cause severe, life-threatening disease, particularly in elderly people or people with asplenia. Severe infection can be associated with marked hemolysis, disseminated intravascular coagulation, and multiorgan system failure. Serosurveys using indirect immunofluorescent antibody assays in areas of Connecticut and New York have revealed seropositivity rates for *B microti* of approximately 1% and 4%, respectively. In a study of blood donors in Connecticut, 19 (56%) of 34 seropositive donors had positive polymerase chain reaction assay results.

No licensed test is available to screen donors for evidence of *Babesia* infection. Donors with a history of babesiosis are indefinitely deferred from donating blood. Although people with acute illness or fever are not suitable to donate blood, people infected with *Babesia* species commonly are asymptomatic or experience only mild and nonspecific symptoms. In addition, *Babesia* species can cause asymptomatic infection for months and even years in untreated, otherwise healthy people. Questioning donors about recent tick bites has been shown to be ineffective, in part because donors who are seropositive for antibody to tickborne agents are no more likely than seronegative donors to recall tick bites. In 2009, the Transfusion Transmitted Diseases Committee of the AABB identified *Babesia* species as an emerging pathogens posing a major potential risk of transmission by transfusion, and investigations on donor testing in areas with endemic infection are ongoing. In 2010, the FDA Blood Products Advisory Committee supported the concept of regional donor testing for *Babesia* species.

TRANSMISSIBLE SPONGIFORM ENCEPHALOPATHIES: PRION DISEASE CAUSING CREUTZFELDT-JAKOB AND VARIANT CREUTZFELDT-JAKOB DISEASE

Creutzfeldt-Jakob disease (CJD) and variant CJD (vCJD) are fatal neurologic illnesses caused by unique infectious agents known as prions (see Prion Diseases: Transmissible Spongiform Encephalopathies, p 653).

SPORADIC CJD. The risk of transmitting most forms of CJD through blood has been considered theoretical. No cases of CJD resulting from receipt of blood transfusion from donors who later developed sporadic, familial, or iatrogenic forms of CJD have been documented, and case-control studies have not found an association between receipt of blood and development of CJD.

Nevertheless, because blood of animals with a number of naturally acquired and experimental transmissible spongiform encephalopathies (TSEs) may be infective, concerns have remained about the theoretical risk of transmitting CJD by blood transfusion. Since 1987, the FDA has recommended that certain people at increased risk of having CJD be deferred as blood donors. Concern increased after 4 reports of transfusion-transmitted vCJD (see below) infection and 1 infection attributed to injections of plasma-derived coagulation factor VIII. People with signs of sporadic CJD or who are at increased risk of iatrogenic or inherited forms of CJD (eg, receipt of pituitary-derived growth hormone or dura mater transplant or family history of CJD, unless TSE-associated mutation is ruled out) should be deferred as donors. In addition, if post-donation information reveals that a donor should have been rejected because of increased CJD risk, in-date Whole Blood and components, including unpooled Plasma remaining from previous donations, should be retrieved and discarded; if those units already have been distributed, a biological product deviation report should be submitted to the FDA by the blood establishment. However, since 1998, withdrawal of plasma derivatives no longer has been recommended in such a situation, because epidemiologic and laboratory data suggest that most plasma derivatives are much less likely to transmit TSE agents than are blood components because Plasma undergoes extensive processing during fraction-ation. The FDA continues to recommend retrieval of derivatives from any plasma pool to which a person subsequently diagnosed with vCJD donated—something that has not occurred in the United States—and case-by-case decisions, in consultation with the CDC, when a person younger than 55 years with a diagnosis of any other form of CJD is subse-quently reported to have donated to a plasma pool.

VARIANT CJD. In 1996, cases of a new clinically and histopathologically distinct variant form of CJD (vCJD) were reported in the United Kingdom. Evidence indicates that the agent responsible for the outbreak of prion disease in cows, bovine spongiform encepha-lopathy (BSE), is the same agent responsible for the outbreak of vCJD in humans. BSE in cattle first was recognized in the United Kingdom in 1986 and later in 24 other countries.

Transmission of vCJD infections to 4 elderly people in the United Kingdom has been attributed presumptively to transfusions received years earlier with nonleukoreduced Red Blood Cells from healthy donors who became ill with vCJD 16 months to 3.5 years after the donations. Three of the recipients had typical vCJD, and a fourth had evidence of preclinical or subclinical infection. The asymptomatic incubation periods in the clinically ill recipients lasted from 6.3 to 8.5 years; the patient with evidence of preclinical infection died of an unrelated illness approximately 5 years after receiving the implicated trans-fusion. Recipients of blood components from other donors later diagnosed with vCJD remain under surveillance in the United Kingdom and France. The magnitude of the risk of acquiring vCJD from transfusion is uncertain. To date, no case of vCJD presump-tively has been attributed to treatment with a plasma derivative. However, one 73-year-old United Kingdom resident with hemophilia who died without neurologic symptoms had evidence of a vCJD infection in his spleen at autopsy; his infection was attributed to receipt of plasma products from the United Kingdom.

In the United States, the following categories of potential blood and plasma donors are permanently deferred: people who received a blood or blood component transfusion in the United Kingdom or in France after January 1, 1980, when the BSE epidemic is believed to have begun; people who have lived in the United Kingdom for any combined period of 3 months or more from the beginning of 1980 until the end of 1996 (after which rigorous food-protection measures were implemented fully throughout the United Kingdom); people who spent a total of 5 years or more in other European countries (excluding countries of the former Soviet Union) from 1980 to the present; people who have received a bovine insulin injection, unless it is confirmed that the insulin was not manufactured from cattle in the United Kingdom; and military personnel, civilian employees, and dependents who resided or worked on US military bases from 1980 through the end of 1990 in northern Europe or through the end of 1996 in southern Europe (as defined by the US Department of Defense). Policies regarding CJD donor deferral may change, and blood and Plasma programs are expected to remain informed about such changes, which are announced promptly by trade organizations and the FDA. In 2009, the Transfusion Transmitted Diseases Committee of the AABB identified the vCJD agent as emerging pathogen posing a major potential risk of transmission by transfusion.

Improving Blood Safety

A number of strategies have been proposed or implemented to further decrease the risk of transmission of infectious agents through blood and blood products. Various safety strategies are as follows.

ELIMINATION OF INFECTIOUS AGENTS

AGENT INACTIVATION. Virtually all plasma derivatives, including Immune Globulin Intravenous (IGIV) and clotting factors, are treated to eliminate infectious agents that may be present despite screening measures. Methods used include wet and dry heat and treatment with a solvent/detergent. Solvent/detergent-treated pooled Plasma for transfusion no longer is marketed in the United States, but methods of treating single-donor Plasma are under study. Solvent/detergent treatment dissolves the lipid envelope of HIV, HBV, and HCV but is not effective against non–lipid-enveloped viruses, such as HAV and parvovirus B19. Transmission of HIV through administration of IGIV has not been documented.

Because of the fragility of Red Blood Cells and Platelets, pathogen inactivation is more difficult. However, several methods have been developed, such as addition of psoralens followed by exposure to ultraviolet A, which binds nucleic acids and blocks replication of bacteria and viruses. This intercept system has been shown to be effective in reducing bacterial contamination while offering protection from a wide variety of viruses, protozoa, and leukocytes. Clinical trials of these treated components are underway.

AGENT REMOVAL. Leukoreduction, in which filters are used to remove donor white blood cells, is performed increasingly in the United States. Benefits of this process include decreasing febrile transfusion reactions, decreasing HLA alloimmunization, and reducing CMV transmission. There are also other less well-described benefits, such as decreasing the immune modulation associated with transfusion. Leukoreduction also decreases cell-associated agents (eg, intracellular viruses, such as CMV, Epstein-Barr virus, HHV-8, and HTLV). Several countries have adopted the practice of universally leukoreducing all cellular products.

DECREASING EXPOSURE TO BLOOD PRODUCTS

Current screening policies have decreased the risk of transfusion-associated infections dramatically, but blood products remain a source of known and potentially unknown infectious agents.

ALTERNATIVES TO HUMAN BLOOD PRODUCTS. Many alternatives to human blood products have been developed. Established alternatives include recombinant clotting factors for patients with hemophilia, and factors such as erythropoietin used to stimulate red blood cell production. Physicians should use the lowest erythropoiesis-stimulating agent dose that will increase the hemoglobin level gradually to a concentration not exceeding 12 g/dL. Increased risks of death and serious cardiovascular and thrombotic events have been described when erythropoiesis-stimulating agents were administered to achieve a target hemoglobin concentration greater than 12 g/dL in people with chronic kidney failure or surgical candidates. Adverse safety outcomes and a shortened time to tumor progression have been observed in certain cancer patients who have chemotherapy-related anemia, such as patients with advanced head and neck cancer receiving radiation therapy and patients with metastatic breast cancer.

Other agents currently in early clinical trials include hemoglobin-based oxygen carriers; red blood cell substitutes, such as human hemoglobin extracted from red blood cells; recombinant human hemoglobin; animal hemoglobin; and various oxygen-carrying chemicals.

AUTOLOGOUS TRANSFUSION. Another means of decreasing recipient exposure is autologous transfusion. Blood may be donated by the patient several weeks before a surgical procedure (preoperative autologous donation) or, alternatively, donated immediately before surgery and replaced with a volume expander (acute normovolemic hemodilution).

In either case, the patient's blood then can be reinfused if needed. Autologous blood is not completely risk free, because bacterial contamination may occur.

Blood-recycling techniques, such as intraoperative blood recovery, also are included in this category. During surgery, patient blood lost may be collected, processed, and reinfused into the patient. When performing this type of intraoperative blood collection, quality-control measurements are required for ensuring the safety of reinfused blood into the recipient.

SURVEILLANCE FOR TRANSFUSION-TRANSMITTED INFECTION

Transfusion-transmitted infection surveillance is crucial and must be coupled with the capacity to rapidly investigate reported cases and to implement measures needed to prevent additional infections. The CDC has developed a Hemovigilance Module in the National Healthcare Safety Network for transfusion-related adverse events of both infectious and noninfectious causes and quality-control incidents (eg, errors and accidents). The National Healthcare Safety Network is a secure Internet-based surveillance system that collects data from voluntary participating health care facilities in the United States. The CDC also has had a blood safety monitoring system since 1998, the Universal Data Collection Program, for recipients of processed plasma factors. The program provides annual testing for hepatitis and HIV, and stores blood specimens in a serum bank for use in blood safety investigations. A similar system has been established in several centers in the United States that treat patients with thalassemia who depend on frequent blood transfusions. For regulatory purposes, transfusion-related fatalities must be reported to the FDA, and product problems must be reported to the manufacturer (or, alternatively, to the supplier for transmission to the manufacturer). Health care professionals also may report such information directly to the FDA through MedWatch. Reports can be made by telephone (1-800-FDA-1088), fax (1-800-FDA-0178), Internet (**www.fda.gov/medwatch/report/hcp.htm**), or mail (see MedWatch, p 957). Voluntary reporting is considered vital for monitoring product safety. The AABB also has formed a patient safety organization through its US Biovigilance Network program, with the intent to analyze data about adverse reactions including that collected through the National Healthcare Safety Network, for the purposes of improved patient safety and prevention.

ORGAN AND TISSUE TRANSPLANTATION

Each year, more than 25 000 organs and 2 000 000 tissues (eg, musculoskeletal allografts, cornea, and skin) are distributed for transplantations, and numerous cell therapy infusions (eg, bone marrow and peripheral stem cell transplants) occur in the United States. The proliferation of these products also has increased the opportunities for transmission of infectious pathogens, including bacteria, viruses, and parasites. Transmission of Chagas disease, *Strongyloides* species, *Mycobacterium tuberculosis*, lymphocytic choriomeningitis virus, rabies, WNV, HIV, and HCV has been reported through solid organ transplantation. CJD transmission has occurred through corneal transplantation. Infectious disease testing for solid organ transplantation is different than for blood (and bone marrow) donation; many standard tests, such as NAATs for HIV, HCV, or WNV, are not required. Individual organ procurement agencies may elect to perform such testing, but requirements may vary by region.

In 2005, the FDA final rule, Current Good Tissue Practice for Human Cells, Tissues, and Cellular and Tissue-Based Products (HCT/Ps), became effective for transplantations other than solid organs. The purpose of this rule was to improve the safety of HCT/Ps by preventing introduction, transmission, and spread of communicable disease through transplantation of HCT/Ps.[1] The Joint Commission adopted some of these standards, which also apply to accredited organizations that store or use tissue. Solid organs for transplantation are overseen by the Health Resources and Services Administration through the Organ Procurement and Transplant Network, which also compiles donor-derived disease reports. All suspected disease-transmission cases, notifiable diseases, and clusters should be reported to public health agencies. A Transplantation Transmission Sentinel Network has been piloted by the CDC to facilitate recognition of adverse events associated with transplanted allografts (organs, tissues, and eyes), but standard tissue nomenclature and tracking is needed for national implementation. Along with receiving mandatory reports of adverse events from HCT/P establishments that manufacture tissue, the FDA encourages direct voluntary reporting through its MedWatch program using MedWatch Form FDA-3500 (**www.fda.gov/medwatch**). Additional information about the FDA and HCT/Ps is available (**www.fda.gov/cber/tiss.htm**).

HUMAN MILK

Breastfeeding provides numerous health benefits to infants, including protection against morbidity and mortality from infectious diseases of bacterial, viral, and parasitic origin. In addition to providing an optimal source of infant nutrition, human milk contains immune-modulating factors, including secretory antibodies, glycoconjugates, anti-inflammatory components, and antimicrobial compounds such as lysozyme and lactoferrin, which contribute to the formation of a health-promoting microbiota and an optimally functioning immune system. Breastfed infants have high concentrations of protective bifidobacteria and lactobacilli in their gastrointestinal tracts, which diminish the risk of colonization and infection with pathogenic organisms. Protection by human milk is established most clearly for pathogens causing gastrointestinal tract infection. In addition, human milk likely provides protection against otitis media, invasive *Haemophilus influenzae* type b infection, and other causes of upper and lower respiratory tract infections. Human milk also decreases the severity of upper and lower respiratory tract respiratory infections, resulting in more than a 70% reduction in hospitalizations. Evidence also indicates that human milk may modulate the development of the immune system of infants.

The American Academy of Pediatrics (AAP) publishes policy statements and a manual on infant feeding[2] that provide further information about the benefits of breastfeeding, recommended feeding practices, and potential contaminants of human milk. In the *Pediatric Nutrition Handbook*[3] and in the AAP policy statement on human milk,[4] issues

---

[1] Centers for Disease Control and Prevention. Notice to readers: FDA rule for current good tissue practice for human cells, tissues, and cellular and tissue-based products. *MMWR Morb Mortal Wkly Rep.* 2005;54(19):490

[2] American Academy of Pediatrics. *Breastfeeding Handbook for Physicians.* Schanler RJ, Gartner LM, Krebs NF, Dooley S, Mass SB, eds. Elk Grove Village, IL: American Academy of Pediatrics; 2006

[3] American Academy of Pediatrics, Committee on Nutrition. *Pediatric Nutrition Handbook.* Kleinman RE, Greer FR, eds. 7th ed. Elk Grove Village, IL: American Academy of Pediatrics; 2014

[4] American Academy of Pediatrics, Section on Breastfeeding. Breastfeeding and the use of human milk. *Pediatrics.* 2012;129(3):e827-e841

regarding immunization of lactating mothers and breastfeeding infants, transmission of infectious agents via human milk, and potential effects on breastfed infants of antimicrobial agents administered to lactating mothers are addressed.

Immunization of Mothers and Infants

EFFECT OF MATERNAL IMMUNIZATION

Women who have not received recommended immunizations before or during pregnancy may be immunized during the postpartum period, regardless of lactation status. Women known to be pregnant or attempting to become pregnant should not receive MMR. No evidence exists to validate any concern about the presence of live vaccine viruses in maternal milk if the mother is immunized during lactation. Lactating women may be immunized as recommended for adults and adolescents (**www.cdc.gov/vaccines** [see adult immunization schedule]). If previously unimmunized or if traveling to an area with endemic poliovirus circulation, a lactating mother may be given inactivated poliovirus vaccine (IPV). Attenuated rubella virus can be detected in human milk and transmitted to breastfed infants, with subsequent seroconversion and subclinical infection in the infant. Rubella-seronegative mothers who could not be immunized during pregnancy should be immunized with measles-mumps-rubella (MMR) vaccine during the early postpartum period. In lactating women who receive live-attenuated varicella vaccine, neither varicella DNA in human milk (by polymerase chain reaction assay) nor varicella antibody in the infant can be detected. Women should receive a dose of tetanus toxoid, reduced diphtheria toxoid, and acellular pertussis (Tdap) vaccine during each pregnancy,[1] preferably between 27 and 36 weeks' gestation. If not administered during pregnancy, Tdap should be administered immediately postpartum.[2,3] If not already vaccinated, pregnant women should receive their annual inactivated influenza vaccine for the current influenza season during pregnancy. Nonimmunized breastfeeding women should receive a seasonal influenza vaccine for the current season as soon as the vaccine is available; either inactivated or live-attenuated influenza vaccine may be administered during the postpartum period.[4,5] Breastfeeding is not a contraindication to administration of live-attenuated influenza vaccine. Pregnancy and breastfeeding are precautions to yellow fever vaccine

---

[1] Centers for Disease Control and Prevention. Updated recommendations for use of tetanus toxoid, reduced diphtheria toxoid, and acellular pertussis vaccine (Tdap) in pregnant women-Advisory Committee on Immunization Practices (ACIP), 2012. *MMWR Morb Mortal Wkly Rep.* 2013;62(7):131-135

[2] American Academy of Pediatrics, Committee on Infectious Diseases. Additional recommendations for use of tetanus toxoid, reduced-content diphtheria toxoid, and acellular pertussis (Tdap) vaccine. *Pediatrics.* 2011;128(4):809-812

[3] Centers for Disease Control and Prevention. Updated recommendations for use of tetanus toxoid, reduced diphtheria toxoid and acellular pertussis vaccine (Tdap) in pregnant women and persons who have or anticipate having close contact with an infant aged <12 months-Advisory Committee on Immunization Practices (ACIP), 2011. *MMWR Morb Mortal Wkly Rep.* 2011;60(41):1424-1426

[4] Centers for Disease Control and Prevention. Prevention and control of influenza with vaccines. Recommendations of the Advisory Committee on Immunization Practices (ACIP), 2011. *MMWR Morb Mortal Wkly Rep.* 2011;60(33):1128-1132. For annual updates, see **www.cdc.gov/vaccines**

[5] American Academy of Pediatrics, Committee on Infectious Diseases. Recommendations for prevention and control of influenza, 2014-2015. *Pediatrics.* 2014;134(5):e1503-e1519. For updates, see **www.aapredbook. aappublications.org/flu/**

administration, because rare cases of in utero or breastfeeding transmission of the vaccine virus have been documented.[1]

EFFICACY OF IMMUNIZATION IN BREASTFED INFANTS

Infants should be immunized according to the recommended childhood and adolescent immunization schedule, regardless of the mode of infant feeding. The immunogenicity of some recommended vaccines is enhanced by breastfeeding, but data are limited as to whether the efficacy of these vaccines also is enhanced. Theoretically, high concentrations of poliovirus antibody in human milk could interfere with the immunogenicity of oral poliovirus vaccine; this is not a concern with IPV, which is the only poliovirus vaccine used in the United States. There is in vitro evidence that human milk from women who live in areas with endemic rotavirus contains antibodies that can neutralize live rotavirus vaccine virus. However, in licensing trials, the effectiveness of rotavirus vaccine in breastfed infants was comparable to that in nonbreastfed infants. Furthermore, breastfeeding reduced the likelihood of rotavirus disease in infancy.

Transmission of Infectious Agents via Human Milk

BACTERIA

Maternal colonization of skin or mucous membrane sites with pathogens such as group B *Streptococcus* and *Staphylococcus aureus* potentially could result in transmission to an infant during breastfeeding, although this scenario rarely results in illness in the infant. Postpartum mastitis occurs in one third of breastfeeding women in the United States and leads to breast abscesses in up to 10% of cases. Both mastitis and breast abscesses have been associated with the presence of bacterial pathogens in human milk. Breast abscesses have the potential to rupture into the ductal system, releasing large numbers of organisms into milk. Although an increase in mastitis attributable to community-associated methicillin-resistant *S aureus* (MRSA) has been noted, cases of infant infection with MRSA were not increased in a single-center cohort study from 1998–2005. Risk factors for postpartum breast abscess attributable to *S aureus* do not seem to have changed with the increased prevalence of community-associated MRSA. In cases of breast abscess or cellulitis, temporary discontinuation of breastfeeding on the affected breast for 24 to 48 hours after surgical drainage and appropriate antimicrobial therapy may be necessary. In general, infectious mastitis resolves with continued lactation during appropriate antimicrobial therapy and does not pose a significant risk for the healthy term infant. Breastfeeding on the affected side in cases of mastitis generally is recommended; however, even when breastfeeding is interrupted on the affected breast, breastfeeding may continue on the unaffected breast.

Women with tuberculosis who have been treated appropriately for 2 or more weeks and who are not considered contagious (negative sputum) may breastfeed. Women with tuberculosis disease suspected of being contagious should refrain from breastfeeding and from other close contact with the infant because of potential spread of *Mycobacterium tuberculosis* through respiratory tract droplets or airborne transmission (see Tuberculosis, p 804). *M tuberculosis* rarely causes mastitis or a breast abscess, but if a breast abscess caused

---

[1]Centers for Disease Control and Prevention. Yellow fever vaccine. Recommendations of the Advisory Committee on Immunization Practices (ACIP). *MMWR Recomm Rep.* 2010;59(RR-7):1-27

by *M tuberculosis* is present, breastfeeding should be discontinued until the mother has received treatment and no longer is considered to be contagious.

Expressed human milk can become contaminated with a variety of bacterial pathogens, including *Staphylococcus* species and gram-negative bacilli. Outbreaks of gram-negative bacterial infections in neonatal intensive care units occasionally have been attributed to contaminated human milk specimens that have been collected or stored improperly. Expressed human milk may be a reservoir for multiresistant *S aureus* and other pathogens. Powdered human milk fortifiers and powdered infant formula receipt has been associated with invasive bacteremia and meningitis attributable to *Cronobacter* species (formerly *Enterobacter sakazakii*), resulting in death in approximately 40% of cases. Routine culturing or heat treatment of a mother's milk fed to her infant has not been demonstrated to be necessary or cost-effective (see Human Milk Banks, p 131). Because of the immune-protective factors in human milk, there is a hierarchical preference for the mother's freshly expressed milk, followed by the mother's previously refrigerated or frozen milk, followed by pasteurized donor milk as the third best option for feeding of sick and/or preterm infants.

VIRUSES

CYTOMEGALOVIRUS. Cytomegalovirus (CMV) may be shed intermittently in human milk. Although CMV has been found in human milk of women who delivered preterm infants, case reviews of preterm babies acquiring CMV postnatally have not demonstrated long-term clinical sequelae over several years of follow-up after infants were discharge from the neonatal intensive care unit (NICU). Very low birth weight preterm infants, however, are at greater potential risk of developing symptomatic disease shortly after acquiring CMV, including through human milk. Decisions about breastfeeding of preterm infants by mothers known to be CMV seropositive should include consideration of the potential benefits of human milk and the risk of CMV transmission. Mothers who deliver infants at <32 weeks' gestation can be screened for CMV. Holder pasteurization (62.5°C [144.5°F] for 30 minutes) and short-term pasteurization (72°C [161.6°F] for 5 seconds) of human milk seems to inactivate CMV; short-term pasteurization may be less harmful to the beneficial constituents of human milk. Freezing milk at −20°C (−4°F) for 24 to 72 hours will decrease viral titers but does not inactivate CMV reliably.

HEPATITIS B VIRUS. Hepatitis B surface antigen (HBsAg) has been detected in milk from HBsAg-positive women. However, studies from Taiwan and England have indicated that breastfeeding by HBsAg-positive women does not increase significantly the risk of infection among their infants. In the United States, infants born to known HBsAg-positive women should receive the initial dose of hepatitis B vaccine within 12 hours of birth, and Hepatitis B Immune Globulin should be administered concurrently but at a different anatomic site. This effectively will eliminate any theoretical risk of transmission through breastfeeding (see Hepatitis B, p 400). There is no need to delay initiation of breastfeeding until after the infant is immunized.

HEPATITIS C VIRUS. Hepatitis C virus (HCV) RNA and antibody to HCV have been detected in milk from mothers infected with HCV. Transmission of HCV via breastfeeding has not been documented in mothers who have positive test results for anti-HCV but negative test results for human immunodeficiency virus (HIV) antibody. Mothers infected with HCV should be counseled that transmission of HCV by breastfeeding theoretically is possible but has not been documented. Mothers infected with HCV should consider abstaining from breastfeeding from a breast with cracked or bleeding nipples. According to current guidelines of the US Public Health Service, maternal HCV infection is not a contraindication to breastfeeding. The decision to breastfeed should be based on an informed discussion between a mother and her health care professional.

HUMAN IMMUNODEFICIENCY VIRUS. HIV has been isolated from human milk and can be transmitted through breastfeeding. The risk of transmission is higher for women who acquire HIV infection during lactation (ie, postpartum) than for women with preexisting infection. In populations such as those in the United States, in which the risk of infant mortality from infectious diseases and malnutrition is low and in which safe and effective alternative sources of feeding are available readily, HIV-infected women, including women receiving antiretroviral therapy, should be counseled not to breastfeed their infants or donate their milk. Randomized clinical trials have demonstrated that infant prophylaxis with daily nevirapine or nevirapine/zidovudine during breastfeeding significantly decreases the risk of postnatal transmission via human milk. Observational data suggest that maternal antiretroviral therapy (ART) during breastfeeding may decrease postnatal infection. However, neither maternal nor infant postpartum antiretroviral therapy is sufficient to eliminate the risk of HIV transmission through breastfeeeding.[1] Available data indicate that various antiretroviral drugs have differential penetration into human milk, with some antiretroviral drugs having concentrations in human milk that are much higher than concentrations in maternal plasma, and other drugs having concentrations in human milk that are much lower than concentrations in plasma or are undetectable. This raises potential concerns regarding infant toxicity, as well as the potential for selection of antiretroviral-resistant virus within human milk.

All pregnant women in the United States should be screened for HIV infection to allow implementation of effective interventions to prevent mother-to-child HIV transmission (eg, antiretroviral prophylaxis and elective cesarean delivery). Women found to have HIV infection should receive appropriate counseling regarding breastfeeding.[2] HIV screening should occur as part of a panel of prenatal testing unless evaluation is declined (see Human Immunodeficiency Virus Infection, p 453).

In areas where infectious diseases and malnutrition are important causes of infant mortality and where safe, affordable, and sustainable replacement feeding may not be available, infant feeding decisions are more complex. In resource-poor locations, women for whom HIV status is unknown are encouraged to continue breastfeeding, because the morbidity associated with formula feeding is unacceptably high. For HIV-infected mothers, studies in Africa revealed that exclusive breastfeeding for the first 3 to 6 months after birth appeared to lower the risk of HIV transmission through human milk compared with infants who received mixed feedings (breastfeeding and other foods or milks). Exclusive breastfeeding by HIV-infected women does not eliminate postnatal transmission, and HIV transmission among exclusively breastfed infants by HIV infected mothers is higher than in HIV-exposed infants who receive only replacement feeding from birth. Current World Health Organization, UNICEF, and UNAIDS infant feeding guidelines state that if replacement

---

[1] Perinatal HIV Guidelines Working Group. Public Health Service Task Force Recommendations for use of Antiretroviral Drugs in Pregnant HIV-Infected Women for Maternal Health and Interventions to Reduce Perinatal HIV Transmission in the United States. September 14, 2011:1-207. Available at: **http://aidsinfo. nih.gov/ContentFiles/PerinatalGL.pdf**

[2] Centers for Disease Control and Prevention. Revised recommendations for HIV testing of adults, adolescents, and pregnant women in health-care settings. *MMWR Recomm Rep.* 2006;55(RR-14):1-17

(formula) feeding is affordable, feasible, acceptable, sustainable, and safe, replacement of human milk from HIV-infected women with nutritional substitutes is recommended to decrease the risk of HIV transmission. If these criteria are not met, HIV-infected women are recommended to breastfeed exclusively for the first 6 months of life, with weaning after that time when replacement feeding meets the affordable, feasible, acceptable, sustainable, and safe criteria. Thus, in resource-poor countries, the most appropriate feeding option for an HIV-infected mother needs to be based on her individual circumstances and should consider the benefits of breastfeeding against the risk of breastfeeding associated transmission of HIV (see Human Immunodeficiency Virus Infection, p 453).

HUMAN T-LYMPHOTROPIC VIRUS TYPE 1. Human T-lymphotropic virus type 1 (HTLV-1), which is endemic in Japan, the Caribbean, and parts of South America, is associated with development of malignant neoplasms and neurologic disorders among adults. Epidemiologic and laboratory studies suggest that mother-to-infant transmission of human HTLV-1 occurs primarily through breastfeeding, although freezing/thawing of expressed human milk may decrease infectivity of human milk. Women in the United States who are HTLV-1 seropositive should be advised not to breastfeed and not to donate to human milk banks.

HUMAN T-LYMPHOTROPIC VIRUS TYPE 2. HTLV-2 is a retrovirus that has been detected among American and European injection drug users and some American Indian/Alaska Native groups. Although apparent maternal-infant transmission has been reported, the rate and timing of transmission have not been established. Until additional data about possible transmission through breastfeeding become available, women in the United States who are HTLV-2 seropositive should be advised not to breastfeed and not to donate to human milk banks. Routine screening for both HTLV-1 or HTLV-2 during pregnancy is not recommended.

HERPES SIMPLEX VIRUS TYPE 1. Women with herpetic lesions may transmit herpes simplex virus (HSV) to their infants by direct contact with the lesions. Transmission may be reduced with hand hygiene and covering of lesions with which the infant might come into contact. Women with herpetic lesions on a breast or nipple should refrain from breastfeeding an infant from the affected breast until lesions have resolved but may breastfeed from the unaffected breast when lesions on the affected breast are covered completely to avoid transmission.

RUBELLA. Wild and vaccine strains of rubella virus have been isolated from human milk. However, the presence of rubella virus in human milk has not been associated with significant disease in infants, and transmission is more likely to occur via other routes. Women with rubella or women who have been immunized recently with a live-attenuated rubella virus-containing vaccine may continue to breastfeed.

VARICELLA. Secretion of attenuated varicella vaccine virus in human milk resulting in infection of an infant of a mother who received varicella vaccine has not been noted in the few instances where it has been studied. Varicella vaccine may be considered for a susceptible breastfeeding mother if the risk of exposure to natural varicella-zoster virus is high. Recommendations for use of passive immunization and varicella vaccine for breastfeeding mothers who have had contact with people in whom varicella has developed, or for contacts of a breastfeeding mother in whom varicella has developed, are available (see Varicella-Zoster Infections, p 846).

WEST NILE VIRUS. West Nile virus RNA has been detected in human milk collected from a woman with disease attributable to West Nile virus; her breastfed infant developed West Nile virus immunoglobulin M antibodies but remained asymptomatic. Animal experiments have shown that West Nile virus can be transmitted in animal milk, and other related flaviviruses can be transmitted to humans via unpasteurized milk from ruminants. The degree to which West Nile virus is transmitted in human milk and the extent to which breastfeeding infants become infected are unknown. Because the health benefits of breastfeeding have been established and the risk of West Nile virus transmission through breastfeeding is unknown, women who reside in an area with endemic West Nile virus infection should continue to breastfeed.

HUMAN MILK BANKS

Some circumstances, such as preterm delivery, may preclude breastfeeding, but infants in these circumstances still may be fed human milk collected from their own mothers or from individual donors. The potential for transmission of infectious agents through donor human milk requires appropriate selection and screening of donors, and careful collection, processing, and storage of human milk. Currently, US donor milk banks that belong to the Human Milk Banking Association of North America (**www.hmbana.org/**) voluntarily follow guidelines drafted in consultation with the US Food and Drug Administration and the Centers for Disease Control and Prevention. Other pasteurization methods are also acceptable, but use of nonpasteurized donor milk should be avoided. These guidelines include screening of all donors for HBsAg and antibodies to HIV-1, HIV-2, HTLV-1, HTLV-2, hepatitis C virus, and syphilis. Donor milk is dispensed only by prescription after it is heat treated at 62.5°C (144.5°F) for 30 minutes and prepasteurization bacterial cultures reveal no growth of pathogenic organisms (*S aureus*, group B *Streptococcus*, and lactose-fermenting coliforms) and no more than 100 000 colony-forming units/mL of normal skin bacteria, and no viable bacteria are present after pasteurization.

INADVERTENT HUMAN MILK EXPOSURE

Policies to deal with occasions when an infant inadvertently is fed expressed human milk not obtained from his or her mother have been developed. These policies require documentation, counseling, and observation of the affected infant for signs of infection and potential testing of the source mother for infections that could be transmitted via human milk. Recommendations for management of a situation involving an accidental exposure may be found on the CDC Web site (**www.cdc.gov/breastfeeding/recommendations/other_mothers_milk.htm**). A summary of the recommendations includes the following:
1. Inform the donor mother about the inadvertent exposure, and ask:
   - Whether she has had a recent HIV test and, if so, would she agree to have the results shared anonymously with the parent(s) of the infant given her milk?
   - If the donor mother does not know her HIV status, would she be willing to be tested and have the results shared anonymously with parent(s) of the recipient infant?
2. Discuss inadvertent administration of the donor milk with the parent(s) of the recipient infant.
   - Inform the parent(s) of the recipient infant that the risk of transmission of HIV infection via this exposure is low. Explain that factors present in human milk act, together with time and cold temperatures, to destroy HIV if present in expressed human milk. Also explain that transmission of HIV from single human milk exposure has never been documented.
   - Recommend that a baseline HIV antibody test be performed from blood of the recipient infant.

Collection of milk from the birth mother of a preterm infant does not require processing if fed to her infant, but proper collection and storage procedures should be followed. Heat treatment at 56°C or greater (133°F or greater) for 30 minutes reliably eliminates bacteria, inactivates HIV, and decreases titers of other viruses but may not eliminate CMV completely. Holder pasteurization (62.5°C [144.5°F] for 30 minutes) reliably inactivates HIV and CMV and eliminates or decreases significantly titers of most other viruses. Short-term pasteurization (72°C [161.6°F] for 5 seconds) also appears to inactivate CMV.

Freezing at −20°C (−4°F) eliminates HTLV-1 and decreases the concentration of CMV but does not destroy most other viruses or bacteria. Microbiologic quality standards for fresh, unpasteurized, expressed milk are not available. If the clinical situation warrants culture, the presence of gram-negative bacteria, *S aureus*, or alpha- or beta-hemolytic streptococci may preclude use of expressed human milk. Routine culture of milk that a birth mother provides to her own infant is not warranted.

Antimicrobial Agents in Human Milk

Antimicrobial agents often are prescribed for lactating women. Although these drugs may be detected in milk, the potential risk to an infant must be weighed against the known benefits of continued breastfeeding. As a general guideline, an antimicrobial agent is safe to administer to a lactating woman if the drug is safe to administer to an infant. Only in rare cases will interruption of breastfeeding be necessary because of maternal antimicrobial use.

The amount of drug an infant receives from a lactating mother depends on a number of factors, including maternal dose, frequency and duration of administration, absorption, timing of medication administration and breastfeeding, and distribution characteristics of the drug. When a lactating woman receives appropriate doses of an antimicrobial agent, the concentration of the compound in her milk usually is less than the equivalent of a therapeutic dose for the infant. A breastfed infant who requires antimicrobial therapy should receive the recommended doses, independent of administration of the agent to the mother.

Current information about drugs and lactation can be found at the Toxicology Data Network Web site (**www.toxnet.nlm.nih.gov/help/LactMedRecordFormat.htm**). Data for drugs, including antimicrobial agents, administered to lactating women are provided in several categories, including maternal and infant drug levels, effects in breastfed infants, possible effects on lactation, the category into which the drug has been placed by the American Academy of Pediatrics, alternative drugs to consider, and references.

....
CHILDREN IN OUT-OF-HOME CHILD CARE[1]

Infants and young children who are cared for in group settings have an increased rate of communicable infectious diseases, including infections from antimicrobial-resistant organisms. Prevention and control of infection in out-of-home child care settings is influenced by several factors, including: (1) care providers' health status, personal hygiene practices, and immunization status; (2) environmental sanitation; (3) food-handling procedures; (4) age and immunization status of children; (5) ratio of children to care providers; (6) physical space and quality of facilities; (7) frequency of use of antimicrobial agents for

---

[1]American Academy of Pediatrics. Managing *Infectious Diseases in Child Care and Schools: A Quick Reference Guide.* Aronson SS, Shope TR, eds. 3rd ed. Elk Grove Village, IL: American Academy of Pediatrics; 2013

children in child care; and (8) adherence to Standard Precautions for infection prevention and control. Collaborative efforts of public health officials, licensing agencies, child care providers, child care health consultants, physicians, nurses, parents, employers, and other members of the community are necessary to address problems of infection prevention in child care settings.

Child care programs should require that all enrollees and staff members receive age-appropriate immunizations as recommended by the American Academy of Pediatrics (AAP) and the Advisory Committee on Immunization Practices (ACIP) of the Centers for Disease Control and Prevention (CDC). The child enrollees should receive routine health care according to AAP *Bright Futures* guidelines, because these programs have the opportunity to provide parents with ongoing instruction in hygiene practices that address predictable issues related to child development and management of minor illnesses. Other resources that can assist providers and parents with these issues include the Healthy Child Care America Web site (**www.healthychildcare.org/contacts. html**). People involved with early education and child care can use the published national standards[1] related to these topics to provide specific education and implementation measures.

Classification of Care Service

Child care services commonly are classified by the type of setting, number of children in care, and age and health status of the children. **Small family child care homes** provide care and education for up to 6 children simultaneously, including any preschool-aged relatives of the care provider, in a setting that usually is the home of the care provider. **Large family child care homes** provide care and education for between 7 and 12 children at a time, including any preschool-aged relatives of the care provider, in a setting that usually is the home of one of the care providers. A **child care center** is a facility that provides care and education to any number of children in a nonresidential setting, or to 13 or more children in any setting if the facility is open on a regular basis. A **facility for ill children** provides care for 1 or more children who are excluded temporarily from their regular child care setting for health reasons. A facility for children with special needs provides specialized care and education for 1 child or more who cannot be accommodated in a setting with normally developing children. All 50 states regulate out-of-home child care; however, efforts to enforce regulations are usually directed toward center-based child care; few states or municipalities license or enforce regulations as carefully for small or large child care homes. Regulatory requirements for every state can be accessed through the Web site of the National Resource Center for Health and Safety in Child Care and Early Education (**www.nrckids.org**).

Grouping of children by age varies, but in child care centers, common groups consist of **infants** (birth through 12 months of age), **toddlers** (13 through 35 months of age), **preschoolers** (36 through 59 months of age), and **school-aged children** (5 through 12 years of age). Age grouping reflects developmental status. Infants and toddlers who require diapering or assistance in using a toilet have significant hands-on contact with

[1]American Academy of Pediatrics, American Public Health Association, National Resource Center for Health and Safety in Child Care and Early Education. *Caring for Our Children: National Health and Safety Performance Standards: Guidelines for Out-of-Home Child Care.* 3rd ed. Elk Grove Village, IL: American Academy of Pediatrics; and Washington, DC: American Public Health Association; 2011

care providers. Furthermore, they have oral contact with the environment, have poor control over their secretions and excretions, and have limited immunity to common pathogens. Toddlers also have frequent direct contact with each other and with secretions of other toddlers.

Management and Prevention of Illness

Appropriate hand hygiene and adherence to immunization recommendations are the most important factors for decreasing transmission of infectious diseases in child care settings. In most instances, the risk of introducing an infectious agent into a child care group is directly related to prevalence of the agent in the population of children and child care providers and to the number of susceptible children in that group. In addition, transmission of an agent within the group depends on the following: (1) characteristics of the organism, such as mode of spread, infective dose, and survival in the environment; (2) frequency of asymptomatic infection or carrier state; and (3) immunity to the respective pathogen. Transmission also can be affected by the age and immunization status of children enrolled and when child care providers do not meticulously use appropriate hand hygiene, respiratory etiquette, and/or practices to minimize the spread of fecal organisms. Children infected in a child care group can transmit organisms not only within the group but also within their households and the community. Modes of transmission of bacteria, viruses, parasites, and fungi within child care settings are listed in Table 2.5 (p 135).

Options for interrupting transmission of pathogens include: (1) hand hygiene; (2) exclusion of ill or infected children from the facility when appropriate; (3) provision of care for ill children at a separate site; (4) cohorting to provide care (eg, segregation of infected children in a group with separate staff and facilities); (5) limiting new admissions; (6) closing the facility (a rarely exercised option); (7) antimicrobial treatment or prophylaxis, when appropriate; and (8) immunization, when appropriate. Recommendations for controlling spread of specific infectious agents differ according to the epidemiology of the pathogen (see disease-specific chapters in Section 3) and characteristics of the setting.

Infection-prevention and -control procedures in child care programs that decrease acquisition and transmission of communicable diseases include: (1) periodic (at least annual) review of facility-maintained child and employee immunization status and established standards to ensure tetanus toxoid, reduced diphtheria toxoid, and acellular pertussis (Tdap) vaccine and seasonal influenza vaccine provision for staff; (2) hygienic and sanitary procedures for toilet use, toilet training, and diaper changing; (3) review and enforcement of hand-hygiene procedures; (4) environmental sanitation; (5) personal hygiene for children and staff; (6) sanitary preparation and handling of food; (7) communicable disease surveillance and reporting; and (8) appropriate handling of animals in the facility. Policies that include education about and implementation of infection-prevention and -control measures for full- and part-time employees and volunteers, as well as exclusion policies for ill children and staff, aid in control of infectious diseases. Health departments should have plans for responding to reportable and nonreportable outbreaks of communicable diseases in child care programs and should provide training, written information, and technical consultation to child care programs when requested or alerted. Evaluation of the well-being of each child should be performed by a trained staff member each day as the child enters the site and throughout the day as needed. Parents should be required to report their child's immunization status on an ongoing basis and should be encouraged to share information with child care staff about their child's acute

Table 2.5. Modes of Transmission of Organisms in Child Care Settings

Usual Route of Transmission[a]	Bacteria	Viruses	Other[b]
Fecal-oral	*Campylobacter* species; *Clostridium difficile*; Shiga toxin-producing *Escherichia coli*, including *E coli* O157:H7, *Salmonella* species; *Shigella* species	Astrovirus, norovirus, enteric adenovirus, enteroviruses, hepatitis A virus, rotaviruses	*Cryptosporidium* species, *Enterobius vermicularis*, *Giardia intestinalis*
Respiratory	*Bordetella pertussis, Haemophilus influenzae* type b, *Mycobacterium tuberculosis, Neisseria meningitidis, Streptococcus pneumoniae*, group A streptococcus, *Kingella kingae*	Adenovirus, influenza virus, human metapneumovirus, measles virus, mumps virus, parainfluenza virus, parvovirus B19, respiratory syncytial virus, rhinovirus, coronavirus, rubella virus, varicella-zoster virus	...
Person-to-person contact	Group A streptococcus, *Staphylococcus aureus*	Herpes simplex virus, varicella-zoster virus	Agents causing pediculosis, scabies, and ringworm[c]
Contact with blood, urine, and/or saliva	...	Cytomegalovirus, herpes simplex virus, hepatitis C virus	...
Bloodborne	...	Hepatitis B virus, hepatitis C virus, HIV	...

[a]The potential for transmission of microorganisms in the child care setting by food and animals also exists (see Appendix VII, Clinical Syndromes Associated With Foodborne Diseases, p 1008, Appendix VIII, Diseases Transmitted by Animals, p 1014, and Diseases Transmitted by Animals [Zoonoses]: Household Pets, Including Nontraditional Pets, and Exposure to Animals in Public Settings, p 219).

[b]Parasites, fungi, mites, and lice.

[c]Transmission also may occur from contact with objects in the environment.

and chronic illnesses and medication use utilizing a formal care plan that is signed by the child's health care provider.

Recommendations for Inclusion or Exclusion

Mild illness is common among children. Most minor illnesses do not constitute a reason for excluding a child from child care, unless the illness prevents the child from participating in normal activities, as determined by the child care staff, or the illness requires a need for care that is greater than staff can provide. Examples of illnesses and conditions that do not necessitate exclusion include:

• Common cold
• Diarrhea, as long as stools are contained in the diaper (for infants), there are no accidents using the toilet (for older children), and stool frequency is less than 2 stools above normal for that child
• Rash without fever and without behavioral change
• Parvovirus B19 infection in an immunocompetent child
• Cytomegalovirus (CMV) infection
• Chronic hepatitis B virus (HBV) infection (see p 145 for possible exceptions)
• Conjunctivitis without fever and without behavioral change (if 2 or more children in a group care setting develop conjunctivitis in the same time period, advice should be sought from the program's health consultant or public health authority)
• Human immunodeficiency virus (HIV) infection (see p 146 for possible exceptions)
• Colonization with methicillin-resistant *Staphylococcus aureus* (MRSA) (in children who do not have active lesions or illness that would otherwise require exclusion)

Asymptomatic children who excrete an enteropathogen usually do not need to be excluded (exceptions include children in whom Shiga toxin-producing *Escherichia coli* (STEC), *Shigella* species, or *Salmonella* serotype Typhi or Paratyphi is confirmed).

Exclusion of sick children and adults from out-of-home child care settings has been recommended when such exclusion could decrease the likelihood of secondary cases. In many situations, the expertise of the program's health consultant and that of the responsible local and state public health authorities are helpful for determining the benefits and risks of excluding children from their usual care program. Most states have laws about isolation of people with specific communicable diseases. Local or state health departments should be contacted for information about these laws, and public health authorities in these areas should be notified about cases of nationally notifiable infectious diseases and unusual outbreaks of other illnesses involving children or adults in the child care environment (see Appendix IV, Nationally Notifiable Infectious Diseases in the United States, p 992).

General recommendations for exclusion of children in out-of-home care are shown in Table 2.6 (p 136). Disease- or condition-specific recommendations for exclusion from out-of-home care and management of contacts are shown in Table 2.7 (p 137).

During the course of an identified outbreak of a nonreportable or reportable communicable illness in a child care setting (see Nationally Notifiable Infectious Diseases, Appendix IV, p 992), a child determined to be contributing to transmission of organisms causing the illness at the program should be excluded. The child may be readmitted when the risk of transmission no longer is present. For most outbreaks of vaccine-preventable illnesses, unvaccinated children should be excluded until they are vaccinated and the risk of transmission no longer exists.

Table 2.6. General Recommendations for Exclusion of Children in Out-of-Home Child Care

Symptom(s)	Management
Illness preventing participation in activities, as determined by child care staff	Exclusion until illness resolves and able to participate in activities
Illness that requires a need for care that is greater than staff can provide without compromising health and safety of others	Exclusion or placement in care environment where appropriate care can be provided, without compromising care of others
Severe illness suggested by fever with behavior changes, lethargy, irritability, persistent crying, difficulty breathing, progressive rash with above symptoms	Medical evaluation and exclusion until symptoms have resolved
Persistent abdominal pain (2 hours or more) or intermittent abdominal pain associated with fever, dehydration, or other systemic signs and symptoms	Medical evaluation and exclusion until symptoms have resolved
Vomiting 2 or more times in preceding 24 hours	Exclusion until symptoms have resolved, unless vomiting is determined to be caused by a noncommunicable condition and child is able to remain hydrated and participate in activities
Diarrhea if stool not contained in diaper or if fecal accidents occur in a child who is normally continent; if stool frequency exceeds 2 or more stools above normal for that child or stools containing blood or mucus	Medical evaluation for stools with blood or mucus; exclusion until stools are contained in the diaper or when toilet-trained children no longer have accidents using the toilet and when stool frequency becomes less than 2 stools above that child's normal frequency/24 hours.
Oral lesions	Exclusion if unable to contain drool or if unable to participate because of other symptoms or until child or staff member is considered to be noninfectious (lesions smaller or resolved).
Skin lesions	Keep lesions on exposed skin surfaces covered with a waterproof dressing

Infectious Diseases—Epidemiology and Control

(Also see disease-specific chapters in Section 3.)

ENTERIC DISEASES

The close interactive personal contact and typically suboptimal hygiene of young children provide ready opportunities for spread of enteric bacteria, viruses, and parasites in child care settings. Enteropathogens transmitted by the fecal oral route, especially those for which infection requires a low infective dose or for which fomites like toys provide a vector for transmission, tend to be the principal organisms implicated in outbreaks. Such pathogens include noroviruses, enteric adenoviruses, astroviruses, *Shigella* species, *E coli*

Table 2.7. Disease- or Condition-Specific Recommendations for Exclusion of Children in Out-of-Home Child Care

Condition	Management of Case	Management of Contacts
Hepatitis A virus (HAV) infection	Serologic testing to confirm HAV infection in suspected cases. Exclusion until 1 week after onset of illness.	In facilities with diapered children, if 1 or more cases confirmed in child or staff attendees or 2 or more cases in households of staff or attendees, HAV vaccine (HepA) or Immune Globulin (IG) should be administered within 14 days of exposure to all unimmunized staff and attendees. In centers without diapered children, HepA or IG should be given to unimmunized classroom contacts of index case. Asymptomatic IG recipients may return after receipt of IG (see Hepatitis A, p 391).
Impetigo	Exclusion until 24 hours after treatment has been initiated. Lesions on exposed skin should be covered with waterproof dressing when possible.	No intervention unless additional lesions develop.
Measles	Exclusion until 4 days after beginning of rash and when the child is able to participate.	Immunize exposed children without evidence of immunity within 72 hours of exposure. Children who do not receive vaccine within 72 hours or who remain unimmunized after exposure should be excluded until at least 2 weeks after onset of rash in the last case of measles. For use of IG, see Measles (p 535).
Mumps	Exclusion until 5 days after onset of parotid gland swelling.	In outbreak setting, people without documentation of immunity should be immunized or excluded. Immediate readmission may occur following immunization. Unimmunized people should be excluded for 26 or more days following onset of parotitis in last case.
Pediculosis capitis (head lice) infestation	Treatment at end of program day and readmission on completion of first treatment.	Household and close contacts should be examined and treated if infested. No exclusion necessary.

Table 2.7. Disease- or Condition-Specific Recommendations for Exclusion of Children in Out-of-Home Child Care, continued

Condition	Management of Case	Management of Contacts
Pertussis	Exclusion until completion of 5 days of the recommended course of antimicrobial therapy if pertussis is suspected; untreated children and providers should be excluded until 21 days have elapsed from cough onset (see Pertussis, p 608).	Immunization and chemoprophylaxis should be administered as recommended for household contacts. Symptomatic children and staff should be excluded until completion of 5 days of antimicrobial therapy. Untreated adults should be excluded until 21 days after onset of cough (see Pertussis, p 608).
Rubella	Exclusion for 7 days after onset of rash for postnatal infection.	Pregnant contacts should be evaluated (see Rubella, p 688).
Infection with *Salmonella* serotypes Typhi or Paratyphi	Exclusion until diarrhea resolves and 3 consecutive stool cultures obtained at least 48 hours after cessation of antimicrobial therapy are negative.	When *Salmonella* serovar Typhi infection is identified in a child care staff member, local or state health departments may be consulted regarding regulations for length of exclusion and testing, which may vary by jurisdiction.
Infection with nontyphoidal *Salmonella, Salmonella* of unknown serotype, *or Clostridium difficile*	Exclusion until diarrhea resolves. Negative stool culture results **not** required for non-serotype Typhi *Salmonella* species, and repeat testing should not be performed for asymptomatic children previously diagnosed with *C difficile.*	Symptomatic contacts should be excluded until symptoms resolve. Stool cultures are not required for asymptomatic contacts.
Scabies	Exclusion until after treatment given.	Close contacts with prolonged skin-to-skin contact should have prophylactic therapy. Bedding and clothing in contact with skin of infected people should be laundered (see Scabies, p 702).

Table 2.7. Disease- or Condition-Specific Recommendations for Exclusion of Children in Out-of-Home Child Care, continued

Condition	Management of Case	Management of Contacts
Infection with Shiga toxin-producing *Escherichia coli* (STEC), including *E coli* O157:H7	Exclusion until diarrhea resolves and 2 stool cultures (obtained at least 48 hours after any antimicrobial therapy has been discontinued) are negative. Some state health departments have less stringent exclusion policies for children who have recovered from less virulent STEC infection.	Meticulous hand hygiene; stool cultures should be performed for any symptomatic contacts. In outbreak situations involving virulent STEC strains, stool cultures of asymptomatic contacts may aid controlling spread. Center(s) with cases should be closed to new admissions during STEC outbreak (see *Escherichia coli* Diarrhea, p 343).
Shigellosis	Exclusion until 24 or more hours after diarrhea has ceased. State regulations may require one or more stool cultures to be negative for *Shigella* species before returning to care.	Meticulous hand hygiene; stool cultures should be performed for any symptomatic contacts (see *Shigella* Infections, p 706).
Staphylococcus aureus skin infections	Exclusion only if skin lesions are draining and cannot be covered with a watertight dressing.	Meticulous hand hygiene; cultures of contacts are not recommended.
Streptococcal pharyngitis	Exclusion until 24 hours after treatment has been initiated.	Symptomatic contacts of documented cases of group A streptococcal infection should be tested and treated if test results are positive.
Tuberculosis	For active disease, exclusion until determined to be non-infectious by physician or health department authority. May return to activities after therapy is instituted, symptoms have diminished, and adherence to therapy is documented. No exclusion for latent tuberculosis infection (LTBI).	Local health department personnel should be informed for contact investigation (see Tuberculosis, p 804).
Varicella (see Varicella-Zoster Infections, p 846)	Exclusion until all lesions have crusted or, in immunized people without crusts, until no new lesions appear within a 24-hour period.	For people without evidence of immunity, varicella vaccine should be administered within 3 days but up to 5 days after exposure, or when indicated, Varicella-Zoster Immune Globulin (VariZig; see Varicella Zoster Virus, p 846) should be administered up to 10 days after exposure.

O157:H7, *Giardia intestinalis, Cryptosporidium* species, and hepatitis A virus (HAV). Rotavirus vaccination has decreased outbreaks attributable to this virus dramatically. *Salmonella* species, *Clostridium difficile*, and *Campylobacter* species infrequently have been associated with outbreaks of disease in children in child care.

Young children who are not toilet trained increase the frequency of environmental fecal contamination. Enteropathogen spread is common in child care programs and is highest in infant and toddler areas, especially among attendees who are not fully toilet trained. Enteropathogens are spread by the fecal-oral route, either directly by person-to-person transmission or indirectly via fomites, environmental surfaces, and food, resulting in transmission of disease. The risk of food contamination can be increased when staff members who assist with toilet use and diaper-changing activities also prepare or serve food. Several enteropathogens, including rotaviruses, norovirus, HAV, *Giardia intestinalis* cysts, *Cryptosporidium* oocysts, and *C difficile* spores survive on environmental surfaces for periods ranging from hours to weeks.

Because infections with *Salmonella* serotypes Typhi or Paratyphi or organisms that produce Shiga toxin (STEC O157:H7) are transmitted easily and can be severe, exclusion of an infected child is warranted until results of 3 stool samples obtained at least 48 hours after cessation of antimicrobial therapy have negative culture results for *Salmonella* serotypes Typhi or Paratyphi (see *Salmonella* Infections, p 695), and results of 2 stool samples have negative culture results for STEC; some state health departments have less stringent exclusion policies for children who have recovered from less virulent STEC infection (see *Escherichia coli* Diarrhea, p 343). Other *Salmonella* serotypes do not require negative culture results from stool samples, and children can return to child care facilities once the diarrhea has resolved. Although not typically severe, infections caused by *Shigella* species can be transmitted easily. State health authorities may require one or more convalescent stool samples to have negative culture results for *Shigella* before readmission to a child care facility. Child care staff and families of enrolled children need to be fully informed about exclusion and readmittance criteria.

Immunization of children 12 through 23 months of age against HAV reduces the spread of HAV within the community attributable to child care programs. HAV infection differs from most other diseases in child care facilities because symptomatic illness occurs primarily among adult contacts of infected asymptomatic children. To recognize outbreaks of HAV infection and initiate appropriate control measures, health care professionals and child care providers should be aware of this epidemiologic characteristic (see Hepatitis A, p 391). Hepatitis A vaccine is routinely recommended for all children 12 months and older and should be considered for staff of child care centers with ongoing or recurrent outbreaks and in communities where cases in a child care center are a major source of HAV infection. Hepatitis A vaccine is not routinely recommended for people working in a child care setting outside of an outbreak situation, and hepatitis A vaccine is not required for attendance at licensed child care or Head Start programs in several states. A child in whom jaundice develops should be evaluated by a pediatrician and should not have contact with other children or staff until a cause is determined and risk of transmission is eliminated.

Human-animal contact involving family and classroom pets, animal displays, and petting zoos exposes children to pathogens harbored by these animals. Reptiles, amphibians, baby poultry, and rodents (eg, hamsters, mice, rats) are not considered appropriate pets for children younger than 5 years, and these children should not have contact with these animals or their habitats because such animals are commonly colonized with *Salmonella* organisms, lymphocytic choriomeningitis virus, and other viruses that may be transmitted to children via contact (see Diseases Transmitted by Animals [Zoonoses]: Household Pets, Including Nontraditional Pets, and Exposure to Animals in Public Settings, p 219). Management of contact between young children and animals known to transmit disease to children is difficult in group child care settings. Optimal hand hygiene, especially after contact with animals and before eating or drinking, is essential to prevent transmission of zoonoses in the child care setting.

The single most important procedure to minimize fecal-oral transmission of pathogenic organisms is frequent use of hand hygiene measures combined with staff training and monitoring of staff implementation. Exclusion criteria are provided in Table 2.6 (p 137) and Table 2.7 (p 138).

RESPIRATORY TRACT DISEASES

Organisms spread by the respiratory route include viruses causing acute upper respiratory tract infections and bacterial organisms associated with invasive infections, such as *Haemophilus influenzae, Streptococcus pneumoniae, Neisseria meningitidis, Bordetella pertussis, Mycobacterium tuberculosis*, and *Kingella kingae*. Possible modes of spread of respiratory tract viruses include aerosols, respiratory droplets, and direct contact with secretions or indirect contact with contaminated fomites. The viral pathogens responsible for respiratory tract disease in child care settings are those that cause disease in the community, including respiratory syncytial virus, parainfluenza virus, influenza virus, human metapneumovirus, adenovirus, and rhinovirus. The incidence of viral infections of the respiratory tract is increased in child care settings. Hand hygiene measures can decrease the incidence of acute respiratory tract disease among children in child care (see Recommendations for Inclusion and Exclusion, p 136). Influenza virus and rhinovirus have been detected on samples from toys, indicating that environmental sanitation, as well as respiratory etiquette, may be important in decreasing the incidence of acute respiratory tract disease in children in child care.

The occurrence of invasive disease attributable to *H influenzae* type b (Hib) is rare since the routine immunization of infants and children with Hib conjugate vaccine was recommended (see *Haemophilus influenzae* Infections, p 368). Infections caused by *N meningitidis* occur in all age groups. Children younger than 1 year experience the highest incidence of invasive meningococcal disease. Extended close contact between children and staff exposed to an index case of meningococcal disease predisposes to secondary transmission. Because outbreaks may occur in child care settings, chemoprophylaxis is indicated for exposed child care contacts regardless of the meningococcal serogroup, and vaccine should be provided if the outbreak is related to a meningococcal serogroup contained in the available meningococcal conjugate vaccine(s) (see Meningococcal Infections, p 547).

In the prevaccine era, the risk of primary invasive disease attributable to *S pneumoniae* among children in child care settings was increased compared with children not in child care settings. Secondary spread of *S pneumoniae* in child care centers has been reported, but the degree of risk of secondary spread in child care facilities is unknown. Available data are insufficient to recommend any antimicrobial regimen for preventing or interrupting the carriage or transmission of pneumococcal infection in out-of-home child care settings. Antimicrobial chemoprophylaxis is not recommended for contacts of children with invasive pneumococcal disease, regardless of their immunization status. Use of *S pneumoniae* conjugate vaccine has decreased dramatically the incidence of both invasive disease and pneumonia among children and other age groups not targeted for vaccination, and has decreased carriage of serotypes of *S pneumoniae* contained in the pneumococcal conjugate vaccine. In 2010, the US Food and Drug Administration (FDA) licensed the 13-valent pneumococcal conjugate vaccine (PCV13), which replaced the heptavalent pneumococcal conjugate vaccine (PCV7). PCV13 added coverage for 6 additional serotypes, potentially providing protection for two thirds of the most common pneumococcal serotypes causing invasive disease in children younger than 5 years (see Pneumococcal Infections, p 626).

Spread of group A streptococcal infection among children in child care has been reported, including in association with varicella outbreaks. A child with proven group A streptococcal infection should be excluded from the classroom until 24 hours after initiation of antimicrobial therapy. Although outbreaks of streptococcal pharyngitis in child care settings have occurred, the risk of secondary transmission after a single case of mild mucosal or even severe invasive group A streptococcal infection remains low. Chemoprophylaxis for contacts after group A streptococcal infection in child care facilities generally is not recommended (see Group A Streptococcal Infections, p 732).

Infants and young children with tuberculosis disease generally are not considered contagious, because younger children are less likely to have cavitary pulmonary lesions and are unable to expel large numbers of organisms into the air forcefully. If approved by health care officials, a child with tuberculosis disease may attend group child care if the following criteria are met: (1) chemotherapy has begun; (2) ongoing adherence to therapy is documented; (3) clinical symptoms have diminished; (4) the child is considered noninfectious to others; and (5) the child is able to participate in activities. Children with latent tuberculosis infection do not need to be excluded from child care.

Because an adult with tuberculosis disease poses a hazard to children in group child care, tuberculin screening with a tuberculin skin test (TST) or an interferon-gamma release blood assay (IGRA) of all staff who have contact with children in a child care setting is recommended before caregiving activities are initiated. Screening should also include other people present in family child care homes who are not care providers. Expert consultation should be obtained for situations in which screening for tuberculosis is undertaken in adults with diminished or altered immunologic function, because tuberculosis testing may be inconclusive in this population (see Tuberculosis, p 804). The need for periodic subsequent tuberculin screening for people without clinically important reactions should be determined on the basis of their risk of acquiring a new infection and local or state health department recommendations. Adults with symptoms compatible with tuberculosis should be evaluated for the disease as soon as possible. Child care providers with suspected or confirmed tuberculosis disease should be excluded from the child care facility and should not be allowed to care for children until their evaluation is negative or chemotherapy has rendered them noninfectious (see Tuberculosis, p 804).

OTHER CONDITIONS

PARVOVIRUS B19. Isolation or exclusion of immunocompetent people with parvovirus B19 infection in child care settings is unwarranted, because little or no virus is present in respiratory tract secretions at the time of occurrence of the rash of erythema infectiosum (see Parvovirus B19, p 593).

VARICELLA-ZOSTER VIRUS. The epidemiology of varicella has changed dramatically since licensure of the varicella vaccine in 1995. In the prevaccine era, attendance in child care was a described risk factor for children acquiring varicella at earlier ages. However, varicella is now an uncommon disease in childhood and in child care settings. Children with varicella who have been excluded from child care may return after all lesions have crusted, which usually occurs on the sixth day after onset of rash. Varicella in vaccinated people usually is less severe clinically. Immunized children with breakthrough varicella with only maculo-papular lesions can return to child care or school if no new lesions have appeared within a 24-hour period. All staff members and parents should be notified when a case of varicella occurs; they should be informed about the greater likelihood of serious infection in suscep-tible adults and adolescents and in susceptible immunocompromised people, in addition to the potential for fetal sequelae if infection occurs in a pregnant woman. Less than 5% of adults born in the United States may be susceptible to varicella-zoster virus. Adults without evidence of immunity should be offered 2 doses of varicella vaccine unless contraindicated. Susceptible child care staff members who are pregnant and exposed to children with vari-cella should be referred promptly to a qualified physician or other health care professional for counseling and management. The American Academy of Pediatrics and Centers for Disease Control and Prevention (CDC) recommend use of varicella vaccine in nonpregnant immunocompetent people 12 months or older without evidence of immunity within 3 days, but up to 5 days, after exposure to varicella (see Varicella-Zoster Infections, p 846). During a varicella outbreak, people who have received 1 dose of varicella vaccine should, resources permitting, receive a second dose of vaccine, provided the appropriate interval has elapsed since the first dose (3 months for children 12 months through 12 years of age and at least 28 days for people 13 years and older).

The decision to exclude staff members or children with herpes zoster infection (shin-gles) whose lesions cannot be covered should be made on the basis of criteria similar to criteria for varicella. In immunocompetent people, herpes zoster lesions that can be cov-ered pose a minimal risk because transmission usually occurs as a result of direct contact with fluid from lesions (see Varicella-Zoster Infections, p 846).

HERPES SIMPLEX VIRUS. Children with HSV gingivostomatitis (ie, primary infection) who do not have control of oral secretions (drooling) should be excluded from child care. Exclusion of children with cold sores (ie, recurrent infection) from child care or school is not indicated. Maternal HSV infections that pose a risk to the neonate usually are acquired by the infant during birth from the mother's genital tract infection. Exposure of a pregnant woman to HSV in a child care setting carries little or no risk for her fetus. Child care providers should be educated on the importance of hand hygiene and other measures for limiting contact with infected material from children with varicella-zoster virus or HSV infection (eg, saliva, tissue fluid, or fluid from a skin lesion).

CYTOMEGALOVIRUS INFECTION. Spread of CMV from an asymptomatic infected child in child care to his or her pregnant mother or to a pregnant child care provider, with subsequent transmission to the fetus, is the most important consequence of child care-related CMV infection (see Cytomegalovirus Infection, p 317). Children enrolled in child care programs are more likely to acquire CMV than are children primarily cared for at home. Excretion rates from urine or saliva in children 1 to 3 years of age who attend child care centers usually range from 30% to 40% but can be as high as 70%, and intermittent excretion commonly continues for years. Studies of CMV seroconversion among female child care providers have found annualized seroconversion rates of 8% to 20%. Women who are or who may become pregnant and who are CMV naïve are at risk of being infected during pregnancy and transmitting CMV to their fetus.

In view of the risk of CMV infection in child care staff and the potential consequences of gestational CMV infection, female child care staff members should be counseled about these risks. This counseling includes discussion between the woman and her health care provider. In utero fetal infection can occur in women with no preexisting CMV immunity (maternal primary infection) or in women with preexisting antibody to CMV (maternal nonprimary infection) by either acquisition of a different viral strain during pregnancy or from reactivation of an existing maternal infection. CMV excretion is so prevalent that attempts at isolation or segregation of children who excrete CMV are impractical and inappropriate. Similarly, testing of children to detect CMV excretion is inappropriate, because excretion often is intermittent and results of testing can be misleading. Therefore, use of Standard Precautions and hand hygiene are the optimal methods of prevention of transmission of infection.

BLOODBORNE VIRUS INFECTIONS

HBV, HIV, and hepatitis C virus (HCV) are bloodborne pathogens. Although risk of contact with blood containing one of these viruses is low in the child care setting, appropriate infection-control practices will prevent transmission of bloodborne pathogens if exposure occurs. All child care providers should receive regular training on how to prevent transmission of bloodborne infections and how to respond should an exposure occur (**www. osha.gov/SLTC/bloodbornepathogens/index.html**).

HEPATITIS B VIRUS. Transmission of HBV in the child care setting has been described but occurs rarely. Because of the low risk of transmission, high immunization rates against HBV in children, and implementation of infection-control measures, children known to have chronic HBV infection (hepatitis B surface antigen [HBsAg] positive) may attend child care in most circumstances. Children who have no behavioral or medical risk factors, such as unusually aggressive behavior (eg, frequent biting), generalized dermatitis, or a bleeding problem, should be admitted to child care without restrictions. The risk of disease transmission from such children is minimal and usually does not justify exclusion of a child who has chronic HBV infection from child care, because all or most of the other children should already should be protected by previous HBV immunization. Admission of HBsAg-positive children with behavioral or medical risk factors should be assessed on an individual basis by the child's physician. Routine screening of children for HBsAg before admission to child care is not justified. Consultation should be sought with the child's physician when admission of a child previously identified to have chronic HBV infection is identified and the child has one or more behavioral or medical risk factors for transmission of bloodborne pathogens. The responsible public health authority or child care health consultant should be consulted when appropriate. Regular assessment of behavioral risk factors and medical conditions of enrolled children with chronic HBV infection is necessary.

Transmission of HBV in a child care setting is most likely to occur through direct exposure to blood after an injury or from bites or scratches that break the skin and introduce blood or body secretions from an HBV carrier into a susceptible person. Indirect transmission through environmental contamination with blood or saliva is possible, but this occurrence has not been documented in a child care setting in the United States.

Existing data in humans suggest a small risk of HBV transmission from the bite of a child with chronic HBV infection. For a susceptible child (not fully immunized with HBV vaccine) who is bitten by a child with chronic HBV infection, prophylaxis with Hepatitis B Immune Globulin (HBIG) and hepatitis B immunization is recommended (see Hepatitis B, p 400).

The risk of HBV acquisition when a susceptible child bites a child who has chronic HBV infection is unknown. A theoretical risk exists if HBsAg-positive blood enters the oral cavity of the biter, but transmission by this route has not been reported. Most experts would initiate or complete the hepatitis B vaccine series but not give HBIG to a susceptible biting child (not fully immunized with HBV vaccine) who does not have oral mucosal disease when the amount of blood transferred from a child with chronic HBV infection is small.

In the common circumstance in which the HBsAg status of both the biting child and the victim is unknown, the risk of HBV transmission is extremely low because of the expected low seroprevalence of HBsAg in most groups of preschool-aged children, the low efficiency of disease transmission from bites, and routine hepatitis B immunization of preschool children. Serologic testing generally is not warranted for the biting child or the recipient of the bite, but each situation should be evaluated individually.

Efforts to decrease the risk of HBV transmission in child care through hygienic and environmental standards generally should focus on precautions for blood exposures and limiting potential saliva contamination of the environment. Toothbrushes and pacifiers should be labeled and stored individually and should not be shared among children. Accidents that lead to bleeding or contamination with blood-containing body fluids by any child should be handled as follows: (1) disposable gloves should be used when cleaning or removing any blood or blood-containing body fluid spills; (2) the material should be absorbed using disposable towels or tissues; (3) the area should be disinfected with a disinfectant registered by the Environmental Protection Agency (EPA) and applied in the manner and time recommended; (4) people involved in cleaning contaminated surfaces should avoid exposure of open skin lesions or mucous membranes to blood or blood-containing body fluids and to wound or tissue exudates; (5) hands should be washed thoroughly after exposure to blood or blood-containing body fluids after gloves are removed and discarded properly; (6) disposable towels or tissues should be used and discarded properly, and mops should be rinsed in disinfectant; (7) blood-contaminated paper towels, diapers, gloves, and other materials should be placed in a leak-proof plastic bag with a secure tie for disposal; and (8) staff members should be educated about Standard Precautions for handling blood or blood-containing material.

HIV INFECTION (ALSO SEE HUMAN IMMUNODEFICIENCY VIRUS INFECTION, P 453).
Transmission of HIV has not been documented in child care settings in the United States. Children who enter child care should not be required to be tested for HIV or to disclose their HIV status. There is no need to restrict placement of HIV-infected children without risk factors for transmission of bloodborne pathogens in child care facilities to protect other children or staff members in these settings. However, a diagnosis of immunodeficiency, regardless of cause, should be disclosed to care providers in case of certain disease exposures (eg, measles or varicella) so that provision of postexposure immunoprophylaxis can be instituted as soon as possible (see Measles, p 535, and Varicella-Zoster Infections, p 846). Because HIV-infected children whose status is unknown may be attending child care, Standard Precautions should be adopted for handling all spills of blood and blood-containing body fluids and wound exudates of all children, as described in the preceding HBV section.

The decision to admit known HIV-infected children to child care is best made on an individual basis by qualified people, including the child's physician, who are able to evaluate whether the child will receive optimal care in the program and whether an HIV-infected child poses a significant risk to others. Consultation with the child's physician should be undertaken if an HIV-infected child has one or more potential risk factors for transmission of bloodborne pathogens (eg, biting behavior, frequent scratching, generalized dermatitis, or bleeding problems). Local or state public health experts should be consulted as appropriate. If a bite results in blood exposure to either person involved, the US Public Health Service recommends evaluation, including consideration of postexposure prophylaxis (see Human Immunodeficiency Virus Infection, p 453).

HIV-infected adults who do not have open and uncoverable skin lesions, other conditions that would allow contact with their body fluids, or a transmissible infectious disease may care for children in child care programs. However, immunosuppressed adults with HIV infection may be at increased risk of acquiring infectious agents from children and should consult their physician about the safety of continuing to work in child care. All child care providers, especially providers known to be HIV infected, should be notified immediately if they have been exposed to varicella, parvovirus B19, tuberculosis, diarrheal disease, or measles through children or other adults in the facility.

HEPATITIS C VIRUS. Transmission risks of HCV infection in child care settings are unknown. Exclusion of children with HCV infection from out-of-home child care is not indicated. The general risk of HCV infection from percutaneous exposure to infected blood is estimated to be 10 times greater than that of HIV but lower than that of HBV. The risk of transmission of HCV via contamination of mucous membranes or broken skin probably is between the risk of transmission of HIV and the risk of transmission of HBV via contaminated blood. Standard Precautions (see Hepatitis C, p 423) should be followed to prevent infection with HCV.

IMMUNIZATIONS

Routine immunization at appropriate ages is important for children in child care, because preschool-aged children can be protected from vaccine-preventable diseases including measles, rubella, Hib, HAV, varicella, pertussis, rotavirus, influenza, and invasive *S pneumoniae* disease, all of which had high incidence rates in the prevaccine era.

Age-appropriate immunization documentation should be provided by parents or guardians of all children in out-of-home child care. Unless contraindications exist or children have received medical, religious, or philosophic exemptions (depending on state immunization laws), immunization records should demonstrate complete immunization for age as shown in the recommended childhood and adolescent immunization schedules (**http://redbook.solutions.aap.org/SS/immunization_Schedules.aspx**). Immunization mandates by state for children in child care can be found online (**www.immunize.org/laws**).

Children who have not received recommended age-appropriate immunizations before enrollment should be immunized as soon as possible, and the series should be completed according to the recommended childhood and adolescent immunization schedules (**http://redbook.solutions.aap.org/SS/immunization_Schedules.aspx**), using the catchup schedule as appropriate. In the interim, permitting unimmunized or inadequately immunized children to attend child care, assuming there is no current outbreak of a vaccine-preventable infection, should depend on medical and legal counsel received regarding how to handle the risk and whether to inform parents of enrolled infants and children about potential exposure to this risk. Unimmunized or underimmunized children place appropriately immunized children and children with vaccine contraindications at risk of contracting a vaccine-preventable disease. If a vaccine-preventable disease to which children may be susceptible occurs in the child care program, all unimmunized and underimmunized children should be excluded for the duration of possible exposure or until they have completed their immunizations.

All adults who work in a child care facility should have received all immunizations routinely recommended for adults (see adult immunization schedule at **www.cdc.gov/ vaccines**). Child care providers should be immunized against influenza annually and should be immunized appropriately against measles as shown in the adult immunization schedule. Requirements of the Occupational Safety and Health Administration (OSHA) state that employers must offer employees hepatitis B vaccine if they are likely, as a part of their duties, to come in contact with blood. All child care providers should receive written information about hepatitis B disease and its complications as well as means of prevention with immunization.

Child care providers should be asked to document evidence of varicella immunity. Child care providers born after 1980 with a negative or uncertain history of varicella and no history of immunization should be immunized with 2 doses of varicella vaccine or undergo serologic testing for susceptibility; providers who are not immune should be offered 2 doses of varicella vaccine, unless it is contraindicated medically. All child care providers should receive written information about varicella, particularly disease manifestations in adults, complications, and means of prevention.

Because the prevalence of HAV infection does not seem to be significantly increased in staff members of child care centers compared with the prevalence in the general population and because HAV immunization of children 12 through 23 months of age is now routine, routine immunization of staff members is not recommended. However, because HAV can cause symptomatic illness in adult contacts and because child care programs have been a source of infection in the community, administering hepatitis A vaccine to staff members in some circumstances may be justified (see Hepatitis A, p 391). During HAV outbreaks, immunization of staff members should be considered (see Hepatitis A, p 391).

All adults who work in child care facilities should receive a 1-time dose of Tdap (tetanus toxoid, reduced diphtheria toxoid, and acellular pertussis) vaccine for booster immunization against tetanus, diphtheria, and pertussis regardless of how recently they received their last dose of Td. Pregnant women should be immunized with Tdap vaccine during each pregnancy, preferably between 27 and 36 weeks' gestation. For other recommendations for Tdap vaccine use in adults, including unimmunized or partially immunized adults, see Pertussis (p 608) and the adult immunization schedule.

General Practices

The following practices are recommended to decrease transmission of infectious agents in a child care setting:

- Each child care facility should have **written policies** for managing child and provider illness in child care.

- **Toilet areas and toilet-training equipment** should be cleaned and disinfected daily and additionally as needed to maintain sanitary conditions.
- **Diaper-changing surfaces** should be nonporous and disinfected between uses. The changing surface should be covered with nonabsorbent paper liners large enough to cover the surface from the child's shoulders to beyond the child's feet. The liner should be discarded after each use. If the surface becomes wet or soiled, it should be cleaned. The changing surface should be cleaned and disinfected after each use.
- **Diaper-changing procedures** should be posted at the changing area. Soiled disposable diapers, training pants, and soiled disposable wiping cloths should be discarded in a secure, hands-free, plastic-lined container with a lid. Diapers should contain all urine and stool and should minimize fecal contamination of children, child care providers, environmental surfaces, and objects in the child care environment. Children should be diapered with disposable diapers containing absorbent gelling material or carboxymethylcellulose or with cloth diapers that have an absorbent inner layer completely covered by an outer waterproof layer with a waist closure (ie, not pull-on pants) that are changed as a unit. Clothes should be worn over diapers while the child is in the child care facility. Clothing, including shoes and socks, should be removed as needed to expose the diaper and prevent contact with diaper contents during the diaper change. Soiled clothing should be bagged and sent home for laundering. Both the child's and caregiver's hands should be washed with soap after the diaper change is complete.
- **Diaper-changing areas** never should be located in or in proximity to food preparation areas and never should be used for temporary placement of food, drinks, or eating utensils. Sinks used to wash hands after diaper changing should not be in the food preparation area.
- The use of **child-sized toilets** or access to steps and modified toilet seats that provide for easier maintenance should be encouraged. The use of potty chairs should be discouraged, but if used, potty chairs should be emptied into a toilet, cleaned in a utility sink, and disinfected after each use. Staff members should disinfect potty chairs, toilets, and diaper-changing areas with an EPA-registered disinfectant and applied in the manner and time recommended.
- **Written procedures for hand hygiene** should be established and enforced.[1] Handwashing sinks should be adjacent to all diaper-changing and toilet areas. These sinks should be washed and disinfected at least daily and should not be used for food preparation. Food and drinking utensils should not be washed in sinks in diaper-changing areas. Handwashing sinks should not be used for rinsing soiled clothing or for cleaning potty chairs. Children should have access to height-appropriate sinks, soap dispensers, and disposable paper towels. Children younger than 5 years should not have independent access to alcohol-based hand sanitizing gels or use them without adult supervision, because they have a high alcohol content and are toxic if ingested and flammable. Alcohol-based sanitizing gels may be used as an adjunct to handwashing with soap or as an option in settings (eg, playgrounds, field trips) where there are no sinks. For certain enteropathogens (eg, *C difficile*), alcohol-based gels are known to

---

[1]Centers for Disease Control and Prevention. Guideline for hand hygiene in health-care settings. Recommendations of the Healthcare Infection Control Practices Advisory Committee and the HICPAC/SHEA/APIC/IDSA Hand Hygiene Task Force. *MMWR Recomm Rep.* 2002;51(RR-16):1-45

be ineffective in killing spores, and use of soap and water is recommended. Soap and water also is preferred in the control of norovirus infections.

- Written **personal hygiene policies** for staff and children are necessary.
- Written **environmental sanitation policies and procedures** should include daily cleaning of floors, covering sandboxes, and cleaning and sanitizing play tables, and cleaning and disinfecting spills of blood or body fluids and wound or tissue exudates at the time of the event. In general, routine housekeeping procedures using a freshly prepared solution of commercially available cleaner (eg, detergents, disinfectant detergents, or chemical germicides) compatible with most surfaces are satisfactory for cleaning spills of vomitus, urine, and feces.
- For **spills of blood** or blood-containing body fluids and of wound and tissue exudates, the material should be removed using gloves to avoid contamination of hands, and the area then should be disinfected using an EPA-registered disinfectant and applied in the manner and time recommended.
- Each **item of sleep equipment** should be used only by a single child and should be cleaned weekly and before being used by another child. Crib mattresses should have a nonporous easy-to-wipe surface and should be cleaned and sanitized when soiled or wet. Sleeping cots should be stored so that contact with the sleeping surface of another mat does not occur. Bedding (sheets and blankets) should be assigned to each child and cleaned and sanitized when soiled or wet.
- Optimally, **toys** that are placed in children's mouths or otherwise contaminated by body secretions should be cleaned with water and detergent, sanitized, rinsed if the manufacturer's label on the product used allows it, and air-dried before handling by another child. All frequently touched toys in rooms that house infants and toddlers should be cleaned and sanitized daily. Toys in rooms for older continent children should be cleaned at least weekly and when soiled. Soft, nonwashable toys should not be used in infant and toddler areas of child care programs. Plush toys and stuffed animals should be laundered frequently.
- **Food** should be handled safely and appropriately to prevent growth of bacteria and to prevent contamination by enteropathogens, insects, or rodents.[1] Hands should be washed using soap and water before handling food. Tables and countertops used for food preparation, food service, and eating should be cleaned and sanitized between uses and between preparation of raw and cooked food. People with signs or symptoms of illness, including vomiting, diarrhea, jaundice, or infectious skin lesions that cannot be covered or with suspected asymptomatic infection with a foodborne pathogen should not be responsible for food handling. Because of their frequent exposure to feces and children with enteric diseases, staff members who change diapers ideally should not prepare or serve food. Except in home-based care, staff members who work with diapered children should not prepare food for, or serve food to, groups of older children. Staff members should not be permitted to change diapers and prepare or serve food on the same day. If doing both is necessary, staff members should prepare food before changing diapers, do both tasks for as few children as possible, and handle food only for the infants and toddlers in their own group and only after thoroughly washing their hands. Facilities should serve only pasteurized milk, cheeses, and juice products (see Appendix VI, Potentially Contaminated Food Products, p 1004).

---

[1]Centers for Disease Control and Prevention. Surveillance for foodborne disease outbreaks—United States, 2011. *MMWR Morb Mortal Wkly Rep.* 2011;60(35):1197-1202

- The living quarters of **pets** should be enclosed and kept clean of waste to decrease the risk of human contact with the waste. Hands should be washed after handling all animals or animal wastes, cages, or food. Dogs and cats should be in good health and immunized appropriately for age, and they should be kept away from child play areas and handled only with staff supervision. Such animals should be given flea-, tick-, and worm-control programs. Reptiles, rodents, amphibians, and baby poultry and their habitats should not be handled by children younger than 5 years (see Diseases Transmitted by Animals [Zoonoses]: Household Pets, Including Nontraditional Pets, and Exposure to Animals in Public Settings, p 219).[1]
- Written policies that comply with local and state regulations for filing and regularly updating **immunization records** of each child and child care provider should be maintained. Children in group child care settings should receive all recommended immunizations, not just those that are required by state law for licensed child care and Head Start programs, including annual influenza vaccine. The immunization of each child enrolled should be updated annually.
- Each child care program should use the services of a **health consultant** to assist in development and implementation of written policies for prevention and control of communicable diseases and provision of related health education to children, staff, and parents. The health consultant should conduct program observations to correct hazards and risky practices.
- The child care provider should, when registering each child, **inform parents of exclusion and readmittance policies and of the requirement to share information about nationally notifiable infectious diseases** affecting the child or any member of the immediate household to facilitate prompt reporting of diseases and institution of control measures. The child care provider or program director, after consulting with the program's health consultant or the responsible public health official, should follow recommendations of the consultant or public health official for **notification of parents** of children who attend the program about exposure of their child to a communicable disease.
- Local and/or state **public health authorities should be contacted** about cases of nationally notifiable diseases involving children or care providers in the child care setting.
- In settings where **human milk** is stored and delivered to infants, there should be a written policy to ensure administration of human milk to the designated infant. Human milk policies should emphasize meticulous labeling, storage, and verification of recipient identity before providing human milk. A monitoring program should be instituted with policies to deal with incidents when human milk inadvertently is fed to an infant other than the designated infant (see Human Milk Banks, p 131). Health care facilities have developed policies that could be adapted to the child care setting to address such incidents. These policies require documentation, counseling, observation of the affected infant for signs of infection, and verification of the donor mother's infectious disease status.

---

[1]National Association of State Public Health Veterinarians, Animal Contact Compendium Committee 2013. Compendium of measures to prevent disease associated with animals in public settings, 2013. *JAVMA*. 2013;243(9):1270-1288

School Health

The clustering of children together that occurs in a school setting provides opportunities for transmission of infectious diseases. Determining the likelihood that infection in one or more children will pose a risk for schoolmates depends on an understanding of several factors: (1) the mechanism of pathogen transmission; (2) the ease with which the organism is spread (contagion); and (3) the likelihood that classmates are immune because of immunization or previous infection. Decisions to intervene to prevent spread of infection within a school should be made through collaboration among school officials, local public health officials, and health care professionals, considering the availability and effectiveness of specific methods of prevention and risk of serious complications from infection.

The United States relies on child care and elementary and secondary school entry immunization requirements to achieve and sustain high levels of immunization coverage. All states require immunization of children at the time of entry into school, and many states require immunization of children throughout grade school, of older children in upper grades, and of young adults entering college. The most up-to-date information about which vaccines are required in a specific state, permissible exemptions, and minor's consent to immunization can be obtained from the immunization program manager of each state health department, from a number of local health departments, from **www. immunize.org/laws**, and from the National Network for Immunization Information (**www.immunizationinfo.org**).

General methods for control and prevention of spread of infection in the school setting include:

- Meticulous hand and environmental hygiene.
- Documentation of the immunization status of enrolled children should be reviewed at the time of enrollment and at regularly scheduled intervals thereafter, in accordance with state requirements. Although specific laws vary by state, most states require proof of protection against poliomyelitis, tetanus, pertussis, diphtheria, *Haemophilus influenzae* type b, measles, mumps, rubella, and varicella. Immunizations against hepatitis B virus (HBV) and meningococcal disease are mandatory in many states (**www.immunize. org/laws**). Hepatitis A virus (HAV) immunization is required for school entry in some states; seasonal influenza vaccination is recommended but not required. Policies established by state health departments concerning exclusion of unimmunized children and exemptions for children with certain underlying medical conditions and families with religious or philosophic objection to immunization should be followed. Exemption rates by state can be found at **www2.cdc.gov/nip/schoolsurv/rptgmenu.asp**.
- Infected children should be excluded from school until they no longer are considered contagious (for recommendations on specific diseases, see relevant disease-specific chapters in Section 3).
- Unimmunized or underimmunized children place other appropriately immunized children at risk of contracting a vaccine-preventable disease. If a vaccine-preventable disease to which children may be susceptible occurs in the school, all unimmunized and underimmunized children should be excluded for the duration of possible exposure or until they have completed their immunizations (for recommendations on specific diseases, see relevant disease-specific chapters in Section 3).

- In some instances, administration of appropriate antimicrobial therapy will limit further spread of infection (eg, streptococcal pharyngitis, pertussis).
- Antimicrobial prophylaxis administered to close contacts of children with infections caused by specific pathogens may be warranted in some circumstances (eg, meningococcal infection, pertussis). Decisions about postexposure prophylaxis after an in-school exposure are best made in conjunction with local public health authorities.
- Temporary school closings can be used in limited circumstances: (1) to prevent spread of infection; (2) when an infection is expected to affect a large number of susceptible students and available control measures are considered inadequate; or (3) when an infection is expected to have a high rate of morbidity or mortality.
- Schools should maintain a clean environment and enforce high standards of personal hygiene, provide appropriate education for school staff, and ensure that the school has a reliable process for notification and education of parents during an exposure or outbreak.

Physicians involved with school health should be aware of current public health guidelines to prevent and control infectious diseases. Close collaboration between the school and physician also is encouraged, helping to ensure that the school receives appropriate guidance and is stocked with the necessary materials to deal with outbreaks and limit spread of infections. In all circumstances requiring intervention to prevent spread of infection within the school setting, the privacy of children who are infected should be protected.

Diseases Preventable by Routine Childhood Immunization

Children and adolescents who have been fully immunized according to the recommended childhood and adolescent immunization schedule (**http://redbook.solutions.aap. org/SS/Immunization_Schedules.aspx**) should be considered to be protected against diseases for which they were immunized. Disease-specific chapters should be consulted for details.

Measles and varicella vaccines have been demonstrated to provide protection in some susceptible people if administered within 72 hours after exposure, and up to 5 days after exposure in the case of varicella vaccine. Measles or varicella immunization should be recommended immediately for all nonimmune people during a measles or varicella outbreak, respectively, except for people with a contraindication to immunization. Many people without evidence of immunity may not yet have been exposed; therefore, vaccinating at any stage of an outbreak can prevent disease. In regard to measles, vaccination efforts should also be considered at unaffected schools that may be at risk during an outbreak. Students immunized against measles or varicella for the first time under these circumstances should be allowed to return to school after immunization, although they will need to be observed for the onset of wild-type disease during the interval before induction of protective immunity is afforded from vaccination (typically 2-3 weeks). Although measles vaccination should be delayed in people with moderate to severe febrile illnesses until resolution of the acute phase of the illness, an outbreak is an exception to this rule. Susceptible children 12 months or older exposed to HAV should receive single-antigen hepatitis A vaccine (HepA) or Immune Globulin (IG) within 14 days after exposure; for healthy people 12 months through 40 years of age, HAV vaccine at the age-appropriate dose is preferred to Immune Globulin Intramuscular (IGIM) because of vaccine advantages, including long-term protection and ease of administration. For people older than 40 years, IGIM is preferred for postexposure prophylaxis because of the absence of data regarding vaccine performance in this age group and the increased risk of severe manifestations of hepatitis A with increasing age. However, HAV vaccine can be used if IGIM is unavailable. People who are immunocompromised, are younger than 12 months, or have chronic liver disease should receive IGIM (see Hepatitis A, p 391).[1]

Mumps and rubella vaccines administered after exposure have not been demonstrated to prevent infection among susceptible contacts, but unimmunized students should receive the vaccines to protect them from infection from subsequent exposure. People who receive mumps immunization should be provided with information on symptoms and signs of illness and be instructed to contact their medical provider should they become sick. As an additional prevention measure, it is imperative that any child diagnosed with mumps stay home from school for 5 days after onset of parotid gland swelling. Those with rubella should be excluded from school for 7 days after the onset of rash.

Students and staff members with documented pertussis should be excluded from school and related activities until they have received at least 5 days of the recommended course of azithromycin; public health authorities should be contacted to assist with outbreak investigation and control. Symptomatic contacts should be tested and treated for pertussis; they also should also be excluded until they have completed 5 days of appropriate antimicrobial treatment. Children and staff members who refuse appropriate antimicrobial treatment should be excluded for 21 days after last contact with the infected person. Chemoprophylaxis should be given to all household contacts and to school contacts who are at risk of severe illness or adverse outcomes (eg, women in the third trimester of pregnancy, people with severe asthma or cystic fibrosis) or who have close contact with such people. Unimmunized or underimmunized contacts should be immunized (see Pertussis, p 608). Tetanus toxoid, reduced diphtheria toxoid, and acellular pertussis (Tdap) vaccine should be substituted for a single dose of tetanus and diphtheria toxoids vaccine for children 7 years or older and adults (Td) in the primary catch-up series or as a booster dose if age appropriate (**http://redbook.solutions.aap.org/SS/Immunization_Schedules.aspx**).

Bacterial meningitis in school-aged children may be caused by *Neisseria meningitidis*. Infected people are not considered contagious after 24 hours of appropriate antimicrobial therapy. After discharge from the hospital, they pose no risk to classmates and may return to school. Prophylactic antimicrobial therapy is not recommended for school contacts in most circumstances. Close observation of contacts is recommended, and they should be evaluated promptly if a febrile illness develops. Students who have been exposed to oral secretions of an infected student, such as through kissing or sharing of food and drink, should receive chemoprophylaxis (see Meningococcal Infections, p 547). Immunization of school contacts with meningococcal conjugate vaccine (MCV4), which in the United States contains antigens for serogroups A, C, Y, and W-135, should be considered in consultation with local public health authorities if evidence suggests an outbreak within a school attributable to one of the meningococcal serogroups contained in the vaccine. A single dose of vaccine should be administered to all children at 11 or 12 years of age

---

[1] Advisory Committee on Immunization Practices (ACIP) Centers for Disease Control and Prevention (CDC). Update: Prevention of hepatitis A after exposure to hepatitis A virus and in international travelers. Updated recommendations of the Advisory Committee on Immunization Practices (ACIP). *MMWR Morb Mortal Wkly Rep.* 2007;56(41):1080-1084

followed by a booster dose at 16 years of age; previously unimmunized adolescents 16 through 18 years of age should receive a single dose. MCV4 administration is not recommended for postexposure prophylaxis following exposure to a single case. Certain high-risk groups 2 through 10 years of age and 19 through 55 years of age also should be vaccinated (see Meningococcal Infections, p 547). For outbreaks related to serogroup B, provision of the serogroup B meningococcal vaccine currently licensed for use in Europe and Australia could be considered after consultation with public health authorities (see Meningococcal Infections, p 547).

Infections Spread by the Respiratory Route

Some pathogens that cause severe lower respiratory tract disease in infants and toddlers, such as respiratory syncytial virus and metapneumovirus, are of less concern in healthy school-aged children. Respiratory tract viruses, however, are associated with exacerbations of reactive airway disease and an increase in the incidence of otitis media and can cause significant complications for children with chronic respiratory tract disease, such as cystic fibrosis, or for children who are immunocompromised. Infection-control principles of respiratory etiquette hand hygiene and covering mouth and nose with tissue when coughing or sneezing (if no tissue is available, use the upper shoulder or elbow area rather than hands) should be taught and implemented in schools.

Influenza virus infection is a common cause of febrile respiratory tract disease and school absenteeism. Annual influenza vaccine should be administered to children 6 months and older and adults (see Influenza Vaccine, p 476). It is recommended that all children diagnosed with an influenza-like illness be fever free for 24 hours before returning to school, whether or not the child received antiviral therapy.

Mycoplasma pneumoniae causes upper and lower respiratory tract infection in school-aged children, and outbreaks of *M pneumoniae* infection occur in communities and schools. The nonspecific symptoms and signs associated with this organism make distinguishing *M pneumoniae* infection from other causes of respiratory tract illness difficult. Antimicrobial therapy does not necessarily eradicate the organism or prevent spread. Thus, intervention to prevent secondary infection in the school setting is difficult. *Mycoplasma* outbreaks in schools should be reported to the local health department.

Students with pharyngitis caused by group A *Streptococcus* may return to school 24 hours after initiation of antimicrobial therapy. Students who have negative results for group A *Streptococcus* on a rapid antigen test but who are awaiting results of culture and not receiving antimicrobial therapy may attend school during the culture incubation period unless the infection involves a child with poor hygiene and poor control of secretions. Symptomatic contacts of students with pharyngitis attributable to group A streptococcal infection should be evaluated and treated if streptococcal infection is demonstrated. Asymptomatic contacts usually require neither evaluation nor therapy.

Before adolescence, children with tuberculosis generally are not contagious, but students who are in close contact with an older child, teacher, or other adult with infectious tuberculosis should be evaluated for infection, including tuberculin skin testing or interferon-gamma release assay (see Tuberculosis, p 804). An adolescent or adult with infectious tuberculosis almost always is the source of infection for young children. If an adult source outside the school is identified (eg, parent or grandparent of a student), efforts should be made to determine whether other students have been exposed to the same source and whether they warrant evaluation for infection.

Children with erythema infectiosum should be allowed to attend school, because the period of contagion occurs before a rash is evident. Parvovirus B19 infection poses no risk of significant illness for healthy classmates, although aplastic crisis can develop in infected children and adults with sickle cell disease or other hemoglobinopathies. Pregnant women exposed to an infected child 5 to 10 days before rash onset should be referred to their physician for counseling and possible serologic testing.

Infections Spread by Direct Contact

Infection and infestation of skin, eyes, and hair can spread through direct contact with the infected area or through contact with contaminated hands or fomites, such as hair brushes, hats, and clothing. *Staphylococcus aureus* (including methicillin-resistant *S aureus* [MRSA]) and group A streptococcal organisms may colonize the skin, oropharynx, or nasal mucosa of asymptomatic people. Clinical disease (lesions) may develop when these organisms are passed from a person with colonized or infected skin to another person. Shared fomites, such as towels, athletic equipment, and razors, also have been implicated in the spread of MRSA within school settings. Although most skin infections attributable to *S aureus* and group A streptococcal organisms are minor and require only topical or oral antimicrobial therapy, person-to-person spread should be interrupted by appropriate treatment whenever skin infections are recognized. Local and systemic infections associated with MRSA pose a diagnostic and therapeutic challenge (see Staphylococcal Infections, p 715). Exclusion is recommended for any child with an open or draining lesion that cannot be covered.

Herpes simplex virus (HSV) infection of the mouth and skin is common among school-aged children. Infection is spread through direct contact with herpetic lesions or via asymptomatic shedding of virus from oral or genital secretions. "Cold sore" lesions of herpes labialis represent active infection, but no evidence suggests that students with active orolabial lesions pose any greater risk to their classmates than do unidentified asymptomatic shedders. For immunocompromised children and for children with open skin lesions (eg, severe eczema), exposure to another child with HSV infection may pose an increased risk of HSV acquisition and of severe or disseminated infection. Because of the frequency of symptomatic and asymptomatic shedding of HSV among classmates and staff members, careful hygienic practices are the best means of preventing infection (see Herpes Simplex, p 432).

Infectious conjunctivitis can be caused by bacterial (eg, nontypable *Haemophilus influenzae* and *Streptococcus pneumoniae*) or viral (eg, adenoviruses, enteroviruses, and HSV) pathogens. Bacterial conjunctivitis is less common in children older than 5 years. Infection occurs through direct contact or through contamination of hands followed by autoinoculation. Respiratory tract spread from large droplets also may occur. Topical antimicrobial therapy is indicated for bacterial conjunctivitis, which usually is distinguished by a purulent exudate. HSV conjunctivitis usually is unilateral and may be accompanied by vesicles on adjacent skin and preauricular adenopathy. Evaluation of HSV conjunctivitis by an ophthalmologist and administration of specific antiviral therapy are indicated. Conjunctivitis attributable to adenoviruses or enteroviruses is self-limited and requires no specific antiviral therapy. Spread of infection is minimized by careful hand hygiene, and infected people should be presumed contagious until symptoms have resolved. Except when viral or bacterial conjunctivitis is accompanied by systemic signs of illness, infected children should be allowed to remain in school once any indicated therapy is implemented, unless their behavior is such that close contact with other students cannot be avoided. The local health department should be notified of an outbreak of conjunctivitis.

Fungal infections of the skin and hair are spread by direct person-to-person contact and through contact with contaminated surfaces or objects. *Trichophyton tonsurans,* the predominant cause of tinea capitis, remains viable for long periods on combs, hair brushes, furniture, and fabric. The fungi that cause tinea corporis (ringworm) are transmissible by direct contact. Tinea cruris (jock itch) and tinea pedis (athlete's foot) occur in adolescents and young adults. The fungi that cause these infections have a predilection for moist areas and are spread through direct contact and contact with contaminated surfaces.

Students with fungal infections of the skin or scalp should be encouraged to receive treatment both for their benefit and to prevent spread of infection. However, lack of treatment does not necessitate exclusion from school unless the nature of their contact with other students could potentiate spread. Students with tinea capitis should be instructed not to share combs, hair brushes, hats, or hair ornaments with classmates until they have been treated. Students with tinea pedis should be excluded from swimming pools and discouraged from walking barefoot on locker room and shower floors until treatment has been initiated. Sharing of towels and shower shoes during sports activities should be discouraged.

Sarcoptes scabiei (scabies) and *Pediculus capitis* (head lice) are transmitted primarily through person-to-person contact. The scabies parasite survives on clothing for only 3 to 4 days without skin contact. Combs, hair brushes, hats, and hair ornaments can transmit head lice, but away from the scalp, lice do not remain viable.

Children identified as having scabies or head lice should be referred for treatment at the end of the school day and subsequently excluded from school only until treatment recommended by the child's health care professional has been started. School contacts generally should not be treated prophylactically. Caregivers who have prolonged skin-to-skin contact with students infested with scabies may benefit from prophylactic treatment (see Scabies, p 702).

Shampooing with an appropriate pediculicide and manually removing nits by combing usually are effective in eradicating viable lice. Manual removal of nits after successful treatment with a pediculicide is helpful, because none of the pediculicides are 100% ovicidal. Fine-toothed nit combs designed for this purpose are available. Removal of nits is tedious and time consuming but may be attempted for aesthetic reasons, to decrease diagnostic confusion, or to improve efficacy (see Pediculosis Capitis, p 597).

Infections Spread by the Fecal-Oral Route

Pathogens spread via the fecal-oral route constitute a risk if the infected person fails to maintain good hygiene, including hand hygiene after toilet use, or if contaminated food is shared between or among schoolmates.

Outbreaks attributable to HAV can occur in schools, but these outbreaks usually are associated with community outbreaks. Schoolroom exposure generally does not pose an appreciable risk of infection, and administration of HepA vaccine or IGIM to susceptible people for postexposure prophylaxis is not indicated following an individual case. However, if transmission within a school is documented, HepA vaccine should be considered as a means of prophylaxis and prolonged protection for immunocompetent people 12 months through 40 years of age (see Hepatitis A, p 391). If an outbreak occurs, consultation with local public health authorities is indicated before initiating interventions. Implementation of the recommended universal immunization of preschool-aged children with HepA vaccine reduced school outbreaks of disease.

Enteroviruses and noroviruses are spread by the fecal-oral route and transmission can be difficult to control. Noroviruses are currently the most common cause of foodborne illness and foodborne disease outbreaks in the United States, and school outbreaks have been reported. Consultation with local public health authorities is indicated for norovirus outbreaks.

Person-to-person spread of bacterial and parasitic enteropathogens within school settings occurs infrequently, but foodborne outbreaks attributable to enteric pathogens can occur. People with gastroenteritis attributable to an enteric pathogen should be excluded until symptoms resolve.

Children in diapers constitute a far greater risk of spread of enteric pathogens compared with fully continent children. Guidelines for control of these infections in child care settings should be applied for diapered school-aged students with developmental disabilities (see Children in Out-of-Home Child Care, p 132).

Infections Spread by Blood and Body Fluids

Contact with blood or body fluids from another person requires more intimate exposure than usually occurs in the school setting. However, care required for children with developmental disabilities may result in exposure of caregivers to urine, saliva, and in some cases, blood. Cytomegalovirus (CMV) may be chronically shed in saliva or urine; however, children who are shedding CMV do not require exclusion or isolation. The application of Standard Precautions and use of hand hygiene, as recommended for children in out-of-home child care, is the optimal means to prevent spread of infection from these exposures (see Children in Out-of-Home Child Care, p 132).

School staff members should be educated on proper procedures for handling blood and body fluid that may be contaminated with blood. For children with epistaxis or bleeding from injury, staff should wear disposable gloves and use appropriate hand hygiene measures immediately after glove removal for protection from bloodborne pathogens. Staff members at the scene of an injury or bleeding incident who do not have access to gloves need to use some type of barrier to avoid exposure to blood or blood-containing materials, use appropriate hand hygiene measures, and adhere to proper protocols for handling contaminated material, including feminine hygiene products.

Students infected with HIV, HBV, or HCV do not need to be identified to school personnel. Because HIV-, HBV-, and HCV-infected children and adolescents will not be identified, policies and procedures to manage all potential exposures to blood or blood-containing materials should be established and implemented. Parents and students should be educated about the types of exposure that present a risk for school contacts. Although a student's right to privacy should be maintained, decisions about activities at school should be made by parents or guardians together with a physician, on a case-by-case basis, keeping the health needs of the infected student and the student's classmates in mind.

Prospective studies to aid in determining the risk of transmission of HIV, HBV, or HCV during contact sports among high school students have not been performed, but the available evidence indicates that the risk is low. Guidelines for management of bleeding injuries have been developed for college and professional athletes in recognition of the possibility of unidentified HIV, HBV, or HCV infection in any competitor. The American Academy of Pediatrics (AAP) has published recommendations for prevention of transmission of HIV and other bloodborne pathogens in the athletic setting.[1,2]

- Athletes infected with HIV, HBV, or HCV should be allowed to participate in competitive sports.
- Physicians should respect the rights of infected athletes to confidentiality. The infection status of patients should not be disclosed to other participants or the staff of athletic programs.
- Testing for bloodborne pathogens should not be mandatory for athletes or sports participants.
- Pediatricians are encouraged to counsel athletes who are infected with HIV, HBV, or HCV and assure them that they have a low risk of infecting other competitors. Infected athletes should consider choosing a sport in which this risk is minimal. This may be protective for other participants and for infected athletes themselves, decreasing their possible exposure to bloodborne pathogens other than the one(s) with which they are infected. Wrestling and boxing probably have the greatest potential for contamination of injured skin by blood. The AAP opposes boxing as a sport for youth for other reasons.[3]
- Athletic programs should inform athletes and their parents that the program is operating under the policies of the aforementioned recommendations and that the athletes have a low risk of becoming infected with a bloodborne pathogen.
- Clinicians and staff of athletic programs should promote HBV immunization among all athletes and among coaches, athletic trainers, equipment handlers, laundry personnel, and any other people at risk of exposure to blood of athletes as an occupational hazard.
- Each coach and athletic trainer must receive training in first aid and emergency care and in prevention of transmission of bloodborne pathogens in the athletic setting. These staff members then can help implement these recommendations.
- Coaches and members of the health care team should educate athletes about precautions described in these recommendations. Such education should include the greater risks of transmission of HIV and other bloodborne pathogens through sexual activity and needle sharing during the use of injection drugs, including anabolic steroids. Athletes should be told not to share personal items, such as razors, toothbrushes, and nail clippers, that might be contaminated with blood.
- Depending on the law in some states, schools may need to comply with Occupational Safety and Health Administration (OSHA) regulations[4] for prevention of bloodborne

[1]American Academy of Pediatrics, Committee on Sports Medicine and Fitness. Human immunodeficiency virus and other blood-borne viral pathogens in the athletic setting. *Pediatrics*. 1999;104(6):1400-1403 (Reaffirmed November 2011)

[2]Rice SG; American Academy of Pediatrics, Council on Sports Medicine and Fitness. Medical conditions affecting sports participation. *Pediatrics*. 2008;121(4):841-848 (Reaffirmed May 2011)

[3]American Academy of Pediatrics, Council on Sports Medicine and Fitness; Canadian Paediatric Society, Healthy Active Living and Sports Medicine Committee. Boxing participation by children and adolescents. *Pediatrics*. 2011;128(3):617-623

[4]Occupational Safety and Health Administration (**www.osha.gov**).

pathogens. The athletic program must determine what rules apply. Compliance with OSHA regulations is a reasonable and recommended precaution even if this is not required specifically by the state.

- The following precautions should be adopted in sports with direct body contact and other sports in which an athlete's blood or other body fluids visibly tinged with blood may contaminate the skin or mucous membranes of other participants or staff members of the athletic program. Even if these precautions are adopted, the risk that a participant or staff member may become infected with a bloodborne pathogen in the athletic setting will not be eliminated entirely.

  - Athletes must cover existing cuts, abrasions, wounds, or other areas of broken skin with an occlusive dressing before and during participation. Caregivers should cover their own damaged skin to prevent transmission of infection to or from an injured athlete.

  - Disposable, waterproof vinyl or latex gloves should be worn to avoid contact with blood or other body fluids visibly tinged with blood and any objects, such as equipment, bandages, or uniforms, contaminated with these fluids. Hands should be cleaned with soap and water or an alcohol-based antiseptic agent as soon as possible after gloves are removed.

  - Athletes with active bleeding should be removed from competition as soon as possible until bleeding is stopped. Wounds should be cleaned with soap and water. Skin antiseptic agents may be used if soap and water are not available. Wounds must be covered with an occlusive dressing that will remain intact and not become soaked through during further play before athletes return to competition.

  - Athletes should be advised to report injuries and wounds in a timely fashion before or during competition.

  - Minor cuts or abrasions that are not bleeding do not require interruption of play but can be cleaned and covered during scheduled breaks. During these breaks, if an athlete's equipment or uniform fabric is wet with blood, the equipment should be cleaned and disinfected (see next bullet), or the uniform should be replaced.

  - Equipment and playing areas contaminated with blood must be cleaned using gloves and disposable absorbent material until all visible blood is gone and then disinfected with a disinfectant registered with the Environmental Protection Agency and applied in the manner and time recommended.[1] The decontaminated equipment or area should be in contact with the bleach solution for at least 30 seconds. The area then may be wiped with a disposable cloth after the minimum contact time or allowed to air dry.

  - Emergency care must not be delayed because gloves or other protective equipment are not available. If the caregiver does not have appropriate protective equipment, a towel may be used to cover the wound until an off-the-field location is reached where gloves can be used during more definitive treatment.

  - Breathing bags (eg, Ambu manual resuscitators) and oropharyngeal airways should be available for use during resuscitation.

---

[1]Centers for Disease Control and Prevention. Guidelines for environmental infection control in health-care facilities. Recommendations of CDC and the Healthcare Infection Control Practices Advisory Committee (HICPAC). *MMWR Recomm Rep.* 2003;52(RR-10):1-42

- Equipment handlers, laundry personnel, and janitorial staff must be educated in proper procedures for handling washable or disposable materials contaminated with blood.
- For guidelines on control and prevention of MRSA in athletes and other school settings, see Staphylococcal Infections (p 715).

INFECTION CONTROL AND PREVENTION FOR HOSPITALIZED CHILDREN

Health care-associated infections (HAIs) are a cause of substantial morbidity and some mortality in hospitalized children, particularly children in intensive care units. Hand hygiene before and after each patient contact remains the single most important practice in prevention and control of HAIs. A comprehensive set of guidelines for preventing and controlling HAIs, including isolation precautions, personnel health recommendations, and guidelines for prevention of postoperative and device-related infections, can be found on the Centers for Disease Control and Prevention (CDC) Web site (**www.cdc. gov/hicpac/pubs.html**). Guidelines for prevention of intravascular catheter-related infections also are available.[1] Additional guidelines are available from the principal infection-control societies in the United States, the Society for Healthcare Epidemiology of America and the Association for Professionals in Infection Control and Epidemiology, as well as subspecialty societies and regulatory agencies, such as the Occupational Safety and Health Administration (OSHA). The Cystic Fibrosis Foundation published an evidence-based guideline for prevention of transmission of infectious agents among cystic fibrosis patients in 2003. The Joint Commission also has established infection control standards. Physicians and infection-control professionals should be familiar with this increasingly complex array of guidelines, regulations, and standards. To accomplish this goal, infection-control programs run by pediatric infectious diseases specialists increasingly are used in hospital settings; to be sustainable over time, these programs require adequate institutional support. Ongoing infection-prevention and -control programs should include education, implementation, reinforcement, documentation, and evaluation of recommendations on a regular basis. Such activities should include conducting surveillance for high-risk HAIs, participating in improvement projects to reduce the incidence of HAIs, sharing data describing the incidence of specifically targeted HAIs, and complying with key prevention activities such as hand hygiene.

Isolation Precautions

Isolation precautions are designed to protect hospitalized children, health care personnel, and visitors by limiting transmission of potential pathogens within the health care setting. The Healthcare Infection Control Practices Advisory Committee in 2007 updated evidence-based isolation guidelines for preventing transmission of infectious agents in

---

[1] O'Grady NP, Alexander M, Burns LA, et al; Healthcare Infection Control Practices Advisory Committee. Guidelines for the prevention of intravascular catheter-related infections. *Am J Infect Control*. 2011;39(4 Suppl 1):S1-S34

health care settings.[1] Adherence to these isolation policies, supplemented by health care facility policies and procedures for other aspects of infection and environmental control and occupational health, should result in reduced transmission and safer patient care. Adaptations should be made according to the conditions and populations served by each facility.

Routine and optimal performance of **Standard Precautions** is appropriate for care of all patients, regardless of diagnosis or suspected or confirmed infection status. In addition to Standard Precautions, **Transmission-Based Precautions** are used when caring for patients who are infected or colonized with pathogens transmitted by airborne, droplet, or contact routes.

STANDARD PRECAUTIONS

Standard Precautions are used to prevent transmission of all infectious agents through contact with any body fluid except sweat (regardless of whether these fluids contain visible blood), nonintact skin, or mucous membranes. Barrier techniques are recommended to decrease exposure of health care personnel to body fluids. Standard Precautions are used with all patients when exposure to blood and body fluids is anticipated and are designed to decrease transmission of microorganisms from patients who are not recognized as harboring potential pathogens, such as bloodborne pathogens and antimicrobial-resistant bacteria. See Table 2.8, p 163, for elements of Standard Precautions (respiratory hygiene/cough etiquette). Standard Precautions include the following practices:

- **Hand hygiene** is necessary before and after all patient contact and after touching blood, body fluids, secretions, excretions, and contaminated items, whether gloves are worn or not. Hand hygiene should be performed either with alcohol-based agents or soap and water before donning and immediately after removing gloves, between patient contacts, and when otherwise indicated to avoid transfer of microorganisms to other patients and to items in the environment. When hands are visibly dirty or contaminated with proteinaceous material, such as blood or other body fluids, hands should be washed with soap and water for at least 20 seconds. The best means of preventing transmission of spores (eg, *Clostridium difficile*) or norovirus is not clear, but handwashing with soap and water currently is preferred over alcohol-based agents.
- **Gloves** (clean, nonsterile) should be worn when touching blood, body fluids, secretions, excretions, and items contaminated with these fluids, except for wiping a child's tears or nose or for routine wet diaper changing. Hand hygiene should be performed before donning gloves. Clean gloves should be used before touching mucous membranes and nonintact skin or if contact with body fluids is possible. Gloves should be changed between tasks and procedures on the same patient after contact with material that may contain a high concentration of microorganisms (eg, purulent drainage). Hand hygiene also should be performed after removal of gloves, even if visible soiling did not occur.
- **Masks, eye protection, and face shields** should be worn to protect mucous membranes of the eyes, nose, and mouth during procedures and patient care activities likely to generate splashes or sprays of blood, body fluids, secretions, or excretions.

---

[1]Centers for Disease Control and Prevention. Guideline for isolation precautions: preventing transmission of infectious agents in healthcare settings 2007. Recommendations of the Healthcare Infection Control Practices Advisory Committee. Atlanta, GA: Centers for Disease Control and Prevention; 2007. Available at: **www.cdc. gov/hicpac/pdf/isolation/Isolation2007.pdf**

Table 2.8. Recommendations for Application of Standard Precautions for Care of All Patients in All Health Care Settings

Component	Recommendations
Hand hygiene	Before and after each patient contact, regardless of whether gloves are used. After touching blood, body fluids, secretions, excretions, or contaminated items; immediately after removing gloves. Alcohol-containing antiseptic hand rubs preferred, except when hands are soiled visibly or if exposure to spores (eg, *Clostridium difficile, Bacillus anthracis*) or norovirus is likely to have occurred.
Personal protective equipment (PPE)	
Gloves	For touching blood, body fluids, secretions, excretions, or contaminated items; for touching mucous membranes and nonintact skin.
Gown	During procedures and patient-care activities when contact of clothing/exposed skin with blood/body fluids, secretions, and excretions is anticipated.
Mask, eye protection (goggles), face shield	During procedures and patient-care activities likely to generate splashes or sprays of blood, body fluids, or secretions, especially suctioning and endotracheal intubation, to protect health care personnel. For patient protection, use of a mask by the person inserting an epidural anesthesia needle or performing myelograms when prolonged exposure of the puncture site is likely to occur.
Soiled patient-care equipment	Handle in a manner that prevents transfer of microorganisms to others and to the environment; wear gloves if visibly contaminated; perform hand hygiene after contact with soiled items and after glove removal.
Environmental control	Develop procedures for routine care, cleaning, and disinfection of environmental surfaces, especially frequently touched surfaces in patient care areas.
Used textiles (linens) and laundry	Handle in a manner that prevents transfer of microorganisms to others and the environment.
Injection practices (use of needles and other sharps)	Do not recap, bend, break, or hand manipulate used needles; if recapping is required, use a one-handed scoop technique only; use needle-free safety devices when available; place used sharps in conveniently placed, puncture-resistant container. Use a sterile, single-use, disposable needle and syringe for each injection given. Single-dose medication vials are preferred when medications are administered to more than one patient.
Patient resuscitation	Use mouthpiece, resuscitation bag, or other ventilation devices to prevent contact with mouth and oral secretions.
Patient placement	Prioritize for single-patient room if patient is at increased risk of transmission, is likely to contaminate the environment, does not maintain appropriate hygiene, or is at increased risk of acquiring infection or developing adverse outcome following infection.

Table 2.8. Recommendations for Application of Standard Precautions for Care of All Patients in All Health Care Settings, continued

Component	Recommendations
Respiratory hygiene/cough etiquette (source containment of infectious respiratory tract secretions in symptomatic patients) beginning at the initial point of encounter (eg, triage and reception areas in emergency departments and physician offices)	Instruct symptomatic people to cover mouth/nose when sneezing/coughing; use tissues and dispose in no-touch receptacle; observe hand hygiene after soiling of hands with respiratory tract secretions; wear surgical mask if tolerated or maintain spatial separation more than 3 feet, if possible.

Masks should be worn when placing catheter or injecting material into the spinal canal or subdural space (eg, during myelograms and spinal or epidural anesthesia).

- **Nonsterile gowns** that are fluid-resistant will protect skin and prevent soiling of clothing during procedures and patient care activities likely to generate splashes or sprays of blood, body fluids, secretions, or excretions. Soiled gowns should be removed promptly and carefully to avoid contamination of clothing.
- **Patient care equipment** that has been used should be handled in a manner that prevents skin or mucous membrane exposures and contamination of clothing or the environment.
- **All used textiles (linens)** are considered to be contaminated and should be handled, transported, and processed in a manner that prevents aerosolization of microorganisms, skin and mucous membrane exposure, and contamination of clothing.
- **Safe injection practices:** Bloodborne pathogen exposure of health care personnel should be avoided by taking precautions to prevent injuries caused by needles, scalpels, and other sharp instruments or devices during procedures; when handling sharp instruments after procedures; when cleaning used instruments; and during disposal of used needles. To prevent needlestick injuries, safety devices should be used whenever they are available. Needles should not be recapped, purposely bent or broken by hand, removed from disposable syringes, or otherwise manipulated by hand. After use, disposable syringes and needles, scalpel blades, and other sharp items should be placed in puncture-resistant containers for disposal; puncture-resistant containers should be located as close as practical to the use area. Large-bore reusable needles should be placed in a puncture-resistant container located close to the site of use for transport to the reprocessing area to ensure maximal patient safety. Sharp devices with safety features are preferred whenever such devices have equivalent function to conventional sharp devices. Single-dose vials of medication are preferred.
- **Mouthpieces, resuscitation bags, and other ventilation devices** should be available in all patient care areas and used instead of mouth-to-mouth resuscitation.

TRANSMISSION-BASED PRECAUTIONS

Transmission-Based Precautions are designed for patients documented or suspected to have colonization or infection with pathogens for which additional precautions beyond **Standard Precautions** are recommended to prevent transmission. The 3 types of transmission routes on which these precautions are based are: airborne, droplet, and contact.

- **Airborne transmission** occurs by dissemination of airborne droplet nuclei (small-particle residue [≤5 μm in size] of evaporated droplets containing microorganisms that remain suspended in the air for long periods) or small respirable particles containing the infectious agent or spores. Microorganisms transmitted by the airborne route can be dispersed widely by air currents and can be inhaled by a susceptible host within the same room or a long distance from the source patient, depending on environmental factors. Special air handling and ventilation are required to prevent airborne transmission. Examples of microorganisms transmitted by airborne droplet nuclei are *Mycobacterium tuberculosis*, rubeola (measles) virus, and varicella-zoster virus. Specific recommendations for **Airborne Precautions** are as follows:
  - Provide infected or colonized patients with a single-patient room (if unavailable, consult an infection-control professional) and keep the door closed at all times.
  - Use special ventilation, including 6 to 12 air changes per hour, air flow direction from surrounding area to the room, and room air exhausted directly to the outside or recirculated through a high-efficiency particulate air (HEPA) filter.
  - If infectious pulmonary tuberculosis is suspected or proven, respiratory protective devices (ie, National Institute for Occupational Safety and Health-certified personally "fitted" and "sealing" respirator, such as N95 or N100 respirators, powered air-purifying respirators) should be worn while inside the patient's room.
  - Susceptible health care personnel should not enter rooms of patients with measles or varicella-zoster virus infections. If susceptible people must enter the room of a patient with measles or varicella infection or an immunocompromised patient with local or disseminated zoster infection, a mask or a respiratory protective device (eg, N95 respirator) that has been fit-tested should be worn. People with proven immunity to these viruses need not wear a mask.
- **Droplet transmission** occurs when droplets containing microorganisms generated from an infected person, primarily during coughing, sneezing, or talking, and during the performance of certain procedures, such as suctioning and bronchoscopy, are propelled a short distance (3-6 feet or less) and deposited into conjunctivae, nasal mucosa, or the mouth of a susceptible person. Because these relatively large droplets do not remain suspended in air, special air handling and ventilation are not required to prevent droplet transmission. Droplet transmission should not be confused with airborne transmission via droplet nuclei, which are much smaller. Specific recommendations for **Droplet Precautions** are as follows:
  - Provide the patient with a single-patient room if possible. If unavailable, consider cohorting patients infected with the same organism. Spatial separation of more than 3 to 6 feet should be maintained between the bed of the infected patient and the beds of the other patients in multiple bed rooms. Standard precautions plus a mask should be used.
  - Wear a mask on entry into the room or into the cubical space and adherence with droplet precautions should be maintained when within 3 to 6 feet of the patient.

Specific illnesses and infections requiring **Droplet Precautions** include the following:

- Adenovirus pneumonia
- Diphtheria (pharyngeal)
- *Haemophilus influenzae* type b (invasive)
- Influenza
- Middle East respiratory syndrome (MERS) (in addition to airborne and contact)
- Mumps
- *Mycoplasma pneumoniae*
- *Neisseria meningitidis* (invasive)
- Parvovirus B19 during the phase of illness before onset of rash in immunocompetent patients (see Parvovirus B19, p 593)
- Pertussis
- Plague (pneumonic)
- Rhinovirus
- Rubella
- Severe acute respiratory syndrome (SARS) (in addition to airborne and contact)
- Group A streptococcal pharyngitis or pneumonia (until appropriate antimicrobial agents have been administered for 24 hours)
- Viral hemorrhagic fevers (eg, Ebola, Lassa, Marburg)

- **Contact Transmission** is the most common route of transmission of HAIs. *Direct contact* transmission involves a direct body surface-to-body surface contact and physical transfer of microorganisms between a person with infection or colonization and a susceptible host, such as occurs when a health care professional examines a patient, turns a patient, gives a patient a bath, or performs other patient care activities that require direct personal contact. Direct contact transmission also can occur between 2 patients when one serves as the source of the infectious microorganisms and the other serves as a susceptible host. *Indirect contact* transmission involves contact of a susceptible host with a contaminated intermediate object, usually inanimate, such as contaminated instruments, needles, dressings, toys, or contaminated hands that are not cleansed or gloves that are not changed between patients.

Specific recommendations for **Contact Precautions** are as follows:

- Provide the patient with a single-patient room if possible. If unavailable, cohorting patients likely to be infected with the same organism and use of Standard and Contact Precautions are permissible.
- Gloves (clean, nonsterile) should be used at all times.
- Hand hygiene should be performed after glove removal.
- Gowns should be used during direct contact with a patient, environmental surfaces, or items in the patient room. Gowns should be worn on entry into the room and should be removed before leaving the patient's room or area.

Specific illnesses and infections with organisms requiring **Contact Precautions** include the following:

- Colonization or infection with multidrug-resistant bacteria judged by the infection-control practitioner on the basis of current state, regional, or national recommendations to be of special clinical and epidemiologic significance (eg, vancomycin-resistant enterococci, methicillin-resistant *Staphylococcus aureus,* multidrug-resistant gram-negative bacilli) or other epidemiologically important susceptible bacteria
- *C difficile*

- Conjunctivitis, viral and hemorrhagic
- Diphtheria (cutaneous)
- Enteroviruses
- *Escherichia coli* O157:H7 and other Shiga toxin-producing *E coli*
- Hepatitis A virus
- Herpes simplex virus (neonatal, mucocutaneous, or cutaneous)
- Herpes zoster (localized with no evidence of dissemination)
- Human metapneumovirus
- Impetigo
- Draining abscess, decubitus ulcer
- Parainfluenza virus
- *Pediculosis capitis, Pediculosis corporis,* and *Pediculosis pubis* (lice)
- Respiratory syncytial virus
- Rotavirus
- *Salmonella* species
- Scabies
- *Shigella* species
- *S aureus* (cutaneous or draining wounds, regardless of susceptibility to methicillin)
- Viral hemorrhagic fevers (eg, Ebola, Lassa, Marburg)

Airborne, Droplet, and **Contact Precautions** should be combined for diseases caused by organisms that have multiple routes of transmission. When used alone or in combination, these **Transmission-Based Precautions** always are to be used in addition to **Standard Precautions**, which are recommended for all patients. The specifications for these categories of isolation precautions are summarized in Table 2.9, and Table 2.10 (p 168) lists syndromes and conditions that are suggestive of contagious

Table 2.9. Transmission-Based Precautions for Hospitalized Patients[a]

Category of Precautions	Single-Patient Room	Respiratory Tract/ Mucous Membrane Protection	Gowns	Gloves
Airborne	Yes, with negative air-pressure ventilation, 6–12 air exchanges per hour, ± HEPA filtration	Respirators: N95 or higher level[b]	No[c]	No[c]
Droplet	Yes[d]	Surgical masks[e]	No[c]	No[c]
Contact	Yes[d]	No	Yes	Yes

HEPA indicates high-efficiency particulate air.

[a]These recommendations are in addition to those for **Standard Precautions** for all patients.

[b]For tuberculosis and select emerging pathogens; otherwise, surgical mask acceptable.

[c]Gowns and gloves may be required as a component of **Standard Precautions** (eg, for blood collection or during procedures likely to cause blood splashes or if there are skin lesions containing transmissible infectious agents).

[d]Preferred. Cohorting of children infected with the same pathogen is acceptable if a single-patient room is not available, a distance of more than 3 feet between patients can be maintained, and precautions are observed between all contacts with different patients in the room.

[e]Masks should be donned for all health care contact within 3 to 6 feet of the patient.

Table 2.10. Clinical Syndromes or Conditions Warranting Precautions in Addition to Standard Precautions to Prevent Transmission of Epidemiologically Important Pathogens Pending Confirmation of Diagnosis[a]

Clinical Syndrome or Condition[b]	Potential Pathogens[c]	Empiric Precautions[d]
Diarrhea		
Acute diarrhea with a likely infectious cause	Enteric pathogens[e]	Contact
Diarrhea in patient with a history of recent antimicrobial use	*Clostridium difficile*	Contact; use soap and water for handwashing
Meningitis	*Neisseria meningitidis, Haemophilus influenzae* type b	Droplet
	Enteroviruses	Contact
Rash or exanthems, generalized, cause unknown		
Petechial or ecchymotic with fever	*N meningitidis*	Droplet
	Hemorrhagic fever viruses	Contact plus Airborne
	Enteroviruses	Contact
Vesicular	Varicella-zoster virus	Airborne and Contact
Maculopapular with coryza and fever	Measles virus	Airborne
Respiratory tract infections		
Pulmonary cavitary disease	*Mycobacterium tuberculosis*	Airborne
Paroxysmal or severe persistent cough during periods of pertussis activity in the community	*Bordetella pertussis*	Droplet
Viral infections, particularly bronchiolitis and croup, in infants and young children	Respiratory viral pathogens	Contact and Droplet until adenovirus, rhinovirus, and influenza virus excluded

Table 2.10. Clinical Syndromes or Conditions Warranting Precautions in Addition to Standard Precautions to Prevent Transmission of Epidemiologically Important Pathogens Pending Confirmation of Diagnosis,[a] continued

Clinical Syndrome or Condition[b]	Potential Pathogens[c]	Empiric Precautions[d]
Risk of multidrug-resistant microorganisms[f]		
History of infection or colonization with multidrug-resistant organisms	Resistant bacteria	Contact
Skin, wound, or urinary tract infection in a patient with a recent stay in a hospital or chronic care facility	Resistant bacteria	Contact until resistant organism is excluded by cultures
Skin or wound infection		
Abscess or draining wound that cannot be covered	*Staphylococcus aureus*, group A *Streptococcus*	Contact

[a] Infection-control professionals are encouraged to modify or adapt this table according to local conditions. To ensure that appropriate empiric precautions are implemented, hospitals must have systems in place to evaluate patients routinely according to these criteria as part of their preadmission and admission care.

[b] Patients with the syndromes or conditions listed may have atypical signs or symptoms (eg, pertussis in neonates may present with apnea, paroxysmal or severe cough may be absent in pertussis in adults). The clinician's index of suspicion should be guided by the prevalence of specific conditions in the community and clinical judgment.

[c] The organisms listed in this column are not intended to represent the complete or even most likely diagnoses but, rather, possible causative agents that require additional precautions beyond **Standard Precautions** until a causative agent can be excluded.

[d] Duration of isolation varies by agent and the antimicrobial treatment administered.

[e] These pathogens include Shiga toxin–producing *Escherichia coli* including *E coli* O157:H7, *Shigella* organisms, *Salmonella* organisms, *Campylobacter* organisms, hepatitis A virus, enteric viruses including rotavirus, *Cryptosporidium* organisms, and *Giardia* organisms. Use masks when cleaning vomitus or stool during norovirus outbreak.

[f] Resistant bacteria judged by the infection control program on the basis of current state, regional, or national recommendations to be of special clinical or epidemiologic significance.

infection and require empiric isolation precautions pending identification of a specific pathogen. When the specific pathogen is known, isolation recommendations and duration of isolation are given in the pathogen- or disease-specific chapters in Section 3.

PEDIATRIC CONSIDERATIONS

Unique differences in pediatric care necessitate modifications of these guidelines, including the following: (1) diaper changing and wiping a child's tears or nose; (2) use of single-patient room isolation; and (3) use of common areas, such as hospital waiting rooms, playrooms, and schoolrooms.

Because diapering or wiping a child's nose or tears does not soil hands routinely, wearing gloves is not mandatory except when gloves are required as part of **Transmission-Based Precautions**. If gloves are worn for diaper changing—for example, for women who are pregnant or likely to be pregnant, and in cases in which soiling of hands is likely—hand hygiene should be performed before and after the diaper changing.

Single-patient rooms are recommended for all patients for **Transmission-Based Precautions** (ie, **Airborne, Droplet,** and **Contact**). Patients placed on **Transmission-Based Precautions** should not leave their rooms to use common areas, such as child life playrooms, schoolrooms, or waiting areas, except under special circumstances as defined by the facility infection-control personnel. The guidelines for **Standard Precautions** state that patients who cannot control body excretions should be in single-patient rooms. Because most young children are incontinent, this recommendation does not apply to routine care of uninfected children.

CDC isolation guidelines were developed for preventing transmission of infection in hospitals and other settings in which health care is delivered. These recommendations do not apply to schools, out-of-home child care centers, and other settings in which healthy children congregate in shared space, including ambulatory care settings.

Strategies to Prevent Health Care-Associated Infections

HAIs in patients in acute care hospitals are associated with substantial morbidity and some mortality. Important infections include central line-associated bloodstream infections, central nervous system shunt infections, surgical site infections, urinary catheter-associated urinary tract infections, ventilator-associated pneumonias, infections caused by viruses (eg, respiratory syncytial virus, rotavirus), and colitis attributable to *C difficile*. Infection-prevention strategies exist for each of these infections. The occurrence of these preventable infections is viewed as a patient safety issue, and there has been an increased emphasis on prevention. Evidence-based protocols have been shown to reduce HAIs by using "bundled strategies" (when multiple prevention activities are implemented simultaneously) and with multidisciplinary participation and collaboration with members of the health care team, including administrators, physicians, nurses, therapists, and housekeeping services. Most studies documenting a favorable effect of implementation of infection-prevention "bundles" have been performed in adult populations, and studies of infection-prevention strategies in pediatric patients are limited. Best-practice bundles in pediatrics have been developed to target reducing central line-associated bloodstream infections and ventilator-associated pneumonias.

Prevention of central line-associated bloodstream infections has been studied in pediatric patients in a multicenter investigation, and a greater than 50% reduction of infections in pediatric intensive care units has been demonstrated.[1] "Bundles" to prevent such infections include processes directed at catheter insertion and at catheter mainte- nance. Such bundles may include the following elements:

- Educate health care personnel in central venous catheter insertion and maintenance techniques relevant to infection prevention, typically with a course or video.
- Insertion practices:
  - Hand hygiene before the procedure.
  - Use of maximal sterile barrier precautions, including a large sterile drape to fully cover the patient and a mask and cap and sterile gown and gloves for the person inserting the catheter.
  - Chlorhexidine-based antiseptic scrub at the insertion site (2 minute scrub at groin; 30 second scrub for all other sites) and air drying. Although chlorhexidine is not approved for use in children younger than 2 months because of absence of safety data, a growing number of institutions are using it routinely on neonates and young infants; use of chlorhexidine in preterm infants is controversial. For neonates weigh- ing less than 1500 g at birth, an iodine-based antiseptic is recommended.
  - Use of a catheter insertion checklist and a trained observer who is empowered to halt the procedure if there is a break in the sterile technique protocol.
- Maintenance practices:
  - Catheter site care:
    - Use a chlorhexidine gluconate scrub to sites for dressing changes (scrub for 30 seconds, air dry for 30 seconds); an iodine-based antiseptic is recommended for smaller infants
    - Use a semi-permeable, transparent dressing over the catheter insertion site
    - Change clear dressings every 7 days, or more frequently if soiled, dampened, or loosened
    - Use a prepackaged dressing-change kit or gather supplies into a cart that can be positioned adjacent to the patient at the time a dressing is to be changed
    - If gauze dressings must be used because of bleeding, change every 2 days, or more frequently if soiled, dampened, or loosened
  - Disinfect catheter hubs, injection ports, and needleless connectors by vigorous rub- bing with an alcohol swab or pad for at least 15 seconds before accessing the cath- eter, a procedure sometimes called "scrub the hub"; allow hub to air dry fully before accessing.
- Evaluate patients daily to determine whether there is a continued need for the central venous catheter and remove catheter if not needed.
- Monitor infection rates and adherence to infection-prevention measures.
- Participate in transinstitutional quality improvement learning collaboratives.

Occupational Health

Transmission of infectious agents within health care settings is facilitated by close con- tact between patients and health care personnel and by lack of hygienic practices by infants and young children. **Standard Precautions** and **Transmission-Based**

---

[1]Miller MR, Niedner MF, Huskins C, et al. Reducing PICU central line-associated bloodstream infections: 3-year results. *Pediatrics*. 2011;128(5):e1077-e1083

Precautions are designed to prevent transmission of infectious agents in health care settings to limit transmission among patients and health care personnel. To further limit risks of transmission of organisms between children and health care personnel, health care facilities should have established personnel health policies and services. Specifically, personnel should be protected against vaccine-preventable diseases by establishing appropriate screening and immunization policies (see adult immunization schedule at **www.cdc. gov/vaccines/schedules/hcp/adult.html**). Guidelines for immunization of health care personnel have been published.[1]

For infections that are not vaccine preventable, personnel should be counseled about exposures and the possible need for leave from work if they are exposed to, ill with, or a carrier of a specific pathogen, whether the exposure occurs in the home, community, or health care setting.

The frequency and need for screening of health care personnel for tuberculosis should be determined by local epidemiologic data, as described in the CDC guideline for prevention of transmission of tuberculosis in health care settings.[2] People with commonly occurring infections, such as gastroenteritis, dermatitis, herpes simplex virus lesions on exposed skin, or upper respiratory tract infections, should be evaluated to determine the resulting risk of transmission to patients or to other health care personnel.

Health care personnel education, including understanding of hospital policies, is of paramount importance in infection control. Pediatric health care personnel should be knowledgeable about the modes of transmission of infectious agents, proper hand hygiene techniques, and serious risks to children from certain mild infections in adults. Frequent educational sessions will reinforce safe techniques and the importance of infection-control policies. Written policies and procedures relating to needlestick or sharp injuries are mandated by OSHA.[3] Recommendations for postinjury prophylaxis are available (see Human Immunodeficiency Virus Infection, p 453, and Table 3.31, p 463).[4,5]

Pregnant health care personnel who follow recommended precautions should not be at increased risk of infections that have possible adverse effects on the fetus (eg, parvovirus B19, cytomegalovirus, rubella, and varicella). The risk of severe influenza infection for pregnant health care personnel can be reduced by influenza immunization and adherence to appropriate infection-control precautions.

Personnel who are immunocompromised and at increased risk of severe infection (eg, *M tuberculosis*, measles virus, herpes simplex virus, and varicella-zoster virus) should seek advice from their primary health care professional.

---

[1] Centers for Disease Control and Prevention. Immunization of health-care personnel: recommendations of the Advisory Committee on Immunization Practices (ACIP). *MMWR Recomm Rep.* 2011;60(RR-7):1-44

[2] Centers for Disease Control and Prevention. Guidelines for preventing the transmission of *Mycobacterium tuberculosis* in health-care settings, 2005. *MMWR Recomm Rep.* 2005;54(RR-17):1-141

[3] Occupational Safety and Health Administration (**www.osha.gov**)

[4] Centers for Disease Control and Prevention. Updated US Public Health Service guidelines for the management of occupational exposures to HIV and recommendations for postexposure prophylaxis. *MMWR Recomm Rep.* 2005;54(RR-9):1-17

[5] Centers for Disease Control and Prevention. Guidance for evaluating health-care personnel for hepatitis B virus protection and for administering postexposure management. *MMWR Recomm Rep.* 2013;62(RR10):1-19

The consequences to pediatric patients of acquiring infections from adults can be significant. Mild illness in adults, such as viral gastroenteritis, upper respiratory tract viral infection, pertussis, or herpes simplex virus infection, can cause life-threatening disease in infants and children. People at greatest risk are preterm infants, children who have heart disease or chronic pulmonary disease, and people who are immunocompromised.

Sibling Visitation

Sibling visits to birthing centers, postpartum rooms, pediatric wards, and intensive care units are encouraged, although some institutions are choosing to restrict visitation of young children during times of peak respiratory viral activity because of their relatively high frequency of asymptomatic viral shedding and difficulties adhering to basic respiratory etiquette and hand hygiene practices. Neonatal intensive care, with its increasing sophistication, often results in long hospital stays for the preterm or sick newborn, making family visits important.

Sibling visits may benefit hospitalized children. Guidelines for sibling visits should be established to maximize opportunities for visiting and to minimize the risks of transmission of pathogens brought into the hospital by young visitors. Guidelines may need to be modified by local nursing, pediatric, obstetric, and infectious diseases staff members to address specific issues in their hospital settings. Basic guidelines for sibling visits to pediatric patients are as follows:

- Before the visit, a trained health care professional should interview the parents at a site outside the unit to assess the health of each sibling visitor. These interviews should be documented, and approval for each sibling visit should be noted. No child with fever or symptoms of an acute infection, including upper respiratory tract infection, gastroenteritis, or cellulitis, should be allowed to visit. Siblings who recently have been exposed to a person with a known communicable disease and are susceptible should not be allowed to visit.
- Siblings who are visiting should have received all recommended immunizations for their age. Before and during influenza season, siblings who visit should have received influenza vaccine.
- Asymptomatic siblings who recently have been exposed to varicella but have been immunized previously can be assumed to be immune.
- The visiting sibling should visit only his or her sibling and not be allowed in playrooms with groups of patients.
- Children should perform recommended hand hygiene before entry into the health care setting and before any patient contact.
- Throughout the visit, sibling activity should be supervised by parents or a responsible adult and limited to the mother's or patient's room or other designated areas where other patients are not present.

Adult Visitation

Guidelines should be established for visits by other relatives and close friends. Anyone with fever or contagious illnesses ideally should not visit. Medical and nursing staff members should be vigilant about potential communicable diseases in parents and other adult visitors (eg, a relative with a cough who may have pertussis or tuberculosis; a parent with a cold visiting a highly immunosuppressed child). Before and during influenza season, all visitors should be encouraged to have received the influenza vaccine. Adherence to these guidelines is especially important for oncology, hematopoietic stem cell transplant, and neonatal intensive care units.

Pet Visitation

Pet visitation in the health care setting includes visits by a child's personal pet and pet visitation as a part of child life therapeutic programs. Guidelines for pet visitation should be established to minimize risks of transmission of pathogens from pets to humans or injury from animals. The specific health care setting and the level of concern for zoonotic disease will influence establishment of pet visitation policies. The pet visitation policy should be developed in consultation with pediatricians, infection-control professionals, nursing staff, the hospital epidemiologist, and veterinarians. Basic principles for pet visitation policies in health care settings are as follows[1]:

- Personal pets other than cats and dogs should be excluded from the hospital. No reptiles (eg, iguanas, turtles, snakes), amphibians, birds, primates, ferrets, or rodents should be allowed to visit. Exceptions may be made for end-of-life patients who are in single-patient rooms.
- Visiting pets should have a certificate of immunization from a licensed veterinarian and verification that the pet is healthy. Some institutions require an assessment of temperament (eg, Canine Good Citizen certificate).
- The pet should be bathed and groomed for the visit.
- Pet visitation should be discouraged in an intensive care unit or hematology-oncology unit, but individual circumstances can be considered.
- The visit of a pet should be approved by an appropriate personnel member (eg, the director of the child life therapy program), who should observe the pet for temperament and general health at the time of visit. The pet should be free of obvious bacterial skin infections, infections caused by superficial dermatophytes, and ectoparasites (fleas and ticks).
- Pet visitation should be confined to designated areas. Contact should be confined to the petting and holding of animals, as appropriate. All contact should be supervised throughout the visit by appropriate personnel and should be followed by hand hygiene performed by the patient and all who had contact with the pet. Supervisors should be familiar with institutional policies for managing animal bites and cleaning pet urine, feces, or vomitus.
- Patients having contact with pets must have approval from a physician or physician representative before animal contact. Documented allergy to dogs or cats should be considered before approving contact. For patients who are immunodeficient or for people receiving immunosuppressive therapy, the risks of exposure to the microflora of pets may outweigh the benefits of contact. Contact of children with pets should be approved on a case-by-case basis.
- Care should be taken to protect indwelling catheter sites (eg, central venous catheters, peritoneal dialysis catheters) and other medical devices. These sites should have dressings that provide an effective barrier to pet contact, including licking, and be covered

[1]Writing Panel of Working Group; Lefebvre SL, Golab GC, Christensen E, et al. Guidelines for animal-assisted interventions in health care facilities. *Am J Infect Control.* 2008;36(2):78-85

with clothing or gown. Concern for contamination of other body sites should be considered on a case-by-case basis.

The pet policy should not apply to professionally trained service animals. These animals are not pets, and separate policies should govern their uses and presence in the hospital, according to the requirements of the Americans with Disabilities Act.

INFECTION CONTROL AND PREVENTION IN AMBULATORY SETTINGS

Infection prevention and control is an integral part of pediatric practice in ambulatory care settings as well as in hospitals. All health care personnel should be aware of the routes of transmission and techniques to prevent transmission of infectious agents. Written policies and procedures for infection prevention and control should be developed, implemented, and reviewed at least every 2 years. **Standard Precautions**, as outlined for the hospitalized child (see Infection Control and Prevention for Hospitalized Children, p 161) and by the Centers for Disease Control and Prevention (CDC),[1] with a modification by the American Academy of Pediatrics exempting the use of gloves for routine diaper changes and wiping a child's nose or tears,[2] are appropriate for most patient encounters. In addition, to help curb ambulatory health care-associated infections, the CDC has created a guideline (**www.cdc.gov/HAI/pdfs/guidelines/standatds-of-ambulatory-care-7-2011.pdf**) and checklist (**www.cdc.gov/HAI/settings/outpatient/checklist/outpatient-care-checklist.html**) that clinicians working in outpatient settings can use to help ensure that appropriate infection-control practices are being followed. Key principles of infection prevention and control in an outpatient setting are as follows:

- Infection prevention and control should begin when the child's appointment is scheduled and initiated when the child enters the office or clinic.
- Standard Precautions should be used when caring for all patients.
- Contact between contagious children and uninfected children should be minimized. Policies for children who are suspected of having contagious infections, such as varicella or measles, should be implemented. Immunocompromised children and neonates should be kept away from people with potentially contagious infections.
- In waiting rooms of ambulatory care facilities, use of respiratory hygiene/cough etiquette should be implemented for patients and accompanying people with suspected respiratory tract infection.[3]
- All health care personnel should perform hand hygiene before and after each patient contact. In health care settings, alcohol-based hand products are preferred for decontaminating hands routinely. Soap and water are preferred when hands are visibly dirty

---

[1]Centers for Disease Control and Prevention. Guideline for isolation precautions: preventing transmission of infectious agents in health care settings 2007. Recommendations of the Healthcare Infection Control Practices Advisory Committee. Atlanta, GA: Centers for Disease Control and Prevention; 2007. Available at: **www.cdc.gov/hicpac/2007IP/2007isolationPrecautions.html**

[2]American Academy of Pediatrics, Committee on Infectious Diseases. Infection prevention and control in pediatric ambulatory settings. *Pediatrics.* 2007;120(3):650-665 (Reaffirmed August 2010)

[3]Centers for Disease Control and Prevention. Respiratory Hygiene/Cough Etiquette in Healthcare Settings. Available at: **www.cdc.gov/flu/professionals/infectioncontrol/resphygiene.htm**

or contaminated with proteinaceous material, such as blood or other body fluids, and after caring for a patient with known or suspected infectious diarrhea (eg, *Clostridium difficile* or norovirus). Parents and children should be taught the importance of hand hygiene. Guidelines on hand hygiene can be found on the CDC Web site (**www.cdc. gov/handhygiene/Guidelines.html**).

- Health care personnel should receive influenza immunization annually as well as immunizations against other vaccine-preventable infections that can be transmitted in an ambulatory setting to patients or to other health care personnel. Other recommended vaccines include tetanus toxoid, reduced diphtheria toxoid, and acellular pertussis (Tdap), measles-mumps-rubella (MMR), varicella, hepatitis A, and hepatitis B.[1]
- Health care personnel should be familiar with aseptic technique, particularly regarding insertion or manipulation of intravascular catheters, performance of other invasive procedures, and preparation and administration of parenteral medications. This includes selection and use of appropriate skin antiseptics. Alcohol is preferred for skin preparation before immunization or routine venipuncture. Skin preparation for incision, suture, or collection of blood for culture requires 70% alcohol, alcohol tinctures of iodine (10%), or alcoholic chlorhexidine (>0.5%) preparations that may be superior to povidone iodine.
- Needles and sharps should be handled with great care. The use of safer medical devices designed to reduce the risk of needle sticks should be implemented. Sharps disposal containers that are impermeable and puncture resistant should be available adjacent to the areas where sharps are used (eg, areas where injections or venipunctures are performed). Sharps containers should be replaced before they become overfilled and kept out of reach of young children. Policies should be established for removal and the disposal of sharps containers consistent with state and local regulations. Guidance on safe injection practices is available on the CDC Web site (**www.cdc.gov/hicpac/pdf/ isolation/Isolation2007.pdf**).
- A written bloodborne pathogen exposure control plan that includes policies for management of exposures to blood and body fluids, such as through needlesticks and exposures of nonintact skin and mucous membranes, should be developed, readily available to all staff, and reviewed regularly (see Hepatitis B, p 400; Hepatitis C, p 423; and Human Immunodeficiency Virus Infection, p 453).
- Standard guidelines for decontamination, disinfection, and sterilization should be followed meticulously.
- Appropriate use of antimicrobial agents is essential to limit the emergence and spread of drug-resistant bacteria (see Antimicrobial Stewardship, p 874).
- Policies and procedures should be developed for communication with local and state health authorities about reportable diseases and suspected outbreaks.
- Ongoing educational programs that encompass appropriate aspects of infection control should be implemented, reinforced, documented, and evaluated on a regular basis.
- Outpatient facilities should employ or have access to an individual with training in infection prevention.
- Physicians should be aware of requirements of government agencies, such as the Occupational Safety and Health Administration, as they relate to the operation of physicians' offices.

---

[1]Centers for Disease Control and Prevention. Immunization of healthcare personnel. Recommendations of the Advisory Committee on Immunization Practices (ACIP). *MMWR Recomm Rep.* 2011;60(RR-7):1-45

SEXUALLY TRANSMITTED INFECTIONS IN ADOLESCENTS AND CHILDREN

Physicians and other health care professionals perform a critical role in preventing and treating sexually transmitted infections (STIs) in the pediatric population. STIs are a major problem for adolescents; an estimated 25% of adolescent females will acquire an STI by 19 years of age. Although an STI in an infant or child early in life can be the result of vertical transmission or autoinoculation, certain STIs (eg, gonorrhea, syphilis, chlamydia, herpes simplex virus [HSV] type 2) are indicative of sexual abuse if acquired after the neonatal period. The detection of *any* STI in an infant or child should lead the clinician to consider the possibility of sexual abuse. Whenever sexual abuse is suspected, appropriate social service and law enforcement agencies must be involved to evaluate the situation further, to ensure the child's or adolescent's protection, and to provide appropriate counseling.

STIs in Adolescents

EPIDEMIOLOGY

Adolescents and young adults have the highest rates of several STIs when compared with any other age group. Adolescents are at greater risk of STIs because they frequently have unprotected intercourse, may be more susceptible biologically to infection, often are engaged in multiple sequential monogamous partnerships of varying durations, and face several potential obstacles in accessing health education and confidential health care services.[1] Public health officials and medical professional organizations recommend routine screening of sexually active adolescent and young adult females for certain STIs, such as chlamydia and gonorrhea, but routine STI screening recommendations for males do not exist. Hence, the rates of these reported STIs are much higher in adolescent females, where routine testing is recommended, compared with males. Care must be taken when interpreting reported STI rates among adolescents because *all* adolescents, including those who have never had sexual intercourse, are included in the denominators used to calculate age-specific STI rates. Rates among sexually experienced adolescents are higher because the denominators are lower. Furthermore, many sexually active adolescents are not tested for STIs, so infections often are not diagnosed or reported.

EVALUATION

At each well-child and sick visit, the health care provider should allow some private time to speak with the adolescent confidentially, apart from the parent(s) or guardian(s). Health care providers can prepare patients and families by educating both parents and preadolescents about the need for confidentiality as adolescence approaches. Pediatricians should screen for STI risk by *routinely* asking all adolescent and young adult patients apart from their parents whether they ever have had sexual intercourse, currently are sexually active, or are planning to be sexually active in the near future. Pediatricians must be sure to define the terms "sexual intercourse" and "sexually active," because these terms can

---

[1]Centers for Disease Control and Prevention. *Sexually Transmitted Disease Surveillance 2012.* Atlanta, GA: US Department of Health and Human Services; 2013

Table 2.11. The Five P's: Partners, Prevention of Pregnancy, Protection from Sexually Transmitted Infections (STIs), Practices, and Past History of STIs: Approaches to Clinical STI Prevention[a]

1. **Partners**
   - "Do you have sex with men, women, or both?"
   - "In the past 2 months, how many partners have you had sex with?"
   - "In the past 12 months, how many partners have you had sex with?"
   - "Is it possible that any of your sex partners in the past 12 months had sex with someone else while they were still in a sexual relationship with you?"

2. **Prevention of Pregnancy**
   - "What are you doing to prevent pregnancy?"

3. **Protection From STIs**
   - "What do you do to protect yourself from STIs and HIV?"

4. **Practices**
   - "To understand your risks for STIs, I need to understand the kind of sex you have had recently."
   - "Have you had vaginal sex, meaning 'penis in vagina sex'?" If yes, "Do you use condoms: never, sometimes, or always?"
   - "Have you had anal sex, meaning 'penis in rectum/anus sex'?" If yes, "Do you use condoms: never, sometimes, or always?"
   - "Have you had oral sex, meaning 'mouth on penis/vagina'?"

   For Condom Answers:
   - If "never:" "Why don't you use condoms?"
   - If "sometimes:" "In what situations (or with whom) do you not use condoms?"

5. **Past history of STIs**
   - "Have you ever had an STI?"
   - "Have any of your partners had an STI?"

   Additional Questions to Identify HIV and Viral Hepatitis Risk Include:
   - "Have you or any of your partners ever injected drugs?"
   - "Have any of your partners exchanged money or drugs for sex?"
   - "Is there anything else about your sexual practices that I need to know about?"

HIV indicates human immunodeficiency virus.
[a]From Centers for Disease Control and Prevention. Sexually transmitted diseases treatment guidelines, 2014. *MMWR Morb Mortal Wkly Rep.* 2015; in press

have different meanings for adolescents. If a patient indicates a history of sexual activity, the health care provider must further define the type of sex (eg, vaginal, oral, or anal) and partner gender to determine what type(s) of STI testing to perform. It is important that adolescents and young adults recognize that oral and anal intercourse, as well as vaginal intercourse, put them at risk of STIs. Although some groups of adolescents and young adults are at increased risk of STIs, all should be fully immunized, screened for risk, and appropriately tested and treated (see Table 2.11). More detailed recommendations for preventive health care for adolescents and young adults are available from the American

Academy of Pediatrics (AAP)[1] and Centers for Disease Control and Prevention (CDC).[2] Despite the high prevalence of STIs among adolescents and young adults, health care professionals frequently fail to take the time to confidentially inquire about sexual behaviors, assess for STI risks, counsel about risk reduction, and screen for STIs.

Sexually active adolescent and young adult females should be screened at least annually for chlamydia and gonorrhea. The AAP and CDC suggest that providers may consider chlamydia screening for sexually active adolescent and young adult males with a history of multiple partners in settings with high chlamydia prevalence rates, such as jails or juvenile correctional facilities, national job training programs, STI clinics, high school clinics, or adolescent clinics. Because asymptomatic gonorrhea infection among males is uncommon and substantial disparities in disease prevalence exist, providers should consider gonorrhea screening of sexually active adolescent and young adult males annually on the basis of individual and population-based risk factors, such as disparities by race and neighborhoods. The AAP and CDC also recommend screening males who have sex with males (MSM) at least annually for urethral and rectal chlamydia and gonorrhea infection and for oropharyngeal gonorrhea infection on the basis of reported sexual practices and screening every 3 to 6 months if the male adolescent is considered high risk because of multiple or anonymous partners, sex in conjunction with illicit drug use, or having sex partners who participate in these activities. Sex partners of chlamydia- or gonorrhea-infected individuals during the 2 months before the diagnosis should also be targeted for testing and treatment because of their high likelihood of infection.

Highly sensitive nucleic acid amplification tests (NAATs) are available that enable testing for gonorrhea and chlamydia with less-invasive specimens, such as vaginal swab specimens or urine specimens; an invasive genital examination is not necessary for an asymptomatic adolescent or young adult.[3] Chlamydia and gonorrhea NAATs are cleared by the US Food and Drug Administration (FDA) to test urine, urethral, vaginal (provider or patient collected), cervical, and liquid cytology specimens. Package inserts for individual NAAT products must be reviewed, however, because the particular specimens approved for use with each test may vary. Female vaginal swab specimens and male urine specimens are the CDC-recommended specimen types. Female urine remains an acceptable chlamydia and gonorrhea NAAT specimen but may have slightly reduced performance when compared with cervical or vaginal swab specimens. Although chlamydia and gonorrhea NAATs are not FDA approved for nongenital (eg, oral or rectal swab specimen) testing, laboratories that have met Clinical Laboratory Improvement Amendment (CLIA) and other regulatory requirements and have validated performance on rectal and oral swab specimens may offer these tests. Large clinical laboratories and many local clinic laboratories offer nongenital chlamydia and gonorrhea NAATs.

Although the AAP and CDC do not recommend routine *Trichomonas vaginalis* screening of asymptomatic adolescents, screening may be considered for adolescent and young adult females at high risk of infection. Factors that may put females at higher risk of

---

[1]American Academy of Pediatrics, Committee on Adolescence and Society for Adolescent Health and Medicine. Screening for nonviral sexually transmitted infections in adolescents and young adults. *Pediatrics* 2014;134(1):e302-e311

[2]Centers for Disease Control and Prevention. Sexually transmitted diseases treatment guidelines, 2014. *MMWR Morb Mortal Wkly Rep.* 2015; in press

[3]Centers for Disease Control and Prevention. Recommendations for the laboratory-based detection of *Chlamydia trachomatis* and *Neisseria gonorrhoeae*—2014. *MMWR Recomm Rep.* 2014;63(RR-2):1-19

T vaginalis infection include new or multiple partners and a history of STIs. Two NAATs are FDA cleared for *T vaginalis* testing. In addition, point-of-care tests, a DNA probe test, and culture are available to test for *T vaginalis*. Although convenient and inexpensive, microscopic evaluation of wet preparations of genital secretions has suboptimal sensitivity (51%–65%) in females and even less sensitive in males, and test sensitivity declines if the evaluation is delayed.[1]

Routine syphilis screening of nonpregnant, heterosexual adolescents and young adults is not recommended. However, the AAP recommends screening for all sexually active adolescent and young adult MSM annually or every 3 to 6 months if high risk, and screening can be considered for youth whose behaviors put them at higher risk.

In the evaluation of the postpubertal adolescent and young adult sexual assault victim, gonorrhea and chlamydia diagnostic evaluation from any sites of penetration or attempted penetration should be performed per CDC guidance. However, local legal authorities will determine acceptance of specific test results in court. Some jurisdictions may prefer *C trachomatis* and *N gonorrhoeae* culture from all sites in lower-prevalence populations because of greater specificity, although sensitivity may be compromised. In addition, the CDC recommends performing a wet mount and culture or point-of-care testing of a vaginal swab specimen for *T vaginalis* infection and a serum sample for immediate evaluation for human immunodeficiency virus (HIV) infection, hepatitis B, and syphilis.

In the evaluation of prepubescent children for possible sexual assault, the CDC recommends cultures for *C trachomatis* collected from the rectum in both boys and girls and from the vagina in girls. A meatal specimen should be obtained from boys for chlamydia testing if urethral discharge is present. Specimen collection for *N gonorrhoeae* culture should include the pharynx and rectum in boys and girls, the vagina in girls, and the urethra in boys. If urethral discharge is present, a meatal specimen is an adequate substitute for an intra-urethral swab specimen. The CDC indicates that NAATs can be used as alternative to culture with vaginal swab or urine specimens from girls only, although consultation with an expert is necessary before use of NAATs in children to minimize the possibility of positive reactions with nongonococcal *Neisseria* species and other commensals. Culture and wet mount of a vaginal swab specimen should also be tested for *T vaginalis* infection and bacterial vaginosis (BV).[2,3]

The CDC also recommends, for the prepubescent sexual assault evaluation, collection of serum samples that can be tested for *T pallidum*, HIV, and hepatitis B virus (HBV) antibodies. Decisions regarding the agents for which to perform serologic tests immediately, specimens preserved for subsequent analysis, and specimens used as a baseline for comparison with follow-up serologic tests should be made on a case-by-case basis.

Sexually active adolescents should receive HIV- and syphilis-prevention counseling at least annually and HIV screening, with frequency of additional testing based on individual risk factors. Papanicolaou (Pap) tests to screen for cervical dysplasia associated with human papillomavirus (HPV) infection should be delayed until the 21st birthday in immunocompetent females, regardless of sexual history. For adolescent females who are

[1]Centers for Disease Control and Prevention. Sexually transmitted diseases treatment guidelines, 2014. *MMWR Morb Mortal Wkly Rep.* 2015; in press

[2]Centers for Disease Control and Prevention. *Sexually Transmitted Disease Surveillance 2012.* Atlanta, GA: US Department of Health and Human Services; 2013

[3]American Academy of Pediatrics, Committee on Adolescence and Society for Adolescent Health and Medicine. Screening for nonviral sexually transmitted infections in adolescents and young adults. *Pediatrics* 2014;134(1):e302-e311

immunosuppressed or immunocompromised, yearly Pap tests should begin with the initiation of sexual intercourse. All adolescents should receive hepatitis B virus immunization if they were not immunized earlier in childhood. HPV vaccine is recommended routinely for 11- or 12-year-olds. Following sexual victimization, the HPV vaccine series should be started as early as 9 years of age (see Human Papillomaviruses, p 576). HPV vaccine is recommended for females 13 through 26 years of age and for males 13 through 21 years of age who have not yet received or completed the vaccine series. Males 22 through 26 years of age may be vaccinated. However, MSM and immunocompromised 22- through 26-year-olds should receive HPV vaccine. Hepatitis A vaccine (HepA) should be offered to adolescents and young adults who have not previously received the HepA vaccine series if immunity against hepatitis A virus is desired or for those at increased risk of infection, such as MSM, patients who live in areas in which older children are targeted for HepA vaccination (see Recommended Childhood and Adolescent Immunization Schedules, **http://redbook.solutions.aap.org/SS/Immunization_Schedules.aspx**), and others at high risk of hepatitis A virus infection (see Hepatitis A, p 391).

MANAGEMENT

All 50 states allow minors to give their own consent for confidential STI testing, diagnosis, and treatment. Pediatricians should consult their own state laws for further guidance. For treatment recommendations for specific STIs, see the disease-specific chapters in Section 3 and Table 4.4, Guidelines for Treatment of Sexually Transmitted Infections in Children and Adolescents According to Syndrome (p 896). Single-dose therapies are available for many STIs, offering the advantage of high patient adherence; directly observed therapy should be provided where feasible. Patients and their partners treated for *N gonorrhoeae*, *C trachomatis*, pelvic inflammatory disease, and trichomoniasis should be advised to refrain from sexual intercourse for 1 week after completion of appropriate treatment.

People diagnosed with uncomplicated urogenital or rectal gonorrhea who are treated with any of the recommended or alternative regimens do not need a test-of-cure. However, any person with pharyngeal gonorrhea who is treated with an alternative regimen should return 14 days after treatment for a test-of cure, using either culture or NAAT. If the NAAT result is positive, every effort should be made to perform a confirmatory culture. All positive cultures for test-of-cure should undergo antimicrobial susceptibility testing. Symptoms that persist after treatment should be evaluated by culture for *N gonorrhoeae* (with or without simultaneous NAAT), and any gonococci isolated should be tested for antimicrobial susceptibility. Persistent urethritis, cervicitis, or proctitis also might be caused by other organisms.[1]

Retesting of people in whom urogenital chlamydia is diagnosed who are treated with a recommended or alterative regimens is not recommended unless therapeutic adherence is in question, symptoms persist, or reinfection is suspected. Moreover, the use of chlamydial NAAT testing at <3 weeks after completion of therapy is not recommended, because false-positive results might occur as a result of the continued presence of nonviable organisms.[1]

Because reinfection by an untreated partner or a new sexual partner is common, pediatricians should rescreen all males and females treated for chlamydia and gonorrhea, as well as for *T vaginalis* in females, approximately 3 months after treatment. If retesting at

---

[1]Centers for Disease Control and Prevention. *Sexually Transmitted Disease Surveillance 2012.* Atlanta, GA: US Department of Health and Human Services; 2013

3 months is not possible, retest whenever patients next present for health care in the 12 months after initial treatment.

Partner treatment is essential, both from a public health perspective and to protect the index patient from reinfection. Sexual partners during the past 60 days should be informed of the infection and encouraged to seek out comprehensive STI evaluation and treatment. If it appears unlikely that partners of patients treated for gonococcal or chlamydial infections will seek care, pediatricians may consider providing expedited partner therapy (EPT) to patients.[1] EPT is the clinical practice of treating the sex partners of patients with diagnosed chlamydia or gonorrhea by providing prescriptions or medications to the patient to take to his/her partner without the health care provider first examining the partner. Information should be provided warning about the low risk of potential adverse events and allergic reactions to EPT, with instructions to seek medical attention in the event that an adverse reaction occurs. The legality of prescribing EPT varies by state. Guidance on the legal status of EPT by jurisdiction is available from CDC (**www.cdc.gov/std/ept**).

PREVENTION

Pediatricians can contribute to primary prevention of STIs by encouraging and supporting a teenager's decision to postpone initiating sexual intercourse. For teenagers who become sexually active, pediatricians should discuss methods of protecting against STIs and unwanted pregnancies, including the correct and consistent use of condoms with all forms of sexual intercourse (vaginal, oral, and anal). Teenagers need to consider the possible association between alcohol or drug use and failure to appropriately use barrier methods correctly when either partner is impaired. Clinicians also should discuss other ways to decrease risk of acquiring STIs, including limiting the number of partners and choosing to abstain even if initiation of sexual intercourse already has occurred.

Preadolescents should be vaccinated against HPV (see Human Papillomaviruses, p 576).[2] Adolescents who have not previously been vaccinated against HPV or hepatitis B should complete the immunization series.

Diagnosis and Treatment of STIs in Children

Because of social and legal implications of a positive STI test result, STIs in children must be diagnosed using tests with high specificity. Therefore, tests that allow for isolation of the organism and have the highest specificities should be used whenever possible. There is increasing evidence that NAATs can be used for this purpose, as the newest technology has shown increased sensitivity compared with culture, and there are patient advantages to single-specimen collection and specimen stability.[3]

Specimens for *N gonorrhoeae* culture should be collected from the pharynx and anus in boys and girls, the vagina in girls and the urethra in boys. Cervical specimens are not recommended for prepubertal girls.[1] Because of the legal implications of a diagnosis of

---

[1] Centers for Disease Control and Prevention. *Sexually Transmitted Disease Surveillance 2012*. Atlanta, GA: US Department of Health and Human Services; 2013

[2] Centers for Disease Control and Prevention. Human papillomavirus vaccination: recommendations of the Advisory Committee on Immunization Practices (ACIP). *MMWR Recomm Rep.* 2014;63(RR-5):1–30

[3] American Academy of Pediatrics, Committee on Adolescence and Society for Adolescent Health and Medicine. Screening for nonviral sexually transmitted infections in adolescents and young adults. *Pediatrics* 2014:134(1):e302–e311

N gonorrhoeae infection in a child, if culture for the isolation of *N gonorrhoeae* is performed, only standard culture procedures should be performed. Data on use of NAATs for detection of *N gonorrhoeae* in children are limited, and performance is test dependent.[1] Consultation with an expert is necessary before using NAATs in this context, both to minimize the possibility of cross-reaction with nongonococcal *Neisseria* species and other commensals (eg, *N meningitidis*, *Neisseria sicca*, *Neisseria lactamica*, *Neisseria cinerea*, and *Moraxella catarrhalis*), and to ensure appropriate interpretation of positive results. NAATs can be used as an alternative to culture with vaginal specimens or urine from girls, whereas culture remains the preferred method for urethral specimens or urine from boys and for extragenital specimens (pharynx and rectum) from all children.[1,2] All positive specimens should be retained for additional testing. Specimens for *C trachomatis* culture should be collected from the anus in both boys and girls and from the vagina in girls. NAATs can be used for detection of *C trachomatis* in vaginal specimens or urine from girls. All specimens should be retained for additional testing. No data are available regarding the use of NAATs in boys or for extragenital specimens (eg, those obtained from the rectum) in boys and girls. Culture remains the preferred method for extragenital sites.

If vaginal discharge is present, specimens for wet mount, NAAT, or culture for *T vaginalis* and wet mount or Gram stain for bacterial vaginosis may be obtained as well. Serum specimens for syphilis and HIV testing should be obtained. Completion of the hepatitis B immunization series should be documented, or the patient should be screened for hepatitis B surface antibody. Completion of the HPV immunization series for children 9 years and older should be documented. Because of the serious implications of the diagnosis of an STI in a child suspected of being the victim of sexual abuse, antimicrobial therapy may need to be withheld until the diagnostic testing for STIs has been performed. For more detailed diagnosis and treatment recommendations for specific STIs, see the disease-specific chapters in Section 3 and Table 4.4, Guidelines for Treatment of Sexually Transmitted Infections in Children and Adolescents According to Syndrome (p 896).

Social Implications of STIs in Children

Children can acquire STIs through vertical transmission, by autoinoculation, or by sexual contact. Each of these mechanisms should be given appropriate consideration in evaluation of a preadolescent child with an STI. Evaluation for the possibility of sexual abuse solely on the basis of suspicion of an STI should not proceed until the STI diagnosis has been confirmed. Factors to be considered in assessing the likelihood of sexual abuse in a child with an STI include the biological characteristics of the STI in question, the age of the child, and whether the child reports a history of sexual victimization (see Table 2.12, p 184). When victimization is reported by a child or adolescent, the risk factors for STIs in a possible assailant (when available), as well as the history of type of sexual contact, may also guide testing and treatment.

Anogenital gonorrhea in a prepubertal child is indicative of sexual abuse. All confirmed cases of gonorrhea in prepubertal children beyond the neonatal period should be reported to the local child protective services agency for investigation.

---

[1]American Academy of Pediatrics, Committee on Adolescence and Society for Adolescent Health and Medicine. Screening for nonviral sexually transmitted infections in adolescents and young adults. *Pediatrics* 2014:134(1):e302–e311

[2]Centers for Disease Control and Prevention. *Sexually Transmitted Disease Surveillance 2012*. Atlanta, GA: US Department of Health and Human Services; 2013

Table 2.12. Implications of Commonly Encountered Sexually Transmitted (ST) or Sexually Associated (SA) Infections for Diagnosis and Reporting of Sexual Abuse Among Infants and Prepubertal Children

ST/SA Confirmed	Evidence for Sexual Abuse	Suggested Action
Neisseria gonorrhoeae[a]	Diagnostic	Report[b]
Syphilis[a]	Diagnostic	Report[b]
Human immunodeficiency virus[c]	Diagnostic	Report[b]
Chlamydia trachomatis[a]	Diagnostic	Report[b]
Trichomonas vaginalis[a]	Highly suspicious	Report[b]
Genital herpes	Highly suspicious (HSV-2 especially)	Report[b,d]
Condylomata acuminata (anogenital warts)[a]	Suspicious	Consider report[b,d,e]
Bacterial vaginosis	Inconclusive	Medical follow-up

[a]If not likely to be perinatally acquired and rare nonsexual, vertical transmission is excluded.
[b]Reports should be made to the agency in the community mandated to receive reports of suspected child abuse or neglect.
[c]If not likely to be acquired perinatally or through transfusion.
[d]Unless there is a clear history of autoinoculation.
[e]Report if there is additional evidence to suspect abuse, including history, physical examination or other infections identified.

Table adapted from Kellogg N; American Academy of Pediatrics, Committee on Child Abuse and Neglect. The evaluation of sexual abuse in children. *Pediatrics.* 2005;116(2):506–512. Updated 2013 Clinical Report available at **http://pediatrics.aap-publications.org/content/132/2/e558.full.pdf+html**

First-episode symptomatic HSV infection has a short incubation period. HSV can be transmitted by sexual or nonsexual contact with another person or by self-inoculation. In an infant or toddler in diapers, genital herpes may result through any of these mechanisms. Viral typing for HSV-1 and HSV-2 will yield additional helpful information. In a prepubertal child, the new occurrence of genital herpes attributable to HSV-2 should prompt a careful investigation, including a child protective services investigation, for suspected sexual abuse. A significant percentage of genital herpes acquired sexually in adolescent and adult populations now is caused by HSV-1, but when HSV-1 genital infection occurs in a prepubertal child, it can be challenging to differentiate sexual abuse from autoinoculation (from the patient's own mouth via their hand, for example).

Trichomoniasis is transmitted perinatally or by sexual contact. In a perinatally infected infant, vaginal discharge can persist for several weeks; accordingly, intense social investigation may not be warranted. However, a new diagnosis of trichomoniasis in an older infant or child should prompt a careful investigation, including a child protective services investigation, for suspected sexual abuse.

Infections that have long incubation periods (eg, HPV infection) and that can be asymptomatic for a period of time after vertical transmission (eg, syphilis, HIV infection, and *C trachomatis* infection) are more problematic. The possibility of vertical transmission should be considered in these cases, but an evaluation of the patient's circumstances by the local child protective services agency usually is warranted. With the exception of HPV, these infections raise a very high suspicion for sexual abuse.

Although hepatitis B virus, hepatitis C virus, scabies, and pediculosis pubis may be transmitted sexually, other modes of transmission can occur. The discovery of any of these conditions in a prepubertal child does not warrant child protective services involvement unless the clinician finds other information that suggests abuse.

Sexual Victimization and STIs

GENERAL CONSIDERATIONS

Child sexual abuse has been defined as the exploitation of a child, either by physical contact or by other interactions, for the sexual gratification of an adult or a minor who is in a position of power over the child. Physicians are required by law to report known or suspected abuse to their local state child protective services agency. Approximately 5% of sexually abused children acquire an STI as a result of the victimization.

SCREENING ASYMPTOMATIC SEXUALLY VICTIMIZED CHILDREN FOR STIs

Factors that influence the likelihood that a sexually victimized child will acquire an STI include the regional prevalence of STIs in the adult population, the number of assailants, the type and frequency of physical contact between the perpetrator(s) and the child, the infectivity of various microorganisms, the child's susceptibility to infection, and whether the child has received antimicrobial treatment. The time interval between a child's physical contact with an assailant and the medical evaluation influences the likelihood that an exposed child will demonstrate signs or symptoms of an STI.

The decision to obtain specimens from genital or other areas from a child who has been victimized sexually to conduct an STI evaluation must be made on an individual basis. The following situations involve a high risk of STIs and constitute a strong indication for testing:
• The child has or has had signs or symptoms of an STI or an infection that can be transmitted sexually, even in the absence of suspicion of sexual abuse.
• A sibling, another child, or an adult in the household or child's immediate environment has an STI.
• A suspected assailant is known to have an STI or to be at high risk of STIs (eg, has had multiple sexual partners or a history of STIs) or has an unknown history.
• The patient or family requests testing.
• Evidence of genital, oral, or anal penetration or ejaculation is present.
See Table 2.13 (p 186) if STI testing of a child is to be performed.

Most experts recommend universal screening of postpubertal patients who have been victims of sexual abuse or assault because of the possibility of a preexisting asymptomatic infection. When STI screening is performed, it should focus on likely anatomic sites of infection as determined by the patient's history and physical examination or by epidemiologic considerations and should include assessment for HIV infection if the patient, family, or both consent to serologic screening; assessment for bacterial vaginosis and trichomoniasis for female patients; and testing for *N gonorrhoeae* infection, *C trachomatis* infection, and syphilis. To preserve the "chain of custody" for information that may later constitute legal evidence, specimens for laboratory analysis obtained from sexually victimized patients should be labeled carefully, and standard hospital procedures for transferring specimens from site to site should be followed carefully. Tests with high specificities should

Table 2.13. Sexually Transmitted Infection (STI) Testing in a Child[a] When Sexual Abuse Is Suspected

Organism/Syndrome	Specimens
Neisseria gonorrhoeae[b]	Rectal, throat, urethral (male), and/or vaginal cultures[c]
Chlamydia trachomatis[b]	Rectal, urethral (male), and vaginal cultures[c]
Syphilis	Darkfield examination of chancre fluid, if present; blood for serologic tests at time of abuse and 6, 12, and 24 wk later
Human immunodeficiency virus	Serologic testing of abuser (if possible); serologic testing of child at time of abuse and 6, 12, and 24 wk later
Hepatitis B virus	Serum hepatitis B surface antigen testing of abuser or hepatitis B surface antibody testing of child, unless the child has received 3 doses of hepatitis B vaccine
Herpes simplex virus (HSV)	Culture of lesion specimen; in addition, polymerase chain reaction assay of lesion specimen if lesion crusted; all virologic specimens should be typed (HSV-1 vs HSV-2)
Bacterial vaginosis	Wet mount, pH, and potassium hydroxide testing of vaginal discharge or Gram stain in pubertal and postmenarcheal girls
Human papillomavirus	Clinical examination, with biopsy of lesion specimen if diagnosis unclear
Trichomonas vaginalis	Wet mount and culture of vaginal discharge[b]
Pediculosis pubis	Identification of eggs, nymphs, and lice with naked eye or using hand lens

[a]See text for indications for testing for STIs (Screening Asymptomatic Sexually Victimized Children for STIs, p 185).
[b]Nucleic acid amplification tests can be used as an alternative to culture with vaginal specimens or urine from girls.
[c]Cervical specimens are not recommended or necessary for prepubertal girls, but cervical specimens must be obtained in pubertal premenarchal and pubertal postmenarcheal girls.

be used, and whenever possible, specimens should be obtained by health care professionals with experience in the evaluation of children who have been sexually abused or assaulted. Consultation with an expert is necessary before using NAATs for gonorrhea in this context to minimize the possibility of cross-reaction with nongonococcal *Neisseria* species and to ensure appropriate interpretation of test results.[1] NAATs can be used for detection of *C trachomatis* in vaginal specimens or urine from girls. All specimens should be retained for additional testing. No data are available regarding the use of NAATs in boys or for extragenital specimens (eg, those obtained from the rectum) in boys and girls. Culture remains the preferred method for extragenital sites. A follow-up visit approximately 2 to 6 weeks after the most recent sexual exposure may include a repeat physical examination and collection of additional specimens. Another follow-up visit at 3 and 6 months after the most recent sexual exposure may be necessary to obtain convalescent sera to test for hepatitis B (if indicated), syphilis, and HIV infection.

---

[1]American Academy of Pediatrics, Committee on Adolescence and Society for Adolescent Health and Medicine. Screening for nonviral sexually transmitted infections in adolescents and young adults. *Pediatrics* 2014;134(1):e302–e311

PROPHYLAXIS AFTER SEXUAL VICTIMIZATION

Presumptive treatment for children who have been sexually assaulted or abused is not recommended, because their incidence of STIs is low, the risk of spread to the upper genital tract in prepubertal girls is low, and follow-up usually can be ensured. If a test result for an STI is positive, treatment then can be given. Factors that may increase the likelihood of infection or that constitute an indication for prophylaxis are the same as those listed under Screening Asymptomatic Sexually Victimized Children for STIs (p 185).

Many experts believe that prophylaxis is warranted for **postpubertal** female patients who seek care after an episode of sexual victimization because of the possibility of a preexisting asymptomatic infection, the potential risk for acquisition of new infections with the assault, the substantial risk of pelvic inflammatory disease in this age group, and poor compliance with follow-up visits for sexual assault.[1] All patients who receive prophylaxis should be tested for relevant STIs (see Table 2.13, p 186) before treatment begins. The decision regarding which specimens and tests to obtain can be made on an individual basis depending on local STI prevalence, prior risk factors, the nature of the sexual assault (ie, sexual abuse over time or one-time assault), or the type of sexual exposure (ie, oral, vaginal, or anal exposure). Postmenarcheal patients should be tested for pregnancy before antimicrobial treatment or emergency contraception is provided. Regimens for prophylaxis are presented in Table 2.14.

Because of the demonstrated effectiveness of prophylaxis to prevent HIV infection after perinatal and occupational exposures, the question arises whether HIV prophylaxis is warranted for children and adolescents after sexual assault (also see Human Immunodeficiency Virus Infection, Control Measures, p 470, and Table 3.32, p 472). The risk of HIV transmission from a single sexual assault that involves transfer of secretions and/or blood is low. Prophylaxis may be considered for patients who seek care within 72 hours after an assault if the assault involved mucosal exposure to secretions; repeated abuse; multiple assailants; oral, vaginal, and/or anal trauma; and particularly if the alleged perpetrator(s) is known to have or is at high risk of having HIV infection (see Human Immunodeficiency Virus Infection, p 453).[2]

The following are recommendations for postexposure assessment of children within 72 hours of sexual assault:

- Review HIV/acquired immunodeficiency syndrome (AIDS) local epidemiology and assess risk of HIV infection in the assailant.
- Evaluate circumstances of assault that may affect risk of HIV transmission.
- Consult with a specialist in treating HIV-infected children if postexposure prophylaxis is considered.
- If the child appears to be at risk of HIV transmission from the assault, discuss postexposure prophylaxis with the caregiver(s), including toxicity and unknown efficacy.

---

[1]Kaufmann M; American Academy of Pediatrics, Committee on Adolescence. Care of the adolescent sexual assault victim. *Pediatrics*. 2008;122(2):462-470

[2]Centers for Disease Control and Prevention. Antiretroviral postexposure prophylaxis after sexual, injection-drug use, or other nonoccupational exposure to HIV in the United States: recommendations from the US Department of Health and Human Services. *MMWR Recomm Rep*. 2005;54(RR-2):1-20

Table 2.14. Prophylaxis After Sexual Victimization: Postpubertal Adolescents

Antimicrobial prophylaxis[a] is recommended to include an empiric regimen to prevent chlamydia, gonorrhea, trichomoniasis, and bacterial vaginosis. Vaccination against hepatitis B and HPV is recommended if not fully immunized.

For gonorrhea	Ceftriaxone, 250 mg, intramuscularly, in a single dose
	PLUS
For dual therapy for gonorrhea and chlamydia	Azithromycin, 1 g, orally, in a single dose
	OR
	Doxycycline, 100 mg, orally, twice a day for 7 days (for those ≥8 y and not pregnant)
	PLUS
For trichomoniasis and bacterial vaginosis	Metronidazole,[b] 2 g, orally, in a single dose or tinidazole, 2 g, orally, in a single dose
	PLUS
For hepatitis B virus infection	Hepatitis B virus immunization at time of initial examination, if not fully immunized. Follow-up doses of vaccine should be administered 1–2 and 4–6 mo after the first dose
	PLUS
For human immunodeficiency virus (HIV) infection[a]	Consider offering prophylaxis for HIV, depending on circumstances (see Table 3.32, p 472)
	PLUS
For HPV	HPV vaccine series should be initiated at ≥9 y if not already given or completed if not fully immunized (3 doses)

Emergency contraception[c]

Levonorgestrel, 1.5 mg, orally, in a single dose

OR

Ulipristal acetate, 30 mg, orally, in a single dose

OR

Oral contraceptive pills, each containing 20 or 30 μg of ethinyl estradiol plus 0.1 mg or 0.15 mg of levonorgestrel or 0.3 mg of norgestrel: each of 2 doses must be given 12 h apart. Each dose must contain at least 100 to 120 μg of ethinyl estradiol and 0.5 to 0.6 mg of levonorgestrel or 1 mg of norgestrel.

HPV indicates human papillomavirus.

Source: Centers for Disease Control and Prevention. Sexually transmitted diseases treatment guidelines, 2014. *MMWR Morb Mortal Wkly Rep.* 2015; in press

[a]See text for discussion of prophylaxis for human immunodeficiency virus (HIV) infection after sexual abuse or assault.

[b]Metronidazole or tinidazole can be taken by the patient at home rather than as directly observed therapy to minimize potential side effects and drug interactions, especially if emergency contraception is provided or alcohol has been recently ingested.

[c]The patient should have a negative pregnancy test result before emergency contraception is given. Although levonorgestrel emergency contraception is most effective if taken within 72 hours of event, data suggest it is effective up to 120 hours. Ulipristal acetate is effective up to 120 hours after unprotected intercourse.

- If caregivers choose for the child to receive antiretroviral postexposure prophylaxis, provide enough medication until the return visit at 3 to 7 days after initial assessment to reevaluate the child and to assess tolerance of medication; dosages should not exceed those for adults.
- Perform HIV antibody test at original assessment, 6 weeks, and 3 months.

HEPATITIS AND YOUTH IN CORRECTIONAL SETTINGS[1]

Pediatricians should work with state and local public health agencies and administrators of correctional facilities to address the health needs of youth in detention and to protect the community. The number of arrests of juveniles (younger than 18 years) in the United States reached a historic low of 1.64 million in 2010, 9% less than the number of arrests in 2009 and 21% less than in 2001.[2] Juveniles accounted for 14% of all violent crime arrests and 22% of all property crime arrests in 2010. On any given day, approximately 120 000 adolescents are held in juvenile correctional facilities or adult prisons or jails. Incarceration periods of at least 90 days await 60% of juvenile inmates, and 15% can expect to be confined for a year or more behind bars.[3] Males account for approximately 85% of juvenile offenders in residential placement, and 61% of juveniles in correctional facilities are members of ethnic or racial minority groups. Female juveniles in custody represent a much larger proportion of "status" offenders, with offenses including ungovernability, running away, truancy, curfew violation, and underage drinking, than "delinquent" offenders who have committed offenses against other people or property (40% vs 14%, respectively).

Juvenile offenders commonly lack regular access to preventive health care in their communities and suffer significantly greater health deficiencies, including psychosocial disorders, chronic illness, exposure to illicit drugs, and physical trauma when compared with adolescents who are not in the juvenile justice system. Detained youth are more likely to have contracted sexually transmitted infections (STIs) early in adolescence, and delayed or incomplete treatment places them at increased risk of chronic complications of chlamydia, gonorrhea, syphilis, and human papillomavirus infections. Tuberculosis (TB) is more common in correctional populations, and although current juvenile detainees continue to have a low prevalence of human immunodeficiency virus (HIV) infection, their high-risk behaviors place them at significant risk. Hepatitis A virus (HAV), hepatitis B virus (HBV), and hepatitis C virus (HCV) infections are of particular concern for juvenile detainees because of their increased frequency of alcohol and injection drug use and increased rate of unprotected sex with multiple partners early in life. While the rate of juvenile arrests for drug abuse violations decreased 15% between 2001 and 2010, a history of injection drug use has played a major role in explaining the increased incidence of HCV infections in adolescent offenders. Infected juveniles place their communities at risk after their release from detention. Personal knowledge of an infection and its transmissibility may allow youth to take preventive measures to reduce their risk of transmitting infection to others.

Up to 15% of all chronic HBV infections and more than 30% of all HCV infections known to exist in the United States are found among people with a history of

---

[1] Centers for Disease Control and Prevention. Prevention and control of infections with hepatitis viruses in correctional settings. *MMWR Recomm Rep.* 2003;52(RR-1):1-33

[2] Puzzanchera C. Juvenile arrests 2010. *Juvenile Offenders and Victims: National Report Series.* Washington, DC: US Department of Justice, Office of Justice Programs, Office of Juvenile Justice and Delinquency Prevention; December 2013. Available at: **www.ojjdp.gov/pubs/242770.pdf**

[3] Puzzanchera C. Juvenile arrests 2008. *Juvenile Justice Bulletin.* Washington, DC: US Department of Justice, Office of Justice Programs, Office of Juvenile Justice and Delinquency Prevention; December 2009. Available at: **www.ncjrs.gov/pdffiles1/ojjdp/228479.pdf**

incarceration. High-risk behaviors make adolescents particularly vulnerable to HAV, HBV, and HCV infections well before their first incarceration. Less than 3% of new hepatitis virus infections of all types are acquired once incarceration has occurred. Most juvenile offenders ultimately are returned to their community and, without intervention, resume a high-risk lifestyle. High recidivism rates lead many juvenile offenders to adult prisons, where the prevalence of HBV and HCV infections may be significantly higher than those found in juvenile correctional facilities. Viral hepatitis also can be a comorbid condition with other diseases, including TB and HIV infection. HIV-infected adolescents should be tested for hepatitis B surface antigen (HBsAg) as soon as possible after their diagnosis. Correctional facilities, in partnership with public health departments and other community resources, have the opportunity to assess, contain, control, and prevent liver infection in a highly vulnerable segment of the population. HCV presents the greatest challenge to correctional facilities overall because of the lack of a vaccine to protect prisoners and the public. The extremely high rate of chronic carriage after infection increases the risk of transmission when youth are released into their communities. The controlled nature of the correctional system facilitates initiation of many hepatitis-prevention (eg, education and counseling) and -treatment strategies for an adolescent population that otherwise is difficult to reach.

Hepatitis A

Correctional facilities in the United States rarely report cases of hepatitis A, and national prevalence data for incarcerated populations are not available. States that have assessed prevalence of past infection in incarcerated populations younger than 20 years show a similar ethnic distribution of predominance in American Indian/Alaska Native and Hispanic inmates and documented and undocumented people from Mexico, as is reflected in the population as a whole. Some estimates suggest an overall seroprevalence of antibody to HAV between 22% and 39% in the adult prison population, with up to a 43% prevalence found in older prisoners between 40 and 49 years of age. Risk factors that could contribute to outbreaks of hepatitis A among adolescents include using injection and noninjection street drugs, having multiple sexual partners, and participating in male-with-male sexual activity.

RECOMMENDATIONS FOR CONTROL OF HAV INFECTIONS IN INCARCERATED YOUTH

Routine screening of incarcerated youth for HAV serologic markers is not recommended. However, adolescents who have signs or symptoms of hepatitis should be tested for acute hepatitis A, acute hepatitis B, and hepatitis C. Hepatitis A vaccine (HepA; see Hepatitis A Vaccine, p 394) should be given to all adolescents who have acknowledged identified risk behaviors (eg, use of injection and noninjection street drugs, having multiple sexual partners, and participating in male-with-male sexual activity) or who have not previously received the HepA vaccine series if immunity against HAV is desired. Correctional facilities in all states should consider routine HepA immunization of all adolescents under their care because of the likelihood that most adolescents in the juvenile correctional system have indications for HepA immunization. If this is not possible, HepA vaccine should be provided to juveniles with high-risk profiles, including illicit drug users and male adolescents who may engage in sex with males. Routine postimmunization serologic testing is not recommended. There is no contraindication to giving HepA vaccine to a person who may be immune as the result of a previous HAV infection or immunization. Incarcerated juveniles found to have acute hepatitis A disease should be reported to the local health department, and appropriate postexposure prophylaxis with HAV vaccine should be given to other susceptible residents who may have been exposed (see Hepatitis A, p 391).

Hepatitis B

HBV in the United States is transmitted mainly through exposure to blood, semen, and vaginal fluid; chronic infection with HBV mainly is found among people born in countries with prevalence higher than 2%, where most infections are transmitted in the perinatal period or during early childhood (see Hepatitis B, p 400). Adolescents in correctional facilities may include foreign-born (eg, Asia, Africa) residents who are more likely to have chronic infection and can transmit infection to susceptible residents. Resident adolescents also can include people with high-risk behaviors, including adolescents engaged in injection drug use with needle sharing; inmates who have had early initiation of sexual intercourse, unprotected sexual activity, multiple sexual partners, or history of STIs; and male adolescents who engage in sex with males. Although no published national studies have determined HBV infection prevalence rates for incarcerated juveniles, rates of HBV seroprevalence in homeless and high-risk street youth are higher when compared with peers lacking risk factors. Studies investigating hepatitis B outbreaks in prison settings also suggest that horizontal transmission may occur when people with chronic HBV infection are present. Adolescent female inmates present additional challenges for hepatitis B assessment and management if they are pregnant during incarceration, in which case coordination of care for mother and infant becomes paramount.

RECOMMENDATIONS FOR CONTROL OF HBV INFECTIONS IN INCARCERATED YOUTH

Routine screening of juvenile inmates for HBV markers generally is not recommended, although testing for chronic infection is recommended in certain populations (see Hepatitis B, p 400). However, in states with school entry laws (**www.immunize.org/laws**) where high levels of adolescent HBV immunization have been achieved, adolescents who entered school when a law was in effect may be considered immunized. In other states, in the absence of proof of immunization, initial testing for HBV immunity may save vaccine costs, provided the timing of testing does not delay HBV immunization should the patient lack immunity. Correctional facilities may wish to survey juvenile inmates periodically for HBV immunity as they enter the institution to approximate HBV infection prevalence and determine the desirability of preimmunization testing. Adolescent detainees with signs and symptoms of hepatitis disease should be tested for serologic markers for acute hepatitis A, acute hepatitis B, and hepatitis C to determine the presence of acute or chronic infection and coinfection.

All adolescents receiving medical evaluation in a correctional facility should begin the hepatitis B (HepB) vaccine series or complete a previously begun series unless they have proof of completion of a previous HepB immunization series. Beginning a HepB vaccine series is critical, because a single dose of vaccine may confer protection from infection and subsequent complications of chronic carriage in a high-risk adolescent who may be lost to follow-up. Routine preimmunization and postimmunization serologic screening is not recommended. In states where HepB vaccine school entry requirements are in place, correctional facilities may use a combination of immunization history, immunization registry data, school entry immunization laws, and serologic testing to develop institutional policies regarding the need for HepB immunization in specific age groups of adolescents. Correctional facilities should have mechanisms in place for completion of the HepB vaccine series in the community after release of the juvenile. Immunization information should be made available to the inmate, the parents or legal guardian, the state immunization registry, and the patient's future medical home in the community.

Postexposure hepatitis B prophylaxis regimens for unimmunized incarcerated adolescents after potential percutaneous or sexual exposures to HBV are available (see Hepatitis B, Care of Exposed People, p 419). Should the source of the exposure be found to be HBsAg positive, the unimmunized inmate exposed percutaneously should receive Hepatitis B Immune Globulin (HBIG) as soon as possible after exposure (preferably within 24 hours and not more than 14 days after exposure), and the HepB vaccine series should be initiated. Exposed juveniles who have begun but not completed their HepB vaccine series should receive an appropriate dose of HBIG and complete the remainder of the series as scheduled (see Hepatitis B, p 400). If the source of exposure is unknown and not available for HBsAg testing, the exposed person should receive HepB vaccine or complete a vaccine series already initiated.

All pregnant adolescents should be tested for HBsAg at the time a pregnancy is discovered, regardless of HepB immunization history and previous results of tests for HBsAg and antibody to HBsAg. Unimmunized pregnant adolescents who are HBsAg negative should begin the HepB vaccine series as soon as possible during the course of pregnancy. Pregnancy is not a contraindication to receiving HepB vaccine in any trimester. The HBsAg status of a pregnant adolescent should be reported to the patient's prenatal care facility, the hospital where she will deliver her infant, and the state health department where case-management assistance will occur. Infants born to HBsAg-positive mothers must receive a dose of HepB vaccine and HBIG within 12 hours of birth (see Hepatitis B, Care of Exposed People, p 419).

Incarcerated adolescents who are found to have evidence of chronic HBV infection should be evaluated by a specialist to determine the extent of their liver disease and their eligibility for antiviral therapy. Detainees who are HBsAg positive should be reported to the local health department to facilitate long-term follow-up after release.

All adolescents with chronic liver disease, including those attributable to HBV, should be immunized with HepA vaccine to prevent fulminant liver disease should infection with HAV occur. Chronically infected adolescents with HBV should be counseled against the use and abuse of alcohol and street drugs, both of which can degrade liver function in patients with HBV-induced cirrhosis. Chronically infected people may remain infectious to sexual and household contacts for life and must be counseled accordingly to protect sexual partners and household contacts.

Hepatitis C

Of the nearly 4 million people chronically infected with HCV in the United States, approximately 30% have been incarcerated in a correctional institution. The most common mode of acquisition of HCV is injection drug use; exposure to multiple sexual partners is a distant second. Up to 80% of inmates who use illicit injection drugs will be infected with HCV within 5 years after onset of their drug use. Tattooing and body piercing in regulated settings are not thought to be significant sources of transmission of HCV, but tattoos received in a correctional facility can be associated with hepatitis C. Prevalence studies of HCV infection in incarcerated youth are limited but show an approximate two- to fourfold increase over youth who are not in the juvenile justice system. Injection drug use is the predominant HCV infection risk factor for detained juveniles.

Testing inmates for HCV infection has created conflicts for administrators of correctional facilities. Many do not view the diagnosis and potential treatment of their residents with HCV infection as part of the correctional mission. Inmates commonly refuse testing, even when at high risk of hepatitis, to avoid persecution from fellow prisoners. The lack of a vaccine for hepatitis C places a substantial burden on prevention counseling to elicit changes in high-risk behaviors and health maintenance counseling to decrease health risks in people already infected. This includes lifestyle alterations and avoidance of street drug and alcohol abuse, which increase morbidity and mortality from hepatitis C.

RECOMMENDATIONS FOR CONTROL OF HCV INFECTIONS IN INCARCERATED YOUTH

Routine screening of incarcerated adolescents for HCV infection is not recommended. Focused screening of adult inmates on the basis of risk criteria has proven reliable and cost-effective for correctional facilities that use it consistently. Risk factor assessments of newly admitted juvenile inmates being considered for HCV testing might include (1) self-reported history of injection drug use; (2) history of liver disease; (3) presence of antibody to hepatitis B core antigen; or (4) increased alanine transaminase concentration. Testing of detainees with one or more of these factors for antibody to HCV can detect more than 90% of HCV infections in correctional facilities. Some juvenile offenders may withhold reporting risk behaviors and yet express interest in HCV testing when offered. These requests, in most instances, should be accommodated. Adolescents with signs or symptoms of hepatitis should undergo diagnostic testing for acute hepatitis A, acute hepatitis B, and HCV infection.

Adolescents who test positive for antibody to HCV should receive ongoing medical attention to determine the likelihood of chronic infection, and cases should be reported to the local health department. The presence of HCV antibody and the absence of HCV RNA do not preclude the possibility of active liver disease, although it is rare if the transaminases also are normal. HCV antigenemia is variable from day to day and occurs in the presence of circulating HCV antibody. Juveniles found to be chronically infected with HCV should receive ongoing medical evaluation (in consultation with an expert in caring for chronic live disease) to monitor the course of their liver disease and to determine their suitability for therapeutic interventions (see Hepatitis C, p 423). Incarcerated adolescents with HCV infection should be enrolled in a risk-reduction program for drug and alcohol avoidance as indicated and should receive counseling for safe sex practices for the safety of their sexual partners and the protection of the community at large (**www.cdc.gov/ hepatitis/Resources/index.htm**). Incarcerated adolescents with hepatitis C-related chronic liver disease or with ongoing risk behaviors should receive HepA and HepB vaccines if not already immunized.

MEDICAL EVALUATION FOR INFECTIOUS DISEASES FOR INTERNATIONALLY ADOPTED, REFUGEE, AND IMMIGRANT CHILDREN[1,2]

Annually, thousands of children from other countries are adopted by families in the United States. In recent years, more than 90% of international adoptees were from Asian (China, South Korea, Taiwan, India, and Philippines), Latin American and Caribbean (Guatemala and Colombia), Eastern European (Russia and the Ukraine), and African (Ethiopia, Nigeria) countries. The diverse birth countries of these children, their unknown medical histories before adoption or immigration, their previous living circumstances (eg, orphanages and/or foster care), and the limited availability of reliable health care in some resource-limited countries make the medical evaluation of these children a challenging and important task. The child should be seen by his or her pediatrician or a physician who specializes in adoption medicine as soon as possible after arrival in the United States to begin all preventive health services, including immunizations. In addition to evaluation of children, it is important that the immunization status of adoptive family members and close contacts is reviewed and immunizations administered as appropriate by US schedules for age.

Prevention of illness in refugee and immigrant children presents special challenges because of the infectious diseases to which they may have been exposed and the different immunization practices in their native countries. The Centers for Disease Control and Prevention (CDC) has issued recommendations for screening of refugees (**www.cdc. gov/immigrantrefugeehealth/guidelines/domestic/domestic-guidelines. html**). Recommended screening tests for infectious diseases are listed in Table 2.15 (also see disease-specific chapters in Section 3). In addition to these infectious disease screening tests, other medical and developmental issues should be part of the initial evaluation of internationally adopted, refugee, and immigrant children.[3]

Children who resided in refugee-processing camps for a few months often have had access to medical and treatment services, which may have included some immunizations. Only written documentation of testing results, treatment, or administration of immunizations should be considered for acceptance. See Children Who Received Immunizations Outside the United States or Whose Immunization Status is Unknown or Uncertain (p 98) for recommendations regarding immunizations. Internationally adopted children typically differ from refugee children in terms of their access to medical care and treatment before arrival in the United States and in the frequency of certain infectious diseases. The history of access to and quality of medical care for international adoptees can be variable. Internationally adopted children are considered legally as a type of immigrant and are required to have a medical examination performed by a physician designated by the US Department of State in their country of origin. However, this

---

[1] For additional information, see Canadian Paediatric Society. *Children and Youth New to Canada: Health Care Guide.* Ottawa, Ontario: Canadian Paediatric Society; 2000; and the CDC (**www.cdc.gov/travel/default.aspx**) and World Health Organization (**www.who.int**) Web sites.

[2] Information for parents can be found at **www.cdc.gov/immigrantrefugeehealth/adoption/index.html/**.

[3] American Academy of Pediatrics, Council on Community Pediatrics. Providing care for immigrant, migrant, and border children. *Pediatrics.* 2013;131(6):e2028-e2034

Table 2.15. Screening Tests for Infectious Diseases in International Adoptees, Refugees, and Immigrants[a]

Hepatitis B virus serologic testing:
   Hepatitis B surface antigen (HBsAg); the panel should be performed to include hepatitis B surface antibody (anti-HBs) and hepatitis B core antibody (anti-HBc)

Hepatitis C virus serologic testing

Syphilis serologic testing:
   Nontreponemal test (eg, RPR, VDRL, or ART)
   Treponemal test (eg, MHA-TP, FTA-ABS, EIA, CIA, or TPPA)

Human immunodeficiency virus (HIV) 1 and 2 serologic testing

Complete blood cell count with red blood cell indices and differential

Stool examination for ova and parasites (3 specimens)[b] with specific request for *Giardia intestinalis* and *Cryptosporidium* species testing

Tuberculin skin test[b] or interferon-gamma release assay

In children from countries with endemic infection[b]:
   Trypanosoma cruzi serologic testing

In children with eosinophilia (absolute eosinophil count exceeding 450 cells/mm^3) and negative stool ova and parasite examinations[c]:
   Strongyloides species serologic testing
   Schistosoma species serologic testing for children from sub-Saharan African, Southeast Asian, and certain Latin American countries

Lymphatic filariasis serologic testing for children older than 2 years from countries with endemic infection[b]

RPR indicates rapid plasma reagin; VDRL, Venereal Disease Research Laboratories; ART, automated reagin test; MHA-TP, microhemagglutination test for *Treponema pallidum;* FTA-ABS, fluorescent treponemal antibody absorption; EIA, enzyme immunoassay; CIA, chemiluminescence assay; TPPA, *T pallidum* particle agglutination.
[a]For evaluation of noninfectious disease conditions, see American Academy of Pediatrics, Council on Community Pediatrics. Providing care for immigrant, migrant, and border children. *Pediatrics.* 2013;131(6):e2028-e2034.
[b]See text.
[c]Some experts would perform serologic tests for schistosomiasis in children from areas with high endemicity regardless of eosinophil count because of its poor positive- and negative-predictive values.

examination usually is limited to completing legal requirements for screening for certain communicable diseases and to examination for serious physical or mental disorders that would prevent the issue of an immigrant visa. Information about this required health assessment is available at **www.cdc.gov/immigrantrefugeehealth/.** Such an evaluation is not a comprehensive assessment of the child's health. During preadoption visits, pediatricians can stress to prospective parents the importance of acquiring immunization and other health records. Adopting parents generally have limited information about a child before adoption. Optimally, parents should obtain all information available for that child and meet with the child's physician before their child arrives to review available information and to discuss common medical issues regarding internationally adopted children. Parents who have not met with a physician before adoption should notify their physician when their child arrives so that a timely medical evaluation can be arranged. Children should be examined as soon as possible after arrival in the United States, preferably within the first 2 weeks. A list of pediatricians with special interest in adoption and foster care medicine is available on the American Academy of Pediatrics Web site (**www2.aap.org/sections/adoption/directory/map-adoption.cfm**).

Infectious diseases are among the most common medical diagnoses identified in immigrant children after arrival in the United States. Children may be asymptomatic, and the diagnoses must be made by laboratory or other tests in addition to history and physical examination. Because of inconsistent use of the birth dose of hepatitis B (HepB) vaccine; inconsistent perinatal screening for hepatitis B virus (HBV), syphilis, and human immunodeficiency virus (HIV); and the high prevalence of certain intestinal parasites and tuberculosis (TB), all international adoptees should be screened for these infections on arrival in the United States.

Consideration of Certain Pathogens and Conditions

HEPATITIS A

Hepatitis A virus (HAV) is endemic in most countries of origin of internationally adopted, refugee and immigrant children. Some children may have acquired HAV infection early in life in their country of origin and may be immune, but others may be incubating HAV or remain susceptible at the time of entry into the United States. Serologic testing for acute infection (hepatitis A immunoglobulin [Ig] M) and immunity (total hepatitis A IgG and IgM antibody) can be performed at the initial visit to determine whether the child is susceptible to HAV, has current HAV infection, or is immune. Children incubating HAV infection at the time of adoption could transmit the virus to their adoptive families and others on arrival in the United States. Adoptive parents and any accompanying family members should ensure that they are immunized or otherwise immune to HAV infection before traveling to adopt their child. In addition, hepatitis A (HepA) vaccine should be administered before the arrival of the adoptee to all susceptible nontraveling people who anticipate having close personal contact with the child adopted internationally from a country with high or intermediate hepatitis A endemicity. Children without HAV immunity who are 12 months and older should receive HepA vaccine as recommended according to the routine immunization schedule (**http://redbook.solutions.aap.org/SS/Immunization_Schedules.aspx**).

HEPATITIS B AND HEPATITIS D

In studies conducted primarily during the 1990s, the prevalence of hepatitis B surface antigen (HBsAg) positivity in internationally adopted children ranged from 1% to 5%, depending on the country of origin and the year studied. Hepatitis B virus (HBV) infection was prevalent in adoptees from regions of high endemicity, including Asia and Africa and some countries of central and eastern Europe (eg, Romania and Bulgaria) and states of the former Soviet Union (eg, Russia and the Ukraine). Over the past 5 to 10 years, the number of countries with routine infant hepatitis B (HepB) immunization programs has increased markedly. By 2006, 163 countries, encompassing 84% of the world's population, had implemented routine infant HepB immunization nationwide. However, administration of a birth dose of HepB vaccine, needed to prevent perinatal transmission from an infected mother, is not routine in many countries, and coverage among infants can be suboptimal. Even when a birth dose is administered, efficacy of postexposure prophylaxis is lower among infants born to pregnant women with high

HBV viral load. Therefore, **all** children should be tested for HBsAg to identify cases of chronic infection, regardless of immunization status (see Hepatitis B, p 400). Although HBV serologic tests may be performed in the country of origin, testing is not required for the immigration examination, testing may be incomplete, and children may become infected after testing. Unimmunized children with negative HBsAg and negative hepatitis B surface antibody (HBsAb) test results should be immunized according to the recommended childhood and adolescent immunization schedules **(http://redbook. solutions.aap.org/SS/Immunization_Schedules.aspx;** also see Children Who Received Immunizations Outside the United States or Whose Immunization Status is Unknown or Uncertain, p 98).

Children with a positive HBsAg test result should be reported to the local or state health department. To distinguish between acute and chronic HBV infection, HBsAg-positive children should be retested. The absence of IgM antibody to hepatitis B core antigen (IgM anti-HBc) or the persistence of HBsAg for at least 6 months indicates chronic HBV infection (see Hepatitis B, p 400). Children with chronic HBV infection should be tested for biochemical evidence of liver disease and followed by a specialist who cares for patients with chronic HBV infection (see Hepatitis B, p 400). All unimmunized household contacts of children with chronic HBV infection should be immunized (see Hepatitis B, p 400).

Hepatitis D virus (HDV), which occurs only in conjunction with the presence of HBsAg, can infect international adoptees, particularly those from North Africa, parts of South America, and the Mediterranean Basin. Serologic tests for diagnosis of HDV infection are not available widely (see Hepatitis D, p 430). Routine testing is recommended as part of further clinical evaluation only for children found to have chronic HBV infection.

HEPATITIS C

Routine testing for hepatitis C virus (HCV) infection is recommended for all children, given that most international adoptees in recent years have been adopted from countries with elevated rates of prevalence (China, Russia, southeast Asia) and because risk factors for infection are rarely known. A serum enzyme immunoassay (EIA) should be used as the initial screening test. Passively transferred maternal antibody can remain detectable by EIA for up to 18 months (see Hepatitis C, p 423); therefore, in young children, a positive EIA result may be attributable to maternal antibody. A positive EIA result should be confirmed with a more specific assay, such as a recombinant immunoblot assay or polymerase chain reaction testing for HCV, and those with positive results should be evaluated and followed by a specialist who cares for patients with chronic hepatitis (see Hepatitis C, p 423).

INTESTINAL PATHOGENS

Fecal examinations for ova and parasites tested in a laboratory experienced in parasitology will identify a pathogen in 15% to 35% of internationally adopted and refugee children. Presence or absence of symptoms is not predictive of parasitosis. The prevalence of intestinal parasites varies by age of the child and country of origin. Additionally, for refugees, guidelines differ depending on whether the child received presumptive therapy overseas **(www.cdc.gov/immigrantrefugeehealth/guidelines/overseas/ interventions/interventions.html).** The most common pathogens identified are *Giardia intestinalis, Dientamoeba fragilis, Hymenolepis* species, *Ascaris lumbricoides,* and *Trichuris trichiura. Strongyloides stercoralis, Entamoeba histolytica,* and hookworm are recovered less commonly. In addition, *Cryptosporidium* species is a leading cause of moderate to severe diarrhea in infants in sub-Saharan Africa and South Asia.[1] Regardless of nutritional status or presence of symptoms, 3 stool specimens collected on separate days should be examined for ova and parasites, and direct fluorescent antibody or EIA testing performed for *Giardia* species and *Cryptosporidium* species. Therapy for intestinal parasites generally will be successful, but complete eradication may not occur. Proof of eradication is not recommended for individuals who are asymptomatic following therapy. If symptoms persist after treatment, however, ova and parasite testing should be repeated to ensure successful elimination of parasites. Children who fail to demonstrate adequate catch-up growth, who have unexplained anemia, or who have gastrointestinal tract symptoms or signs that occur or recur months or even years after arrival in the United States should be reevaluated for intestinal parasites. In addition, when newly arrived adoptees have acute onset of diarrhea, stool specimens also should be tested for *Salmonella* species, *Shigella* species, *Campylobacter* species, and Shiga toxin-producing *Escherichia coli,* including *E coli* O157:H7. Antimicrobial susceptibility testing should be performed if bacterial pathogens are isolated to inform decisions regarding possible treatment and public health measures.

SYPHILIS

Congenital syphilis, especially with involvement of the central nervous system, may not have been diagnosed or may have been treated inadequately in children from some resource-limited countries. Children 15 years and older should have had serologic testing for syphilis as part of the required overseas medical assessment. Children who had positive test results are required to complete treatment before arrival in the United States. After arrival in the United States, clinicians should screen children for syphilis by reliable nontreponemal and treponemal serologic tests, regardless of history or a report of treatment (see Syphilis, p 755). Children with positive nontreponemal or treponemal serologic test results should be evaluated by a health care professional with specific expertise to assess the differential diagnosis of pinta, yaws, and syphilis and to determine the stage of infection so that appropriate treatment can be administered (see Syphilis, p 755).

TUBERCULOSIS

Infection with an organism of the *Mycobacterium tuberculosis* complex commonly is encountered in international adoptees from all countries, although incidence rates of tuberculosis (TB) vary by country and by age within countries. The screening requirements for immigrants for TB underwent a major revision in 2007 and have been fully implemented as of October 2013. For immigrants from countries with TB prevalence ≥20 cases per 100 000 population, requirements include: chest radiograph for all people 15 years and older; tuberculin skin test (TST or, in some instances, interferon-gamma release assay [IGRA]) for children 2 to 14 years of age; sputum cultures and drug susceptibility testing; and completion of directly observed treatment for TB before immigration for people with pulmonary disease. Children younger than 2 years are not tested unless it is brought to attention of screening physicians overseas that they are a known contact of an active case, have HIV infection, or have signs or symptoms suggestive of TB. Testing overseas for

---

[1]Kotloff KL, Nataro JP, Blackwelder WC, et al. Burden and aetiology of diarrhoeal disease in infants and young children in developing countries (the Global Enteric Multicenter Study, GEMS): a prospective, case-control study. *Lancet.* 2013;382(9888):209-222

adoptees (a special class of immigrants) and refugees is unlikely. Information about the screening and implementation requirements is available at **www.cdc.gov/immigrantrefugeehealth/pdf/tuberculosis-ti-2009.pdf.**

Because TB can be more severe in young children and can reactivate in later years, testing for latent *M tuberculosis* infection (LTBI) in this high-risk population of immigrants, adoptees, and refugees is important. TST is preferred for children younger than 5 years. Either TST or IGRA can be used for children 5 years or older (see Tuberculosis, p 804, for further guidance).[1] Some experts use IGRA for children as young as 3 years of age. Presence or absence of a bacille Calmette-Guérin (BCG) vaccine scar should be noted. BCG coverage in most countries where the vaccine is used is very high, and clinicians should be prepared to discuss the limitations of BCG when questioned by caregivers. BCG protects children from lethal forms of TB (eg, meningitis) with approximately 80% efficacy, but its efficacy against pulmonary TB or LTBI is much lower. Receipt of BCG vaccine is not a contraindication to a TST, and a positive TST result usually should not be attributed to BCG vaccine. Some international adoptees initially may be anergic because of malnutrition or HIV infection. If malnutrition is suspected, the test for LTBI should be repeated when the child is nourished appropriately. In these children, further investigation is necessary to determine whether LTBI or tuberculosis disease is present, for which therapy, albeit different, is needed in both instances (see Tuberculosis, p 804). Some experts repeat the TST in 3 to 6 months for all international adoptees if the initial TST result had <10 mm of induration, because the initial test may have been falsely negative because of recent infection. However, a boosting phenomenon attributable to BCG vaccination can confound interpretation, yielding a false-positive TST result. In BCG-vaccinated children 5 years and older, IGRA can be performed to help determine whether a "positive" TST result is attributable to LTBI or to the previous BCG vaccine.[1] Some experts would use the IGRA for children as young as 3 years of age. Routine chest radiography is not indicated in asymptomatic children in whom the TST or IGRA result is negative. In children with a positive test result for TB infection, further investigation, including a chest radiograph and physical examination, is necessary to determine whether tuberculosis disease is present (see Tuberculosis, p 804). When tuberculosis disease is suspected in an international child, efforts to isolate and test the organism for drug susceptibilities are imperative because of the high prevalence of drug resistance in many countries. Physicians expert in management of TB should be consulted when preventive therapy or therapy for TB disease is indicated for children from countries with prevalent isoniazid resistance.

HIV INFECTION

The risk of HIV infection in internationally adopted children depends on the country of origin and on individual risk factors. Because adoptees may come from populations at high risk of infection, screening for HIV should be performed for **all** internationally adopted children. The decision to screen immigrant children for HIV depends on findings from the history and physical examination. Although some children will have HIV test results documented in their referral information, test results from the child's country of origin may not be reliable. Since 2010, refugees and immigrants no longer are required

---

[1] Starke JR; American Academy of Pediatrics, Committee on Infectious Diseases. Technical report: interferon-γ release assays for diagnosis of tuberculosis infection and disease in children. *Pediatrics.* 2014;134(6):e1763–e1773

to have HIV testing as part of immigration medical assessments (as previously was required for all people 15 years and older and for younger children if history or examination raised concern about possible HIV infection—eg, maternal history of HIV infection, history of rape or sexual assault; **www.cdc.gov/immigrantrefugeehealth/laws-regs/hiv-ban-removal/index.html**). HIV testing still is recommended for people who are diagnosed with active tuberculosis as part of the overseas medical assessment. HIV testing after arrival in the United States is recommended for refugees 13 through 64 years of age and encouraged for refugees 12 years or younger and older than 64 years of age (**www.cdc.gov/immigrantrefugeehealth/guidelines/domestic/screening-hiv-infection-domestic.html**). The decision to screen immigrant children for HIV after arrival in the United States should depend on history and risk factors (eg, receipt of blood products, maternal drug use), physical examination findings, and prevalence of HIV infection in the child's country of origin. If there is a suspicion of HIV infection, testing should be performed before administration of live vaccines. (**http://aidsinfo.nih.gov/contentfiles/lvguidelines/oi_guidelines_pediatrics.pdf**).

CHAGAS DISEASE (AMERICAN TRYPANOSOMIASIS)

Chagas disease is endemic throughout much of Mexico and Central and South America (see American Trypanosomiasis, p 803). Risk of Chagas disease varies by region within countries with endemic infection. The risk of Chagas disease is low in internationally adopted children from countries with endemic infection, and treatment of infected children is highly effective. Countries with endemic Chagas disease include Argentina, Belize, Bolivia, Brazil, Chile, Colombia, Costa Rica, Ecuador, El Salvador, French Guiana, Guatemala, Guyana, Honduras, Mexico, Nicaragua, Panama, Paraguay, Peru, Suriname, Uruguay, and Venezuela. Transmission within countries with endemic infection is focal, but if a child comes from a country with endemic Chagas disease or has received a blood transfusion in a country with endemic disease, testing for *Trypanosoma cruzi* should be considered. Serologic testing should be performed only in children 12 months or older because of the potential presence of maternal antibody.

TISSUE PARASITES

Eosinophilia is commonly but not universally present in people with tissue parasites. In international adoptees and refugees who did not receive albendazole or ivermectin for presumptive therapy of intestinal helminths who have negative stool ova and parasite test results and in whom eosinophilia (absolute eosinophil count exceeding 450 cells/mm^3) is found on review of complete blood cell count, serologic testing for strongyloidiasis, schistosomiasis, and lymphatic filariasis should be considered. Although logistically attractive to perform all tests at first encounter, predictive values of many serologic tests for parasites are suboptimal; common treatable causes of eosinophilia usually should be considered first. Serologic testing for *Strongyloides stercoralis* should be performed on all international adoptees (and refugees as noted above) with eosinophilia and no identified pathogen commonly associated with an increased eosinophil count, regardless of country of origin. Testing for *Schistosoma* species and lymphatic filariasis is limited to people from endemic countries. Serologic testing for *Schistosoma* species should be performed for **all** children with eosinophilia and no identified pathogen commonly associated with eosinophilia who are from Sub-Saharan Africa, South East Asia, or areas of Latin America where schistosomiasis is endemic. Serologic testing for lymphatic filariasis should be considered in children older than 2 years with eosinophilia who are from countries with endemic lymphatic filariasis (**www.cdc.gov/parasites/lymphaticfilariasis/index.html**). A positive serologic result will need to be confirmed in a reference laboratory (CDC or National Institutes of Health) for release of drugs for treatment from the CDC Drug Service.

OTHER INFECTIOUS DISEASES

Skin infections that occur commonly in international adoptees include bacterial (eg, impetigo) and fungal (eg, candidiasis) infections and ectoparasitic infestations (eg, scabies and pediculosis). Adoptive parents should be instructed on how to examine their child for signs of scabies, pediculosis, and tinea so that treatment can be initiated and transmission to others can be prevented (see Scabies, p 702, and Pediculosis, p 597–603).

Diseases such as typhoid fever, malaria, leprosy, or melioidosis are encountered infrequently in internationally adopted children. Although routine screening for these diseases is not recommended, findings of fever, splenomegaly, respiratory tract infection, anemia, or eosinophilia should prompt an appropriate evaluation on the basis of the epidemiology of infectious diseases that occur in the child's country of origin. If the child came from a country where malaria is present, malaria should be considered in the differential diagnosis (see Malaria, p 528).

In the United States, multiple outbreaks of measles have been reported in children adopted from China and in their US contacts. Measles elimination has been achieved only in the Americas; transmission continues in other parts of the world. From January 1 through May 23, 2014, measles importation into the United States occurred from more than 18 countries and affected 288 people. Prospective parents who are traveling internationally to adopt children, as well as their household contacts, should ensure that they have a history of natural disease or have been immunized adequately for measles according to US recommendations. All people born after 1957 should receive 2 doses of measles-containing vaccine after the age of 12 months in the absence of documented measles infection or contraindication to the vaccine (see Measles, p 535).

Clinicians should be aware of potential diseases in internationally adopted children and their clinical manifestations. Some diseases, such as central nervous system cysticercosis, can have incubation periods as long as several years and, thus, may not be detected during initial screening. On the basis of findings at the initial evaluation, consideration should be given to a repeat evaluation 6 months after adoption. In most cases, the longer the interval from adoption to development of a clinical syndrome, the less likely the syndrome can be attributed to a pathogen acquired in the country of origin.

···

INJURIES FROM DISCARDED NEEDLES IN THE COMMUNITY

Contact with and injuries from hypodermic needles and syringes discarded in public places, presumably by injection drug users, may pose a risk of transmission of bloodborne pathogens, including human immunodeficiency virus (HIV), hepatitis B virus (HBV), and hepatitis C virus (HCV). An epidemiologic study of 274 pediatric-aged children (mean age, 7.4 years) identified with a community-acquired needlestick injury over a

19-year period observed no seroconversions, confirming that the risk of transmission of bloodborne viruses in these events is low.[1] Infection risks and options for postexposure prophylaxis (PEP) vary depending on the virus and type of injury and exposure. Although nonoccupational needlestick injuries may pose a lower risk of infection transmission than do occupational needlestick injuries, a person injured by a needle in a nonoccupational setting needs evaluation, counseling, and in some cases, PEP. Even if the potential for the discarded syringe to contain a specific bloodborne pathogen can be estimated from the background prevalence rates of these infections in the local community, the need to test the injured or exposed person usually is not influenced significantly by this assessment.

Wound Care and Tetanus Prophylaxis

Management of people with needlestick injuries includes acute wound care and consideration of the need for antimicrobial prophylaxis. Standard wound cleansing and care is indicated; such wounds rarely require closure. A tetanus toxoid containing vaccine, with or without Tetanus Immune Globulin, should be considered as appropriate for the age, the severity of the injury, the immunization status of the exposed person, and the potential for dirt or soil contamination of the needle (see Tetanus, p 773). Tetanus and diphtheria toxoids (Td) vaccine should be used if the patient has already received all necessary doses of pertussis containing vaccine. DTaP or Tdap should be given if pertussis vaccine is needed (see Pertussis, p 608).

Bloodborne Pathogens

Consideration of the need for prophylaxis for HBV and HIV is the next step in exposure management; currently, there is no recommended PEP for HCV. Risk of acquisition of various pathogens depends on the nature of the wound, the ability of the pathogens to survive on environmental surfaces, the volume of source material, the concentration of virus in the source material, prevalence rates among local injection drug users, the probability that the syringe and needle were used by a local injection drug user, and the immunization status of the exposed person. Unlike an occupational blood or body fluid exposure, in which the status of the exposure source for HBV, HCV, and HIV often is known, these data usually are not available to help in the decision-making process in a nonoccupational exposure.[2,3]

HEPATITIS B VIRUS

HBV is the hardiest of the major bloodborne pathogens and can survive on environmental surfaces at room temperature for at least 7 days. Transmission occurs at a rate of 23% to 62% during needlestick injury between health care personnel and HBV-positive sources. Prompt and appropriate PEP intervention reduces this risk. The effectiveness

---

[1] Papenburg J, Blais D, Moore D, et al. Pediatric injuries from needles discarded in the community: epidemiology and risk of seroconversion. *Pediatrics.* 2008;122(2):e487-e487

[2] Centers for Disease Control and Prevention. Updated US Public Health Service guidelines for the management of occupational exposures to HBV, HCV, and HIV and recommendations for postexposure prophylaxis. *MMWR Recomm Rep.* 2001;50(RR-11):1-52

[3] US Department of Health and Human Services. Antiretroviral postexposure prophylaxis after sexual, injection-drug use, or other nonoccupational exposure to HIV in the United States: recommendations from the US Department of Health and Human Services. *MMWR Recomm Rep.* 2005;54(RR-2):1-20

of PEP diminishes the longer after exposure it is initiated. Children who have needle-stick injuries and who have not completed the 3-dose hepatitis B (HepB) vaccine series should receive a dose of HepB vaccine and, if indicated, should be scheduled to receive the remaining doses required to complete the schedule. Administration of Hepatitis B Immune Globulin usually is not indicated if the child has received the 3-dose regimen of HepB vaccine. If the child has received 2 doses of HepB vaccine 4 or more months previously, the immediate administration of the third dose of vaccine alone should be sufficient in most cases. Experts differ in opinion about the need for Hepatitis B Immune Globulin at the time of an injury of an incompletely immunized child. If the needle is from a person known to be hepatitis B surface antigen (HBsAg) positive, consideration could be given to testing the child for hepatitis B surface antibody and providing Hepatitis B Immune Globulin in addition to continuing with the HepB vaccination series.

HUMAN IMMUNODEFICIENCY VIRUS

Infection with HIV usually is the greatest concern of the victim and family. The risk of HIV transmission from a needle discarded in public is low. To date, no cases in which HIV was transmitted by needlestick injury outside a health care setting have been reported to the Centers for Disease Control and Prevention. Risk of HIV transmission from a puncture wound caused by a needle found in the community is lower than the 0.3% risk of HIV transmission to a health care professional from a needlestick injury from a person with known HIV infection. In most reports of occupational HIV transmission by percutaneous injury, needlestick injury occurred shortly after needle withdrawal from the vein or artery of the source patient with HIV infection. HIV RNA was detected in only 3 (3.8%) of 80 discarded disposable syringes that had been used by health care professionals for intramuscular or subcutaneous injection of patients with HIV infection, indicating that most syringes will not contain transmissible HIV even after being used to draw blood from a person with HIV infection.[1] HIV is susceptible to drying, and when HIV is placed on a surface exposed to air, the 50% tissue culture infective dose decreases by approximately 1 log every 9 hours.[2]

Despite the low risk, there may be rare situations (eg, large-bore needle with fresh blood) in which HIV testing in the child who suffered the needlestick is appropriate. HIV antibody testing should be performed at baseline, and follow-up testing should be performed at 4 to 6 weeks and 12 weeks after injury. Because concurrent acquisition of HCV and HIV infection may be associated with delayed HIV seroconversion,[3] a child whose HCV antibody test is negative at baseline but seroconverts to positive at 4 to 6 weeks after exposure should undergo HIV follow-up testing at 3, 6, and 12 months to rule out delayed seroconversion. Testing also is indicated if an illness consistent with acute HIV-related syndrome develops before the 6-week testing. Negative results from these initial tests support the conclusion that any subsequent positive test result likely reflects infection acquired from the needlestick. A positive initial test result in a pediatric patient requires further investigation of the cause,

[1] Rich JD, Dickinson BP, Carney JM, Fisher A, Heimer R. Detection of HIV-1 nucleic acid and HIV-1 antibodies in needles and syringes used for non-intravenous injection. *AIDS*. 1998;12(17):2345-2350

[2] Resnick L, Veren K, Salahuddin SZ, Tondreau S, Markham PD. Stability and inactivation of HTLV-III/LAV under clinical and laboratory environments. *JAMA*. 1986;255(14):1887-1891

[3] Terzi R, Niero F, Iemoli E, Capetti A, Coen M, Rizzardini G. Late HIV seroconversion after non-occupational postexposure prophylaxis against HIV with concomitant hepatitis C virus seroconversion. *AIDS*. 2007;21(2):262-263

such as perinatal transmission, sexual abuse or activity, or drug use. An alternative option is to obtain and save a baseline serum specimen for later testing for HIV antibody in the unlikely event that a subsequent test result is positive. Counseling is necessary before and after testing (see Human Immunodeficiency Virus Infection, p 453).

A specialist in HIV infection should be consulted before deciding whether to initiate PEP (PEP Hotline 888-448-4911). Antiretroviral therapy is not without risk and often is associated with significant adverse effects (see Human Immunodeficiency Virus Infection, p 453). In the rare event that the needle user is known to be HIV positive, PEP should be started immediately. If the needle user is known and has a low risk of being HIV-infected, most experts agree that PEP does not need to be administered pending test results of the user. In most situations, the needle user is not known. Data are not available on the efficacy of PEP with antiretroviral drugs in these circumstances for adults or children, and as a result, the US Public Health Service is unable to recommend for or against PEP in this circumstance.[1] PEP should be considered on a case-by-case basis, taking into consideration type of exposure and prevalence in the geographic area. Some experts recommend that antiretroviral chemoprophylaxis be considered if the needle and/or syringe are available and found to contain visible blood; testing the syringe for HIV is not practical or reliable and is not recommended. If the decision to begin prophylaxis is made, any delay before starting the medications should be minimized (see Human Immunodeficiency Virus Infection, p 453). Medication should begin within 72 hours and should continue for 28 days as a combination of 3 antiretroviral drugs. The suggested medication options are the same for the HIV occupational exposure (see Human Immunodeficiency Virus Infection, p 453).

HEPATITIS C VIRUS

The third bloodborne pathogen of concern is HCV, which can last in the environment for at least 16 to 23 hours. The prevalence of chronic HCV infection in the United States varies by race/ethnicity, age group, geographic location, and individual history of risk behaviors. Although transmission by sharing syringes among injection drug users is efficient, the risk of transmission from a discarded syringe is likely to be low. Testing for HCV is not recommended routinely in the absence of a risk factor for infection or a known exposure to a HCV-positive source. If performed, antibody to HCV (anti-HCV) can be detected in 80% of newly infected patients within 15 weeks after exposure and in 97% of newly infected patients by 6 months after exposure. If earlier diagnosis is desired, testing for HCV RNA may be performed at 4 to 6 weeks after exposure. Positive test results should be confirmed by supplemental confirmatory laboratory tests (see Hepatitis C, p 423). There is no recommended PEP for HCV using antiviral drugs or Immune Globulin preparations, because any HCV antibody-positive donor is excluded from the pool from which Immune Globulin products are prepared.

Preventing Needlestick Injuries

Needlestick injuries of both children and adults can be minimized by implementing public health programs on safe needle disposal and programs for exchange of used syringes and needles from injection drug users for sterile needles. Syringe and needle exchanges

---

[1]Centers for Disease Control and Prevention. Antiretroviral postexposure prophylaxis after sexual injection-drug-use, or other nonoccupational exposure to HIV in the United States: recommendations from the US Department of Health and Human Services. *MMWR Recomm Rep.* 2005;54(RR-2):1-20

decrease improper disposal and spread of bloodborne pathogens without increasing the rate of injection drug use. The American Academy of Pediatrics supports needle-exchange programs in conjunction with drug treatment and within the context of continuing research to assess their effectiveness. In addition, children should be educated to avoid playing in areas known to be frequented by injecting drug users and to avoid playing with discarded needles and syringes.

BITE WOUNDS

As many as 1% of all pediatric visits to emergency departments during summer months are for treatment of human or animal bite wounds. An estimated 5 million bites occur annually in the United States; dog bites account for approximately 90% of those wounds. The rate of infection after cat bites is as high as 50%; rates of infection after dog or human bites are 10% to 15%. Although postinjury rates of infection can be minimized through early administration of proper wound care principles, the bites of humans, wild animals, or nontraditional pets potentially are sources of serious morbidity. Parents should be informed to teach children to avoid contact with wild animals and should secure garbage containers so that raccoons and other animals will not be attracted to the home and places where children play. Nontraditional pets, including ferrets, iguanas and other reptiles, and wild animals also pose an infection as well as an injury risk for children, and their ownership should be discouraged in households with young children. Potential transmission of rabies is increased when a bite is from a wild animal (especially a bat or a carnivore) or from a domestic animal with uncertain immunization status that cannot be captured for adequate quarantine (see Rabies, p 658). Dead animals should be avoided, because they can be infested with arthropods (fleas or ticks) infected with a variety of bacterial, rickettsial, protozoan, or viral agents.

Recommendations for bite wound management are provided in Table 2.16. Because of the small number of prospective controlled studies of the topic, the consideration of whether to suture closed bite wounds remains controversial except when

Table 2.16. Management of Human or Animal Bite Wounds

Category of Management	Management
Cleansing	Remove visible foreign material
	Cleanse the wound surface with clean water or saline. Cleansers 1% povidone–iodine or 1% benzalkonium chloride can be used for particularly soiled wounds
	Irrigate open wounds with a copious volume of sterile water or saline solution by moderate-pressure irrigation[a]
	Avoid blind high-pressure irrigation of puncture wounds
	Standard Precautions should be used
Wound culture	No for fresh wounds,[b] unless signs of infection exist
	Yes for wounds that appear infected[c]
Diagnostic imaging	Indicated for penetrating injuries overlying bones or joints, for suspected fracture, or to assess foreign body inoculation
Débridement	Remove superficial devitalized tissue and foreign material

Table 2.16. Management of Human or Animal Bite Wounds, continued

Category of Management	Management
Operative débridement and exploration	Yes if any of the following: • Extensive wounds with devitalized tissue or mechanical dysfunction • Penetration of joints (clenched fist injury) or cranium • Plastic or other repairs requiring general anesthesia
Assess mechanical function	Assess and address mechanical function of injured structures
Wound closure	Yes for selected fresh,[b] nonpuncture bite wounds (see text)
Assess tetanus immunization status[d]	Yes for all wounds
Assess risk of rabies	Yes if bite by any rabies-prone, unobservable wild or domestic animal with unknown immunization status[e]
Assess risk of hepatitis B virus infection	Yes for human bite wounds[f]
Assess risk of human immunodeficiency virus	Yes for human bite wounds[g]
Initiate antimicrobial therapy[h]	Yes for: • Moderate or severe bite wounds, especially if edema or crush injury is present • Puncture wounds, especially if penetration of bone, tendon sheath, or joint has occurred • Deep or surgically closed facial bite wounds • Hand and foot bite wounds • Genital area bite wounds • Wounds in immunocompromised and asplenic people • Wounds with signs of infection • Cat bite wounds
Follow-up	Inspect wound for signs of infection within 48 hours

[a]Use of an 18-gauge needle with a large-volume syringe is effective. Antimicrobial or anti-infective solutions offer no advantage and may increase tissue irritation.
[b]Wounds less than 12 hours old.
[c]Both aerobic and anaerobic bacterial culture should be performed.
[d]See Tetanus, p 773.
[e]See Rabies, p 658.
[f]See Hepatitis B, p 400.
[g]See Human Immunodeficiency Virus Infection, p 453.
[h]See Table 2.17 (p 208) for suggested drug choices.

rabies is suspected. Bites from a rabid animal should not be sutured closed. However, published data support surgical closure with interrupted sutures or adhesive strips of recent, apparently uncontaminated, low-risk lesions after thorough wound cleansing, irrigation, removal of foreign materials, and débridement. Although high pressure irrigation should not be used for puncture wounds, thorough wound cleansing before surgical closure has been demonstrated to bring the rate of secondary infection of these wounds to well below 10%. Use of local anesthesia can facilitate these procedures. Sedation can also be helpful in certain circumstances. Bite wounds on the face seldom become bacterially infected, but if a wound has important cosmetic considerations, it should be closed whenever possible. Surgical closures can be performed at the time of initial management (primary) or delayed until the patient has received a brief course of antibiotic therapy (delayed primary closure). Smaller, cosmetically unimportant wounds can be cleansed and allowed to heal by secondary intent. Hand and foot wounds have a higher risk of infection. More complicated injuries should be managed in consultation with an appropriate surgical specialist. Approximation of margins and closure by delayed primary or secondary intent is prudent for infected nonfacial wounds. To minimize risk of infection, bite wounds should not be sealed with a tissue adhesive, no matter their age or appearance. Elevation of injured areas to minimize swelling will enhance wound healing.

Published evidence indicates that most infected mammalian bite wounds are polymicrobial in nature, often involving a mixture of mouth flora from the biting animal and, likely, skin flora from the victim. Specimens for aerobic and anaerobic culture should be obtained from wounds that appear infected. Limited data exist to guide short-term antimicrobial therapy for patients with wounds that do not appear infected. It takes at least 12 hours for the signs of infection to manifest clinically. Patients with mild injuries in which the skin is abraded do not need to be treated with antimicrobial agents. For those injuries, cleansing is sufficient. For fresh wounds, including all penetrating cat bite wounds (which are particularly prone to secondary infection), a 3- to 5-day course of therapy with a broad-spectrum antimicrobial agent may decrease the rate of infection. Children at high risk of infection (eg, children who are immunocompromised or who have crush injuries or deep tissue, compartment, or joint penetration) should receive preemptive antimicrobial therapy. Guidelines for initial choice of antimicrobial therapy for human and animal bites are provided in Table 2.17 (p 208). In the child with a confirmed bite wound-associated infection, initial therapy should be modified when culture results become available. Methicillin-resistant *Staphylococcus aureus* (MRSA) is a potential bite wound pathogen; empiric therapy may require modification if MRSA is isolated from an infected wound (see Staphylococcal Infections, p 715). Coverage for MRSA should be considered in severe bite wound infections while cultures are pending. Likewise, MRSA should be considered in a fresh or otherwise uninfected-appearing wound of a patient known to be colonized with that agent.

The treatment of choice following most bite wounds for which therapy is provided is amoxicillin-clavulanic acid (Table 2.17, p 208). Treatment of the child with a serious allergy to penicillin and a human or animal bite wound is problematic. Oral or parenteral treatment with trimethoprim-sulfamethoxazole, which is effective against *S aureus* (including MRSA), *Pasteurella multocida*, and *Eikenella corrodens*, in conjunction with clindamycin, which is active in vitro against anaerobic bacteria, streptococci, and many strains of *S aureus*, may be effective for preventing or treating bite wound infections. Extended-spectrum cephalosporins, such as cefotaxime or ceftriaxone parenterally or cefpodoxime orally, do not have good anaerobic spectra of activity but can be used in conjunction with clindamycin as alternative therapy for penicillin-allergic patients who can tolerate cephalosporins. Doxycycline is an alternative agent that has activity against *P multocida;* use of doxycycline in children younger than 8 years must be weighed against the risk of dental staining. Tetracycline-based antimicrobial agents,

Table 2.17. Antimicrobial Agents for Human or Animal Bite Wounds

Source of Bite	Organism(s) Likely to Cause Infection	Antimicrobial Agent			
		Oral Route	Oral Alternatives for Penicillin-Allergic Patients[a]	Intravenous Route[b,c]	Intravenous Alternatives for Penicillin-Allergic Patients[a,b,c]
Dog, cat, or mammal[d]	*Pasteurella* species, *Staphylococcus aureus*, streptococci, anaerobes, *Capnocytophaga* species, *Moraxella* species, *Corynebacterium* species, *Neisseria* species	Amoxicillin-clavulanate	Extended-spectrum cephalosporin or trimethoprim-sulfamethoxazole[e] **PLUS** Clindamycin	Ampicillin-sulbactam[f]	Extended-spectrum cephalosporin or trimethoprim-sulfamethoxazole **PLUS** Clindamycin **OR** Carbapenem
Reptile[g]	Enteric gram-negative bacteria, anaerobes	Amoxicillin-clavulanate	Extended-spectrum cephalosporin or trimethoprim-sulfamethoxazole[e] **PLUS** Clindamycin	Ampicillin-sulbactam[f] **PLUS** Gentamicin	Extended spectrum cephalosporin or gentamicin or aztreonam or quinolone **PLUS** Clindamycin **OR** Carbapenem

Table 2.17. Antimicrobial Agents for Human or Animal Bite Wounds, continued

Source of Bite	Organism(s) Likely to Cause Infection	Antimicrobial Agent			
		Oral Route	Oral Alternatives for Penicillin-Allergic Patients[a]	Intravenous Route[b,c]	Intravenous Alternatives for Penicillin-Allergic Patients[a,b,c]
Human	Streptococci, S aureus, Eikenella corrodens, Haemophilus species, anaerobes	Amoxicillin-clavulanate	Extended-spectrum cephalosporin or trimethoprim-sulfamethoxazole[e] **PLUS** Clindamycin	Ampicillin-sulbactam[f]	Extended spectrum cephalosporin or trimethoprim-sulfamethoxazole **PLUS** Clindamycin **OR** Carbapenem

[a]For patients with history of allergy to penicillin or one of its congeners, alternative drugs are recommended. In patients without a history of anaphylaxis, wheezing, angioedema, or urticaria, an extended-spectrum cephalosporin or other beta-lactam–class drug may be acceptable. For example, ceftriaxone, rather than trimethoprim-sulfamethoxazole, could be used intravenously.

[b]Coverage for methicillin-resistant S aureus with vancomycin should be considered for severe bite wounds.

[c]Note that use of ampicillin-sulbactam or carbapenem monotherapy will not include activity against methicillin-resistant S aureus isolates.

[d]Data are lacking to guide antimicrobial use for bites that are not overtly infected from small mammals, such as guinea pigs and hamsters.

[e]Doxycycline is an alternative for children 8 years and older.

[f]Piperacillin-tazobactam or ticarcillin-clavulanate can be used as alternatives.

[g]The role of empirical antimicrobial use for noninfected snake bite wounds is not well-defined. Therapy should be chosen on the basis of results of cultures from infected wounds.

including doxycycline, may cause permanent tooth discoloration for children younger than 8 years if used for repeated treatment courses. However, doxycycline binds less readily to calcium compared with older tetracyclines, and in some studies doxycycline was not associated with visible teeth staining in younger children (see Tetracyclines, p 873). Azithromycin and fluoroquinolones display good in vitro activity against organisms that commonly cause bite wound infections, but clinical trial data are lacking and fluoroquinolones are not approved for this indication in children. Carbapenems are an option for children with penicillin allergy, but cross-reactions with penicillins can occur infrequently. If a carbapenem is used as monotherapy, it should be noted that carbapenems do not have activity against MRSA. A 7- to 10-day course usually is sufficient for soft tissue infections. Longer courses of treatment may be indicated, depending on severity of infection, feasibility of draining abscesses if they occur, and patient's clinical responses. The duration of treatment for bite wound-associated bone infections is based on location, severity, and pathogens isolated.

PREVENTION OF TICKBORNE INFECTIONS

Tickborne infectious diseases in the United States include diseases caused by bacteria (eg, tularemia), spirochetes (Lyme disease, relapsing fever), rickettsiae (eg, Rocky Mountain spotted fever, ehrlichiosis, anaplasmosis), viruses (eg, Colorado tick fever, Powassan virus, Heartland virus), and protozoa (eg, babesiosis) (see Table 2.18, p 211, and disease-specific chapters in Section 3). Different species of ticks transmit different infectious agents (eg, brown dog ticks and American dog ticks are vectors of the agent that causes Rocky Mountain spotted fever; lone star ticks transmit the agents of ehrlichiosis and southern tick-associated rash illness or STARI), and some species of ticks (eg, the black-legged tick) may transmit several agents (Lyme disease, babesiosis, anaplasmosis). Physicians should be aware of the epidemiology of tickborne infections in their local areas. Prevention of tickborne diseases is accomplished by avoiding tick-infested habitats, decreasing tick populations in the environment, using personal protection against tick bites, and limiting the length of time ticks remain attached to the human host. Control of tick populations in the wider environment often is not practical but can be effective in more defined areas, such as around places where children reside. Using consumer-applied acaricides (pesticides targeting ticks), using veterinary treatments of pets, or contracting with a licensed pest-control operator can be efficient approaches to reducing tick populations and, therefore, the risk of tickborne disease in highly tick-infested areas. Specific measures for prevention are as follows:

- Physicians, parents, and children should be made aware that ticks can transmit pathogens that cause human and animal diseases.
- Tick-infested areas should be avoided whenever possible. Most ticks prefer dense woods with thick growth of shrubs and small trees as well as along the edges of the woods, where the woods abut lawns. Ticks require humidity to survive, and drier areas usually are less infested. For homes located in tick-prone areas, risk of exposure can be reduced by locating play equipment in sunny, dry areas away from forest edges, by creating a barrier of dry wood chips or gravel between recreation areas and forest, by mowing vegetation, and by keeping leaves raked and underbrush cleared. The brown dog tick is able to survive in more arid environments and can be

Table 2.18. Some Tick-Transmitted Pathogens
(Domestic and Imported)

Human Disease Type	Pathogens in the United States	Pathogens in Other Countries
Bacteria		
Human anaplasmosis	*Anaplasma phagocytophilum*	*A phagocytophilum*
Human ehrlichiosis	*Ehrlichia chaffeensis, Ehrlichia ewingii, Ehrlichia muris*-like species	*E muris, Ehrlichia canis, Ehrlichia ruminantium,* other species
Lyme disease, Lyme borreliosis	*Borrelia burgdorferi sensu stricto*	*Borrelia burgdorferi sensu lato,* including *Borrelia afzelii, Borrelia garinii, B burgdorferi sensu stricto,* and other genomospecies in Europe
Q fever (uncommon tick transmission)	*Coxiella burnetii*	*C burnetii*
Spotted fever group of rickettsioses	*Rickettsia rickettsii, Rickettsia parkeri, Rickettsia* species serotype 364D, other species	*R rickettsii, Rickettsia conorii, Rickettsia africae, Rickettsia honei, Rickettsia japonica, Rickettsia massiliae, Rickettsia sibirica, Rickettsia slovaca,* other species
Tickborne relapsing fever	*Borrelia hermsii, Borrelia turicatae, Borrelia parkeri, Borrelia miyamotoi,* and other species	*Borrelia duttonii, Borrelia miyamotoi,* other species
Tularemia	*Francisella tularensis*	*F tularensis*
Protozoa		
Human babesiosis	*Babesia microti, Babesia* species (MO1), *Babesia duncani* (WA1, CA2)	*B microti, Babesia divergens,* other species
Viruses		
Coltivirus infection	Colorado tick fever virus	Eyach virus
Flavivirus infection	Powassan virus, Deer tick virus	Powassan virus, tickborne encephalitis virus, louping-ill virus, Kyasanur Forest disease virus, Omsk hemor-rhagic fever virus
Phlebovirus infection	Heartland virus	Bhanja virus, severe fever with thrombocytopenia syndrome (SFTS) virus

introduced indoors. This species may be found in cracks and crevices of housing or in animal housing or bedding.

• If a tick-infested area is entered, clothing should be worn that covers the arms, legs, head, and neck and other exposed skin areas. Pants should be tucked into boots or socks, and long-sleeved shirts should be buttoned at the cuff. Additional protection includes use of topical DEET (N,N-diethyl-meta-toluamide), permethrin, and other products (see descriptions that follow). DEET is excellent protection against mosquitoes; permethrin is superior for ticks.

- **Permethrin.** Permethrin (a synthetic pyrethroid) is a contact pesticide and tick and insect repellent and can be sprayed onto clothes to decrease tick attachment. Permethrin should not be sprayed directly onto skin, and treated clothing should be dried before wearing. The US Environmental Protection Agency (EPA) has approved commercial sale of outdoor clothing treated with permethrin for children of all ages and for pregnant women. Permethrin-treated clothing remains effective for many launderings and has been shown repeatedly to reduce tick bites and reduce exposure to tickborne pathogens.
- **DEET.** Products containing from 5% to 30% DEET provide up to 2 to 6 hours protection but may require reapplication for maximum effectiveness. Higher DEET concentrations (up to 98%) and some newer DEET formulations with lower concentrations that are microencapsulated provide protection times up to 12 hours. Although there have been rare reports of serious neurologic complications in children possibly associated with exposure to DEET-containing insect repellents, the risk is extremely low when these products are used properly. Products containing DEET should be applied as recommended (see Prevention of Mosquitoborne Infections, p 213). For children 2 months and older, products with no more than 30% DEET are recommended. Products containing DEET are not recommended for use on infants younger than 2 months. Repellents should not be used on skin, clothing, or mosquito nets on which young children may chew or suck.
- **Picaridin and other products.** Picaridin (KBR 3023), the plant-based oil of eucalyptus, IR3535 (3-[N-Butyl-N-acetyl]-aminopropionic acid, ethyl ester), 2-undecanone, and other active ingredients have been registered for use as tick repellents by the EPA. These products are readily available and provide protection times similar to the DEET repellents, ranging from 2 to 12 hours, depending on the concentration of active ingredient and formulation. Check the product labels for information on duration of protection. The non-DEET products may be more acceptable to some families because they do not damage certain synthetic fabrics and plastics as may DEET-containing products.
- People should inspect themselves and their children's bodies, clothing, and equipment used daily after possible tick exposure. As soon as possible after potential tick exposure, it is important to remove clothes as they may still harbor crawling ticks. Bathing or showering after coming indoors (preferably within 2 hours) can help with finding attached ticks and washing off any unattached ticks that may have gone unnoticed.
- Placing outdoor clothing in the dryer on high heat for 1 hour will kill unattached ticks. When conducting tick checks, special attention should be given to the exposed regions of the body where ticks often attach, including the head, neck, and behind the ears on children. Ticks also may attach at areas of tight clothing (eg, sock line, belt line, axillae, groin).
- Ticks should be removed from skin as soon as they are discovered, because risk of transmission of pathogens increases with time of tick attachment. For removal, it is most important to grasp the tick close to the skin. Curved forceps or tweezers are recommended; grasp close to the skin and gently pull straight out without twisting motions. Care must be taken not to break mouthparts (These often are cemented into the skin by the tick) as the tick is removed. Tweezers also can be used to remove

mouthparts or "cement" left on the skin. If fingers are used to remove ticks, they should be protected with a barrier, such as tissue, and washed after removal of the tick. The bite site should be washed with soap and water to reduce the risk of secondary skin infections.

- Testing ticks removed from animals or humans for infectious diseases is not recommended.
- Maintaining tick-free pets also will decrease tick exposure in and around the home. Daily inspection of pets and removal of ticks are indicated, as is the routine use of appropriate veterinary products to prevent ticks on pets. Consult a veterinarian for information on suitable effective products.
- Chemoprophylaxis to prevent Lyme disease may be considered under certain circumstances and certain age groups in areas with highly endemic Lyme disease (see Lyme Disease, p 516).

PREVENTION OF MOSQUITOBORNE INFECTIONS

Mosquitoborne infectious diseases in the United States are caused by arboviruses (eg, West Nile, La Crosse, St. Louis encephalitis, eastern equine encephalitis, and western equine encephalitis viruses [see Arboviruses, p 240]). International travelers may encounter other arboviral (eg, yellow fever, dengue, Chikungunya, Japanese encephalitis) or other mosquitoborne infections (eg, malaria) during travel (also see disease-specific chapters in Section 3). Physicians should be aware of the epidemiology of arbovirus infections in their local areas. Prevention involves protection from the bite of an infected mosquito. In areas with arbovirus transmission, protection of children is recommended during outdoor activities, including activities related to school, child care, or camping. Education of families and other caregivers is an important component of prevention. Specific measures include:

- **Eliminate local mosquito breeding sites.** Mosquitoes develop in standing water. Often, large numbers of mosquitoes are produced from sources at or very near the home. Measures to limit mosquito breeding sites around the home include drainage or removal of receptacles for standing water (old tires, toys, flower pots, cans, buckets, barrels, other containers that collect rain water); keeping swimming pools, decorative pools, children's wading pools, and bird-baths clean; and cleaning clogged rain gutters. Under certain circumstances, large-scale mosquito-control measures may be conducted by communities or public health officials. These efforts include drainage of standing water, use of larvicides in waters that are sources of mosquitoes, and use of pesticides to control biting adult mosquitoes.
- **Reduce exposure to mosquitoes.** Avoiding mosquito bites by limiting outdoor activities at times of high mosquito activity, which primarily occur at dusk and dawn, and screening of windows and doors can help reduce exposure to mosquitoes. Many parts of the United States also have mosquitoes that bite during the day, and some of these have been found to transmit La Crosse, dengue, and West Nile viruses. Mosquito traps, electrocutors (bug zappers), ultrasonic repellers, and other devices marketed to prevent mosquitoes from biting people are not effective and should not be relied on to reduce mosquito bites. Mosquitoes that transmit malaria are active at night.

- **Use barriers to protect skin.** Barriers include mosquito nets and screens for baby strollers or other areas where immobile children are placed. Additional protection can be gained, when practical, by using clothing to cover exposed skin (ie, long sleeves, long pants, socks, shoes, and hats).
- **Discourage mosquitoes from biting.** Mosquitoes are attracted to people by odors on the skin and by carbon dioxide and other volatile chemicals from the breath. The active ingredients in repellents make the user unattractive for feeding, but they do not kill the mosquitoes. Repellents should be used during outdoor activities when mosquitoes are present, especially in regions with arbovirus transmission and when traveling to areas with endemic malaria, and should always be used according to the label instructions. Repellents are synthetic compounds or derivatives of plant oils. The most effective repellents for use on skin are products that contain either DEET (N,N-diethyl-meta-toluamide), picaridin (KBR 3023), IR3535 (3-[N-Butyl-N-acetyl]-aminopropionic acid, ethyl ester), or the plant-based oil of lemon eucalyptus (OLE) and its synthetic equivalent p-menthane-3,8-diol (PMD). Products containing these active ingredients have been shown to have good repellent activity. Products with a higher concentration of active ingredients generally protect longer and are appropriate for people who will be exposed to mosquitoes during outdoor activities lasting many hours. Products with lower concentrations of active ingredients may be used when more transient protection is required and can be reapplied as needed. Studies in human volunteers document the association of active ingredient concentration with duration of repellent activity. The US Environmental Protection Agency (EPA) reports that protection times range from as low as 2 hours for products containing 5% DEET to 10 hours or more for products containing 40% or more DEET. However, time-released DEET formulations are available that provide 11 to 12 hours protection with concentrations of 20% to 30% DEET. Products containing 5% picaridin provide 3 to 4 hours of protection, and products with 20% picaridin can provide protection for 8 to 12 hours. IR3535 is available in formulations ranging from 7.5% to 20%, with estimated protection times ranging from 2 hours for the lower concentrations to up to 10 hours with the higher concentrations. Products containing 30% to 40% OLE provide 6 hours of protection, and products with 8% to 10% PMD protect for up to 2 hours but are not recommended for children younger than 3 years. All other products studied, including those based on citronella, catnip oil, and other essential plant oils, provide minimal protection and are not recommended. Ingestion of garlic or vitamin B_1, wearing devices that emit sounds, and impregnated wristbands are ineffective measures.

DEET has been used worldwide since 1957, has been studied more extensively than any other repellent, and has a good safety profile. Concerns about potential toxicity, especially in children, are unfounded. Adverse effects are rare; are most often associated with ingestions, chronic use, or excessive use; and do not appear to be related to DEET concentration used. Urticaria and contact dermatitis have been reported in a small number of people. Although rare, adverse systemic effects including encephalopathy have been reported after skin application in children. Encephalopathy also has been reported after unintentional ingestion. DEET is irritating to eyes and mucous membranes. Concentrated formulations can damage plastic and certain fabrics. If used appropriately, DEET does not present a health problem.

Although concentrations of 10% to 15% DEET or lower have been recommended for children, there is no evidence that these concentrations are safer than 30% DEET. There is no evidence that repellents that do not contain DEET are safer for children.

The EPA has approved DEET for use on children with no age restriction and no restrictions on the percentage of DEET contained in the product. The American Academy of Pediatrics recommends that repellents used on children should contain no more than 30% DEET and that insect repellents are not recommended for use in children younger than 2 months.[1] The Centers for Disease Control and Prevention currently recommends DEET at concentrations up to 50% for both adults and children and suggests an infant carrier drape with mosquito netting for protection for infants younger than 2 months.

Picaridin-containing compounds have been used as an insect repellent for years in Europe, and Australia as a 20% formulation with no serious toxicity reported. Except for eye irritation, products containing OLE appear safe, although the EPA specifies that they should not be used on children younger than 3 years.

Permethrin-containing repellents are registered by the EPA for use on clothing, shoes, bed nets, and camping gear. Permethrin is a synthetic pyrethroid that is highly effective both as an insecticide and as a repellent for ticks, mosquitoes, and other arthropods. Permethrin can be sprayed onto clothes but should not be sprayed onto skin. Some manufacturers now offer permethrin-treated clothing, and beginning in 2003, the EPA approved commercial sale of outdoor clothing treated with permethrin for children of all ages and for pregnant women. Repellents should not be used on clothing or mosquito nets on which young children may chew or suck.

The EPA recommends the following precautions when using insect repellents. Recommendations for use of any of these insect repellents should be followed for children:

- Do not apply over cuts, wounds, or irritated or sunburned skin. Avoid areas around eyes and mouth.
- Do not spray onto the face; apply with hands.
- Use just enough to cover exposed skin.
- Do not apply to young children's hands, because they may rub it into their eyes or mouth.
- Do not allow young children to apply a product themselves.
- Do not apply under clothing.
- Do not use sprays in enclosed areas or near food.
- Repellents containing DEET, applied according to label instructions, can be used along with a separate sunscreen. No data are available regarding the use of other active repellent ingredients in combination with a sunscreen.
- Reapply if washed off by sweating or by getting wet.
- After returning indoors, wash treated skin with soap and water or bathe. Also, wash treated clothing before wearing again (unless product instructions for permethrin clothing treatments state otherwise).
- If a child develops a rash or other reaction from any insect repellent, wash the repellent off with soap and water and contact the child's physician or the US poison control center (800-222-1222) for guidance.

Spatial repellent devices that release a repellent material into an area in the form of a vapor are becoming more widely available. These products release volatile active ingredients, such as metofluthrin and allethrin, and are approved by the EPA for use outdoors. Although many of these products have documented repellent activity, their ability to provide protection from mosquito bites has not been evaluated thoroughly.

[1] American Academy of Pediatrics, Committee on Environmental Health. Pesticides. In: Etzel RA, Balk SJ, eds. *Pediatric Environmental Health. 3rd* ed. Elk Grove Village, IL: American Academy of Pediatrics; 2012:515-548

PREVENTION OF ILLNESSES ASSOCIATED WITH RECREATIONAL WATER USE

Pathogen transmission via recreational water (eg, swimming pools, interactive fountains, lakes, oceans) is an increasingly recognized source of illness in the United States. Since the mid-1980s, the number of outbreaks related to recreational water activities has increased substantially, particularly outbreaks associated with treated recreational water venues (eg, swimming pools).[1] Therefore, preventing recreational water-associated illness (RWI) is becoming increasingly important for the health of children and adults. RWIs are caused by infectious pathogens transmitted by ingesting, inhaling aerosols of, or having contact with contaminated water from swimming pools, interactive fountains, water parks, hot tubs/spas, lakes, rivers, or oceans. RWIs also can be caused by chemicals in the water or chemicals that volatilize from the water and cause indoor air quality problems. Illnesses caused by recreational water exposure can involve the gastrointestinal tract, respiratory tract, central nervous system, skin, ears, or eyes. During 2009–2010, 81 waterborne disease outbreaks associated with recreational water were reported.[1] Of the 81 outbreaks, 54% involved only the gastrointestinal tract, 26% involved only the skin, and 10% involved only the respiratory tract. The leading etiologic agent of outbreaks associated with treated recreational water venues was *Cryptosporidium* species, associated with 24 (69%) of 35 treated recreational water-associated outbreaks with identified infectious causes[1] (see Cryptosporidiosis, p 312). Cryptosporidiosis may cause life-threatening infection in immunocompromised children and adolescents.

Swimming is a communal bathing activity by which the same water is shared by dozens to thousands of people each day, depending on venue size (eg, small wading pools, municipal pools, water parks). Fecal contamination of recreational water venues is a common occurrence because of the high prevalence of diarrhea and fecal incontinence (particularly in young children) and the presence of residual fecal material on bodies of swimmers (up to 10 g on young children). The largest outbreaks of waterborne disease tend to affect children younger than 5 years disproportionately, occur during the summer months, and result in gastroenteritis.

To protect swimmers from pathogens, water in public treated recreational water venues is chlorinated to oxidize fecal matter and pathogens. Although this is sufficient for most, some pathogens are moderately to highly tolerant to chlorination and can survive for extended periods of time in chlorinated water. *Cryptosporidium* oocysts can remain infectious for more than 10 days in chlorine concentrations typically mandated in swimming pools, thus contributing to the role of *Cryptosporidium* species as the leading cause of treated recreational water-associated outbreaks. *Giardia intestinalis* has been shown to survive for up to 45 minutes in water chlorinated at concentrations typically used in swimming pools and is well documented as a cause of recreational water-associated disease outbreaks.

Recreational water use is an ideal means of amplifying pathogen transmission within a community because of extremely chlorine-tolerant pathogens, coupled with low infectious doses, high pathogen-excretion concentrations, and poor swimmer hygiene (eg,

---

[1]Centers for Disease Control and Prevention. Recreational water-associated disease outbreaks—United States, 2009-2010. *MMWR Morb Mortal Wkly Rep.* 2014;63(1):6-10. Available at: **www.cdc.gov/mmwr/pdf/wk/mm6301.pdf**

swimming when ill with diarrhea, swallowing recreational water). As a result, one or more swimmers ill with diarrhea can contaminate large volumes of water and expose large numbers of swimmers to pathogens, particularly if pool disinfection is inadequate or the pathogen is chlorine tolerant. However, RWI outbreaks generally can be prevented and controlled through a combination of water disinfection, proper pool maintenance, and improved swimmer hygiene and behavior.

Control Measures

Swimming continues to be a safe and effective means of physical activity. Transmission of infectious pathogens that cause RWIs can be prevented by reducing contamination of swimming venues and exposure to contaminated water. Pediatricians should counsel families:

- Do not go into recreational water (eg, swim) when ill with diarrhea.
  - After cessation of symptoms, people who had diarrhea attributable to *Cryptosporidium* also should avoid recreational water activities for an additional 2 weeks. This is because of prolonged excretion of infectious *Cryptosporidium* oocysts after cessation of symptoms, the potential for intermittent exacerbations of diarrhea, and the increased transmission potential in treated venues (eg, swimming pools) because of the parasite's high chlorine tolerance.
  - After cessation of symptoms, children who had diarrhea attributable to other potential waterborne pathogens (eg, *Shigella* species, norovirus) and who are incontinent should avoid recreational water activities for 1 additional week.
- Do not go into recreational water (eg, swim) if you have open wounds or sores until the wounds or sores heal. Open wounds can serve as portals of entry for pathogens.
- Avoid ingestion of recreational water.
- Practice good swimming hygiene by:
  - Taking a cleansing shower, using soap and water, before going into recreational water.
  - Washing children thoroughly, especially the perianal area, with soap and water before allowing them to go into recreational water.
  - Taking children on bathroom breaks every 60 minutes or checking their diapers every 30 to 60 minutes.
  - Washing hands with soap and water after toilet use and diaper-changing activities. Toilet use and diaper changing should occur away from the recreational water source and food preparation activities.
  - Washing hands with soap and water before consumption of food and drink.
  - Implementing seasonal educational campaigns to maximize awareness of healthy swimming behaviors (**www.cdc.gov/healthywater/swimming/protection/triple-a-healthy-swimming.html**).

Recommendations for responding to fecal incidents in treated recreational water venues have been published.[1]

---

[1]Centers for Disease Control and Prevention. Notice to readers: revised recommendations for responding to fecal accidents in disinfected swimming venues. *MMWR Morb Mortal Wkly Rep.* 2008;57(6):151-152. Available at: **www.cdc.gov/mmwr/preview/mmwrhtml/mm5706a5.htm**

"Swimmer's Ear"/Acute Otitis Externa

Participation in recreational water activities can predispose children to infections of the external auditory canal. Acute otitis externa (AOE) or "swimmer's ear" is diffuse inflammation of the external auditory canal and usually is attributed to bacterial infection. Recreational water activities, showering, and bathing can introduce water into the ear canal, wash away protective ear wax, and cause maceration of the thin skin of the ear canal, predisposing the ear canal to bacterial infection. AOE is most common among children 5 to 14 years of age but can occur in all age groups, including adults. A marked seasonality is observed, with cases peaking during the summer months. Warm, humid environments and frequent submersion of the head while swimming are risk factors for AOE.

The 2 bacteria most commonly associated with AOE are *Pseudomonas aeruginosa* and *Staphylococcus aureus*. Many cases are polymicrobial. *Aspergillus* species and *Candida* species have been identified rarely in AOE. Cultures of swab specimens taken from the external ear canal in AOE might reflect normal ear canal flora or pathogenic organisms.

AOE readily responds to treatment with topical antimicrobial agents with or without a topical steroid. Unless the infection has spread to surrounding tissues or the patient has complicating factors (eg, diabetes or immunosuppression), topical treatment alone should be sufficient and systemic antimicrobials are usually not required. Polymyxin B sulfate/ neomycin sulfate, gentamicin sulfate, and ciprofloxacin for 7 to 10 days are topical antibiotic agents used commonly. If clinical improvement is not noted by 48 to 72 hours, foreign body obstruction of the canal, noncompliance with therapy, or alternate diagnoses such as contact dermatitis or traumatic cellulitis should be considered. Topical agents that have the potential for ototoxicity (eg, gentamicin, neomycin, agents with a low pH, hydrocortisone-neomycin-polymyxin) should not be used in children with tympanostomy tubes or a perforated tympanic membrane. Patients with AOE should avoid submerging their head in water for 7 to 10 days, but competitive swimmers might be able to return to the pool if pain has resolved and they use well-fitting ear plugs.

Swimmers should be instructed to keep their ear canals as dry as possible. This can be accomplished by covering the opening of the external auditory canal with a bathing cap or by using ear plugs or swim molds. Following swimming or showering, the ears should be dried thoroughly.

If a person experiences recurring episodes of AOE, consideration can be given to use of antimicrobial otic drops after recreational water exposure as an additional preventive measure. Commercial ear-drying agents are available for use as directed, or a 1:1 mixture of acetic acid (white vinegar) and isopropanol (rubbing alcohol) may be placed in the external ear canal after swimming or showering to restore the proper acidic pH to the ear canal and to dry residual water. Otic drying agents should not be used in the presence of tympanostomy tubes, tympanic membrane perforation, acute external ear infection, or ear drainage.

For additional information on otitis externa prevention, visit **www.cdc.gov/ healthywater/swimming/rwi/illnesses/swimmers-ear-prevention- guidelines.html.**

DISEASES TRANSMITTED BY ANIMALS (ZOONOSES): HOUSEHOLD PETS, INCLUDING NONTRADITIONAL PETS, AND EXPOSURE TO ANIMALS IN PUBLIC SETTINGS[1,2]

Animals can provide wonderful opportunities for education and entertainment. However, disease transmission between animals and humans is possible for children who interact with pets or other domestic or wild animals. Important zoonoses that may be encountered in North America, the common animal source or vector, and major modes of transmission are reviewed in disease-specific chapters in Section 3 and are listed in Appendix VIII (p 1014). Most households in the United States contain 1 or more pets. The number of families with nontraditional pets, defined as (1) imported, nonnative species or species that originally were nonnative but now are bred in the United States; (2) indigenous wildlife; or (3) wildlife hybrids (offspring of wildlife crossbred with domestic animals), has increased in recent years. Infants and children also come in contact with animals at many venues outside the home, including agricultural fairs, farms, zoos, petting zoos, schools or child care centers, hospitals, and animal swap meets. Examples of nontraditional pets and animals commonly encountered in public settings are listed in Table 2.19, p 220.

Exposure to animals can pose significant infection risks to all people, but children younger than 5 years, pregnant women, people older than 65 years, and people of all ages with immunodeficiencies are at higher risk of serious infections. The increased infection risk for children younger than 5 years is attributable, in part, to children's less-than-optimal hygiene practices and developing immune systems. Children younger than 5 years also are at increased risk of injury from animals because of their size and behavior. Bites, scratches, kicks, falls, and crush injuries to hands or feet from being pinned between an animal and a fixed object can occur.

Nontraditional pets pose a potential risk of infection and injury. Most imported nonnative animal species are caught in the wild rather than bred in captivity. These animals are held and transported in close contact with multiple other species, thus increasing the transmission risk of potential pathogens for humans and domestic animals. Some nonnative animals are brought into the United States illegally, thus bypassing rules established to reduce introduction of disease and potentially dangerous animals. Some species of nonnative animals may also be bred in captivity in North America. In addition, as an animal matures, its physical and behavioral characteristics can result in an increased risk of injuries to children. The behavior of captive indigenous wildlife and wildlife hybrids cannot be predicted. These potential risks are enhanced when there is an inadequate

---

[1]Pickering LK; Marano N; Bocchini JA; Angulo FJ; American Academy of Pediatrics, Committee on Infectious Diseases. Exposure to nontraditional pets at home and to animals in public settings: risks to children. *Pediatrics.* 2008;122(4):876-886 (Reaffirmed December 2011)

[2]National Association of State Public Health Veterinarians. Compendium of measures to prevent disease associated with animals in public settings, 2011. *MMWR Recomm Rep.* 2011;60(RR-04):1-24

Table 2.19. Nontraditional Pets and/or Animals That May Be Encountered in Public Settings[a]

Category	Examples
Amphibians	Frogs, toads, newts, salamanders
Reptiles	Turtles, lizards, iguanas, snakes, alligators, crocodiles
Birds	Poultry (chicks, chickens, ducks, geese, and turkeys), parakeets and other parrots
Aquatic animals	Many types of fish, rays, sharks
Mammals	
Domesticated livestock/farm animals	Cattle, pigs, goats, sheep
Equines	Horses, mules, donkeys
Small, exotic animals	Ferrets, hedgehogs, sugar gliders
Lagomorphs	Rabbits, hares, pikas
Rodents	Mice, rats, hamsters, gerbils, guinea pigs, chinchillas
Wildlife	Raccoons, kinkajous, skunks, foxes, coyotes, deer, chipmunks, squirrels, prairie dogs, civet cats, tigers, lions, bobcats, bears, nonhuman primates
Feral animals	Cats, dogs, horses, swine

[a]Adapted from Pickering LK; Marano N; Bocchini JA; Angulo FJ; American Academy of Pediatrics, Committee on Infectious Diseases. Exposure to nontraditional pets at home and to animals in public settings: risks to children. *Pediatrics.* 2008;122(4):876–886 (Reaffirmed June 2013).

understanding of disease transmission and methods to prevent transmission; animal behavior; or how to maintain appropriate facilities, environment, or nutrition for captive animals. Among nontraditional pets, reptiles, amphibians, and poultry pose a particular risk because of high asymptomatic carriage rates of *Salmonella* species, the intermittent shedding of *Salmonella* organisms in their feces, and persistence of *Salmonella* organisms in the environment. In recent years, multiple large outbreaks of zoonotic salmonellosis have been linked to these species and are described on the Centers for Disease Control and Prevention's Gastrointestinal (Enteric) Zoonoses Web site (**www.cdc.gov/zoonotic/ gi/**). The US Food and Drug Administration's ban on commercial distribution of turtles with shells less than 4 inches long in 1975 resulted in a sustained reduction of human *Salmonella* infections. *Salmonella* infections also have been described as a result of contact with aquatic frogs, iguanas, hedgehogs, hamsters, mice, and other rodents and with poultry or backyard flocks, including chicks, chickens, ducks, ducklings, geese, goslings, and turkeys. Lymphocytic choriomeningitis infections also have been described as a result of contact with pet rodents (eg, hamsters). Additionally, pet products, such as dry dog and cat food, and pet treats, such as pig ears and feeder rodents (both live and frozen) used to feed reptiles and amphibians, have been sources of *Salmonella* infections, especially among young children.

Infectious diseases, injuries, and other health problems can occur after contact with animals in public settings. Enteric bacteria and parasites pose the highest infection risk. Individual cases and outbreaks associated with *Salmonella* species, *Escherichia coli* O157:H7, and *Cryptosporidium* species are most commonly reported. Many recent outbreaks of enteric zoonoses have been linked to contact with ruminant livestock (cattle, sheep, and goats); poultry, including chicks, chickens, and ducks; reptiles, especially small turtles; amphibians; and rodents. However, other domestic and wild animals also are potential sources of illness. Infected animals often are asymptomatic carriers of potential human pathogens. Direct contact with animals (especially young animals), contamination of the environment or food or water sources, and inadequate hand hygiene facilities at animal exhibits all have been implicated as reasons for infection in these public settings. Indirect contact with animals can also be a source of illness to people, including water in a reptile or amphibian tank or contaminated barriers or fencing. Unusual infection or exposure has been reported occasionally. Rabies has occurred in animals in a petting zoo, pet store, animal shelter, and county fair, necessitating prophylaxis of adults and children.

Contact with animals has numerous positive benefits, including opportunities for education and entertainment. However, many pet owners and people in the process of choosing a pet are unaware of the potential risks posed by pets. Additionally, most people are unaware that animals that appear healthy may carry pathogenic microbes. Pediatricians, veterinarians, and other health care professionals are in a unique position to offer advice on proper pet selection, to provide information about safe pet ownership and responsibility, and to minimize risks to infants and children. Pet size and temperament should be matched to the age and behavior of an infant or child. Acquisition and ownership of nontraditional pets should be discouraged in households with young children or other high-risk individuals. Information brochures and posters in multiple languages are available for display in physician and veterinarian offices so parents can be educated about the guidelines available for safe pet selection and appropriate handling (**www.cdc.gov/zoonotic/gi/, www.cdc.gov/healthypets/index.htm, www.cdc.gov/Features/ HealthyPets/,** and **https://ebusiness.avma.org/ebusiness50/ productcatalog/ProductCategory.aspx?ID=132).**

Young children should always be supervised closely when in contact with animals at home or in public settings, including child care centers or schools, and children should be educated about appropriate human-animal interactions. Parents should be made aware of recommendations for prevention of human diseases and injuries from exposure to pets, including nontraditional pets and animals in the home, animals in public settings, and pet products including food and pet treats (Table 2.20). Pets and other animals should receive appropriate veterinary care from a licensed veterinarian who can provide preventive care, including vaccinations and parasite control, appropriate for the species.

Questions regarding pet and animal contact should be part of well-child evaluations and the evaluation of a suspected infectious disease.

Table 2.20. Guidelines for Prevention of Human Diseases From Exposure to Pets, Nontraditional Pets, and Animals in Public Settings[a,b]

General

- Always supervise children, especially children younger than 5 years, during interaction with animals
- Wash hands immediately after contact with animals, animal products, feed or treats, or animal environments and after taking off dirty clothes or shoes; hands should be washed even when direct contact with an animal did not occur
- Supervise hand washing for children younger than 5 years
- Do not allow children to kiss animals or to eat, drink, or put objects or hands into their mouths after handling animals or while in animal areas
- Do not permit nontraditional pets to roam or fly freely in the house or allow nontraditional or domestic pets to have contact with wild animals
- Do not permit animals in areas where food or drink are stored, prepared, served, or consumed
- Never bring wild animals home, and never adopt wild animals as pets
- Teach children never to handle unfamiliar, wild, or domestic animals, even if animals appear friendly
- Avoid rough play with animals to prevent scratches or bites
- Pets and other animals should receive appropriate veterinary care from a licensed veterinarian who can provide preventive care, including vaccination and parasite control, appropriate for the species
- Administer rabies vaccine to all dogs, cats, horses, and ferrets; livestock animals and horses with frequent human contact also should be up to date with all immunizations
- Keep animals clean and free of intestinal parasites, fleas, ticks, mites, and lice
- People at increased risk of infection or serious complications of salmonellosis and other enteric infections (eg, children younger than 5 years, people older than 65 years, and immunocompromised people) should avoid contact with high-risk animals (turtles and other reptiles; poultry, including chicks, chickens, ducklings, and ducks in backyard flocks; aquatic frogs and other amphibians; and farm animals) and animal-derived pet treats and pet foods
- People at increased risk of infection or serious complications of lymphocytic choriomeningitis virus infections (eg, pregnant women and immunocompromised people) should avoid contact with rodents and rodent housing and bedding.

Animals Visiting Schools and Child-Care Facilities

- Designate specific areas for animal contact
- Display animals in enclosed cages or under appropriate restraint
- Do not allow food in animal-contact areas
- Always supervise children, especially those younger than 5 years, during interaction with animals
- Obtain a certificate of veterinary inspection for visiting animals and/or proof of rabies immunization according to local or state requirements
- Properly clean and disinfect all areas where animals have been present

Table 2.20. Guidelines for Prevention of Human Diseases From Exposure to Pets, Nontraditional Pets, and Animals in Public Settings,[a,b] continued

- Consult with parents or guardians to determine special considerations needed for children who are immunocompromised or who have allergies or asthma
- Animals not recommended in schools, child-care settings, hospitals, or nursing homes include nonhuman primates; inherently dangerous animals (lions, tigers, cougars, bears, wolf/dog hybrids), mammals at high risk of transmitting rabies (bats, raccoons, skunks, foxes, coyotes, and mongooses), aggressive animals or animals with unpredictable behavior; stray animals with unknown health history; venomous or toxin-producing spiders, insects, reptiles, and amphibians; and animals at higher risk for causing serious illness or injury, including reptiles, amphibians, or chicks, ducks, or other live poultry; and ferrets. Additionally, children younger than 5 years should not be allowed to have direct contact with these animals.
- Farm animals are not appropriate in facilities with children younger than 5 years and should not be displayed to older children in school settings unless meticulous attention to personal hygiene can be ensured.
- Ensure that people who provide animals for educational purposes are knowledgeable regarding animal handling and zoonotic disease issues

Public Settings

- Venue operators must know about risks of disease and injury
- Venue operators and staff must maintain a safe environment
- Venue operators and staff must educate visitors about the risk of disease and injury and provide appropriate preventive measures
- Venue operators and staff should be familiar with the recommendations detailed in the Compendium of Measures to Prevent Diseases Associated with Animals in Public Settings[b]

Animal Specific

- Know that healthy animals can carry germs that can make people sick. People can become ill when they touch an animal, pick up an animal's dropping, or enter an animal environment even if they don't touch the animal
- Children younger than 5 years, pregnant women, and immunocompromised people should avoid contact with reptiles, amphibians, rodents, ferrets, baby poultry (chicks, ducklings), preweaned calves, and any items that have been in contact with these animals or their environments
- Reptiles, amphibians, rodents, ferrets, and baby poultry (chicks, ducklings) should be kept out of households that contain children younger than 5 years, pregnant women, immunocompromised people, people older than 65 years, or people with sickle cell disease and should not be allowed in child care centers or other facilities that house high-risk individuals (eg, nursing homes).
- Reptiles, amphibians, rodents, and baby poultry should not be permitted to roam freely throughout a home or living area and should not be permitted in kitchens or other areas where food and drink is prepared, stored, served, or consumed
- Animal cages or enclosures should not be cleaned in sinks or other areas used to store, prepare, serve, or consume food and drinks; These items should be cleaned outside the house if possible

Table 2.20. Guidelines for Prevention of Human Diseases From Exposure to Pets, Nontraditional Pets, and Animals in Public Settings,[a,b] continued

- Mammals at high risk of transmitting rabies (bats, raccoons, skunks, foxes, and coyotes) should not be touched

- Disposable gloves should be used when cleaning fish aquariums, and aquarium water should not be disposed in sinks used for food preparation or for obtaining drinking water

- Pregnant women and immunocompromised people should avoid contact with cat feces or soil contaminated with cat feces

[a]Pickering LK, Marano N, Bocchini JA, Angulo FJ; American Academy of Pediatrics, Committee on Infectious Diseases. Exposure to nontraditional pets at home and to animals in public settings: risks to children. *Pediatrics.* 2008;122(4):876–886 (Reaffirmed June 2013).

[b]For complete recommendations, see: National Association of State Public Health Veterinarians, Animal Contact Compendium Committee 2013. Compendium of measures to prevent disease associated with animals in public settings, 2013. *J Am Vet Med Assoc.* 2013;243(9):1270-1288.

Summaries of Infectious Diseases

Actinomycosis

CLINICAL MANIFESTATIONS: Actinomycosis results from pathogen introduction following a breakdown in mucocutaneous protective barriers. Spread within the host is by direct invasion of adjacent tissues, typically forming sinus tracts that cross tissue planes. The most common species causing human disease is *Actinomyces israelii*.

There are 3 common anatomic sites. **Cervicofacial** is most common, often occurring after tooth extraction, oral surgery, other oral/facial trauma, or even from carious teeth. Localized pain and induration may progress to cervical abscess and "woody hard" nodular lesions ("lumpy jaw"), which can develop draining sinus tracts, usually at the angle of the jaw or in the submandibular region. Infection may contribute to chronic tonsillar airway obstruction. **Thoracic** disease most commonly is secondary to aspiration of oropharyngeal secretions but may be an extension of cervicofacial infection. It occurs rarely after esophageal disruption secondary to surgery or nonpenetrating trauma. Thoracic presentation includes pneumonia, which can be complicated by abscesses, empyema, and rarely, pleurodermal sinuses. Focal or multifocal mediastinal and pulmonary masses may be mistaken for tumors. **Abdominal** actinomycosis usually is attributable to penetrating trauma or intestinal perforation. The appendix and cecum are the most common sites; symptoms are similar to appendicitis. Slowly developing masses may simulate abdominal or retroperitoneal neoplasms. Intra-abdominal abscesses and peritoneal-dermal draining sinuses occur eventually. Chronic localized disease often forms draining sinus tracts with purulent discharge. **Other sites** of infection include the liver, pelvis (which, in some cases, has been linked to use of intrauterine devices), heart, testicles, and brain (which usually is associated with a primary pulmonary focus). Noninvasive primary cutaneous actinomycosis has occurred.

ETIOLOGY: *A israelii* and at least 5 other *Actinomyces* species cause human disease. All are slow-growing, microaerophilic or facultative anaerobic, gram-positive, filamentous branching bacilli. They can be part of normal oral, gastrointestinal tract, or vaginal flora. *Actinomyces* species frequently are copathogens in tissues harboring multiple other anaerobic and/or aerobic species. Isolation of *Aggregatibacter (Actinobacillus) actinomycetemcomitans*, frequently detected with *Actinomyces* species, may predict the presence of actinomycosis.

EPIDEMIOLOGY: *Actinomyces* species occur worldwide, being components of endogenous oral and gastrointestinal tract flora. *Actinomyces* species are opportunistic pathogens (reported in patients with human immunodeficiency virus [HIV] and chronic granulomatous disease), with disease usually following penetrating (including human bite wounds) and nonpenetrating trauma. Infection is uncommon in infants and children, with 80% of cases occurring in adults. The male-to-female ratio in children is 1.5:1. Overt, microbiologically confirmed, monomicrobial disease caused by *Actinomyces* species has become rare in the era of antimicrobial agents.

The **incubation period** varies from several days to several years.

DIAGNOSTIC TESTS: Microscopic demonstration of beaded, branched, gram-positive bacilli in purulent material or tissue specimens suggests the diagnosis. Only specimens from normally sterile sites should be submitted for culture. Specimens must be obtained, transported, and cultured anaerobically on semiselective (kanamycin/vancomycin) media. Acid-fast staining can distinguish *Actinomyces* species, which are acid-fast negative, from *Nocardia* species, which are variably acid-fast positive. Yellow "sulfur granules" visualized microscopically or macroscopically in drainage or loculations of purulent material suggest the diagnosis. A Gram stain of "sulfur granules" discloses a dense aggregate of bacterial filaments mixed with inflammatory debris. Immunofluorescent stains for *Actinomyces* species are available. *Actinomyces israelii* forms "spiderlike" microcolonies on culture medium after 48 hours. *Actinomyces* species can be identified in tissue specimens using the 16s rRNA sequencing and polymerase chain reaction assay.

TREATMENT: Initial therapy should include intravenous penicillin G or ampicillin for 4 to 6 weeks followed by high doses of oral penicillin (up to 2 g/day for adults), usually for a total of 6 to 12 months. Exclusively oral therapy has been reported as effective as intravenous therapy for cases of cervicofacial disease. Amoxicillin, erythromycin, clindamycin, doxycycline, and tetracycline are alternative antimicrobial choices. Amoxicillin/clavulanate, piperacillin/tazobactam, ceftriaxone, clarithromycin, linezolid, and meropenem also show high activity in vitro. All *Actinomyces* appear resistant to ciprofloxacin and metronidazole. Tetracyclines are not recommended for pregnant women or children younger than 8 years of age. Tetracycline-based antimicrobial agents, including doxycycline, may cause permanent tooth discoloration for children younger than 8 years if used for repeated treatment courses. However, doxycycline binds less readily to calcium compared with older tetracyclines, and in some studies, doxycycline was not associated with visible teeth staining in younger children (see Tetracyclines, p 873).

Surgical drainage often is a necessary adjunct to medical management and may allow for a shorter duration of antimicrobial treatment.

ISOLATION OF THE HOSPITALIZED PATIENT: Standard precautions are recommended. There is no person-to-person spread.

CONTROL MEASURES: Appropriate oral hygiene, regular dental care, and careful cleansing of wounds, including human bite wounds, can prevent infection.

Adenovirus Infections

CLINICAL MANIFESTATIONS: Adenovirus infections of the upper respiratory tract are common and, although often subclinical, can result in symptoms of the common cold, pharyngitis, tonsillitis, otitis media, and pharyngoconjunctival fever. Life-threatening disseminated infection, severe pneumonia, hepatitis, meningitis, and encephalitis occur occasionally, especially among young infants and immunocompromised people. Adenoviruses occasionally cause a pertussis-like syndrome, croup, bronchiolitis, exudative tonsillitis, pneumonia, and hemorrhagic cystitis. Ocular adenovirus infections may present as follicular conjunctivitis or as epidemic keratoconjunctivitis. Enteric adenoviruses are an important cause of childhood gastroenteritis.

ETIOLOGY: Adenoviruses are double-stranded, nonenveloped DNA viruses; at least 51 distinct serotypes and multiple genetic variants divided into 7 species (A through G) infect humans. Some adenovirus types are associated primarily with respiratory tract disease (types 1-5, 7, 14, and 21), and others are associated primarily with gastroenteritis (types 40 and 41). During 2007, adenovirus type 14 emerged in the United States, where it caused severe and sometimes fatal respiratory tract illness in mostly adults, both civilian and military, and has now spread to Europe and Asia. Infection with one adenovirus type confers type-specific immunity, which forms the basis of adenovirus vaccines used in new military recruits (see Control Measures).

EPIDEMIOLOGY: Infection in infants and children can occur at any age. Adenoviruses causing respiratory tract infections usually are transmitted by respiratory tract secretions through person-to-person contact, airborne droplets, and fomites. Adenoviruses are hardy viruses, can survive on environmental surfaces for long periods, and are not inactivated by many disinfectants. The conjunctiva can provide a portal of entry. Outbreaks of febrile respiratory tract illness can be a common and significant problem in military trainees. Community outbreaks of adenovirus-associated pharyngoconjunctival fever have been attributed to water exposure from contaminated swimming pools and fomites, such as shared towels. Health care-associated transmission of adenoviral respiratory tract, conjunctival, and gastrointestinal tract infections can occur in hospitals, residential institutions, and nursing homes from exposures to infected health care personnel, patients, or contaminated equipment. Adenovirus infections in transplant recipients can occur from donor tissues. Epidemic keratoconjunctivitis commonly occurs by direct contact, has been associated with equipment used during eye examinations, and is caused principally by serotypes 8, 19, and 37. Enteric strains of adenoviruses are transmitted by the fecal-oral route. Adenoviruses do not demonstrate the marked seasonality of other respiratory tract viruses and circulate throughout the year. Whether individual adenovirus serotypes demonstrate seasonality is not clear. Enteric disease occurs year-round and primarily affects children younger than 4 years. Adenovirus infections are most communicable during the first few days of an acute illness, but persistent and intermittent shedding for longer periods, even months, is common. Asymptomatic infections are common. Reinfection can occur.

The **incubation period** for respiratory tract infection varies from 2 to 14 days; for gastroenteritis, the **incubation period** is 3 to 10 days.

DIAGNOSTIC TESTS: Methods for diagnosis of adenovirus infection include isolation in cell culture, antigen detection, and molecular detection. Adenoviruses associated with respiratory tract disease can be isolated from pharyngeal and eye secretions and from feces by inoculation of specimens into susceptible cell cultures. A pharyngeal or ocular isolate is more suggestive of recent infection than is a fecal isolate, which may indicate either recent infection or prolonged carriage. Rapid detection of adenovirus antigens is possible in a variety of body fluids by commercial immunoassay, including direct fluorescent assay. These rapid assays can be useful for the diagnosis of respiratory tract infections, ocular disease, and diarrheal disease. Enteric adenovirus types 40 and 41 usually cannot be isolated in standard cell cultures. Adenoviruses can be identified by electron microscopic examination of respiratory and stool specimens, but this modality lacks sensitivity. Polymerase chain reaction assays for adenovirus DNA are replacing other detection methods because of improved sensitivity and increasing commercial availability; however, the persistent and intermittent shedding that commonly follows an acute adenoviral infection can complicate the clinical interpretation of a positive molecular diagnostic test result. Adenovirus typing is available from some reference and research laboratories, although its clinical utility is limited; typing can be determined by hemagglutination inhibition or serum neutralization tests with selected antisera or by molecular methods. Serodiagnosis is used primarily for epidemiologic studies.

TREATMENT: Treatment of adenovirus infection is supportive. Randomized clinical trials evaluating specific antiviral therapy have not been performed. However, case reports of the successful use of cidofovir in immunocompromised patients with severe adenoviral disease have been published, albeit without a uniform dose or dosing strategy. An oral lipid conjugate of cidofovir, brincidofovir (CMX001), is being evaluated for the treatment of adenoviral disease in immunocompromised patients but is not commercially available at this time.

ISOLATION OF THE HOSPITALIZED PATIENT: In addition to standard precautions for young children with respiratory tract infections, contact and droplet precautions are indicated for the duration of hospitalization. In immunocompromised patients, contact and droplet precautions should be extended because of possible prolonged shedding of the virus. For patients with conjunctivitis and for diapered and incontinent children with adenoviral gastroenteritis, contact precautions are indicated for the duration of illness.

CONTROL MEASURES: Appropriate hand hygiene, respiratory hygiene, and cough etiquette should be followed. Children who are in group child care, particularly children from 6 months through 2 years of age, are at increased risk of adenoviral respiratory tract infections and gastroenteritis. Effective measures for preventing spread of adenovirus infection in this setting have not been determined, but frequent hand hygiene is recommended. If 2 or more children in a group child care setting develop conjunctivitis in the same period, advice should be sought from the health consultant of the program or the state health department.

Adequate chlorination of swimming pools is recommended to prevent pharyngoconjunctival fever. Epidemic keratoconjunctivitis associated with ophthalmologic practice can be difficult to control and requires use of single-dose medication dispensing and strict attention to hand hygiene and instrument sterilization procedures. Health care professionals with known or suspected adenoviral conjunctivitis should avoid direct patient contact for 14 days after onset of disease in the most recently involved eye. Adenoviruses are difficult to inactivate with alcohol-based gels because they lack an envelope, and may remain viable on skin, fomites, and environmental surfaces for extended periods. Thus, assiduous adherence to hand hygiene and use of disposable gloves when caring for infected patients are recommended.

A live, nonattenuated, oral adenovirus vaccine for types 4 and 7 (2 oral tablets, 1 for each of the 2 strains) has been licensed by the US Food and Drug Administration for prevention of febrile, acute respiratory tract disease. Tablets should be swallowed whole and not chewed. This vaccine is licensed for people 17 through 50 years of age who do not have contraindications and primarily is used in military personnel.

Amebiasis

CLINICAL MANIFESTATIONS: The majority of individuals with *Entamoeba histolytica* have asymptomatic noninvasive intestinal tract infection. When symptomatic, the clinical syndromes associated with *Entamoeba histolytica* infection generally include cramps, watery or bloody diarrhea, and weight loss. Occasionally the parasite may spread to other organs, most commonly the liver (liver abscess), and cause fever and right upper quadrant pain.

Disease is more severe in very young people, elderly people, malnourished people, and pregnant women. People with symptomatic intestinal amebiasis generally have a gradual onset of symptoms over 1 to 3 weeks. The mildest form of intestinal tract disease is nondysenteric colitis. However, amebic dysentery is the most common clinical manifestation of amebiasis and generally includes diarrhea with either gross or microscopic blood in the stool, lower abdominal pain, and tenesmus. Weight loss is common because of the gradual onset, but fever occurs only in a minority of patients (8%–38%). Symptoms may be chronic, characterized by the presence of periods of diarrhea and intestinal spasms alternating with periods of constipation, and may mimic those of inflammatory bowel disease. Progressive involvement of the colon may produce toxic megacolon, fulminant colitis, ulceration of the colon and perianal area, and rarely, perforation. Colonic progression may occur at multiples sites and carries a high fatality rate. Progression may occur in patients inappropriately treated with corticosteroids or antimotility drugs. An ameboma may occur as an annular lesion of the colon and may present as a palpable mass on physical examination. Amebomas can occur in any area of the colon but are more common in the cecum. They may be mistaken for colonic carcinoma. Amebomas usually resolve with antiamebic therapy and do not require surgery.

In a small proportion of patients, extraintestinal disease may occur. The liver is the most common extraintestinal site, and infection may spread from there to the pleural space, lungs, and pericardium. Liver abscess may be acute, with fever, abdominal pain, tachypnea, liver tenderness, and hepatomegaly, or may be chronic, with weight loss, vague abdominal symptoms, and irritability. Rupture of abscesses into the abdomen or chest may lead to death. Evidence of recent intestinal tract infection usually is absent in extraintestinal disease. Infection also may spread from the colon to the genitourinary tract and the skin. The organism may spread hematogenously to the brain and other areas of the body.

ETIOLOGY: The genus *Entamoeba* includes 6 species that live in the human intestine. Three of these species are identical morphologically: *E histolytica, Entamoeba dispar, and Entamoeba moshkovskii.* Not all *Entamoeba* species are equally virulent. *E dispar* and *E moshkovskii*, generally believed to be nonpathogenic, recently have been associated with intestinal and extraintestinal pathology, putting their avirulent status in question. The *Entamoeba* species are excreted as cysts or trophozoites in stool of infected people.

EPIDEMIOLOGY: *E histolytica* can be found worldwide but is more prevalent in people of lower socioeconomic status who live in resource-limited countries, where the prevalence of amebic infection may be as high as 50% in some communities. Groups at increased risk of infection in industrialized countries include immigrants from or long-term visitors to areas with endemic infection, institutionalized people, and men who have sex with men. *E histolytica* is transmitted via amebic cysts by the fecal-oral route. Ingested cysts, which are unaffected by gastric acid, undergo excystation in the alkaline small intestine and produce trophozoites that infect the colon. Cysts that develop subsequently are the source of transmission, especially from asymptomatic cyst excreters. Infected patients excrete cysts intermittently, sometimes for years if untreated. Transmission has been associated with contaminated food or water. Fecal-oral transmission also can occur in the setting of anal sexual practices or direct rectal inoculation through colonic irrigation devices.

The **incubation period** is variable, ranging from a few days to months or years, but commonly is 2 to 4 weeks.

DIAGNOSTIC TESTS: A definitive diagnosis of intestinal tract infection depends on identifying trophozoites or cysts in stool specimens. Examination of serial specimens may be necessary. Specimens of stool may be examined microscopically by wet mount within 30 minutes of collection or may be fixed in formalin or polyvinyl alcohol (available in kits) for concentration, permanent staining, and subsequent microscopic examination. Microscopy does not differentiate between *E histolytica* and less pathogenic strains. Antigen test kits are available for routine laboratory testing of *E histolytica* directly from stool specimens. Biopsy specimens and endoscopy scrapings (not swabs) may be examined using similar methods. *E histolytica* is not distinguished easily from the more prevalent *E dispar* and *E moshkovskii*, although trophozoites containing ingested red blood cells are more likely to be *E histolytica*. Polymerase chain reaction assay and isoenzyme analysis can differentiate *E histolytica* from *E dispar*, *E moshkovskii*, and other *Entamoeba* species; some monoclonal antibody-based antigen detection assays also can differentiate *E histolytica* from *E dispar*.

The indirect hemagglutination (IHA) test has been replaced by commercially available enzyme immunoassay (EIA) kits for routine serodiagnosis of amebiasis. The EIA detects antibody specific for *E histolytica* in approximately 95% or more of patients with extraintestinal amebiasis, 70% of patients with active intestinal tract infection, and 10% of asymptomatic people who are passing cysts of *E histolytica*. Patients may continue to have positive serologic test results even after adequate therapy. Diagnosis of an *E histolytica* liver abscess and other extraintestinal infections is aided by serologic testing, because stool tests and abscess aspirates frequently are not revealing.

Ultrasonography, computed tomography, and magnetic resonance imaging can identify liver abscesses and other extraintestinal sites of infection. Aspirates from a liver abscess usually show neither trophozoites nor leukocytes.

TREATMENT: Treatment involves elimination of the tissue-invading trophozoites as well as organisms in the intestinal lumen. *E dispar* and *E moshkovskii* infections often are considered to be nonpathogenic and do not necessarily require treatment. Corticosteroids and antimotility drugs administered to people with amebiasis can worsen symptoms and the disease process. In settings where tests to distinguish species are not available, treatment should be given to symptomatic people on the basis of positive results of microscopic examination. The following regimens are recommended:

- **Asymptomatic cyst excreters (intraluminal infections):** treat with a luminal amebicide, such as iodoquinol or paromomycin. Metronidazole is not effective against cysts.
- **Patients with mild to moderate or severe intestinal tract symptoms or extraintestinal disease (including liver abscess):** treat with metronidazole or tinidazole, followed by a therapeutic course of a luminal amebicide (iodoquinol or, in absence of intestinal obstruction, paromomycin). Nitazoxanide also may be effective for mild to moderate intestinal amebiasis, although it is not approved by the US Food and Drug Administration for this indication. An alternate treatment for liver abscess is chloroquine phosphate administered concomitantly with metronidazole or tinidazole, followed by a therapeutic course of a luminal amebicide.

Percutaneous or surgical aspiration of large liver abscesses occasionally may be required when response of the abscess to medical therapy is unsatisfactory or there is risk of rupture. In most cases of liver abscess, however, drainage is not required and does not speed recovery.

Follow-up stool examination is recommended after completion of therapy, because no pharmacologic regimen is completely effective in eradicating intestinal tract infection. Household members and other suspected contacts also should have adequate stool examinations performed and should be treated if results are positive for *E histolytica*.

ISOLATION OF THE HOSPITALIZED PATIENT: In addition to standard precautions, contact precautions are recommended for the duration of illness.

CONTROL MEASURES: Careful hand hygiene after defecation, sanitary disposal of fecal material, and treatment of drinking water will control spread of infection. Sexual transmission may be controlled by use of condoms and avoidance of sexual practices that may permit fecal-oral transmission. Because of the risk of shedding infectious cysts, people diagnosed with amebiasis should refrain from using recreational water venues (eg, swimming pools, water parks) until after their course of luminal chemotherapy is completed and any diarrhea they might have been experiencing has resolved.

Amebic Meningoencephalitis and Keratitis
(*Naegleria fowleri, Acanthamoeba* species, and *Balamuthia mandrillaris*)

CLINICAL MANIFESTATIONS: *Naegleria fowleri* can cause a rapidly progressive, almost always fatal, primary amebic meningoencephalitis (PAM). Early symptoms include fever, headache, vomiting, and sometimes disturbances of smell and taste. The illness progresses rapidly to signs of meningoencephalitis, including nuchal rigidity, lethargy, confusion, personality changes, and altered level of consciousness. Seizures are common, and death generally occurs within a week of onset of symptoms. No distinct clinical features differentiate this disease from fulminant bacterial meningitis.

Granulomatous amebic encephalitis (GAE) caused by *Acanthamoeba* species and *Balamuthia mandrillaris* has a more insidious onset and develops as a subacute or chronic disease. In general, GAE progresses more slowly than PAM, leading to death several weeks to months after onset of symptoms. Signs and symptoms may include personality changes, seizures, headaches, ataxia, cranial nerve palsies, hemiparesis, and other focal neurologic deficits. Fever often is low grade and intermittent. The course may resemble that of a bacterial brain abscess or a brain tumor. Chronic granulomatous skin lesions (pustules, nodules, ulcers) may be present without central nervous system (CNS) involvement, particularly in patients with acquired immunodeficiency syndrome, and lesions may be present for months before brain involvement in immunocompetent hosts.

The most common symptoms of amebic keratitis, a vision-threatening infection usually caused by *Acanthamoeba* species, are pain (often out of proportion to clinical signs), photophobia, tearing, and foreign body sensation. Characteristic clinical findings include radial keratoneuritis and stromal ring infiltrate. *Acanthamoeba* keratitis generally follows an indolent course and initially may resemble herpes simplex or bacterial keratitis; delay in diagnosis is associated with worse outcomes.

ETIOLOGY: *N fowleri, Acanthamoeba* species, and *B mandrillaris* are free-living amebae that exist as motile, infectious trophozoites and environmentally hardy cysts.

EPIDEMIOLOGY: *N fowleri* is found in warm fresh water and moist soil. Most infections with *N fowleri* have been associated with swimming in natural bodies of warm fresh water, such as ponds, lakes, and hot springs, but other sources have included tap water from geothermal sources and contaminated and poorly chlorinated swimming pools. Disease has been reported worldwide but is uncommon. In the United States, infection occurs primarily in the summer and usually affects children and young adults. Disease has followed inappropriate use of tap water for sinus rinses. The trophozoites of the parasite invade the brain directly from the nose along the olfactory nerves via the cribriform plate. In infections with *N fowleri*, trophozoites, but not cysts, can be visualized in sections of brain or in cerebrospinal fluid (CSF).

The **incubation period** for *N fowleri* infection typically is 3 to 7 days.

Acanthamoeba species are distributed worldwide and are found in soil; dust; cooling towers of electric and nuclear power plants; heating, ventilating, and air conditioning units; fresh and brackish water; whirlpool baths; and physiotherapy pools. The environmental niche of *B mandrillaris* is not delineated clearly, although it has been isolated from soil. CNS infection attributable to *Acanthamoeba* occurs primarily in debilitated and immunocompromised people. However, some patients infected with *B mandrillaris* have had no demonstrable underlying disease or defect. CNS infection by both amebae probably occurs most commonly by inhalation or direct contact with contaminated soil or water. The primary foci of these infections most likely are skin or respiratory tract, followed by hematogenous spread to the brain. Fatal encephalitis caused by *Balamuthia* and transmitted by the organ donor has been reported in recipients of organ transplants. *Acanthamoeba* keratitis occurs primarily in people who wear contact lenses, although it also has been associated with corneal trauma. Poor contact lens hygiene and/or disinfection practices as well as swimming with contact lenses are risk factors.

The **incubation periods** for *Acanthamoeba* and *Balamuthia* GAE are unknown. It is thought to take several weeks or months to develop the first symptoms of CNS disease following exposure to the amebae. However, patients exposed to *Balamuthia* through solid organ transplantation can develop symptoms of *Balamuthia* GAE more quickly—within a few weeks. The **incubation period** for *Acanthamoeba* keratitis also is unknown but thought to range from several days to several weeks.

DIAGNOSTIC TESTS: In *N fowleri* infection, computed tomography scans of the head without contrast are unremarkable or show only cerebral edema but with contrast might show meningeal enhancement of the basilar cisterns and sulci. However, these changes are not specific for amebic infection. CSF pressure usually is elevated (300 to >600 mm water), and CSF indices may show a polymorphonuclear pleocytosis, an increased protein concentration, and a normal to very low glucose concentration; Gram stains are negative for bacteria. *N fowleri* infection can be documented by microscopic demonstration of the motile trophozoites on a wet mount of centrifuged CSF. Smears of CSF should be stained with Giemsa, Trichome, or Wright stains to identify the trophozoites, if present; Gram stain is not useful in ruling in *N fowleri* CNS infection. The organism also can be cultured on nonnutrient agar plates layered with *Escherichia coli* or on monolayers of E6 and human lung fibroblast cells. Trophozoites can be visualized in sections of the brain. Immunofluorescence and polymerase chain reaction (PCR) assays performed on CSF and biopsy material to identify the organism are available through the Centers for Disease Control and Prevention (CDC).

In infection with *Acanthamoeba* species and *B mandrillaris*, trophozoites and cysts can be visualized in sections of brain, lungs, and skin; in cases of *Acanthamoeba* keratitis, they also can be visualized in corneal scrapings and by confocal microscopy in vivo in the cornea. In GAE infections, CSF indices typically reveal a lymphocytic pleocytosis and an increased protein concentration, with normal or low glucose but no organisms. Computed tomography and magnetic resonance imaging of the head may show single or multiple space-occupying, ring-enhancing lesions that can mimic brain abscesses, tumors, cerebro-vascular accidents, or other diseases. *Acanthamoeba* species, but not *Balamuthia* species, can be cultured by the same method used for *N fowleri*. *B mandrillaris* can be grown using mammalian cell culture. Like *N fowleri*, immunofluorescence and PCR assays can be performed on clinical specimens to identify *Acanthamoeba* species and *Balamuthia* species; these tests are available through the CDC.

TREATMENT: If meningoencephalitis caused by *N fowleri* is suspected because of the presence of amebic organisms in CSF, therapy should not be withheld while waiting for results of confirmatory diagnostic tests. Although an effective treatment regimen for PAM has not been identified, amphotericin B is the drug of choice. In vitro testing indicates that *N fowleri* is highly sensitive to amphotericin B. However, treatment usually is unsuccessful, with only a few cases of complete recovery having been documented. Two survivors recovered after treatment with amphotericin B in combination with an azole drug (either miconazole or fluconazole) plus rifampin, although rifampin probably had no additional effect; these patients also received dexamethasone to control cerebral edema. Although these 2 patients did not receive azithromycin, this drug has both in vitro and in vivo efficacy against *Naegleria* species and also may be considered as an adjunct to amphotericin B. Miltefosine, available through the CDC (770-488-7100), also has been used successfully to treat PAM caused by *N fowleri* as well as in other patients with *B mandrillaris* GAE and cutaneous lesions. Early diagnosis and institution of high-dose drug therapy is thought to be important for optimizing outcome.

Effective treatment for infections caused by *Acanthamoeba* species and *B mandrillaris* has not been established. Several patients with *Acanthamoeba* GAE and *Acanthamoeba* cutaneous infections without CNS involvement have been treated successfully with a multidrug regimen consisting of various combinations of pentamidine, sulfadiazine, flucytosine, either fluconazole or itraconazole, trimethoprim-sulfamethoxazole, and topical application of chlorhexidine gluconate and ketoconazole for skin lesions. Voriconazole, miltefosine, and azithromycin also might be of some value in treating *Acanthamoeba* infections. Three patients survived *B mandrillaris* infection following treatment with pentamidine, sulfadiazine, fluconazole, and either azithromycin or clarithromycin, in addition to surgical resection of the CNS lesions; in 2 of these cases, flucytosine was used as well. Of these 3 survivors, all had GAE and 1 had an accompanying cutaneous lesion. Recently, the CDC has received reports of additional survivors. The most up-to-date guidance for treatment of PAM can be found on the CDC Web site (**www.cdc.gov/naegleria**). Unlike with *Acanthamoeba* species, voriconazole has virtually no effect on *Balamuthia* species in vitro.

Patients with *Acanthamoeba* keratitis should be evaluated by an ophthalmologist. Early diagnosis and therapy are important for a good outcome.

ISOLATION OF THE HOSPITALIZED PATIENT: Standard precautions are recommended.

CONTROL MEASURES: People should assume that there is always a slight risk of developing PAM caused by *N fowleri* when entering warm fresh water. Only avoidance of such water-related activities can prevent *Naegleria* infection, although the risk might be reduced by taking measures to limit water exposure through known routes of entry, such as getting water up the nose. Water for sinus rinses should be either previously boiled or properly filtered, or labeled as sterile or distilled (additional information available at **www.cdc.gov/naegleria**). Presently, no clearly defined recommendations are available to prevent GAE attributable to *Acanthamoeba* species or *B mandrillaris*. To prevent *Acanthamoeba* keratitis, steps should be taken to avoid corneal trauma, such as the use of protective eyewear during high-risk activities, and contact lens users should maintain good contact lens hygiene and disinfection practices, use only sterile solutions as applicable, change lens cases frequently, and avoid swimming and showering while wearing contact lenses. Advice for people who wear contact lenses can be found on the CDC Web site (**www.cdc.gov/contactlenses**).[1]

Anthrax[2,3]

CLINICAL MANIFESTATIONS: Anthrax can occur in 4 forms, depending on the route of infection: cutaneous, inhalation, gastrointestinal, and injection. **Cutaneous** anthrax begins as a pruritic papule or vesicle after an incubation period of 5 to 7 days (range of 1 to 12 days) and progresses over 2 to 6 days to an ulcerated lesion with subsequent formation of a central black eschar. The lesion itself characteristically is painless, with surrounding edema, hyperemia, and painful regional lymphadenopathy. Patients may have associated fever, lymphangitis, and extensive edema.

Inhalation anthrax is a frequently lethal form of the disease and is a medical emergency. The initial presentation is nonspecific and may include fever, sweats, nonproductive cough, chest pain, headache, myalgia, malaise, nausea, and vomiting, but illness progresses to the fulminant phase 2 to 5 days later. In some cases, the illness is biphasic with a period of improvement between prodromal symptoms and overwhelming illness. Fulminant manifestations include hypotension, dyspnea, hypoxia, cyanosis, and shock occurring as a result of hemorrhagic mediastinal lymphadenitis, hemorrhagic pneumonia, hemorrhagic pleural effusions, bacteremia, and toxemia. A widened mediastinum is the classic finding on imaging of the chest. Chest radiography also may show pleural effusions and/or infiltrates, both of which may be hemorrhagic in nature.

Gastrointestinal tract disease can present as one of 2 distinct clinical syndromes—intestinal or oropharyngeal. Patients with the intestinal form have symptoms of nausea, anorexia, vomiting, and fever progressing to severe abdominal pain, massive ascites, hematemesis, and bloody diarrhea, related to the development of edema and ulceration of the bowel, primarily in the region of the ileum and cecum. Patients with oropharyngeal anthrax also may have dysphagia with posterior oropharyngeal necrotic ulcers, which may be associated with marked, often unilateral neck swelling, regional adenopathy, fever, and sepsis. **Injection** anthrax has not been reported to date in children; it has been reported primarily as occurring among injecting heroin users; however, smoking and snorting of heroin also have been identified as exposure routes. Systemic illness can result from hematogenous and lymphatic dissemination and can occur with any form of anthrax. Most patients with inhalation, gastrointestinal, and injection anthrax have systemic illness. Patients with cutaneous anthrax also should be considered to have systemic illness if they have tachycardia, tachypnea, hypotension, hyperthermia, hypothermia, or leukocytosis, or have lesions that involve the head, neck, or upper torso or that are large, bullous, multiple,

---

[1]Centers for Disease Control and Prevention. Estimated burden of keratitis—United States, 2010. *MMWR Morb Mortal Wkly Rep.* 2014;63(45):1027-1030

[2]Center for Infectious Disease Research and Policy, University of Minnesota. Anthrax: Current, comprehensive information on pathogenesis, microbiology, epidemiology, diagnosis, treatment, and prophylaxis. Available at: **www.cidrap.umn.edu/cidrap/content/bt/anthrax/index.html**

[3]Stern EJ, Uhde KB, Shadomy SV, Messonnier N. Conference report on public health and clinical guidelines for anthrax. *Emerg Infect Dis.* 2008;14(4). Available at: **wwwnc.cdc.gov/eid/article/14/4/07-0969_article**

or surrounded by edema. Anthrax meningitis can occur in any patient with systemic illness regardless of origin; it also can occur in patients lacking any other apparent clinical presentation. The case-fatality rate for patients with appropriately treated cutaneous anthrax usually is less than 1%. Even with antimicrobial treatment and supportive care, the mortality rate for inhalation or gastrointestinal tract disease is between 40% and 45% and approaches 100% for meningitis.

ETIOLOGY: *Bacillus anthracis* is an aerobic, gram-positive, encapsulated, spore-forming, nonhemolytic, nonmotile rod. *B anthracis* has 3 major virulence factors: an antiphagocytic capsule and 2 exotoxins, called lethal and edema toxins. The toxins are responsible for the substantial morbidity and clinical manifestations of hemorrhage, edema, and necrosis.

EPIDEMIOLOGY: Anthrax is a zoonotic disease most commonly affecting domestic and wild herbivores that occurs in many rural regions of the world. *B anthracis* spores can remain viable in the soil for decades, representing a potential source of infection for livestock or wildlife through ingestion of spore-contaminated vegetation or water. In susceptible hosts, the spores germinate to become viable bacteria. Natural infection of humans occurs through contact with infected animals or contaminated animal products, including carcasses, hides, hair, wool, meat, and bone meal. Outbreaks of gastrointestinal tract anthrax have occurred after ingestion of undercooked or raw meat from infected animals. Historically, the vast majority (more than 95%) of cases of anthrax in the United States were cutaneous infections among animal handlers or mill workers. Severe disseminated anthrax following soft tissue infection among heroin users has been reported. The incidence of naturally occurring human anthrax decreased in the United States from an estimated 130 cases annually in the early 1900s to 0 to 2 cases per year from 1979 through 2013. Recent cases of inhalation, cutaneous, and gastrointestinal tract anthrax have occurred in drum makers working with animal hides contaminated with *B anthracis* spores or in people participating in events where spore-contaminated drums were played.[1] Severe soft tissue infections among heroin users, including cases with disseminated systemic infection, have been reported, though to date such cases have only been reported in Northern Europe.

B anthracis is one of the most likely agents to be used as a biological weapon, because (1) its spores are highly stable; (2) spores can infect via the respiratory route; and (3) the resulting inhalation anthrax has a high mortality rate. In 1979, an accidental release of *B anthracis* spores from a military microbiology facility in the former Soviet Union resulted in at least 68 deaths. In 2001, 22 cases of anthrax (11 inhalation, 11 cutaneous) were identified in the United States after intentional contamination of the mail; 5 (45%) of the inhalation anthrax cases were fatal. In addition to aerosolization, there is a theoretical health risk associated with *B anthracis* spores being introduced into food products or water supplies. Use of *B anthracis* in a biological attack would require immediate response and mobilization of public health resources. Anthrax meets the definition of a nationally and immediately notifiable condition, as specified by the US Council of State and Territorial Epidemiologists; therefore, every suspected case should be reported immediately to the local or state health department (see Biological Terrorism, p 109).

The **incubation period** typically is 1 week or less for cutaneous or gastrointestinal tract anthrax. However, because of spore dormancy and slow clearance of spores from the lungs, the **incubation period** for inhalation anthrax may be prolonged and has

---

[1]Centers for Disease Control and Prevention. Gastrointestinal anthrax after an animal-hide drumming event— New Hampshire and Massachusetts, 2009. *MMWR Morb Mortal Wkly Rep.* 2010;59(28):872-877

been reported to range from 2 to 43 days in humans and up to 2 months in experimental nonhuman primates. Discharge from cutaneous lesions potentially is infectious, but person-to-person transmission rarely has been reported, and other forms of anthrax are not associated with person-to-person transmission. Both inhalation and cutaneous anthrax have occurred in laboratory workers.

DIAGNOSTIC TESTS: Depending on the clinical presentation, Gram stain, culture, and polymerase chain reaction (PCR) testing for anthrax should be performed on specimens of blood, pleural fluid, cerebrospinal fluid (CSF), and tissue biopsy specimens and on swabs of vesicular fluid or eschar material from cutaneous or oropharyngeal lesions, rectal swabs, or stool. Whenever possible, specimens for these tests should be obtained before initiating antimicrobial therapy, because previous treatment with antimicrobial agents makes isolation by culture unlikely. Gram-positive bacilli seen on unspun peripheral blood smears or in vesicular fluid or CSF can be an important initial finding, and polychrome methylene blue-stained smears showing bacilli stained blue with the capsule visualized in red (M'Fadyean reaction) are considered a presumptive identification of *B anthracis*. Traditional microbiologic methods can presumptively identify *B anthracis* from cultures. Definitive identification of suspect *B anthracis* isolates can be performed through the Laboratory Response Network (LRN) in each state. Additional diagnostic tests for anthrax can be accessed through state health departments, including bacterial DNA detection in blood, CSF, or exudates by PCR assay, tissue immunohistochemistry, an enzyme immunoassay that measures immunoglobulin G antibodies against *B anthracis* protective antigen in paired sera, or a MALDI-TOF mass spectrometry assay measuring lethal factor activity in serum samples. The sensitivity of DNA or antigen detection methods may decline after antimicrobial treatment has been initiated. The commercially available QuickELISA Anthrax-PA Kit can be used as a screening test. Clinical evaluation of patients with suspected inhalation anthrax should include a chest radiograph and/or computed tomography scan to evaluate for widened mediastinum, pleural effusion, and/or pulmonary infiltrates.

TREATMENT[1,2]: A high index of suspicion and rapid administration of appropriate antimicrobial therapy to people suspected of being infected, along with access to critical care support, are essential for effective treatment of anthrax. No controlled trials in humans have been performed to validate current treatment recommendations for anthrax, and there is limited clinical experience. Case reports suggest that naturally occurring localized or uncomplicated cutaneous disease can be treated effectively with 7 to 10 days of a single oral antimicrobial agent. First-line agents include ciprofloxacin or an equivalent fluoroquinolone and doxycycline; clindamycin is an alternative, as are penicillins if the isolate is known to be penicillin-susceptible. For bioterrorism-associated cutaneous disease in adults or children, ciprofloxacin (30 mg/kg per day, orally, divided 2 times/day for children, not to exceed 1000 mg every 24 hours) or doxycycline (100 mg, orally, 2 times/day for children 8 years or older; or 4 mg/kg per day, orally, divided 2 times/day for children younger than 8 years [see Tetracyclines, p 875]) are recommended for initial treatment

---

[1]Bradley JS, Peacock G, Krug SE, et al; American Academy of Pediatrics, Committee on Infectious Diseases, Disaster Preparedness Advisory Council. Clinical report: pediatric anthrax clinical management. *Pediatrics.* 2014;133(5):e1411-e1436

[2]Hendricks KA, Wright ME, Shadomy SV, et al. Centers for Disease Control and Prevention expert panel meetings on prevention and treatment of anthrax in adults. *Emerg Infect Dis.* 2014;20(2). Available at: **wwwnc.cdc.gov/eid/article/20/2/13-0687_intro**

until antimicrobial susceptibility data are available. Because of the risk of concomitant inhalational exposure and subsequent spore dormancy in the lungs, the antimicrobial regimen in cases of bioterrorism-associated cutaneous anthrax or that were exposed to other sources of aerosolized spores should be continued for a total of 60 days to provide post-exposure prophylaxis (PEP), in conjunction with administration of vaccine (see Control Measures).

On the basis of in vitro data and animal studies, ciprofloxacin (30 mg/kg/day, intravenously, divided every 8 hours, not to exceed 400 mg/dose) is recommended as the primary antimicrobial component of an initial multidrug regimen for treatment of all forms of systemic anthrax until results of antimicrobial susceptibility testing are known.[1,2] Levofloxacin and moxifloxacin are considered equivalent alternatives to ciprofloxacin. Meningeal involvement should be suspected in all cases of inhalation anthrax and other systemic anthrax infections; thus, treatment of systemic anthrax should include at least 2 other agents with known central nervous system (CNS) penetration in conjunction with ciprofloxacin. There is a theoretical benefit to the use of both a bactericidal and a protein synthesis-inhibiting agent as the additional drugs in this combination. Meropenem is recommended as the second bactericidal antimicrobial, and if meropenem is not available, doripenem and imipenem/cilastatin are considered alternatives; if the strain is known to be susceptible, penicillin G or ampicillin are equivalent alternatives. Linezolid is recommended as the preferred protein synthesis inhibitor if meningeal involvement is suspected.

If CNS penetration is less important because meningitis has been ruled out, treatment may consist of 2 antimicrobial agents, including a bactericidal and a protein synthesis-inhibiting agent. In such an instance, clindamycin is the preferred protein synthesis inhibitor, and linezolid, doxycycline, and rifampin are acceptable alternatives. Ciprofloxacin is the preferred bactericidal agent, with meropenem, levofloxacin, imipenem/cilastatin, and vancomycin being acceptable alternatives; if the strain is known to be susceptible, penicillin G or ampicillin are equivalent alternatives. Because of intrinsic resistance, cephalosporins and trimethoprim-sulfamethoxazole should not be used.

Treatment should continue for at least 14 days or longer, depending on patient condition. Intravenous therapy can be changed to oral therapy when progression of symptoms cease and it is clinically appropriate. There is the risk of spore dormancy in the lungs in people with bioterrorism-associated cutaneous or systemic anthrax or people who were exposed to other sources of aerosolized spores. In these cases, the antimicrobial regimen should be continued for a total of 60 days to provide PEP, in conjunction with administration of vaccine (see Control Measures); antimicrobial drug options are the same as those for PEP.

Neither ciprofloxacin nor tetracyclines are used routinely in young children or pregnant women because of safety concerns. However, ciprofloxacin or doxycycline should be used for treatment of life-threatening anthrax infections in children until antimicrobial susceptibility patterns are known. Tetracycline-based antimicrobial agents, including doxycycline, may cause permanent tooth discoloration for children younger than 8 years

---

[1]Hendricks KA, Wright ME, Shadomy SV, et al. Centers for Disease Control and Prevention expert panel meetings on prevention and treatment of anthrax in adults. *Emerg Infect Dis.* 2014;20(2). Available at: **wwwnc.cdc.gov/eid/article/20/2/13-0687_intro**

[2]Bradley JS, Peacock G, Krug SE, et al; American Academy of Pediatrics, Committee on Infectious Diseases, Disaster Preparedness Advisory Council. Clinical report: pediatric anthrax clinical management. *Pediatrics.* 2014;133(5):e1411-e1436

if used for repeated treatment courses. However, doxycycline binds less readily to calcium compared with older tetracyclines, and in some studies, doxycycline was not associated with visible teeth staining in younger children (see Tetracyclines, p 873). Although no prospective data exist on staining of teeth in children younger than 8 years taking a 60-day course of doxycycline, the benefits of preventing life-threatening anthrax infection outweigh the potential risks of injury to teeth. Similarly, although no prospective data exist on the risks of cartilage toxicity with ciprofloxacin, particularly for a 60-day course, the benefits of an extended course for prophylaxis in children outweigh the concerns for potential cartilage toxicity.

For anthrax with evidence of systemic illness, including fever, shock, and dissemination to other organs, Anthrax Immune Globulin (AIG) or Raxibacumab (GlaxoSmithKline, Research Triangle Park, NC), a humanized monoclonal antibody, should be considered in consultation with the Centers for Disease Control and Prevention (CDC). Raxibacumab is approved by the US Food and Drug Administration (FDA); AIG requires use under a CDC-sponsored investigational new drug (IND) protocol. Supportive symptomatic (intensive care) treatment also is important. Aggressive pleural fluid or ascites drainage is critical if effusions exist, because drainage appears to be associated with improved survival. Obstructive airway disease resulting from associated edema may complicate cutaneous anthrax of the face or neck and can require aggressive monitoring for airway compromise.

ISOLATION OF THE HOSPITALIZED PATIENT: Standard precautions are recommended. In addition, contact precautions should be implemented when draining cutaneous lesions are present. Cutaneous lesions become sterile within 24 hours of starting appropriate antimicrobial therapy. Patient care does not appear to be a risk for transmission. Contaminated dressings and bedclothes should be incinerated or steam sterilized (121°C for 30 minutes) to destroy spores. Terminal cleaning of the patient's room can be accomplished with an Environmental Protection Agency-registered hospital-grade disinfectant and should follow standard facility practices typically used for all patients. Autopsies performed on patients with systemic anthrax require special precautions.

CONTROL MEASURES: BioThrax (Anthrax Vaccine Adsorbed [AVA]), the only vaccine licensed in the United States for use in humans, is prepared from a cell-free culture filtrate. The vaccine's efficacy for prevention of anthrax is based on animal studies, a single placebo-controlled human trial of the alum-precipitated precursor of the current AVA, observational data from humans, and immunogenicity data from humans and other mammals. In the human trial in adult mill workers, the alum-precipitated precursor to AVA had a demonstrated 93% efficacy for preventing cutaneous and inhalation anthrax. Multiple reviews and publications evaluating AVA safety have found adverse events usually are local injection site reactions, with rare systemic symptoms, including fever, chills, muscle aches, and hypersensitivity.

The CDC updated its recommendations on exposure to anthrax through bioterrorism in 2014. In the event of a bioterrorism event, information of importance to health care providers and the public will be posted on the CDC Anthrax Web site **(http://emergency.cdc.gov/agent/anthrax/index.asp).** Within 48 hours of exposure to *B anthracis* spores, public health authorities plan to provide a 10-day course of antimicrobial prophylaxis to the local population, including children likely to have been exposed to spores. Within 10 days of exposure, public health authorities plan to further define those who have had a clear and significant exposure and will require an additional 50 days of antimicrobial PEP and begin the 3-dose anthrax vaccine (AVA) series for children. Either AIG or Raxibacumab antitoxin is indicated in patients with anthrax systemic disease.[1]

The general procedure for AVA vaccination in the pre-event or pre-exposure setting is a priming series of three 0.5-mL intramuscular (IM) injections at 0, 1, and 6 months with boosters at 12 and 18 months and annually thereafter for those at continued risk of infection. People with medical contraindications to intramuscular administration (eg, people with coagulation disorders) may receive the vaccine by subcutaneous administration. Pre-event immunization is recommended for people at risk of repeated exposures to aerosolized *B anthracis* spores, including selected laboratory workers, environmental investigators and remediation workers, military personnel, and some emergency and other responders.

Postexposure management for previously unvaccinated people older than 18 years who have been exposed to aerosolized *B anthracis* spores consists of 60 days of appropriate antimicrobial prophylaxis combined with 3 subcutaneous doses of AVA (administered at 0, 2, and 4 weeks postexposure). AVA is not licensed for use in pregnant women; however, in a postevent setting that poses a high risk of exposure to aerosolized *B anthracis* spores, pregnancy is neither a precaution nor a contraindication to its use in PEP. AVA is not licensed for use in pediatric populations and has not been studied in children; however, there is no reason to suggest an increased risk of adverse events associated with the use of anthrax vaccine in pediatric populations. Until there are sufficient data to support FDA approval, AVA will be made available for children at the time of an event as an investigational vaccine through an expedited process that will require institutional review board approval, including the use of appropriate consent documents. Information on the process required for use of AVA in children will be available on the CDC Web site at the time of an event (**www.cdc.gov/anthrax**), as well as through the American Academy of Pediatrics (AAP) and the FDA.[2] All exposed children 6 weeks and older should receive 3 doses of AVA at 0, 2, and 4 weeks in addition to 60 days of antimicrobial chemoprophylaxis. The recommended route of vaccine administration in children is subcutaneous, although both subcutaneous and intramuscular injections appear to achieve similar levels of immunogenicity in 60 days. Children younger than 6 weeks should immediately begin antimicrobial prophylaxis but delay starting the vaccine series until they reach 6 weeks of age.

When no information is available about antimicrobial susceptibility of the implicated strain of *B anthracis*, ciprofloxacin and doxycycline are equivalent first-line antimicrobial agents for initial PEP for adults or children (see Tetracyclines, p 873). Levofloxacin and clindamycin are second-line antimicrobial agents for PEP. Safety data on extended use of levofloxacin in any population for longer than 28 days are limited; therefore, levofloxacin should only be used when the benefit outweighs the risk. Although fluoroquinolones and tetracyclines are not normally recommended as first-choice drugs in children because of safety concerns, these concerns are outweighed by the need for prophylaxis to prevent disease in pregnant women and children exposed to *B anthracis* after a biological terrorism event. When the antimicrobial susceptibility profile demonstrates appropriate sensitivity

[1]Hendricks KA, Wright ME, Shadomy SV, et al. Centers for Disease Control and Prevention expert panel meetings on prevention and treatment of anthrax in adults. *Emerg Infect Dis.* 2014;20(2). Available at: **wwwnc.cdc.gov/eid/article/20/2/13-0687_intro**

[2]Bradley JS, Peacock G, Krug SE, et al; American Academy of Pediatrics, Committee on Infectious Diseases, Disaster Preparedness Advisory Council. Clinical report: pediatric anthrax clinical management. *Pediatrics.* 2014;133(5):e1411-e1436

to amoxicillin (minimum inhibitory concentration ≤0.125 µg/mL), public health authorities may recommend changing PEP antimicrobial therapy for children to oral amoxicillin. Because of the lack of data on amoxicillin dosages for treating anthrax (and the associated high mortality rate), the AAP recommends a higher dosage of oral amoxicillin, 80 mg/kg per day, divided into 3 daily doses administered every 8 hours (each dose not to exceed 500 mg). Because of intrinsic resistance, cephalosporins and trimethoprim-sulfamethoxazole should not be used for prophylaxis.

Arboviruses (also see Dengue, p 322, and West Nile Virus, p 865)

(Including California serogroup, chikungunya, Colorado tick fever, eastern equine encephalitis, Japanese encephalitis, Powassan, St. Louis encephalitis, tickborne encephalitis, Venezuelan equine encephalitis, Western equine encephalitis, and yellow fever viruses)

CLINICAL MANIFESTATIONS: More than 100 arthropodborne viruses (arboviruses) are known to cause human disease. Although most infections are subclinical, symptomatic illness usually manifests as 1 of 3 primary clinical syndromes: generalized febrile illness, neuroinvasive disease, or hemorrhagic fever (Table 3.1, p 241).

- **Generalized febrile illness.** Most arboviruses are capable of causing a systemic febrile illness that often includes headache, arthralgia, myalgia, and rash. Some viruses also can cause more characteristic clinical manifestations, such as severe joint pain (eg, chikungunya virus) or jaundice (yellow fever virus). With some arboviruses, fatigue, malaise, and weakness can linger for weeks following the initial infection.

  The majority of people infected with chikungunya virus become symptomatic. The incubation period typically is 3 to 7 days (range, 1–12 days). The disease most often is characterized by acute onset of fever (typically >39°C [102°F]) and polyarthralgia. Joint symptoms usually are bilateral and symmetric and can be severe and debilitating. Other symptoms may include headache, myalgia, arthritis, conjunctivitis, nausea/vomiting, or maculopapular rash. Clinical laboratory findings can include lymphopenia, thrombocytopenia, elevated creatinine, and elevated hepatic transaminases. Acute symptoms typically resolve within 7 to 10 days. Rare complications include uveitis, retinitis, myocarditis, hepatitis, nephritis, bullous skin lesions, hemorrhage, meningoencephalitis, myelitis, Guillain-Barré syndrome, and cranial nerve palsies. People at risk for severe disease include neonates exposed intrapartum, older adults (eg, >65 years), and people with underlying medical conditions (eg, hypertension, diabetes, or cardiovascular disease). Some patients might have relapse of rheumatologic symptoms (polyarthralgia, polyarthritis, tenosynovitis) in the months following acute illness. Studies report variable proportions of patients with persistent joint pains for months to years. Mortality is rare.

- **Neuroinvasive disease.** Many arboviruses cause neuroinvasive diseases, including aseptic meningitis, encephalitis, or acute flaccid paralysis. Illness usually presents with a prodrome similar to the systemic febrile illness followed by neurologic symptoms. The specific symptoms vary by virus and clinical syndrome but can include vomiting, stiff neck, mental status changes, seizures, or focal neurologic deficits. The severity and long-term outcome of the illness vary by etiologic agent and the underlying characteristics of the host, such as age, immune status, and preexisting medical condition.

Table 3.1. Clinical Manifestations for Select Domestic and International Arboviral Diseases

Virus	Systemic Febrile Illness	Neuroinvasive Disease[a]	Hemorrhagic Fever
Domestic			
Chikungunya	Yes[b]	Rare	No
Colorado tick fever	Yes	Rare	No
Dengue	Yes	Rare	Yes
Eastern equine encephalitis	Yes	Yes	No
La Crosse	Yes	Yes	No
Powassan	Yes	Yes	No
St. Louis encephalitis	Yes	Yes	No
Western equine encephalitis	Yes	Yes	No
West Nile	Yes	Yes	No
International			
Japanese encephalitis	Yes	Yes	No
Tickborne encephalitis	Yes	Yes	No
Venezuelan equine encephalitis	Yes	Yes	No
Yellow fever	Yes	No	Yes

[a] Aseptic meningitis, encephalitis, or acute flaccid paralysis.
[b] Most often characterized by sudden onset of high fever and severe joint pain.

- **Hemorrhagic fever.** Hemorrhagic fevers can be caused by dengue or yellow fever viruses. After several days of nonspecific febrile illness, the patient may develop overt signs of hemorrhage (eg, petechiae, ecchymoses, bleeding from the nose and gums, hematemesis, and melena) and septic shock (eg, decreased peripheral circulation, azotemia, tachycardia, and hypotension). Hemorrhagic fever caused by dengue and yellow fever viruses may be confused with hemorrhagic fevers transmitted by rodents (eg, Argentine hemorrhagic fever, Bolivian hemorrhagic fever, and Lassa fever) or those caused by Ebola or Marburg viruses. For information on other potential infections causing hemorrhagic manifestations, see Hemorrhagic Fevers Caused by Arenaviruses (p 381), Hemorrhagic Fevers Caused by Bunyaviruses (p 383), and Hemorrhagic Fevers Caused by Filoviruses: Ebola and Marburg (p 386).

ETIOLOGY: Arboviruses are RNA viruses that are transmitted to humans primarily through bites of infected arthropods (mosquitoes, ticks, sand flies, and biting midges). The viral families responsible for most arboviral infections in humans are *Flaviviridae* (genus *Flavivirus*), *Togaviridae* (genus *Alphavirus*), and *Bunyaviridae* (genus *Orthobunyavirus* and *Phlebovirus*). *Reoviridae* (genus *Coltivirus*) also are responsible for a smaller number of human arboviral infections (eg, Colorado tick fever) (Table 3.2, p 242).

EPIDEMIOLOGY: Most arboviruses maintain cycles of transmission between birds or small mammals and arthropod vectors. Humans and domestic animals usually are infected incidentally as "dead-end" hosts (Table 3.2, p 242). Important exceptions are dengue, yellow fever, and chikungunya viruses, which can be spread from person-to-arthropod-to-person

Table 3.2. Genus, Geographic Location, Vectors, and Average Number of Annual Cases Reported in the United States for Selected Domestic and International Arboviral Diseases

Virus	Genus	Predominant Geographic Locations		Vectors	Number of US Cases/Year (Range)[a]
		United States	Non-United States		
Domestic					
Chikungunya	*Alphavirus*	Imported, and local transmission in Florida[b]	Asia, Africa, Indian Ocean, Western Pacific, Caribbean, South America, North America[c]	Mosquitoes	2006–2013: 28 (5–65) 2014: >1500[c]
Colorado tick fever	*Coltivirus*	Rocky Mountain states	Western Canada	Ticks	7 (4–14)
Dengue	*Flavivirus*	Puerto Rico, Florida, Texas, and Hawaii	Worldwide in tropical areas	Mosquitoes	273 (2–720)[d]
Eastern equine encephalitis	*Alphavirus*	Eastern and gulf states	Canada, Central and South America	Mosquitoes	9 (4–22)
La Crosse	*Orthobunyavirus*	Midwest and Appalachia	Canada	Mosquitoes	82 (50–130)
Powassan	*Flavivirus*	Northeast and Midwest	Canada, Russia	Ticks	5 (0–16)
St. Louis encephalitis	*Flavivirus*	Widespread	Canada, Caribbean, Mexico, Central and South America	Mosquitoes	14 (1–49)
Western equine encephalitis	*Alphavirus*	Central and West	Central and South America	Mosquitoes	Less than 1
West Nile	*Flavivirus*	Widespread	Canada, Europe, Africa, Asia	Mosquitoes	3278 (712–9862)
International					
Japanese encephalitis	*Flavivirus*	Imported only	Asia	Mosquitoes	Less than 1
Tickborne encephalitis	*Flavivirus*	Imported only	Europe, northern Asia	Ticks	Less than 1
Venezuelan equine encephalitis	*Alphavirus*	Imported only	Mexico, Central and South America	Mosquitoes	Less than 1
Yellow fever	*Flavivirus*	Imported only	South America, Africa	Mosquitoes	Less than 1

[a] Average annual number of domestic and/or imported cases from 2003 through 2012.

[b] As of December 2, 2014, 11 cases of local transmission documented in Florida.

[c] From 2006–2013, studies identified an average of 28 people per year in the United States with positive tests for recent chikungunya virus infection (range 5–65 per year). All were travelers visiting or returning to the United States from affected areas, mostly Asia. As of December 2, 2014, a total of 1911 chikungunya virus disease cases have been reported during 2014 to ArboNET from US states. Eleven locally transmitted cases have been reported from Florida. All other cases occurred in travelers returning from affected areas in the Americas (n=1880), the Pacific Islands (n=9), or Asia (n=11). Updated information on chikungunya in the Americas can be found at **www.cdc.gov/chikungunya/geo/united-states.html** and **www.paho.org/hq/index.php?Itemid=40931**.

[d] Domestic and imported cases reported to ArboNET excluding indigenous transmission in Puerto Rico; dengue became nationally notifiable in 2010.

(anthroponotic transmission). For other arboviruses, humans usually do not develop a sustained or high enough level of viremia to infect biting arthropod vectors. Direct person-to-person spread of arboviruses can occur through blood transfusion, organ transplantation, intrauterine transmission, and possibly human milk (see Blood Safety, p 112, and Human Milk, p 125). Transmission through percutaneous, mucosal, or aerosol exposure to some arboviruses has occurred rarely in laboratory and occupational settings.

In the United States, arboviral infections primarily occur from late spring through early autumn, when mosquitoes and ticks are most active. The number of domestic or imported arboviral disease cases reported in the United States varies greatly by specific etiology and year (Table 3.2, p 242). Underreporting and underdiagnosis of milder disease makes a true determination of the number of cases difficult.

Overall, the risk of severe clinical disease for most arboviral infections in the United States is higher among adults than among children. One notable exception is La Crosse virus infection, for which children are at highest risk of severe neurologic disease and possible long-term sequelae. Eastern equine encephalitis virus causes a low incidence of disease but high case-fatality rate (40%) across all age groups.

Outbreaks of chikungunya have occurred in countries in Africa, Asia, Europe, and the Indian and Pacific Oceans. In late 2013, chikungunya virus was found for the first time in the Americas on islands in the Caribbean, with attack rates of up to 80% on some islands. It has spread rapidly throughout the Caribbean, and local transmission has occurred recently in Florida and in South America. As of December 12, 2014, more than 1 million cases of suspected chikungunya have been reported in the Americas.[1] Current case estimates in the Americas can be found at **www.paho.org/hq/index.php?Itemid=40931.** Chikungunya virus primarily is transmitted to humans through the bites of infected mosquitoes, predominantly *Aedes aegypti* and *Aedes albopictus*. Humans are the primary host of chikungunya virus during epidemic periods. Bloodborne transmission is possible; cases have been documented among laboratory personnel handling infected blood and a health care worker drawing blood from an infected patient. Rare in utero transmission has been documented mostly during the second trimester. Intrapartum transmission also has been documented when the mother was viremic around the time of delivery. Studies have not found chikungunya virus in human milk.

The **incubation periods** for arboviral diseases typically range between 2 and 15 days. Longer incubation periods can occur in immunocompromised people and for tickborne viruses, such as tickborne encephalitis and Powassan viruses.

DIAGNOSTIC TESTS: Arboviral infections are confirmed most frequently by measurement of virus-specific antibody in serum or cerebrospinal fluid (CSF), usually using an enzyme immunoassay (EIA). Acute-phase serum specimens should be tested for virus-specific immunoglobulin (Ig) M antibody. With clinical and epidemiologic correlation, a positive IgM test result has good diagnostic predictive value, but cross-reaction with related arboviruses from the same viral family can occur (eg, West Nile and St. Louis encephalitis viruses, which both are flaviviruses). For most arboviral infections, IgM is detectable 3 to 8 days after onset of illness and persists for 30 to 90 days, but longer persistence has been documented. Therefore, a positive IgM test result on serum occasionally may reflect a

---

[1]Centers for Disease Control and Prevention. Chikungunya cases identified through passive surveillance and household investigations—Puerto Rico, May 5—August 12, 2014. *MMWR Morb Mortal Wkly Rep.* 2014;63(48):1121-1128

past infection. Serum collected within 10 days of illness onset may not have detectable IgM, and the test should be repeated on a convalescent sample. IgG antibody generally is detectable in serum shortly after IgM and persists for years. A plaque-reduction neutralization test can be performed to measure virus-specific neutralizing antibodies and to discriminate between cross-reacting antibodies in primary arboviral infections. A fourfold or greater increase in virus-specific neutralizing antibodies between acute- and convalescent-phase serum specimens collected 2 to 3 weeks apart may be used to confirm recent infection. In patients who have been immunized against or infected with another arbovirus from the same virus family in the past, cross-reactive antibodies in both the IgM and neutralizing antibody assays may make it difficult to identify which arbovirus is causing the patient's illness. For some arboviral infections (eg, Colorado tick fever), the immune response may be delayed, with IgM antibodies not appearing until 2 to 3 weeks after onset of illness and neutralizing antibodies taking up to a month to develop. Immunization history, date of symptom onset, and information regarding other arboviruses known to circulate in the geographic area that may cross-react in serologic assays should be considered when interpreting results.

Viral culture and nucleic acid amplification tests (NAATs) for RNA can be performed on acute-phase serum, CSF, or tissue specimens. Arboviruses that are more likely to be detected using culture or NAATs early in the illness include chikungunya, Colorado tick fever, dengue, and yellow fever viruses. For other arboviruses, results of these tests often are negative even early in the clinical course because of the relatively short duration of viremia. Immunohistochemical staining can detect specific viral antigen in fixed tissue.

Antibody testing for common domestic arboviral diseases is performed in most state public health laboratories and many commercial laboratories. Confirmatory plaque-reduction neutralization tests, viral culture, NAATs, immunohistochemical staining, and testing for less common domestic and international arboviruses are performed at the Centers for Disease Control and Prevention (CDC; telephone: 970-221-6400) and selected other reference laboratories. Confirmatory testing typically is arranged through local and state health departments.

TREATMENT: The primary treatment for all arboviral disease is supportive. Although various therapies have been evaluated for several arboviral diseases, none have shown specific benefit.

ISOLATION OF THE HOSPITALIZED PATIENT: Standard precautions are recommended.

CONTROL MEASURES: Reduction of vectors in areas with endemic transmission is important to reduce risk of infection. Use of certain personal protective strategies can help decrease the risk of human infection. These strategies include using insect repellent, wearing long pants and long-sleeved shirts while outdoors, conducting a full-body check for ticks after outdoor activities, staying in screened or air-conditioned dwellings, and limiting outdoor activities during peak vector feeding times (see Prevention of Mosquitoborne Infections, p 213, and Prevention of Tickborne Infections, p 210). Select arboviral infections also can be prevented through screening of blood and organ donations and through immunization. The blood supply in the United States has been screened for West Nile virus since 2003. Blood donations from areas with endemic transmission also are screened for dengue virus. Although some arboviruses can be transmitted through human milk, transmission appears rare. Because the benefits of breastfeeding seem to outweigh the risk of illness in breastfeeding infants, mothers should be encouraged to breastfeed even in areas of active arboviral transmission.

Vaccines are available in the United States to protect against travel-related yellow fever and Japanese encephalitis.

Yellow Fever Vaccine.[1] Live-attenuated (17D strain) yellow fever vaccine is available at state-approved immunization centers. A single dose provides protection for 10 years or longer. Unless contraindicated, yellow fever immunization is recommended for all people 9 months or older living in or traveling to areas with endemic disease and is required by international regulations for travel to and from certain countries (**wwwnc.cdc.gov/travel/**). Infants younger than 6 months should not be immunized, because they have an increased risk of vaccine-associated encephalitis. The decision to immunize infants between 6 and 9 months of age must balance the infant's risk of exposure with the risk of vaccine-associated encephalitis.

Yellow fever vaccine is a live-virus vaccine produced in embryonic chicken eggs and, thus, is contraindicated in people who have an allergic reaction to eggs or chicken proteins and in people who are immunocompromised. Procedures for immunizing people with egg allergy are described in the vaccine package insert. Pregnancy and breastfeeding are precautions to yellow fever vaccine administration, because rare cases of in utero or breastfeeding transmission of the vaccine virus have been documented. Whenever possible, pregnant and breastfeeding women should defer travel to areas where yellow fever is endemic. If travel to an area with endemic disease is unavoidable and the risks for yellow fever virus exposure are believed to outweigh the vaccination risks, a pregnant or breastfeeding woman should be vaccinated. If the risks of vaccination are believed to outweigh the risks for yellow fever virus exposure, a pregnant or breastfeeding woman should be excused from immunization and issued a medical waiver letter to fulfill health regulations. For more detailed information on the yellow fever vaccine, including adverse events, precautions, and contraindications, visit **wwwnc.cdc.gov/travel/** or see Required or Recommended Travel-Related Immunizations (p 103).

Japanese Encephalitis Vaccine.[2] The risk of Japanese encephalitis for most travelers to Asia is low but varies on the basis of destination, duration, season, and activities. All travelers to countries with endemic Japanese encephalitis should be informed of the risks and should use personal protective measures to reduce the risk of mosquito bites. For some travelers who will be in high-risk settings, Japanese encephalitis vaccine can further reduce the risk for infection. The CDC recommends Japanese encephalitis vaccine for travelers who plan to spend a month or longer in areas with endemic infection during the Japanese encephalitis virus transmission season. Japanese encephalitis vaccine also should be considered for shorter-term travelers if they plan to travel outside of an urban area and have an itinerary or activities that will increase their risk of Japanese encephalitis virus exposure. Information on the location of Japanese encephalitis virus transmission and detailed information on vaccine recommendations and adverse events can be obtained from the CDC (**wwwnc.cdc.gov/travel/**).

An inactivated Vero cell culture-derived Japanese encephalitis vaccine (IXIARO [JE-VC]) is licensed and available in the United States for use in adults and children 2 months

[1]Centers for Disease Control and Prevention. Yellow fever vaccine: recommendations of the Advisory Committee on Immunization Practices (ACIP). *MMWR Recomm Rep.* 2010;59(RR-7):1-27

[2]Centers for Disease Control and Prevention. Inactivated Japanese encephalitis vaccines: recommendations of the Advisory Committee on Immunization Practices (ACIP). *MMWR Recomm Rep.* 2010;59(RR-1):1-27

and older.[1] The primary vaccination series is 2 doses administered 28 days apart. The dose is 0.25 mL for children 2 months through 2 years of age and 0.5 mL for adults and children 3 years and older. For adults, a booster dose may be given at 1 year or longer after the primary series and prior to potential Japanese encephalitis virus exposure. Data are not yet available on the need for a booster dose in children, the response to a booster dose administered more than 2 years after the primary series, or the need for and timing of additional booster doses.

No efficacy data exist for JE-VC. The vaccine was licensed on the basis of its ability to induce Japanese encephalitis virus-neutralizing antibodies as a surrogate for protection and its safety profile. No safety concerns have been identified in passive postmarketing surveillance of more than 400 000 doses distributed in the United States.

Other Arboviral Vaccines. An inactivated vaccine for tickborne encephalitis virus is licensed in Canada and some countries in Europe where the disease is endemic, but this vaccine is not available in the United States. Experimental vaccines exist against chikungunya, eastern equine encephalitis, Venezuelan equine encephalitis, and western equine encephalitis viruses, but are used primarily to protect laboratory workers and other people with occupational exposure to these viruses and are not available for public use. Dengue and West Nile virus vaccines are under development.

Public Health Reporting. Most arboviral diseases are nationally notifiable conditions and should be reported to the appropriate local and state health authorities. For select arboviruses (eg, chikungunya, dengue, and yellow fever viruses), patients may remain viremic during their acute illness. Such patients pose a risk for further person-to-mosquito-to-person transmission, increasing the importance of timely reporting.

Arcanobacterium haemolyticum Infections

CLINICAL MANIFESTATIONS: Acute pharyngitis attributable to *Arcanobacterium haemolyticum* often is indistinguishable from that caused by group A streptococci. Fever, pharyngeal exudate, lymphadenopathy, rash, and pruritus are common, but palatal petechiae and strawberry tongue are absent. In almost half of all reported cases, a maculopapular or scarlatiniform exanthem is present, beginning on the extensor surfaces of the distal extremities, spreading centripetally to the chest and back, and sparing the face, palms, and soles. Rash is associated primarily with cases presenting with pharyngitis and typically develops 1 to 4 days after onset of sore throat, although cases have been reported with rash preceding pharyngitis. Respiratory tract infections that mimic diphtheria, including membranous pharyngitis, sinusitis, and pneumonia; and skin and soft tissue infections, including chronic ulceration, cellulitis, paronychia, and wound infection, have been attributed to *A haemolyticum*. Invasive infections, including septicemia, peritonsillar abscess, Lemierre syndrome, brain abscess, orbital cellulitis, meningitis, endocarditis, pyogenic arthritis, osteomyelitis, urinary tract infection, pneumonia, spontaneous bacterial peritonitis, and pyothorax have been reported. No nonsuppurative sequelae have been reported.

ETIOLOGY: *A haemolyticum* is a catalase-negative, weakly acid-fast, facultative, hemolytic, anaerobic, gram-positive, slender, sometimes club-shaped bacillus formerly classified as *Corynebacterium haemolyticum*.

---

[1] Centers for Disease Control and Prevention. Use of Japanese encephalitis vaccine in children: recommendations of the Advisory Committee on Immunization Practices, 2013. *MMWR Morb Mortal Wkly Rep.* 2013;62(45):898-910

EPIDEMIOLOGY: Humans are the primary reservoir of *A haemolyticum*, and spread is person to person, presumably via droplet respiratory tract secretions. Severe disease occurs almost exclusively among immunocompromised people. Pharyngitis occurs primarily in adolescents and young adults and is very unusual in young children. Although long-term pharyngeal carriage with *A haemolyticum* has been described after an episode of acute pharyngitis, isolation of the bacterium from the nasopharynx of asymptomatic people is rare. Case reports also document isolation of *A haemolyticum* in combination with other pathogens. Person-to-person spread is inferred from studies of families and epidemiologic reports.

The **incubation period** is unknown.

DIAGNOSTIC TESTS: *A haemolyticum* grows on blood-enriched agar, but colonies are small, have narrow bands of hemolysis, and may not be visible for 48 to 72 hours. The organism is not detected on routine evaluation of pharyngitis by a rapid antigen test for group A streptococci. Detection is enhanced by culture on rabbit or human blood agar rather than on more commonly used sheep blood agar because of larger colony size and wider zones of hemolysis. Presence of 5% carbon dioxide enhances growth. Routine throat cultures are inoculated onto sheep blood agar, and *A haemolyticum* will be missed if laboratory personnel are not trained to identify the organism. Pits characteristically form under the colonies on blood agar plates. Two biotypes of *A haemolyticum* have been identified: a rough biotype predominates in respiratory tract infections, and a smooth biotype is most commonly associated with skin and soft-tissue infections.

TREATMENT: Erythromycin is the drug of choice for treating tonsillopharyngitis attributable to *A haemolyticum*, but no prospective therapeutic trials have been performed. *A haemolyticum* generally is susceptible in vitro to azithromycin, erythromycin, clindamycin, cefuroxime, vancomycin, and tetracycline. Failures in treatment of pharyngitis with penicillin have been reported. Resistance to trimethoprim-sulfamethoxazole is common. In rare cases of disseminated infection, susceptibility tests should be performed. In disseminated infection, parenteral penicillin plus an aminoglycoside may be used initially as empiric treatment.

ISOLATION OF THE HOSPITALIZED PATIENT: Standard precautions are recommended.

CONTROL MEASURES: None.

Ascaris lumbricoides Infections

CLINICAL MANIFESTATIONS: Most infections with *Ascaris lumbricoides* are asymptomatic, although moderate to heavy infections may lead to malnutrition and nonspecific gastrointestinal tract symptoms. During the larval migratory phase, an acute transient pneumonitis (Löffler syndrome) associated with fever and marked eosinophilia may occur. Acute intestinal obstruction has been associated with heavy infections. Children are prone to this complication because of the small diameter of the intestinal lumen and their propensity to acquire large worm burdens. Worm migration can cause peritonitis secondary to intestinal wall perforation and common bile duct obstruction resulting in biliary colic, cholangitis, or pancreatitis. Adult worms can be stimulated to migrate by stressful conditions (eg, fever, illness, or anesthesia) and by some anthelmintic drugs. *A lumbricoides* has been found in the appendiceal lumen in patients with acute appendicitis.

ETIOLOGY: *A lumbricoides* is the most prevalent of all human intestinal nematodes (roundworms), with more than 1 billion people infected worldwide.

EPIDEMIOLOGY: Adult worms live in the lumen of the small intestine. Female worms produce approximately 200 000 eggs per day, which are excreted in stool and must incubate in soil for 2 to 3 weeks for an embryo to become infectious. Following ingestion of embryonated eggs, usually from contaminated soil, larvae hatch in the small intestine, penetrate the mucosa, and are transported passively by portal blood to the liver and lungs. After migrating into the airways, larvae ascend through the tracheobronchial tree to the pharynx, are swallowed, and mature into adults in the small intestine. Infection with *A lumbricoides* is most common in resource-limited countries, including rural and urban communities characterized by poor sanitation. Adult worms can live for 12 to 18 months, resulting in daily fecal excretion of large numbers of ova. Female worms are longer than male worms and can measure 40 cm in length and 6 mm in diameter. Direct person-to-person transmission does not occur.

The **incubation period** (interval between ingestion of eggs and development of egg-laying adults) is approximately 8 weeks.

DIAGNOSTIC TESTS: Ova routinely are detected by examination of a fresh stool specimen using light microscopy. Infected people also may pass adult worms from the rectum, from the nose after migration through the nares, and from the mouth, usually in vomitus. Adult worms may be detected by computed tomographic scan of the abdomen or by ultrasonographic examination of the biliary tree.

TREATMENT: Albendazole (taken with food in a single dose), mebendazole for 3 days, or ivermectin (taken on an empty stomach in a single dose) are recommended for treatment of ascariasis (see Drugs for Parasitic Infections, p 927). Nitazoxanide taken twice a day for 3 days also is effective against *A lumbricoides*. Although widely accepted for treatment of ascariasis, albendazole is not labeled for this indication. Although the safety of albendazole in children younger than 6 years is not certain, studies in children as young as one year old suggest that its use is safe. Ivermectin and nitazoxanide also are not labeled for use for treatment of ascariasis. The safety of ivermectin in children weighing less than 15 kg has not been established. Reexamination of stool specimens can be performed 2 weeks after therapy to determine whether the worms have been eliminated.

Conservative management of small bowel obstruction, including nasogastric suction and intravenous fluids, may result in resolution of major symptoms before administration of anthelmintic therapy. Use of mineral oil or diatrizoate meglumine and diatrizoate sodium solution (Gastrografin), either orally or by nasogastric tube, may also cause relaxation of the bolus of worms. Piperazine, which is not available in the United States, causes worms to be paralyzed, allows them to be eliminated in stool, and may relieve intestinal obstruction caused by heavy worm burden. Surgical intervention occasionally is necessary to relieve intestinal or biliary tract obstruction or for volvulus or peritonitis secondary to perforation. Endoscopic retrograde cholangiopancreatography has been used successfully for extraction of worms from the biliary tree.

ISOLATION OF THE HOSPITALIZED PATIENT: Standard precautions are recommended.

CONTROL MEASURES: Sanitary disposal of human feces prevents transmission. Vegetables cultivated in areas where uncomposted human feces are used as fertilizer must be thoroughly cooked before eating.

Mass drug administration of benzimidazoles to high-risk groups is recommended by the World Health Organization for the community-based control of ascariasis and other soil-transmitted helminth infections, although evidence of sustained benefit or reductions in prevalence of infection is limited.

Aspergillosis

CLINICAL MANIFESTATIONS: Aspergillosis manifests as 3 principal clinical entities: invasive aspergillosis, pulmonary aspergilloma, and allergic disease. Colonization of the respiratory tract is common. The clinical manifestations and severity depend on the immune status of the host.

* Invasive aspergillosis occurs almost exclusively in immunocompromised patients with prolonged neutropenia (eg, cytotoxic chemotherapy), graft-versus-host disease, impaired phagocyte function (eg, chronic granulomatous disease), or receipt of T-lymphocyte-immunosuppressive therapy (eg, corticosteroids, calcineurin inhibitors, tumor necrosis factor [TNF]-alpha inhibitors). Children at highest risk include those with new-onset acute myelogenous leukemia, with relapse of hematologic malignancy, and recipients of allogeneic hematopoietic stem cell and solid organ transplantation. Invasive infection usually involves pulmonary, sinus, cerebral, or cutaneous sites. Rarely, endocarditis, osteomyelitis, meningitis, infection of the eye or orbit, and esophagitis occur. The hallmark of invasive aspergillosis is angioinvasion with resulting thrombosis, dissemination to other organs, and occasionally erosion of the blood vessel wall with catastrophic hemorrhage. Aspergillosis in patients with chronic granulomatous disease rarely displays angioinvasion.

* Aspergillomas and otomycosis are 2 syndromes of nonallergic colonization by *Aspergillus* species in immunocompetent children. Aspergillomas ("fungal balls") grow in preexisting pulmonary cavities or bronchogenic cysts without invading pulmonary tissue; almost all patients have underlying lung disease, such as cystic fibrosis or tuberculosis. Patients with otomycosis have chronic otitis media with colonization of the external auditory canal by a fungal mat that produces a dark discharge.

* Allergic bronchopulmonary aspergillosis is a hypersensitivity lung disease that manifests as episodic wheezing, expectoration of brown mucus plugs, low-grade fever, eosinophilia, and transient pulmonary infiltrates. This form of aspergillosis occurs most commonly in immunocompetent children with asthma or cystic fibrosis and can be a trigger for asthmatic flares.

* Allergic sinusitis is a far less common allergic response to colonization by *Aspergillus* species than is allergic bronchopulmonary aspergillosis. Allergic sinusitis occurs in children with nasal polyps or previous episodes of sinusitis or in children who have undergone sinus surgery. Allergic sinusitis is characterized by symptoms of chronic sinusitis with dark plugs of nasal discharge.

ETIOLOGY: *Aspergillus* species are ubiquitous molds that grow on decaying vegetation and in soil. *Aspergillus fumigatus* is the most common cause of invasive aspergillosis, with *Aspergillus flavus* being the next most common. Several other species, including *Aspergillus terreus, Aspergillus nidulans,* and *Aspergillus niger,* also cause invasive human infections.

EPIDEMIOLOGY: The principal route of transmission is inhalation of conidia (spores) originating from multiple environmental sources (eg, plants, vegetables, dust from construction or demolition), soil, and water supplies (eg, shower heads). Incidence of disease in stem cell transplant recipients is highest during periods of neutropenia or during treatment for graft-versus-host disease. In solid organ transplant recipients, the risk is highest 1 to 6 months after transplantation or during periods of increased immunosuppression. Disease has followed use of contaminated marijuana in the immunocompromised host. Health care-associated outbreaks of invasive pulmonary aspergillosis in susceptible hosts have occurred in which the probable source of the fungus was a nearby construction site or faulty ventilation system; however, frequently, the source of health care-associated aspergillosis is not known. Outbreaks of colonization related to construction have been reported and may be a marker of high environmental fungal burden. Cutaneous aspergillosis occurs less frequently and usually involves sites of skin injury, such as intravenous catheter sites, sites of traumatic inoculation, and sites associated with occlusive dressings, burns, or surgery. Transmission by direct inoculation of skin abrasions or wounds is less likely. Person-to-person spread does not occur.

The **incubation period** is unknown and may be variable.

DIAGNOSTIC TESTS: Dichotomously branched and septate hyphae, identified by microscopic examination of 10% potassium hydroxide wet preparations or of Gomori methenamine-silver nitrate stain of tissue or bronchoalveolar lavage specimens, are suggestive of the diagnosis. Isolation of *Aspergillus* species or molecular testing with specific reagents is required for definitive diagnosis. The organism usually is not recoverable from blood (except *A terreus*) but is isolated readily from lung, sinus, and skin biopsy specimens when cultured on Sabouraud dextrose agar or brain-heart infusion media (without cycloheximide). *Aspergillus* species can be a laboratory contaminant, but when evaluating results from ill, immunocompromised patients, recovery of this organism frequently indicates infection. Biopsy of a lesion usually is required to confirm the diagnosis, and care should be taken to distinguish aspergillosis from mucormycosis, which appears similar by diagnostic imaging studies. An enzyme immunosorbent assay serologic test for detection of galactomannan, a molecule found in the cell wall of *Aspergillus* species, from the serum or bronchoalveolar lavage (BAL) fluid is available commercially and has been found to be useful in children and adults. A test result of ≥0.5 from the serum or ≥1.0 from BAL fluid supports a diagnosis of invasive aspergillosis, and serum monitoring of serum antigen concentrations twice weekly in periods of highest risk (eg, neutropenia and active graft-versus-host disease) may be useful for early detection of invasive aspergillosis in at-risk patients. False-positive test results have been reported and can be related to consumption of food products containing galactomannan (eg, rice and pasta), colonization of the gut of neonates with *Bifidobacterium* species, or cross-reactivity with antimicrobial agents derived from fungi (eg, penicillins, especially piperacillin-tazobactam). A negative galactomannan test result does not exclude diagnosis of invasive aspergillosis, and the greatest utility may be in monitoring response to disease rather than in its use as a diagnostic marker. False-negative galactomannan test results consistently occur in patients with chronic granulomatous disease, so the test should not be used in these patients. Limited data suggest that other nonspecific fungal biomarkers, such as 1,3-β-D glucan testing, may be useful in the diagnosis of aspergillosis. Unlike adults, children frequently do not manifest cavitation or the air crescent or halo signs on chest radiography, and lack of these characteristic signs does not exclude the diagnosis of invasive aspergillosis.

In allergic aspergillosis, diagnosis is suggested by a typical clinical syndrome with elevated total concentrations of immunoglobulin (Ig) E (≥1000 ng/mL) and *Aspergillus*-specific serum IgE, eosinophilia, and a positive result from a skin test for *Aspergillus* antigens. In people with cystic fibrosis, the diagnosis is more difficult, because wheezing, eosinophilia, and a positive skin test result not associated with allergic bronchopulmonary aspergillosis often are present.

TREATMENT[1]: Voriconazole is the drug of choice for invasive aspergillosis, except in neonates, for whom amphotericin B deoxycholate in high doses is recommended (see Antifungal Drugs for Systemic Fungal Infections, p 905). Voriconazole has been shown to be superior to amphotericin B in a large, randomized trial in adults. Therapy is continued for at least 12 weeks, but treatment duration should be individualized. Monitoring of serum galactomannan concentrations in those with significant elevation at onset, on a twice weekly basis, may be useful to assess response to therapy concomitant with clinical and radiologic evaluation. Voriconazole is metabolized in a linear fashion in children (nonlinear in adults), so the recommended adult dosing (per kg) is too low for children. The optimal dose for children 2 to 12 years of age is to load with 9 mg/kg intravenously, every 12 hours, for 1 day and then continue with 8 mg/kg/dose intravenously, every 12 hours. Children 12 years and older who weigh ≥50 kg should receive the adult dose of 6 mg/kg intravenously, every 12 hours, for 1 day and then continue with 4 mg/kg/dose intravenously, every 12 hours. Conversion to oral voriconazole requires a dose increase to 9 mg/kg orally every 12 hours. Close monitoring of voriconazole serum trough concentrations is critical for both efficacy and safety, and most experts agree that for children voriconazole trough concentrations should be between 2 μg/mL and 6 μg/mL,[2,3] whereas for adults they should be ≥1 μg/mL. It is important to individualize dosing in patients following initiation of voriconazole therapy, because there is high interpatient variability in metabolism. Itraconazole alone is an alternative for mild to moderate cases of aspergillosis, although extensive drug interactions and poor absorption (capsular form) limit its utility.

Lipid formulations of amphotericin B can be considered as alternative primary therapy in some patients, but *A terreus* is resistant to all amphotericin B products. In refractory disease, treatment may include posaconazole, caspofungin, or micafungin. Caspofungin has been studied in pediatric patients older than 3 months as salvage therapy for invasive aspergillosis. The pharmacokinetics of caspofungin in adults differ from those in children, in whom a body-surface area dosing scheme is preferred to a weight-based dosing regimen. Limited data from a predominantly adult population are available but suggest that micafungin and caspofungin have similar efficacy in treatment of refractory aspergillosis. The pharmacokinetics and safety of posaconazole have not been evaluated in younger children. Posaconazole absorption often is erratic and the patient must be fully feeding or tolerating oral liquid supplementation.

The efficacy and safety of combination antifungal therapy for invasive aspergillosis is uncertain, but the most promising combination is a broad-spectrum azole combined with an echinocandin. Immune reconstitution can occur during treatment in some patients. Decreasing immunosuppression if possible (specifically decreasing corticosteroid dose) is critical to disease control.

Surgical excision of a localized invasive lesion (eg, cutaneous eschars, a single pulmonary lesion, sinus debris, accessible cerebral lesions) usually is warranted. In pulmonary disease, surgery is indicated only when a mass is impinging on a great vessel. Allergic bronchopulmonary aspergillosis is treated with corticosteroids and adjunctive antifungal

[1]Walsh TJ, Anaissie EJ, Denning DW, et al. Treatment of aspergillosis: clinical practice guidelines of the Infectious Diseases Society of America. *Clin Infect Dis.* 2008;46(3):327-360

[2]Chen J, Chan C, Colantonio D, et al. Therapeutic drug monitoring of voriconazole in children. *Ther Drug Monit.* 2012;34(1):77-84

[3]Choi SH, Lee SY, Hwang JY, et al. Importance of voriconazole therapeutic drug monitoring in pediatric cancer patients with invasive aspergillosis. *Pediatr Blood Cancer.* 2013;60(1):82-87

therapy is recommended. Allergic sinus aspergillosis also is treated with corticosteroids, and surgery has been reported to be beneficial in many cases. Antifungal therapy has not been found to be useful.

ISOLATION OF THE HOSPITALIZED PATIENT: Standard precautions are recommended.

CONTROL MEASURES: Outbreaks of invasive aspergillosis and *Aspergillus* colonization have occurred among hospitalized patients during construction in hospitals or at nearby sites. Environmental measures reported to be effective include erecting suitable barriers between patient care areas and construction sites, routine cleaning of air-handling systems, repair of faulty air flow, and replacement of contaminated air filters. High-efficiency particulate air filters and laminar flow rooms markedly decrease the risk of exposure to conidia in patient care areas. These latter measures may be expensive and difficult for patients to tolerate.

Posaconazole has been shown to be effective in 2 randomized controlled trials as prophylaxis against invasive aspergillosis for patients 13 years and older who have undergone hematopoietic stem cell transplantation and have graft-versus-host disease, and in patients with hematologic malignancies with prolonged neutropenia. Low-dose amphotericin B, itraconazole, voriconazole, or posaconazole prophylaxis have been reported for other high-risk patients, but controlled trials have not been completed in pediatric patients.

Patients at risk of invasive infection should avoid environmental exposure (eg, gardening) following discharge from the hospital. People with allergic aspergillosis should take measures to reduce exposure to *Aspergillus* species in the home.

Astrovirus Infections

CLINICAL MANIFESTATIONS: Illness is characterized by diarrhea accompanied by low-grade fever, malaise, and nausea, and less commonly, vomiting and mild dehydration. Illness in an immunocompetent host is self-limited, lasting a median of 5 to 6 days. Asymptomatic infections are common.

ETIOLOGY: Astroviruses are nonenveloped, single-stranded RNA viruses with a characteristic starlike appearance when visualized by electron microscopy. Eight human antigenic types originally were described, and several novel species have been identified in recent years.

EPIDEMIOLOGY: Human astroviruses have a worldwide distribution. Multiple antigenic types cocirculate in the same region. Astroviruses have been detected in as many as 5% to 17% of sporadic cases of nonbacterial gastroenteritis among young children in the community but appear to cause a lower proportion of cases of more severe childhood gastroenteritis requiring hospitalization (2.5% to 9%). Astrovirus infections occur predominantly in children younger than 4 years and have a seasonal peak during the late winter and spring in the United States. Transmission is via the fecal-oral route through contaminated food or water, person-to-person contact, or contaminated surfaces. Outbreaks tend to occur in closed populations of the young and the elderly, particularly among hospitalized children (health care-associated infections) and children in child care centers. Excretion lasts a median of 5 days after onset of symptoms, but asymptomatic excretion after illness can last for several weeks in healthy children. Persistent excretion may occur in immunocompromised hosts.

The **incubation period** is 3 to 4 days.

DIAGNOSTIC TESTS: Commercial tests for diagnosis are not available in the United States, although enzyme immunoassays are available in many other countries. The following tests are available in some research and reference laboratories: electron microscopy for detection of viral particles in stool, enzyme immunoassay for detection of viral antigen in stool or antibody in serum, latex agglutination in stool, and reverse transcriptase-polymerase chain reaction (RT-PCR) assay for detection of viral RNA in stool. Of these tests, RT-PCR assay is the most sensitive.

TREATMENT: No specific antiviral therapy is available. Oral or parenteral fluids and electrolytes are given to prevent and correct dehydration.

ISOLATION OF THE HOSPITALIZED PATIENT: In addition to standard precautions, contact precautions are recommended for diapered or incontinent children for the duration of illness.

CONTROL MEASURES: No specific control measures are available. The spread of infection in child care settings can be decreased by using general measures for control of diarrhea, such as training care providers in infection-control procedures, maintaining cleanliness of surfaces, keeping food preparation duties and areas separate from child care activities, exercising adequate hand hygiene, cohorting ill children, and excluding ill child care providers, food handlers, and children (see Children in Out-of-Home Child Care, p 132).

Babesiosis

CLINICAL MANIFESTATIONS: *Babesia* infection often is asymptomatic or associated with mild, nonspecific symptoms. The infection also can be severe and life threatening, particularly in people who are asplenic, immunocompromised, or elderly. In general, babesiosis, like malaria, is characterized by the presence of fever and hemolytic anemia; however, some infected people who are immunocompromised or at the extremes of age (eg, preterm infants) are afebrile. Infected people may have a prodromal illness, with gradual onset of symptoms, such as malaise, anorexia, and fatigue, followed by development of fever and other influenza-like symptoms (eg, chills, sweats, myalgia, arthralgia, headache, anorexia, nausea). Less common findings include sore throat, nonproductive cough, abdominal pain, vomiting, weight loss, conjunctival injection, photophobia, emotional lability, and hyperesthesia. Congenital infection with manifestation as severe sepsis syndrome has been reported.

Clinical signs generally are minimal, often consisting only of fever and tachycardia, although hypotension, respiratory distress, mild hepatosplenomegaly, jaundice, and dark urine may be noted. Thrombocytopenia is common; disseminated intravascular coagulation can be a complication of severe babesiosis. If untreated, illness can last for several weeks or months; even asymptomatic people can have persistent low-level parasitemia, sometimes for longer than 1 year.

ETIOLOGY: *Babesia* species are intraerythrocytic protozoa. The etiologic agents of babesiosis in the United States include *Babesia microti*, which is the cause of most reported cases, and several other genetically and antigenically distinct organisms, such as *Babesia duncani* (formerly the WA1-type parasite).

EPIDEMIOLOGY: Babesiosis predominantly is a tickborne zoonosis. *Babesia* parasites also can be transmitted by blood transfusion and through congenital/perinatal routes. In the United States, the primary reservoir host for *B microti* is the white-footed mouse *(Peromyscus leucopus)*, and the primary vector is the tick *Ixodes scapularis*, which also can transmit *Borrelia* *burgdorferi,* the causative agent of Lyme disease, and *Anaplasma phagocytophilum,* the causative agent of human granulocytic anaplasmosis. Humans become infected through tick bites, which typically are not noticed. The white-tailed deer *(Odocoileus virginianus)* is an important host for blood meals for the tick but is not a reservoir host of *B microti.* An increase in the deer population in some geographic areas, including some suburban areas, during the past few decades is thought to be a major factor in the spread of *I scapularis* and the increase in numbers of reported cases of babesiosis. The reported vectorborne cases of *B microti* infection have been acquired in the Northeast (particularly, but not exclusively, in Connecticut, Massachusetts, New Jersey, New York, and Rhode Island) and in the upper Midwest (Wisconsin and Minnesota). Occasional human cases of babesiosis caused by other species have been described in various regions of the United States; tick vectors and reservoir hosts for these agents typically have not yet been identified. Whereas most US vectorborne cases of babesiosis occur during late spring, summer, or autumn, transfusion-associated cases can occur year round.

The **incubation period** typically ranges from approximately 1 week to 5 weeks following a tick bite and from approximately 1 to 9 weeks after a contaminated blood transfusion but occasionally is longer (eg, latent infection might become symptomatic after splenectomy).

DIAGNOSTIC TESTS: Acute, symptomatic cases of babesiosis typically are diagnosed by microscopic identification of the organism on Giemsa- or Wright-stained blood smears. If the diagnosis of babesiosis is being considered, manual (nonautomated) review of blood smears for parasites should be requested explicitly. If seen, the tetrad (Maltese-cross) form is pathognomonic. *B microti* and other *Babesia* species can be difficult to distinguish from *Plasmodium falciparum;* examination of blood smears by a reference laboratory should be considered for confirmation of the diagnosis. Adjunctive molecular and serologic testing is performed at the Centers for Disease Control and Prevention and at some other laboratories. If indicated, the possibility of concurrent *B burgdorferi* or *Anaplasma* infection should be considered.

TREATMENT: Clindamycin plus oral quinine for 7 to 10 days or atovaquone plus azithromycin for 7 to 10 days had comparable efficacy in a controlled clinical trial conducted among adult patients who did not have life-threatening babesiosis (see Drugs for Parasitic Infections, p 927). Therapy with atovaquone plus azithromycin is associated with fewer adverse effects. However, the combination of clindamycin and quinine remains the standard of care for severely ill patients. Exchange blood transfusions should be considered for patients who are critically ill (eg, hemodynamically unstable), especially but not exclusively for patients with parasitemia levels of 10% or higher.

ISOLATION OF THE HOSPITALIZED PATIENT: Standard precautions are recommended.

CONTROL MEASURES: Specific recommendations concern prevention of tick bites and are similar to those for prevention of Lyme disease and other tickborne infections (see Prevention of Tickborne Infections, p 210). People with a known history of *Babesia* infection are deferred indefinitely from donating blood. To date, no *Babesia* tests have been licensed for screening blood donors, but screening for *Babesia microti* currently is under investigation for donor screening in select areas in the United States and its territories. Babesiosis is a nationally notifiable disease and is a reportable disease in many states.

Bacillus cereus Infections

CLINICAL MANIFESTATIONS: *Bacillus cereus* is associated primarily with 2 toxin-mediated foodborne illnesses, emetic and diarrheal, but it also can cause invasive extraintestinal infection. The emetic syndrome develops after a short incubation period, similar to staphylococcal foodborne illness. It is characterized by nausea, vomiting, and abdominal cramps, and diarrhea can follow in up to a third of patients. The diarrheal syndrome has a longer incubation period, is more severe, and resembles *Clostridium perfringens* foodborne illness. It is characterized by moderate to severe abdominal cramps and watery diarrhea, vomiting in approximately 25% of patients, and occasionally low-grade fever. Both illnesses usually are short-lived, but the emetic toxin has been associated with fulminant liver failure.

Invasive extraintestinal infection can be severe and can include a wide range of diseases, including wound and soft tissue infections; bacteremia, including central line-associated bloodstream infection; endocarditis; osteomyelitis; purulent meningitis and ventricular shunt infection; pneumonia; and ocular infections. Along with staphylococci, *B cereus* is a significant cause of bacterial endophthalmitis. Ocular involvement includes panophthalmitis, endophthalmitis, and keratitis. *B cereus* constitutes a large proportion of organisms that cause endophthalmitis that follow penetrating trauma. Endogenous endophthalmitis can result from bacteremic seeding.

ETIOLOGY: *B cereus* is an aerobic and facultatively anaerobic, spore-forming, gram-positive bacillus.

EPIDEMIOLOGY: *B cereus* is ubiquitous in the environment and commonly is present in small numbers in raw, dried, and processed foods. The organism is a common cause of foodborne illness in the United States but may be under-recognized because few people seek care for mild illness and physicians or clinical laboratories do not routinely test for *B cereus*.

Spores of *B cereus* are heat resistant and can survive pasteurization, brief cooking, or boiling. Vegetative forms can grow and produce enterotoxins over a wide range of temperatures, both in foods and in the gastrointestinal tract; the latter results in the diarrheal syndrome. A wide variety of food vehicles have been implicated. The emetic syndrome occurs after eating contaminated food containing preformed emetic toxin. The best known association of the emetic syndrome is with ingestion of fried rice made from boiled rice stored at room temperature overnight, but illness has been associated with a wide variety of foods. Foodborne illness caused by *B cereus* is not transmissible from person to person

Risk factors for invasive disease attributable to *B cereus* include history of injection drug use, presence of indwelling intravascular catheters or implanted devices, neutropenia or immunosuppression, and preterm birth. *B cereus* endophthalmitis has occurred after penetrating ocular trauma and injection drug use. The **incubation period** for foodborne illness is 0.5 to 6 hours for the emetic syndrome and 6 to 24 hours for the diarrheal syndrome.

DIAGNOSTIC TESTS: For foodborne outbreaks, isolation of *B cereus* from the stool or vomitus of 2 or more ill people and not from control patients, or isolation of 10^5 colony-forming units/g or greater from epidemiologically implicated food, suggests that *B cereus* is the cause of the outbreak. Because the organism can be recovered from stool specimens from some well people, the presence of *B cereus* in feces or vomitus of ill people is not definitive evidence of infection. Food samples must be tested for both enterotoxins, because either alone can cause illness. The most commonly used and informative subtyping method for *B cereus* is multilocus sequence typing.

In patients with risk factors for invasive disease, isolation of *B cereus* from wounds, blood, or other usually sterile body fluids is significant. The common perception of *Bacillus* species as "contaminants" may delay recognition and treatment of serious *B cereus* infections.

TREATMENT: *B cereus* foodborne illness usually requires only supportive treatment, including rehydration. Antimicrobial therapy is indicated for patients with invasive disease. Prompt removal of any potentially infected foreign bodies, such as central lines or implants, is essential. For intraocular infections, an ophthalmologist should be consulted regarding use of intravitreal vancomycin therapy in addition to systemic therapy. *B cereus* usually is resistant to beta-lactam antibiotics and clindamycin but is susceptible to vancomycin, which is the drug of choice. Alternative drugs, including linezolid and fluoroquinolones, may be considered depending on susceptibility results.

ISOLATION OF THE HOSPITALIZED PATIENT: Standard precautions are recommended.

CONTROL MEASURES: Proper cooking and appropriate storage of foods, particularly rice cooked for later use, will help prevent foodborne outbreaks. Information on recommended safe food handling practices, including time and temperature requirements during cooking, storage, and reheating, can be found at **www.foodsafety.gov.** Hand hygiene and strict aseptic technique in caring for immunocompromised patients or patients with indwelling intravascular catheters are important to minimize the risk of invasive disease.

Bacterial Vaginosis

CLINICAL MANIFESTATIONS: Bacterial vaginosis (BV) is a polymicrobial clinical syndrome characterized by changes in vaginal flora, with replacement of normally abundant *Lactobacillus* species by high concentrations of anaerobic bacteria. BV is diagnosed primarily in sexually active postpubertal females, but women who have never been sexually active also can be affected. BV is asymptomatic in 50% to 75% of females with microbiologic evidence of infection. Symptoms include vaginal discharge and/or vaginal odor. Classic signs, when present, include a thin white or grey, homogenous, adherent vaginal discharge with a fishy odor often noted to increase after addition of potassium hydroxide. Symptoms of vulvovaginal irritation, pruritus, dysuria, or abdominal pain are not associated with BV but are suggestive of mixed vaginitis. In pregnant women, BV has been associated with adverse outcomes, including chorioamnionitis, premature rupture of membranes, preterm delivery, and postpartum endometritis. Vaginitis and vulvitis in prepubertal girls rarely, if ever, are manifestations of BV. Vaginitis in prepubertal girls frequently is nonspecific, but possible causes include foreign bodies and infections attributable to group A streptococci, *Escherichia coli*, herpes simplex virus, *Neisseria gonorrhoeae*, *Chlamydia trachomatis*, *Trichomonas vaginalis*, or enteric bacteria, including *Shigella* species.

ETIOLOGY: The microbiologic cause of BV has not been delineated fully. Hydrogen peroxide-producing *Lactobacillus* species predominate among vaginal flora and play a protective role. In females with BV, these species largely are replaced by commensal anaerobes. Typical microbiologic findings of vaginal specimens show increased concentrations of *Gardnerella vaginalis, Mycoplasma hominis, Prevotella* species, *Mobiluncus* species, and *Ureaplasma* species. Numerous other fastidious organisms have been associated with BV as well. These organisms are collectively referred to as BV-associated bacteria.

EPIDEMIOLOGY: BV is the most common cause of vaginal discharge in sexually active adolescent and adult females. In this population, BV may be the sole cause of the symptoms, or it may accompany other conditions associated with vaginal discharge, such as trichomoniasis or mucopurulent cervicitis secondary to other sexually transmitted infections (STIs). BV occurs more frequently in females with a new sexual partner or a higher number of sexual partners and in those who engage in douching. Although evidence of sexual transmission of BV is inconclusive, the correct and consistent use of condoms reduces the risk of acquisition. BV increases the risk of infectious complications following gynecologic surgery as well as pregnancy complications and the acquisition of other STIs, including human immunodeficiency virus (HIV), herpes simplex virus-2, *N gonorrhoeae*, and *C trachomatis*. Because BV is a polymicrobial infection, an **incubation period** has not been defined. Recurrence is common.

DIAGNOSTIC TESTS: BV most commonly is diagnosed clinically using the Amsel criteria, requiring that 3 or more of the following symptoms or signs are present:
- Homogenous, thin grey or white vaginal discharge that smoothly coats the vaginal walls
- Vaginal fluid pH greater than 4.5
- A fishy (amine) odor of vaginal discharge before or after addition of 10% potassium hydroxide (ie, the "whiff test")
- Presence of clue cells (squamous vaginal epithelial cells covered with bacteria, which cause a stippled or granular appearance and ragged "moth-eaten" borders) representing at least 20% of the total vaginal epithelial cells seen on microscopic evaluation of vaginal fluid.

An alternative method for diagnosing BV is the Nugent score, which is used widely as the gold standard for making the diagnosis in the research setting. A Gram stain of the vaginal fluid is evaluated, and a numerical score is generated on the basis of the apparent quantity of lactobacilli relative to BV-associated bacteria. The score is interpreted as normal (0-3), intermediate (4-6), or frank BV (7-10). Douching, recent intercourse, menstruation, and coexisting infection can alter findings on Gram stain.

The Affirm VPIII test is a DNA probe test that detects *G vaginalis* and can be used when symptoms and signs are suggestive of BV but microscopy is unavailable. Clinical Laboratory Improvement Amendments (CLIA)-waived rapid tests for BV that measure the activity of sialidase, an enzyme generated by several BV-associated bacteria, such as Diagnosit BVBlue (Gryphus Diagnostics, Knoxville, TN) and OSOM BVBlue Test (Sekisui Diagnostics, Lexington, MA), have strong clinical performance compared with the Nugent criteria. The FemExam *G vaginalis* PIP Activity TestCard (Litmus Concepts Inc, Santa Clara, CA) detects proline iminopeptidase activity of anaerobes and can be performed as a point-of-care test in less than 2 minutes. A CLIA waiver for use as a point-of-care test is pending. Papanicolaou (Pap) testing is not recommended for the diagnosis of BV because of its low sensitivity.

Sexually active females with BV should be evaluated for coinfection with other STIs, including syphilis, gonorrhea, chlamydia, trichomoniasis, and HIV infection. Completion of the hepatitis B immunization series and the human papillomavirus immunization series should be confirmed.

TREATMENT: Symptomatic patients should be treated. The goals of treatment are to relieve the symptoms and signs of infection and potentially to decrease the risk of infectious complications and acquisition of other STIs. Treatment considerations should include patient preference for oral versus intravaginal treatment, possible adverse effects, and the presence of coinfections. Nonpregnant patients may be treated orally with metronidazole 500 mg twice daily for 7 days or topically with metronidazole gel 0.75% once daily for 5 days or clindamycin cream 2% once daily for 7 days intravaginally at bedtime. Alternative regimens include oral tinidazole, oral clindamycin, or clindamycin intravaginal ovules (see Table 4.4, p 896). Patients who are treated with metronidazole should not consume alcohol during therapy and for 1 day after completion of therapy. Patients should refrain from sexual intercourse or use condoms appropriately during treatment, keeping in mind that clindamycin cream is oil-based and can weaken latex condoms and diaphragms for up to 5 days after completion of therapy. There is no demonstrated benefit of treating sexual partners. Follow-up is not necessary if symptoms resolve.

Approximately 30% of appropriately treated females have a recurrence within 3 months. Retreatment with the same regimen or an alternative regimen are both reasonable options. For patients with frequent recurrences, limited data support the use of metronidazole gel twice weekly for 4 to 6 months after completion of a BV treatment course. Experts also recommend use of intravaginal boric acid for 3 weeks or a prolonged course of metronidazole (10-14 days with vaginal gel or oral tablets) or tinidazole (for a week) before starting the course of metronidazole gel to increase the likelihood of remaining BV free. Studies of intravaginal lactobacillus preparations have shown inconsistent results, and their routine use is not recommended at this time.

Pregnant or breastfeeding females with symptoms of BV should be treated. Metronidazole, 500 mg twice daily for 7 days or 250 mg orally 3 times daily for 7 days, or clindamycin, 300 mg orally twice daily for 7 days, are the preferred treatments during pregnancy. Oral therapies are preferred in pregnancy to treat possible upper genital tract infection. Treatment of BV in asymptomatic pregnant females has not consistently been shown to reduce the incidence of preterm delivery in females with or without additional risk factors (such as prior history of a preterm birth); some studies demonstrate an increase in adverse events among treated females. Intravaginal clindamycin given during the latter half of pregnancy has been associated with adverse outcomes in the newborn. More research in this population is needed before definitive screening and treatment recommendations may be made.

ISOLATION OF THE HOSPITALIZED PATIENT: Standard precautions are recommended.

CONTROL MEASURES: None.

Bacteroides and Prevotella Infections

CLINICAL MANIFESTATIONS: *Bacteroides* and *Prevotella* organisms from the oral cavity can cause chronic sinusitis, chronic otitis media, dental infection, peritonsillar abscess, cervical adenitis, retropharyngeal space infection, aspiration pneumonia, lung abscess, pleural empyema, or necrotizing pneumonia. Species from the gastrointestinal tract are recovered in patients with peritonitis, intra-abdominal abscess, pelvic inflammatory disease, postoperative wound infection, or vulvovaginal and perianal infections. Invasion of the bloodstream from the oral cavity or intestinal tract can lead to brain abscess, meningitis, endocarditis, arthritis, or osteomyelitis. Skin and soft tissue infections include synergistic bacterial gangrene and necrotizing fasciitis; omphalitis in newborn infants; cellulitis at the site of fetal monitors, human bite wounds, or burns; infections adjacent to the mouth or rectum; and infected decubitus ulcers. Neonatal infections, including conjunctivitis, pneumonia, bacteremia, or meningitis, rarely occur. In most settings where *Bacteroides* and *Prevotella* are implicated, the infections are polymicrobial.

ETIOLOGY: Most *Bacteroides* and *Prevotella* organisms associated with human disease are pleomorphic, non-spore–forming, facultatively anaerobic, gram-negative bacilli.

EPIDEMIOLOGY: *Bacteroides* species and *Prevotella* species are part of the normal flora of the mouth, gastrointestinal tract, and female genital tract. Members of the *Bacteroides fragilis* group predominate in the gastrointestinal tract flora; members of the *Prevotella melaninogenica* (formerly *Bacteroides melaninogenicus*) and *Prevotella oralis* (formerly *Bacteroides oralis*) groups are more common in the oral cavity. These species cause infection as opportunists, usually after an alteration in skin or mucosal membranes in conjunction with other endogenous species. Endogenous infection results from aspiration, bowel perforation, or damage to mucosal surfaces from trauma, surgery, or chemotherapy. Enterotoxigenic *B fragilis* may be a cause of diarrhea. Mucosal injury or granulocytopenia predispose to infection. Except in infections resulting from human bites, no evidence of person-to-person transmission exists.

The **incubation period** is variable and depends on the inoculum and the site of involvement but usually is 1 to 5 days.

DIAGNOSTIC TESTS: Anaerobic culture media are necessary for recovery of *Bacteroides* or *Prevotella* species. Because infections usually are polymicrobial, aerobic cultures also should be obtained. A putrid odor suggests anaerobic infection. Use of an anaerobic transport tube or a sealed syringe is recommended for collection of clinical specimens.

TREATMENT: Abscesses should be drained when feasible; abscesses involving the brain, liver, and lungs may resolve with effective antimicrobial therapy. Necrotizing soft tissue lesions should be débrided surgically.

The choice of antimicrobial agent(s) is based on anticipated or known in vitro susceptibility testing. *Bacteroides* infections of the mouth and respiratory tract generally are susceptible to penicillin G, ampicillin, and extended-spectrum penicillins, such as ticarcillin or piperacillin. Clindamycin is active against virtually all mouth and respiratory tract *Bacteroides* and *Prevotella* isolates and is recommended by some experts as the drug of choice for anaerobic infections of the oral cavity and lungs but is not recommended for central nervous system infections. Some species of *Bacteroides* and almost 50% of *Prevotella* species produce beta-lactamase. A beta-lactam penicillin active against *Bacteroides* species combined with a beta-lactamase inhibitor (ampicillin-sulbactam, amoxicillin-clavulanate, ticarcillin-clavulanate, or piperacillin-tazobactam) can be useful to treat these infections. *Bacteroides* species of the gastrointestinal tract usually are resistant to penicillin G but are susceptible predictably to metronidazole, beta-lactam plus beta-lactamase inhibitors, chloramphenicol, and sometimes, clindamycin. Tigecycline has demonstrated in vitro activity against *Prevotella* species and *Bacteroides* species but is not approved by the US Food and Drug Administration for use in people younger than 18 years. More than 80% of isolates are susceptible to cefoxitin, ceftizoxime, linezolid, imipenem, and meropenem. Cefuroxime, cefotaxime, and ceftriaxone are not reliably effective.

ISOLATION OF THE HOSPITALIZED PATIENT: Standard precautions are recommended.

CONTROL MEASURES: None.

Balantidium coli Infections
(Balantidiasis)

CLINICAL MANIFESTATIONS: Most human infections are asymptomatic. Acute symptomatic infection is characterized by rapid onset of nausea, vomiting, abdominal discomfort or pain, and bloody or watery mucoid diarrhea. In some patients, the course is chronic with intermittent episodes of diarrhea, anorexia, and weight loss. Rarely, organisms spread to mesenteric nodes, pleura, lung, liver, or genitourinary sites. Inflammation of the gastrointestinal tract and local lymphatic vessels can result in bowel dilation, ulceration, perforation, and secondary bacterial invasion. Colitis produced by *Balantidium coli* often is indistinguishable from colitis produced by *Entamoeba histolytica.* Fulminant disease can occur in malnourished or otherwise debilitated or immunocompromised patients.

ETIOLOGY: *B coli*, a ciliated protozoan, is the largest pathogenic protozoan known to infect humans.

EPIDEMIOLOGY: Pigs are the primary host reservoir of *B coli*, but other sources of infection have been reported. Infections have been reported in most areas of the world but are rare in industrialized countries. Cysts excreted in feces can be transmitted directly from hand to mouth or indirectly through fecally contaminated water or food. Excysted trophozoites infect the colon. A person is infectious as long as cysts are excreted in stool. Cysts may remain viable in the environment for months.

The **incubation period** is not established, but may be several days.

DIAGNOSTIC TESTS: Diagnosis of infection is established by scraping lesions via sigmoidoscopy, histologic examination of intestinal biopsy specimens, or ova and parasite examination of stool. The diagnosis usually is established by demonstrating trophozoites (or less frequently, cysts) in stool or tissue specimens. Stool examination is less sensitive, and repeated stool examination may be necessary to diagnose infection, because shedding of organisms can be intermittent. Microscopic examination of fresh diarrheal stools must be performed promptly, because trophozoites degenerate rapidly.

TREATMENT: The drug of choice is a tetracycline, which may cause permanent tooth discoloration for children younger than 8 years if used for repeated treatment courses (see Tetracyclines, p 873). Alternative drugs are metronidazole and iodoquinol (see Drugs for Parasitic Infections, p 927). Successful use of nitazoxanide also has been reported.

ISOLATION OF THE HOSPITALIZED PATIENT: In addition to standard precautions, contact precautions are recommended, because human-to-human transmission can occur rarely.

CONTROL MEASURES: Control measures include sanitary disposal of human feces and avoidance of contamination of food and water with porcine feces. Travelers should avoid ingestion of potentially contaminated food or water. Despite chlorination of water, waterborne outbreaks of disease have occurred.

Baylisascaris Infections

CLINICAL MANIFESTATIONS: *Baylisascaris* worms are intestinal parasites found in a large number of animals. *Baylisascaris procyonis,* a raccoon roundworm, is a rare cause of acute eosinophilic meningoencephalitis. *Baylisacaris columnaris* is an intestinal parasite found in skunks. In a young child, acute central nervous system (CNS) disease (eg, altered mental status and seizures) accompanied by peripheral and/or cerebrospinal fluid (CSF) eosinophilia can occur 2 to 4 weeks after infection. Severe neurologic sequelae or death are usual outcomes. *B procyonis* also is a rare cause of extraneural disease in older children and adults. Ocular larva migrans can result in diffuse unilateral subacute neuroretinitis; direct visualization of worms in the retina sometimes is possible. Visceral larval migrans can present with nonspecific signs, such as macular rash, pneumonitis, and hepatomegaly. Similar to visceral larva migrans caused by *Toxocara*, subclinical or asymptomatic infection is thought to be the most common outcome of infection.

ETIOLOGY: *B procyonis* is a 10- to 25-cm long roundworm (nematode) with a direct life cycle usually limited to its definitive host, the raccoon. Domestic dogs and some exotic pets, such as kinkajous and ringtails, can serve as definitive hosts and a potential source of human disease.[1]

EPIDEMIOLOGY: *B procyonis* is distributed focally throughout the United States; in areas where disease is endemic, an estimated 22% to 80% of raccoons can harbor the parasite in their intestine. Reports of infections in dogs raise concern that infected dogs may be able to spread the disease. Embryonated eggs containing infective larvae are ingested from the soil by raccoons, rodents, and birds. When infective eggs or an infected host is eaten by a raccoon, the larvae grow to maturity in the small intestine, where adult female worms shed millions of eggs per day. Eggs become infective after 2 to 4 weeks in the environment and may persist long-term in the soil. Cases of raccoon infection have been reported throughout the United States. Risk is greatest in areas where significant raccoon populations live near humans. Fewer than 25 cases of *Baylisascaris* disease have been document-ment in the United States, although cases may be undiagnosed or underreported.

Risk factors for *Baylisascaris* infection include contact with raccoon latrines (bases of trees, unsealed attics, or flat surfaces such as logs, tree stumps, rocks, decks, and rooftops) and uncovered sand boxes, geophagia/pica, age younger than 4 years, and in older children, developmental delay. Nearly all reported cases have been in males.

DIAGNOSTIC TESTS: *Baylisascaris* infection is confirmed by identification of larvae in biopsy specimens. Serologic testing (serum, CSF) is available at the Centers for Disease Control and Prevention. A presumptive diagnosis can be made on the basis of clinical (meningoencephalitis, diffuse unilateral subacute neuroretinitis, pseudotumor), epidemiologic (raccoon exposure), and laboratory (blood and CSF eosinophilia) findings. Neuroimaging results can be normal initially, but as larvae grow and migrate through CNS tissue, focal abnormalities are found in periventricular white matter and elsewhere. In ocular disease, ophthalmologic examination can reveal characteristic chorioretinal lesions or rarely larvae. Because eggs are not shed in human feces, stool examination is not helpful. The disease is not transmitted from person to person.

TREATMENT: On the basis of CNS and CSF penetration and in vitro activity, alben-dazole, in conjunction with high-dose corticosteroids, has been advocated most widely. Treatment with anthelmintic agents and corticosteroids may not affect clinical outcome once severe CNS disease manifestations are evident. If the infection is suspected, treat-ment should be started while the diagnostic evaluation is being completed. Some experts advocate use of additional anthelmintic agents. Limited data are available regarding safety and efficacy of these therapies in children. Preventive therapy with albendazole

---

[1]Centers for Disease Control and Prevention. Raccoon roundworms in pet kinkajous—three states, 1999 and 2010. *MMWR Morb Mortal Wkly Rep.* 2011;60(10):302-305

should be considered for children with a history of ingestion of soil potentially contaminated with raccoon feces; however, no definitive preventive dosing regimen has been established. Worms localized to the retina may be killed by direct photocoagulation (see Drugs for Parasitic Infections, p 927).

ISOLATION OF THE HOSPITALIZED PATIENT: Standard precautions are recommended.

CONTROL MEASURES: *Baylisascaris* infections are prevented by avoiding ingestion of soil contaminated with stool of infected animal reservoirs, primarily raccoons; avoiding raccoon defecation sites, such as flat tree stumps and rocks; washing hands after contact with soil or with pets or other animals; discouraging raccoon presence by limiting access to human or pet food sources; and decontaminating raccoon latrines (especially if located near homes) by treating the area with boiling water or a propane torch, in keeping with local fire safety regulations, or through proper removal if located within the home (eg, attic).

Infections With *Blastocystis hominis* and Other Subtypes

CLINICAL MANIFESTATIONS: The importance of *Blastocystis* species as a cause of gastrointestinal tract disease is controversial. The asymptomatic carrier state is well documented. Clinical symptoms reported include bloating, flatulence, mild to moderate diarrhea without fecal leukocytes or blood, abdominal pain, nausea, and poor growth. When *Blastocystis hominis* is identified in stool from symptomatic patients, other causes of this symptom complex, particularly *Giardia intestinalis* and *Cryptosporidium parvum*, should be investigated before assuming that *B hominis* is the cause of the signs and symptoms. Polymerase chain reaction fingerprinting suggests that some *B hominis* organisms are disease associated but others are not.

ETIOLOGY: *B hominis* previously has been classified as a protozoan, but molecular studies have characterized it as a stramenopile (a eukaryote). Multiple forms have been described: vacuolar, which is observed most commonly in clinical specimens; granular; which is seen rarely in fresh stools; ameboid; and cystic.

EPIDEMIOLOGY: *Blastocystis* species are recovered from 1% to 20% of stool specimens examined for ova and parasites. Because transmission is believed to be via the fecal-oral route, presence of the organism may be a marker for presence of other pathogens spread by fecal contamination. Transmission from animals occurs.

The **incubation period** has not been established.

DIAGNOSTIC TESTS: Stool specimens should be preserved in polyvinyl alcohol and stained with trichrome or iron-hematoxylin before microscopic examination. The parasite may be present in varying numbers, and infections may be reported as light to heavy. The presence of 5 or more organisms per high-power (×400 magnification) field can indicate heavy infection with many organisms, which to some experts suggests causation when other enteropathogens are absent. Other experts consider the presence of 10 or more organisms per 10 oil immersion fields (×1000 magnification) to represent many organisms.

TREATMENT: Indications for treatment are not established. Some experts recommend that treatment should be reserved for patients who have persistent symptoms and in whom no other pathogen or process is found to explain the gastrointestinal tract symptoms. Randomized controlled treatment trials with both nitazoxanide and metronidazole have demonstrated benefit in symptomatic patients. Trimethoprim-sulfamethoxazole and iodoquinol have been used with limited success (see Drugs for Parasitic Infections, p 927). Notably, other experts believe that *B hominis* does not cause symptomatic disease and recommend only a careful search for other causes of symptoms.

ISOLATION OF THE HOSPITALIZED PATIENT: In addition to standard precautions, contact precautions are recommended for diapered or incontinent children.

CONTROL MEASURES: Personal hygiene measures, including hand washing with soap and warm water after using the toilet, after changing diapers, and before preparing food, should be practiced.

Blastomycosis

CLINICAL MANIFESTATIONS: Infections can be acute, chronic, or fulminant but are asymptomatic in up to 50% of infected people. The most common clinical manifestation of blastomycosis in children is prolonged pulmonary disease, with fever, chest pain, and nonspecific symptoms such as fatigue and myalgia. Rarely, patients may develop acute respiratory distress syndrome (ARDS). Typical radiographic patterns include patchy pneumonitis, a mass-like infiltrate, or nodules. Blastomycosis can be misdiagnosed as bacterial pneumonia, tuberculosis, sarcoidosis, or malignant neoplasm. Disseminated blastomycosis, which can occur in up to 25% of cases, most commonly involves the skin, osteoarticular structures, and the genitourinary tract. Cutaneous manifestations can be verrucous, nodular, ulcerative, or pustular. Abscesses usually are subcutaneous but can involve any organ. Central nervous system infection is less common, and intrauterine or congenital infection is rare.

ETIOLOGY: Blastomycosis is caused by *Blastomyces dermatitidis*, a thermally dimorphic fungus existing in the yeast form at 37°C (98°F) in infected tissues and in a mycelial form at room temperature and in soil. Conidia, produced from hyphae of the mycelial form, are infectious.

EPIDEMIOLOGY: Infection is acquired through inhalation of conidia from soil and can occur in both immunocompetent and immunocompromised hosts. Increased mortality rates for patients with pulmonary blastomycosis have been associated with advanced age, chronic obstructive pulmonary disease, cancer, and African American race. Person-to-person transmission does not occur. Blastomycosis is endemic in areas of the central United States, with most cases occurring in the Ohio and Mississippi river valleys, the southeastern states, and states that border the Great Lakes. Sporadic cases also have been reported in Hawaii, Israel, India, Africa, and Central and South America.

The **incubation period** ranges from 2 weeks to 3 months.

DIAGNOSTIC TESTS: Definitive diagnosis of blastomycosis is based on identification of characteristic thick-walled, broad-based, single budding yeast cells either by culture or in histopathologic specimens. The organism may be seen in sputum, tracheal aspirates, cerebrospinal fluid, urine, or histopathologic specimens from lesions processed with 10% potassium hydroxide or a silver stain. Children with pneumonia who are unable to produce sputum may require bronchoalveolar lavage or open biopsy to establish the diagnosis. Bronchoalveolar lavage is high yield, even in patients with bone or skin manifestations. Organisms can be cultured on brain-heart infusion media and Sabouraud dextrose agar at room temperature. Chemiluminescent DNA probes are available for identification of *B dermatitidis*. Because serologic tests (immunodiffusion and complement fixation) lack adequate sensitivity, effort should be made to obtain appropriate specimens for culture. An assay that detects *Blastomyces* antigen in urine is available commercially, but significant cross-reactivity occurs in patients with other endemic mycoses; clinical and epidemiologic considerations often aid with interpretation.

TREATMENT[1]: Because of the high risk of dissemination, some experts recommend that all cases of blastomycosis in children should be treated. Amphotericin B deoxycholate or lipid formulation is recommended for initial therapy of severe disease. Oral itraconazole is recommended for step-down therapy and for mild to moderate infection. Liposomal amphotericin B is recommended for central nervous system infection and may be followed by a prolonged course of azole therapy with fluconazole, voriconazole, or itraconazole (see Antifungal Drugs for Systemic Fungal Infections, p 905). Itraconazole is indicated for treatment of non–life-threatening infection outside of the central nervous system in adults and is recommended in children; however, the safety and efficacy of this agent in children with blastomycosis has not been established.[1] Serum trough concentrations of itraconazole should be ≥ 1 but <10 μg/mL. Concentrations should be checked after 2 weeks of therapy to ensure adequate drug levels.

Therapy for severe or central nervous system infections usually is continued for at least 12 months. Therapy for mild to moderate pulmonary and extrapulmonary disease usually involves at least 6 to 12 months of therapy. Some experts suggest 1 year of therapy for patients with osteomyelitis.

ISOLATION OF THE HOSPITALIZED PATIENT: Standard precautions are recommended.

CONTROL MEASURES: None.

Bocavirus

CLINICAL MANIFESTATIONS: Human bocavirus (HBoV) first was identified in 2005 from a cohort of children with acute respiratory tract symptoms. Cough, rhinorrhea, wheezing, and fever have been attributed to HBoV. HBoV has been identified in 5% to 33% of all children with acute respiratory tract infections in various settings (eg, inpatient facilities, outpatient facilities, child care centers). High rates of HBoV subclinical infections have also been documented in children of similar age, complicating etiologic association with disease. The role of HBoV as a pathogen in human infection is further confounded by simultaneous detection of other viral pathogens in patients from whom HBoV is identified, with coinfection rates as high as 80%. HBoV has been detected in stool samples from children with acute gastroenteritis; however, further studies are needed to better understand the role of HBoV in gastroenteritis. Infection with HBoV appears to be ubiquitous, because nearly all children develop serologic evidence of previous HBoV infection by 5 years of age.

ETIOLOGY: HBoV is a nonenveloped, single-stranded DNA virus classified in the family *Parvoviridae*, genus *Bocavirus*, on the basis of its genetic similarity to the closely related **bo**vine parvovirus 1 and **ca**nine minute virus, from which the name "**boca**virus" was derived. Four distinct genotypes have been described (HBoV types 1–4), although there are no data regarding antigenic variation or distinct serotypes. HBoV1 replicates primarily in the respiratory tract and has been associated with upper and lower respiratory tract

[1]Chapman SW, Dismukes WE, Proia LA, et al. Clinical guidelines for the management of blastomycosis: 2008 update by the Infectious Diseases Society of America. *Clin Infect Dis.* 2008;46(12):1801-1812

illness. HBoV2, HBoV3, and HBoV4 have been found predominantly in stool, without clear association with any clinical illness, except a few reports that associated HBoV2 with gastroenteritis.

EPIDEMIOLOGY: Detection of HBoV has been described only in humans. Transmission is presumed to be from respiratory tract secretions, although fecal-oral transmission may be possible on the basis of the finding of HBoV in stool specimens from children, including symptomatic children with diarrhea.

The frequent codetection of other viral pathogens of the respiratory tract in association with HBoV has led to speculation about the role played by HBoV; it may be a true copathogen, it may be shed for long periods after primary infection, or it may reactivate during subsequent viral infections. Extended and intermittent shedding of HBoV has been reported for up to 75 days after initial detection.

HBoV circulates worldwide and throughout the year. In temperate climates, seasonal clustering in the spring associated with increased transmission of other respiratory tract viruses has been reported.

DIAGNOSTIC TESTS: Commercial molecular diagnostic assays for HBoV are available. HBoV polymerase chain reaction and detection of HBoV-specific antibody also are used by research laboratories to detect the presence of virus and infection, respectively.

TREATMENT: No specific therapy is available.

ISOLATION OF THE HOSPITALIZED PATIENT: The presence of virus in respiratory tract secretions and stool suggests that, in addition to standard precautions, contact precautions should be effective in limiting the spread of infection for the duration of the symptomatic illness in infants and young children. Prolonged shedding of virus in respiratory tract secretions and in stool may occur after resolution of symptoms, particularly in immune-compromised hosts and therefore the duration of contact precautions should be extended in these situations.

CONTROL MEASURES: Appropriate respiratory hygiene and cough etiquette should be followed. Although possible health care-associated transmission of HBoV has been described, investigations of transmissibility of HBoV in the community or health care settings have not been published. Appropriate hand hygiene, particularly when handling respiratory tract secretions or diapers of ill children, is recommended. The presence of HBoV in serum also raises the possibility of transmission by transfusion, although this mode of transmission has not been documented.

Borrelia Infections
(Relapsing Fever)

CLINICAL MANIFESTATIONS: Two types of relapsing fever occur in humans: tickborne and louseborne. Both are characterized by sudden onset of high fever, shaking chills, sweats, headache, muscle and joint pain, altered sensorium, nausea, and diarrhea. A fleeting macular rash of the trunk and petechiae of the skin and mucous membranes sometimes occur. Findings and complications can differ between types of relapsing fever and include hepatosplenomegaly, jaundice, thrombocytopenia, iridocyclitis, cough with pleuritic pain, pneumonitis, meningitis, and myocarditis. Mortality rates can exceed 30% in untreated louseborne relapsing fever (possibly related to comorbidities in refugee-type settings where this disease typically is found) and 4% to 10% in untreated tickborne relapsing fever. Death occurs predominantly in people with underlying illnesses, infants, and elderly people. Early treatment reduces mortality to less than 5%. Untreated, an initial febrile period of 2 to 7 days terminates spontaneously by crisis. The initial febrile episode is followed by an afebrile period of several days to weeks, then by one relapse or more (0–13 for tickborne, 1–5 for louseborne). Relapses typically become shorter and progressively milder, as afebrile periods lengthen. Relapse is associated with expression of new borrelial antigens, and resolution of symptoms is associated with production of antibody specific to those new antigenic determinants. Infection during pregnancy often is severe and can result in spontaneous abortion, preterm birth, stillbirth, or neonatal infection.

ETIOLOGY: Relapsing fever is caused by certain spirochetes of the genus *Borrelia*. Worldwide, at least 14 *Borrelia* species cause tickborne (endemic) relapsing fever, including *Borrelia hermsii*, *Borrelia turicatae*, and *Borrelia parkeri* in North America. *Borrelia recurrentis* is the only species that causes louseborne (epidemic) relapsing fever and has no animal reservoir.

EPIDEMIOLOGY: Endemic tickborne relapsing fever is distributed widely throughout the world, is transmitted by soft-bodied ticks (*Ornithodoros* species), and occurs sporadically and in small clusters, often within families or cohabiting groups. In the United States, tickborne relapsing fever can be acquired only in western states but has been diagnosed in other states in travelers returning from these areas. Ticks become infected by feeding on rodents or other small mammals and transmit infection via their saliva and other fluids when they take subsequent blood meals. Ticks may serve as reservoirs of infection as a result of transovarial and trans-stadial transmission. Soft-bodied ticks inflict painless bites and feed briefly (15-90 minutes), usually at night, so people often are unaware of bites.

Most tickborne relapsing fever in the United States is caused by *B hermsii*. Infection typically results from tick exposures in rodent-infested cabins in western mountainous areas, including state and national parks. However, infection also has occurred in primary residences and luxurious rental properties. *B turicatae* infections occur less frequently; most cases have been reported from Texas and often are associated with tick exposures in rodent-infested caves. A single human infection has been reported with *B parkeri*; the tick infected with this *Borrelia* species is associated with arid areas or grasslands in the western United States.

Louseborne epidemic relapsing fever has been reported in Ethiopia, Eritrea, Somalia, and the Sudan, especially in refugee and displaced populations. Epidemic transmission occurs when body lice *(Pediculus humanus)* become infected by feeding on humans with spirochetemia; infection is transmitted when infected lice are crushed and their body fluids contaminate a bite wound or skin abraded by scratching.

Infected body lice and ticks may remain alive and infectious for several years without feeding. Relapsing fever is not transmitted between individual humans, but perinatal transmission from an infected mother to her infant does occur and can result in preterm birth, stillbirth, and neonatal death.

The **incubation period** is 2 to 18 days, with a mean of 7 days.

DIAGNOSTIC TESTS: Spirochetes can be observed by dark-field microscopy and in Wright-, Giemsa-, or acridine orange-stained preparations of thin or dehemoglobinized thick smears of peripheral blood or in stained buffy-coat preparations. Organisms often can be visualized in blood obtained while the person is febrile, particularly during initial febrile episodes; organisms are less likely to be recovered from subsequent relapses. Spirochetes can be cultured from blood in Barbour-Stoenner-Kelly medium or by intraperitoneal inoculation of immature laboratory mice, although these tests are not widely available. Serum antibodies to *Borrelia* species can be detected by enzyme immunoassay and Western immunoblot analysis at some reference and commercial specialty laboratories; a fourfold increase in titer is considered confirmatory. These antibody tests are not standardized and are affected by antigenic variations among and within *Borrelia* species and strains. Serologic cross-reactions occur with other spirochetes, including *Borrelia burgdorferi, Treponema pallidum,* and *Leptospira* species. Biological specimens for laboratory testing can be sent to the Division of Vector-Borne Diseases, Centers for Disease Control and Prevention, 3156 Rampart Rd, Fort Collins, CO 80521 (telephone: 970-221-6400).

TREATMENT: Treatment of tickborne relapsing fever with a 5- to 10-day course of one of the tetracyclines, usually doxycycline, produces prompt clearance of spirochetes and remission of symptoms. Tetracycline-based antimicrobial agents, including doxycycline, may cause permanent tooth discoloration for children younger than 8 years if used for repeated treatment courses. However, doxycycline binds less readily to calcium compared with older tetracyclines, and in some studies, doxycycline was not associated with visible teeth staining in younger children (see Tetracyclines, p 873). For children younger than 8 years and for pregnant women, penicillin and erythromycin are the preferred drugs. Penicillin G procaine or intravenous penicillin G is recommended as initial therapy for people who are unable to take oral therapy, although low-dose penicillin G has been associated with a higher frequency of relapse. A Jarisch-Herxheimer reaction (an acute febrile reaction accompanied by headache, myalgia, respiratory distress in some cases, and an aggravated clinical picture lasting less than 24 hours) commonly is observed during the first few hours after initiating antimicrobial therapy. Because this reaction sometimes is associated with transient hypotension attributable to decreased effective circulating blood volume (especially in louseborne relapsing fever), patients should be hospitalized and monitored closely, particularly during the first 4 hours of treatment. However, the Jarisch-Herxheimer reaction in children typically is mild and usually can be managed with antipyretic agents alone.

Single-dose treatment using a tetracycline, penicillin, erythromycin, or chloramphenicol is effective for curing louseborne relapsing fever.

ISOLATION OF THE HOSPITALIZED PATIENT: Standard precautions are recommended. If louse infestation is present, contact precautions also are indicated until delousing (see Pediculosis, p 597–603).

CONTROL MEASURES: Soft ticks often can be found in rodent nests; exposure is reduced most effectively by preventing rodent infestations of homes or cabins by blocking rodent access to foundations and attics and other forms of rodent control. Dwellings infested with soft ticks should be rodent-proofed and treated professionally with chemical agents. When in a louse-infested environment, body lice can be controlled by bathing, washing clothing at frequent intervals, and use of pediculicides (see Pediculosis, p 597–603). Reporting of suspected cases of relapsing fever to health authorities is required in most western states and is important for initiation of prompt investigation and institution of control measures.

Brucellosis

CLINICAL MANIFESTATIONS: Onset of brucellosis in children can be acute or insidious. Manifestations are nonspecific and include fever, night sweats, weakness, malaise, anorexia, weight loss, arthralgia, myalgia, abdominal pain, and headache. Physical findings may include lymphadenopathy, hepatosplenomegaly, and arthritis. Abdominal pain and peripheral arthritis are reported more frequently in children than in adults. Neurologic deficits, ocular involvement, epididymo-orchitis, and liver or spleen abscesses are reported. Anemia, leukopenia, thrombocytopenia or, less frequently, pancytopenia are hematologic findings that might suggest the diagnosis. Serious complications include meningitis, endocarditis, and osteomyelitis and, less frequently, pneumonitis and aortic involvement. A detailed history including travel, exposure to animals and food habits, including ingestion of raw milk, should be obtained if brucellosis is considered. Chronic disease is less common among children than among adults, although the rate of relapse has been found to be similar. Brucellosis in pregnancy is associated with risk of spontaneous abortion, preterm delivery, miscarriage, and intrauterine infection with fetal death.

ETIOLOGY: *Brucella* bacteria are small, nonmotile, gram-negative coccobacilli. The species that are known to infect humans are *Brucella abortus, Brucella melitensis, Brucella suis,* and rarely, *Brucella canis.* Three recently identified species, *Brucella ceti, Brucella pinnipedialis,* and *Brucella inopinata,* are potential human pathogens.

EPIDEMIOLOGY: Brucellosis is a zoonotic disease of wild and domestic animals. It is transmissible to humans by direct or indirect exposure to aborted fetuses or tissues or fluids of infected animals. Transmission occurs by inoculation through mucous membranes or cuts and abrasions in the skin, inhalation of contaminated aerosols, or ingestion of undercooked meat or unpasteurized dairy products.[1] People in occupations such as farming, ranching, and veterinary medicine, as well as abattoir workers, meat inspectors, and laboratory personnel, are at increased risk. Clinicians should alert the laboratory if they anticipate *Brucella* might grow from microbiologic specimens so that appropriate laboratory precautions can be taken. In the United States, approximately 100 to 200 cases of brucellosis are reported annually, and 3% to 10% of cases occur in people younger than 19 years. The majority of pediatric cases reported in the United States result from ingestion of unpasteurized dairy products. Although human-to-human transmission is rare, in utero transmission has been reported, and infected mothers can transmit *Brucella* to their infants through breastfeeding.

The **incubation period** varies from less than 1 week to several months, but most people become ill within 3 to 4 weeks of exposure.

DIAGNOSTIC TESTS: A definitive diagnosis is established by recovery of *Brucella* species from blood, bone marrow, or other tissue specimens. A variety of media will support growth of *Brucella* species, but the physician should contact laboratory personnel and ask them to incubate cultures for a minimum of 4 weeks. Newer BACTEC systems have greater reliability and can detect *Brucella* species within 5 to 7 days. In patients with a clinically compatible illness, serologic testing using the serum agglutination test can confirm the diagnosis with a fourfold or greater increase in antibody titers between acute

---

[1] American Academy of Pediatrics, Committee on Infectious Diseases, Committee on Nutrition. Consumption of raw or unpasteurized milk and milk products by pregnant women and children. *Pediatrics.* 2014;133(1):175-179

and convalescent serum specimens collected at least 2 weeks apart. The serum agglutination test, the gold standard test for serologic diagnosis, will detect antibodies against *B abortus*, *B suis*, and *B melitensis* but not *B canis*, which requires use of *B canis*-specific antigen. Although a single titer is not diagnostic, most patients with active infection in an area without endemic infection will have a titer of 1:160 or greater within 2 to 4 weeks of clinical disease onset. Lower titers may be found early in the course of infection. Immunoglobulin (Ig) M antibodies are produced within the first week, followed by a gradual increase in IgG synthesis. Low IgM titers may persist for months or years after initial infection. Increased concentrations of IgG agglutinins are found in acute infection, chronic infection, and relapse. When interpreting serum agglutination test results, the possibility of cross-reactions of *Brucella* antibodies with antibodies against other gram-negative bacteria, such as *Yersinia enterocolitica* serotype 09, *Francisella tularensis*, and *Vibrio cholerae*, should be considered. Enzyme immunoassay is a sensitive method for determining IgG, IgA, and IgM anti-*Brucella* antibody titers. Until better standardization is established, enzyme immunoassay should be used only for suspected cases with negative serum agglutination test results or for evaluation of patients with suspected chronic brucellosis, reinfection, or complicated cases. Polymerase chain reaction tests have been developed but are not available in most clinical laboratories. If a laboratory is not available to perform diagnostic testing for *Brucella*, physician should contact the state health department for assistance.

TREATMENT: Prolonged antimicrobial therapy is imperative for achieving a cure. Relapses generally are not associated with development of *Brucella* resistance but rather with premature discontinuation of therapy. Because monotherapy is associated with a high rate of relapse, combination therapy is recommended as standard treatment. Most combination regimens include oral doxycycline or trimethoprim-sulfamethoxazole plus rifampin.

Oral doxycycline (2–4 mg/kg per day, maximum 200 mg/day, in 2 divided doses) or, alternatively, oral tetracycline (30–40 mg/kg per day, maximum 2 g/day, in 4 divided doses) is the drug of choice and should be administered for a minimum of 6 weeks in children older than 8 years. However, because of the longer duration of therapy, tetracyclines, including doxycycline, should be avoided, if possible, in children younger than 8 years (see Tetracyclines, p 873). Oral trimethoprim-sulfamethoxazole (trimethoprim, 10 mg/kg per day, maximum 480 mg/day; and sulfamethoxazole, 50 mg/kg per day, maximum 2.4 g/day), divided in 2 doses for at least 4 to 6 weeks, is appropriate therapy for younger children.

In combination therapy regimens, rifampin (15–20 mg/kg per day, maximum 600–900 mg/day, in 1 or 2 divided doses) should be added to doxycycline (or trimethoprim-sulfamethoxazole). Because of the potential emergence of rifampin resistance, rifampin monotherapy is not recommended. Failure to complete the full 6-week course of therapy may result in relapse.

For treatment of serious infections or complications, including endocarditis, meningitis, spondylitis, and osteomyelitis, a 3-drug regimen should be used with gentamicin included for the first 7 to 14 days of therapy, in addition to tetracycline (or trimethoprim-sulfamethoxazole, if tetracyclines are not used) and rifampin for a minimum of 6 weeks. For life-threatening complications of brucellosis, such as meningitis or endocarditis, the duration of therapy often is extended for 4 to 6 months. Surgical intervention should be considered in patients with complications, such as deep tissue abscesses, endocarditis, mycotic aneurysm, and foreign body infections.

The benefit of corticosteroids for people with neurobrucellosis is unproven. Occasionally, a Jarisch-Herxheimer-like reaction (an acute febrile reaction accompanied by headache, myalgia, and an aggravated clinical picture lasting less than 24 hours) occurs shortly after initiation of antimicrobial therapy, but this reaction rarely is severe enough to require corticosteroids.

ISOLATION OF THE HOSPITALIZED PATIENT: In addition to standard precautions, contact precautions are indicated for patients with draining wounds.

CONTROL MEASURES: The control of human brucellosis depends on eradication of *Brucella* species from cattle, goats, swine, and other animals. Contact with infected animals should be avoided, especially female animals that have aborted or are giving birth. Pasteurization of dairy products for human consumption is important to prevent disease, especially in children.[1] The certification of raw milk does not eliminate the risk of transmission of *Brucella* organisms.

Burkholderia Infections

CLINICAL MANIFESTATIONS: *Burkholderia cepacia* complex has been associated with infections in individuals with cystic fibrosis, chronic granulomatous disease, hemoglobinopathies, or malignant neoplasms and in preterm infants. Airway infections in people with cystic fibrosis usually occur later in the course of disease, after respiratory epithelial damage and bronchiectasis has occurred. Cystic fibrosis patients can become chronically infected with no change in the rate of pulmonary decompensation or can experience an accelerated decline in pulmonary function or an unexpectedly rapid deterioration in clinical status that results in death. In patients with chronic granulomatous disease, pneumonia is the most common manifestation of *B cepacia* complex infection; lymphadenitis also occurs. Disease onset is insidious, with low-grade fever early in the course and systemic effects occurring 3 to 4 weeks later. Pleural effusions are common, and lung abscesses can occur. Health care-associated infections including wound and urinary tract infections and pneumonia also have been reported, and clusters of disease have been associated with contaminated nasal sprays, mouthwash, and sublingual probes.

Burkholderia pseudomallei is the cause of melioidosis. Its geographic range is expanding, and disease now is known to be endemic in Southeast Asia, northern Australia, areas of the Indian Subcontinent, southern China, Hong Kong, Taiwan, several Pacific and Indian Ocean Islands, and some areas of South and Central America. Melioidosis can occur in the United States, usually among travelers returning from areas with endemic disease. Melioidosis can be asymptomatic or can manifest as a localized infection or as fulminant septicemia. More than half of individuals with melioidosis are bacteremic at presentation. Pneumonia is the most commonly reported clinical manifestation of melioidosis. Genitourinary infections including prostatic abscesses, skin infections, septic arthritis and osteomyelitis, and central nervous system involvement including brain abscesses also are frequently identified. Acute suppurative parotitis is a manifestation that occurs frequently in children in Thailand and Cambodia but is less commonly seen in other endemic areas. Localized infection usually is nonfatal. In severe cutaneous infection,

---

[1] American Academy of Pediatrics, Committee on Infectious Diseases, Committee on Nutrition. Consumption of raw or unpasteurized milk and milk products by pregnant women and children. *Pediatrics.* 2014;133(1):175-179

necrotizing fasciitis has been reported. In disseminated infection, hepatic and splenic abscesses can occur, and relapses are common without prolonged therapy.

ETIOLOGY: The *Burkholderia* genus comprises more than 40 species that are nutritionally diverse, oxidase- and catalase-producing, non–lactose-fermenting, gram-negative bacilli. *B cepacia* complex comprises at least 17 species. Additional members of the complex continue to be identified but are rare human pathogens. Other clinically important species of *Burkholderia* include *Burkholderia pseudomallei, Burkholderia gladioli,* and *Burkholderia mallei* (the agent responsible for glanders). *Burkholderia thailandensis* and *Burkholderia oklahomensis* are rare human pathogens.

EPIDEMIOLOGY: *Burkholderia* species are environmentally derived waterborne and soilborne organisms that can survive for prolonged periods in a moist environment. Depending on the species, transmission may occur from other people (person to person), from contact with contaminated fomites, and from exposure to environmental sources. Epidemiologic studies of recreational camps and social events attended by people with cystic fibrosis from different geographic areas have documented person-to-person spread of *B cepacia* complex. The source of acquisition of *B cepacia* complex by patients with chronic granulomatous disease has not been identified. Health care-associated spread of *B cepacia* complex most often is associated with contamination of disinfectant solutions used to clean reusable patient equipment, such as bronchoscopes and pressure transducers, or to disinfect skin. Contaminated medical products, including mouthwash and inhaled medications, have been identified as a cause of multistate outbreaks of colonization and infection. *B gladioli* has been isolated from sputum of people with cystic fibrosis and may be mistaken for *B cepacia*. The clinical significance of *B gladioli* in cystic fibrosis is not known.

In areas with highly endemic infection, *B pseudomallei* is acquired early in life, with the highest seroconversion rates between 6 and 42 months of age. Melioidosis is seasonal, with more than 75% of cases occurring during the rainy season. Disease can be acquired by direct inhalation of aerosolized organisms or dust particles containing organisms, by percutaneous or wound inoculation with contaminated soil or water, or by ingestion of contaminated soil, water, or food. People also can become infected as a result of laboratory exposures when proper techniques and/or proper personal protective equipment guidelines are not followed. Symptomatic infection can occur in children 1 year or younger, with pneumonia and parotitis reported in infants as young as 8 months; in addition, 2 cases of human milk transmission from mothers with mastitis have been reported. Risk factors for melioidosis include frequent contact with soil and water as well as underlying chronic disease, such as diabetes mellitus, renal insufficiency, chronic pulmonary disease, thalassemia, and immunosuppression not related to human immunodeficiency virus (HIV) infection. *B pseudomallei* also has been reported to cause pulmonary infection in people with cystic fibrosis and septicemia in children with chronic granulomatous disease.

The **incubation period** for melioidosis is 1 to 21 days, with a median of 9 days, but can be prolonged (years).

DIAGNOSTIC TESTS: Culture is the appropriate method to diagnose *B cepacia* complex infection. In cystic fibrosis airway infection, culture of sputum on selective agar is recommended to decrease the potential for overgrowth by mucoid *Pseudomonas aeruginosa*. Confirmation of identification of *B cepacia* complex species by polymerase chain reaction assay or mass spectroscopy is recommended. Definitive diagnosis of melioidosis is made by isolation of *B pseudomallei* from blood or other infected sites. The likelihood of successfully isolating the organism is increased by culture of sputum, throat, rectum, and ulcer or skin lesion specimens. A direct polymerase chain reaction assay may provide a more rapid result than culture but is less sensitive, especially when performed on blood, and is not recommended for routine use as a diagnostic assay. Serologic testing is not adequate for diagnosis in endemic areas because of high background seropositivity. However, a positive result by the indirect hemagglutination assay for a traveler who has returned from an area with endemic infection may support the diagnosis of melioidosis; definitive diagnosis still requires isolation of *B pseudomallei* from an infected site. Other rapid assays are being developed for diagnosis of melioidosis but are not yet commercially available.

TREATMENT: Meropenem is the agent most active against the majority of *B cepacia* complex isolates, although other drugs that may be effective include imipenem, trimethoprim-sulfamethoxazole, ceftazidime, doxycycline, and chloramphenicol. Some experts recommend combinations of antimicrobial agents that provide synergistic activity against *B cepacia* complex. The majority of *B cepacia* complex isolates are intrinsically resistant to aminoglycosides and polymyxins.

The drugs of choice for initial treatment of melioidosis depend on the type of clinical infection, susceptibility testing, and presence of comorbidities in the patient (eg, diabetes, liver or renal disease, cancer, hemoglobinopathies, cystic fibrosis). Treatment of severe invasive infection should include meropenem, imipenem, or ceftazidime (rare resistance) for a minimum of 10 to 14 days. After acute therapy is completed, oral eradication therapy with trimethoprim-sulfamethoxazole for 3 to 6 months is recommended to reduce recurrence. Amoxicillin clavulanate and doxycycline are considered second-line oral agents and may be associated with a higher rate of relapse.

ISOLATION OF THE HOSPITALIZED PATIENT: In addition to standard precautions, contact and droplet precautions are recommended for cystic fibrosis patients infected with *B cepacia* complex and in other patients infected with multidrug-resistant strains. Human-to-human transmission is extremely rare for *B pseudomallei*, and standard precautions are recommended.

CONTROL MEASURES: Because some strains (sometimes called genomovars) of *B cepacia* complex are highly transmissible and virulence is not well understood, the Cystic Fibrosis Foundation (CFF) mandates that all cystic fibrosis care centers limit contact between *B cepacia* complex-infected and -uninfected patients with cystic fibrosis. This includes inpatient, outpatient, and social settings. For example, patients with cystic fibrosis who are infected with *B cepacia* complex sometimes are seen during different clinic hours than those who are not. Hospitalized patients colonized with *B cepacia* should wear a mask if they leave their room for medical needs. Education of patients and families about hand hygiene and appropriate personal hygiene is recommended.

Prevention of infection with *B pseudomallei* in areas with endemic disease can be difficult, because contact with contaminated water and soil is common. People with diabetes mellitus, renal insufficiency, or skin lesions should avoid contact with soil and standing water in these areas, and it is recommended that they stay inside during weather that could result in aerosolization of the organism. Wearing boots and gloves during agricultural work in areas with endemic disease is recommended. Cystic fibrosis patients should be educated regarding their risk for infection when traveling to regions where *B pseudomallei* is endemic. A human vaccine is not available, but research is ongoing.

Campylobacter Infections

CLINICAL MANIFESTATIONS: Predominant symptoms of *Campylobacter* infections include diarrhea, abdominal pain, malaise, and fever. Stools can contain visible or occult blood. In neonates and young infants, bloody diarrhea without fever can be the only manifestation of infection. Pronounced fevers in children can result in febrile seizures that can occur before gastrointestinal tract symptoms. Abdominal pain can mimic that produced by appendicitis or intussusception. Mild infection lasts 1 or 2 days and resembles viral gastroenteritis. Most patients recover in less than 1 week, but 10% to 20% have a relapse or a prolonged or severe illness. Severe or persistent infection can mimic acute inflammatory bowel disease. Bacteremia is uncommon but can occur in elderly patients and in patients with underlying conditions. Immunocompromised hosts can have prolonged, relapsing, or extraintestinal infections, especially with *Campylobacter fetus* and other *Campylobacter* species. Immunoreactive complications, such as acute idiopathic polyneuritis (Guillain-Barré syndrome) (occurring in 1:1000), Miller Fisher variant of Guillain-Barré syndrome (ophthalmoplegia, areflexia, ataxia), reactive arthritis, Reiter syndrome (arthritis, urethritis, and bilateral conjunctivitis), myocarditis, pericarditis, and erythema nodosum, can occur during convalescence.

ETIOLOGY: *Campylobacter* species are motile, comma-shaped, gram-negative bacilli that cause gastroenteritis. There are 25 species within the genus *Campylobacter*, but *Campylobacter jejuni* and *Campylobacter coli* are the species isolated most commonly from patients with diarrhea. *C fetus* predominantly causes systemic illness in neonates and debilitated hosts. Other *Campylobacter* species, including *Campylobacter upsaliensis, Campylobacter lari,* and *Campylobacter hyointestinalis,* can cause similar diarrheal or systemic illnesses in children.

EPIDEMIOLOGY: Data from the Foodborne Diseases Active Surveillance Network (**www.cdc.gov/foodnet**) indicate that, although incidence decreased in the early 2000s, the 2012 incidence of culture-confirmed cases of 14.3 per 100 000 population represented a 14% increase over a 2006-2008 baseline. Disease incidence has remained stable since 2010-2012, with 13.8 cases per 100 000 population in 2013.[1] The highest rates of infection occur in children younger than 5 years (24.08 per 100 000 in 2009). The majority of *Campylobacter* infections are acquired domestically, but it is also the most common cause of laboratory-confirmed diarrhea in returning international travelers. In susceptible people, as few as 500 *Campylobacter* organisms can cause infection.

The gastrointestinal tracts of domestic and wild birds and animals are reservoirs of the bacteria. *C jejuni* and *C coli* have been isolated from feces of 30% to 100% of healthy chickens, turkeys, and water fowl. Poultry carcasses commonly are contaminated. Many farm animals, pets, and meat sources can harbor the organism and are potential sources of infection. Transmission of *C jejuni* and *C coli* occurs by ingestion of contaminated food or water or by direct contact with fecal material from infected animals or people. Improperly cooked poultry, untreated water, and unpasteurized milk have been the main vehicles of transmission. *Campylobacter* infections usually are sporadic; outbreaks are rare but have occurred among school children who drank unpasteurized milk,[2] including

---

[1]Centers for Disease Control and Prevention. Incidence and trends of infection with pathogens transmitted commonly through food—Foodborne Diseases Active Surveillance Network, 10 U.S. Sites, 2006–2013. *MMWR Morb Mortal Wkly Rep.* 2014;63(15):328-332

[2]American Academy of Pediatrics, Committee on Infectious Diseases and Committee on Nutrition. Consumption of raw or unpasteurized milk and milk products by pregnant women and children. *Pediatrics.* 2014;133(1):175-179

children who participated in field trips to dairy farms. Person-to-person spread occurs occasionally, particularly among very young children, and risk is greatest during the acute phase of illness. Uncommonly, outbreaks of diarrhea in child care centers have been reported. Person-to-person transmission also has occurred in neonates of infected mothers and has resulted in health care-associated outbreaks in nurseries. In perinatal infection, *C jejuni* and *C coli* usually cause neonatal gastroenteritis, whereas *C fetus* often causes neonatal septicemia or meningitis. Enteritis occurs in people of all ages. Excretion of *Campylobacter* organisms typically lasts 2 to 3 weeks without treatment and can be as long as 7 weeks.

The **incubation period** usually is 2 to 5 days but can be longer.

DIAGNOSTIC TESTS: *C jejuni* and *C coli* can be cultured from feces, and *Campylobacter* species, including *C fetus*, can be cultured from blood. Isolation of *C jejuni* and *C coli* from stool specimens requires selective media, microaerobic conditions, and an incubation temperature of 42°C. Although other *Campylobacter* species occasionally are isolated using routine culture methods, additional methods that use nonselective isolation techniques and increased hydrogen microaerobic conditions usually are required for isolation of species other than *C jejuni* and *C coli*. *C upsaliensis*, *C hyointestinalis*, *C lara*, and *C fetus* may not be isolated because of susceptibility to antimicrobial agents present in the *Campylobacter* selective media used routinely to isolate *C jejuni* and *C coli*. Direct-examination, culture-independent methods also are available, in addition to culture, but all have the major drawback of not providing an opportunity to determine antibiotic susceptibilities for the infecting organism. The presence of motile curved, spiral, or S-shaped rods resembling *Vibrio cholerae* by stool phase contrast or darkfield microscopy can provide rapid, presumptive evidence for *Campylobacter* species infection directly from fresh stool samples. However, this is less sensitive than culture, requires significant microscopic expertise, and is not performed routinely. *C jejuni* and *C coli* can be detected directly (but not differentiated) by commercially available enzyme immunoassays. These immunologic assays provide rapid diagnosis of enteric infection with *C jejuni* and *C coli* but have variable performance. False-positive results from these non-culture-based techniques have been reported, and given that *Campylobacter* infection is a low-incidence disease, raise concern regarding the specificity of these tests. Two multiplex nucleic acid amplification tests (NAATs) that detect *Campylobacter* species and other gastrointestinal pathogens, including *Salmonella*, *Shigella*, *Campylobacter*, and Shiga toxin-producing *Escherichia coli*, recently became available commercially. Limited data on their performance characteristics are available at this time. For serious infection, isolation of the organism is preferred to confirm diagnosis, and the patient samples should be retained for antimicrobial susceptibility testing.

TREATMENT: Rehydration is the mainstay of treatment for all children with diarrhea. Azithromycin and erythromycin shorten the duration of illness and excretion of susceptible organisms and prevent relapse when given early in gastrointestinal tract infection. Treatment with azithromycin (10 mg/kg/day, for 3 days) or erythromycin (40 mg/kg/day, in 4 divided doses, for 5 days) usually eradicates the organism from stool within 2 or 3 days. A fluoroquinolone, such as ciprofloxacin, may be effective, but resistance to ciprofloxacin is common (31% of *C coli* isolates and 22% of *C jejuni* isolates in the United States in 2010 **[www.cdc.gov/NARMS]**), and fluoroquinolones are not approved for this indication by the US Food and Drug Administration for people younger than 18 years (see Fluoroquinolones, p 872). If antimicrobial therapy is given for treatment of gastroenteritis, the recommended duration is 3 to 5 days. Antimicrobial agents for bacteremia should be selected on the basis of antimicrobial susceptibility tests. *C fetus* generally is susceptible to aminoglycosides, extended-spectrum cephalosporins, meropenem, imipenem, ampicillin, and erythromycin. Antimotility agents should not be used, because they have been shown to prolong symptomatology and may be associated with an increased risk of death.

ISOLATION OF THE HOSPITALIZED PATIENT: In addition to standard precautions, contact precautions are recommended for diapered and incontinent children for the duration of illness.

CONTROL MEASURES:
- Hand hygiene should be performed after handling raw poultry, cutting boards and utensils should be washed with soap and water after contact with raw poultry, and contact of fruits and vegetables with juices of raw poultry should be avoided.
- Poultry should be cooked thoroughly.
- Hand hygiene should be performed after contact with feces of dogs and cats, particularly stool of puppies and kittens with diarrhea.
- People should not drink raw milk.
- Chlorination of water supplies is important.
- People with diarrhea should be excluded from food handling, care of patients in hospitals, and care of people in custodial care and child care centers.
- Infected food handlers and hospital employees who are asymptomatic need not be excluded from work if proper personal hygiene measures, including hand hygiene, are maintained.
- Outbreaks are uncommon in child care centers. General measures for interrupting enteric transmission in child care centers are recommended (see Children in Out-of-Home Child Care, p 132). Infants and children in diapers who have symptomatic infection should be excluded from child care or cared for in a separate area until diarrhea has subsided. Azithromycin or erythromycin treatment may further limit the potential for transmission.
- Stool cultures of asymptomatic exposed children are not recommended.

Candidiasis

CLINICAL MANIFESTATIONS: Mucocutaneous infection results in oral-pharyngeal (thrush) or vaginal or cervical candidiasis; intertriginous lesions of the gluteal folds, buttocks, neck, groin, and axilla; paronychia; and onychia. Dysfunction of T lymphocytes, other immunologic disorders, and endocrinologic diseases are associated with chronic mucocutaneous candidiasis. Chronic or recurrent oral candidiasis can be the presenting sign of human immunodeficiency virus (HIV) infection or primary immunodeficiency. Esophageal and laryngeal candidiasis can occur in immunocompromised patients. Disseminated or invasive candidiasis occurs in very low birth weight neonates, and in immunocompromised or debilitated hosts can involve virtually any organ or anatomic site and can be rapidly fatal. Candidemia can occur with or without systemic disease in patients with indwelling central vascular catheters, especially patients receiving prolonged intravenous infusions with parenteral alimentation or lipids. Peritonitis can occur in patients undergoing peritoneal dialysis, especially in patients receiving prolonged broad-spectrum antimicrobial therapy. Candiduria can occur in patients with indwelling urinary catheters, focal renal infection, or disseminated disease.

ETIOLOGY: *Candida* species are yeasts that reproduce by budding. *Candida albicans* and several other species form long chains of elongated yeast forms called pseudohyphae. *C albicans* causes most infections, but in some regions and patient populations the non-albicans *Candida* species now account for more than half of invasive infections. Other species, including *Candida tropicalis, Candida parapsilosis, Candida glabrata, Candida krusei, Candida guilliermondii, Candida lusitaniae,* and *Candida dubliniensis,* also can cause serious infections, especially in immunocompromised and debilitated hosts. *C parapsilosis* is second only to *C albicans* as a cause of systemic candidiasis in very low birth weight neonates.

EPIDEMIOLOGY: Like other *Candida* species, *C albicans* is present on skin and in the mouth, intestinal tract, and vagina of immunocompetent people. Vulvovaginal candidiasis is associated with pregnancy, and newborn infants can acquire the organism in utero, during passage through the vagina, or postnatally. Mild mucocutaneous infection is common in healthy infants. Person-to-person transmission occurs rarely. Invasive disease typically occurs in people with impaired immunity, with infection usually arising endogenously from colonized sites. Factors such as extreme prematurity, neutropenia, or treatment with corticosteroids or cytotoxic chemotherapy increases the risk of invasive infection. People with diabetes mellitus generally have localized mucocutaneous lesions. In clinical studies, 5% to 20% of newborn infants weighing less than 1000 g at birth develop invasive candidiasis. Patients with neutrophil defects, such as chronic granulomatous disease or myeloperoxidase deficiency, also are at increased risk. Patients undergoing intravenous alimentation or receiving broad-spectrum antimicrobial agents, especially extended-spectrum cephalosporins, carbapenems, and vancomycin, or requiring long-term indwelling central venous or peritoneal dialysis catheters have increased susceptibility to infection. Postsurgical patients can be at risk, particularly after cardiothoracic or abdominal procedures.

The **incubation period** is unknown.

DIAGNOSTIC TESTS: The presumptive diagnosis of mucocutaneous candidiasis or thrush usually can be made clinically, but other organisms or trauma also can cause clinically similar lesions. Yeast cells and pseudohyphae can be found in *C albicans*-infected tissue and are identifiable by microscopic examination of scrapings prepared with Gram, calcofluor white, or fluorescent antibody stains or in a 10% to 20% potassium hydroxide suspension. Endoscopy is useful for diagnosis of esophagitis. Although ophthalmologic examination can reveal typical retinal lesions attributable to hematogenous dissemination, the yield of routine ophthalmologic evaluation in affected patients is low. Lesions in the brain, kidney, liver, or spleen can be detected by ultrasonography, computed tomography, or magnetic resonance imaging; however, these lesions typically are not detected by imaging until late in the course of disease or after neutropenia has resolved.

A definitive diagnosis of invasive candidiasis requires isolation of the organism from a normally sterile body site (eg, blood, cerebrospinal fluid, bone marrow) or demonstration of organisms in a tissue biopsy specimen. Negative results of culture for *Candida* species do not exclude invasive infection in immunocompromised hosts; in some settings, blood culture is only 50% sensitive. Recovery of the organism is expedited using automated blood culture systems or a lysis-centrifugation method. Special fungal culture media are not needed to grow *Candida* species. A presumptive species identification of *C albicans* can be made by demonstrating germ tube formation, and molecular fluorescence in situ hybridization testing rapidly can distinguish *C albicans* from non-albicans *Candida* species.

Patient serum can be tested using the assay for (1,3)-beta-D-glucan from fungal cell walls, which does not distinguish *Candida* species from other fungi. Data on use of this assay for children are more limited than for adult patients, but test results may be helpful when evaluating immunocompromised patients for invasive fungal disease.

TREATMENT[1]:

Mucous Membrane and Skin Infections. Oral candidiasis in immunocompetent hosts is treated with oral nystatin suspension or clotrimazole troches applied to lesions. Troches should not be used in infants. Fluconazole may be more effective than oral nystatin or clotrimazole troches and may be considered if other treatments fail. Fluconazole or itraconazole can be beneficial for immunocompromised patients with oropharyngeal candidiasis. Voriconazole or posaconazole (in children 13 years and older) are alternative drugs. Although cure rates with fluconazole are greater than with nystatin, relapse rates are comparable. Safety and efficacy of itraconazole in HIV-infected children with oropharyngeal candidiasis have been demonstrated.

Esophagitis caused by *Candida* species is treated with oral fluconazole. Intravenous fluconazole, an echinocandin, or amphotericin B should be used for patients who cannot tolerate oral therapy. For disease refractory to fluconazole, itraconazole solution, voriconazole, or posaconazole (in children 13 years and older) is recommended. The recommended duration of therapy is 14 to 21 days. However, the duration of treatment depends on severity of illness and patient factors, such as age and degree of immunocompromise. Suppressive therapy with fluconazole is recommended for recurrent infections.

Skin infections are treated with topical nystatin, miconazole, clotrimazole, naftifine, ketoconazole, econazole, or ciclopirox (see Topical Drugs for Superficial Fungal Infections, p 913). Nystatin usually is effective and is the least expensive of these drugs.

Vulvovaginal candidiasis is treated effectively with many topical formulations, including clotrimazole, miconazole, butoconazole, terconazole, and tioconazole. Such topically applied azole drugs are more effective than nystatin. Oral azole agents (fluconazole, itraconazole, and ketoconazole) also are effective and should be considered for recurrent or refractory cases (see Recommended Doses of Parenteral and Oral Antifungal Drugs, p 909).

For chronic mucocutaneous candidiasis, fluconazole, itraconazole, and voriconazole are effective drugs. Low-dose amphotericin B administered intravenously is effective in severe cases. Relapses are common with any of these agents once therapy is terminated, and treatment should be viewed as a lifelong process, hopefully using only intermittent pulses of antifungal agents. Invasive infections in patients with this condition are rare.

Keratomycosis is treated with corneal baths of voriconazole (1%) in conjunction with systemic therapy. Patients with cystitis caused by *Candida*, especially patients with neutropenia, patients with renal allographs, and patients undergoing urologic manipulation, should be treated with fluconazole for 7 days because of the concentrating effect of fluconazole in the urinary tract. An alternative is a short course (7 days) of low-dose amphotericin B intravenously (0.3 mg/kg per day). Repeated bladder irrigations with amphotericin B (50 μg/mL of sterile water) have been used to treat patients with candidal cystitis, but this does not treat disease beyond the bladder and is not recommended routinely. A urinary catheter in a patient with candidiasis should be removed or replaced promptly.

[1]Infectious Diseases Society of America. Clinical practice guidelines for the management of candidiasis: 2009 update by the Infectious Diseases Society of America. *Clin Infect Dis.* 2009;48(5):503–535

Invasive Disease

General Recommendations. Most *Candida* species are susceptible to amphotericin B, although *C lusitaniae* and some strains of *C glabrata* and *C krusei* exhibit decreased susceptibility or resistance. Among patients with persistent candidemia despite appropriate therapy, investigation for a deep focus of infection should be conducted. Lipid-associated preparations of amphotericin B can be used as an alternative to amphotericin B deoxycholate in patients who experience significant toxicity during therapy.

Fluconazole is not an appropriate choice for therapy before the infecting *Candida* species has been identified, because *C krusei* is resistant to fluconazole, and more than 50% of *C glabrata* isolates also can be resistant. Although voriconazole is effective against *C krusei*, it is often ineffective against *C glabrata*. The echinocandins (caspofungin, micafungin, and anidulafungin) all are active in vitro against most *Candida* species and are appropriate first-line drugs for *Candida* infections in severely ill or neutropenic patients (see Antifungal Drugs for Systemic Fungal Infections, p 905). The echinocandins should be used with caution against *C parapsilosis* infection, because some decreased in vitro susceptibility has been reported. If an echinocandin is initiated empirically and *C parapsilosis* is isolated in a recovering patient, then the echinocandin can be continued.

Neonates. Neonates are more likely than older children and adults to have meningitis as a manifestation of candidiasis. Although meningitis can be seen in association with candidemia, approximately half of neonates with candida meningitis do not have a positive blood culture. Central nervous system disease in the neonate typically manifests as meningoencephalitis and should be assumed to be present in the neonate with candidemia and signs and symptoms of meningoencephalitis because of the high incidence of this complication. A lumbar puncture is recommended for all neonates with candidemia.

Amphotericin B deoxycholate is the drug of choice for treating neonates with systemic candidiasis, including meningitis. For patients with CNS infection, flucytosine is not recommended routinely for use with amphotericin B deoxycholate for *C albicans* infection involving the central nervous system because of difficulty in maintaining appropriate serum concentrations and the risk of toxicity. However, the addition of flucytosine (25 mg/kg/dose, administered orally every 6 hours) may be considered in patients who do not demonstrate a clinical response to initial therapy. For susceptible *Candida* species, step-down treatment with fluconazole (12 mg/kg/day administered once daily) may be considered after the patient with *Candida* meningitis has responded to initial treatment. Therapy for CNS infection is at least 3 weeks and should continue until all signs and symptoms and CSF and radiologic abnormalities have resolved. Echinocandins should be used with caution in neonates, because dosing and safety have not been established; they currently are not recommended for treatment of CNS candidal infections in neonates.

For candidemia without CNS infection, therapy with fluconazole (12 mg/kg/day, administered once daily) is an alternative to amphotericin B deoxycholate if the species is susceptible. The duration of therapy for uncomplicated candidemia is 2 weeks.

Lipid formulations of amphotericin B should be used with caution in neonates, particularly in patients with urinary tract involvement. Recent evidence suggests that treatment of neonates with lipid formulations of amphotericin may be associated with worse outcomes when compared with amphotericin B deoxycholate or fluconazole. Published reports in adults and anecdotal reports in preterm infants indicate that lipid-associated amphotericin B preparations have failed to eradicate renal candidiasis, because these large-molecule drugs may not penetrate well into the renal parenchyma. It is unclear whether this is the reason for the inferior outcomes reported with the lipid formulations.

Older Children and Adolescents. In nonneutropenic and clinically stable children and adults, fluconazole or an echinocandin (caspofungin, micafungin, anidulafungin) is the recommended treatment; amphotericin B deoxycholate or lipid formulations are alternative therapies (see Antifungal Drugs for Systemic Fungal Infections, p 905). In nonneutropenic patients with candidemia and no metastatic complications, treatment should continue for 2 weeks after documented clearance of *Candida* from the bloodstream and resolution of clinical manifestations associated with candidemia.

In critically ill neutropenic patients, an echinocandin or a lipid formulation of amphotericin B is recommended because of the fungicidal nature of these agents when compared with fluconazole, which is fungistatic. In less seriously ill neutropenic patients, fluconazole is the alternative treatment for patients who have not had recent azole exposure, but voriconazole can be considered in situations in which additional mold coverage is desired. The duration of treatment for candidemia without metastatic complications is 2 weeks after documented clearance of *Candida* organisms from the bloodstream and resolution of symptoms attributable to candidemia. Avoidance or reduction of systemic immunosuppression also is advised when feasible.

Management of Indwelling Catheters. In neonates and nonneutropenic children, prompt removal of any infected vascular or peritoneal catheters is strongly recommended. For neutropenic children, catheter removal should be considered. The recommendation in this population is weaker because the source of candidemia in the neutropenic child is more likely to be gastrointestinal, and it is difficult to determine the relative contribution of the catheter. Immediate replacement of a catheter over a wire in the same catheter site is not recommended. Replacement can be attempted once the infection is controlled.

In the situation in which prompt removal of an infected catheter and rapid clearance is established, treatment could be limited for a shorter course. If there is concern about invasive or metastatic disease in this situation, treatment should continue for 2 weeks after documented clearance of *Candida* from the bloodstream and resolution of clinical manifestations associated with candidemia.

Additional Assessments. Ophthalmologic evaluation is recommended for all patients with candidemia, although the yield is noted to be low. Evaluation should occur once candidemia is controlled, and in patients with neutropenia, evaluation should be deferred until recovery of the neutrophil count.

Chemoprophylaxis. Invasive candidiasis in neonates is associated with prolonged hospitalization and neurodevelopmental impairment or death in almost 75% of affected infants with extremely low birth weight (less than 1000 g). The poor outcomes, despite prompt diagnosis and therapy, make prevention of invasive candidiasis in this population desirable. Four prospective randomized controlled trials and 10 retrospective cohort studies of fungal prophylaxis in neonates with birth weight less than 1000 g or less than 1500 g have demonstrated significant reduction of *Candida* colonization, rates of invasive candidiasis, and *Candida*-related mortality in nurseries with a moderate or high incidence of invasive candidiasis. Besides birth weight, other risk factors for invasive candidiasis in neonates include inadequate infection-prevention practices and prolonged use of antimicrobial agents. Adherence to optimal infection-control practices, including "bundles" for intravascular catheter insertion and maintenance and antimicrobial stewardship, can diminish infection rates and should be optimized before implementation of chemoprophylaxis as standard practice in a neonatal intensive care unit. On the basis of current data, fluconazole is the preferred agent for prophylaxis, because it has been shown to be effective and safe. Fluconazole prophylaxis is recommended for extremely low birth weight infants cared for in neonatal intensive care units with moderate (5%–10%) or high (≥10%) rates of invasive candidiasis. The recommended regimen for extremely low birth weight neonates is to initiate fluconazole treatment intravenously during the first 48 to 72 hours after birth at a dose of 3 mg/kg, and administer it twice a week for 4 to 6 weeks, or until intravenous access no longer is required for care. For infants who are tolerating enteral feeds, fluconazole oral absorption is good, even in preterm infants. This chemoprophylaxis dosage, dosing interval, and duration has not been associated with emergence of fluconazole-resistant *Candida* species.

Fluconazole prophylaxis also can decrease the risk of mucosal (eg, oropharyngeal and esophageal) candidiasis in patients with advanced HIV disease. However, an increased incidence of infections attributable to *C krusei* (which intrinsically is resistant to fluconazole) has been reported in non–HIV-infected patients receiving prophylactic fluconazole. Adults undergoing allogeneic hematopoietic stem cell transplantation had significantly fewer *Candida* infections when given fluconazole, but limited data are available for children. Prophylaxis should be considered for children undergoing allogenic hematopoietic stem cell transplantation and other highly myelosuppressive chemotherapy during the period of neutropenia. Prophylaxis is not recommended routinely for other immunocompromised children, including children with HIV infection.

ISOLATION OF THE HOSPITALIZED PATIENT: Standard precautions are recommended.

CONTROL MEASURES: Prolonged broad-spectrum antimicrobial therapy and use of systemic corticosteroids in susceptible patients promote overgrowth of *Candida* and predispose to invasive infection. Meticulous care of central intravascular catheters is recommended for any patient requiring long-term intravenous access.

Cat-Scratch Disease
(Bartonella henselae)

CLINICAL MANIFESTATIONS: Infections with *Bartonella henselae* can be asymptomatic, but the predominant clinical manifestation of cat-scratch disease (CSD) in an immunocompetent person is regional lymphadenopathy/lymphadenitis. Most people with CSD are afebrile or have low grade fever with mild systemic symptoms such as malaise, anorexia, fatigue, and headache. Fever and mild systemic symptoms occur in approximately 30% of patients.

A skin papule or pustule often is found at the presumed site of inoculation and usually precedes development of lymphadenopathy by approximately 1 to 2 weeks (range, 7–60 days). Lymphadenopathy involves nodes that drain the site of inoculation, typically axillary, but cervical, submental, epitrochlear, or inguinal nodes can be involved. The skin overlying affected lymph nodes if often tender, warm, erythematous, and indurated. Most *Bartonella*-infected lymph nodes will resolve spontaneously within 4 to 6 weeks, but approximately 10% to 25% of affected nodes suppurate spontaneously.

Inoculation of the periocular tissue can result in Parinaud oculoglandular syndrome, which consists of follicular conjunctivitis and ipsilateral preauricular lymphadenopathy. Less common manifestations of *Bartonella henselae* infection likely reflect bloodborne disseminated disease and include endocarditis, encephalopathy, osteolytic lesions, granulomata in the liver and spleen, glomerulonephritis, pneumonia, thrombocytopenic purpura, and erythema nodosum. CSD also may present with fevers for 1 to 3 weeks (ie, fever of unknown origin) and may be associated with nonspecific symptoms, such as malaise, abdominal pain, headache, and myalgias. Ocular manifestations occur in 5% to 10% of patients and include oculoglandular syndrome, and rarely, retinochoroiditis, anterior uveitis, vitritis, pars planitis, retinal vasculitis, retinitis, branch retinal arteriolar or venular occlusions, macular hole, or serous retinal detachments (extraordinarily rare).

The most classic and frequent presentation of ocular *Bartonella* infection is neuroretinitis, characterized by unilateral painless vision impairment, granulomatous optic disc swelling, and macular edema, with lipid exudates (macular star); simultaneous bilateral involvement has been reported but is less common.

ETIOLOGY: *B henselae*, the causative organism of CSD, is a fastidious, slow-growing, gram-negative bacillus that also is the causative agent of bacillary angiomatosis (vascular proliferative lesions of skin and subcutaneous tissue) and bacillary peliosis (reticuloendothelial lesions in visceral organs, primarily the liver). The latter 2 manifestations of infection are reported among immunocompromised patients, primarily those with human immunodeficiency virus infection. *B henselae* is related closely to *Bartonella quintana*, the agent of louseborne trench fever that caused significant illness and disease among troops during World War I and also is a causative agent of bacillary angiomatosis. *B quintana* also can cause endocarditis.

EPIDEMIOLOGY: CSD is a common infection, although its true incidence is unknown. *B henselae* is a common causes of regional lymphadenopathy/lymphadenitis in children. Cats are the natural reservoir for *B henselae*, with a seroprevalence of 13% to 90% in domestic and stray cats in the United States. Other animals, including dogs, can be infected and occasionally are associated with human infection. Cat-to-cat transmission occurs via the cat flea *(Ctenocephalides felis)*, with feline infection resulting in bacteremia that usually is asymptomatic and lasts weeks to months. Fleas acquire the organism when feeding on a bacteremic cat and then shed infectious organisms in their feces. The bacteria are transmitted to humans by inoculation through a scratch or bite from a bacteremic cat or by hands contaminated by flea feces touching an open wound or the eye. Kittens (more often than cats) and animals from shelters or adopted as strays are more likely to be bacteremic. Most reported cases occur in people younger than 20 years of age, with most patients having a history of recent contact with apparently healthy cats, typically kittens. Infection occurs more often during the autumn and winter. There is no convincing evidence to date that ticks are a competent vector for transmission of *Bartonella* organisms to humans. No evidence of person-to-person transmission exists.

The **incubation period** from the time of the scratch to appearance of the primary cutaneous lesion is 7 to 12 days; the period from the appearance of the primary lesion to the appearance of lymphadenopathy is 5 to 50 days (median, 12 days).

DIAGNOSTIC TESTS: *B henselae* is a fastidious organism; recovery by routine culture rarely is successful. Specialized laboratories experienced in isolating *Bartonella* organisms are recommended for processing of cultures. The indirect immunofluorescent antibody (IFA) assay for detection of serum antibodies to antigens of *Bartonella* species is useful for diagnosis of CSD. The IFA test is available at many commercial laboratories and through the Centers for Disease Control and Prevention (CDC), but because of cross-reactivity with other infections and a high seroprevalence in the general population, clinical correlation is essential. Enzyme immunoassays for detection of antibodies to *B henselae* have been developed; however, further investigation is required to determine whether they are more sensitive or specific than the IFA test. Convalescent titers 2 weeks following a negative initial result can be performed if strong clinical suspicion persists, because immunoglobulin (Ig) M may return to normal before IgG titers increase. There is limited association between serological titer and clinical manifestations or duration of symptoms. Polymerase chain reaction (PCR) assays are available in some commercial and research laboratories and at the CDC for testing of tissue or body fluids. Clinicians are cautioned against using newly developed diagnostic tests that have not been independently validated or cleared by the US Food and Drug Administration (eg, preenrichment culture, then PCR assay).

If tissue (eg, lymph node) specimens are available, bacilli occasionally may be visualized using a silver stain (eg, Warthin-Starry or Steiner stain); however, this test is not specific for *B henselae*. Early histologic changes in lymph node specimens consist of lymphocytic infiltration with epithelioid granuloma formation. Later changes consist of polymorphonuclear leukocyte infiltration with granulomas that become necrotic and resemble granulomas from patients with tularemia, brucellosis, and mycobacterial infections.

TREATMENT: Management of localized uncomplicated CSD primarily is aimed at relief of symptoms, because the disease usually is self-limited, resolving spontaneously in 2 to 4 months. Azithromycin has been shown to have a modest clinical benefit in treating localized CSD, with a significantly greater decrease in lymph node volume after 1 month of therapy compared with placebo; however, symptomatic improvement was not demonstrated. Painful suppurative nodes can be treated with needle aspiration for relief of symptoms; incision and drainage should be avoided, because this may facilitate fistula formation, and surgical excision generally is unnecessary.

Many experts recommend antimicrobial therapy in acutely or severely ill immunocompetent patients with systemic symptoms, particularly people with retinitis, hepatic or splenic involvement, or painful adenitis. Antimicrobial therapy is recommended for all immunocompromised people. Reports suggest that several oral antimicrobial agents (azithromycin, clarithromycin, ciprofloxacin, doxycycline, trimethoprim-sulfamethoxazole, and rifampin) and parenteral gentamicin are effective. The optimal duration of therapy is not known but may be several weeks for systemic disease.

Although evidence is lacking, neuroretinitis often is treated with both systemic antibiotics and corticosteroids to decrease the optic disc swelling and promote a more rapid return of vision. Doxycycline is preferred for neuroretinitis. Tetracycline-based antimicrobial agents, including doxycycline, may cause permanent tooth discoloration for children younger than 8 years if used for repeated treatment courses. However, doxycycline binds less readily to calcium compared with older tetracyclines, and in some studies, doxycycline was not associated with visible teeth staining in younger children (see Tetracyclines, p 873). A macrolide agent may be used for children younger than 8 years. Reports in the literature note that a large majority of such patients experience significant visual recovery to 20/40 or better.

Antimicrobial therapy for patients with bacillary angiomatosis and bacillary peliosis has been shown to be beneficial and is recommended. Azithromycin or doxycycline are effective for treatment of these condition; therapy should be administered for several months to prevent relapse in immunocompromised people.

ISOLATION OF THE HOSPITALIZED PATIENT: Standard precautions are recommended.

CONTROL MEASURES: Effort should be undertaken to avoid scratches and bites from cats or kittens. Immunocompromised people should avoid contact with cats that scratch or bite and should avoid cats younger than 1 year or stray cats. Sites of cat scratches or bites should be washed immediately. Care of cats should include flea control. Testing or treatment of cats for *Bartonella* infection is not recommended, nor is removal of the cat from the household or declawing.

Chancroid

CLINICAL MANIFESTATIONS: Chancroid is an acute ulcerative disease of the genitalia. An ulcer begins as an erythematous papule that becomes pustular and erodes over several days, forming a sharply demarcated, somewhat superficial lesion with a serpiginous border. The base of the ulcer is friable and can be covered with a gray or yellow, purulent exudate. Single or multiple ulcers can be present. Unlike a syphilitic chancre, which is painless and indurated, the chancroid ulcer often is painful and nonindurated and can be associated with a painful, unilateral inguinal suppurative adenitis (bubo). Without treatment, ulcer(s) can spontaneously resolve, cause extensive erosion of the genitalia, or lead to scarring and phimosis, a painful inability to retract the foreskin.

In most males, chancroid manifests as a genital ulcer with or without inguinal tenderness; edema of the prepuce is common. In females, most lesions are at the vaginal introitus and symptoms include dysuria, dyspareunia, vaginal discharge, pain on defecation, or anal bleeding. Constitutional symptoms are unusual.

ETIOLOGY: Chancroid is caused by *Haemophilus ducreyi*, which is a gram-negative coccobacillus.

EPIDEMIOLOGY: Chancroid is a sexually transmitted infection associated with poverty, prostitution, and illicit drug use. Chancroid is endemic in Africa and the tropics but is rare in the United States, and when it does occur, it usually is associated with sporadic outbreaks. Coinfection with syphilis or herpes simplex virus (HSV) occurs in as many as 17% of patients. Chancroid is a well-established cofactor for transmission of human immunodeficiency virus (HIV). *H ducreyi* also causes a chronic limb ulceration syndrome that is spread by nonsexual contact in older children and adults in the Western Pacific islands; to date, this syndrome is restricted to that region. Because sexual contact is the major primary route of transmission, the diagnosis of chancroid in infants and young children is strong evidence of sexual abuse.

The **incubation period** is 1 to 10 days.

DIAGNOSTIC TESTS: Chancroid usually is diagnosed on the basis of clinical findings (1 or more painful genital ulcers with tender suppurative inguinal adenopathy) and by excluding other genital ulcerative diseases, such as syphilis, HSV infection, or lymphogranuloma venereum. Confirmation is made by isolation of *H ducreyi* from a genital ulcer or lymph node aspirate, although sensitivity is less than 80%. Because special culture media and conditions are required for isolation, laboratory personnel should be informed of the suspicion of chancroid. Buboes almost always are sterile. Polymerase chain reaction assays can provide a specific diagnosis but are not available in most clinical laboratories.

TREATMENT: *H ducreyi* has been uniformly susceptible to third-generation cephalosporins, macrolides, and quinolones. The prevalence of antibiotic resistance is unknown because of syndromic management of genital ulcers and the lack of diagnostic testing. Recommended regimens include azithromycin or ceftriaxone. Alternatives include erythromycin or ciprofloxacin (see Table 4.4, p 896). Ciprofloxacin is not approved by the US Food and Drug Administration for people younger than 18 years for this indication and should not be administered to pregnant or lactating women (see Antimicrobial Agents and Related Therapy, p 873). Patients with HIV infection may need prolonged therapy. Syndromic management usually includes treatment for syphilis.

Clinical improvement occurs 3 to 7 days after initiation of therapy, and healing is complete in approximately 2 weeks. Adenitis often is slow to resolve and can require needle aspiration or surgical incision. Patients should be reexamined 3 to 7 days after initiating therapy to verify healing. If healing has not begun, the diagnosis may be incorrect or the patient may have an additional sexually transmitted infection, both of which necessitate further testing. Slow clinical improvement and relapses can occur after therapy, especially in HIV-infected people. Close clinical follow-up is recommended; retreatment with the original regimen usually is effective in patients who experience a relapse.

Patients should be evaluated for other sexually transmitted infections, including syphilis, herpes simplex virus, chlamydia, gonorrhea, and HIV infection, at the time of diagnosis. Because chancroid is a risk factor for HIV infection and facilitates HIV transmission, if the initial HIV test result is negative, it should be repeated 3 months later. Because syphilis and *H ducreyi* frequently are cotransmitted, serologic testing for syphilis also should be repeated if initially negative. All people having sexual contact with patients with chancroid within 10 days before onset of the patient's symptoms need to be examined and treated, even if they are asymptomatic.

ISOLATION OF THE HOSPITALIZED PATIENT: Standard precautions are recommended.

CONTROL MEASURES: Identification, examination, and treatment of sexual partners of patients with chancroid are important control measures. Regular condom use may decrease transmission, and male circumcision is thought to be partially protective. Immunization status for hepatitis B and human papillomavirus should be reviewed and updated if necessary.

CHLAMYDIAL INFECTIONS

Chlamydophila (formerly *Chlamydia*) *pneumoniae*

CLINICAL MANIFESTATIONS: Patients may be asymptomatic or mildly to moderately ill with a variety of respiratory tract diseases caused by *Chlamydophila pneumoniae*, including pneumonia, acute bronchitis, prolonged cough, and less commonly, pharyngitis, laryngitis, otitis media, and sinusitis. In some patients, a sore throat precedes the onset of cough by a week or more. The clinical course can be biphasic, culminating in atypical pneumonia. *C pneumoniae* can present as severe community-acquired pneumonia in immunocompromised hosts and has been associated with acute exacerbation of respiratory symptoms in patients with cystic fibrosis and in acute chest syndrome in children with sickle cell disease.

Physical examination may reveal nonexudative pharyngitis, pulmonary rales, and bronchospasm. Chest radiography may reveal a variety of findings ranging from pleural effusion and bilateral infiltrates to a single patchy subsegmental infiltrate. Illness can be prolonged, and cough can persist for 2 to 6 weeks or longer.

ETIOLOGY: *C pneumoniae* is an obligate intracellular bacterium. *C pneumoniae* is distinct antigenically, genetically, and morphologically from *Chlamydia* species, so it is grouped in the genus *Chlamydophila*. All isolates of *C pneumoniae* appear serologically to be closely related.

EPIDEMIOLOGY: *C pneumoniae* infection is presumed to be transmitted from person to person via infected respiratory tract secretions. It is unknown whether there is an animal reservoir. The disease occurs worldwide, but in tropical and less developed areas, disease occurs earlier in life than in industrialized countries in temperate climates. The timing of initial infection peaks between 5 and 15 years of age. In the United States, approximately 50% of adults have *C pneumoniae*-specific serum antibody by 20 years of age, indicating previous infection by the organism. Recurrent infection is common, especially in adults. Clusters of infection have been reported in groups of children and young adults. There is no evidence of seasonality.

The mean **incubation period** is 21 days.

DIAGNOSTIC TESTS: Serologic testing has been the primary laboratory means of diagnosis of *C pneumoniae* infection but is problematic in many respects. The microimmunofluorescent antibody test is the most sensitive and specific serologic test for acute infection. A fourfold increase in immunoglobulin (Ig) G titer between acute and convalescent sera or an IgM titer of 1:16 or greater are evidence of acute infection; use of acute and convalescent titers is preferred to a single elevated IgM titer. Use of a single IgG titer in diagnosis of acute infection is not recommended, because during primary infection, IgG antibody may not appear until 6 to 8 weeks after onset of illness during primary infection and increases within 1 to 2 weeks with reinfection. In primary infection, IgM antibody appears approximately 2 to 3 weeks after onset of illness, but caution is advised when interpreting a single IgM antibody titer for diagnosis, because a single result can be either falsely positive because of cross-reactivity with other *Chlamydia* species or falsely negative in cases of reinfection, when IgM may not appear. Early antimicrobial therapy also may suppress antibody response. Past exposure is indicated by a stable IgG titer of 1:16 or greater.

C pneumoniae can be isolated from swab specimens obtained from the nasopharynx or oropharynx or from sputum, bronchoalveolar lavage, or tissue biopsy specimens. Specimens should be placed into appropriate transport media and stored at 4°C until inoculation into cell culture; specimens that cannot be processed within 24 hours should be frozen and stored at −70°C. Culturing *C pneumoniae* is difficult and often fails to detect the organism. A positive culture is confirmed by propagation of the isolate or a positive polymerase chain reaction assay result. Nasopharyngeal shedding can occur for months after acute disease, even with treatment. Immunohistochemistry, used to detect *C pneumoniae* in tissue specimens, requires control antibodies and tissues in addition to skill in recognizing staining artifacts to avoid false-positive results.

Because of the difficulty of accurately detecting *C pneumoniae* via culture, serologic testing, or immunohistochemistry testing, several types of polymerase chain reaction (PCR) assays, including multiplex, hybridization probe methods, and fluorescent probe-based method, have been developed. Sensitivity and specificity of these different PCR techniques remain largely unknown, and reliability of results has been reported to vary widely between laboratories using the same PCR assay. A multiplex PCR assay has been cleared by the US Food and Drug Administration for the diagnosis of *C pneumoniae* using nasopharyngeal samples. The test appears to have high sensitivity and specificity.[1]

---

[1]US Food and Drug Administration. FDA expands use for Film Array Respiratory Panel [news release]. May 15, 2012. Available at: **www.fda.gov/NewsEvents/Newsroom/PressAnnouncements/ucm304177.htm**

TREATMENT: Most respiratory tract infections thought to be caused by *C pneumoniae* are treated empirically. For suspected *C pneumoniae* infections, treatment with macrolides (eg, azithromycin, erythromycin, or clarithromycin) is recommended. Tetracycline or doxycycline may be used but should not be given routinely to children younger than 8 years. Tetracycline-based antimicrobial agents, including doxycycline, may cause permanent tooth discoloration for children younger than 8 years if used for repeated treatment courses. However, doxycycline binds less readily to calcium compared with older tetracyclines, and in some studies, doxycycline was not associated with visible teeth staining in younger children (see Tetracyclines, p 873). Newer fluoroquinolones (levofloxacin and moxifloxacin) are alternative drugs for patients who are unable to tolerate macrolide antibiotics but should not be used as first-line treatment. In vitro data suggest that *C pneumoniae* is not susceptible to sulfonamides.

Duration of therapy typically is 10 to 14 days for erythromycin, clarithromycin, tetracycline, or doxycycline. With azithromycin, the treatment duration typically is 5 days. However, with all of these antimicrobial agents, the optimal duration of therapy has not been established.

ISOLATION OF THE HOSPITALIZED PATIENT: In addition to standard precautions, droplet precautions are recommended for the duration of symptomatic illness.

CONTROL MEASURES: Recommended prevention measures include minimizing crowding, maintaining personal hygiene, employing respiratory hygiene (or cough etiquette), and frequent hand hygiene.

Chlamydophila (formerly *Chlamydia*) psittaci
(Psittacosis, Ornithosis, Parrot Fever)

CLINICAL MANIFESTATIONS: Psittacosis (ornithosis) is an acute respiratory tract infection with systemic symptoms and signs that often include fever, nonproductive cough, headache, and malaise. Less common symptoms include pharyngitis, diarrhea, and altered mental status. Extensive interstitial pneumonia can occur, with radiographic changes characteristically more severe than would be expected from physical examination findings. Endocarditis, myocarditis, pericarditis, thrombophlebitis, nephritis, hepatitis, and encephalitis are rare complications. Recent studies have suggested an association with ocular adnexal marginal zone lymphomas involving orbital soft tissue, lacrimal glands, and conjunctiva.

ETIOLOGY: *Chlamydophila psittaci* is an obligate intracellular bacterial pathogen that is distinct antigenically, genetically, and morphologically from *Chlamydia* species and, following reclassification, is grouped in the genus *Chlamydophila*.

EPIDEMIOLOGY: Birds are the major reservoir of *C psittaci*. The term psittacosis commonly is used, although the term ornithosis more accurately describes the potential for nearly all domestic and wild birds to spread this infection, not just psittacine birds (eg, parakeets, parrots, macaws). In the United States, psittacine birds, pigeons, and turkeys are important sources of human disease. Importation and illegal trafficking of exotic birds is associated with an increased incidence of disease in humans because shipping, crowding, and other stress factors may increase shedding of the organism among birds with latent infection. Infected birds, whether asymptomatic or obviously ill, may transmit the organism. Infection usually is acquired by inhaling aerosolized excrement or respiratory secretions from the eyes or beaks of infected birds. Handling of plumage and mouth-to-beak contact are the modes of exposure described most frequently, although transmission has been reported through exposure to aviaries, bird exhibits, and lawn mowing. Excretion of *C psittaci* from birds may be intermittent or continuous for weeks or months. Pet owners and workers at poultry slaughter plants, poultry farms, and pet shops are at increased risk of infection. Laboratory personnel working with *C psittaci* also are at risk. Psittacosis is worldwide in distribution and tends to occur sporadically in any season. Although rare, severe illness and abortion have been reported in pregnant women.

The **incubation period** usually is 5 to 14 days but may be longer.

DIAGNOSTIC TESTS: A confirmed case of psittacosis requires a clinically compatible illness with fever, chills, headache, cough, and myalgias, plus laboratory confirmation by one of the following: (1) isolation of *C psittaci* from respiratory tract specimens or blood, or (2) fourfold or greater increase in immunoglobulin (Ig) G by complement fixation (CF) or a titer of 1:32 with microimmunofluorescence (MIF) against *C psittaci* between paired acute- and convalescent-phase serum specimens obtained at least 2 to 4 weeks apart. A probable case of psittacosis requires a clinically compatible illness and either: (1) supportive serologic test results (eg, *C psittaci* IgM ≥1:16 in at least 1 serum specimen obtained after onset of symptoms), or (2) detection of *C psittaci* DNA in a respiratory tract specimen by polymerase chain reaction (PCR) assay. For serologic testing, MIF is more sensitive and specific than CF for *C psittaci*; however, both CF and MIF can cross-react with other chlamydial species and should be interpreted cautiously. Additionally, nucleic acid amplification tests (NAATs) have been developed that can distinguish *C psittaci* from other chlamydial species and are under investigation for detection of *C psittaci* from human clinical samples. Treatment with antimicrobial agents may suppress the antibody response, and in such cases a third serum sample obtained 4 to 6 weeks after the acute-phase sample may be useful in confirming the diagnosis. Culturing the organism is recommended; however, it is difficult and should be attempted only by experienced personnel in laboratories where strict containment measures to prevent spread of the organism are used during collection and handling of all specimens because of occupational and laboratory safety concerns.

TREATMENT: Tetracycline or doxycycline is the drug of choice. Tetracycline-based antimicrobial agents, including doxycycline, may cause permanent tooth discoloration for children younger than 8 years if used for repeated treatment courses. However, doxycycline binds less readily to calcium compared with older tetracyclines, and in some studies, doxycycline was not associated with visible teeth staining in younger children (see Tetracyclines, p 873). Erythromycin and azithromycin are alternative agents and are recommended for younger children and pregnant women. Therapy should be for a minimum of 10 days and should continue for 10 to 14 days after fever abates. In patients with severe infection, intravenous doxycycline (4 mg/kg/day, divided into 2 infusions, maximum 100 mg/dose) may be considered.

ISOLATION OF THE HOSPITALIZED PATIENT: Standard precautions are recommended, because person-to-person transmission has been theorized but not proven.

CONTROL MEASURES: Human psittacosis is a nationally notifiable disease and should be reported to public health authorities. All birds suspected to be the source of human infection should be seen by a veterinarian for evaluation and management. Birds with *C psittaci* infection should be isolated and treated with appropriate antimicrobial agents for at least

30 to 45 days.[1] Birds suspected of dying from *C psittaci* infection should be sealed in an impermeable container and transported on dry ice to a veterinary laboratory for testing. All potentially contaminated caging and housing areas should be disinfected thoroughly before reuse to eliminate any infectious organisms. People cleaning cages or handling possibly infected birds should wear personal protective equipment including gloves, eyewear, a disposable hat, and a respirator with N95 or higher rating. *C psittaci* is susceptible to many but not all household disinfectants and detergents. Effective disinfectants include 1:1000 dilutions of quaternary ammonium compounds and freshly made 1:32 dilutions of household bleach (1/2 cup per gallon). People exposed to common sources of infection should be observed for development of fever or respiratory tract symptoms; early diagnostic tests should be performed, and therapy should be initiated if symptoms appear.

Chlamydia trachomatis

CLINICAL MANIFESTATIONS: *Chlamydia trachomatis* is associated with a range of clinical manifestations, including neonatal conjunctivitis, nasopharyngitis, and pneumonia in young infants, genital tract infection, lymphogranuloma venereum (LGV), and trachoma.

- **Neonatal chlamydial conjunctivitis** is characterized by ocular congestion, edema, and discharge developing a few days to several weeks after birth and lasting for 1 to 2 weeks and sometimes longer. In contrast to trachoma, scars and pannus formation are rare.
- **Pneumonia** in young infants usually is an afebrile illness of insidious onset occurring between 2 and 19 weeks after birth. A repetitive staccato cough, tachypnea, and rales in an afebrile 1-month-old infant are characteristic but not always present. Wheezing is uncommon. Hyperinflation usually accompanies infiltrates seen on chest radiographs. Nasal stuffiness and otitis media may occur. Untreated disease can linger or recur. Severe chlamydial pneumonia has occurred in infants and some immunocompromised adults.
- **Genitourinary tract** manifestations, such as vaginitis in prepubertal girls; urethritis, cervicitis, endometritis, salpingitis, proctitis, and perihepatitis (Fitz-Hugh-Curtis syndrome) in postpubertal females; urethritis, epididymitis, and proctitis in males; and Reiter syndrome (arthritis, urethritis, and bilateral conjunctivitis) also can occur. Infection can persist for months to years. Reinfection is common. In postpubertal females, chlamydial infection can progress to pelvic inflammatory disease and can result in ectopic pregnancy, infertility, or chronic pelvic pain.
- **LGV** classically is an invasive lymphatic infection with an initial ulcerative lesion on the genitalia accompanied by tender, suppurative inguinal and/or femoral lymphadenopathy that typically is unilateral. The ulcerative lesion often has resolved by the time the patient seeks care. Proctocolitis may occur in women or men who engage in anal intercourse. Symptoms can resemble those of inflammatory bowel disease, including mucoid or hemorrhagic rectal discharge, constipation, tenesmus, and/or anorectal pain. Stricture or fistula formation can follow severe or inadequately treated infection.
- **Trachoma** is a chronic follicular keratoconjunctivitis with neovascularization of the cornea that results from repeated and chronic infection. Blindness secondary to extensive local scarring and inflammation occurs in 1% to 15% of people with trachoma.

---

[1]National Association of State Public Health Veterinarians. *Compendium of Measures to Control* Chlamydophila psittaci *Infection Among Humans (Psittacosis) and Pet Birds (Avian Chlamydiosis), 2008.* Available at: **www.nasphv .org/Documents/Psittacosis.pdf**

ETIOLOGY: *C trachomatis* is an obligate intracellular bacterial agent with at least 18 serologic variants (serovars) divided between the following biologic variants (biovars): oculogenital (serovars A–K) and LGV (serovars L1, L2, and L3). Trachoma usually is caused by serovars A through C, and genital and perinatal infections are caused by B and D through K.

EPIDEMIOLOGY: *C trachomatis* is the most common reportable sexually transmitted infection (STI) in the United States, with high rates among sexually active adolescents and young adult females. A significant proportion of patients are asymptomatic, providing an ongoing reservoir for infection. Prevalence of the organism consistently is highest among adolescent and young adult females. Among all 14- to 25-year-old people participating in the 2008 National Health and Nutrition Examination Survey, prevalence was 3.3% among females and 1.7% among males. Racial disparities are significant. The estimated prevalence among non-Hispanic black people (6.7%) was higher than the estimated prevalence among non-Hispanic white people (0.3%) and Mexican American people (2.4%). Among males who have sex with males (MSM) screened for rectal chlamydial infection, positivity ranges from 3% to 10%.[1] Oculogenital serovars of *C trachomatis* can be transmitted from the genital tract of infected mothers to their infants during birth. Acquisition occurs in approximately 50% of infants born vaginally to infected mothers and in some infants born by cesarean delivery with membranes intact. The risk of conjunctivitis is 25% to 50% and the risk of pneumonia is 5% to 30% in infants who contract *C trachomatis*. The nasopharynx is the anatomic site most commonly infected.

Genital tract infection in adolescents and adults is transmitted sexually. The possibility of sexual abuse always should be considered in prepubertal children beyond infancy who have vaginal, urethral, or rectal chlamydial infection. Sexual abuse is not limited to prepubertal children, and chlamydial infections can result from sexual abuse/assault in postpubertal adolescents as well.

Asymptomatic infection of the nasopharynx, conjunctivae, vagina, and rectum can be acquired at birth. Nasopharyngeal cultures have been observed to remain positive for as long as 28 months and vaginal and rectal cultures for more than 1 year in infants with infection acquired at birth. Infection is not known to be communicable among infants and children. The degree of contagiousness of pulmonary disease is unknown but seems to be low.

LGV biovars are worldwide in distribution but particularly are prevalent in tropical and subtropical areas. Although disease occurs rarely in the United States, outbreaks of LGV have been reported among men who have sex with men. Infection often is asymptomatic in females. Perinatal transmission is rare. LGV is infectious during active disease. Little is known about the prevalence or duration of asymptomatic carriage.

Although rarely observed in the United States since the 1950s, trachoma is the leading infectious cause of blindness worldwide, causing up to 3% of the world's blindness. It generally is confined to poor populations in resource-limited nations of Africa, the Middle East, Asia, Latin America, the Pacific Islands, and remote aboriginal communities in Australia. Trachoma is transmitted by transfer of ocular discharge. Predictors of scarring and blindness for trachoma include increasing age and constant, severe trachoma.

---

[1]Centers for Disease Control and Prevention. CDC Grand Rounds: chlamydia prevention challenges and strategies for reducing disease burden and sequelae. *MMWR Morb Mortal Wkly Rep.* 2011;60(12):370-373

The **incubation period** of chlamydial illness is variable, depending on the type of infection, but usually is at least 1 week.

DIAGNOSTIC TESTS[1]: *C trachomatis* urogenital infection in females can be diagnosed by testing first catch urine or by collecting swab specimens from the endocervix or vagina. Diagnosis of *C trachomatis* urethral infection in males can be made by testing a urethral swab or first catch urine specimen. Nucleic acid amplification tests (NAATs) are the most sensitive tests for these specimens and are the recommended tests for *C trachomatis* detection.[2] NAATs are the preferred tests for these specimens and are the recommended tests for *C trachomatis* detection.

For detecting *C trachomatis* infections of the genital tract among **postpubescent individuals**, older nonculture tests and non-NAATs, such as DNA probe, DFA tests, or EIA, have inferior sensitivity and specificity characteristics and no longer are recommended for *C trachomatis* testing.[2] Commercial NAATs have been approved by the FDA for testing of vaginal (provider or patient-collected), endocervical, and male intraurethral swabs and male and female urine specimens and liquid cytology specimens. Package inserts for individual NAAT products must be reviewed, however, because the particular specimens approved for use with each test may vary. The Centers for Disease Control and Prevention (CDC) recommends vaginal swab as the preferred means of screening females and urine as the preferred means for screening males for *C trachomatis* infection. Female urine remains an acceptable chlamydia NAAT specimen but may have slightly reduced performance when compared with cervical or vaginal swab specimens. NAATs have not been approved by the FDA for use with rectal specimens, but laboratories that have met Clinical Laboratory Improvement Amendments (CLIA) and other regulatory requirements and have validated chlamydia NAAT performance on rectal swab specimens may perform this test. *C trachomatis* testing of pharyngeal specimens from asymptomatic postpubescent individuals generally is not recommended, because the clinical significance of oropharyngeal *C trachomatis* infection is unclear. NAATs also permit dual testing of specimens for *C trachomatis* and *Neisseria gonorrhoeae*.

NAATs have not been approved by the FDA for testing of conjunctival specimens from infants with suspected *C trachomatis* **conjunctivitis** or for testing of nasopharyngeal swab, tracheal aspirate, or lung biopsy specimens from infants with suspected *C trachomatis* **pneumonia**. Published evaluations of NAATs for these indications are limited, but sensitivity and specificity is expected to be at least as high as those for culture or the selected nonamplified direct detection methods, because they have shown superior performance with other specimen types.

In the **evaluation of prepubescent children for possible sexual assault**, the CDC recommends culture for *C trachomatis* of a specimen collected from the rectum in both boys and girls and from the vagina in girls. A meatal specimen should be obtained from boys for chlamydia testing if urethral discharge is present. NAATs are not approved by the FDA for this indication but are available more widely and are more sensitive than culture in limited published evaluations. Test specificity, which is of critical concern

---

[1] American Academy of Pediatrics, Committee on Adolescence; Society for Adolescent Health and Medicine. Screening for nonviral sexually transmitted infections in adolescents and young adults. *Pediatrics.* 2014;134(1):e302-e311

[2] Centers for Disease Control and Prevention. Recommendations for the laboratory-based detection of *Chlamydia trachomatis* and *Neisseria gonorrhoeae*—2014. *MMWR Recomm Rep.* 2014;63(RR-2):1-19

because of the potential legal consequences of positive test results, has been high in limited published evaluations of NAATs for this indication.

Serum anti-*C trachomatis* antibody concentrations are difficult to determine, and only a few clinical laboratories perform this test. In **children with pneumonia**, an acute microimmunofluorescent serum titer of *C trachomatis*-specific immunoglobulin (Ig) M of 1:32 or greater is diagnostic. Diagnosis of **LGV** can be supported but not confirmed by a positive result (ie, titer >1:64) on a complement-fixation test for chlamydia or a high titer (typically >1:256, but this can vary by laboratory) on a microimmunofluorescent serologic test for *C trachomatis*. However, most available serologic tests in the United States are based on EIAs and might not provide a quantitative "titer-based" result.

Diagnosis of genitourinary tract chlamydial disease in a child should prompt examination for **other STIs**, including syphilis, gonorrhea, and human immunodeficiency virus (HIV) infection, and investigation of sexual abuse/assault. In the case of an infant, because cultures can be positive for at least 12 months after infection acquired at birth, evaluation of the mother also is advisable.

Diagnosis of **ocular trachoma** usually is made clinically in countries with endemic infection.

TREATMENT[1]:

* Infants with **chlamydial conjunctivitis** or **pneumonia** are treated with oral erythromycin base or ethylsuccinate (50 mg/kg/day in 4 divided doses daily) for 14 days or with azithromycin (20 mg/kg as a single daily dose) for 3 days. Because the efficacy of erythromycin therapy is approximately 80% for both of these conditions, a second course may be required, and follow-up of infants is recommended. A diagnosis of *C trachomatis* infection in an infant should prompt treatment of the mother and her sexual partner(s). The need for treatment of infants can be avoided by screening pregnant females to detect and treat *C trachomatis* infection before delivery.

    An association between orally administered erythromycin and infantile hypertrophic pyloric stenosis (IHPS) has been reported in infants younger than 6 weeks. The risk of IHPS after treatment with other macrolides (eg, azithromycin and clarithromycin) is unknown, although IHPS has been reported after use of azithromycin. Because confirmation of erythromycin as a contributor to cases of IHPS will require additional investigation and because alternative therapies are not as well studied, the American Academy of Pediatrics continues to recommend use of erythromycin for treatment of diseases caused by *C trachomatis*. Physicians who prescribe erythromycin to newborn infants should inform parents about the signs and potential risks of developing IHPS. Cases of pyloric stenosis after use of oral erythromycin or azithromycin should be reported to MedWatch (see MedWatch, p 957).

* Infants born to mothers known to have untreated chlamydial infection are at high risk of infection; however, prophylactic antimicrobial treatment is not indicated, because the efficacy of such treatment is unknown. Infants should be monitored clinically to ensure appropriate treatment if infection develops. If adequate follow-up cannot be ensured, preemptive therapy should be considered.

* For uncomplicated *C trachomatis* **anogenital tract infection in adolescents or adults**, oral doxycycline (100 mg, twice daily) for 7 days or azithromycin (in a single 1-g

---

[1]Centers for Disease Control and Prevention. Sexually transmitted diseases treatment guidelines, 2014. *MMWR Recomm Rep.* 2014; in press

oral dose) is recommended. Alternatives include oral erythromycin base (500 mg, 4 times/day) for 7 days, erythromycin ethylsuccinate (800 mg, 4 times/day) for 7 days, ofloxacin (300 mg, twice daily) for 7 days, levofloxacin (500 mg, once daily) for 7 days, or doxycycline delayed-release (200-mg tablet, once daily) for 7 days. **For children who weigh <45 kg,** the recommended regimen is oral erythromycin base or ethylsuccinate, 50 mg/kg/day, divided into 4 doses daily for 14 days. **For children who weigh ≥45 kg but who are younger than 8 years,** the recommended regimen is azithromycin, 1 g, orally, in a single dose. **For children 8 years and older**, the recommended regimen is azithromycin, 1 g, orally, in a single dose, or doxycycline, 100 mg, orally, twice a day for 7 days. **For pregnant females**, the recommended treatment is azithromycin (1 g, orally, as a single dose). Amoxicillin (500 mg, orally, 3 times/day) for 7 days or erythromycin base (500 mg, orally, 4 times/day) for 7 days are alternative regimens. Doxycycline, ofloxacin, and levofloxacin are contraindicated during pregnancy.

Follow-up Testing. Test-of cure is not recommended for nonpregnant adult or adolescent patients treated for uncomplicated chlamydial infection unless compliance is in question, symptoms persist, or reinfection is suspected. Test-of-cure (preferably by NAAT) is recommended 3 to 4 weeks after treatment of pregnant females. Because some of these regimens for pregnant women may not be highly efficacious, a second course of therapy may be required. A NAAT conducted less than 3 weeks after completion of therapy can yield false-positive results because of continued presence of dead organisms. Reinfection is common after initial infection and treatment, and all infected adolescents and adults should be tested for *C trachomatis* in the next 3 months following initial treatment. If retesting at 3 months is not possible, retest whenever patients next present for health care in the 12 months after initial treatment, regardless of whether patients believe their sexual partners were treated.

• For **LGV**, doxycycline (100 mg, orally, twice daily) for 21 days is the preferred treatment for children 8 years and older, and erythromycin, 500 mg, orally, 4 times daily for 21 days, is an alternative regimen; azithromycin (1 g, once weekly for 3 weeks) probably is effective but has not been as well studied.

• Treatment of **trachoma** is azithromycin, orally, as a single dose of 20 mg/kg (maximum dose of 1000 mg) as recommended by the World Health Organization for all people diagnosed with trachoma as well as for all of their household contacts.

ISOLATION OF THE HOSPITALIZED PATIENT: Standard precautions are recommended.

CONTROL MEASURES:

Pregnancy. Identification and treatment of females with *C trachomatis* genital tract infection during pregnancy can prevent disease in the infant. Pregnant females at high risk of *C trachomatis* infection, in particular females 24 years or younger and females with new or multiple sexual partners, should be targeted for screening. The CDC recommends routine testing of all pregnant women during the first trimester and advises retesting of all pregnant females younger than 25 years during the third trimester to prevent perinatal complications. Pregnant females diagnosed with a chlamydial infection during the first trimester not only should receive a test to document chlamydial eradication 3 to 4 weeks after treatment but also should be tested 3 months after treatment as well as in the third trimester.

Neonatal Chlamydial Conjunctivitis. Recommended topical prophylaxis with erythromycin or tetracycline for all newborn infants for prevention of gonococcal ophthalmia will not prevent neonatal chlamydial conjunctivitis or extraocular infection (see Prevention of Neonatal Ophthalmia, p 972).

Contacts of Infants With C trachomatis ***Conjunctivitis or Pneumonia.*** Mothers of infected infants and mothers' sexual partners should be treated for *C trachomatis.*

Routine Screening Tests.[1] All sexually experienced adolescent and young adult females (25 years or younger) should be tested at least annually for *Chlamydia* infection, even if no symptoms are present or barrier contraception is reported. Sexually experienced adolescent and young adult MSM should be screened routinely for rectal and urethral chlamydia annually if they engaged in receptive or insertive anal intercourse, respectively. MSM should be screened every 3 to 6 months if at high risk because of multiple or anonymous sex partners, sex in conjunction with illicit drug use, or sex with partners who participate in these activities. Annual screening may be considered for sexually active males who have sex with females in settings with high prevalence rates, such as jails or juvenile corrections facilities, national job training programs, STI clinics, high school clinics, and adolescent clinics for patients who have a history of multiple partners.

Management of Sex Partners. All people with sexual contact in the 60 days preceding diagnosis or onset of symptoms of patients with *C trachomatis* infection (whether symptomatic or asymptomatic), nongonococcal urethritis, mucopurulent cervicitis, epididymitis, or pelvic inflammatory disease should be evaluated and treated for *C trachomatis* infection. The patient's last sex partner should be treated even if last sexual contact was more than 60 days before diagnosis in the index case. Among females or heterosexual male patients, if concerns exist that sex partners who are referred for evaluation and treatment will not seek care, expedited partner therapy (EPT, which is the practice of treating the sex partners of patients diagnosed with chlamydia or gonorrhea by providing prescriptions or medications to the index patient to take to his or her partner without the health care provider first examining the partner) can be considered but is not optimal. To clarify the legal status of EPT in each state, refer to the CDC Web site (**www.cdc.gov/std/ept/**). EPT should include efforts to educate partners about symptoms of chlamydia and gonorrhea and to encourage partners to seek clinical evaluation. EPT should not be considered a routine partner management strategy in MSM because of the high risk of coexisting undiagnosed STIs or HIV infection. Integrated recommendations for services provided to partners of people with STIs, including *C trachomatis,* are available.[2,3]

LGV. Nonspecific preventive measures for LGV are the same as measures for STIs in general and include education, case reporting, condom use, and avoidance of sexual contact with infected people. Partners exposed to an LGV-infected person within the 60 days before the patient's symptom onset should be tested and treated.

Trachoma. Although rarely observed in the United States since the 1950s, trachoma is the leading infectious cause of blindness worldwide. Prevention methods recommended by the World Health Organization for global elimination of blindness attributable to trachoma by 2020 include surgery, antibiotic agents, face washing, and environmental improvement (SAFE). Azithromycin (20 mg/kg, maximum 1 g), once a year as a

---

[1]American Academy of Pediatrics, Committee on Adolescence; Society for Adolescent Health and Medicine. Screening for nonviral sexually transmitted infections in adolescents and young adults. *Pediatrics.* 2014;134(1):e302-e311

[2]Centers for Disease Control and Prevention. Recommendations for partner services programs for HIV infection, syphilis, gonorrhea, and chlamydial infection. *MMWR Recomm Rep.* 2008;57(RR-9):1-63

[3]Centers for Disease Control and Prevention. Sexually transmitted diseases treatment guidelines, 2014. *MMWR Recomm Rep.* 2014; in press

single oral dose, is used in mass drug administration campaigns for trachoma control. Azithromycin typically is given to children in a community up to 14 years of age to decrease the reservoir of active trachoma.[1]

CLOSTRIDIAL INFECTIONS

Botulism and Infant Botulism
(Clostridium botulinum)

CLINICAL MANIFESTATIONS: Botulism is a neuroparalytic disorder characterized by an acute, afebrile, symmetric, descending, flaccid paralysis. Paralysis is caused by blockade of neurotransmitter release at the voluntary motor and autonomic neuromuscular junctions. Four naturally occurring forms of human botulism exist: infant, foodborne, wound, and adult intestinal colonization. Cases of iatrogenic botulism, which result from injection of excess therapeutic botulinum toxin, have been reported. Onset of symptoms occurs abruptly within hours or evolves gradually over several days and includes diplopia, dysphagia, dysphonia, and dysarthria. Cranial nerve palsies are followed by symmetric, descending, flaccid paralysis of somatic musculature in patients who remain fully alert. Infant botulism, which occurs predominantly in infants younger than 6 months (range, 1 day to 12 months), is preceded by or begins with constipation and manifests as decreased movement, loss of facial expression, poor feeding, weak cry, diminished gag reflex, ocular palsies, loss of head control, and progressive descending generalized weakness and hypotonia. Some reports suggest that sudden infant death could result from rapidly progressing infant botulism.

ETIOLOGY: Botulism occurs after absorption of botulinum toxin into the circulation from a mucosal or wound surface. Seven antigenic toxin types (A-G) of *Clostridium botulinum* have been identified. Non-*botulinum* species of *Clostridium* rarely may produce these neurotoxins and cause disease. Of the 7 recognized serotypes of botulinum toxin, the most common serotypes associated with naturally occurring illness are types A, B, E, and rarely, F. Most cases of infant botulism result from toxin types A and B, but a few cases of types E and F have been caused by *Clostridium butyricum* (type E), *C botulinum* (type E), and *Clostridium baratii* (type F) (especially in very young infants). *C botulinum* spores are ubiquitous in soils and dust worldwide and have been isolated from the home vacuum cleaner dust of infant botulism patients.

EPIDEMIOLOGY: Infant botulism (annual average, 96 laboratory-confirmed cases in 2006-2011; age range, <1 to 60 weeks; median age, 16 weeks) results after ingested spores of *C botulinum* or related neurotoxigenic clostridial species germinate, multiply and produce botulinum toxin in the large intestine through transient colonization of the intestinal microflora. Cases may occur in breastfed infants at the time of first introduction of non-human milk substances; the source of spores usually is not identified. Honey has been

---

[1]Northern Territory Government, Centre for Disease Control. *Guidelines for Management of Trachoma in the Northern Territory 2008.* Alice Springs, Northern Territory, Australia: Department of Health and Families; 2008. Available at: **www.k4health.org/sites/default/files/Guidelines%20for%20Management%20 of%20Trachoma%20-%20CDC.pdf**

identified as an avoidable source of spores. No case of infant botulism has been proven to be attributable to consumption of corn syrup. Rarely, intestinal botulism can occur in older children and adults, usually after intestinal surgery and exposure to antimicrobial agents.

Foodborne botulism (annual average, 17 cases in 2006-2010; age range, 3–91 years; median age, 53 years) results when food that carries spores of *C botulinum* is preserved or stored improperly under anaerobic conditions that permit germination, multiplication, and toxin production. Illness follows ingestion of the food containing preformed botulinum toxin. Home-processed foods are by far the most common cause of foodborne botulism in the United States, followed by rare outbreaks associated with commercially processed foods and restaurant-associated foods.

Wound botulism (annual average, 26 laboratory-confirmed cases in 2006-2010; age range, 14–66 years; median age, 46 years) results when *C botulinum* contaminates traumatized tissue, germinates, multiplies, and produces toxin. Gross trauma or crush injury can be a predisposing event. During the last decade, self-injection of contaminated black tar heroin has been associated with most cases.

Immunity to botulinum toxin does not develop in botulism. Botulism is not transmitted from person to person. The usual **incubation period** for foodborne botulism is 12 to 48 hours (range, 6 hours–8 days). In infant botulism, the **incubation period** is estimated at 3 to 30 days from the time of ingestion of spores. For wound botulism, the **incubation period** is 4 to 14 days from time of injury until onset of symptoms.

DIAGNOSTIC TESTS: A toxin neutralization bioassay in mice[1] is used to detect botulinum toxin in serum, stool, enema fluid, gastric aspirate, or suspect foods. Enriched selective media is required to isolate *C botulinum* from stool and foods. The diagnosis of infant botulism is made by demonstrating botulinum toxin or botulinum toxin-producing organisms in feces or enema fluid or toxin in serum. Wound botulism is confirmed by demonstrating organisms in the wound or tissue or toxin in the serum. To increase the likelihood of diagnosis in foodborne botulism, all suspect foods should be collected, and serum and stool or enema specimens should be obtained from all people with suspected illness. In foodborne cases, serum specimens may be positive for toxin as long as 12 days after admission. Although toxin can be demonstrated in serum in some infants with botulism (eg, 13% in one large study), stool is the best specimen for diagnosis; enema effluent also can be useful. If constipation makes obtaining a stool specimen difficult, an enema of sterile, nonbacteriostatic water should be given promptly. Because results of laboratory bioassay testing may require several days, treatment with antitoxin should be initiated urgently for all forms of botulism on the basis of clinical suspicion. The most prominent electromyographic finding is an incremental increase of evoked muscle potentials at high-frequency nerve stimulation (20–50 Hz). In addition, a characteristic pattern of brief, small-amplitude, overly abundant motor action potentials may be seen after stimulation of muscle, but its absence does not exclude the diagnosis; this test is infrequently needed for diagnosis.

TREATMENT:
Meticulous Supportive Care. Meticulous supportive care, in particular respiratory and nutritional support, constitutes a fundamental aspect of therapy in all forms of botulism. Recovery from botulism may take weeks to months.

---

[1]For information, consult your state health department.

Antitoxin for Infant Botulism. Human-derived antitoxin should be given immediately. Human Botulism Immune Globulin for intravenous use (BIG-IV; BabyBIG) is licensed by the US Food and Drug Administration (FDA) for treatment of infant botulism caused by *C botulinum* type A or type B. BabyBIG is produced and distributed by the California Department of Public Health (24-hour telephone number: 510-231-7600; **www.infantbotulism.org**). BabyBIG significantly decreases days of mechanical ventilation, days of intensive care unit stay, and total length of hospital stay by almost 1 month and is cost saving. BabyBIG is first-line therapy for naturally occurring infant botulism. Equine-derived heptavalent botulinum antitoxin (BAT; see below) was licensed by the FDA in 2013 for treatment of adult and pediatric botulism and is available through the Centers for Disease Control and Prevention (CDC). BAT has been used to treat type F infant botulism patients where the antitoxin is not contained in BabyBIG, on a case-by-case basis.

As with other Immune Globulin Intravenous preparations, routine live-virus vaccines should be delayed for 6 months after receipt of BabyBIG because of potential interference with immune responses (see Table 1.10).

Antitoxin for Noninfant Forms of Botulism. Immediate administration of antitoxin is the key to successful therapy, because antitoxin treatment ends the toxemia and stops further uptake of toxin. However, because botulinum neurotoxin becomes internalized in the nerve ending, administration of antitoxin does not reverse paralysis. On suspicion of foodborne botulism, the state health department should be contacted immediately to discuss and report the case; all states maintain a 24-hour telephone service. If contact cannot be made with the state health department, the CDC Emergency Operations Center should be contacted at 770-488-7100 for botulism case consultation and antitoxin. Since 2010, BAT is the only botulinum antitoxin released in the United States for treatment of non-infant botulism. BAT contains antitoxin against all 7 (A-G) botulinum toxin types and has been "de-speciated" by enzymatic removal of the Fc immunoglobulin fragment, resulting in a product that is >90% Fab and F(ab')$_2$ immunoglobulin fragments. BAT is provided by the CDC with a treatment protocol that includes specific, detailed instructions for intravenous administration of antitoxin and return of required paperwork to the CDC. Additional information may be found on the CDC Web site (**www.cdc.gov/nczved/ divisions/dfbmd/diseases/botulism/**).

Antimicrobial Agents. Antimicrobial therapy is not prescribed in infant botulism unless clearly indicated for a concurrent infection. Aminoglycoside agents can potentiate the paralytic effects of the toxin and should be avoided. Antibiotic agents may be given to patients with wound botulism after antitoxin has been administered. The role of antimicrobial therapy in the adult intestinal colonization form of botulism, if any, has not been established.

ISOLATION OF THE HOSPITALIZED PATIENT: Standard precautions are recommended.

CONTROL MEASURES:
- Any case of suspected botulism is a nationally notifiable disease and is required by law to be reported immediately (ie, by phone or fax) to local and state health departments. Immediate reporting of suspect cases is particularly important, because a single case could be the harbinger of many more cases, as with foodborne botulism, and because of possible use of botulinum toxin as a bioterrorism weapon.
- Honey should not be given to children younger than 12 months because of the possibility of contaminating spores.

- Prophylactic antitoxin is not recommended for asymptomatic people who have ingested a food known to contain botulinum toxin. Physicians treating a patient who has been exposed to toxin or is suspected of having any type of botulism should contact their state health department immediately. People exposed to toxin who are asymptomatic should have close medical observation in nonsolitary settings.
- Education regarding safe practices in food preparation and home-canning methods should be promoted. Use of a pressure cooker (at 116°C [240.8°F]) is necessary to kill spores of *C botulinum*. Bringing the internal temperature of foods to 85°C (185°F) for 10 minutes will destroy the toxin. Time, temperature, and pressure requirements vary with altitude and the product being heated. Food containers that appear to bulge may contain gas produced by *C botulinum* and should be discarded. Other foods that appear to have spoiled should not be eaten or tasted (**http://nchfp.uga.edu/publications/publications_usda.html**).
- The investigational pentavalent botulinum toxoid vaccine (types A, B, C, D, and E) has been discontinued by the CDC for immunization of laboratory workers at high risk of exposure to botulinum toxin and no longer is available.[1]

Clostridial Myonecrosis
(Gas Gangrene)

CLINICAL MANIFESTATIONS: Disease onset is heralded by acute pain at the site of the wound, followed by edema, increasing exquisite tenderness, exudate, and progression of pain. Systemic findings initially include tachycardia disproportionate to the degree of fever, pallor, diaphoresis, hypotension, renal failure, and later, alterations in mental status. Crepitus is suggestive but not pathognomonic of *Clostridium* infection and is not always present. Diagnosis is based on clinical manifestations, including the characteristic appearance of necrotic muscle at surgery. Untreated gas gangrene can lead to disseminated myonecrosis, suppurative visceral infection, septicemia, and death within hours.

ETIOLOGY: Clostridial myonecrosis is caused by *Clostridium* species, most often *Clostridium perfringens*. These organisms are large, gram-positive, spore-forming, anaerobic bacilli with blunt ends. Other *Clostridium* species (eg, *Clostridium sordellii*, *Clostridium septicum*, *Clostridium novyi*) also have been associated with myonecrosis. Disease manifestations are caused by potent clostridial exotoxins (eg, *C sordellii* with medical abortion and *C septicum* with malignancy). Mixed infection with other gram-positive and gram-negative bacteria is common.

EPIDEMIOLOGY: Clostridial myonecrosis usually results from contamination of open wounds involving muscle. The sources of *Clostridium* species are soil, contaminated foreign bodies, and human and animal feces. Dirty surgical or traumatic wounds, particularly those with retained foreign bodies or significant amounts of devitalized tissue, predispose to disease. Nontraumatic gas gangrene occurs rarely in immunocompromised people and most often is described in those with underlying malignancy, neutrophil dysfunction, or diseases associated with bowel ischemia.

The **incubation period** from the time of injury is 1 to 4 days.

---

[1] Centers for Disease Control and Prevention. Notice of CDC's discontinuation of investigational pentavalent (ABCDE) botulinum toxoid vaccine for workers at high risk for occupational exposure to botulinum toxins. *MMWR Morb Mortal Wkly Rep.* 2011;60(42):1454-1455

DIAGNOSTIC TESTS: Anaerobic cultures of wound exudate, involved soft tissue and muscle, and blood should be performed. Because *Clostridium* species are ubiquitous, their recovery from a wound is not diagnostic unless typical clinical manifestations are present. A Gram-stained smear of wound discharge demonstrating characteristic gram-positive bacilli and few, if any, polymorphonuclear leukocytes suggests clostridial infection. Tissue specimens (not swab specimens) for anaerobic culture must be obtained to confirm the diagnosis. Because some pathogenic *Clostridium* species are exquisitely oxygen sensitive, care should be taken to optimize anaerobic growth conditions. A radiograph of the affected site can demonstrate gas in the tissue, but this is a nonspecific finding and is not always present. Occasionally, blood cultures are positive and are considered diagnostic.

TREATMENT:
- Prompt and complete surgical excision of necrotic tissue and removal of foreign material is essential. Repeated surgical débridement may be required to ensure complete removal of all infected tissue. Vacuum-assisted wound closure can be used following multiple débridements.
- Management of shock, fluid and electrolyte imbalance, hemolytic anemia, and other complications is crucial.
- High-dose penicillin G (250 000–400 000 U/kg per day) should be administered intravenously. Clindamycin, metronidazole, meropenem, ertapenem, and chloramphenicol can be considered as alternative drugs for patients with a serious penicillin allergy or for treatment of polymicrobial infections. The combination of penicillin G and clindamycin may be superior to penicillin alone because of the theoretical benefit of clindamycin inhibiting toxin synthesis.
- Hyperbaric oxygen may be beneficial, but efficacy data from adequately controlled clinical studies are not available.

ISOLATION OF THE HOSPITALIZED PATIENT: Standard precautions are recommended.

CONTROL MEASURES: Prompt and careful débridement, flushing of contaminated wounds, and removal of foreign material should be performed.

Penicillin G (50 000 U/kg per day) or clindamycin (20-30 mg/kg per day) has been used for prophylaxis in patients with grossly contaminated wounds, but efficacy is unknown.

Clostridium difficile

CLINICAL MANIFESTATIONS: *Clostridium difficile* is associated with several syndromes as well as with asymptomatic carriage. Mild to moderate illness is characterized by watery diarrhea, low-grade fever, and mild abdominal pain. Pseudomembranous colitis is characterized by diarrhea with mucus in feces, abdominal cramps and pain, fever, and systemic toxicity. Occasionally, children have marked abdominal tenderness and distention with minimal diarrhea (toxic megacolon). The colonic mucosa often contains 2- to 5-mm, raised, yellowish plaques. Disease often begins while the child is hospitalized receiving antimicrobial therapy but can occur up to 10 weeks after therapy cessation. Community-associated *C difficile* disease is less common but is occurring with increasing frequency. The illness usually, but not always, is associated with antimicrobial therapy or prior hospitalization. Complications, which occur more commonly in older adults, can include toxic megacolon, intestinal perforation, systemic inflammatory response syndrome, and death. Severe or fatal disease is more likely to occur in neutropenic children with leukemia, infants with Hirschsprung disease, and patients with inflammatory bowel disease. Asymptomatic colonization with *C difficile*, including toxin-producing strains, occurs in children younger than 5 years and is most common in infants younger than 1 year. It is unclear how frequently *C difficile* causes disease in infants.

ETIOLOGY: *C difficile* is a spore-forming, obligate anaerobic, gram-positive bacillus. Disease is related to A and B toxins produced by these organisms.

EPIDEMIOLOGY: *C difficile* can be isolated from soil and is found commonly in the hospital environment. *C difficile* is acquired from the environment or from stool of other colonized or infected people by the fecal-oral route. Intestinal colonization rates in healthy infants can be as high as 50% but usually are less than 5% in children older than 5 years and adults. Hospitals, nursing homes, and child care facilities are major reservoirs for *C difficile*. Risk factors for acquisition of the bacteria include prolonged hospitalization and exposure to an infected person either in the hospital or the community. Risk factors for *C difficile* disease include antimicrobial therapy, repeated enemas, gastric acid suppression therapy, prolonged nasogastric tube placement, gastrostomy and jejunostomy tubes, underlying bowel disease, gastrointestinal tract surgery, renal insufficiency, and humoral immunocompromise. *C difficile* colitis has been associated with exposure to almost every antimicrobial agent. Hospitalization of children for *C difficile* colitis is increasing. The NAP-1 strain, a more virulent strain of *C difficile* with variations in toxin genes, is associated with severe disease, has emerged as a cause of outbreaks among adults, and has been reported in children.

The **incubation period** is unknown; colitis usually develops 5 to 10 days after initiation of antimicrobial therapy but can occur on the first day and up to 10 weeks after therapy cessation.

DIAGNOSTIC TESTS: The diagnosis of *C difficile* disease is based on the presence of liquid stools/diarrhea and detection of *C difficile* toxins in a diarrheal stool specimen.[1]

Attempts to isolate the organism or toxins from the stool of a patient who is not having liquid stools (unless toxic megacolon is suspected) is not a useful test and should not be performed. Endoscopic findings of pseudomembranes and hyperemic, friable rectal mucosa suggest pseudomembranous colitis. The most common testing method for *C difficile* toxins is the commercially available enzyme immunoassay (EIA), which detects toxins A and B. Although EIAs are rapid and performed easily, their sensitivity is relatively low. The cell culture cytotoxicity assay, which also tests for toxin in stool, is more sensitive than the EIA but requires more labor and has a slow turnaround time, limiting its usefulness in the clinical setting. Two-step testing algorithms that use the sensitive but nonspecific (detects both toxigenic and nontoxigenic strains) glutamate dehydrogenase EIA combined with confirmatory toxin testing of positive results also can be used. Molecular assays using nucleic acid amplification tests (NAATs) have been developed and are cleared by the US Food and Drug Administration. NAATs combine good sensitivity and specificity, provide results to clinicians in times comparable to EIAs, and are not required to be part of a 2- or 3-step algorithm. Many children's hospitals are converting to NAAT technology to diagnose *C difficile* infection, but more data are needed in children before this technology can be used routinely as a standalone test. The predictive value of a positive test result in a child younger than 5 years is unknown, because asymptomatic carriage of toxigenic

---

[1]American Academy of Pediatrics, Committee on Infectious Diseases. *Clostridium difficile* infection in infants and children. *Pediatrics.* 2013;131(1):196-200

strains often occurs in these children. *C difficile* toxin degrades at room temperate and can be undetectable within 2 hours after collection of a stool specimen. Stool specimens not tested promptly or maintained at 4°C can yield false-negative results. Because colonization with *C difficile* in infants is common, testing for other causes of diarrhea always is recommended in these patients. Tests of cure are not recommended and should not be performed.

TREATMENT:
- Precipitating antimicrobial therapy should be discontinued as soon as possible.
- Antimicrobial therapy for *C difficile* infection is indicated for symptomatic patients.
- *C difficile* is susceptible to metronidazole and vancomycin. Metronidazole (30 mg/kg per day, orally, in 4 divided doses, maximum 2 g/day) is the drug of choice for the initial treatment of children and adolescents with mild to moderate diarrhea and for first relapse.
- Oral vancomycin (40 mg/kg per day, orally, in 4 divided doses, to a maximum daily dose not to exceed 2 g) or vancomycin administered by enema plus intravenous metronidazole is indicated as initial therapy for patients with severe disease (hospitalized in an intensive care unit, pseudomembranous colitis by endoscopy, or significant underlying intestinal tract disease) and for patients who do not respond to oral metronidazole. Vancomycin for intravenous use can be prepared for oral use as a lower-cost alternative. Intravenously administered vancomycin is not effective for *C difficile* infection.
- Therapy with either metronidazole or vancomycin or the combination should be administered for at least 10 days.
- Up to 25% of patients experience a relapse after discontinuing therapy, but infection usually responds to a second course of the same treatment. Metronidazole should not be used for treatment of a second recurrence or for chronic therapy, because neurotoxicity is possible. Tapered or pulse regimens of vancomycin are recommended under this circumstance.
- Fidaxomicin has been approved for treatment of *C difficile*-associated diarrhea in adults, including those with mild-moderate and severe disease, and reports suggest it is noninferior when compared with oral vancomycin. No comparisons to metronidazole are available, and no pediatric data are available.
- Nitazoxanide also is an effective therapy in adults.
- Drugs that decrease intestinal motility should not be administered.
- Follow-up testing for toxin is not recommended.
- Fecal transplant (intestinal microbiota transplantation) appears to be effective in adults, but there are limited data in pediatrics.
- Investigational therapies include other antimicrobial agents (rifaximin, tinidazole), Immune Globulin therapy, toxin binders, and probiotics.[1]

ISOLATION OF THE HOSPITALIZED PATIENT: In addition to standard precautions, contact precautions and a private room (if feasible) are recommended for the duration of illness.

CONTROL MEASURES:
- Exercising meticulous hand hygiene, properly handling contaminated waste (including diapers), disinfecting fomites, and limiting use of antimicrobial agents are the best available methods for control of *C difficile* infection. Alcohol-based hand hygiene products

[1]Thomas DW, Greer FR; American Academy of Pediatrics, Committee on Nutrition. Probiotics and prebiotics in pediatrics. *Pediatrics.* 2010;126(6):1217-1231

do not inactivate *C difficile* spores. Washing hands with soap and water is considered to be more effective in removing *C difficile* spores from contaminated hands and should be performed after each contact with a *C difficile* infected patient in outbreak settings or an increased *C difficile* infection rate,[1] but there is disagreement among experts about when and whether soap-and-water hand hygiene should be used preferentially over alcohol hand gel in nonoutbreak settings. The most effective means of preventing hand contamination is the use of gloves when caring for infected patients or their environment, followed by hand hygiene after glove removal.

- Thorough cleaning of hospital rooms and bathrooms of patients with *C difficile* disease is essential. Because *C difficile* spores are difficult to kill, organisms can resist action of many common hospital disinfectants, and many hospitals have instituted the use of disinfectants with sporicidal activity (eg, hypochlorite).

- Children with *C difficile* diarrhea should be excluded from child care settings for the duration of diarrhea, and infection-control measures should be enforced (see Children in Out-of-Home Child Care, p 132).

Clostridium perfringens Food Poisoning

CLINICAL MANIFESTATIONS: *Clostridium perfringens* foodborne illness is characterized by a sudden onset of watery diarrhea and moderate to severe, cramping, mid-epigastric pain. Vomiting and fever are uncommon. Symptoms usually resolve within 24 hours. The shorter incubation period, shorter duration, and absence of fever in most patients differentiate *C perfringens* foodborne disease from shigellosis and salmonellosis, and the infrequency of vomiting and longer incubation period contrast with the clinical features of foodborne disease associated with heavy metals, *Staphylococcus aureus* enterotoxins, *Bacillus cereus* emetic toxin, and fish and shellfish toxins. Diarrheal illness caused by *B cereus* diarrheal enterotoxins can be indistinguishable from that caused by *C perfringens* (see Appendix VII, Clinical Syndromes Associated With Foodborne Diseases, p 1008). Enteritis necroticans (also known as pigbel) results from hemorrhagic necrosis of the midgut and is a cause of severe illness and death attributable to *C perfringens* food poisoning caused by contamination with *Clostridium* strains carrying a β toxin. Rare cases have been reported in the Highlands of Papua, in New Guinea, and in Thailand; malnutrition is an important risk factor. Necrotizing colitis and death have been described in patients with Type A *Clostridium* taking medications resulting in constipation.

ETIOLOGY: Typical food poisoning is caused by a heat-labile *C perfringens* enterotoxin, produced during sporulation in the small intestine. *C perfringens* type A, which produces a toxin and enterotoxin, commonly causes foodborne illness. Enteritis necroticans is caused by *C perfringens* type C, which produces α and β toxins and enterotoxin. *C perfringens* type B, which produces e toxin, a neurotoxin, has been proposed as an environmental trigger for multiple sclerosis.

EPIDEMIOLOGY: *C perfringens* is a gram-positive, spore-forming bacillus that is ubiquitous in the environment, the intestinal tracts of humans and animals, and commonly present in raw meat and poultry. Spores of *C perfringens* that survive cooking can germinate and multiply rapidly during slow cooling, when stored at temperatures from 20°C to 60°C

[1]Cohen SH, Gerding DN, Johnson S, et al. Clinical practice guidelines for *Clostridium difficile* infection in adults: 2010 update by the Society for Healthcare Epidemiology of America (SHEA) and the Infectious Diseases Society of America (IDSA). *Infect Control Hosp Epidemiol.* 2010;31(5):431-455

(68°C–140°F), and during inadequate reheating. At an optimum temperature, *C perfringens* has one of the fastest rates of growth of any bacterium. Illness results from consumption of food containing high numbers of vegetative organisms ($>10^5$ colony forming units/g) followed by enterotoxin production in the intestine.

Beef, poultry, gravies, and dried or precooked foods are common sources. Ingestion of the organism is most commonly associated with foods prepared by restaurants or caterers or in institutional settings (eg, schools and camps) where food is prepared in large quantities, cooled slowly, and stored inappropriately for prolonged periods. Illness is not transmissible from person to person.

The **incubation period** is 6 to 24 hours, usually 8 to 12 hours.

DIAGNOSTIC TESTS: Because the fecal flora of healthy people commonly includes *C perfringens*, counts of *C perfringens* of 10^6 colony forming units (CFU)/g of feces or greater obtained within 48 hours of onset of illness are required to support the diagnosis in ill people. The diagnosis also can be supported by detection of enterotoxin in stool. *C perfringens* can be confirmed as the cause of an outbreak if 10^6 CFU/g are isolated from stool or enterotoxin is demonstrated in the stool of 2 or more ill people or when the concentration of organisms is at least 10^5/g in the epidemiologically implicated food. Although *C perfringens* is an anaerobe, special transport conditions are unnecessary. Stool specimens, rather than rectal swab specimens, should be obtained, transported in ice packs, and tested within 24 hours.

TREATMENT: Oral rehydration or, occasionally, intravenous fluid and electrolyte replacement may be indicated to prevent or treat dehydration. Antimicrobial agents are not indicated.

ISOLATION OF THE HOSPITALIZED PATIENT: Standard precautions are recommended.

CONTROL MEASURES: Preventive measures depend on limiting proliferation of *C perfringens* in foods by cooking foods thoroughly and maintaining food at warmer than 60°C (140°F) or cooler than 7°C (45°F). Meat dishes should be served hot shortly after cooking. Foods never should be held at room temperature to cool; they should be refrigerated after removal from warming devices or serving tables as soon as possible and with 2 hours of preparation. Information on recommended safe food handling practices, including time and temperature requirements during cooking, storage, and reheating, can be found at **www.foodsafety.gov.**

Coccidioidomycosis

CLINICAL MANIFESTATIONS: Primary pulmonary infection is acquired by inhaling fungal conidia and is asymptomatic or self-limited in 60% of infected children. Constitutional symptoms, including extreme fatigue and weight loss, are common and can persist for weeks or months. Symptomatic disease can resemble influenza or community-acquired pneumonia, with malaise, fever, cough, myalgia, arthralgia, headache, and chest pain. Pleural effusion, empyema, and mediastinal involvement are more common in children.

Acute infection may be associated only with cutaneous abnormalities, such as erythema multiforme, an erythematous maculopapular rash, or erythema nodosum. Chronic pulmonary lesions are rare, but approximately 5% of infected people develop asymptomatic pulmonary radiographic residua (eg, cysts, nodules, cavitary lesions, coin lesions). Nonpulmonary primary infection is rare and usually follows trauma associated with contamination of wounds by arthroconidia. Cutaneous lesions and soft tissue infections often are accompanied by regional lymphadenitis.

Disseminated (extrapulmonary) infection occurs in less than 0.5% of infected people; common sites of dissemination include skin, bones and joints, and the central nervous system (CNS). Meningitis invariably is fatal if untreated. Congenital infection is rare.

ETIOLOGY: *Coccidioides* species are dimorphic fungi. In soil, *Coccidioides* organisms exist in the mycelial phase as mold growing as branching, septate hyphae. Infectious arthroconidia (ie, spores) produced from hyphae become airborne, infecting the host after inhalation or, rarely, inoculation. In tissues, arthroconidia enlarge to form spherules; mature spherules release hundreds to thousands of endospores that develop into new spherules and continue the tissue cycle. Molecular studies have divided the genus *Coccidioides* into 2 species: *Coccidioides immitis,* confined mainly to California, and *Coccidioides posadasii,* encompassing the remaining areas of distribution of the fungus within certain deserts of the southwestern United States, northern Mexico, and areas of Central and South America.

EPIDEMIOLOGY: *Coccidioides* species are found mostly in soil in areas of the southwestern United States with endemic infection, including California, Arizona, New Mexico, west and south Texas, southern Nevada, and Utah; northern Mexico; and throughout certain parts of Central and South America. In areas with endemic coccidioidomycosis, clusters of cases can follow dust-generating events, such as storms, seismic events, archaeologic digging, or recreational activities. The majority of cases occur without a known preceding event. The incidence of reported coccidioidomycosis cases has increased substantially over the past decade and a half, rising from 5.3 per 100 000 population in the area of endemicity (Arizona, California, Nevada, New Mexico, and Utah) in 1998 to 42.6 per 100 000 in 2011.[1] Infection is thought to provide lifelong immunity. Person-to-person transmission of coccidioidomycosis does not occur except in rare instances of cutaneous infection with actively draining lesions, donor-derived transmission via an infected organ, and congenital infection following in utero exposure. Preexisting impairment of T-lymphocyte–mediated immunity is a major risk factor for severe primary coccidioidomycosis, disseminated disease, or relapse of past infection. Other people at risk of severe or disseminated disease include people of African or Filipino ancestry, women in the third trimester of pregnancy, and children younger than 1 year. Cases may occur in people who do not reside in regions with endemic infection but who previously have visited these areas. In regions without endemic infection, careful travel histories should be obtained from people with symptoms or findings compatible with coccidioidomycosis. Because the signs and symptoms of infection are nonspecific, the diagnosis is not considered, and therefore, most infections are not identified. *Coccidioides* species are listed by the Centers for Disease Control and Prevention as agents of bioterrorism.

The **incubation period** typically is 1 to 4 weeks in primary infection; disseminated infection may develop years after primary infection.

DIAGNOSTIC TESTS: Diagnosis of coccidioidomycosis is best established using serologic, histopathologic, and culture methods. Serologic tests are useful in the diagnosis and management of infection. The immunoglobulin (Ig) M response can be detected

---

[1]Centers for Disease Control and Prevention. Increase in reported coccidioidomycosis—United States, 1998–2011. *MMWR Morb Mortal Wkly Rep.* 2013;62(12):217-221

by enzyme immunoassay (EIA) or immunodiffusion methods. In approximately 50% and 90% of primary infections, IgM is detected in the first and third weeks, respectively. IgG response can be detected by immunodiffusion, EIA, or complement fixation (CF) tests. Immunodiffusion and CF tests are highly specific. CF antibodies in serum usually are of low titer and are transient if the disease is asymptomatic or mild. Persistent high titers (≥1:16) occur with severe disease and almost always in disseminated infection. Cerebrospinal fluid (CSF) antibodies also are detectable by immunodiffusion or CF testing. Increasing serum and CSF titers indicate progressive disease, and decreasing titers usually suggest improvement. CF titers may not be reliable in immunocompromised patients; low or nondetectable titers in immunocompromised patients should be interpreted with caution. Because clinical laboratories use different diagnostic test kits, positive results should be confirmed in a reference laboratory.

Spherules are as large as 80 μm in diameter and can be visualized with 100 to 400 × magnification in infected body fluid specimens (eg, pleural fluid, bronchoalveolar lavage) and biopsy specimens of skin lesions or organs. For biopsy specimens, use of silver or period-acid Schiff staining is helpful. The presence of a mature spherule with endospores is pathognomonic of infection. Isolation of *Coccidioides* species in culture establishes the diagnosis, even in patients with mild symptoms. Culture of organisms is possible on a variety of artificial media but potentially is hazardous to laboratory personnel, because spherules can convert to arthroconidia-bearing mycelia on culture plates. Clinicians should inform the laboratory if there is suspicion of coccidioidomycosis. Suspect cultures should be sealed and handled using appropriate safety equipment and procedures. A DNA probe can identify *Coccidioides* species in cultures, thereby decreasing risk of exposure to infectious fungi.

An EIA test for urine, serum, plasma, or bronchoalveolar lavage fluid is available from 1 US laboratory for detection of *Coccidioides* antigen. Antigen can be positive in patients with more severe forms of disease (sensitivity 71%). Cross reactions occur in patients with histoplasmosis, blastomycosis, or paracoccidioidomycosis.

TREATMENT: Antifungal therapy for uncomplicated primary infection in people without risk factors for severe disease is controversial. Although most cases will resolve without therapy, some experts believe that treatment may reduce illness duration or risk for severe complications. Most experts recommend treatment of coccidioidomycosis for people at risk of severe disease or people with severe primary infection. Severe primary infection is manifested by complement fixation titers of 1:16 or greater, infiltrates involving more than half of one lung or portions of both lungs, weight loss of greater than 10%, marked chest pain, severe malaise, inability to work or attend school, intense night sweats, or symptoms that persist for more than 2 months. In such cases, fluconazole or itraconazole (200–400 mg daily) is recommended for 3 to 6 months. If itraconazole is administered, measurement of a trough serum concentration (or a random sample obtained 8 or more hours after a dose) is recommended to ensure that absorption is satisfactory; levels of ≥1 μg/mL should be targeted. Repeated patient encounters every 1 to 3 months for up to 2 years, either to document radiographic resolution or to identify pulmonary or extrapulmonary complications, are recommended. For diffuse pneumonia, defined as bilateral reticulonodular or military infiltrates, amphotericin B or high-dose fluconazole is recommended. Amphotericin B is more frequently used in the presence of severe hypoxemia or rapid clinical deterioration. The total length of therapy for diffuse pneumonia should be 1 year.

Oral itraconazole or fluconazole is the recommended initial therapy for disseminated infection not involving the CNS. Amphotericin B is recommended as alternative therapy if lesions are progressing or are in critical locations, such as the vertebral column. In patients experiencing failure of conventional amphotericin B deoxycholate therapy or experiencing drug-related toxicities, a lipid formulation of amphotericin B can be substituted.

Consultation with a specialist for treatment of patients with CNS disease caused by *Coccidioides* species is recommended. Oral fluconazole (adult dose: 400 mg/day, up to 800 or 1000 mg/day) is recommended for treatment of patients with CNS infection. Patients who respond to azole therapy should continue this treatment indefinitely. For CNS infections that are unresponsive to oral azoles or are associated with severe basilar inflammation, intrathecal amphotericin B deoxycholate therapy (0.1–1.5 mg per dose) can be used to augment the azole therapy. A subcutaneous reservoir can facilitate administration into the cisternal space or lateral ventricle.

The role of newer azole antifungal agents, such as voriconazole and posaconazole, in treatment of coccidiomycosis has not been established. These newer agents may be administered in certain clinical settings, such as therapeutic failure in severe coccidioidal disease (eg, meningitis). When used, these newer azoles should be administered in consultation with experts experienced with their use in treatment of coccidioidomycosis.

The duration of antifungal therapy is variable and depends on the site(s) of involvement, clinical response, and mycologic and immunologic test results. In general, therapy is continued until clinical and laboratory evidence indicates that active infection has resolved. Treatment for disseminated coccidioidomycosis is at least 6 months but for some patients may be extended to 1 year or longer. The role of subsequent suppressive azole therapy is uncertain, except for patients with CNS infection, osteomyelitis, or underlying human immunodeficiency virus (HIV) infection or solid organ transplant recipients, for whom suppressive therapy is lifelong.[1] Women should be advised to avoid pregnancy while receiving fluconazole, which may be teratogenic.

Surgical débridement or excision of lesions in bone, pericardium, and lung has been advocated for localized, symptomatic, persistent, resistant, or progressive lesions. In some localized infections with sinuses, fistulae, or abscesses, amphotericin B has been instilled locally or used for irrigation of wounds. Antifungal prophylaxis for solid organ transplant recipients may be considered if they reside in endemic areas and have a prior serologic test result or a history of coccidiomycosis.

ISOLATION OF THE HOSPITALIZED PATIENT: Standard precautions are recommended. Care should be taken in handling, changing, and discarding dressings, casts, and similar materials in which arthroconidial contamination could occur.

CONTROL MEASURES: Measures to control dust are recommended in areas with endemic infection, including construction sites, archaeologic project sites, or other locations where activities cause excessive soil disturbance. Immunocompromised people residing in or traveling to areas with endemic infection should be counseled to avoid exposure to activities that may aerosolize spores in contaminated soil.

---

[1]Panel on Opportunistic Infections in HIV-Exposed and HIV-Infected Children. Guidelines for the Prevention and Treatment of Opportunistic Infections in HIV-Exposed and HIV-Infected Children. Rockville, MD: US Department of Health and Human Services; 2013. Available at: **http://aidsinfo.nih.gov/contentfiles/lvguidelines/oi_guidelines_pediatrics.pdf**

Coronaviruses, Including SARS and MERS

CLINICAL MANIFESTATIONS: Human coronaviruses (HCoVs) 229E, OC43, NL63, and HKU1 are associated most frequently with the common cold, an upper respiratory tract infection characterized by rhinorrhea, nasal congestion, sore throat, sneezing, and cough that may be associated with fever. Symptoms are self-limiting and typically peak on day 3 or 4 of illness. These HCoV infections also may be associated with acute otitis media or asthma exacerbations. Less frequently, they are associated with lower respiratory tract infections, including bronchiolitis, croup, and pneumonia, primarily in infants and immunocompromised children and adults.

SARS-CoV, the HCoV responsible for the 2002-2003 global outbreak of severe acute respiratory syndrome (SARS), was associated with more severe symptoms, although a spectrum of disease including asymptomatic infections and mild disease occurred. SARS-CoV disproportionately affected adults, who typically presented with fever, myalgia, headache, malaise, and chills followed by a nonproductive cough and dyspnea generally 5 to 7 days later. Approximately 25% of infected adults developed watery diarrhea. Twenty percent developed worsening respiratory distress requiring intubation and ventilation. The overall associated mortality rate was approximately 10%, with most deaths occurring in the third week of illness. The case-fatality rate in people older than 60 years approached 50%. Typical laboratory abnormalities include lymphopenia and increased lactate dehydrogenase and creatine kinase concentrations. Most have progressive unilateral or bilateral ill-defined airspace infiltrates on chest imaging. Pneumothoraces and other signs of barotrauma are common in critically ill patients receiving mechanical ventilation.

SARS-CoV infections in children are less severe than in adults; notably, no infant or child deaths from SARS-CoV infection were documented in the 2002-2003 global outbreak. Infants and children younger than 12 years who develop SARS typically present with fever, cough, and rhinorrhea. Associated lymphopenia is less severe, and radiographic changes are milder and generally resolve more quickly than in adolescents and adults. Adolescents who develop SARS have clinical courses more closely resembling those of adult disease, presenting with fever, myalgia, headache, and chills. They also are more likely to develop dyspnea, hypoxemia, and worsening chest radiographic findings. Laboratory abnormalities are comparable to those in adult disease.

MERS-CoV, the HCoV associated with the Middle East respiratory syndrome (MERS), also can cause severe disease. On the basis of what is known to date, MERS-CoV is associated with a severe respiratory illness similar to that noted with SARS-CoV, although a spectrum of disease including asymptomatic infections and mild disease may occur. Patients commonly present with fever, myalgia, chills, shortness of breath, and cough. Approximately 25% of patients may also experience vomiting, diarrhea, or abdominal pain. Rapid deterioration of oxygenation with progressive unilateral or bilateral airspace infiltrates on chest imaging may follow, requiring mechanical ventilation. The case-fatality rate is high, estimated at nearly 50%. To date, most infections have been reported in male adults, and most cases have been reported with comorbidities, such as diabetes, chronic renal disease, hypertension, and chronic cardiac disease.

ETIOLOGY: Coronaviruses are enveloped, nonsegmented, single-stranded, positive-sense RNA viruses named after their corona- or crown-like surface projections observed on electron microscopy that correspond to large surface spike proteins. Coronaviruses are classified in the Nidovirales order. Coronaviruses are host specific and can infect humans as well as a variety of different animals, causing diverse clinical syndromes. Four distinct genera have been described: *Alphacoronavirus, Betacoronavirus, Gammacoronavirus,* and *Deltacoronavirus.* HCoVs 229E and NL63 belong to the genus *Alphacoronavirus,* HCoVs OC43 and HKU1 belong to lineage A of the genus *Betacoronavirus,* SARS-CoV belongs to lineage B of the genus *Betacoronavirus,* and MERS-CoV belongs to lineage C of the genus *Betacoronavirus.*

EPIDEMIOLOGY: Coronaviruses first were recognized as animal pathogens in the 1930s. Thirty years later, 229E and OC43 were identified as human pathogens, along with other coronavirus strains that were not investigated further and for which little is known regarding their prevalence and associated disease syndromes. In 2003, SARS-CoV was identified as a novel virus responsible for the 2002-2003 global outbreak of SARS, which lasted for 9 months and resulted in 8096 reported cases and 774 deaths. No SARS-CoV infections have been reported worldwide since early 2004. Most experts believe SARS-CoV evolved from a natural reservoir of SARS-CoV-like viruses in bats through civet cats or other wet market intermediate hosts in China. Whether or not a large-scale reemergence of SARS will occur is unknown. Finding a novel HCoV sparked a renewed interest in HCoV research, and 2 years later NL63 and HKU1 were identified as newly recognized HCoVs. Investigations have revealed that NL63 was present in archived human respiratory tract specimens as early as 1981 and HKU1 as early as 1995. In 2012, MERS-CoV was identified as a novel virus associated with the death of a 60-year-old man from Saudi Arabia with acute pneumonia and renal failure. As of June 11, 2014, 699 laboratory-confirmed cases of human infection with MERS-CoV have been reported, with 209 deaths. Updated figures on global cases can be found on the World Health Organization Web site (**www.who.int/csr/disease/coronavirus_infections/archive_updates/en/**). MERS-CoV is thought to have evolved from a natural reservoir of MERS-CoV-like viruses in bats. An animal source for MERS-CoV has not yet been determined. However, recent studies have demonstrated MERS-CoV genetic sequences and presence of neutralizing antibodies to CoV in dromedary camels. How this relates to transmission to humans is unclear at this time.

The HCoVs 229E, OC43, NL63, and HKU1 can be found worldwide. They cause most disease in the winter and spring months in temperate climates. Seroprevalence data for these HCoVs suggest that exposure is common in early childhood, with approximately 90% of adults being seropositive for 229E, OC43, and NL63 and 60% being seropositive for HKU1. In contrast, SARS-CoV infection has not been detected in humans since early 2004, when 4 isolated cases of SARS with no associated transmission were identified in China and 2 isolated cases and a cluster of 11 cases (1 death) were identified in South East Asia that was related to breaches in biosafety practices in different laboratories culturing the virus. MERS-CoV has been reported to date in people who reside in or have traveled to the Middle East or who have had contact with a case from the Middle East, including travel-related cases in the United States. Human-to-human transmission, including clusters of cases, has been observed. On the basis of available information from all recently affected countries, there is no evidence of sustained human-to-human transmission in the community. Whether ongoing transmission is going to continue with spread to other regions is not yet clear.

The modes of transmission for 229E, OC43, NL63, and HKU1 have not been well studied. However, on the basis of studies of other respiratory tract viruses, it is likely that transmission occurs primarily via a combination of droplet and direct and indirect contact spread. Which of these modes are most important remains to be determined, and the possible role of aerosol spread requires further study. For SARS-CoV, studies suggest that droplet and direct contact spread are likely the most common modes of transmission, although evidence of indirect contact spread and aerosol spread also exist. Fecal droplet and fecal-oral transmission have also been proposed as possible routes of SARS-CoV transmission. Some people with SARS-CoV were super spreaders and played a major role in the geographic dissemination. There is no evidence of vertical transmission of SARS-CoV. The modes of transmission for MERS-CoV are still being studied.

HCoV 229E and OC43 are most likely to be transmitted during the first few days of illness, when symptoms and respiratory viral loads are at their highest. Further study is needed to confirm that this holds true for the NL63 and HKU1 viruses. SARS-CoV is most likely to be transmitted during the second week of illness, when both symptoms and respiratory viral loads peak. The peak communicable period or kinetics for MERS-CoV are not yet known.

The **incubation period** for HCoV infections, other than SARS-CoV and MERS-CoV, is estimated to be 2 to 5 days (median 3 days), primarily on the basis of studies with 229E. The **incubation period** for SARS-CoV is estimated to be 2 to 10 days (median, 4 days). The **incubation period** for MERS-CoV is estimated to be 2 to 14 days (median, approximately 5 days).

DIAGNOSTIC TESTS: The 2002-2003 SARS global outbreak garnered renewed interest in better understanding the etiology of respiratory tract infections, and some clinical laboratories have since started offering comprehensive respiratory molecular diagnostic testing for HCoVs using reverse transcriptase-polymerase chain reaction (RT-PCR) assays. Diagnostic laboratory and clinical guidance for SARS is available on the Centers for Disease Control and Prevention (CDC) SARS Web site (**www.cdc.gov/sars/index .html**). Given the potential for false-positive test results and the associated public health implications, testing for SARS-CoV in the absence of known person-to-person transmission of SARS must be performed with caution and only in consultation with regional public health departments when there is a high degree of suspicion in a patient with no alternative diagnosis. Guidance regarding testing for MERS-CoV is available on the CDC MERS Web site (**www.cdc.gov/coronavirus/MERS/index.html**).

Specimens obtained from the upper and lower respiratory tract are the most appropriate samples for HCoV detection. The yield from lower respiratory tract specimens is higher for SARS-CoV and MERS-CoV. Stool and serum samples also frequently are positive using RT-PCR in patients with SARS-CoV and have been positive in some patients with MERS-CoV. For 229E and OC43, specimens are most likely to be positive during the first few days of illness; whether this also is true for NL63 and HKU1 requires further study. For SARS-CoV, respiratory and stool specimens may not be positive until the second week of illness when symptoms and viral loads peak; serum samples are most likely positive in the first week of illness. Compared with adults, infants and children with SARS-CoV infections are less likely to have positive specimens, consistent with the milder symptoms and presumed corresponding lower viral loads seen in this age group. The optimal timing of specimen collection for MERS-CoV still is being studied.

Serologic testing is a useful tool for diagnosis for SARS and MERS, although these tests are not available widely. Although acute and convalescent sera are optimal, a single serum specimen collected 2 or more weeks from symptom onset may help with the diagnosis of SARS or MERS, because these infections are so rare. The CDC should be contacted for additional information on serologic testing.

A diagnosis of SARS or MERS should not be based on a single positive laboratory test. Any positive test result should be validated by an approved laboratory and must be evaluated in the context of clinical findings, exposure risk factors, laboratory test results for other common respiratory pathogens, and epidemiologic data.

TREATMENT: Infections attributable to HCoVs generally are treated with supportive care. SARS-CoV and MERS-CoV infections are more serious. Steroids, type 1 interferons, convalescent plasma, ribavirin, and lopinavir/ritonavir all were used clinically to treat patients with SARS, albeit without benefit of controlled data and, thus, no evidence of efficacy. Because of these limitations of trial designs, no definitive conclusions regarding efficacy of any treatment can be made. There are reports of patients who were treated with supportive care only who recovered uneventfully. In the event that SARS-CoV reemerges, clarification of the effectiveness of treatments through controlled clinical trials is required. In vitro data document that cyclosporin A and alpha interferon inhibit MERS-CoV replication. However, treatment efficacy of any antiviral agent for MERS-CoV has yet to be established.

ISOLATION OF THE HOSPITALIZED PATIENT: In addition to standard precautions, health care professionals should use airborne, droplet, and contact precautions when examining and caring for infants and young children with signs and symptoms of a respiratory tract infection for the duration of their illness (**www.cdc.gov/hicpac/2007IP/2007 isolationPrecautions.html**). Airborne, droplet, and contact precautions are recommended for patients with suspected SARS-CoV infection for the duration of illness plus 10 days after resolution of fever, provided respiratory symptoms are absent or improving. Airborne, droplet, and contact precautions are recommended as well for patients with suspected MERS-CoV infection. Recommendations regarding when to discontinue these precautions have not yet been established but are expected once more is learned about MERS-CoV. It would be prudent to maintain isolation precautions for the duration of Illness pending formal recommendations. (**www.cdc.gov/coronavirus/mers/ infection-prevention-control.html**).

CONTROL MEASURES: Practicing appropriate hand and respiratory hygiene likely is the most useful and easily implemented control measure to curb spread of all respiratory tract viruses, including HCoVs. For hospitalized patients, following additional infection-control practices is recommended. Public health departments should be notified of any suspected cases of SARS-CoV and MERS-CoV as soon as possible. The control of the 2002-2003 SARS global outbreak was credited to the rapid identification of cases and early implementation of infection-control and public-health measures, such as contact tracing, isolation, and quarantine.

Cryptococcus neoformans and *Cryptococcus gattii* Infections (Cryptococcosis)

CLINICAL MANIFESTATIONS: Primary infection is acquired by inhalation of aerosolized *Cryptococcus* fungal elements found in contaminated soil and often is asymptomatic or mild in degree. Pulmonary disease, when symptomatic, is characterized by cough, chest pain, and constitutional symptoms. Chest radiographs may reveal solitary or multiple masses; patchy, segmental, or lobar consolidation, which often is multifocal; or nodular or reticulonodular interstitial changes. Pulmonary cryptococcosis may present as acute respiratory distress syndrome and may mimic *Pneumocystis* pneumonia. Hematogenous dissemination to the central nervous system (CNS), bones, skin, and other sites can occur, is uncommon, and almost always occurs in children with defects in T-lymphocyte–mediated immunity (eg, children with leukemia or lymphoma, children taking corticosteroids, children with congenital immunodeficiency or acquired immunodeficiency syndrome [AIDS], or children who have undergone solid organ transplantation). Usually several sites are infected, but manifestations of involvement at 1 site predominate. Cryptococcal meningitis, the most common and serious form of cryptococcal disease, often follows an indolent course. Symptoms are characteristic of meningitis, meningoencephalitis, or space-occupying lesions but can sometimes manifest only as subtle, nonspecific findings such as fever, headache, or behavioral changes. Cryptococcal fungemia without apparent organ involvement occurs in patients with human immunodeficiency virus (HIV) infection but is rare in children.

ETIOLOGY: Although there are more than 30 species of *Cryptococcus*, only 2 species, *Cryptococcus neoformans* (var *neoformans* and var *grubii*) and *Cryptococcus gattii* are regarded as human pathogens.

EPIDEMIOLOGY: *C neoformans* var *neoformans* and *C neoformans* var *grubii* are isolated primarily from soil contaminated with pigeon or other bird droppings and cause most human infections, especially infections in immunocompromised hosts. *C neoformans* infects 5% to 10% of adults with AIDS, but infection is rare in HIV-infected children. *C gattii* (formerly *C neoformans* var *gattii*) is associated with trees and surrounding soil and has emerged as a pathogen producing a respiratory syndrome with or without neurologic findings in individuals from British Columbia, Canada, the Pacific Northwest region of the United States, and occasionally other regions of the United States. A high frequency of disease has also been reported in Aboriginal people in Australia and in the central province of Papua New Guinea. *C gattii* causes disease in immunocompetent and immunocompromised people, and cases have been reported in children. Person-to-person transmission does not occur.

The **incubation period** for *C neoformans* is unknown but likely variable; dissemination often represents reactivation of latent disease acquired previously. For *C gattii*, the **incubation period** is 8 weeks to 13 months.

DIAGNOSTIC TESTS: The latex agglutination test, lateral flow assay, and enzyme immunoassay for detection of cryptococcal capsular polysaccharide antigen in serum or CSF specimens are excellent rapid diagnostic tests for those with suspected meningitis. Antigen is detected in cerebrospinal fluid (CSF) or serum specimens from more than 98% of patients with cryptococcal meningitis. In patients with cryptococcal meningitis, antigen test results can be falsely negative when antigen concentrations are low or very high (prozone effect), if infection is caused by unencapsulated strains, or if the patient is less severely immunocompromised.

Definitive diagnosis requires isolation of the organism from body fluid or tissue specimens. Blood should be cultured by lysis-centrifugation. Media containing cycloheximide, which inhibits growth of *C neoformans*, should not be used. Most laboratories confirm the production of urease by *Cryptococcus* species, noting that virtually all other fungi are urease negative (exceptions being *Trichosporon* species and some *Candida* species). The production of melanin by *Cryptococcus* species can be confirmed using Niger seed agar or using the caffeic acid disk test. Differentiation between *C neoformans* and *C gattii* can be made by the use of the selective medium L-canavanine glycine bromothymol blue (CGB) agar. *C gattii* will grow in the presence of L-canavanine, utilizing the glycine and causing the bromothymol indicator to turn the agar blue. *C neoformans* will not grow in presence of L-canavanine, and the agar remains unchanged. Sabouraud dextrose agar is useful for isolation of *Cryptococcus* organisms from sputum, bronchopulmonary lavage, tissue, or CSF specimens. In refractory or relapse cases, susceptibility testing can be helpful, although antifungal resistance is uncommon. CSF specimens may contain only a few organisms, and a large quantity of CSF may be needed to recover the organism. In children with central nervous system disease, CSF cell count and protein and glucose concentrations can be normal. Polymerase chain reaction assays are investigational. Encapsulated yeast cells can be visualized using India ink or other stains of CSF and bronchoalveolar lavage specimens, but this method has limited sensitivity. Focal pulmonary or skin lesions can be biopsied for fungal staining and culture.

TREATMENT: The Infectious Diseases Society of America has published practice management guidelines for cryptococcal disease.[1,2] Amphotericin B deoxycholate, 1 mg/kg/day (see Antifungal Drugs for Systemic Fungal Infections, p 905), in combination with oral flucytosine, 25 mg/kg/dose, 4 times/day, is indicated as initial therapy for patients with meningeal and other serious cryptococcal infections. Serum flucytosine concentrations should be maintained between 30 and 80 µg/mL. Patients with meningitis should receive combination therapy for at least 2 weeks followed by consolidation therapy with fluconazole (10-12 mg/kg, divided in 2 doses [maximum dose, 800 mg] daily) for a minimum of 8 weeks or until CSF culture is sterile. Alternatively, the amphotericin B deoxycholate and flucytosine combination can be continued for 6 to 10 weeks. Lipid formulations of amphotericin B can be used as a substitute for conventional amphotericin B in children with renal impairment. If flucytosine cannot be administered, amphotericin B alone is an acceptable alternative and is administered for 4 to 6 weeks. A lumbar puncture should be performed after 2 weeks of therapy to document microbiologic clearance. The 20% to 40% of patients in whom culture is positive after 2 weeks of therapy will require a more prolonged treatment course. When infection is refractory to systemic therapy, intraventricular amphotericin B can be administered. Monitoring of serum cryptococcal antigen is not useful to monitor response to therapy in patients with cryptococcal meningitis. Patients with less severe disease can be treated with fluconazole or itraconazole, but data on use of these drugs for children with *C neoformans* infection are limited. Another potential treatment option for HIV-infected patients with less severe disease or patients in whom amphotericin B treatment is not possible is combination therapy with fluconazole and flucytosine. The combination of fluconazole and flucytosine has superior efficacy compared with fluconazole alone. Echinocandins are not active against cryptococcal infections and should not be used.

Increased intracranial pressure occurs frequently despite microbiologic response and often is associated with clinical deterioration. Significant elevation of intracranial pressure

[1]Perfect J, Dismukes WE, Dromer F, et al. Clinical practice guidelines for the management of cryptococcal disease: 2010 update by the Infectious Diseases Society of America. *Clin Infect Dis.* 2010;50(3):291-322

[2]Panel on Opportunistic Infections in HIV-Exposed and HIV-Infected Children. Guidelines for the Prevention and Treatment of Opportunistic Infections in HIV-Exposed and HIV-Infected Children. Rockville, MD: US Department of Health and Human Services; 2013. Available at: **http://aidsinfo.nih.gov/contentfiles/lvguidelines/oi_guidelines_pediatrics.pdf**

is a major source of morbidity and should be managed with frequent repeated lumbar punctures or placement of a lumbar drain.

Children with HIV infection who have completed initial therapy for cryptococcosis should receive long-term suppressive therapy with fluconazole (6 mg/kg daily). Oral itraconazole daily or amphotericin B deoxycholate, 1 to 3 times weekly, are alternatives. Data regarding discontinuing this secondary prophylaxis after immune reconstitution as a consequence of antiretroviral therapy are available for adults but not for children. Discontinuing chronic suppressive therapy for cryptococcosis (after 1 year or longer of secondary prophylaxis) can be considered in asymptomatic children 6 years or older who are receiving antiretroviral therapy, have sustained ($\geq$6 months) increases in CD4+ T-lymphocyte counts to $\geq$100 cells/mm^3, and have an undetectable viral load for at least 3 months. Secondary prophylaxis should be reinstituted if the CD4+ T-lymphocyte count decreases to <100/mm^3. Most experts would not discontinue secondary prophylaxis for patients younger than 6 years.[1]

ISOLATION OF THE HOSPITALIZED PATIENT: Standard precautions are recommended.

CONTROL MEASURES: None.

Cryptosporidiosis

CLINICAL MANIFESTATIONS: Frequent, nonbloody, watery diarrhea is the most common manifestation of cryptosporidiosis, although infection can be asymptomatic. Other symptoms include abdominal cramps, fatigue, fever, vomiting, anorexia, and weight loss. In infected immunocompetent adults and children, diarrheal illness is self-limited, usually lasting 2 to 3 weeks. Infected immunocompromised hosts, such as children who have received solid organ transplants or who have advanced human immunodeficiency virus (HIV) disease, may experience profuse diarrhea lasting weeks to months; this can lead to malnutrition and wasting and, as such, could be a significant contributing factor leading to death. Extraintestinal cryptosporidiosis (ie, disease in the pulmonary or biliary tract or rarely in the pancreas) has been reported in immunocompromised people.

The diagnosis of cryptosporidiosis should be considered in any solid organ transplant or HIV patient with diarrhea. Delay in diagnosis and treatment can be associated with prolonged diarrhea and weight loss. Elevated tacrolimus concentrations have been reported in solid organ transplant patients, thought to be related to altered drug metabolism in the small intestine and resulting in acute kidney injury.

ETIOLOGY: *Cryptosporidium* species are oocyst-forming coccidian protozoa. Oocysts are excreted in feces of an infected host and are transmitted via the fecal-oral route. *Cryptosporidium hominis*, which predominantly infects people, and *Cryptosporidium parvum*, which infects people, preweaned calves, and other mammals, are the primary *Cryptosporidium* species that infect humans. *Cryptosporidium* has been detected in raw or unpasteurized milk or milk products.[2]

---

[1]Panel on Opportunistic Infections in HIV-Exposed and HIV-Infected Children. Guidelines for the Prevention and Treatment of Opportunistic Infections in HIV-Exposed and HIV-Infected Children. Rockville, MD: US Department of Health and Human Services; 2013. Available at: **http://aidsinfo.nih.gov/contentfiles/lvguidelines/oi_guidelines_pediatrics.pdf**

[2]American Academy of Pediatrics, Committee on Infectious Diseases, Committee on Nutrition. Consumption of raw or unpasteurized milk and milk products by pregnant women and children. *Pediatrics.* 2014;133(1):175-179

EPIDEMIOLOGY: Extensive waterborne disease outbreaks have been associated with contamination of drinking water and recreational water (eg, swimming pools, lakes, and interactive fountains). The incidence of cryptosporidiosis has been increasing since 2005 in the United States, culminating in the total (confirmed and probable) number of cases of cryptosporidiosis reported annually increasing 16.9% from 7656 for 2009 to 8951 for 2010.[1] A total (confirmed and probable) of 7956 cases were reported in 2012.[2] In children, the incidence of cryptosporidiosis is greatest during summer and early fall, corresponding to the outdoor swimming season. Cases are most frequently reported in children 1 to 4 years of age, followed by those 5 to 9 years of age. Disease in children with immune dysfunction, especially solid organ transplant patients or HIV infection, may be protracted and refractory to therapy.

Because oocysts are extremely chlorine tolerant, multistep treatment processes often are used to remove (eg, filter) and inactivate (eg, ultraviolet treatment) oocysts to protect public drinking water supplies. Typical filtration systems used for swimming pools are only partially effective in removing oocysts from contaminated water. As a result, *Cryptosporidium* species have become the leading cause of recreational water-associated outbreaks, being associated with 24 (69%) of 35 treated recreational water-associated outbreaks with identified infectious causes.[3]

In addition to waterborne transmission, humans can acquire infections from livestock; from animals found in petting zoos, particularly preweaned calves; or from pets. Person-to-person transmission occurs as well and can cause outbreaks in child care centers, in which up to 70% of attendees reportedly have been infected. *Cryptosporidium* species also can cause traveler's diarrhea (**www.cdc.gov/parasites/crypto/travelers.html**).

The **incubation period** usually is 3 to 14 days. Recurrence of symptoms after seeming resolution has been reported frequently. In immunocompetent people, oocyst shedding usually ceases within 2 weeks after complete symptom resolution. In immunocompromised people, the period of oocyst shedding can continue for months.

DIAGNOSTIC TESTS: Routine laboratory examination of stool for ova and parasites might not include testing for *Cryptosporidium* species, so testing for the organism should be requested specifically. The direct immunofluorescent antibody (DFA) method for detection of oocysts in stool is the current test of choice for diagnosis of cryptosporidiosis. The detection of oocysts on microscopic examination of stool specimens also is diagnostic. The formalin ethyl acetate stool concentration method is recommended before staining the stool specimen with a modified Kinyoun acid-fast stain. Oocysts generally are small (4–6 μm in diameter) and can be missed in a rapid scan of a slide.

Enzyme immunoassays (EIAs) and immune chromatographic tests (point-of-care rapid tests) for detecting antigen in stool are available commercially. When using rapid tests, follow the manufacturer's directions and consider confirmation by microscopy.

---

[1]Centers for Disease Control and Prevention. Cryptosporidiosis surveillance—United States, 2009–2010. *MMWR Surveill Summ.* 2012;61(SS–5):1–12. Available at **www.cdc.gov/mmwr/preview/mmwrhtml/ss6105a1.htm**

[2]Centers for Disease Control and Prevention. Summary of notifiable diseases, 2012. *MMWR Morb Mortal Wkly Rep.* 2014;61(53):1-121

[3]Centers for Disease Control and Prevention. Recreational water–associated disease outbreaks—United States, 2009–2010. *MMWR Morb Mortal Wkly Rep.* 2014;63(1):6–10. Available at: **www.cdc.gov/mmwr/pdf/wk/mm6301.pdf**

Because shedding can be intermittent, at least 3 stool specimens collected on separate days should be examined before considering test results to be negative. Organisms also can be identified in intestinal biopsy tissue or sampling of intestinal fluid.

TREATMENT: Generally, immunocompetent people need no specific therapy. A 3-day course of nitazoxanide oral suspension has been approved by the US Food and Drug Administration (FDA) for treatment of all people 1 year and older with diarrhea associated with cryptosporidiosis. The nitazoxanide dose for healthy children not infected with human immunodeficiency virus (HIV) is age based: 1 through 3 years of age, 100 mg orally, twice daily; 4 through 11 years, 200 mg orally, twice daily; ≥12 years, 500 mg orally, twice daily.

The appropriate treatment of cryptosporidiosis in children who are solid organ transplant recipients is not known, but longer courses of nitazoxanide (generally >14 days) have been recommended.

In HIV-infected patients, improvement in CD4+ T-lymphocyte count associated with antiretroviral therapy can lead to symptom resolution and cessation of oocyst shedding. For this reason, administration of combination antiretroviral therapy (cART) is the primary treatment for cryptosporidiosis in patients with HIV infection. In vitro and observational studies suggest cART containing a protease inhibitor might be preferable because of a direct effect of the protease inhibitor on the parasite. Given the seriousness of this infection in immunocompromised individuals, use of nitazoxanide can be considered in immunocompromised HIV-infected children in conjunction with cART for immune restoration. The recommended nitazoxanide dosing is the same as for immunocompetent people mentioned previously.[1]

Paromomycin, or a combination of paromomycin and azithromycin, might be effective, but few data regarding efficacy are available.

ISOLATION OF THE HOSPITALIZED PATIENT: In addition to standard precautions, contact precautions are recommended for diapered or incontinent people for the duration of illness or to control institutional outbreaks.

CONTROL MEASURES: The following measures should be provided for parents and can help prevent and control cryptosporidiosis:

- Wash hands with soap and water for at least 20 seconds, rubbing hands together vigorously and scrubbing all surfaces:
  - before preparing or eating food;
  - after using the toilet or assisting someone with using the toilet;
  - after changing a diaper or having a diaper changed;
  - after caring for someone who is ill with diarrhea; and
  - after handling an animal or its waste.
- Do not participate in recreational water activities, such as swimming, while ill with diarrhea and for 2 weeks after symptoms have completely resolved.
- Avoid ingestion of recreational water. For additional information, see Prevention of Illnesses Associated with Recreational Water Use (p 216).

---

[1]Panel on Opportunistic Infections in HIV-Exposed and HIV-Infected Children. Guidelines for the Prevention and Treatment of Opportunistic Infections in HIV-Exposed and HIV-Infected Children. Department of Health and Human Services. Available at: **http://aidsinfo.nih.gov/contentfiles/lvguidelines/oi _guidelines_pediatrics.pdf**

- The families of immunocompromised children should be educated about risk of swimming in recreational water.
- Exclude children ill with diarrhea from child care settings until diarrhea has resolved. (also see Children in Out-of-Home Child Care, p 132).
- Do not consume inadequately treated water or ice. This includes water or ice from lakes, rivers, springs, ponds, streams, or shallow wells.
- When traveling in countries where the drinking water supply might be unsafe, do not consume inadequately treated water or ice.
  - If the safety of drinking water is questionable:
    - Drink bottled water from an unopened, factory-sealed container.
    - Disinfect water by heating it to a rolling boil for 1 minute. The time of boiling (1 minute at sea level) will depend on altitude.
    - Use a filter that has been tested and rated by NSF Standard 53 or 58 for cyst and oocyst reduction/removal or has an absolute pore size of 1 mm or smaller; filtered water will need additional treatment to kill or inactivate bacteria and viruses.

For additional information on cryptosporidiosis prevention, visit the CDC Web site (**www.cdc.gov/parasites/crypto/prevention**).

Cutaneous Larva Migrans

CLINICAL MANIFESTATIONS: Nematode larvae produce pruritic, reddish papules at the site of skin entry, a condition referred to as creeping eruption. As the larvae migrate through skin, advancing several millimeters to a few centimeters a day, intensely pruritic serpiginous tracks or bullae are formed. This condition most often is caused by larvae of the dog and cat hookworm *Ancylostoma braziliense* but can be caused by other nematodes, including *Strongyloides* and human hookworm species. Larval activity can continue for several weeks or months, but the infection is self-limiting. The incubation period for cutaneous larva migrans typically is short, with signs and symptoms developing several days after larval penetration of the skin. However, in some cases, onset of disease may be delayed for weeks to months. Cutaneous larva migrans is a clinical diagnosis based on advancing serpiginous tracks in the skin with associated intense pruritus. Rarely, in infections with certain species of parasites, larvae may penetrate deeper tissues and cause pneumonitis (Löeffler syndrome), which can be severe. Occasionally, the larvae of *Ancylostoma caninum* can reach the intestine and may cause eosinophilic enteritis.

ETIOLOGY: Infective larvae of cat and dog hookworms (ie, *Ancylostoma braziliense* and *Ancylostoma caninum*) are the usual causes. Other skin-penetrating nematodes are occasional causes.

EPIDEMIOLOGY: Cutaneous larva migrans is a disease of children, utility workers, gardeners, sunbathers, and others who come in contact with soil contaminated with cat and dog feces. In the United States, the disease is most prevalent in the Southeast. Cases in the United States also can be imported by travelers returning from tropical and subtropical areas.

DIAGNOSTIC TESTS: The diagnosis is made clinically, and biopsies are not indicated. Biopsy specimens typically demonstrate an eosinophilic inflammatory infiltrate, but the migrating parasite is not visualized. Eosinophilia and increased immunoglobulin (Ig) E serum concentrations occur in some cases. Larvae have been detected in sputum and gastric washings in patients with the rare complication of pneumonitis. Enzyme immu-noassay or Western blot analysis using antigens of *A caninum* have been developed in research laboratories, but these assays are not available for routine diagnostic use.

TREATMENT: The disease usually is self-limited, with spontaneous cure after several weeks or months. Orally administered albendazole or ivermectin is the recommended therapy (see Drugs for Parasitic Infections, p 927).

ISOLATION OF THE HOSPITALIZED PATIENT: Standard precautions are recommended.

CONTROL MEASURES: Skin contact with moist soil contaminated with animal feces should be avoided. In warm climates, beaches should be kept free of dog and cat feces.

Cyclosporiasis

CLINICAL MANIFESTATIONS: Watery diarrhea is the most common symptom of cyclo-sporiasis and can be profuse and protracted. Anorexia, nausea, vomiting, substantial weight loss, flatulence, abdominal cramping, myalgia, and prolonged fatigue can occur. Low-grade fever occurs in approximately 50% of patients. Biliary tract disease has been reported. Infection usually is self-limited, but untreated people may have remitting, relaps-ing symptoms for weeks to months. Asymptomatic infection has been documented most commonly in settings where cyclosporiasis is endemic.

ETIOLOGY: *Cyclospora cayetanensis* is a coccidian protozoan; oocysts (rather than cysts) are passed in stools.

EPIDEMIOLOGY: *C cayetanensis* is known to be endemic in many resource-limited coun-tries and has been reported as a cause of traveler's diarrhea. Both foodborne and water-borne outbreaks have been reported. Most of the outbreaks in the United States and Canada have been associated with consumption of imported fresh produce. Humans are the only known hosts for *C cayetanensis*. Direct person-to-person transmission is unlikely, because excreted oocysts take days to weeks under favorable environmental conditions to sporulate and become infective. The oocysts are resistant to most disinfectants used in food and water processing and can remain viable for prolonged periods in cool, moist environments.

The **incubation period** typically is 1 week but can range from 2 days to 2 weeks.

DIAGNOSTIC TESTS: Diagnosis is made by identification of oocysts (8–10 μm in diam-eter) in stool, intestinal fluid/aspirate, or intestinal biopsy specimens. Oocysts may be shed at low levels, even by people with profuse diarrhea. This constraint underscores the utility of repeated stool examinations, sensitive recovery methods (eg, concentration procedures), and detection methods that highlight the organism. Oocysts are autofluorescent and are variably acid fast after modified acid fast staining of stool specimens. Investigational molecular diagnostic assays (eg, polymerase chain reaction) are available at the Centers for Disease Control and Prevention and some other reference laboratories.

TREATMENT: Trimethoprim-sulfamethoxazole, typically for 7 to 10 days, is the drug of choice. People infected with human immunodeficiency virus may need long-term mainte-nance therapy (see Drugs for Parasitic Infections, p 927).

ISOLATION OF THE HOSPITALIZED PATIENT: In addition to standard precautions, contact precautions are recommended for diapered or incontinent children.

CONTROL MEASURES: Avoiding food or water that may be contaminated with feces is the best way to prevent cyclosporiasis. Fresh produce always should be washed thoroughly before it is eaten. This precaution, however, may not eliminate the risk of transmission. Cyclosporiasis is a nationally notifiable disease and is a reportable disease in many states.

Cytomegalovirus Infection

CLINICAL MANIFESTATIONS: Manifestations of acquired human cytomegalovirus (CMV) infection vary with the age and immunocompetence of the host. Asymptomatic infections are the most common, particularly in children. An infectious mononucleosis-like syndrome with prolonged fever and mild hepatitis, occurring in the absence of heterophile antibody production ("monospot negative"), may occur in adolescents and adults. Pneumonia, colitis, retinitis, and a syndrome characterized by fever, thrombocytopenia, leukopenia, and mild hepatitis may occur in immunocompromised hosts, including people receiving treatment for malignant neoplasms, people infected with human immunodeficiency virus (HIV), and people receiving immunosuppressive therapy for organ or hematopoietic stem cell transplantation. Less commonly, patients treated with biologic response modifiers (see Biologic Response Modifiers Used to Decrease Inflammation, p 83) can exhibit CMV end-organ disease, such as retinitis and hepatitis.

Congenital infection has a spectrum of clinical manifestations but usually is not evident at birth (asymptomatic congenital CMV infection). Approximately 10% of infants with congenital CMV infection exhibit clinical findings that are evident at birth (symptomatic congenital CMV disease), with manifestations including intrauterine growth restriction, jaundice, purpura, hepatosplenomegaly, microcephaly, intracerebral (typically periventricular) calcifications, and retinitis; developmental delays are common among these infants in later infancy and early childhood. Death attributable to congenital CMV is estimated to occur in 3% to 10% of infants with symptomatic infections, or 0.3% to 1.0% of all infants with congenital CMV. Sensorineural hearing loss (SNHL) is the most common sequela following congenital CMV infection, with SNHL occurring in up to 50% of children with congenital infections that are symptomatic at birth and up to 15% of those with asymptomatic infections. Congenital CMV infection is the leading nongenetic cause of SNHL in children in the United States. Progressive SNHL can occur following symptomatic or asymptomatic congenital CMV infection, with 50% of affected children continuing to have further deterioration (progression) of their hearing loss. Between 55% and 75% of symptomatic and asymptomatic children, respectively, who ultimately develop congenital CMV-associated SNHL will not have hearing loss detectable within the first month of life, illustrating the high frequency of late-onset SNHL in these populations. For this reason, targeted CMV testing of infants who fail their universal newborn hearing screen will not detect the majority of infants who are at risk of CMV-associated hearing loss. Approximately 20% of all hearing loss at birth and 25% of all hearing loss at 4 years of age is attributable to congenital CMV infection. As such, children with symptomatic or asymptomatic congenital CMV infection should be evaluated regularly for early detection and appropriate intervention of suspected hearing losses.

Infection acquired from maternal cervical secretions during the intrapartum period, or in the postpartum period from human milk, usually is not associated with clinical illness in term babies. In preterm infants, however, postpartum infection resulting from human milk or from transfusion from CMV-seropositive donors has been associated with systemic infections, including hepatitis, interstitial pneumonia, hematologic abnormalities including thrombocytopenia and leukopenia, and a viral sepsis syndrome.

ETIOLOGY: Human CMV, also known as human herpesvirus 5, is a member of the herpesvirus family (*Herpesviridae*), the beta-herpesvirus subfamily (*Betaherpesvirinae*), and the *Cytomegalovirus* genus. The viral genome contains double-stranded DNA and at 196 000 to 240 000 bp encoding at least 166 proteins, is the largest of the human Herpesvirus genomes.

EPIDEMIOLOGY: CMV is highly species-specific, and only human CMV has been shown to infect humans and cause disease. The virus is ubiquitous, and CMV strains exhibit extensive genetic diversity. Transmission occurs horizontally (by direct person-to-person contact with virus-containing secretions), vertically (from mother to infant before, during, or after birth), and via transfusions of blood, platelets, and white blood cells from infected donors (see Blood Safety, p 112). CMV also can be transmitted with organ or hematopoietic stem cell transplantation. Infections have no seasonal predilection. CMV persists after a primary infection and intermittent virus shedding and symptomatic infection can occur throughout the lifetime of the infected person, particularly under conditions of immunosuppression. Reinfection with other strains of CMV can occur in seropositive hosts.

Horizontal transmission probably is the result of exposure to saliva and genital secretions from infected individuals, but contact with infected urine also can have a role. Spread of CMV in households and child care centers is well documented. Excretion rates from urine or saliva in children 1 to 3 years of age who attend child care centers usually range from 30% to 40% but can be as high as 70%. In addition, these children frequently excrete high quantities of virus. Young children can transmit CMV to their parents, including mothers who may be pregnant, and other caregivers, including child care staff (also see Children in Out-of-Home Child Care, p 132). In adolescents and adults, sexual transmission occurs, as evidenced by detection of virus in seminal and cervical fluids. As such, CMV is considered to be a sexually transmitted infection (STI).

CMV-seropositive healthy people have latent CMV in their leukocytes and tissues; hence, blood transfusions and organ transplantation can result in transmission. Severe CMV disease following transfusion or organ transplantation is more likely to occur if the recipient is immunosuppressed and CMV-seronegative or is a preterm infant. In contrast, among nonautologous hematopoietic stem cell transplant recipients, CMV-seropositive recipients who receive transplants from seronegative donors are at greatest risk of disease when exposed to CMV after transplant, perhaps secondary to the failure of transplanted graft to provide immunity to the recipient. Latent CMV may reactivate in immunosuppressed people and result in disease if immunosuppression is severe (eg, in patients with acquired immunodeficiency syndrome [AIDS] or solid organ or hematopoietic stem cell transplant recipients).

Vertical transmission of CMV to an infant occurs in one of the following time periods: (1) in utero by transplacental passage of maternal bloodborne virus; (2) at birth by passage through an infected maternal genital tract; or (3) postnatally by ingestion of CMV-positive human milk or by transfusion. Between 0.5% and 1% of all live-born infants are infected in utero and excrete CMV at birth, making this the most common congenital viral infection in the United States. In utero fetal infection can occur in women with no preexisting CMV immunity (maternal primary infection) or in women with preexisting antibody to CMV (maternal nonprimary infection) either by acquisition of a different viral strain during pregnancy or by reactivation of an existing maternal infection. Congenital infection and associated sequelae can occur irrespective of the trimester of pregnancy when the mother is infected, but severe sequelae are associated more commonly with primary maternal infection acquired during the first half of gestation. Damaging fetal infections following nonprimary maternal infection have been reported, and acquisition of a different viral strain during pregnancy in women with preexisting CMV antibody can cause symptomatic congenital infection with sequelae. It is estimated that more than two thirds of infants with congenital CMV infection in the United States are born to women with nonprimary infection, and the contribution of nonprimary maternal infection as a cause of damaging congenital CMV infection is believed to be common in populations with higher maternal CMV seroprevalence than that of the United States. Thus, the definition of protective immunity in congenital CMV infection remains contentious and is an active area of research.

Cervical excretion of CMV is common among seropositive women, resulting in exposure of many infants to CMV at birth. Cervical excretion rates are higher among young mothers in lower socioeconomic groups. Similarly, although disease can occur in seronegative infants fed CMV-infected human milk, most infants who acquire CMV from ingestion of infected human milk do not develop clinical illness or sequelae, most likely because of the presence of passively transferred maternal antibody. Among infants who acquire infection from maternal cervical secretions or human milk, preterm infants born before 32 weeks' gestation and with a birth weight less than 1500 g are at greater risk of CMV disease than are full-term infants.

The **incubation period** for horizontally transmitted CMV infections is unknown. Infection usually manifests 3 to 12 weeks after blood transfusions and between 1 and 4 months after organ transplantation. Experimental models have related the variations in incubation period to the size of the virus inoculum and route of infection.

DIAGNOSTIC TESTS: The diagnosis of CMV disease is confounded by the ubiquity of the virus, the high rate of asymptomatic excretion, the frequency of reactivated infections, the development of serum immunoglobulin (Ig) M CMV-specific antibody in some episodes of reactivation, reinfection with different strains of CMV, and concurrent infection with other pathogens.

Virus can be isolated in cell culture from urine, oral fluids, peripheral blood leukocytes, human milk, semen, cervical secretions, and other tissues and body fluids. Recovery of virus from a target organ provides strong evidence that the disease is caused by CMV infection. It is important to note that standard virus cultures must be maintained for >28 days prior to considering such cultures negative. In contrast, shell vial culture and immunofluorescence antibody (IFA) stain for immediate early antigen provides results within days. A presumptive diagnosis of CMV infection beyond the neonatal period has been associated with a fourfold antibody titer increase in paired serum specimens or by demonstration of virus excretion. Viral DNA can be detected by polymerase chain reaction assay in tissues and some fluids, such as cerebrospinal fluid (CSF), urine, and saliva. Detection of CMV DNA by polymerase chain reaction (PCR) assay in blood does not necessarily indicate acute infection or disease, especially in immunocompetent people. Detection of pp65 antigen or quantification of viral DNA (eg, by quantitative PCR assay) in white blood cells often is used to detect infection in immunocompromised hosts.

Various serologic assays, including immunofluorescence assays, latex agglutination assays, and enzyme immunoassays, are available for detecting CMV-specific antibodies.

Amniocentesis has been used in several small series of patients to establish the diagnosis of intrauterine infection. Following delivery, proof of congenital infection requires virologic detection of CMV in urine, oral fluids, respiratory tract secretions, blood, or CSF obtained within 2 to 4 weeks of birth. The analytical sensitivity of CMV DNA detection by PCR assay of dried blood spots is low, limiting use of this type of specimen for widespread screening for congenital CMV infection. A positive PCR assay result from a neonatal dried blood spot confirms congenital infection, but a negative result does not rule out congenital infection. Differentiation between intrauterine and perinatal infection is difficult at later than 2 to 4 weeks of age unless clinical manifestations of the former, such as chorioretinitis or intracranial calcifications, are present. A strongly positive CMV-specific IgM during early infancy can be suggestive of congenital CMV infection; however, IgM serologic methods commonly have reduced specificity and frequently result in false-positive results, making serologic diagnosis of congenital CMV infection problematic.

TREATMENT: Intravenous ganciclovir (see Non-HIV Antiviral Drugs, p 919) is approved for induction and maintenance treatment of retinitis caused by acquired or recurrent CMV infection in immunocompromised adult patients, including HIV-infected patients, and for prophylaxis and treatment of CMV disease in adult transplant recipients. Valganciclovir, the oral prodrug of ganciclovir, also is approved for treatment (induction and maintenance) of CMV retinitis in immunocompromised adult patients, including HIV-infected patients, and for prevention of CMV disease in kidney, kidney-pancreas, or heart transplant recipients at high risk of CMV disease. Valganciclovir also is approved for prevention of CMV disease in pediatric kidney or heart transplant patients 4 months and older. Ganciclovir and valganciclovir also are used to treat CMV infections of other sites (esophagus, colon, lungs) and for preemptive treatment of immunosuppressed adults with CMV antigenemia or viremia. Oral ganciclovir no longer is available in the United States, but oral valganciclovir is available in both tablet and powder for oral solution formulations.

Neonates with symptomatic congenital CMV disease with or without central nervous system (CNS) involvement have improved audiologic and neurodevelopmental outcomes at 2 years of age when treated with oral valganciclovir (16 mg/kg/dose, administered orally twice daily) for 6 months. The dose should be adjusted each month to account for weight gain. If an infant is unable to absorb medications reliably from the gastrointestinal tract (eg, because of necrotizing enterocolitis or other bowel disorders), intravenous ganciclovir at 6 mg/kg/dose provides systemic ganciclovir exposure that is similar to that provided by oral valganciclovir at 16 mg/kg/dose. Significant neutropenia occurs in one fifth of infants treated with oral valganciclovir and in two thirds of infants treated with parenteral ganciclovir. Absolute neutrophil counts should be performed weekly for 6 weeks, then at 8 weeks, then monthly for the duration of antiviral treatment; serum aminotransferase concentration should be measured monthly during treatment. Antiviral therapy should be limited to patients with symptomatic congenital CMV disease who are able to start treatment within the first month of life. Infants with asymptomatic congenital CMV infection should not receive antiviral treatment.

Preterm infants with perinatally acquired CMV infection can have symptomatic, end-organ disease (eg, pneumonitis, hepatitis, thrombocytopenia). Antiviral treatment has not been studied in this population. If such patients are treated with parenteral ganciclovir, a reasonable approach is to treat for 2 weeks and then reassess responsiveness to therapy. If clinical data suggest benefit of treatment, an additional 1 to 2 weeks of parenteral ganciclovir can be considered if symptoms and signs have not resolved.

In hematopoietic stem cell transplant recipients, the combination of Immune Globulin Intravenous (IGIV) or CMV Immune Globulin Intravenous (CMV-IGIV) and ganciclovir, administered intravenously, has been reported to be synergistic in treatment of CMV pneumonia. IGIV products, unlike CMV-IGIV, have varying anti-CMV antibody concentrations from lot to lot, are not tested routinely for their quantities of anti-CMV antibodies, and do not have a specified titer of antibodies to CMV that have correlated with efficacy. Valganciclovir and foscarnet also have been approved for treatment and maintenance of CMV retinitis in adults with acquired immunodeficiency syndrome (see Non-HIV Antiviral Drugs, p 919). Foscarnet is more toxic (with high rates of limiting nephrotoxicity) but may be advantageous for some patients with HIV infection, including people with disease caused by ganciclovir-resistant virus or people who are unable to tolerate ganciclovir. Cidofovir is efficacious for CMV retinitis in adults with AIDS, but cidofovir has not been studied in children and is associated with significant nephrotoxicity.

CMV establishes lifelong persistent infection, and as such, it is not eliminated from the body with antiviral treatment of CMV disease. Until immune reconstitution is achieved with antiretroviral therapy (ART), chronic suppressive therapy should be administered to HIV-infected patients with a history of CMV end-organ disease (eg, retinitis, colitis, pneumonitis) to prevent recurrence. Recognizing limitations of the pediatric data but drawing on the growing experience in adult patients, discontinuing prophylaxis may be considered for pediatric patients 6 years and older with CD4+ T-lymphocyte counts of >100 cells/mm^3 for >6 consecutive months and for children younger than 6 years with CD4+ T-lymphocyte percentages of >15% for >6 consecutive months. For immunocompromised children with CMV retinitis, such decisions should be made in close consultation with an ophthalmologist and should take into account such factors as magnitude and duration of CD4+ T-lymphocyte increase, anatomic location of the retinal lesion, vision in the contralateral eye, and the feasibility of regular ophthalmologic monitoring. All patients who have had anti-CMV maintenance therapy discontinued should continue to undergo regular ophthalmologic monitoring at a minimum of 3- to 6-month intervals for early detection of CMV relapse as well as immune reconstitution uveitis.[1]

ISOLATION OF THE HOSPITALIZED PATIENT: Standard precautions are recommended.

CONTROL MEASURES:

Care of Exposed People. When caring for children, hand hygiene, particularly after changing diapers, is advised to decrease transmission of CMV. Because asymptomatic excretion of CMV is common in people of all ages, a child with congenital CMV infection should not be treated differently from other children.

Although unrecognized exposure to people who are shedding CMV likely is common, concern may arise when immunocompromised patients or nonimmune pregnant women, including health care professionals, are exposed to patients with clinically recognizable CMV infection. Standard precautions should be sufficient to interrupt transmission of CMV (see Infection Control and Prevention for Hospitalized Children, p 161).

---

[1]Siberry GK, Abzug MJ, Nachman S, et al; Panel on Opportunistic Infections in HIV-Exposed and HIV-Infected Children. Guidelines for the prevention and treatment of opportunistic infections in HIV-exposed and HIV-infected children: recommendations from the National Institutes of Health, Centers for Disease Control and Prevention, the HIV Medicine Association of the Infectious Diseases Society of America, the Pediatric Infectious Diseases Society, and the American Academy of Pediatrics. *Pediatr Infect Dis J.* 2013;32(Suppl 2). Available at: **http://journals.lww.com/pidj/toc/2013/11002**

Child Care. Female child care workers in child care centers should be aware of CMV and its potential risks and should have access to appropriate hand hygiene measures to minimize occupationally acquired infection (**www.cdc.gov/cmv/index.html**; see discussion of CMV in Children in Out-of-Home Child Care, p 144).

Immunoprophylaxis. CMV-IGIV has been developed for prophylaxis of CMV disease in seronegative kidney, lung, liver, pancreas, and heart transplant recipients. CMV-IGIV seems to be moderately effective in kidney and liver transplant recipients and has been used in combination with antiviral agents. Results of an initial study of its use in pregnant women to prevent CMV transmission to the fetus were compromised by methodologic difficulties in the conduct of the trial, and a well-designed but relatively small second study failed to demonstrate benefit on decreasing the risk of congenital CMV infection or disease. Therefore, use of CMV-IGIV in pregnant women to prevent CMV transmission is not recommended at this time. The role of CMV-IGIV in the prevention of intrauterine transmission of CMV in pregnant women with primary CMV infection currently is being evaluated in a large prospective randomized clinical trial conducted by the National Institute of Child Health and Human Development Maternal and Fetal Medicine Network. Evaluation of investigational vaccines in healthy volunteers and renal transplant recipients is in progress, and 2 recent studies have provided provocative findings suggesting that such vaccines may be of value.

Prevention of Transmission by Blood Transfusion. Transmission of CMV by blood transfusion to newborn infants or other immune-compromised hosts virtually has been eliminated by use of CMV antibody-negative donors, by freezing red blood cells in glycerol before administration, by removal of the buffy coat, or by filtration to remove white blood cells.

Prevention of Transmission by Human Milk. Pasteurization or freezing of donated human milk can decrease the likelihood of CMV transmission. Holder pasteurization (62.5°C [144.5°F] for 30 minutes) and short-term pasteurization (72°C [161.6°F] for 5 seconds) of milk appear to inactivate CMV; short-term pasteurization may be less harmful to the beneficial constituents of human milk. Freezing milk at −20°C (−4°F) will decrease viral titers but does not eliminate CMV reliably. If fresh donated milk is needed for infants born to CMV antibody-negative mothers, providing these infants with milk from only CMV antibody-negative women should be considered. For further information on human milk banks, see Human Milk (p 125).

Prevention of Transmission in Transplant Recipients. CMV antibody-negative recipients of tissue from CMV-seropositive donors are at high risk of CMV disease. If such circumstances cannot be avoided, prophylactic administration of antiviral therapy or monitoring for viremia and administering preemptive antiviral therapy have been shown to be clearly beneficial in decreasing the incidence of CMV disease in these patients.

Dengue

CLINICAL MANIFESTATIONS: Dengue has a wide range of clinical presentations, from asymptomatic infection to classic dengue fever and severe dengue (ie, dengue hemorrhagic fever or dengue shock syndrome). Approximately 5% of patients develop severe dengue, which is more common with second or other subsequent infections. Less common clinical syndromes include myocarditis, pancreatitis, hepatitis, and neuroinvasive disease.

Dengue begins with a nonspecific, acute febrile illness lasting 2 to 7 days (**febrile phase**), often accompanied by muscle, joint, and/or bone pain, headache, retro-orbital pain, facial erythema, injected oropharynx, macular or maculopapular rash, leukopenia,

and petechiae or other minor bleeding manifestations. During fever defervescence, usually on days 3–7 of illness, an increase in vascular permeability in parallel with increasing
hematocrit (hemoconcentration) may occur. The period of clinically significant plasma
leakage usually lasts 24 to 48 hours (**critical phase**), followed by a **convalescent
phase** with gradual improvement and stabilization of the hemodynamic status. Warning
signs of progression to severe dengue occur in the late febrile phase and include persistent
vomiting, severe abdominal pain, mucosal bleeding, difficulty breathing, early signs of
shock, and a rapid decline in platelet count with an increase in hematocrit. Patients with
nonsevere disease begin to improve during the critical phase, but people with clinically
significant plasma leakage attributable to increased vascular permeability develop severe
disease with pleural effusions and/or ascites, hypovolemic shock, and hemorrhage.

ETIOLOGY: Four related RNA viruses of the genus *Flavivirus* (see Arboviruses, p 240), dengue viruses (DENV)-1, -2, -3, and -4, cause symptomatic (approx 25%) and asymptomatic
(approx 75%) infections. Infection with one DENV type produces lifelong immunity
against that type and a very short period of cross-protection against infection with the
other 3 types of DENV. After this short period of cross-protection, infection with a different strain may predispose to more severe disease. A person has a lifetime risk of up to
4 DENV infections.

EPIDEMIOLOGY: DENV primarily is transmitted to humans through the bite of infected
Aedes aegypti (and less commonly *Aedes albopictus* or *Aedes polynesiensis*) mosquitoes. Humans
are the main amplifying host of DENV and the main source of virus for *Aedes* mosquitoes. A sylvatic nonhuman primate DENV transmission cycle exists in parts of Africa
and Southeast Asia but rarely crosses to humans. Because of the approximately 7 days of
viremia, DENV can be transmitted following receipt of blood products, donor organs, or
tissue; percutaneous exposure to blood; and exposure in utero or at parturition.

   Dengue is a major public health problem in the tropics and subtropics; an estimated
50 to 100 million dengue cases occur annually in more than 100 countries, and 40%
of the world's population lives in areas with DENV transmission. In the United States,
dengue is endemic in Puerto Rico, the Virgin Islands, and American Samoa. In addition,
millions of US travelers, including children, are at risk, because dengue is the leading
cause of febrile illness among travelers returning from the Caribbean, Latin America, and
South Asia. Outbreaks with local DENV transmission have occurred in Texas, Hawaii,
and Florida in the last decade (see Table 3.2, p 242). However, although 16 states have
A aegypti and 35 states have *A albopictus* mosquitoes, local dengue transmission is uncommon because of infrequent contact between people and infected mosquitoes. Dengue
occurs in both children and adults. It is most likely to cause severe disease in young
children and women, especially pregnant women, and in patients with chronic diseases
(asthma, sickle cell anemia, and diabetes mellitus).

   The **incubation period** for DENV replication in mosquitoes is 8 to 12 days (extrin-
sic incubation); mosquitoes remain infectious for life. In humans, the **incubation period**
is 3 to 14 days before symptom onset (intrinsic incubation). Infected people, both symptomatic and asymptomatic, can transmit DENV to mosquitoes 1 to 2 days before symptoms develop and throughout the approximately 7-day viremic period.

DIAGNOSTIC TESTS: Laboratory confirmation of the clinical diagnosis of dengue can be
made on a single serum specimen obtained during the febrile phase of the illness by testing for DENV either by detection of DENV RNA by reverse transcriptase-polymerase

chain reaction (RT-PCR) assay or detection of DENV nonstructural protein 1 (NS-1) antigen by immunoassay and testing for anti-DENV immunoglobulin (Ig) M antibodies by enzyme immunoassay (EIA). DENV is detectable by RT-PCR or NS1 antigen EIAs from the beginning of the febrile phase until day 7 to 10 after illness onset, but anti-DENV IgM antibodies are not detectable until at least 5 days after illness onset. Other tests, such as IgG anti-DENV EIA and hemagglutination inhibition assay, are not as specific for making the diagnosis of dengue. Anti-DENV IgG antibody remains elevated for life after DENV infection and often is falsely positive in people with prior infection with or immunization against other flaviviruses (eg, West Nile, Japanese encephalitis, or yellow fever viruses). A fourfold or greater increase in anti-DENV IgG antibody titers between the acute (≤5 days after onset of symptoms) and convalescent (>15 days after onset of symptoms) samples confirms recent infection. A single anti-DENV IgG antibody titer of ≥ 1:1280 is highly suggestive of a dengue diagnosis. Dengue diagnostic testing is available through commercial reference laboratories and some state public health laboratories; reference testing is available from the Dengue Branch of the Centers for Disease Control and Prevention (**www.cdc.gov/dengue/**).

TREATMENT: No specific antiviral therapy exists for dengue. During the febrile phase, patients should stay well hydrated and avoid use of aspirin (acetylsalicylic acid), salicylate-containing drugs, and other nonsteroidal anti-inflammatory drugs (eg, ibuprofen) to minimize the potential for bleeding. Additional supportive care is required if the patient becomes dehydrated or develops warning signs of severe disease at the time of fever defervescence.

Early recognition of shock and intensive supportive therapy can reduce risk of death from approximately 10% to less than 1% in severe dengue. During the critical phase, maintenance of fluid volume and hemodynamic status is crucial to management of severe cases. Patients should be monitored for early signs of shock, occult bleeding, and resolution of plasma leak to avoid prolonged shock, end organ damage, and fluid overload. Patients with refractory shock may require intravenous colloids and/or blood or blood products after an initial trial of intravenous crystalloids. Reabsorption of extravascular fluid occurs during the convalescent phase with stabilization of hemodynamic status and diuresis. It is important to watch for signs of fluid overload, which may manifest as a decrease in the patient's hematocrit as a result of the dilutional effect of reabsorbed fluid.

ISOLATION OF THE HOSPITALIZED PATIENT: Standard precautions are recommended, with attention to the potential for bloodborne transmission. When indicated, attention should be given to control of *Aedes* mosquitoes to prevent secondary transmission of DENV from patients to others.

CONTROL MEASURES: Vaccines are not available to prevent dengue. A number of candidates are in clinical trials to evaluate immunogenicity, safety, and efficacy, as are innovative approaches to vector control. No chemoprophylaxis or antiviral medication is available to treat patients with dengue. People traveling to areas with endemic dengue (see DengueMap: **www.healthmap.org/dengue/**) are at risk of dengue and should take precautions to protect themselves from mosquito bites. Travelers should select accommodations that are air conditioned and/or have screened windows and doors. *Aedes* mosquitoes bite during the daytime, so bed nets are indicated for children sleeping during the day. Travelers should wear clothing that fully covers arms and legs, especially during early morning and late afternoon. Use of mosquito repellents containing up to 50%

N,N-diethyl-meta-toluamide (DEET) for adults (including pregnant women) and up to 30% DEET for children older than 2 months is recommended when used accordingly to the product directions (see Prevention of Mosquitoborne Infections, p 213).

Dengue, acquired locally in the United States and during travel, became a nationally notifiable disease in 2010. Suspected cases should be reported to state health departments.

Diphtheria

CLINICAL MANIFESTATIONS: Respiratory tract diphtheria usually occurs as membranous nasopharyngitis or obstructive laryngotracheitis. Membranous pharyngitis associated with a bloody nasal discharge should suggest diphtheria. Local infections are associated with a low-grade fever and gradual onset of manifestations over 1 to 2 days. Less commonly, diphtheria presents as cutaneous, vaginal, conjunctival, or otic infection. Cutaneous diphtheria is more common in tropical areas and among the urban homeless. Extensive neck swelling with cervical lymphadenitis (bull neck) is a sign of severe disease. Life-threatening complications of respiratory diphtheria include upper airway obstruction caused by extensive membrane formation; myocarditis, which often is associated with heart block; and cranial and peripheral neuropathies. Palatal palsy, characterized by nasal speech, frequently occurs in pharyngeal diphtheria.

ETIOLOGY: Diphtheria is caused by toxigenic strains of *Corynebacterium diphtheriae*. In industrialized countries, toxigenic strains of *Corynebacterium ulcerans* are emerging as an important cause of a diphtheria-like illness. *C diphtheriae* is an irregularly staining, gram-positive, nonspore-forming, nonmotile, pleomorphic bacillus with 4 biotypes (*mitis, intermedius, gravis,* and *belfanti*). All biotypes of *C diphtheriae* may be either toxigenic or nontoxigenic. The bacteria remain confined to the superficial layers of skin or respiratory mucosa and induce a local inflammatory reaction. Within the first several days of respiratory tract infection, a dense pseudomembrane forms and becomes adherent to the local tissue. Toxigenic strains express an exotoxin that consists of an enzymatically active A domain and a binding B domain, which promotes the entry of A into the cell. The toxin gene, *tox,* is carried by a family of related corynebacteria phages. The toxin, an ADP-ribosylase toxin, inhibits protein synthesis in all cells, including myocardial, renal, and peripheral nerve cells, resulting in myocarditis, acute tubular necrosis, and delayed peripheral nerve conduction. Nontoxigenic strains of *C diphtheriae* can cause sore throat and, rarely, other invasive infections, including endocarditis and foreign body infections.

EPIDEMIOLOGY: Humans are the sole reservoir of *C diphtheriae*. Organisms are spread by respiratory tract droplets and by contact with discharges from skin lesions. In untreated people, organisms can be present in discharges from the nose and throat and from eye and skin lesions for 2 to 6 weeks after infection. Patients treated with an appropriate antimicrobial agent usually are not communicable 48 hours after treatment is initiated. Transmission results from intimate contact with patients or carriers. People who travel to areas where diphtheria is endemic or people who come into contact with infected travelers from such areas are at increased risk of being infected with the organism; rarely, fomites and raw milk or milk products can serve as vehicles of transmission. Severe disease occurs more often in people who are unimmunized or inadequately immunized. Fully immunized people may be asymptomatic carriers or have mild sore throat. The incidence of respiratory diphtheria is greatest during autumn and winter, but summer epidemics can occur in warm climates in which skin infections are prevalent. During the

1990s, epidemic diphtheria occurred throughout the newly independent states of the former Soviet Union, with case-fatality rates ranging from 3% to 23%. Diphtheria remains endemic in these countries as well as in countries in Africa, Latin America, Asia, the Middle East, and parts of Europe, where childhood immunization coverage with diphtheria toxoid-containing vaccines is suboptimal (**www.cdc.gov/travel/yellowbook**). During 2012, one probable case of diphtheria was reported in the United States, representing the first case since 2003.[1] Cases of cutaneous diphtheria likely still occur in the United States, but only respiratory tract cases are included for national notification.

The **incubation period** usually is 2 to 5 days (range, 1–10 days).

DIAGNOSTIC TESTS: Specimens for culture should be obtained from the nose or throat and any mucosal or cutaneous lesion. Material should be obtained from beneath the membrane, or a portion of the membrane itself should be submitted for culture. Because special medium is required for isolation (eg, cystine-tellurite blood agar or modified Tinsdale agar), laboratory personnel should be notified that *C diphtheriae* is suspected. Specimens collected for culture can be placed in any transport medium (eg, Amies, Stuart media) or in a sterile container and transported at 4°C or in silica gel packs to a reference laboratory for culture. When *C diphtheriae* is recovered from a patient with suspected diphtheria, the strain should be tested for toxigenicity at a laboratory recommended by state or local authorities. All *C diphtheriae* isolates should be sent through the state health department to the Centers for Disease Control and Prevention (CDC).

TREATMENT:

Antitoxin. Because the condition of patients with diphtheria may deteriorate rapidly, a single dose of equine antitoxin should be administered on the basis of clinical diagnosis, even before culture results are available. Antitoxin and its indications for use and instructions for administration are available through the CDC (CDC Emergency Operations Center, 770-488-7100; **www.cdc.gov/diphtheria/dat.html**). To neutralize toxin from the organism as rapidly as possible, intravenous administration of the antitoxin is preferred. Before intravenous administration of antitoxin, tests for sensitivity to horse serum should be performed, initially with a scratch test. Allergic reactions of variable severity to horse serum can be expected in 5% to 20% of patients. The dose of antitoxin depends on the site and size of the diphtheria membrane, duration of illness, and degree of toxic effects; presence of soft, diffuse cervical lymphadenitis suggests moderate to severe toxin absorption. Suggested dose ranges are: pharyngeal or laryngeal disease of 2 days' duration or less, 20 000 to 40 000 U; nasopharyngeal lesions, 40 000 to 60 000 U; extensive disease of 3 or more days' duration or diffuse swelling of the neck, 80 000 to 120 000 U. Antitoxin probably is of no value for cutaneous disease, but some experts recommend 20 000 to 40 000 U of antitoxin, because toxic sequelae have been reported. Although the FDA specifies that all Immune Globulin Intravenous (IGIV) preparations must have a minimum concentration of antibodies to *C diphtheriae*, use of IGIV for therapy of cutaneous or respiratory diphtheria has not been approved or evaluated for efficacy.

Antimicrobial Therapy. Erythromycin administered orally or parenterally for 14 days, aqueous penicillin G administered intravenously for 14 days, or penicillin G procaine administered intramuscularly for 14 days constitute acceptable therapy. Antimicrobial

[1]Centers for Disease Control and Prevention. Summary of notifiable diseases, 2012. *MMWR Morb Mortal Wkly Rep.* 2014;61(53):1-121

therapy is required to stop toxin production, to eradicate the *C diphtheriae* organism, and to prevent transmission, but it is not a substitute for antitoxin, which is the primary therapy. Elimination of the organism should be documented 24 hours after completion of treatment by 2 consecutive negative cultures from specimens taken 24 hours apart.

Immunization. Active immunization against diphtheria should be undertaken during convalescence from diphtheria; disease does not necessarily confer immunity.

Cutaneous Diphtheria. Thorough cleansing of the lesion with soap and water and administration of an appropriate antimicrobial agent for 10 days are recommended.

Carriers. If not immunized, carriers should receive active immunization promptly, and measures should be taken to ensure completion of the immunization schedule. If a carrier has been immunized previously but has not received a booster of diphtheria toxoid within 5 years, a booster dose of a vaccine containing diphtheria toxoid (DTaP, Tdap, DT, or Td, depending on age) should be given. Tdap is preferred over Td if the patient is 11 years or older and has not received Tdap previously. Carriers should be given oral erythromycin for 10 to 14 days or a single intramuscular dose of penicillin G benzathine (600 000 U for children weighing less than 30 kg, and 1.2 million U for children weighing 30 kg or more and adults). Two follow-up cultures should be obtained after completing antimicrobial treatment to ensure detection of relapse, which occurs in as many as 20% of patients treated with erythromycin. The first culture should be obtained 24 hours after completing treatment. If results of cultures are positive, an additional 10-day course of oral erythromycin should be given, and follow-up cultures should be performed again. Erythromycin-resistant strains have been identified, but their epidemiologic significance has not been determined. Fluoroquinolones (see Fluoroquinolones, p 872), rifampin, clarithromycin, and azithromycin have good in vitro activity and may be better tolerated than erythromycin, but these drugs have not been evaluated in clinical infection or in carriers.

ISOLATION OF THE HOSPITALIZED PATIENT: In addition to standard precautions, droplet precautions are recommended for patients and carriers with pharyngeal diphtheria until 2 cultures from both the nose and throat collected 24 hours after completing antimicrobial treatment are negative for *C diphtheriae*. Contact precautions are recommended for patients with cutaneous diphtheria until 2 cultures of skin lesions taken at least 24 hours apart and 24 hours after cessation of antimicrobial therapy are negative.

CONTROL MEASURES:

Care of Exposed People. Whenever respiratory diphtheria is suspected or proven, local public health officials should be notified promptly. Cutaneous diphtheria is not included for national notification. All diphtheria isolates should be sent to the CDC through the state health department. Management of exposed people is based on individual circumstances, including immunization status and likelihood of adherence to follow-up and prophylaxis. The following are recommended:

- Close contacts of a person suspected to have diphtheria should be identified promptly. Contact tracing should begin in the household and usually can be limited to household members and other people with a history of direct, habitual close contact (including kissing or sexual contacts), health care personnel exposed to nasopharyngeal secretions, people sharing utensils or kitchen facilities, and people caring for infected children.
- For close contacts, *regardless of their immunization status,* the following measures should be taken: (1) surveillance for 7 days for evidence of disease; (2) culture for *C diphtheriae;* and (3) antimicrobial prophylaxis with oral erythromycin (40–50 mg/kg per day for 7 to

10 days, maximum 1 g/day) or a single intramuscular injection of penicillin G benzathine (600 000 U for children weighing less than 30 kg, and 1.2 million U for children weighing 30 kg or more and adults). The efficacy of antimicrobial prophylaxis is presumed but not proven. Follow-up cultures of pharyngeal specimens should be performed after completion of therapy for contacts proven to be carriers after completion of therapy (see Carriers, p 327). If cultures are positive, an additional 10-day course of erythromycin should be given, and follow-up cultures of pharyngeal specimens again should be performed.

- Asymptomatic, previously immunized close contacts should receive a booster dose of an age-appropriate diphtheria toxoid-containing vaccine (DTaP [or DT], Tdap, or Td) if they have not received a booster dose of a diphtheria toxoid-containing vaccine within 5 years (Tdap [11 years older] is preferred over Td, if the person previously has not received pertussis booster vaccine).
- Asymptomatic close contacts who have had fewer than 3 doses of a diphtheria toxoid-containing vaccine, children younger than 7 years of age in need of their fourth dose of DTaP (or DT), or people whose immunization status is not known should be immunized with an age-appropriate diphtheria toxoid-containing vaccine (DTaP [or DT], Tdap, or Td, as indicated).
- Contacts who cannot be kept under surveillance should receive penicillin G benzathine but not erythromycin, because adherence to an oral regimen is less likely, and if not fully immunized or if immunization status is not known they should be immunized with DTaP, Tdap, DT, or Td vaccine, as appropriate for age.
- Use of equine diphtheria antitoxin in unimmunized close contacts is not recommended, because there is no evidence that antitoxin provides additional benefit for contacts who have received antimicrobial prophylaxis.

Immunization. Universal immunization with a diphtheria toxoid-containing vaccine is the only effective control measure. The schedules for immunization against diphtheria are presented in the childhood and adolescent (**http://aapredbook.aappublications .org/site/resources/izschedules.xhtml**) and adult (**www.cdc.gov/vaccines**) immunization schedules. The benefit of diphtheria toxoid immunization is proven by the rarity of disease in countries in which high rates of immunization with diphtheria toxoid-containing vaccines have been achieved. The decreased frequency of endogenous exposure to the organism in countries with high childhood coverage rates implies decreased boosting of immunity. Therefore, ensuring continuing immunity requires regular booster injections of diphtheria toxoid (as Tdap once; see Pertussis, p 609) or as Td vaccine every 10 years after completion of the initial immunization series.

Pneumococcal and meningococcal conjugate vaccines containing diphtheria toxoid or CRM_{197} protein, a nontoxic variant of diphtheria toxin, are not substitutes for diphtheria toxoid immunization.

Immunization of children from 2 months of age to the seventh birthday (**http:// aapredbook.aappublications.org/site/resources/izschedules.xhtml**) routinely consists of 5 doses of diphtheria and tetanus toxoid-containing and acellular pertussis vaccines (DTaP vaccine). Immunization against diphtheria and tetanus for children younger than 7 years in whom pertussis immunization is contraindicated (see Pertussis, p 608) should be accomplished with DT instead of DTaP vaccine (see Tetanus, p 773).

Other recommendations for diphtheria immunization, including recommendations for older children (7 through 18 years of age) and adults, can be found in the recommended childhood and adolescent (**http://aapredbook.aappublications.org/site/resources/izschedules.xhtml**) and adult (**www.cdc.gov/vaccines**) immunization schedules.

When children and adults require tetanus toxoid for wound management (see Tetanus, p 773), the use of preparations containing diphtheria toxoid (DTaP, Tdap, DT, or Td vaccine, as appropriate for age or for a specific contraindication to pertussis immunization) is preferred to tetanus toxoid and will help to maintain diphtheria and, when appropriate, pertussis immunity.

Travelers to countries with endemic or epidemic diphtheria should have their diphtheria immunization status reviewed and updated when necessary.

Precautions and Contraindications. See Pertussis (p 608) and Tetanus (p 773).

Ehrlichia, Anaplasma, and Related Infections
(Human Ehrlichiosis, Anaplasmosis, and Related Infections)

CLINICAL MANIFESTATIONS: Infections by members of the bacterial family *Anaplasmataceae* (genera *Anaplasma*, *Ehrlichia*, *Neorickettsia*, and the proposed genus *Neoehrlichia*) cause human illness with similar signs, symptoms, and clinical courses. All are acute, systemic, febrile illnesses, with common systemic manifestations including fever, headache, chills, malaise, myalgia, and nausea. More variable symptoms include arthralgia, vomiting, diarrhea, cough, and confusion. Rash is more commonly reported for *Ehrlichia* infections than *Anaplasma* infections but still occurs in only a minority of adult patients; it may be more common in children infected with *Ehrlichia* (up to 60% of cases). More severe manifestations of these diseases may include acute respiratory distress syndrome, encephalopathy, meningitis, disseminated intravascular coagulation, spontaneous hemorrhage, and renal failure. Significant laboratory findings in *Anaplasma* and *Ehrlichia* infections may include leukopenia, lymphopenia, thrombocytopenia, hyponatremia, and elevated serum hepatic transaminase concentrations. Cerebrospinal fluid abnormalities (ie, pleocytosis with a predominance of lymphocytes and increased total protein concentration) are common. Neorickettsiosis is characterized by lymphadenopathy, a sign that is not commonly seen with infections by other members of this bacterial family. As also occurs with ehrlichiosis and anaplasmosis, neoehrlichiosis patients often have had leukocytosis and elevated C-reactive protein concentrations, but liver transaminase levels usually are within normal ranges. Most reported cases of neoehrlichiosis have been in people with underlying immunosuppressive conditions.

Without treatment, symptoms typically last 1 to 2 weeks, but prompt antimicrobial therapy will shorten the duration and reduce the risk of serious manifestations and sequelae. Following infection, fatigue may last several weeks; some reports suggest the occurrence of neurologic complications in some children after severe disease, and more commonly with *Ehrlichia* infections. Fatal infections have been reported more commonly for *Ehrlichia chaffeensis* infections (approximately 1%–3% case fatality) than for anaplasmosis (less than 1% case fatality). One fatal case has been reported for *Neoehrlichia* infection. Typically, *E chaffeensis* presents with more severe disease than does *Anaplasma phagocytophilum*. Secondary or opportunistic infections may occur in severe illness, resulting in a delay in recognition and administration of appropriate antimicrobial treatment. People with underlying immunosuppression are at greater risk of severe disease. Severe disease has been reported in people who initially received trimethoprim-sulfamethoxazole before a correct diagnosis was confirmed.

Ehrlichia and *Anaplasma* species do not cause vasculitis or endothelial cell damage characteristic of some other rickettsial diseases. However, because of the nonspecific presenting symptoms, Rocky Mountain spotted fever should be considered in the differential diagnosis of tickborne Anaplasmataceae infections in the United States. The recently discovered, tickborne Heartland virus also can present similarly; health care providers should consider Heartland virus testing in patients who develop fever, leukopenia, and thrombocytopenia without a more likely explanation and who have tested negative for *Ehrlichia* and *Anaplasma* infection or have not responded to doxycycline therapy.[1]

ETIOLOGY: In the United States, human ehrlichiosis and anaplasmosis are caused by at least 4 different species of obligate intracellular bacteria: *E chaffeensis*, *Ehrlichia ewingii*, *Ehrlichia muris*-like agent, and *A phagocytophilum* (Table 3.3). *Ehrlichia* and *Anaplasma* species are gram-negative cocci that measure 0.5 to 1.5 μm in diameter with tropisms for different white blood cell types. In other parts of the world, human *Ehrlichia canis* and *Anaplasma platys* have been reported in only a few cases. *E muris* is suspected to cause disease in Russia and Japan. *Neorickettsia sennetsu* may cause illness in Asia, while the organism designated as *Neoehrlichia mikurensis* has been found in various European and Asian countries.

EPIDEMIOLOGY: In the United States, the reported incidences of *E chaffeensis* and *A phagocytophilum* infections during 2012 were 3.8 and 8.0 cases per million population, respectively. These diseases are underrecognized, and selected active surveillance programs have shown the incidence to be substantially higher in some areas with endemic infection. Most cases of *E chaffeensis* and *E ewingii* infection are reported from the south central and southeastern United States, as well as East Coast states. Ehrlichiosis caused by *E chaffeensis* and *E ewingii* are associated with the bite of the lone star tick *(Amblyomma americanum)*. To date, cases attributable to the new *E muris*-like agent have been reported only from Minnesota and Wisconsin. Most cases of human anaplasmosis have been reported from the upper Midwest and northeast United States (eg, Wisconsin, Minnesota, Connecticut, and New York) and northern California. In most of the United States, *A phagocytophilum* is transmitted by the blacklegged tick *(Ixodes scapularis)*, which also is the vector for Lyme disease *(Borrelia burgdorferi)* and babesiosis *(Babesia microti)*. This tick also is suspected to be a vector for the *E muris*-like agent. In the western United States, the western blacklegged tick *(Ixodes pacificus)* is the main vector for *A phagocytophilum*. Various mammalian wildlife reservoirs for the agents of human ehrlichiosis and anaplasmosis have been identified, including white-tailed deer and wild rodents. In other parts of the world, other bacterial species of this family are transmitted by the endemic tick vectors for that area. An exception is *N sennetsu*, which occurs in Asia and is transmitted through ingestion of infected trematodes residing in fish.

Reported cases of symptomatic ehrlichiosis and anaplasmosis characteristically are in older people, with age-specific incidences greatest in people older than 40 years. However, seroprevalence data indicate that exposure to *E chaffeensis* may be common in children. In the United States, most human infections occur between April and September, and the

---

[1]Centers for Disease Control and Prevention. Notes from the field: heartland virus disease—United States, 2012–2013. *MMWR Morb Mortal Wkly Rep.* 2014;63(12):270-271

Table 3.3. Human Ehrlichiosis, Anaplasmosis, and Related Infections

Disease	Causal Agent	Major Target Cell	Tick Vector	Geographic Distribution
Ehrlichiosis caused by *Ehrlichia chaffeensis* (also known as human monocytic ehrlichiosis, or HME)	*E chaffeensis*	Usually monocytes	Lone star tick *(Amblyomma americanum)*	USA: Predominantly southeast, south central, and east coast states; has been reported outside USA
Anaplasmosis (also known as human granulocytic anaplasmosis, or HGA)	*Anaplasma phagocytophilum*	Usually granulocytes	Blacklegged tick *(Ixodes scapularis)* or Western blacklegged tick *(Ixodes pacificus)*	USA: Northeastern and upper Midwestern states and northern California; Europe and Asia
Ehrlichiosis caused by *Ehrlichia ewingii*	*E ewingii*	Usually granulocytes	Lone star tick *(A americanum)*	USA: Southeastern, south central, and Midwestern states; Africa, Asia
Ehrlichiosis caused by *Ehrlichia muris*-like agent	*E muris*-like agent	Unknown, suspected in monocytes	*I scapularis* is identified as a possible vector	USA: Minnesota, Wisconsin
Ehrlichiosis caused by *Ehrlichia muris*	*Ehrlichia muris sensu stricto*	Unknown, suspected in monocytes	*Ixodes persulcatus, Ixodes ovatus*	Asia
Thrombocytic anaplasmosis	*Anaplasma platys*	Platelets	*Rhipicephalus sanguineus (suspected)*	Venezuela
Ehrlichiosis caused by *Ehrlichia canis*	*E canis*	Monocytes	*Rhipicephalus sanguineus (suspected)*	Venezuela
Neorickettsiosis, sennetsu fever, glandular fever	*Neorickettsia sennetsu*	Monocytes	Ingestion of infected trematodes residing in fish	Japan, Malaysia, Laos
Neoehrlichiosis	Candidatus *Neoehrlichia mikurensis*	Unknown	*Ixodes ricinus, Ixodes persulcatus, Haemaphysalis flava*	Europe and Asia

peak occurrence is from May through July. Coinfections of anaplasmosis with other tick-borne diseases, including babesiosis and Lyme disease, may cause illnesses that are more severe or of longer duration than a single infection. A possible case of perinatal transmission of *A phagocytophilum* has been reported. Ehrlichiosis and anaplasmosis infections may occur after blood transfusion from asymptomatic donors, and several cases have been reported.

The **incubation period** usually is 5 to 14 days for *E chaffeensis* and 5 to 21 days for *A phagocytophilum*.

DIAGNOSTIC TESTS: Detection of specific DNA in a clinical specimen by polymerase chain reaction (PCR) assay is a very sensitive and specific means of early diagnosis for these infections. Whole blood anticoagulated with ethylenediaminetetraacetic acid (EDTA) should be collected at the first presentation to the health care professional and before antibiotic therapy has been initiated. PCR assays for both anaplasmosis and ehrlichiosis are available increasingly at many commercial laboratories and state public health laboratories. Sequence confirmation of the amplified product provides specific identification and often is necessary to identify infection with certain species (eg, *E ewingii* and *E muris*-like agent in the United States). Because these organisms are obligate intracellular organisms, isolation of the bacterium in cell culture requires that appropriate acute clinical samples be sent to specialty research laboratories or the Centers for Disease Control and Prevention (CDC). These must be collected before antimicrobial treatment begins, because the ability to detect the organisms decreases rapidly after doxycycline is initiated. In the case of fatal infections, PCR may be conducted on autopsy specimens, including liver, spleen, and lung. In addition, immunohistochemistry may be used to demonstrate *Ehrlichia* or *Anaplasma* antigen in formalin-fixed, paraffin-embedded tissues.

Identification of stained peripheral blood smears to look for classic clusters of organism known as **morulae** may occasionally indicate infection with Anaplasmataceae, but this method is generally insensitive and is not recommended as a first-line diagnostic tool. In many patients, serologic testing may be used to demonstrate evidence of a fourfold change in immunoglobulin (Ig) G-specific antibody titer by indirect immunofluorescence antibody (IFA) assay between paired serum specimens (the first specimen taken in the first week of illness and a second specimen taken 2–4 weeks later). Specific antigens are available for serologic testing of *E chaffeensis* and *A phagocytophilum* infections, although cross-reactivity between species can make it difficult to interpret the causative agent in areas where geographic distributions overlap. Similarly, because IgM and IgG often increase concurrently and because certain IgM assays may be more prone to false-positive reactions, examination of IgG antibodies is recommended when assessing acutely infected patients but requires both acute and convalescent samples. Because *E ewingii* never has been grown in culture, no antigens are available for diagnostic use; *E ewingii* and *E muris*-like agent infections are best confirmed by molecular detection methods. These organisms share some antigens with *E chaffeensis*, so some cases of these ehrlichioses might be presumptively diagnosed serologically using *E chaffeensis* antigens. These serologic tests are available in reference laboratories, in some commercial laboratories and state health departments, and at the CDC.

TREATMENT: Doxycycline is the drug of choice for treatment of human ehrlichiosis and anaplasmosis, regardless of patient age, and has also been shown to be effective for the other Anaplasmataceae infections (see Tetracyclines, p 873). The recommended pediatric dosage of doxycycline is 4 mg/kg per day, divided every 12 hours, intravenously or orally (maximum 100 mg/dose). Oral dosing is preferred for children who are able take oral medication. For larger children and adults, the dose is 100 mg, every 12 hours. Ehrlichiosis and anaplasmosis can be severe or fatal in untreated patients or patients with predisposing conditions; initiation of therapy early in the course of disease helps minimize complications of illness. Most patients begin to respond within 48 hours of initiating doxycycline treatment. Treatment with trimethoprim-sulfamethoxazole has been linked to more severe outcome and is contraindicated. Treatment should continue for at least 3 days after defervescence; the standard course of treatment is 5 to 10 days.

Clinical manifestations and geographic distributions of ehrlichiosis, anaplasmosis, and Rocky Mountain spotted fever overlap in the United States. As with other rickettsial diseases, when a presumptive diagnosis of ehrlichiosis or anaplasmosis is made, clinical samples should be taken for analysis, and testing may be appropriating for multiple possible etiologies. Doxycycline should be started immediately and should not be delayed pending laboratory confirmation of infection.

ISOLATION OF THE HOSPITALIZED PATIENT: Standard precautions are recommended. Human-to-human transmission via direct contact has not been documented.

CONTROL MEASURES: Specific measures focus on limiting exposures to ticks and tick bites and are similar to those for Rocky Mountain spotted fever and other tickborne diseases (see Prevention of Tickborne Infections, p 210). A risk of blood transfusion infection should be considered in areas with endemic infection. Because of its unique mode of transmission, neorickettsiosis may be prevented by proper cooking of fish. Travel histories to areas with other species of Anaplasmataceae should be evaluated if imported infection is suspected. Prophylactic administration of doxycycline after a tick bite is not indicated because of the low risk of infection and lack of proven efficacy in averting later infection. Cases of ehrlichiosis and anaplasmosis are notifiable diseases in the United States and should be reported to the local/state health department. Additional information is available on the CDC Web site (**www.cdc.gov/ehrlichiosis/**), including a collaborative report providing recommendations for "Diagnosis and Management of Tickborne Rickettsial Diseases" (**www.cdc.gov/mmwr/preview/mmwrhtml/rr5504a1 .htm**).

Enterovirus (Nonpoliovirus)
(Group A and B Coxsackieviruses, Echoviruses, Numbered Enteroviruses)

CLINICAL MANIFESTATIONS: Nonpolio enteroviruses are responsible for significant and frequent illnesses in infants and children and result in protean clinical manifestations. The most common manifestation is nonspecific febrile illness, which in young infants may lead to evaluation for bacterial sepsis. Other manifestations can include the following: (1) respiratory: coryza, pharyngitis, herpangina, stomatitis, bronchiolitis, pneumonia, and pleurodynia; (2) skin: hand-foot-and-mouth disease, onychomadesis (periodic shedding of nails), and nonspecific exanthems; (3) neurologic: aseptic meningitis, encephalitis, and motor paralysis (acute flaccid paralysis); (4) gastrointestinal/genitourinary: vomiting, diarrhea, abdominal pain, hepatitis, pancreatitis, and orchitis; (5) eye: acute hemorrhagic conjunctivitis and uveitis; (6) heart: myopericarditis; and (7) muscle: pleurodynia and other skeletal myositis. Neonates, especially those who acquire infection in the absence of serotype-specific maternal antibody, are at risk of severe disease, including viral sepsis, meningoencephalitis, myocarditis, hepatitis, coagulopathy, and pneumonitis. Infection with enterovirus 71 is associated with hand-foot-and-mouth disease, herpangina, and in a small proportion of cases, severe neurologic disease, including brainstem encephalomyelitis, paralytic disease, other neurologic manifestations; secondary pulmonary edema/hemorrhage and cardiopulmonary collapse can occur, occasionally resulting in fatalities and sequelae. Other noteworthy but not exclusive serotype associations include coxsackieviruses A6 and A16 with hand-foot-and-mouth disease, coxsackievirus A6 with atypical rashes, coxsackievirus A24 variant and enterovirus 70 with acute hemorrhagic conjunctivitis, and coxsackieviruses B1 through B5 with pleurodynia and myopericarditis.

Enterovirus D68 (EV-D68) was first identified in California in 1962 and has been associated with mild to severe respiratory illness in infants, children, and teenagers. In August 2014, clusters of disease caused by EV-D68, prominently associated with exacerbation of asthma, were noted in Kansas City, MO, and Chicago, IL, with subsequent spread throughout the country. By the end of October 2014, EV-D68 had been detected in 48 states, with more than 1100 patients testing positive in the Centers for Disease Control and Prevention laboratory. Almost all of the CDC-confirmed cases were among children, many of whom had asthma or a history of wheezing. Nine children died with EV-D68, although its contribution to the fatal outcome is not fully known at the time of publication. Updated information on the EV-D68 outbreak can be found at **www.cdc.gov/non-polio-enterovirus/outbreaks/EV-D68-activity.html.** Additionally, a polio-like, acute neurologic syndrome was reported in a few children with a history of recent respiratory illnesses, some of which were caused by EV-D68. Illness consisted of spinal fluid pleocytosis and acute onset of limb weakness and changes on magnetic resonance imaging of the spinal cord demonstrating nonenhancing lesions restricted to the gray matter. EV-D68 has not been detectable in these patients' cerebrospinal fluid samples, although there are 2 published reports of children with neurologic illnesses confirmed as EV-D68 infection from cerebrospinal fluid testing. As of December 2014, 94 children with acute flaccid myelitis have been reported in 33 states. These types of neurologic cases were recognized in 2012-2013 as well, prior to the EV-D68 epidemic. EV-D68 has not been proven to be a cause of this neurologic illness, and the full spectrum of disease caused by EV-D68 remains unknown. Updated information on cases of acute flaccid myelitis can be found at **www.cdc.gov/ncird/investigation/viral/sep2014/index.html.**

Patients with humoral and combined immune deficiencies can develop persistent central nervous system infections, a dermatomyositis-like syndrome, and/or disseminated infection. Severe neurologic and/or multisystem disease is reported in hematopoietic stem cell and solid organ transplant recipients, children with malignancies, and patients treated with anti-CD20 monoclonal antibody.

ETIOLOGY: The enteroviruses comprise a genus in the *Picornavirus* family of RNA viruses. The nonpolio enteroviruses include more than 100 distinct serotypes formerly subclassified as group A coxsackieviruses, group B coxsackieviruses, echoviruses, and newer numbered enteroviruses. A more recent classification system groups these nonpolio enteroviruses into 4 species (Enterovirus [EV] A, B, C, and D) on the basis of genetic similarity, although traditional serotype names are retained for individual serotypes; polioviruses are members of EV-C. Echoviruses 22 and 23 have been reclassified as human parechoviruses 1 and 2, respectively (see Human Parechovirus Infections, p 592).

EPIDEMIOLOGY: Humans are the only known reservoir for human enteroviruses, although some primates can become infected. Enterovirus infections are common and distributed worldwide. They are spread by fecal-oral and respiratory routes and from mother to infant prenatally, in the peripartum period, and possibly via breastfeeding. Enteroviruses may survive on environmental surfaces for periods long enough to allow transmission from fomites. Hospital nursery and other institutional outbreaks may occur. Infection incidence, clinical attack rates, and disease severity typically are greatest in young children, and infections occur more frequently in tropical areas and where poor sanitation, poor hygiene, and overcrowding are present. Most enterovirus infections in temperate climates occur in the summer and fall (June through October in the northern hemisphere), but seasonal patterns are less evident in the tropics. Epidemics of enterovirus meningitis, enterovirus 71-associated hand-foot-and-mouth disease with neurologic and cardiopulmonary complications (particularly in south eastern Asia), and enterovirus 70- and coxsackievirus A24-associated acute hemorrhagic conjunctivitis (especially in tropical regions) occur. Fecal viral shedding can persist for several weeks or months after onset of infection, but respiratory tract shedding usually is limited to 1 to 3 weeks or less. Infection and viral shedding can occur without signs of clinical illness.

The usual **incubation period** for enterovirus infections is 3 to 6 days, except for acute hemorrhagic conjunctivitis, in which the **incubation period** is 24 to 72 hours.

DIAGNOSTIC TESTS: Enteroviruses can be detected by reverse transcriptase-polymerase chain reaction (PCR) assay and culture from a variety of specimens, including stool, rectal swabs, throat swabs, nasopharyngeal aspirates, conjunctival swabs, tracheal aspirates, blood, urine, and tissue biopsy specimens and from cerebrospinal fluid (CSF) when meningitis is present. Patients with enterovirus 71 neurologic disease often have negative results of PCR assay and culture of CSF (even in the presence of CSF pleocytosis) and blood; PCR assay and culture of throat or rectal swab and/or vesicle fluid specimens more frequently are positive. PCR assays for detection of enterovirus RNA are available at many reference and commercial laboratories for CSF, blood, and other specimens. PCR assay is more rapid and more sensitive than isolation of enteroviruses in cell culture and can detect all enteroviruses, including serotypes that are difficult to cultivate in viral culture. Sensitivity of culture ranges from 0% to 80% depending on serotype and cell lines used. Many group A coxsackieviruses grow poorly or not at all in vitro. Culture usually requires 3 to 8 days to detect growth. The serotype of enterovirus may be identified either by partial genomic sequencing of the VP1 capsid region from the original specimen or viral isolate or by serotype-specific antibody staining or neutralization assay of the viral isolate at select reference laboratories. Serotyping may be indicated in cases of special clinical interest or for epidemiologic purposes. Acute infection with a known enterovirus serotype can be determined at reference laboratories by demonstration of a change in neutralizing or other serotype-specific antibody titer between acute and convalescent serum specimens or detection of serotype-specific immunoglobulin (Ig) M, but serologic assays are relatively insensitive, may lack specificity, and rarely are used for diagnosis of acute infection.

TREATMENT: No specific therapy is available for enteroviruses infections. Immune Globulin Intravenous (IGIV) may be beneficial for chronic enterovirus meningoencephalitis in immunodeficient patients. IGIV also has been used for life-threatening neonatal enterovirus infections (maternal convalescent plasma has also been used), severe enterovirus infections in transplant recipients and people with malignancies, suspected viral myocarditis, and enterovirus 71 neurologic disease, but proof of efficacy for these uses is lacking. High-titer enterovirus 71 Immune Globulin is being evaluated in areas with epidemic disease. Interferons occasionally have been used for treatment of enterovirus-associated myocarditis, without definitive proof of efficacy. The antiviral drug pleconaril has activity against enteroviruses (but likely not parechoviruses) but is not available commercially at this time. Other agents with activity against enteroviruses are in development (eg, pocapavir).

ISOLATION OF THE HOSPITALIZED PATIENT: In addition to standard precautions, contact precautions are indicated for infants and young children for the duration of enterovirus illness. Cohorting of infected neonates has been effective in controlling hospital nursery enterovirus outbreaks.

CONTROL MEASURES: Hand hygiene, especially after diaper changing, is important in decreasing spread of enteroviruses within families and institutions. Other measures include avoidance of contaminated utensils and fomites and disinfection of surfaces. Recommended chlorination treatment of drinking water and swimming pools may help prevent transmission.

Maintenance administration of IGIV in patients with severe deficits of B-lymphocyte function (eg, severe combined immunodeficiency syndrome, X-linked agammaglobulinemia) may prevent chronic enterovirus infection of the central nervous system. Prophylactic immune globulin has been used to help control hospital nursery outbreaks. Vaccines for virulent enterovirus serotypes, such as enterovirus 71, are under investigation.

Epstein-Barr Virus Infections
(Infectious Mononucleosis)

CLINICAL MANIFESTATIONS: Infectious mononucleosis is the most common presentation of Epstein-Barr virus (EBV) infection. It manifests typically as fever, pharyngitis with petechiae, exudative pharyngitis, lymphadenopathy, hepatosplenomegaly, and atypical lymphocytosis. The spectrum of diseases is wide, ranging from asymptomatic to fatal infection. Infections commonly are unrecognized in infants and young children. Rash can occur and is more common in patients treated with ampicillin or amoxicillin as well as with other penicillins. Central nervous system (CNS) manifestations include aseptic meningitis, encephalitis, myelitis, optic neuritis, cranial nerve palsies, transverse myelitis, Alice in Wonderland syndrome, and Guillain-Barré syndrome. Hematologic complications include splenic rupture, thrombocytopenia, agranulocytosis, hemolytic anemia, and hemophagocytic lymphohistiocytosis (HLH, or hemophagocytic syndrome). Pneumonia, orchitis, and myocarditis are observed infrequently. Early in the course of primary infection, up to 20% of circulating B lymphocytes are infected with EBV, and EBV-specific cytotoxic/suppressor T lymphocytes account for up to 30% of the CD8+ T cells in the blood. Replication of EBV in B lymphocytes results in T-lymphocyte proliferation and inhibition of B-lymphocyte proliferation by T-lymphocyte cytotoxic responses. Fatal disseminated infection or B-lymphocyte or T-lymphocyte lymphomas can occur in children with no detectable immunologic abnormality as well as in children with congenital or acquired cellular immune deficiencies.

EBV is associated with several other distinct disorders, including X-linked lymphoproliferative syndrome, post-transplantation lymphoproliferative disorders, Burkitt lymphoma, nasopharyngeal carcinoma, and undifferentiated B- or T-lymphocyte lymphomas. X-linked lymphoproliferative syndrome occurs in people with an inherited, maternally derived, recessive genetic defect in the SH2DIA gene, which is important in several lymphocyte signaling pathways. The syndrome is characterized by several phenotypic expressions, including occurrence of fatal infectious mononucleosis early in life among boys, nodular B-lymphocyte lymphomas often with CNS involvement, and profound hypogammaglobulinemia.

EBV-associated lymphoproliferative disorders result in a number of complex syndromes in patients who are immunocompromised, such as transplant recipients or people infected with human immunodeficiency virus (HIV). The highest incidence of these disorders occurs in liver and heart transplant recipients, in whom the proliferative states range from benign lymph node hypertrophy to monoclonal lymphomas. Other EBV syndromes are of greater importance outside the United States. EBV is present in virtually 100% of endemic Burkitt lymphoma (a B-lymphocyte tumor predominantly found in head and neck lymph nodes), found primarily in Central Africa versus 20% in sporadic Burkitt lymphoma (found in abdominal lymphoid tissue predominantly in North America and Europe). EBV is found in nasopharyngeal carcinoma in Southeast Asia and the Inuit populations. EBV also has been associated with Hodgkin disease (B-lymphocyte tumor), non-Hodgkin lymphomas (B and T lymphocyte), gastric carcinoma "lymphoepitheliomas," and a variety of common epithelial malignancies.

Chronic fatigue syndrome is not related to EBV infection; however, fatigue lasting weeks to a few months may follow up to 10% of cases of classic infectious mononucleosis.

ETIOLOGY: EBV (also known as human herpesvirus 4) is a gammaherpesvirus of the *Lymphocryptovirus* genus and is the most common cause of infectious mononucleosis (>90% of cases).

EPIDEMIOLOGY: Humans are the only known reservoir of EBV, and approximately 90% of US adults have been infected. Close personal contact usually is required for transmission. The virus is viable in saliva for several hours outside the body, but the role of fomites in transmission is unknown. EBV also may be transmitted by blood transfusion or transplantation. Infection commonly is contracted early in life, particularly among members of lower socioeconomic groups, in which intrafamilial spread is common. Endemic infectious mononucleosis is common in group settings of adolescents, such as in educational institutions. No seasonal pattern has been documented. Intermittent excretion in saliva may be lifelong after infection.

The **incubation period** of infectious mononucleosis is estimated to be 30 to 50 days.

DIAGNOSTIC TESTS: Routine diagnosis depends on serologic testing. Nonspecific tests for heterophile antibody, including the Paul-Bunnell test and slide agglutination reaction test, are available most commonly. The heterophile antibody response primarily is immunoglobulin (Ig) M, which appears during the first 2 weeks of illness and gradually disappears over a 6-month period. The results of heterophile antibody tests often are negative in children younger than 4 years with EBV infection, but heterophile antibody tests identify approximately 85% of cases of classic infectious mononucleosis in older children and adults during the second week of illness. An absolute increase in atypical lymphocytes during the second week of illness with infectious mononucleosis is a characteristic but nonspecific finding. However, the finding of greater than 10% atypical lymphocytes together with a positive heterophile antibody test result in the classical illness pattern is considered diagnostic of acute infection.

Multiple specific serologic antibody tests for EBV infection are available in diagnostic virology laboratories (see Table 3.4 and Fig 3.1). The most commonly performed test is for antibody against the viral capsid antigen (VCA). Because IgG antibodies against VCA occur in high titer early in infection and persist for life, testing of acute and convalescent serum specimens for IgG anti-VCA may not be useful for establishing the presence of active infection. Testing for presence of IgM anti-VCA antibody and the absence of antibodies to Epstein-Barr nuclear antigen (EBNA) is useful for identifying active and recent infections. Because serum antibody against EBNA is not present until several weeks to months after onset of infection, a positive anti-EBNA antibody test typically excludes an active primary infection. Testing for antibodies against early antigen (EA) usually is not required to assess EBV-associated mononucleosis. However, in selected situations, it may be beneficial if it is performed by a laboratory that is proficient with the EA test. Interpretations of EBV serologic testing are based on quantitative immunofluorescent antibody tests performed during various stages of mononucleosis and its resolution, although detection of antibodies by enzyme immunoassays usually is performed by clinical laboratories. Typical patterns of antibody responses to EBV infection are illustrated in Fig 3.1 (p 339).

Serologic testing for EBV is useful, particularly for evaluating patients who have heterophile-negative infectious mononucleosis and for cases in which the infectious mononucleosis syndrome is not present completely. Testing for other agents, especially cytomegalovirus, *Toxoplasma* species, human herpesvirus 6, and HIV, also may be indicated for some of these patients. Diagnosis of the entire range of EBV-associated illness requires use of molecular and antibody techniques, particularly for patients with immune deficiencies.

Isolation of EBV from oropharyngeal secretions by culture in cord blood cells is possible, but techniques for performing this procedure usually are not available in routine diagnostic laboratories, and viral isolation does not necessarily indicate acute infection. Polymerase chain reaction (PCR) assay for detection of EBV DNA in serum, plasma, and tissue and reverse transcriptase-PCR assay for detection of EBV RNA in lymphoid cells,

Table 3.4. Serum Epstein-Barr Virus (EBV) Antibodies in EBV Infection

Infection	VCA IgG	VCA IgM	EA (D)	EBNA
No previous infection	−	−	−	−
Acute infection	+	+	+/−	−
Recent infection	+	+/−	+/−	+/−
Past infection	+	−	+/−	+

VCA IgG indicates immunoglobulin (Ig) G class antibody to viral capsid antigen; VCA IgM, IgM class antibody to VCA; EA (D), early antigen diffuse staining; and EBNA, EBV nuclear antigen.

tissue, and/or body fluids are available commercially and may be useful in evaluation of immunocompromised patients and in complex clinical problems.

TREATMENT: Patients suspected to have infectious mononucleosis should not be given ampicillin or amoxicillin, which cause nonallergic morbilliform rashes in a high proportion of patients with active EBV infection. Although therapy with short-course corticosteroids may have a beneficial effect on acute symptoms, because of potential adverse effects their use should be considered only for patients with marked tonsillar inflammation with impending airway obstruction, massive splenomegaly, myocarditis, hemolytic anemia, or HLH. The dosage of prednisone usually is 1 mg/kg per day, orally (maximum 20 mg/day), for 7 days with subsequent tapering. Life-threatening HLH has been treated with cytotoxic agents and immunomodulators, including cyclosporin and corticosteroids. Although acyclovir has in vitro antiviral activity against EBV, therapy is of no proven value in infectious mononucleosis or in EBV lymphoproliferative syndromes limited to cells with latent viral gene expression. Decreasing immunosuppressive therapy is beneficial for patients with EBV-induced post-transplant lymphoproliferative disorders, whereas an antiviral drug, such as acyclovir, valacyclovir, or ganciclovir, sometimes is used in patients with active replicating EBV

FIG 3.1. SCHEMATIC REPRESENTATION OF THE EVOLUTION OF ANTIBODIES TO VARIOUS EPSTEIN-BARR VIRUS ANTIGENS IN PATIENTS WITH INFECTIOUS MONONUCLEOSIS.

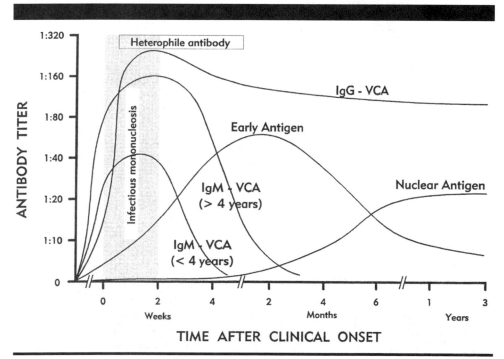

Reproduced with permission from American Society for Microbiology. Epstein-Barr virus. In: Rose NR, de Macario EC, Folds JD, eds. 5th ed. *Manual of Clinical Laboratory Immunology.* Washington, DC: American Society for Microbiology; 1997:Fig 634–643

infection with or without passive antibody therapy provided by IGIV and/or immunosuppression to inhibit immune-mediated injury, such as in HLH.

Contact and collision sports should be avoided until the patient is recovered fully from infectious mononucleosis and the spleen no longer is palpable. In the setting of acute infectious mononucleosis, sport participation in both strenuous and contact situations can result in splenic rupture. In the first 3 weeks following the onset of symptoms, the risk of rupture is related primarily to splenic fragility. Strenuous activity should be avoided for 21 days after onset of symptoms. After 21 days, limited noncontact aerobic activity can be allowed if there are no symptoms and no overt splenomegaly. Clearance to participate in contact or collision sports is appropriate after 4 weeks since the onset of symptoms if the athlete is asymptomatic and has no overt splenomegaly. Imaging modalities rarely are helpful in decisions about clearance to return to contact or collision sports. Because the spleen can vary in size and since a baseline evaluation is rarely available, imaging is not likely to provide evidence for safety clearly to participate in contact sports prior to 28 days following onset of symptoms. Repeat monospot or EBV serologic testing should not be used to determine whether an athlete can safely return to competition in a contact and collision sports. It commonly may take up to 3 months following mononucleosis for the athlete to return to preillness fitness.

ISOLATION OF THE HOSPITALIZED PATIENT: Standard precautions are recommended.

CONTROL MEASURES: None.

Escherichia coli and Other Gram-Negative Bacilli
(Septicemia and Meningitis in Neonates)

CLINICAL MANIFESTATIONS: Neonatal septicemia or meningitis caused by *Escherichia coli* and other gram-negative bacilli cannot be differentiated clinically from septicemia or meningitis caused by other organisms. The early signs of sepsis can be subtle and similar to signs observed in noninfectious processes. Signs of septicemia include fever, temperature instability, heart rate abnormalities, grunting respirations, apnea, cyanosis, lethargy, irritability, anorexia, vomiting, jaundice, abdominal distention, cellulitis, and diarrhea. Meningitis, especially early in the course, can occur without overt signs suggesting central nervous system involvement. Some gram-negative bacilli, such as *Citrobacter koseri*, *Chronobacter* (formerly *Enterobacter*) *sakazakii*, *Serratia marcescens*, and *Salmonella* species, are associated with brain abscesses in infants with meningitis caused by these organisms.

ETIOLOGY: *E coli* strains, often those with the K1 capsular polysaccharide antigen, are the most common cause of septicemia and meningitis in neonates. Other important gram-negative bacilli causing neonatal septicemia include *Klebsiella* species, *Enterobacter* species, *Proteus* species, *Citrobacter* species, *Salmonella* species, *Pseudomonas* species, *Acinetobacter* species, and *Serratia* species. Nonencapsulated strains of *Haemophilus influenzae* and anaerobic gram-negative bacilli are rare causes.

EPIDEMIOLOGY: The source of *E coli* and other gram-negative bacterial pathogens in neonatal infections during the first several days of life typically is the maternal genital tract. Reservoirs for gram-negative bacilli also can be present within the health care environment. Acquisition of gram-negative organisms can occur through person-to-person transmission from hospital nursery personnel and from nursery environmental sites, such as sinks, countertops, powdered infant formula, and respiratory therapy equipment, especially among very preterm infants who require prolonged neonatal intensive care management. Predisposing factors in neonatal gram-negative bacterial infections include maternal intrapartum infection, gestation less than 37 weeks, low birth weight, and prolonged rupture of membranes. Metabolic abnormalities (eg, galactosemia), fetal hypoxia, and acidosis have been implicated as predisposing factors. Neonates with defects in the integrity of skin or mucosa (eg, myelomeningocele) or abnormalities of gastrointestinal or genitourinary tracts are at increased risk of gram-negative bacterial infections. In neonatal intensive care units, systems for respiratory and metabolic support, invasive or surgical procedures, indwelling vascular access catheters, and frequent use of broad-spectrum antimicrobial agents enable selection and proliferation of strains of gram-negative bacilli that are resistant to multiple antimicrobial agents.

Multiple mechanisms of resistance in gram-negative bacilli can be present simultaneously. Resistance resulting from production of chromosomally encoded or plasmid-derived AmpC beta-lactamases or from plasmid-mediated extended-spectrum beta-lactamases (ESBLs), occurring primarily in *E coli, Klebsiella* species, and *Enterobacter* species but reported in many other gram-negative species, has been associated with nursery outbreaks, especially in very low birth weight infants. Organisms that produce ESBLs typically are resistant to penicillins, cephalosporins, and monobactams and can be resistant to aminoglycosides. Carbapenem-resistant strains have emerged among *Enterobacteriaceae*, especially *Klebsiella pneumoniae, Pseudomonas aeruginosa,* and *Acinetobacter* species. ESBL- and carbapenemase-producing bacteria often carry additional genes conferring resistance to aminoglycosides and sulfonamides as well as fluoroquinolones.

The **incubation period** is variable; time of onset of infection ranges from birth to several weeks after birth or longer in very low birth weight, preterm infants with prolonged hospitalizations.

DIAGNOSTIC TESTS: Diagnosis is established by growth of *E coli* or other gram-negative bacilli from blood, cerebrospinal fluid (CSF), or other usually sterile sites. Special screening and confirmatory laboratory procedures are required to detect some multidrug-resistant gram-negative organisms. Molecular diagnostics are being used increasingly for identification of pathogens; specimens should be saved for resistance testing.

TREATMENT:
- Initial empiric treatment for suspected early-onset gram-negative septicemia in neonates is ampicillin and an aminoglycoside. An alternative regimen of ampicillin and an extended-spectrum cephalosporin (such as cefotaxime) can be used, but rapid emergence of cephalosporin-resistant organisms, especially *Enterobacter* species, *Klebsiella* species, and *Serratia* species, and increased risk of colonization or infection with ESBL-producing *Enterobacteriaceae* can occur when use is routine in a neonatal unit. Hence, routine use of an extended-spectrum cephalosporin is not recommended unless gram-negative bacterial meningitis is suspected.
- The proportion of *E coli* bloodstream infections with onset within 72 hours of life that are resistant to ampicillin is high among very low birth weight infants. These *E coli* infections almost invariably are susceptible to gentamicin, although monotherapy with an aminoglycoside is not recommended.
- Once the causative agent and its in vitro antimicrobial susceptibility pattern are known, nonmeningeal infections should be treated with ampicillin, an appropriate aminoglycoside, or an extended-spectrum cephalosporin (such as cefotaxime). Many experts would treat nonmeningeal infections caused by *Enterobacter* species, *Serratia* species, or

Pseudomonas species and some other less commonly occurring gram-negative bacilli with a beta-lactam antimicrobial agent and an aminoglycoside. For ampicillin-susceptible CSF isolates of *E coli*, meningitis can be treated with ampicillin or cefotaxime; meningitis caused by an ampicillin-resistant isolate is treated with cefotaxime with or without an aminoglycoside. Combination therapy with cefotaxime and an aminoglycoside antimicrobial agent is used for empiric therapy and until CSF is sterile. Some experts continue combination therapy for a longer duration. Expert advice from an infectious disease specialist can be helpful for management of meningitis.

- The drug of choice for treatment of infections caused by ESBL-producing organisms is meropenem, which is active against gram-negative aerobic organisms with chromosomally mediated AmpC beta-lactamases or ESBL-producing strains, except carbapenemase-producing strains, especially some *Klebsiella pneumoniae* isolates. Of the aminoglycosides, amikacin retains the most activity against ESBL-producing strains. An aminoglycoside or cefepime can be used if the organism is susceptible. Expert advice from an infectious disease specialist can help in management of ESBL-producing gram-negative infections in neonates.
- The treatment of infections caused by carbapenemase-producing gram-negative organisms is guided by the susceptibility profile and can include an aminoglycoside, especially amikacin, trimethoprim-sulfamethoxazole, or colistin. Isolates often are susceptible to tigecycline, fluoroquinolones, and polymyxin B, for which experience in neonates is limited. Combination therapy often is used. Expert advice from an infectious disease specialist can help in management of carbapenemase-producing gram-negative infections in neonates.
- All infants with gram-negative meningitis should undergo repeat lumbar puncture to ensure sterility of the CSF after 24 to 48 hours of therapy. If CSF remains culture positive, choice and doses of antimicrobial agents should be evaluated, and another lumbar puncture should be performed after 48 to 72 hours.
- Duration of therapy is based on clinical and bacteriologic response of the patient and the site(s) of infection; the usual duration of therapy for uncomplicated bacteremia is 10 to 14 days, and for meningitis, minimum duration is 21 days.
- All infants with gram-negative meningitis should undergo careful follow-up examinations, including testing for hearing loss, neurologic abnormalities, and developmental delay.

ISOLATION OF THE HOSPITALIZED PATIENT: Standard precautions are recommended. Exceptions include hospital nursery epidemics, infants with *Salmonella* infection, and infants with infection caused by gram-negative bacilli that are resistant to multiple antimicrobial agents, including ESBL-producing strains and carbapenemase-producing *Enterobacteriaceae*; in these situations, contact precautions also are indicated.[1]

CONTROL MEASURES: Infection-control personnel should be aware of pathogens causing infections in infants so that clusters of infections are recognized and investigated appropriately. Several cases of infection caused by the same genus and species of bacteria occurring in infants in physical proximity or caused by an unusual pathogen indicate the need for an epidemiologic investigation (see Infection Control and Prevention for Hospitalized Children, p 161). Periodic review of in vitro antimicrobial susceptibility patterns of clinically important bacterial isolates from newborn infants, especially infants in

---

[1]Centers for Disease Control and Prevention. Guidance for control of infections with carbapenem-resistant or carbapenemase-producing Enterobacteriaceae in acute care facilities. *MMWR Morb Mortal Wkly Rep.* 2009;58(10):256-260

the neonatal intensive care unit, can provide useful epidemiologic and therapeutic information. Immune Globulin Intravenous therapy for newborn infants receiving antimicrobial agents for suspected or proven serious infection has been shown to have no effect on outcomes measured and is not recommended.

Escherichia coli Diarrhea
(Including Hemolytic-Uremic Syndrome)

CLINICAL MANIFESTATIONS: At least 5 pathotypes of diarrhea-producing *Escherichia coli* strains have been identified. Clinical features of disease caused by each pathotype are summarized as follows (also see Table 3.5):

- Shiga toxin-producing *E coli* (STEC) organisms are associated with diarrhea, hemorrhagic colitis, and hemolytic-uremic syndrome (HUS). STEC O157:H7 is the serotype most often implicated in outbreaks and consistently is a virulent STEC serotype, but other serotypes also can cause illness. STEC illness typically begins with nonbloody diarrhea. Stools usually become bloody after 2 or 3 days, representing the onset of hemorrhagic colitis. Severe abdominal pain typically is short lived, and low grade fever is present in approximately one third of cases. In people with presumptive diagnoses of intussusception, appendicitis, inflammatory bowel disease, or ischemic colitis, disease caused by *E coli* O157:H7 and other STEC should be considered.
- Diarrhea caused by enteropathogenic *E coli* (EPEC) is watery. Although usually mild, diarrhea can result in dehydration and even death. Illness occurs almost exclusively in children younger than 2 years and predominantly in resource-limited countries, either

Table 3.5. Classification of *Escherichia coli* Associated With Diarrhea

Pathotype	Epidemiology	Type of Diarrhea	Mechanism of Pathogenesis
Shiga toxin-producing *E coli* (STEC)	Hemorrhagic colitis and hemolytic-uremic syndrome in all ages	Bloody or nonbloody	Shiga toxin production, large bowel attachment, coagulopathy
Enteropathogenic *E coli* (EPEC)	Acute and chronic endemic and epidemic diarrhea in infants	Watery	Small bowel adherence and effacement
Enterotoxigenic *E coli* (ETEC)	Infant diarrhea in resource-limited countries and travelers' diarrhea in all ages	Watery	Small bowel adherence, heat stable/heat-labile enterotoxin production
Enteroinvasive *E coli* (EIEC)	Diarrhea with fever in all ages	Bloody or nonbloody; dysentery	Adherence, mucosal invasion and inflammation of large bowel
Enteroaggregative *E coli* (EAEC)	Acute and chronic diarrhea in all ages	Watery, occasionally bloody	Small and large bowel adherence, enterotoxin and cytotoxin production

sporadically or in epidemics. In resource-limited countries, EPEC may be associated with high case fatality. Chronic EPEC diarrhea can be persistent and can result in wasting or growth retardation. EPEC infection is uncommon in breastfed infants.

- Diarrhea caused by enterotoxigenic *E coli* (ETEC) is a 1- to 5-day, self-limited illness of moderate severity, typically with watery stools and abdominal cramps. ETEC is common in infants in resource-limited countries and in travelers to those countries. ETEC infection rarely is diagnosed in the United States. However, outbreaks and studies with small numbers of patients have demonstrated that ETEC infection occasionally is acquired in the United States.
- Diarrhea caused by enteroinvasive *E coli* (EIEC) is similar clinically to diarrhea caused by *Shigella* species. Although dysentery can occur, diarrhea usually is watery without blood or mucus. Patients often are febrile, and stools can contain leukocytes.
- Enteroaggregative *E coli* (EAEC) organisms cause watery diarrhea and are common in people of all ages in industrialized as well as resource-limited countries. EAEC has been associated with prolonged diarrhea (14 days or longer). Asymptomatic infection can be accompanied by subclinical inflammatory enteritis, which can cause growth disturbance.

Sequelae of STEC Infection. HUS is a serious sequela of STEC enteric infection. *E coli* O157:H7 is the STEC serotype most commonly associated with HUS, which is defined by the triad of microangiopathic hemolytic anemia, thrombocytopenia, and acute renal dysfunction. Children younger than 5 years are at highest risk of HUS, which occurs in approximately 15% of those with laboratory-confirmed *E coli* O157:H7 infection, as compared with approximately 6% among people of all ages. HUS occurs in approximately 1% of patients of all ages with laboratory-confirmed non-O157:H7 STEC infection. The term thrombotic thrombocytopenic purpura (TTP) sometimes is used incorrectly for adults with STEC-associated HUS.

HUS typically develops 7 days (up to 2 weeks, and rarely 2-3 weeks) after onset of diarrhea. More than 50% of children with HUS require dialysis, and 3% to 5% die. Patients with HUS can develop neurologic complications (eg, seizures, coma, or cerebral vessel thrombosis). Children presenting with an elevated white blood cell count (>20 × 10^9/mL) or oliguria or anuria are at higher risk of poor outcome, as are, seemingly paradoxically, children with hematocrit close to normal rather than low. Most who survive have a very good prognosis, which can be predicted by normal creatinine clearance and no proteinuria or hypertension 1 or more years after HUS.

ETIOLOGY: Five pathotypes of diarrhea-producing *E coli* have been distinguished by pathogenic and clinical characteristics. Each pathotype comprises characteristic serotypes, indicated by somatic (O) and flagellar (H) antigens.

EPIDEMIOLOGY: Transmission of most diarrhea-associated *E coli* strains is from food or water contaminated with human or animal feces or from infected symptomatic people. STEC is shed in feces of cattle and, to a lesser extent, sheep, deer, and other ruminants. Human infection is acquired via contaminated food or water or via direct contact with an infected person, a fomite, or a carrier animal or its environment. Many food vehicles have caused *E coli* O157 outbreaks, including undercooked ground beef (a major source), raw leafy greens, and unpasteurized milk and juice. Outbreak investigations also have implicated petting zoos, drinking water, and ingestion of recreational water. The infectious dose is low; thus, person-to-person transmission is common in households and has occurred in child care centers. Less is known about the epidemiology of STEC strains other than O157:H7. The non-O157 STEC strains most commonly linked to illness in the United States are O26, O45, O103, O111, O121, and O145. Among children younger than 5 years, the incidence of HUS is highest in 1-year-old children and lowest in infants. A severe outbreak of bloody diarrhea and HUS occurred in Europe in 2011; the outbreak was attributed to an EAEC strain of serotype O104:H4 that had acquired the Shiga toxin 2a-encoding phage. This experience highlights the importance of considering serotypes other than O157:H7 in outbreaks and cases of HUS. There are 2 types of Shiga toxin (Stx), Stx1 and Stx2; several variants of each type exist. In general, STEC strains that produce Stx2, especially variants Stx2a, Stx2c, and Stx2d, are more virulent than strains that only produce Stx1. However, in the clinical setting, there is limited ability to differentiate between Stx variants.

With the exception of EAEC, non-STEC pathotypes most commonly are associated with disease in resource-limited countries, where food and water supplies commonly are contaminated and facilities and supplies for hand hygiene are suboptimal. For young children in resource-limited countries, transmission of ETEC, EPEC, and other diarrheal pathogens via contaminated weaning foods (sometimes by use of untreated drinking water in the foods) also is common. ETEC diarrhea occurs in people of all ages but is especially frequent and severe in infants in resource-limited countries. ETEC is a major cause of travelers' diarrhea. EAEC increasingly is recognized as a cause of diarrhea in the United States.

The **incubation period** for most *E coli* strains is 10 hours to 6 days; for *E coli* O157:H7, the **incubation period** usually is 3 to 4 days (range, 1–8 days).

DIAGNOSTIC TESTS: Diagnosis of infection caused by diarrhea-associated *E coli* other than STEC is difficult, because tests are not widely available to distinguish these pathotypes from normal *E coli* strains present in stool flora. Culture-independent tests are necessary to detect non-O157:H7 STEC infections. Newly licensed multiplex polymerase chain reaction (PCR) assays can detect a variety of enteric infections, including ETEC and STEC. Several commercially available, sensitive, specific, and rapid assays for Shiga toxins in stool or broth culture of stool, including enzyme immunoassays (EIA) and immunochromatographic assays, have been approved by the US Food and Drug Administration.[1] All stool specimens submitted for routine testing from patients with acute community-acquired diarrhea (regardless of patient age, season, or presence or absence of blood in the stool) should be cultured simultaneously for *E coli* O157:H7 and tested with an assay that detects Shiga toxins (or the genes that encode them). Most *E coli* O157:H7 isolates can be identified presumptively when grown on sorbitol-containing selective media, because they cannot ferment sorbitol within 24 hours. All presumptive *E coli* O157:H7 isolates and all Shiga toxin-positive specimens that did not yield a presumptive *E coli* O157 isolate should be sent to a public health laboratory for further characterization, including selective methods to identify non-O157 STEC, serotyping, and pulsed-field gel electrophoresis.

---

[1]Centers for Disease Control and Prevention. Recommendations for diagnosis of Shiga toxin-producing *Escherichia coli* infections by clinical laboratories. *MMWR Recomm Rep.* 2009;58(RR-12):1-14

STEC also should be sought in stool specimens from all patients diagnosed with post-diarrheal HUS. However, the absence of STEC does not preclude the diagnosis of probable STEC-associated HUS, because HUS typically is diagnosed a week or more after onset of diarrhea, when the organism may not be detectable by conventional methods. Selective enrichment followed by immunomagnetic separation can increase markedly the sensitivity of STEC detection, so this testing especially is useful for patients who were not tested early in their diarrheal illness. The test is available at some state public health laboratories and at the Centers for Disease Control and Prevention (CDC). DNA probes also are available in reference and research laboratories. Serologic diagnosis using enzyme immunoassay to detect serum antibodies to *E coli* O157 and O111 lipopolysaccharides is available at the CDC for outbreak investigations and for patients with HUS.

TREATMENT: Orally administered electrolyte-containing solutions usually are adequate to prevent or treat dehydration and electrolyte abnormalities.[1] Antimotility agents should not be administered to children with inflammatory or bloody diarrhea. Patients with proven or suspected STEC infection should be fully but prudently rehydrated as soon as clinically feasible. Careful monitoring of patients with hemorrhagic colitis (including complete blood cell count with smear, blood urea nitrogen, and creatinine concentrations) is recommended to detect changes suggestive of HUS. If patients have no laboratory evidence of hemolysis, thrombocytopenia, or nephropathy 3 days after resolution of diarrhea, their risk of developing HUS is low. In resource-limited countries, nutritional rehabilitation should be provided as part of case management algorithms for diarrhea where feasible. Feeding, including breastfeeding, should be continued for young children with *E coli* enteric infection.

Antimicrobial Therapy. A meta-analysis did not find that children with hemorrhagic colitis caused by STEC have a greater risk of developing HUS if treated with an antimicrobial agent. However, a controlled trial has not been performed, and a beneficial effect of antimicrobial treatment has not been proven. The most recently published observational studies found that treatment of diarrhea with at least some classes of antibiotics was associated with HUS development. Most experts advise not prescribing antimicrobial therapy for children with *E coli* O157:H7 enteritis or a clinical or epidemiologic picture strongly suggestive of STEC infection.

Empiric self-treatment of diarrhea for travelers to a resource-limited country is effective, and azithromycin (not FDA approved for this indication) or a fluoroquinolone have been the most reliable agents for therapy (fluoroquinolones are not approved in people younger than 18 years for this indication; see Fluoroquinolones, p 874); the choice of therapy depends on the pathogen and local antibiotic resistance patterns. Rifaximin may be used for people 12 years and older.

ISOLATION OF THE HOSPITALIZED PATIENT: In addition to standard precautions, contact precautions are indicated for patients with all types of *E coli* diarrhea for the duration of illness. Patients with postdiarrheal HUS should be presumed to have STEC infection.

CONTROL MEASURES:
Escherichia coli *O157:H7 and Other STEC Infection.* All ground beef should be cooked thoroughly until no pink meat remains and the juices are clear or to an internal

---

[1]Centers for Disease Control and Prevention. Managing acute gastroenteritis among children: oral rehydration, maintenance, and nutritional therapy. *MMWR Recomm Rep.* 2003;52(RR-16):1–16

temperature of 160°F (71°C). Raw milk should not be ingested,[1] and only pasteurized apple juice and cider products should be consumed. Because STEC has a low infectious dose and can be waterborne, people with proven or suspected STEC infection should not use recreational water venues (eg, swimming pools, water slides) until 2 weeks after symptoms resolve.

Outbreaks in Child Care Centers. If an outbreak of HUS or diarrhea attributable to STEC occurs in a child care center, immediate involvement of public health authorities is critical. Infection caused by STEC is notifiable, and rapid reporting of cases allows interventions to prevent further disease. Ill children with STEC O157 infection or virulent non-O157 STEC infection (such as those caused by Stx2-producing strains or in the context of an outbreak that includes HUS cases or a high frequency of bloody diarrhea) should not be permitted to reenter the child care center until diarrhea has resolved and 2 stool cultures (obtained at least 48 hours after any antimicrobial therapy has been discontinued) are negative for STEC. Some state health departments have less stringent exclusion policies for children who have recovered from less virulent STEC infection. Stool cultures should be performed for any symptomatic contacts. In outbreak situations involving virulent STEC strains, stool cultures of asymptomatic contacts may aid controlling spread. Strict attention to hand hygiene is important but can be insufficient to prevent transmission. The child care center should be closed to new admissions during an outbreak, and care should be exercised to prevent transfer of exposed children to other centers.

Nursery and Other Institutional Outbreaks. Strict attention to hand hygiene is essential for limiting spread. Exposed patients should be observed closely, their stools should be cultured for the causative organism, and they should be separated from unexposed infants (also see Children in Out-of-Home Child Care, p 132).

Travelers' Diarrhea. Travelers' diarrhea usually is acquired by ingestion of contaminated food or water and is a significant problem for people traveling in resource-limited countries. Diarrhea commonly is caused by ETEC. Diarrhea attributable to *E coli* O157 is rare in US travelers; a much higher proportion of patients with non-O157 STEC infection have traveled internationally in the previous week. Travelers should be advised to drink only bottled or canned beverages and boiled or bottled water; travelers should avoid ice, raw produce including salads, and fruit that they have not peeled themselves. Cooked foods should be eaten hot. Antimicrobial agents are not recommended for prevention of travelers' diarrhea in children. Antimicrobial therapy generally is recommended for travelers in resource-limited areas when diarrhea is moderate to severe or is associated with fever or bloody stools. Several antimicrobial agents, such as azithromycin, rifaximin, and ciprofloxacin, can be effective in treatment of travelers' diarrhea. The drug of first choice for children is azithromycin and for adults is azithromycin or ciprofloxacin. Treatment for no more than 3 days is advised. Packets of oral rehydration salts can be added to boiled or bottled water and ingested to help maintain fluid balance.

Recreational Water. People should avoid ingesting recreational water. People with diarrhea caused by these potentially waterborne pathogens should not use recreational water venues (eg, swimming pools, water slides) for 2 weeks after symptoms resolve.

---

[1] American Academy of Pediatrics, Committee on Infectious Diseases, Committee on Nutrition. Consumption of raw or unpasteurized milk and milk products by pregnant women and children. *Pediatrics.* 2014;133(1):175-179

Fungal Diseases

In addition to the mycoses discussed in individual chapters of Section 3 of the *Red Book* (eg, aspergillosis, blastomycosis, candidiasis, coccidioidomycosis, cryptococcosis, histoplasmosis, paracoccidioidomycosis, and sporotrichosis), uncommonly encountered fungi can cause infection in infants and children with immunosuppression or other underlying conditions. Children can acquire infection with these fungi through inhalation via the respiratory tract or through direct inoculation after traumatic disruption of cutaneous barriers. A list of these fungi and the pertinent underlying host conditions, reservoirs or routes of entry, clinical manifestations, diagnostic laboratory tests, and treatments can be found in Table 3.6 (p 349). Taken as a group, few in vitro antifungal susceptibility data are available on which to base treatment recommendations for these uncommon invasive fungal infections, especially in children (see Antifungal Drugs for Systemic Fungal Infections, p 905). Consultation with a pediatric infectious disease specialist experienced in the diagnosis and treatment of invasive fungal infections should be considered when caring for a child infected with one of these mycoses.

Table 3.6. Additional Fungal Diseases

Disease and Agent	Underlying Host Condition(s)	Reservoir(s) or Route(s) of Entry	Common Clinical Manifestations	Diagnostic Laboratory Test(s)	Treatment
Hyalohyphomycosis					
Fusarium species	Granulocytopenia; hematopoietic stem cell transplantation; severe immunocompromise	Respiratory tract; sinuses; skin	Pulmonary infiltrates; cutaneous lesions, eg ecthyma; sinusitis; disseminated infection	Culture of blood or tissue specimen	Voriconazole or D-AMB[a]
Malassezia species	Immunosuppression; preterm birth; exposure to parenteral nutrition that includes fat emulsions	Skin	Central line-associated bloodstream infection; interstitial pneumonitis; urinary tract infection; meningitis	Culture of blood, catheter tip, or tissue specimen (requires special laboratory handling)	Removal of catheters and temporary cessation of lipid infusion; D-AMB
Penicilliosis					
Penicillium marneffei	Human immunodeficiency virus infection and exposure to southeast Asia	Respiratory tract	Pneumonitis; invasive dermatitis; disseminated infection	Culture of blood, bone marrow, or tissue; histopathologic examination of tissue	Itraconazole[b] or D-AMB
Phaeohyphomycosis					
Alternaria species	None or trauma or immunosuppression	Respiratory tract; skin	Sinusitis; cutaneous lesions	Culture and histopathologic examination of tissue	Voriconazole or high-dose D-AMB[a]
Bipolaris species	None, trauma, immunosuppression, or chronic sinusitis	Environment	Sinusitis; disseminated infection	Culture and histopathologic examination of tissue	Voriconazole, itraconazole,[b] or D-AMB[a]; surgical excision
Curvularia species	Immunosuppression; altered skin integrity; asthma or nasal polyps; chronic sinusitis	Environment	Allergic fungal sinusitis; invasive dermatitis; disseminated infection	Culture and histopathologic examination of tissue	Allergic fungal sinusitis: surgery and corticosteroids Invasive disease: voriconazole, itraconazole,[b] or D-AMB[a]

Table 3.6. Additional Fungal Diseases, continued

Disease and Agent	Underlying Host Condition(s)	Reservoir(s) or Route(s) of Entry	Common Clinical Manifestations	Diagnostic Laboratory Test(s)	Treatment
Exophiala species, *Exserohilum* species	None or trauma or immunosuppression	Environment	Sinusitis; cutaneous lesions; disseminated infection; meningitis associated with contaminated steroid for epidural use	Culture and histopathologic examination of tissue	Voriconazole,[c] itraconazole,[b] D-AMB, or surgical excision
Pseudallescheria boydii (*Scedosporium apiospermum*) *Scedosporium* species	None or trauma or immunosuppression	Environment	Pneumonia; disseminated infection; osteomyelitis or septic arthritis; mycetoma (immunocompetent patients); endocarditis	Culture and histopathologic examination of tissue	Voriconazole[d] or itraconazole
Trichosporonosis					
Trichosporon species	Immunosuppression; central venous catheter	Normal flora of gastrointestinal tract	Bloodstream infection; endocarditis; pneumonitis; disseminated infection	Blood culture; histopathologic examination of tissue; urine culture	D-AMB[a] or voriconazole[d]
Mucormycosis (formerly Zygomycosis)					
Rhizopus; Mucor; Lichtheimia (formerly *Absidia*) species; *Rhizomucor* species	Immunosuppression; hematologic malignant neoplasm; renal failure; diabetes mellitus; iron overload syndromes	Respiratory tract; skin	Rhinocerebral infection; pulmonary infection; disseminated infection; skin and gastrointestinal tract less commonly	Histopathologic examination of tissue and culture	High dose of D-AMB for initial therapy and consider posaconazole[e] for maintenance therapy and surgical excision, as feasible (voriconazole has no activity)

D-AMB indicates deoxycholate amphotericin B; if the patient is intolerant of or refractory to D-AMB, liposomal amphotericin B can be substituted.

[a] Consider use of a lipid-based formulation of amphotericin B.

[b] Itraconazole has been shown to be effective for cutaneous disease in adults, but safety and efficacy have not been established in children younger than 12 years.

[c] Voriconazole demonstrates activity in vitro, but no clinical data are available.

[d] Itraconazole may be the treatment of choice, but data on safety and effectiveness in children are limited.

[e] Posaconazole demonstrates activity in vitro, but few clinical data are available for children.

Fusobacterium Infections
(Including Lemierre Disease)

CLINICAL MANIFESTATIONS: *Fusobacterium necrophorum* and *Fusobacterium nucleatum* can be isolated from oropharyngeal specimens in healthy people, are frequent components of human dental plaque, and may lead to periodontal disease. Invasive disease attributable to *Fusobacterium* species has been associated with otitis media, tonsillitis, gingivitis, and oropharyngeal trauma, including dental surgery. Ten percent of cases of invasive *Fusobacterium* infections are associated with concomitant Epstein-Barr virus infection. Risk may be increased after macrolide use.

Invasive infection with *Fusobacterium* species can lead to life-threatening disease. Otogenic infection is the most frequent primary source in children and can be complicated by meningitis and thrombosis of dural venous sinuses. Invasive infection following tonsillitis was described early in the 20th century and was referred to as postanginal sepsis or Lemierre disease. Lemierre disease occurs most often in adolescents and young adults and is characterized by internal jugular vein septic thrombophlebitis or thrombosis (JVT), evidence of septic embolic lesions in lungs or other sterile sites, and isolation of *Fusobacterium* species from blood or other normally sterile sites. Lemierre-like syndromes also have been reported following infection with *Arcanobacterium haemolyticum*, *Bacteroides* species, anaerobic *Streptococcus* species, other anaerobic bacteria, and methicillin-susceptible and resistant strains of *Staphylococcus aureus*. Fever and sore throat are followed by severe neck pain (anginal pain) that can be accompanied by unilateral neck swelling, trismus, and dysphagia. Patients with classic Lemierre disease have a sepsis syndrome with multiple organ dysfunction. Metastatic complications from septic embolic phenomena associated with suppurative JVT are common and may manifest as disseminated intravascular coagulation, pleural empyema, pyogenic arthritis, or osteomyelitis. Persistent headache or other neurologic signs may indicate the presence of cerebral venous sinus thrombosis (eg, cavernous sinus thrombosis), meningitis, or brain abscess.

JVT can be completely vaso-occlusive. Surgical débridement of necrotic tissue may be necessary for patients who do not respond to antimicrobial therapy. Some children with JVT associated with Lemierre disease have evidence of thrombophilia at diagnosis. These findings often resolve over several months and can indicate response to the inflammatory, prothrombotic process associated with infection rather than an underlying hypercoagulable state.

ETIOLOGY: *Fusobacterium* species are anaerobic, non–spore-forming, gram-negative bacilli. Human infection usually results from *F necrophorum* subspecies *funduliforme*, but infections with other species including *F nucleatum*, *Fusobacterium gonidiaformans*, *Fusobacterium naviforme*, *Fusobacterium mortiferum*, and *Fusobacterium varium* have been reported. Infection with *Fusobacterium* species, alone or in combination with other oral anaerobic bacteria, may result in Lemierre disease.

EPIDEMIOLOGY: *Fusobacterium* species commonly are found in soil and in the respiratory tracts of animals, including cattle, dogs, fowl, goats, sheep, and horses, and can be isolated from the oropharynx of healthy people. *Fusobacterium* infections are most common in adolescents and young adults, but infections, including fatal cases of Lemierre disease, have been reported in infants and young children. Those with sickle cell disease or diabetes mellitus may be at greater risk of infection.

DIAGNOSTIC TESTS: *Fusobacterium* species can be isolated using conventional liquid anaerobic blood culture media. However, the organism grows best on semisolid media for fastidious anaerobic organisms or blood agar supplemented with vitamin K, hemin, menadione, and a reducing agent. Colonies are cream to yellow colored, smooth, and round with a narrow zone of hemolysis on blood agar. Many strains fluoresce chartreuse green under ultraviolet light. Most *Fusobacterium* organisms are indole positive. The accurate identification of anaerobes to the species level has become important with the increasing incidence of microorganisms that are resistant to multiple drugs. Sequencing of the 16S rRNA gene and phylogenetic analysis can identify anaerobic bacteria to the genus or taxonomic group level and frequently to the species level.

The diagnosis of Lemierre disease should be considered in ill-appearing febrile children and adolescents with sore throat and exquisite neck pain over the angle of the jaw. Anaerobic blood culture in addition to aerobic blood culture should be performed to detect invasive *Fusobacterium* species infection. Computed tomography and magnetic resonance imaging are more sensitive than ultrasonography to document thrombosis and thrombophlebitis of the internal jugular vein early in the course of illness and to better identify thrombus extension.

TREATMENT: *Fusobacterium* species may be susceptible to metronidazole, clindamycin, chloramphenicol, carbapenems (meropenem or imipenem), cefoxitin, and ceftriaxone. Resistance to antimicrobial agents has increased in anaerobic bacteria during the last decade, and susceptibility no longer is predictable. Therefore, susceptibility testing is indicated for all clinically significant anaerobic isolates, including *Fusobacterium* species. Metronidazole is the treatment preferred by many experts, because the drug has excellent activity against all *Fusobacterium* species and good tissue penetration. However, metronidazole lacks activity against microaerophilic streptococci that can coinfect some patients. Clindamycin generally is an effective agent. *Fusobacterium* species intrinsically are resistant to gentamicin, fluoroquinolone agents, and typically macrolides. Tetracyclines have limited activity. Up to 50% of *F nucleatum* and 20% of *F necrophorum* isolates produce beta-lactamases, rendering them resistant to penicillin, ampicillin, and some cephalosporins.

Because *Fusobacterium* infections often are polymicrobial, broad-spectrum therapy frequently is necessary. Therapy has been advocated with a penicillin-beta-lactamase inhibitor combination (ampicillin-sulbactam, piperacillin-tazobactam, or ticarcillin-clavulanate) or a carbapenem (meropenem, imipenem, or ertapenem) or combination therapy with metronidazole or clindamycin in addition to other agents active against aerobic oral and respiratory tract pathogens (cefotaxime, ceftriaxone, or cefuroxime). Duration of antimicrobial therapy depends on the anatomic location and severity of infection but usually is several weeks. Surgical intervention involving débridement or incision and drainage of abscesses may be necessary. Anticoagulation therapy has been used in both adults and children with JVT and cavernous sinus thrombosis. In cases with extensive thrombosis, anticoagulation therapy may decrease the risk of clot extension and shorten recovery time.

ISOLATION OF THE HOSPITALIZED PATIENT: Standard precautions are recommended. Person-to-person transmission of *Fusobacterium* species has not been documented.

CONTROL MEASURES: Oral hygiene and dental cleanings may reduce density of oral colonization with *Fusobacterium* species, prevent gingivitis and dental caries, and reduce the risk of invasive disease.

Giardia intestinalis (formerly Giardia lamblia and Giardia duodenalis) Infections
(Giardiasis)

CLINICAL MANIFESTATIONS: Symptomatic infection with *Giardia intestinalis* causes a broad spectrum of clinical manifestations. Children can have occasional days of acute watery diarrhea with abdominal pain, or they may experience a protracted, intermittent, often debilitating disease characterized by passage of foul-smelling stools associated with anorexia, flatulence, and abdominal distention. Anorexia, combined with malabsorption, can lead to significant weight loss, failure to thrive, and anemia. Humoral immunodeficiencies predispose to chronic symptomatic *G intestinalis* infections. Asymptomatic infection is common; approximately 50% to 75% of people who acquired infection in outbreaks occurring in child care settings and in the community were asymptomatic.

ETIOLOGY: *G intestinalis* is a flagellate protozoan that exists in trophozoite and cyst forms; the infective form is the cyst. Infection is limited to the small intestine and biliary tract.

EPIDEMIOLOGY: Giardiasis is the most common intestinal parasitic infection of humans identified in the United States and globally with a worldwide distribution. Approximately 20 000 cases are reported in the United States each year, with highest incidence reported among children 1 to 9 years of age, adults 35 to 44 years of age, and residents of northern states. Peak onset of illness occurs annually during early summer through early fall.[1] Humans are the principal reservoir of infection, but *Giardia* organisms can infect dogs, cats, beavers, rodents, sheep, cattle, nonhuman primates, and other animals. *G intestinalis* assemblages are quite species-specific, such that the organisms that affect nonhumans usually are not infectious to humans. People become infected directly from an infected person or through ingestion of fecally contaminated water or food. Most community-wide epidemics have resulted from a contaminated drinking water supply; outbreaks associated with recreational water also have been reported. Outbreaks resulting from person-to-person transmission occur in child care centers or institutional care settings, where staff and family members in contact with infected children or adults become infected themselves. Although less common, outbreaks associated with food or food handlers also have been reported. Surveys conducted in the United States have identified overall prevalence rates of *Giardia* organisms in stool specimens that range from 5% to 7%, with variations depending on age, geographic location, and seasonality. Duration of cyst excretion is variable but can range from weeks to months. Giardiasis is communicable for as long as the infected person excretes cysts.

The **incubation period** usually is 1 to 3 weeks.

DIAGNOSTIC TESTS: Commercially available, sensitive, and specific enzyme immunoassay (EIA) and direct fluorescence antibody (DFA) assays are the standard tests used for diagnosis of giardiasis in the United States. EIA has a sensitivity of up to 95% and a specificity of 98% to 100% when compared with microscopy. DFA assay has the advantage that organisms are visualized. Laboratories can reduce reagent and personnel costs by pooling specimens from patients before evaluation either by microscopy or EIA.

---

[1] Centers for Disease Control and Prevention Giardiasis surveillance—United States, 2009-2010. *MMWR Surveill Summ.* 2012;61(5):13-23

Traditionally, diagnosis has been based on the microscopic identification of trophozoites or cysts in stool specimens. However, this requires an experienced microscopist, and sensitivity can be suboptimal if the specimen contains low numbers of organisms. Stool needs to be examined as soon as possible or placed immediately in a preservative, such as neutral-buffered 10% formalin or polyvinyl alcohol. A single direct smear examination of stool has a sensitivity of 75% to 95%. Sensitivity is higher for diarrheal stool specimens, because they contain higher concentrations of organisms. Sensitivity of microscopy is increased by examining 3 or more specimens collected every other day. Commercially available stool collection kits in childproof containers are convenient for preserving stool specimens collected at home. When giardiasis is suspected clinically but the organism is not found on repeated stool examination, inspection of duodenal contents obtained by direct aspiration or by using a commercially available string test (Enterotest) may be diagnostic. Rarely, duodenal biopsy is required for diagnosis.

TREATMENT: Some infections are self-limited, and treatment is not required. Dehydration and electrolyte abnormalities can occur and should be corrected. Metronidazole, nitazoxanide, and tinidazole are the drugs of choice. Metronidazole (if used for a 5-day course) is the least expensive of these therapies. A 5- to 10-day course of metronidazole has an efficacy of 80% to 100% in pediatric patients, but poor palatability has been noted for metronidazole suspension. A 1-time dose of tinidazole, a nitroimidazole for children 3 years and older, has a median efficacy of 91% in pediatric patients (range, 80%–100%) and has fewer adverse effects than does metronidazole. A 3-day course of nitazoxanide oral suspension has similar efficacy to metronidazole and has the advantage(s) of treating other intestinal parasites and of being approved for use in children 1 year and older. Paromomycin, a poorly absorbed aminoglycoside that is 50% to 70% effective, is recommended for treatment of symptomatic infection in pregnant women in the second and third trimester.

Symptom recurrence after completing antimicrobial treatment can be attributable to reinfection, post-*Giardia* lactose intolerance (occurs in 20%–40% of patients), immunosuppression, insufficient treatment, or drug resistance. Detailed exposure history and repeat fecal testing is important in determining the cause of recurrence of symptoms. If reinfection is suspected, a second course of the same drug should be effective. Treatment with a different class of drug is recommended for resistant giardiasis. Other treatment options include combination of a nitroimidazole plus quinacrine for at least 2 weeks or high-dose courses of the original agent.

Patients who are immunocompromised because of hypogammaglobulinemia or lymphoproliferative disease are at higher risk of giardiasis, and it is more difficult to treat in these patients. Among human immunodeficiency virus (HIV)-infected children and adults without acquired immunodeficiency syndrome (AIDS), effective combination and antiparasitic therapy are the major initial treatments for these infections. Especially in HIV-infected children, combination antiretroviral therapy should be part of the primary initial treatment for giardiasis. Patients with AIDS often respond to standard therapy; however, in some cases, additional treatment is required. If giardiasis is refractory to standard treatment among HIV-infected patients with AIDS, high doses, longer treatment duration, or combination therapy may be appropriate.

Treatment of asymptomatic carriers is not recommended but could be considered for carriers in households of patients with hypogammaglobulinemia or cystic fibrosis.

ISOLATION OF THE HOSPITALIZED PATIENT: In addition to standard precautions, contact precautions for the duration of illness are recommended for diapered and incontinent children.

CONTROL MEASURES:

- **Handwashing:** Wash hands with soap and water for at least 20 seconds, rubbing hands together vigorously and scrubbing all surfaces:
  - before preparing or eating food,
  - after using the toilet or assisting someone with using the toilet,
  - after changing a diaper or having a diaper changed,
  - after caring for someone who is ill with diarrhea, and
  - after handling an animal or its waste.
- **Child care centers:** In child care centers, improved sanitation and personal hygiene should be emphasized (also see Children in Out-of-Home Child Care, p 132). Hand hygiene by staff and children should be emphasized, especially after toilet use or handling of soiled diapers, which is a key preventive action for control of spread of giardiasis. When an outbreak is suspected, the local health department should be contacted, and an epidemiologic investigation should be undertaken to identify and treat all symptomatic children, child care providers, and family members infected with *G intestinalis.* People with diarrhea should be excluded from the child care center until they become asymptomatic. Treatment or exclusion of asymptomatic carriers is not effective for outbreak control and is not recommended; testing of asymptomatic individuals is not recommended.
- **Drinking water:** Waterborne disease can be prevented by combination of adequate filtration of water from surface water sources (eg, lakes, rivers, streams), chlorination, and maintenance of water distribution systems.
- **Camping/hiking:** Where water might be contaminated, travelers, campers, and hikers should be advised of methods to make water safe for drinking, including boiling, chemical disinfection, and filtration. Boiling is the most reliable method to make water safe for drinking. The time of boiling depends on altitude (1 minute at sea level). Chemical disinfection with iodine is an alternative method of water treatment using either tincture of iodine or tetraglycine hydroperiodide tablets. Chlorine in various forms also can be used for chemical disinfection, but germicidal activity is dependent on several factors, including pH, temperature, and organic content of the water. Commercially available portable water filters provide various degrees of protection. Many commercially available filters are marketed as being able to remove *Giardia* and *Cryptosporidium* species from water. Additional information about water purification, including a traveler's guide for buying water filters, can be found at **www.cdc.gov/crypto/factsheets/filters.html.**
- **Recreational water:** People with diarrhea caused by *Giardia* species should not use recreational water venues (eg, swimming pools, water slides) while symptomatic. People should avoid ingestion of recreational water. For additional information, see Prevention of Illnesses Associated With Recreational Water Use (p 216).
- **Immunosuppressed/HIV-infected people:** For immunosuppressed people, the risk of giardiasis and severity of the infection increases with the severity of immunosuppression. There is no specific preventive course, but combination antiretroviral therapy is the primary method to prevent advanced immunodeficiency.

Gonococcal Infections

CLINICAL MANIFESTATIONS: Gonococcal infections in children and adolescents occur in 3 distinct age groups.

* Infection in the **newborn infant** usually involves the eyes. Other possible manifestations of neonatal gonococcal infection include scalp abscess (which can be associated with fetal scalp monitoring) and disseminated disease with bacteremia, arthritis, or meningitis. Vaginitis and urethritis may occur as well.
* In children beyond the newborn period, including **prepubertal children,** gonococcal infection may occur in the genital tract and almost always is transmitted sexually. Vaginitis is the most common manifestation in prepubertal females. Progression to pelvic inflammatory disease (PID) appears to be less common in this age group than in older adolescents. Gonococcal urethritis is possible but uncommon in prepubertal males. Anorectal and tonsillopharyngeal infection also can occur in prepubertal children and often is asymptomatic.
* In **sexually active adolescent and young adult females,** gonococcal infection of the genital tract often is asymptomatic. Common clinical syndromes include urethritis, endocervicitis, and salpingitis. In males, infection often is symptomatic, and the primary site is the urethra. Infection of the rectum and pharynx can occur alone or with genitourinary tract infection in either gender. Rectal and pharyngeal infections often are asymptomatic. Extension from primary genital mucosal sites in males can lead to epididymitis and in females to bartholinitis, PID with resultant tubal scarring, and perihepatitis (Fitz-Hugh-Curtis syndrome). Even asymptomatic infection in females can progress to PID, with tubal scarring that can result in ectopic pregnancy, infertility, or chronic pelvic pain. Infection involving other mucous membranes can produce conjunctivitis, pharyngitis, or proctitis. Hematogenous spread from mucosal sites can involve skin and joints (arthritis-dermatitis syndrome; disseminated gonococcal infection) and occurs in up to 3% of untreated people with mucosal gonorrhea. Bacteremia can result in a maculopapular rash with necrosis, tenosynovitis, and migratory arthritis. Arthritis may be reactive (sterile) or septic in nature. Meningitis and endocarditis occur rarely.

ETIOLOGY: *Neisseria gonorrhoeae* is a gram-negative, oxidase-positive diplococcus.

EPIDEMIOLOGY: Gonococcal infections occur only in humans. The source of the organism is exudate and secretions from infected mucosal surfaces; *N gonorrhoeae* is communicable as long as a person harbors the organism. Transmission results from intimate contact, such as sexual acts, parturition, and very rarely, household exposure in prepubertal children. Sexual abuse should be considered strongly when genital, rectal, or pharyngeal colonization or infection is diagnosed in prepubertal children beyond the newborn period (see Sexual Victimization and STIs, p 185).

N gonorrhoeae infection is the second most commonly reported sexually transmitted infection (STI) in the United States, following *Chlamydia trachomatis* infection. In 2012, a total of 334 826 cases of gonorrhea were reported in the United States, a rate of 108 cases per 100 000 population, and 58% of reported gonorrhea cases were diagnosed among 15- to 24-year-olds.[1] The reported rate of diagnosis is highest in females

---

[1]Centers for Disease Control and Prevention. *Sexually Transmitted Disease Surveillance 2012.* Atlanta, GA: US Department of Health and Human Services; 2013

15 through 24 years of age. Among males, the rate is highest in those 20 through 24 years of age (Fig 3.2). Racial disparities are remarkable (Fig 3.3). In 2012, the rate of gonorrhea among black people was 15 times the rate among white people. Rates were

FIG 3.2. GONORRHEA. RATES OF DIAGNOSIS BY AGE AND GENDER, 2012.

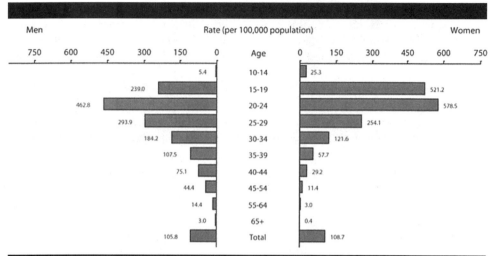

Reproduced from Centers for Disease Control and Prevention. 2012 Sexually Transmitted Diseases Surveillance. Available at **www.cdc.gov/std/stats12/figures/16.htm.**

FIG 3.3. GONORRHEA. RATES BY RACE/ETHNICITY IN THE UNITED STATES, 2008-2012.

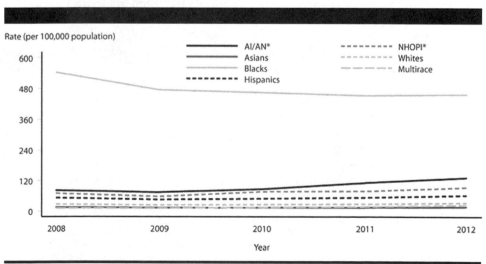

Reproduced from Centers for Disease Control and Prevention. 2012 Sexually Transmitted Diseases Surveillance. Available at **www.cdc.gov/std/stats12/figures/19.htm.**
AI/AN, American Indian/Alaska Native; NHOPI, Native Hawaiian and Other Pacific Islander.

4 times higher among American Indian/Alaska Native people, 3 times higher among Native Hawaiian/Pacific Islander people, and 2 times higher among Hispanic people than among whites. Considering all racial/ethnic and age categories, gonorrhea rates were highest for black people 15 through 19 years of age and 20 through 24 years of age in 2012. Black females 15 through 19 years of age had a gonorrhea rate that was 15 times the rate among white females in the same age group, and black males 15 through 19 years of age had a gonorrhea rate that was 26 times the rate among white males in the same age group. Disparities in gonorrhea rates also are observed by sexual behavior. Surveillance networks that monitor trends in STI prevalence among males who sex with males (MSM) have found very high proportions of positive gonorrhea pharyngeal, urethral, and rectal test results as well as coinfection with other STIs and human immunodeficiency virus (HIV).

The **incubation period** usually is 2 to 7 days. Concurrent infection with *C trachomatis* is common.

Diagnosis of genitourinary tract gonorrhea infection in a child, adolescent, or young adult should prompt investigation for **other STIs**, including chlamydia, syphilis, and HIV infection.

DIAGNOSTIC TESTS[1,2]: Microscopic examination of Gram-stained smears of exudate from the conjunctivae, vagina of prepubertal girls, male urethra, skin lesions, synovial fluid, and when clinically warranted, cerebrospinal fluid (CSF) may be useful in the initial evaluation. Identification of gram-negative intracellular diplococci in these smears can be helpful, particularly if the organism is not recovered in culture. However, because of low sensitivity, a negative smear result should not be considered sufficient for ruling out infection.

N gonorrhoeae can be isolated from normally sterile sites, such as blood, CSF, or synovial fluid, using nonselective chocolate agar with incubation in 5% to 10% carbon dioxide. Selective media that inhibit normal flora and nonpathogenic *Neisseria* organisms are used for cultures from nonsterile sites, such as the cervix, vagina, rectum, urethra, and pharynx. Specimens for *N gonorrhoeae* culture from mucosal sites should be inoculated immediately onto appropriate agar, because the organism is extremely sensitive to drying and temperature changes.

Caution should be exercised when interpreting the significance of isolation of *Neisseria* organisms, because *N gonorrhoeae* can be confused with other *Neisseria* species that colonize the genitourinary tract or pharynx. At least 2 confirmatory bacteriologic tests involving different biochemical principles should be performed by the laboratory. Interpretation of culture of *N gonorrhoeae* from the pharynx of young children necessitates particular caution because of the high carriage rate of nonpathogenic *Neisseria* species and the serious implications of such a culture result.

Nucleic acid amplification tests (NAATs) are far superior in overall performance compared with other *N gonorrhoeae* culture and nonculture diagnostic methods to test

---

[1]American Academy of Pediatrics, Committee on Adolescence; Society for Adolescent Health and Medicine. Screening for nonviral sexually transmitted infections in adolescents and young adults. *Pediatrics.* 2014;134(1):e302-e311

[2]Centers for Disease Control and Prevention. Recommendations for the laboratory-based detection of *Chlamydia trachomatis* and *Neisseria gonorrhoeae*—2014. *MMWR Recomm Rep.* 2014;63(RR-2):1-19

genital and nongenital specimens, but performance varies by NAAT type.[1] These tests include polymerase chain reaction (PCR), transcription-mediated amplification (TMA), and strand-displacement amplification (SDA). Most commercially available products now are approved by the US Food and Drug Administration (FDA) for testing male urethral swab specimens, female endocervical or vaginal swab specimens (provider or patient-collected), male or female urine specimens, or liquid cytology specimens. Package inserts for individual NAAT products must be reviewed, however, because the particular specimens approved for use with each test may vary. Use of less-invasive specimens, such as urine or vaginal swab specimens, increases feasibility of routine testing of sexually active adolescents by their primary care providers and in other clinical settings. NAATs also permit dual testing of specimens for *C trachomatis* and *N gonorrhoeae*. The Centers for Disease Control and Prevention (CDC) recommends the vaginal swab as the preferred means of screening females and urine as the preferred means for screening males for *N gonorrhoeae* infection. Female urine remains an acceptable gonorrhea NAAT specimen but may have slightly reduced performance when compared with cervical or vaginal swab specimens.

For identifying *N gonorrhoeae* from nongenital sites, culture is the most widely used test and allows for antimicrobial susceptibility testing to aid in management should infection persist following initial therapy. NAATs are not cleared by the FDA for *N gonorrhoeae* testing on rectal or pharyngeal swab specimens but are more sensitive compared with *N gonorrhoeae* culture. Many commercial and public health laboratories that have met Clinical Laboratory Improvement Amendment (CLIA) and other regulatory requirements and have validated gonorrhea NAAT performance on rectal and/or pharyngeal swab specimens may perform these tests. Some NAATs have the potential to cross-react with nongonococcal *Neisseria* species that commonly are found in the throat, leading to false-positive test results. A limited number of nonculture tests are approved by the FDA for conjunctival specimens.

Sexual Abuse.[2] In all prepubertal children beyond the newborn period and in adolescents who have gonococcal infection but report no prior sexual activity, sexual abuse must be considered to have occurred until proven otherwise (see Sexual Victimization and STIs, p 185). Health care providers have a responsibility to report suspected sexual abuse to the state child protective services agency. This mandate does not require that the provider is certain that abuse has occurred but only that there is "reasonable cause to suspect abuse." Cultures should be performed on genital, rectal, and pharyngeal swab specimens for all patients before antimicrobial treatment is given. All gonococcal isolates from such patients should be preserved. Nonculture gonococcal tests, including Gram stain, DNA probes, enzyme immunoassays, or NAATs of oropharyngeal, rectal, or genital tract swab specimens in children cannot be relied on as the sole method for diagnosis of gonococcal infection for this purpose, because false-positive results can occur. NAATs can be used as alternative to culture with vaginal swab specimens or urine specimens from prepubertal girls. Culture remains the preferred method for urethral specimens from boys and extragenital specimens (pharynx and rectum) in boys and girls.

[1]Centers for Disease Control and Prevention. Recommendations for the laboratory-based detection of *Chlamydia trachomatis* and *Neisseria gonorrhoeae*—2014. *MMWR Recomm Rep.* 2014;63(RR-2):1-19

[2]Jenny C, Crawford-Jakubiak JE; American Academy of Pediatrics, Committee on Child Abuse and Neglect. The evaluation of children in the primary care setting when sexual abuse is suspected. *Pediatrics.* 2013;132(2):e558-e567

Detection of gonorrhea in a child requires an evaluation for other sexually transmitted infections, such as *C trachomatis* infection, syphilis, and human immunodeficiency virus (HIV) infection. Completion of the series of vaccines for hepatitis B and human papillomavirus should be determined, then offered if not completed and if appropriate for the age group.

TREATMENT[1,2]: The rapid emergence of antimicrobial resistance has led to a limited number of approved therapies for gonococcal infections. Resistance to penicillin and tetracycline is widespread, and as of 2007, the CDC no longer recommends the use of fluoroquinolones for gonorrhea because of the increased prevalence of quinolone-resistant *N gonorrhoeae* in the United States. This leaves the cephalosporins as the only recommended antimicrobial class for the treatment of gonococcal infections. Over the past decade, the minimum inhibitory concentrations (MIC) for oral cefixime activity against *N gonorrhoeae* strains circulating in the United States and other countries has increased, suggesting that resistance to this drug is emerging. Treatment failure following the use of cefixime has been described in North America, Europe, and Asia. Therefore, as of 2012, the CDC no longer recommends the use of cefixime as a first-line treatment for gonococcal infection. Ceftriaxone, 250 mg, intramuscularly, once, with either azithromycin, 1 g orally, once, or doxycycline, 100 mg, twice daily for 7 days, is the recommended treatment for all gonococcal infections, regardless of age (see Table 3.7, p 361). Azithromycin is preferred to doxycycline because of the convenience of single-dose therapy and because gonococcal resistance to tetracyclines appears to be greater than resistance to azithromycin. Although other parenteral extended-spectrum cephalosporins, such as cefotaxime, may be acceptable, they offer no clear advantage over ceftriaxone in most cases, and their efficacy in the treatment of pharyngeal infections has not been well documented. Oral cefixime should only be considered for treatment of an anogenital infection if parenteral treatment with ceftriaxone is not available. Combination therapy using 2 antimicrobials with different mechanisms of action may improve treatment efficacy for *N gonorrhoeae*, potentially delay emergence and spread of resistance to cephalosporins, and ensure treatment of cooccurring pathogens (eg, chlamydia).

Test-of-cure samples are not required in adolescents or adults with uncomplicated gonorrhea who are asymptomatic after being treated with a recommended antimicrobial regimen that includes ceftriaxone alone or with one of the listed alternative regimens. If an alternative regimen is used for treatment of pharyngeal gonorrhea infection, the CDC recommends a test-of-cure 14 days after treatment is completed, ideally using culture so that antimicrobial susceptibility testing may be performed. If culture is not available, the CDC recommends testing with a gonorrhea NAAT. If the NAAT result remains positive, every effort should be made to obtain a culture for susceptibility testing. Children treated with ceftriaxone do not require follow-up cultures unless they remain in an at-risk environment, but if treated with other regimens for pharyngeal infection, follow-up culture is

[1]Centers for Disease Control and Prevention. Sexually transmitted diseases treatment guidelines, 2014. *MMWR Morb Mortal Wkly Rep.* 2014; in press

[2]American Academy of Pediatrics, Committee on Adolescence; Society for Adolescent Health and Medicine. Screening for nonviral sexually transmitted infections in adolescents and young adults. *Pediatrics.* 2014;134(1):e302-e311

Table 3.7. Uncomplicated Gonococcal Infection: Treatment of Children Beyond the Newborn Period and Adolescents[a]

Disease	Prepubertal Children Who Weigh Less Than 100 lb (45 kg)	Disease	Patients Who Weigh 100 lb (45 kg) or More and Who Are 8 Years or Older
Uncomplicated vulvovaginitis, cervicitis, urethritis, proctitis, or pharyngitis	Ceftriaxone, 125 mg, IM, in a single dose[b]	Uncomplicated endocervicitis, urethritis, proctitis, or pharyngitis[c]	Ceftriaxone, 250 mg, IM, in a single dose[b] **PLUS**[a] Azithromycin, 1 g, orally, in a single dose Alternative regimen for patients with severe cephalosporin allergy: Consult an expert in infectious diseases[c]

IM indicates intramuscularly.

[a] For adolescents, azithromycin is recommended in combination with ceftriaxone as dual treatment for gonococcal infection. In addition, azithromycin provides therapy for *Chlamydia trachomatis* on the presumption that the patient has concomitant infection.

[b] Data supporting the use of oral cefixime to treat gonococcal infections in children are very limited. Ceftriaxone is preferred whenever possible. For uncomplicated anogenital infections in adolescents, dual treatment with cefixime, 400 mg, orally, and azithromycin may be used if ceftriaxone is not feasible. Cefixime should not be used to treat pharyngeal infection.

[c] Because data are limited regarding alternative regimens for treating gonorrhea among children and adolescents who have documented cephalosporin allergy, consultation with an expert in infectious diseases is recommended. In adults, dual treatment with single doses of oral gemifloxacin, 320 mg, plus oral azithromycin, 2 g, or dual treatment with single doses of intramuscular gentamicin, 240 mg, plus oral azithromycin, 2 g, are potential therapeutic options. However, there are no data on the efficacy of these regimens in children or adolescents.

Adapted from Centers for Disease Control and Prevention. Sexually transmitted diseases treatment guidelines, 2014. *MMWR Morb Mortal Wkly Rep.* 2014; in press.

indicated. Patients who have symptoms that persist after treatment or whose symptoms recur shortly after treatment should be reevaluated by culture for *N gonorrhoeae*, and any gonococci isolated should be tested for antimicrobial susceptibility. Treatment failures should be reported to the CDC through the local or state health department.

Because patients may be reinfected by a new or untreated partner within a few months after diagnosis and treatment, providers should advise all adolescents and adults diagnosed with gonorrhea to be retested approximately 3 months after treatment. Patients who do not receive a test-of-reinfection at 3 months should be tested whenever they are seen for care within the next 12 months. All patients with presumed or proven gonorrhea should be evaluated for concurrent syphilis, HIV, and *C trachomatis* infections.

Specific recommendations for management and antimicrobial therapy are as follows:

Neonatal Disease. Infants with clinical evidence of ophthalmia neonatorum, scalp abscess, or disseminated infections attributable to *N gonorrhoeae* should be hospitalized. Cultures of blood, eye discharge, and other potential sites of infection, such as CSF, should be performed on specimens from infants to confirm the diagnosis and to determine antimicrobial susceptibility. Tests for concomitant infection with *C trachomatis*, congenital syphilis, and HIV infection should be performed. Results of the maternal test for hepatitis B surface antigen should be confirmed. The mother and her partner(s) also need appropriate examination and treatment for *N gonorrhoeae*.

Ophthalmia Neonatorum. Recommended antimicrobial therapy for ophthalmia neonatorum caused by *N gonorrhoeae* is a single one-time dose of ceftriaxone, 25 to 50 mg/kg, intravenously or intramuscularly, not to exceed 125 mg. Infants with gonococcal ophthalmia should receive eye irrigations with saline solution immediately and at frequent intervals until discharge is eliminated. Topical antimicrobial treatment alone is inadequate and unnecessary when recommended systemic antimicrobial treatment is given. Infants with gonococcal ophthalmia should be hospitalized and evaluated for disseminated infection (sepsis, arthritis, meningitis). Treatment of ophthalmia neonatorum may need to be continued beyond the single treatment dose until systemic infection has been ruled out; in practice, parenteral therapy is likely to be provided for 48 to 72 hours to ensure that bacterial cultures of normally sterile sites are negative.

Disseminated Neonatal Infections and Scalp Abscesses. Recommended therapy for arthritis, septicemia, or abscess is ceftriaxone, 25 to 50 mg/kg/day, intravenously or intramuscularly, in a single daily dose for 7 days. Cefotaxime, 25 mg/kg, every 12 hours, is recommended for infants with hyperbilirubinemia. If meningitis is documented, treatment should be continued for a total of 10 to 14 days.

Gonococcal Infections in Children Beyond the Neonatal Period and Adolescents. Recommendations for treatment of gonococcal infections, by age and weight, are provided in Tables 3.7 (p 361) and 3.8 (p 363).

Special Problems in Treatment of Children (Beyond the Neonatal Period) and Adolescents. Providers treating patients with uncomplicated infections of the vagina, endocervix, urethra, or anorectum and a history of severe **adverse reactions to cephalosporins** (eg, anaphylaxis, ceftriaxone-induced hemolysis, Stevens-Johnson syndrome, toxic epidermal necrolysis) should consult an expert in infectious diseases. In adults, dual treatment with a single dose of gemifloxacin, 320 mg, plus oral azithromycin, 2 g, or dual treatment with a single dose of intramuscular gentamicin, 240 mg, plus oral azithromycin, are potential therapeutic options. However, there are no data on the efficacy of these regimens in children or adolescents. Monotherapy with azithromycin, 2 g orally, as a single dose, has

Table 3.8. Complicated Gonococcal Infection: Treatment of Children Beyond the Newborn Period and Adolescents[a]

Disease[b]	Prepubertal Children Who Weigh Less Than 100 lb (45 kg)	Disease[b]	Patients Who Weigh 100 lb (45 kg) or More and Who Are 8 Years or Older
Disseminated gonococcal infection (eg, arthritis-dermatitis syndrome)	Ceftriaxone, 50 mg/kg/day (maximum 1 g/day), IV or IM, once a day for 7 days **PLUS[a]** Erythromycin base or ethylsuccinate 50 mg/kg/day (maximum 2 g), orally, divided into 4 doses daily for 14 days[c]	Disseminated gonococcal infections	Ceftriaxone, 1 g, IV or IM, given once a day for 7 days[d] **PLUS[a]** Azithromycin, 1 g, orally, in a single dose
Meningitis or endocarditis	Ceftriaxone, 50 mg/kg/day (maximum 2 g/day), IV or IM, given every 12–24 h; for meningitis, duration is 10–14 days; for endocarditis, duration is at least 28 days **PLUS[a]** Erythromycin base or ethylsuccinate, 50 mg/kg/day, orally, divided into 4 doses daily for 14 days[c]	Meningitis or endocarditis	Ceftriaxone, 1–2 g, IV, every 12–24 h; for meningitis, duration is 10–14 days; for endocarditis, duration is at least 28 days **PLUS[a]** Azithromycin, 1 g, orally, in a single dose
Conjunctivitis[e]	Ceftriaxone, 50 mg/kg (maximum 125 mg), IM, in a single dose	Conjunctivitis[e]	Ceftriaxone, 1 g, IM, in a single dose **PLUS[a]** Azithromycin, 1 g, orally, in a single dose
		Epididymitis	Ceftriaxone, 250 mg, IM, in a single dose **PLUS[a]** Doxycycline, 100 mg, orally, twice daily for 10 days

continued

Table 3.8. Complicated Gonococcal Infection: Treatment of Children Beyond the Newborn Period and Adolescents,[a] continued

Disease[b]	Prepubertal Children Who Weigh Less Than 100 lb (45 kg)	Disease[b]	Patients Who Weigh 100 lb (45 kg) or More and Who Are 8 Years of Age or Older
Conjunctivitis,[e] continued		Pelvic inflammatory disease	See Table 3.48 (p 607)

IV indicates intravenously; IM, intramuscularly.

[a]Concomitant therapy for *Chlamydia trachomatis* is recommended in addition to the recommended treatment for gonococcal infection.

[b]Hospitalization should be considered, especially for people treated as outpatients whose infection has failed to respond and people who are unlikely to adhere to treatment regimens. Patients with meningitis or endocarditis should be hospitalized.

[c]Limited evidence suggests that azithromycin, 20 mg/kg (maximum 1 g), orally, in a single dose, is an alternative treatment for chlamydia in children who weigh less than 45 kg.

[d]Patients with a diagnosis of disseminated gonococcal infection should have specimens obtained for culture and antimicrobial susceptibility testing, and treatment should be guided by results of antimicrobial susceptibility testing when available. Pending antimicrobial susceptibility results, patients should be initiated and continued on the recommended regimen to complete at least a 7-day course of therapy.

[e]Eyes should be lavaged with saline solution to clear accumulated secretions.

Adapted from Centers for Disease Control and Prevention. Sexually transmitted diseases treatment guidelines, 2014. *MMWR Morb Mortal Wkly Rep.* 2014; in press.

been demonstrated to be effective against uncomplicated urogenital gonorrhea. However, monotherapy no longer is recommended because of concerns about the ease with which *N gonorrhoeae* can develop resistance to macrolides and because several studies have documented azithromycin treatment failures. Spectinomycin, 40 mg/kg, maximum 2 g, given intramuscularly as a single dose, is an alternative but is not available in the United States. Because data are limited regarding alternative regimens for treating gonorrhea among people who have documented severe cephalosporin allergy, consultation with an expert in infectious diseases may be warranted.

Pharyngeal infection generally is more difficult to treat than anogenital infection. Patients with uncomplicated pharyngeal gonococcal infection should be treated with ceftriaxone, 250 mg, intramuscularly (Table 3.7, p 361), in a single dose, plus azithromycin, 1 g, orally, in a single dose. Cefixime has unacceptably low efficacy for the eradication of *N gonorrhoeae* in the pharynx and should not be used. If ceftriaxone is not used, test-of-cure should be performed, using culture if possible.

Children or adolescents with **HIV infection** should receive the same treatment for gonococcal infection as children without HIV infection.

Acute PID. *N gonorrhoeae* and *C trachomatis* are implicated in many cases of PID; most cases have a polymicrobial etiology. No reliable clinical criteria distinguish gonococcal from nongonococcal-associated PID. Hence, broad-spectrum treatment regimens are recommended (see Pelvic Inflammatory Disease, p 603).

Acute Epididymitis. Sexually transmitted organisms, such as *N gonorrhoeae* or *C trachomatis*, can cause acute epididymitis in sexually active adolescents and young adults but rarely if ever cause acute epididymitis in prepubertal children. The recommended regimen for sexually transmitted epididymitis is ceftriaxone, 250 mg, intramuscularly, once, plus doxycycline, 100 mg, twice daily for 14 days (see Table 3.8, p 363).

ISOLATION OF THE HOSPITALIZED PATIENT: Standard precautions are recommended, including for newborn infants with ophthalmia.

CONTROL MEASURES:

Neonatal Ophthalmia. For routine prophylaxis of infants immediately after birth, 0.5% erythromycin ophthalmic ointment is instilled into each eye; subsequent irrigation should not be performed (see Prevention of Neonatal Ophthalmia, p 972). Also approved for prophylaxis of neonatal ophthalmia are 1% tetracycline ophthalmic ointment and 1% silver nitrate, but these no longer are available in the United States. Prophylaxis may be delayed for up to 1 hour after birth to facilitate parent-infant bonding, but a monitoring system should be in place to ensure that all newborn infants receive prophylaxis no later than 1 hour after birth. Topical prophylaxis for preventing chlamydial ophthalmia does not work, likely because colonization of the nasopharynx is not prevented.

Infants Born to Mothers With Gonococcal Infections. When prophylaxis is administered correctly, infants born to mothers with gonococcal infection rarely develop gonococcal ophthalmia. However, because gonococcal ophthalmia or disseminated infection occasionally can occur in this situation, infants born to mothers known to have gonorrhea should receive ceftriaxone as a single dose of 25 to 50 mg/kg (maximum dose, 125 mg), intravenously or intramuscularly (see Prevention of Neonatal Ophthalmia, p 972). When systemic ceftriaxone therapy is administered prophylactically, topical antimicrobial therapy is not necessary.

Children and Adolescents With Sexual Exposure to a Patient Known to Have Gonorrhea. Exposed people should undergo examination and culture and should receive the same treatment as do people known to have gonorrhea.

Pregnancy. All pregnant women should be screened for syphilis, HIV, chlamydia, and hepatitis B at the first prenatal visit. Pregnant females at risk of gonorrhea, including females younger than 25 years or living in an area in which the prevalence of *N gonorrhoeae* is high, should have a genital gonorrhea test at the time of their first prenatal visit. A repeat test in the third trimester is recommended for females at continued risk of gonococcal infection, including females younger than 25 years. Recommended therapeutic regimens for patients found to be infected are as described previously for gonococcal infection, except that doxycycline should not be used in pregnant females because of the potential toxic effects on the fetus. For pregnant females who are severely allergic to cephalosporins, a consultation with an infectious diseases expert is indicated.

Routine Screening Tests.[1] All sexually active females younger than 25 years, should be tested at least annually for gonorrhea infection, even if no symptoms are present or barrier contraception is reported. Sexually active adolescent and young adult males who have sex with males (MSM) should be screened routinely for oral, rectal, and urethral gonorrhea annually if they engage in receptive oral, anal, or insertive intercourse, respectively. Screening should be performed every 3 to 6 months if the person is at high risk because of multiple or anonymous partners, sex in conjunction with illicit drug use, or having sex partners who participate in these activities. Screening should be considered annually for sexually active males who have sex with females on the basis of individual and population-based risk factors, such as disparities by race and neighborhoods.

Case Reporting and Management of Sexual Partners. All cases of gonorrhea must be reported to local public health officials (see Appendix IV, Nationally Notifiable Infectious Diseases in the United States, p 992). Ensuring that sexual contacts are treated and counseled to use condoms is essential for community control, prevention of reinfection, and prevention of complications in the contact(s). All sexual contacts in the 60 days preceding onset of symptoms in the index case should be evaluated for *N gonorrhoeae* infection and treated if results are positive. If time of the last sexual contact was more than 60 days before symptom onset or patient diagnosis, the most recent sex partner should be evaluated and treated. Recommendations for services provided to partners of people with gonorrhea are available.[2] Cases in prepubertal children must be investigated to determine the source of infection.

Among females or heterosexual male patients, if concerns exist that sex partners who are referred to evaluation and treatment will not seek care, expedited partner therapy (EPT), the clinical practice of treating the sex partners of patients diagnosed with chlamydia or gonorrhea by providing prescriptions or medications to the patient to take to his or her partner without the health care provider first examining the partner, can be considered. However, because the CDC no longer recommends the routine use of a single orally administered antibiotic for the treatment of gonorrhea in the United States, EPT is not possible if treatment involves an injection. If a heterosexual partner of a gonorrhea patient cannot be linked to evaluation and treatment in a timely fashion, EPT with cefixime and azithromycin still should be considered, because not treating partners is significantly more harmful than is practicing EPT for gonorrhea. EPT, especially for

---

[1]American Academy of Pediatrics, Committee on Adolescence, and Society for Adolescent Health and Medicine. Screening for nonviral sexually transmitted infections in adolescents and young adults. *Pediatrics.* 2014;134(1):e302-e311

[2]Centers for Disease Control and Prevention. Recommendations for partner services programs for HIV infection, syphilis, gonorrhea, and chlamydial infection. *MMWR Recomm Rep.* 2008;57(RR-9):1–63

gonorrhea, always should be accompanied by efforts to educate partners about symptoms and to encourage partners to seek clinical evaluation. To clarify the legal status of EPT in each state, refer to the CDC Web site (**www.cdc.gov/std/ept/**). EPT should not be considered a routine partner management strategy in MSM because of the high risk of coexisting undiagnosed STIs or HIV infection.

Granuloma Inguinale
(Donovanosis)

CLINICAL MANIFESTATIONS: Initial lesions of this sexually transmitted infection are single or multiple subcutaneous nodules that gradually ulcerate. These nontender, granulomatous ulcers are beefy red and highly vascular and bleed readily on contact. Lesions usually involve the genitalia without regional adenopathy, but anal infections occur in 5% to 10% of patients; lesions at distant sites (eg, face, mouth, or liver) are rare. Subcutaneous extension into the inguinal area results in induration that can mimic inguinal adenopathy (ie, "pseudobubo"). Verrucous, necrotic, and fibrous lesions may occur as well. Fibrosis manifests as sinus tracts, adhesions, and lymphedema, resulting in extreme genital deformity. Urethral obstruction can occur.

ETIOLOGY: The disease, Donovanosis, is caused by *Klebsiella granulomatis* (formerly known as *Calymmatobacterium granulomatis*), an intracellular gram-negative bacillus.

EPIDEMIOLOGY: Indigenous granuloma inguinale occurs very rarely in the United States and most industrialized nations. The disease is endemic in some tropical and developing areas, including India; Papua, New Guinea; the Caribbean; central Australia; and southern Africa. The incidence of infection seems to correlate with sustained high temperatures and high relative humidity. Infection usually is acquired by sexual intercourse, most commonly with a person with active infection but possibly also from a person with asymptomatic rectal infection. Young children can acquire infection by contact with infected secretions. The period of communicability extends throughout the duration of active lesions or rectal colonization.

The **incubation period** is 8 to 80 days.

DIAGNOSTIC TESTS: The causative organism is difficult to culture, and diagnosis requires microscopic demonstration of dark staining intracytoplasmic Donovan bodies on Wright or Giemsa staining of a crush preparation from subsurface scrapings of a lesion or tissue. The microorganism also can be detected by histologic examination of biopsy specimens. Lesions should be cultured for *Haemophilus ducreyi* to exclude chancroid. Granuloma inguinale often is misdiagnosed as carcinoma, which can be excluded by histologic examination of tissue or by response of the lesion to antimicrobial agents. Culture of *K granulomatis* is difficult to perform and is not available routinely. Diagnosis by polymerase chain reaction assay and serologic testing is available only in research laboratories.

TREATMENT: For people 8 years and older, doxycycline, 100 mg orally, twice daily for at least 21 days and until the lesions are completely healed, is the treatment of choice. Tetracycline-based antimicrobial agents, including doxycycline, may cause permanent tooth discoloration for children younger than 8 years if used for repeated treatment courses. However, doxycycline binds less readily to calcium compared with older tetracyclines, and in some studies, doxycycline was not associated with visible teeth staining in younger children (see Tetracyclines, p 873). Azithromycin, 1 g orally, once per week for at least 3 weeks and until all lesions have completely healed, is an alternative regimen for children younger than 8 years. Trimethoprim-sulfamethoxazole, ciprofloxacin, and erythromycin may be used in appropriate patients as well. Gentamicin can be added if no improvement is evident after several days of therapy. Antimicrobial therapy is continued for at least 3 weeks and until the lesions have resolved. Partial healing usually is noted within 7 days of initiation of therapy. Relapse can occur, especially if the antimicrobial agent is stopped before the primary lesion has healed completely. Complicated or long-standing infection can require surgical intervention. Pregnant and lactating females should be treated with erythromycin base, 500 mg orally, 4 times/day for at least 3 weeks and until all lesions have completely healed, and consideration should be given to adding a parenteral aminoglycoside (eg, gentamicin). Azithromycin might prove useful for treating granuloma inguinale during pregnancy, but published data are lacking.

Patients should be evaluated for other sexually transmitted infections, such as gonorrhea, syphilis, chancroid, chlamydia, hepatitis B virus, and human immunodeficiency virus infections. Completion of the series of vaccines for hepatitis B and human papillomavirus should be determined, then offered if not completed and if appropriate for the age group.

ISOLATION OF THE HOSPITALIZED PATIENT: Standard precautions are recommended.

CONTROL MEASURES: Sexual partners should be examined, counseled to use condoms, and offered antimicrobial therapy if lesions are present. The value of treating asymptomatic sexual partners has not been demonstrated.

Haemophilus influenzae Infections

CLINICAL MANIFESTATIONS: *Haemophilus influenzae* type b (Hib) causes pneumonia, bacteremia, meningitis, epiglottitis, septic arthritis, cellulitis, otitis media, purulent pericarditis, and less commonly, endocarditis, endophthalmitis, osteomyelitis, peritonitis, and gangrene. Non-type b-encapsulated strains present in a similar manner to type b infections. Nontypable strains more commonly cause infections of the respiratory tract (eg, otitis media, sinusitis, pneumonia, conjunctivitis) and, less often, bacteremia, meningitis, chorioamnionitis, and neonatal septicemia.

ETIOLOGY: *H influenzae* is a pleomorphic gram-negative coccobacillus. Encapsulated strains express 1 of 6 antigenically distinct capsular polysaccharides (a through f); nonencapsulated strains lack capsule genes and are designated nontypable.

EPIDEMIOLOGY[1]: The mode of transmission is person to person by inhalation of respiratory tract droplets or by direct contact with respiratory tract secretions. In neonates, infection is acquired intrapartum by aspiration of amniotic fluid or by contact with genital tract secretions containing the organism. Pharyngeal colonization by *H influenzae* is relatively common, especially with nontypable and non-type b capsular type strains. Similar to findings in the pre-Hib vaccine era, in resource-limited countries where Hib vaccine has not been routinely implemented, the major reservoir of Hib is young infants and toddlers, who carry the organism in the upper respiratory tract.

---

[1]Centers for Disease Control and Prevention. Prevention and control of *Haemophilus influenzae* type b disease: recommendations of the Advisory Committee on Immunization Practices (ACIP). *MMWR Recomm Rep.* 2014;63(RR-1):1–14

Before introduction of effective Hib conjugate vaccines, Hib was the most common cause of bacterial meningitis in children in the United States. The peak incidence of invasive Hib infections occurred between 6 and 18 months of age. In contrast, the peak age for Hib epiglottitis was 2 to 4 years of age.

Unimmunized children younger than 4 years are at increased risk of invasive Hib disease. Factors that predispose to invasive disease include sickle cell disease, asplenia, human immunodeficiency virus (HIV) infection, certain immunodeficiency syndromes, and malignant neoplasms. Historically, invasive Hib was more common in black, Alaska Native, Apache, and Navajo children; boys; child care attendees; children living in crowded conditions; and children who were not breastfed.

Since introduction of Hib conjugate vaccines in the United States, the incidence of invasive Hib disease has decreased by 99% to fewer than 1 cases per 100 000 children younger than 5 years. In 2012, 30 cases of invasive type b disease were reported in children younger than 5 years. In the United States, invasive Hib disease occurs primarily in underimmunized children and among infants too young to have completed the primary immunization series. Hib remains an important pathogen in many resource-limited countries where Hib vaccines are not available routinely.

The epidemiology of invasive *H influenzae* disease in the United States has shifted in the postvaccination era. Nontypable *H influenzae* now causes the majority of invasive *H influenzae* disease in all age groups. From 1999 through 2008, the annual incidence of invasive nontypable *H influenzae* disease was 1.73/100 000 in children younger than 5 years and 4.08/100 000 in adults 65 years and older. Nontypable *H influenzae* causes approximately 50% of episodes of acute otitis media and sinusitis in children and is a common cause of recurrent otitis media. The rate of nontypable *H influenzae* infections in boys is twice that in girls and peaks in the late fall.

In some North American indigenous populations, *Haemophilus influenzae* type a (Hia) has emerged as a significant cause of invasive disease. The 2002-2012 incidence of Hia in Alaska Native children younger than 5 years was 18/100 000/year (vs 0.5/100 000 in nonnative children). The incidence was highest in southwestern Alaska Native children younger than 5 years (72/100 000/year). Similarly, Hia has emerged among northern Canadian indigenous children, who experienced an incidence of 102/100 000/year in children younger than 2 years. There has been an ongoing lower level of Hia disease in Navajo children younger than 5 years (20/100 000/year, 1988-2003). Invasive disease has also been caused by other encapsulated non-b strains.

The **incubation period** is unknown.

DIAGNOSTIC TESTS: The diagnosis of invasive disease is established by growth of *H influenzae* from cerebrospinal fluid (CSF), blood, synovial fluid, pleural fluid, or pericardial fluid. Gram stain of an infected body fluid specimen can facilitate presumptive diagnosis. All *H influenzae* isolates associated with invasive infection should be serotyped. Although the potential for suboptimal sensitivity and specificity exists with slide agglutination serotyping (SAST) depending on reagents used, SAST or genotyping by polymerase chain reaction (PCR) are acceptable methods for capsule typing. If PCR capsular typing is not available locally, isolates should be submitted to the state health department or to a reference laboratory for testing.

Otitis media attributable to *H influenzae* is diagnosed by culture of tympanocentesis fluid; organisms isolated from other respiratory tract swab specimens (eg, throat, ear drainage) may not be the same as those from middle-ear culture.

TREATMENT:
- Initial therapy for children with *H influenzae* meningitis is cefotaxime or ceftriaxone. Ampicillin should be substituted if the Hib isolate is susceptible. Beta-lactamase–negative, ampicillin-resistant strains of *H influenzae* have been described, and some experts recommend caution in using ampicillin when minimum inhibitory concentrations (MICs) of 1 to 2 µg/mL are found, especially in the setting of invasive infection or disease in immunocompromised hosts. Treatment of other invasive *H influenzae* infections is similar. Therapy is continued for 7 to 10 days by the intravenous route and longer in complicated infections.
- Dexamethasone is beneficial for treatment of infants and children with Hib meningitis to diminish the risk of hearing loss, if given before or concurrently with the first dose of antimicrobial agent(s).
- Epiglottitis is a medical emergency. An airway must be established promptly via controlled intubation.
- Infected pleural or pericardial fluid should be drained.
- For empiric treatment of acute otitis media in children younger than 2 years or in children 2 years or older with severe disease, oral amoxicillin (see details in Pneumococcal Infections, p 626, and Appropriate Use of Antimicrobial Agents, p 874) is recommended[1] for 10 days. A 7-day course is considered for children 2 through 5 years of age, and a 5-day course may be used for older children. In the United States, approximately 30% to 40% of *H influenzae* isolates produce beta-lactamase, so amoxicillin may fail, necessitating use of a beta-lactamase–resistant agent, such as amoxicillin-clavulanate; an oral cephalosporin, such as cefdinir, cefuroxime, or cefpodoxime; or azithromycin for children with beta-lactam antibiotic allergy. In vitro susceptibility testing of isolates from middle-ear fluid specimens helps guide therapy in complicated or persistent cases.

ISOLATION OF THE HOSPITALIZED PATIENT: In addition to standard precautions, in patients with invasive Hib disease, droplet precautions are recommended for 24 hours after initiation of effective antimicrobial therapy.

CONTROL MEASURES (FOR INVASIVE HIB DISEASE):
Care of Exposed People. Secondary cases of Hib disease have occurred in unimmunized or incompletely immunized children exposed in a child care or household setting to invasive Hib disease. Such children should be observed carefully for fever or other signs/symptoms of disease. Exposed children in whom febrile illness develops should receive prompt medical evaluation.

Chemoprophylaxis.[2] The risk of invasive Hib disease is increased among unimmunized household contacts younger than 4 years. Rifampin eradicates Hib from the pharynx in approximately 95% of carriers and decreases the risk of secondary invasive illness in exposed household contacts. Child care center contacts also may be at increased risk of secondary disease, but secondary disease in child care contacts is rare when all contacts are older than 2 years.

---

[1]Lieberthal AS, Carroll AE, Chonmaitree T, et al; American Academy of Pediatrics, Subcommittee on Diagnosis and Management of Acute Otitis Media. Clinical practice guideline: the diagnosis and management of acute otitis media. *Pediatrics.* 2013;131(3):e964-e999

[2]Centers for Disease Control and Prevention. Prevention and control of *Haemophilus influenzae* type b disease: recommendations of the Advisory Committee on Immunization Practices (ACIP). *MMWR Recomm Rep.* 2014;63(RR-1):1–14

Indications and guidelines for chemoprophylaxis in different circumstances are summarized in Table 3.9.

- **Household.** Chemoprophylaxis is not recommended for contacts of people with invasive disease caused by non-type b or nontypable *H influenzae* strains, because secondary disease is rare. In households with a person with invasive Hib disease and at least 1 household member who is younger than 48 months and unimmunized or incompletely immunized against Hib, rifampin prophylaxis is recommended for all household contacts, regardless of age. In households with an immunocompromised child, even if the child is older than 48 months and fully immunized, all members of the household should receive rifampin because of the possibility that immunization may not have been effective. Similarly, in households with a contact younger than 12 months who has not received the 2- or 3-dose primary series of Hib conjugate vaccine, depending on vaccine product, all household members should receive rifampin prophylaxis. Given that most secondary cases in households occur during the first week after hospitalization of the index case, when indicated, prophylaxis (see Table 3.9) should be initiated as

Table 3.9. Indications and Guidelines for Rifampin Chemoprophylaxis for Contacts of Index Cases of Invasive *Haemophilus influenzae* Type b (Hib) Disease

Chemoprophylaxis Recommended

- For all household contacts[a] in the following circumstances:
  - Household with at least 1 contact younger than 4 years of age who is unimmunized or incompletely immunized[b]
  - Household with a child younger than 12 months of age who has not completed the primary Hib series
  - Household with a contact who is an immunocompromised child, regardless of that child's Hib immunization status or age
- For preschool and child care center contacts when 2 or more cases of Hib invasive disease have occurred within 60 days (see text)
- For index patient, if younger than 2 years of age or member of a household with a susceptible contact and treated with a regimen other than cefotaxime or ceftriaxone, chemoprophylaxis at the end of therapy for invasive infection

Chemoprophylaxis Not Recommended

- For occupants of households with no children younger than 4 years of age other than the index patient
- For occupants of households when all household contacts are immunocompetent, all household contacts 12 through 48 months of age have completed their Hib immunization series, and when household contacts younger than 12 months of age have completed their primary series of Hib immunizations
- For preschool and child care contacts of 1 index case
- For pregnant women

---

[a]Defined as people residing with the index patient or nonresidents who spent 4 or more hours with the index patient for at least 5 of the 7 days preceding the day of hospital admission of the index case.

[b]Complete immunization is defined as having had at least 1 dose of conjugate vaccine at 15 months of age or older; 2 doses between 12 and 14 months of age; or the 2- or 3-dose primary series when younger than 12 months with a booster dose at 12 months of age or older.

soon as possible. Because some secondary cases occur later, initiation of prophylaxis 7 days or more after hospitalization of the index patient still may be of some benefit.

- **Child care and preschool.** When 2 or more cases of invasive Hib disease have occurred within 60 days and unimmunized or incompletely immunized children attend the child care facility or preschool, rifampin prophylaxis for all attendees (irrespective of their age and vaccine status) and child care providers should be considered. In addition to these recommendations for chemoprophylaxis, unimmunized or incompletely immunized children should receive a dose of vaccine and should be scheduled for completion of the recommended age-specific immunization schedule (**http://aapredbook .aappublications.org/site/resources/izschedules.xhtml**). Data are insufficient on the risk of secondary transmission to recommend chemoprophylaxis for attendees and child care providers when a single case of invasive Hib disease occurs; the decision to provide chemoprophylaxis in this situation is at the discretion of the local health department.

- **Index case.** Treatment of Hib disease with cefotaxime or ceftriaxone eradicates Hib colonization, eliminating the need for prophylaxis of the index patient. Patients who do not receive at least 1 dose of cefotaxime or ceftriaxone and who are younger than 2 years should receive rifampin prophylaxis at the end of therapy for invasive infection.

- **Dosage.** For prophylaxis, rifampin should be given orally, once a day for 4 days (20 mg/kg; maximum dose, 600 mg). The dose for infants younger than 1 month is not established; some experts recommend lowering the dose to 10 mg/kg. For adults, each dose is 600 mg.

Immunization.[1] Three single-antigen (monovalent) Hib conjugate vaccine products and 3 combination vaccine products that contain Hib conjugate are available in the United States (see Table 3.10, p 373). The Hib conjugate vaccines consist of the Hib capsular polysaccharide (polyribosylribotol phosphate [PRP]) covalently linked to a carrier protein. Protective antibodies are directed against PRP. Conjugate vaccines vary in composition and immunogenicity, and as a result, recommendations for their use differ.

Depending on the vaccine, the recommended primary series consists of 3 doses given at 2, 4, and 6 months of age or of 2 doses given at 2 and 4 months of age (see Recommendations for Immunization, p 374, and Table 3.11, p 374). The recommended doses can be given as a Hib-hepatitis B (HepB) combination vaccine, as a diphtheria and tetanus toxoids and acellular pertussis (DTaP)-inactivated poliovirus (IPV)/Hib combination vaccine, or as a bivalent meningococcal conjugate/Hib conjugate vaccine. The regimens in Table 3.11 (p 374) likely are to be equivalent in protection after completion of the recommended primary series. For American Indian/Alaska Native children, optimal immune protection is achieved by administration of PRP-OMP (outer membrane protein complex) Hib vaccine (see American Indian/Alaska Native Children, *Haemophilus influenzae* type b, p 91).

Combination Vaccines. Three combination vaccines that contain Hib are licensed in the United States: HepB-Hib combination, DTaP-IPV/Hib, and HibMenCY combination (see Table 3.10, p 373) vaccines. The HepB-Hib combination vaccine is licensed for use at 2, 4, and 12 through 15 months of age and should not be given to infants younger than 6 weeks. The DTaP-IPV/Hib combination vaccine is licensed for children 6 weeks through 4 years of age, given as a 4-dose series at 2, 4, 6, and 15 through 18 months of age. HibMenCY is licensed for children 6 weeks through 18 months of age and is

[1]Centers for Disease Control and Prevention. Prevention and control of Haemophilus influenzae type b disease: recommendations of the Advisory Committee on Immunization Practices (ACIP). *MMWR Recomm Rep.* 2014;63(RR-1):1–14

Table 3.10. *Haemophilus influenzae* Type b (Hib) Conjugate Vaccines Licensed for Use in Infants and Children in the United States[a]

Vaccine	Trade Name	Components	Manufacturer
PRP-T	ActHIB	PRP conjugated to tetanus toxoid	Sanofi Pasteur
PRP-T[b]	Hiberix[b]	PRP conjugated to tetanus toxoid	GlaxoSmithKline Biologicals
PRP-OMP	PedvaxHIB	PRP conjugated to OMP	Merck & Co, Inc
PRP-OMP-HepB[c]	Comvax	PRP-OMP + hepatitis B vaccine	Merck & Co, Inc
DTaP-IPV/PRP-T[d]	Pentacel	DTaP-IPV + PRP-T	Sanofi Pasteur
MenCY/PRP-T[e]	MenHibRix	MenCY + PRP-T	GlaxoSmithKline

PRP-T indicates polyribosylribotol phosphate-tetanus toxoid; DTaP, diphtheria and tetanus toxoids and acellular pertussis; OMP, outer membrane protein complex from *Neisseria meningitidis;* HepB, hepatitis B vaccine.

[a] Hib conjugate vaccines may be given in combination products or as reconstituted products, provided the combination or reconstituted vaccine is licensed by the US Food and Drug Administration (FDA) for the child's age and administration of the other vaccine component(s) also is justified.

[b] PRP-T (Hiberix), manufactured by GlaxoSmithKline Biologicals, is licensed only for the final (booster) dose of the Hib vaccine series and should not be used for primary immunization in infants at 2, 4, or 6 months of age (Centers for Disease Control and Prevention. Licensure of a *Haemophilus influenzae* type b [Hib] vaccine [Hiberix] and updated recommendations for use of Hib vaccines. *MMWR Morb Mortal Wkly Rep.* 2009;58[36]:1008-1009). GlaxoSmithKline no longer is marketing this product.

[c] The combination *H influenzae* type b (PRP-OMP) and HepB (Recombivax, 5 μg) vaccine (Comvax) is licensed for use at 2, 4, and 12 through 15 months of age. Merck has discontinued this product and it will not be available after December 31, 2014.

[d] The DTaP-IPV liquid component is used to reconstitute a lyophilized ActHIB vaccine component to form Pentacel.

[e] MenCY/PRP-T can be used in a 4-dose series for infants at risk of meningococcal disease but does not provide protection against meningococcal serotpyes A and W and should not be used for protection of infants traveling to or residing in areas with hyperendemic or epidemic meningococcal disease (see Meningococcal Infections, p 547). MenCY/PRP-T also may be used in any infant for routine vaccination against Hib.

recommended as a 4-dose series at 2, 4, 6, and 12 through 15 months for infants at increased risk for meningococcal disease. However, HibMenCY does not provide protection against meningococcal serotpyes A and W and should not be used for protection of infants traveling to or residing in areas with hyperendemic or epidemic meningococcal disease (see Meningococcal Infections, p 547). HibMenCY also may be used in any infant for routine vaccination against Hib.

Vaccine Interchangeability. Hib conjugate vaccines licensed within the age range for the primary vaccine series are considered interchangeable as long as recommendations for a total of 3 doses in the first year of life are followed (ie, if 2 doses of Hib-OMP are not given, 3 doses of a Hib-containing vaccine are required).

Dosage and Route of Administration. The dose of each Hib conjugate vaccine is 0.5 mL, given intramuscularly.

Children With Immunologic Impairment. Children at increased risk of Hib disease may have impaired anti-PRP antibody responses to conjugate vaccines. Examples include children with functional or anatomic asplenia, HIV infection, or immunoglobulin deficiency (including an isolated immunoglobulin [Ig] G2 subclass deficiency) or early component complement deficiency); recipients of hematopoietic stem cell transplants; and children undergoing chemotherapy for a malignant neoplasm. Some children with immunologic impairment may benefit from more doses of conjugate vaccine than usually indicated (see Recommendations for Immunization: Indications and Schedule).

Table 3.11. Recommended Regimens for Routine *Haemophilus influenzae* Type b (Hib) Conjugate Immunization for Children Immunized at 2 Months Through 4 Years of Age[a]

Vaccine Product	Primary Series	Booster Dose	Catch-up Doses[b]
PRP-T (ActHIB, Sanofi Pasteur)	2, 4, 6 mo	12 through 15 mo	16 mo through 4 y
PRP-T (Hiberix, GlaxoSmithKline)	Not licensed	12 through 15 mo	16 mo through 4 y
PRP-OMP (PedvaxHIB, Merck)[c,d]	2, 4 mo	12 through 15 mo	16 mo through 4 y
Combination vaccines			
PRP-OMP-HepB (Comvax, Merck)[c,d]	2, 4 mo	12 through 15 mo	Not licensed
DTaP-IPV/PRP-T (Pentacel, Sanofi Pasteur)	2, 4, 6 mo	12 through 15 mo	16 mo through 4 y
MenCY/PRP-T (MenHibRix, GlaxoSmithKline)[e]	2, 4, 6 mo	12 through 15 mo	Not licensed

PRP-T indicates polyribosylribotol phosphate-tetanus toxoid; OMP, outer membrane protein complex from *Neisseria meningitidis*.
[a]See text and Table 3.10 (p 373) for further information about specific vaccines and Table 1.9 (p 37) for information about combination vaccines.
[b]See Catch-up Immunization Schedule (**http://aapredbook.aappublications.org/site/resources/izschedules .xhtml**) for additional information.
[c]If a PRP-OMP vaccine is not administered as both doses in the primary series, a third dose of Hib conjugate vaccine is needed to complete the primary series
[d]Preferred for American Indian/Alaska Native children.
[e]MenCY/PRP-T can be used in a 4-dose series for infants at risk of meningococcal disease but does not provide protection against meningococcal serotpyes A and W and should not be used for protection of infants traveling to or residing in areas with hyperendemic or epidemic meningococcal disease (see Meningococcal Infections, p 547). MenCY/PRP-T also may be used in any infant for routine vaccination against Hib.

Adverse Reactions. Adverse reactions to Hib conjugate vaccines are uncommon. Pain, redness, and swelling at the injection site occur in approximately 25% of recipients, but these symptoms typically are mild and last fewer than 24 hours.

Recommendations for Immunization:

Indications and Schedule

- All children should be immunized with an Hib conjugate vaccine beginning at approximately 2 months of age (see Table 3.11). Other general recommendations are as follows:
  - ◆ Immunization can be initiated as early as 6 weeks of age.
  - ◆ Vaccine can be administered during visits for other childhood immunizations (see Simultaneous Administration of Multiple Vaccines, p 35).
- For routine immunization of children younger than 7 months, the following guidelines are recommended:
  - ◆ **Primary series.** A 3-dose regimen of PRP-T (tetanus toxoid conjugate)-containing or a 2-dose regimen of PRP-OMP-containing vaccine should be administered (see Table 3.11). Doses are administered at approximately 2-month intervals. When sequential doses of different vaccine products are administered or uncertainty exists about which products previously were used, 3 doses of a conjugate vaccine are considered sufficient to complete the primary series, regardless of the regimen used.

- ◆ **Booster immunization at 12 through 15 months of age.** For children who have completed a primary series, an additional dose of conjugate vaccine is recommended at 12 through 15 months of age and at least 2 months after the last dose. Any monovalent or combination Hib conjugate vaccine is acceptable for this dose.
- Children younger than 5 years who did not receive Hib conjugate vaccine during the first 6 months of life should be immunized according to the recommended catch-up immunization schedule (see **http://aapredbook.aappublications.org/site/resources/izschedules.xhtml** and Table 3.11, p 374). For accelerated immunization in infants younger than 12 months, a minimum of a 4-week interval between doses can be used.
- Children with Hib invasive infection younger than 24 months can remain at risk of developing a second episode of disease. These children should be immunized according to the age-appropriate schedule for unimmunized children as if they had received no previous Hib vaccine doses (see Table 3.11, p 374, and Table 1.9, p 37). Immunization should be initiated 1 month after onset of disease or as soon as possible thereafter.
- Immunologic evaluation should be performed in children who experience invasive Hib disease despite 2 to 3 doses of vaccine and in children with recurrent invasive disease attributable to type b strains.
- Special circumstances are as follows (Table 3.12):
  - ◆ **Lapsed immunizations.** Recommendations for children who have had a lapse in the schedule of immunizations are based on limited data. Current recommendations are summarized in the annual immunization schedule (**http://aapredbook.aappublications.org/site/resources/izschedules.xhtml**).

Table 3.12. Use of *Haemophilus influenzae* Type b (Hib) Conjugate Immunization in Special Populations

High-risk Group	Vaccine Recommendations
Patient <12 mo	Follow routine Hib vaccination recommendations
Patients 12 through 59 mo	If unimmunized or received 0 or 1 dose before age 12 mo: 2 doses 2 mo apart If received 2 or more doses before age 12 mo: 1 dose If completed a primary series and received a booster dose at age 12 mo or older: no additional doses
Patients undergoing chemotherapy or radiation therapy, age <59 mo	If routine Hib doses given 14 or more days before starting therapy: revaccination not required If dose given within 14 days of starting therapy or given during therapy: repeat doses starting at least 3 mo following therapy completion
Patients undergoing elective splenectomy, age ≥15 mo	If unimmunized: 1 dose prior to procedure
Asplenic patients >59 mo and adults	If unimmunized: 1 dose
HIV-infected children >59 mo	If unimmunized: 1 dose
HIV-infected adults	Hib vaccination is not recommended
Recipients of hematopoietic stem cell transplant, all ages	Regardless of Hib vaccination history: 3 doses (at least 1 mo apart) beginning 6–12 mo after transplant

- **Preterm infants.** For preterm infants, immunization should be based on chronologic age and should be initiated at 2 months of age according to recommendations in Table 3.11 (p 374).
- **Functional/anatomic asplenia.** Children with decreased or absent splenic function who have received a primary series of Hib immunizations and a booster dose at 12 months or older need not be immunized further. Children who have received a primary series and a booster dose and are undergoing scheduled splenectomy (eg, for Hodgkin disease, spherocytosis, immune thrombocytopenia, or hypersplenism) may benefit from an additional dose of any licensed conjugate vaccine. This dose should be provided at least 14 days before the procedure.
- **Recipients of chemotherapy, radiation therapy, or hematopoietic stem cell transplants.** Because of potential suboptimal antibody response, Hib vaccination during chemotherapy or radiation therapy may not be effective; children younger than 60 months who are vaccinated within 14 days before starting immunosuppressive therapy or while receiving immunosuppressive therapy should be considered unimmunized, and doses should be repeated beginning at least 3 months after completion of chemotherapy. Recipients of hematopoietic stem cell transplants should be revaccinated with a 3-dose series at least 3 months after successful transplant, regardless of vaccination history or age.
- **Other high-risk groups.** Patients with HIV infection or immunoglobulin (Ig) G2 subclass deficiency and children receiving chemotherapy for malignant neoplasms also are at increased risk of invasive Hib disease. Whether these children will benefit from additional doses after completion of the primary series of immunizations and the booster dose at 12 months or older is unknown.
- **Catch-up immunization for high-risk groups (http://aapredbook .aappublications.org/site/resources/izschedules.xhtml)** (Table 3.12):
  - For children 12 through 59 months of age with an underlying condition predisposing to Hib disease who are not immunized or have received only 1 dose of conjugate vaccine before 12 months of age, 2 doses of any conjugate vaccine, separated by 2 months, are recommended. For children in this age group who received 2 doses before 12 months of age, 1 additional dose of conjugate vaccine is recommended.
  - Unimmunized children with HIV infection; children with functional or anatomic asplenia, including sickle cell disease; and children having undergone reconstitution following stem cell transplant and who are older than 59 months of age should receive 1 dose of any licensed Hib conjugate vaccine.

Public Health Reporting. All cases of *H influenzae* invasive disease, including type b, non-type b, and nontypable, should be reported to the Centers for Disease Control and Prevention through the local or state public health department.

Hantavirus Pulmonary Syndrome

CLINICAL MANIFESTATIONS: Hantaviruses cause 2 distinct clinical syndromes: hantavirus pulmonary syndrome (HPS), a noncardiogenic pulmonary edema observed in the New World; and hemorrhagic fever with renal syndrome (HFRS), which occurs worldwide (see Hemorrhagic Fevers Caused by Bunyaviruses, p 383). After an incubation period of 1 to 6 weeks, the prodromal illness of HPS is 3 to 7 days and is characterized by fever; chills; headache; myalgia of the shoulders, lower back, and thighs; nausea; vomiting; diarrhea;

dizziness; and sometimes cough. Respiratory tract symptoms or signs usually do not occur during the first 3 to 7 days, but then pulmonary edema and severe hypoxemia appear abruptly after the onset of cough and dyspnea. The disease then progresses over a number of hours. In severe cases, persistent hypotension caused by myocardial dysfunction is present. In fatal cases, death occurs in 1 to 2 days following hospitalization.

Extensive bilateral interstitial and alveolar pulmonary edema and pleural effusions are the result of a diffuse pulmonary capillary leak and appear to be immune mediated in the endothelial cells of the microvasculature. Intubation and assisted ventilation usually are required for only 2 to 4 days, with resolution heralded by onset of diuresis and rapid clinical improvement.

The severe myocardial depression is different from that of septic shock, with low cardiac indices and stroke volume index, normal pulmonary wedge pressure, and increased systemic vascular resistance. Poor prognostic indicators include persistent hypotension, marked hemoconcentration, a cardiac index of less than 2, and abrupt onset of lactic acidosis with a serum lactate concentration of >4 mmol/L (36 mg/dL).

The mortality rate for patients with HPS is between 30% and 40%. Asymptomatic and milder forms of disease are rare. Limited information suggests that clinical manifestations and prognosis are similar in adults and children. Serious sequelae are uncommon.

ETIOLOGY: Hantaviruses are RNA viruses of the *Bunyaviridae* family. Sin Nombre virus (SNV) is the major cause of HPS in the western and central regions of the United States. Bayou virus, Black Creek Canal virus, Monongahela virus, and New York virus are responsible for sporadic cases in Louisiana, Texas, Florida, New York, and other areas of the eastern United States. Hantavirus serotypes associated with an HPS syndrome in South and Central America include Andes virus, Oran virus, Laguna Negra virus, and Choclo virus. During the past decade, Brazil, Chile, and Argentina have reported most of the HPS cases in the Americas.

EPIDEMIOLOGY: Rodents are the natural hosts for hantaviruses and acquire lifelong, asymptomatic, chronic infection with prolonged viruria and virus in saliva, urine, and feces. Humans acquire infection through direct contact with infected rodents, rodent droppings, or rodent nests or through the inhalation of aerosolized virus particles from rodent urine, droppings, or saliva. Rarely, infection may be acquired from rodent bites or contamination of broken skin with excreta. Person-to-person transmission of hantaviruses has not been demonstrated in the United States but has been reported in Chile and Argentina with the Andes virus. At-risk activities include handling or trapping rodents; cleaning or entering closed or rarely used rodent-infested structures; cleaning feed storage or animal shelter areas; hand plowing; and living in a home with an increased density of mice. For backpackers or campers, sleeping in a structure also inhabited by rodents has been associated with HPS. Weather conditions resulting in exceptionally heavy rainfall and improved rodent food supplies can result in a large increase in the rodent population with more frequent contact between humans and infected mice, resulting in an increase in human disease. Most cases occur during the spring and summer, with the geographic location determined by the habitat of the rodent carrier.

SNV is transmitted by the deer mouse, *Peromyscus maniculatus;* Black Creek Canal virus is transmitted by the cotton rat, *Sigmodon hispidus;* Bayou virus is transmitted by the rice rat, *Oryzomys palustris;* and New York virus is transmitted by the white-footed mouse, *Peromyscus leucopus.*

The **incubation period** may be 1 to 6 weeks after exposure to infected rodents, their saliva, or excreta.

DIAGNOSTIC TESTS: Characteristic laboratory findings include neutrophilic leukocytosis with immature granulocytes, including more than 10% immunoblasts (basophilic cytoplasm, prominent nucleoli, and an increased nuclear-cytoplasmic ratio), thrombocytopenia, and increased hematocrit. SNV RNA has been detected by reverse transcriptase-polymerase chain reaction assay of peripheral blood mononuclear cells and other clinical specimens from the early phase of the disease, frequently before the hospitalization. Viral RNA is not detected readily in bronchoalveolar lavage fluids.

Hantavirus-specific immunoglobulin (Ig) M and IgG antibodies often are present at the onset of clinical disease, and serologic testing is the method of choice for diagnosis. IgG may be negative in rapidly fatal cases. Rapid diagnosis can facilitate immediate appropriate supportive therapy and early transfer to a tertiary care facility. Enzyme immunoassay (available through many state health departments and the Centers for Disease Control and Prevention) and Western blot assays use recombinant antigens and have a high degree of specificity for detection of IgG and IgM antibody. Viral culture is not useful for diagnosis. Finally, immunohistochemistry in tissues (staining of capillary endothelial cells of the lungs and almost every organ in the body) obtained from autopsy can also establish the diagnosis retrospectively.

TREATMENT: Patients with suspected HPS should be transferred immediately to a tertiary care facility where supportive management of pulmonary edema, severe hypoxemia, and hypotension can occur during the first critical 24 to 48 hours.

In severe forms, early mechanical ventilation and inotropic and pressor support are necessary. Extracorporeal membrane oxygenation (ECMO) should be considered when pulmonary wedge pressure and cardiac indices have deteriorated and may provide short-term support for the severe capillary leak syndrome in the lungs.

Ribavirin is active in vitro against hantaviruses, including SNV. However, 2 clinical studies of intravenous ribavirin (1 open-label study and 1 randomized, placebo-controlled, double-blind study) failed to show benefit in treatment of HPS in the cardiopulmonary stage.

ISOLATION OF THE HOSPITALIZED PATIENT: Standard precautions are recommended. HPS has not been associated with health care-associated or person-to-person transmission in the United States.

CONTROL MEASURES:

Care of Exposed People. Serial clinical examinations should be used to monitor individuals at high risk of infection after exposure (see Epidemiology, p 377).

Environmental Control. Hantavirus infections of humans occur primarily in adults and are associated with domestic, occupational, or leisure activities facilitating contact with infected rodents, usually in a rural setting. Eradicating the host reservoir is not feasible. The best available approach for disease control and prevention is risk reduction through environmental hygiene practices that discourage rodents from colonizing the home and work environment and that minimize aerosolization and contact with the virus in rodent saliva and excreta. Measures to decrease exposure in the home and workplace include eliminating food available to rodent, reducing possible nesting sites, sealing holes and other possible entrances for rodents, and using "snap traps" and rodenticides. Before entering areas with potential rodent infestations, doors and windows should be opened to ventilate the enclosure.

Hantaviruses, because of their lipid envelope, are susceptible to most disinfectants, including diluted bleach solutions, detergents, and most general household disinfectants. Dusty or dirty areas or articles should be moistened with 10% bleach or other disinfectant solution before being cleaned. Brooms and vacuum cleaners should not be used to clean rodent-infested areas. Use of a 10% bleach solution to disinfect dead rodents and wearing rubber gloves before handling trapped or dead rodents is recommended. Gloves and traps should be disinfected after use. The cleanup of areas potentially infested with hantavirus-infected rodents should be carried out by knowledgeable professionals using appropriate personal protective equipment. Potentially infected material should be handled according to local regulations for infectious waste.

Chemoprophylaxis measures or vaccines are not available.

Public Health Reporting. Possible hantavirus occurrence should be reported immediately to local and state public health authorities. In addition, HPS is reportable in the United States using the guidelines of the Council of State and Territorial Epidemiologists.

Helicobacter pylori Infections

CLINICAL MANIFESTATIONS: *Helicobacter pylori* causes chronic active gastritis and may result in duodenal, and to a lesser extent gastric, ulcers. Persistent infection with *H pylori* increases the risk of gastric cancer. In children, *H pylori* infection can result in gastroduodenal inflammation that can manifest as epigastric pain, nausea, vomiting, hematemesis, and guaiac-positive stools. Symptoms can resolve within a few days or can wax and wane. Extraintestinal conditions in children that have been associated with *H pylori* infection can include iron-deficiency anemia and short stature. However, most infections are thought to be asymptomatic. Moreover, there is no clear association between infection and recurrent abdominal pain, in the absence of peptic ulcer disease. The organism can persist in the stomach for years or for life. *H pylori* infection is not associated with secondary gastritis (eg, autoimmune or associated with nonsteroidal anti-inflammatory agents).

ETIOLOGY: *H pylori* is a gram-negative, spiral, curved, or U-shaped microaerophilic bacillus that has single or multiple flagella at one end. The organism is catalase, oxidase, and urease positive.

EPIDEMIOLOGY: *H pylori* organisms have been isolated from humans and other primates. An animal reservoir for human transmission has not been demonstrated. Organisms are thought to be transmitted from infected humans by the fecal-oral, gastro-oral, and oral-oral routes. Nearly half of the world's population is infected with *H pylori*, with a disproportionally high prevalence rate in developing countries. Infection rates are low in children in resource-rich, industrialized countries, except in children from lower socioeconomic groups. Most infections are acquired in the first 5 years of life and can reach prevalence rates of up to 80% in resource-limited countries. Approximately 70% of infected people are asymptomatic, 20% of people have macroscopic (ie, visual) and microscopic findings of ulceration, and an estimated 1% have features of neoplasia.

The **incubation period** is unknown.

DIAGNOSTIC TESTS: *H pylori* infection can be diagnosed by culture of gastric biopsy tissue on nonselective media (eg, chocolate agar) or selective media (eg, Skirrow agar) at 37°C (98°F) under microaerobic conditions for 3 to 7 days. Antibiotic susceptibility testing of cultured isolates may be necessary to guide therapy in refractory cases. The organism also can be identified by polymerase chain reaction (PCR) or fluorescence in situ hybridization (FISH) of gastric biopsy tissue. Organisms usually can be visualized on histologic sections with Warthin-Starry silver, Steiner, Giemsa, or Genta staining. Presence of *H pylori* can be confirmed but not excluded on the basis of hematoxylin-eosin stains. Because of production of urease by organisms, urease testing of a gastric specimen can give a rapid and specific microbiologic diagnosis. Each of these tests requires endoscopy and biopsy. Noninvasive, commercially available tests for active infection include breath tests that detect labeled carbon dioxide in expired air after oral administration of iso-topically labeled urea (^{13}C or ^{14}C); these tests are expensive and are not useful in young children. The US Food and Drug Administration cleared the first *H pylori* breath test for children 3 to 17 years of age in 2012. A stool antigen test (by enzyme immunoassay) also is available commercially and can be used for children of any age, especially before and after treatment. Each of these commercially available tests for active infection (ie, breath or stool tests) has a high sensitivity and specificity. Serologic testing for *H pylori* infection by detection of immunoglobulin (Ig) G antibodies specific for *H pylori* may be useful for epidemiologic surveys but does not help clarify the current status of infection and is not recommended for screening children.

TREATMENT: Universal eradication of *H pylori* is not recommended.[1] Treatment is recom-mended for infected patients who have peptic ulcer disease (currently or in the past 1–5 years), gastric mucosa-associated lymphoid tissue-type lymphoma, or early gastric cancer. Screening for and treatment of infection, if found, may be considered for children with one or more primary relatives with gastric cancer, children who are in a high-risk group for gastric cancer (eg, immigrants from resource-limited countries or countries with high rates of gastric cancer), or children who have unexplained iron-deficiency anemia. Treatment also may be considered if infection is found at the time of diagnostic endoscopy for gastro-intestinal tract symptoms, even if gastritis is the only histologic lesion found.

Eradication therapy for *H pylori* consists of at least 7 to 14 days of treatment; eradica-tion rates are higher for regimens of 14 days. A number of treatment regimens have been evaluated and are approved for use in adults; the safety and efficacy of these regimens in pediatric patients have not been established. First-line eradication regimens include: (1) triple therapy with a proton pump inhibitor (PPI) (eg, lansoprazole, omeprazole, esomeprazole, pantoprazole, rabeprazole) plus amoxicillin plus clarithromycin or met-ronidazole; or (2) bismuth salts plus amoxicillin plus metronidazole. An alternative sequential regimen that may be more effective includes dual therapy with amoxicillin and a PPI for 5 days, followed by 5 days of triple therapy (a PPI plus clarithromycin and metronidazole). These regimens are effective in eliminating the organism, healing the ulcer, and preventing recurrence. Alternate therapies in people 8 years and older include: (1) bismuth subsalicylate plus metronidazole plus tetracycline plus either a PPI or an H_2 blocker (eg, cimetidine, famotidine, nizatidine, ranitidine), or (2) bismuth subcitrate potas-sium plus metronidazole plus tetracycline plus omeprazole. Tetracycline products are not recommended in patients younger than 8 years. Tetracycline-based antimicrobial agents, including doxycycline, may cause permanent tooth discoloration for children younger than 8 years if used for repeated treatment courses. However, doxycycline binds less read-ily to calcium compared with older tetracyclines, and in some studies, doxycycline was not associated with visible teeth staining in younger children (see Tetracyclines, p 873). A

[1]Koletzko S, Jones NL, Goodman K, et al. Evidence-based guidelines from ESPGHAN and NASPGHAN for Helicobacter pylori infection in children. *J Pediatr Gastroenterol Nutr.* 2011;53(2):230-243

breath or stool test may be performed as follow-up to document organism eradication 4 to 8 weeks after completion of therapy, although the stool antigen test result may remain positive for up to 90 days after treatment. Salvage therapies for treatment failure include increasing the duration of therapy (ie, 2 to 4 weeks) or bismuth-based quadruple therapy for 1 to 2 weeks (eg, bismuth subsalicylate plus 2 antibiotic agents plus a PPI).

ISOLATION OF THE HOSPITALIZED PATIENT: Standard precautions are recommended.

CONTROL MEASURES: Disinfection of gastroscopes prevents transmission of the organism between patients.

Hemorrhagic Fevers Caused by Arenaviruses[1]

CLINICAL MANIFESTATIONS: Arenaviruses are responsible for several hemorrhagic fevers (HFs): Old World arenavirus HFs include Lassa fever and the recently described Lujo virus infections; New World arenavirus HFs include Argentine, Bolivian, Brazilian, Venezuelan, and Chapare virus infection. Lymphocytic choriomeningitis virus (LCMV) is an arenavirus that generally induces less severe disease, although it can cause HFs in immunosuppressed patients; LCMV is discussed in a separate chapter (p 527). Disease associated with arenaviruses ranges in severity from mild, acute, febrile infections to severe illnesses in which vascular leak, shock, and multiorgan dysfunction are prominent features. Fever, headache, myalgia, conjunctival suffusion, retro-orbital pain, facial flushing, bleeding, and abdominal pain are common early symptoms in all infections. Thrombocytopenia, leukopenia, axillary petechiae, generalized lymphadenopathy, and encephalopathy usually are present in Argentine HF, Bolivian HF, and Venezuelan HF, and exudative pharyngitis often occurs in Lassa fever. Mucosal bleeding occurs in severe cases as a consequence of vascular damage, thrombocytopenia, and platelet dysfunction. Proteinuria is common, but renal failure is unusual. Increased serum concentrations of aspartate transaminase (AST) can portend a severe or possibly fatal outcome of Lassa fever. Shock develops 7 to 9 days after onset of illness in more severely ill patients with these infections. Upper and lower respiratory tract symptoms can develop in people with Lassa fever. Encephalopathic signs, such as tremor, alterations in consciousness, and seizures, can occur in South American HFs and in severe cases of Lassa fever. Transitory deafness is reported in 30% of early convalescents of Lassa fever. The mortality rate in South American HFs is 15% to 30%.

ETIOLOGY: Arenaviruses are segmented, single-stranded RNA viruses. The major New World arenavirus hemorrhagic fevers occurring in the Western hemisphere are caused by the Tacaribe serocomplex of arenaviruses: Argentine HF caused by Junin virus, Bolivian HF caused by Machupo virus, and Venezuelan HF caused by Guanarito virus. A fourth arenavirus, Sabia virus, has been recognized to cause 2 unrelated cases of naturally occurring HF in Brazil and 2 laboratory-acquired cases. Chapare virus has been isolated from a human fatal case in Bolivia. The Old World complex of arenaviruses includes Lassa virus, which causes Lassa fever in West Africa, as well as Lujo virus, which was described in southern Africa during an outbreak characterized by fatal human-to-human transmission. Several other arenaviruses are known only from their rodent reservoirs in the Old and New World.

EPIDEMIOLOGY: Arenaviruses are maintained in nature by association with specific rodent hosts, in which they produce chronic viremia and viruria. The principal routes of infection

---

[1]Does not include lymphocytic choriomeningitis virus, which is reviewed on p 527.

are inhalation and contact of mucous membranes and skin (eg, through cuts, scratches, or abrasions) with urine and salivary secretions from these persistently infected rodents. Ingestion of food contaminated by rodent excrement also may cause disease transmission. All arenaviruses are infectious as aerosols, and arenaviruses causing HF should be considered highly hazardous to people working with any of these viruses in the laboratory. Laboratory-acquired infections have been documented with Lassa, Machupo, Junin, and Sabia viruses. The geographic distribution and habitats of the specific rodents that serve as reservoir hosts largely determine the areas with endemic infection and the populations at risk. Before a vaccine became available in Argentina, several hundred cases of Argentine HF occurred annually in agricultural workers and inhabitants of the Argentine pampas. The Argentine HF vaccine is not licensed in the United States. Epidemics of Bolivian HF occurred in small towns between 1962 and 1964; sporadic disease activity in the countryside has continued since then. Venezuelan HF first was identified in 1989 and occurs in rural north-central Venezuela. Lassa fever is endemic in most of West Africa, where rodent hosts live in proximity with humans, causing thousands of infections annually. Lassa fever has been reported in the United States and Western Europe in people who have traveled to West Africa.

The **incubation periods** are from 6 to 17 days.

DIAGNOSTIC TESTS: Viral nucleic acid can be detected in acute disease by reverse transcriptase-polymerase chain reaction assay. These viruses may be isolated from blood of acutely ill patients as well as from various tissues obtained postmortem, but isolation should be attempted only under Biosafety level-4 (BSL-4) conditions. Virus antigen is detectable by enzyme immunoassay (EIA) in acute specimens and postmortem tissues. Virus-specific immunoglobulin (Ig) M antibodies are present in the serum during acute stages of illness but may be undetectable in rapidly fatal cases. The IgG antibody response is delayed. Diagnosis can be made retrospectively by immunohistochemistry in formalin-fixed tissues obtained from autopsy.

If a viral hemorrhagic fever is suspected, the state/local health department or Centers for Disease Control and Prevention (CDC; Viral Special Pathogens Branch: 404-639-1115) should be contacted to assist with case investigation, diagnosis, treatment, and control measures.

TREATMENT: Intravenous ribavirin substantially decreases the mortality rate in patients with severe Lassa fever, particularly if they are treated during the first week of illness. For Argentine HF, transfusion of immune plasma in defined doses of neutralizing antibodies is the standard specific treatment when administered during the first 8 days from onset of symptoms. Intravenous ribavirin has been used with success to abort a Sabia laboratory infection and to treat Bolivian HF patients and the only Lujo infection survivor. Ribavirin did not reduce mortality when initiated 8 days or more after onset of Argentine HF symptoms. Whether ribavirin treatment initiated early in the course of the disease has a role in the treatment of Argentine HF remains to be seen. Intravenous ribavirin is available only from the manufacturer through an investigational new drug (IND) protocol. Health care providers who need to obtain intravenous ribavirin should contact the US Food and Drug Administration (FDA) or the manufacturer (Valent Pharmaceuticals: 800-548-5100; FDA 24-hour emergency line: 866-300-4374 or 301-796-8240). Meticulous fluid balance is an important aspect of supportive care in each of the HFs.

ISOLATION OF THE HOSPITALIZED PATIENT: In addition to standard precautions, contact and droplet precautions, including careful prevention of needlestick injuries and careful handling of clinical specimens for the duration of illness, are recommended for all HFs caused by arenaviruses. A negative-pressure ventilation room is recommended for patients with prominent cough or severe disease, and people entering the room should wear personal protection respirators. A negative pressure room should be used when aerosol-generating procedures are conducted, such as intubation or airway suctioning. Additional viral HF-specific isolation precautions have been recommended in the event that a viral HF virus is used as a weapon of bioterrorism.[1]

CONTROL MEASURES:
Care of Exposed People. No specific measures are warranted for exposed people unless direct contamination with blood, excretions, or secretions from an infected patient has occurred. If such contamination has occurred, recording body temperature twice daily for 21 days is recommended. Reporting of fever or of symptoms of infection is an indication for intravenous ribavirin treatment for Lassa fever, Bolivian HF, or Sabia or Lujo infections.
Immunoprophylaxis. A live-attenuated Junin vaccine protects against Argentine HF and probably against Bolivian HF. The vaccine is associated with minimal adverse effects in adults; similar findings have been obtained from limited safety studies in children 4 years and older. The vaccine is not available in the United States.
Environmental. In town-based outbreaks of Bolivian HF, rodent control has proven successful. Area rodent control is not practical for control of Argentine HF or Venezuelan HF. Intensive rodent control efforts have decreased the rate of peridomestic Lassa virus infection, but rodents eventually reinvade human dwellings, and infection still occurs in rural settings.
Public Health Reporting. Because of the risk of health care-associated transmission, state health departments and the CDC should be contacted for specific advice about management and diagnosis of suspected cases. Lassa fever and New World Arenavirus HFs are reportable in the United States according to guidelines of the US Council of State and Territorial Epidemiologists.

Hemorrhagic Fevers Caused by Bunyaviruses[2]

CLINICAL MANIFESTATIONS: Bunyaviruses are vectorborne infections (except for hantavirus) that often result in severe febrile disease with multisystem involvement. Human infection by bunyaviruses may be associated with high rates of morbidity and mortality. In the United States, disease attributable to a bunyavirus most likely is caused by either hantavirus or members of the California serogroup.

Hemorrhagic fever with renal syndrome (HFRS) is a complex, multiphasic disease characterized by vascular instability and varying degrees of renal insufficiency. Fever, flushing, conjunctival injection, headache, blurred vision, abdominal pain, and lumbar pain are followed by hypotension, oliguria, and subsequently, polyuria. Petechiae are frequent, but more serious bleeding manifestations are rare. Shock and acute renal insufficiency may occur. Nephropathia epidemica (attributable to Puumala virus) occurs in Europe and presents as a milder disease with acute influenza-like illness, abdominal pain, and proteinuria. Acute renal dysfunction also occurs, but hypotensive shock or

---

[1] National Center for Infectious Diseases. Interim guidance for managing patients with suspected viral hemorrhagic fever in U.S. hospitals [pamphlet]. Atlanta, GA: Centers for Disease Control and Prevention; May 19, 2005. Available at: **http://stacks.cdc.gov/view/cdc/22139**

[2] Does not include hantavirus pulmonary syndrome, which is reviewed on p 376.

requirement for dialysis are rare. However, more severe forms of HFRS (ie, attributable to Dobrava virus) also occur in Europe.

Crimean-Congo hemorrhagic fever (CCHF) is a multisystem disease characterized by hepatitis and profuse bleeding. Fever, headache, and myalgia are followed by signs of a diffuse capillary leak syndrome with facial suffusion, conjunctivitis, icteric hepatitis, proteinuria, and disseminated intravascular coagulation associated with petechiae and purpura on the skin and mucous membranes. A hypotensive crisis often occurs after the appearance of frank hemorrhage from the gastrointestinal tract, nose, mouth, or uterus. Mortality rates range from 20% to 35%.

Rift Valley fever (RVF), in most cases, is a self-limited undifferentiated febrile illness. Occasionally, hemorrhagic fever with shock and icteric hepatitis, encephalitis, or retinitis develops.

ETIOLOGY: *Bunyaviridae* are segmented, single-stranded RNA viruses with different geographic distributions depending on their vector or reservoir. Hemorrhagic fever syndromes are associated with viruses from 3 genera: hantaviruses, nairoviruses (CCHF virus), and phleboviruses (RVF, Heartland virus in the United States, sandfly fever viruses in Europe, and severe fever with thrombocytopenia syndrome [SFTS] virus in China). Old World hantaviruses (Hantaan, Seoul, Dobrava, and Puumala viruses) cause HFRS, and New World hantaviruses (Sin Nombre and related viruses) cause hantavirus pulmonary syndrome (see Hantavirus Pulmonary Syndrome, p 376).

EPIDEMIOLOGY: The epidemiology of these diseases mainly is a function of the distribution and behavior of their reservoirs and vectors. All genera except hantaviruses are associated with arthropod vectors, and hantavirus infections are associated with airborne exposure to infected wild rodents, primarily via inhalation of virus-contaminated urine, droppings, or nesting materials.

Classic HFRS occurs throughout much of Asia and Eastern and Western Europe, with up to 100 000 cases per year. The most severe form of the disease is caused by the prototype Hantaan virus and Dobrava viruses in rural Asia and Europe, respectively; Puumala virus is associated with milder disease (nephropathia epidemica) in Western Europe. Seoul virus is distributed worldwide in association with *Rattus* species and can cause a disease of variable severity. Person-to-person transmission never has been reported with HFRS.

CCHF occurs in much of sub-Saharan Africa, the Middle East, areas in West and Central Asia, and the Balkans. CCHF virus is transmitted by ticks and occasionally by contact with viremic livestock and wild animals at slaughter. Health care-associated transmission of CCHF is a frequent and serious hazard.

RVF occurs throughout sub-Saharan Africa and has caused large epidemics in Egypt in 1977 and 1993–1995, Mauritania in 1987, Saudi Arabia and Yemen in 2000, Kenya in 1997 and 2006–2007, Madagascar in 1990 and 2008, and South Africa in 2010. The virus is arthropodborne and is transmitted from domestic livestock to humans by mosquitoes. The virus also can be transmitted by aerosol and by direct contact with infected aborted tissues or freshly slaughtered infected animal carcasses. Person-to-person transmission has not been reported, but laboratory-acquired cases are well documented.

The **incubation period**s for CCHF and RVF range from 2 to 10 days; for HFRS, incubation periods usually are longer, ranging from 7 to 42 days.

DIAGNOSTIC TESTS: CCHF and RVF viruses can be cultivated readily (restricted to Biosafety level-4 [BSL-4] laboratories) from blood and tissue specimens of infected patients. Polymerase chain reaction (PCR) assays performed with appropriate safety precautions usually are sensitive on samples obtained during the acute phase of CCHF and RVF but less for HFRS. Detection of viral antigen by enzyme immunoassay (EIA) is a useful alternative for CCHF and RVF. Serum immunoglobulin (Ig) M and IgG virus-specific antibodies typically develop early in convalescence in CCHF and RVF but could be absent in rapidly fatal cases of CCHF. In HFRS, IgM and IgG antibodies usually are detectable at the time of onset of illness or within 48 hours, when it is too late for virus isolation and PCR assay. IgM antibodies or rising IgG titers in paired serum specimens, as demonstrated by EIA, are diagnostic; neutralizing antibody tests provide greater virus-strain specificity but rarely are utilized. Diagnosis can be made retrospectively by immunohistochemistry assay of formalin-fixed tissues obtained from necropsy.

TREATMENT: Ribavirin administered intravenously to patients with HFRS within the first 4 days of illness may be effective in decreasing renal dysfunction, vascular instability, and mortality. However, intravenous ribavirin is not available commercially in the United States and is available only from the manufacturer through an investigational new drug (IND) protocol. Health care providers who need to obtain intravenous ribavirin should contact the US Food and Drug Administration (FDA) or the manufacturer (Valent Pharmaceuticals: 800-548-5100; FDA 24-hour emergency line: 866-300-4374 or 301-796-8240). Supportive therapy for HFRS should include: (1) treatment of shock; (2) monitoring of fluid balance; (3) dialysis for complications of renal failure; (4) control of hypertension during the oliguric phase; and (5) early recognition of possible myocardial failure with appropriate therapy.

Oral and intravenous ribavirin given to patients with CCHF has been associated with milder disease, although no controlled studies have been performed. Ribavirin also may be efficacious as postexposure prophylaxis of CCHF. Studies in animals and humans investigating whether ribavirin has potential benefit in treatment of hemorrhagic RVF have been inconclusive.

If a viral hemorrhagic fever is suspected, the state/local health department or Centers for Disease Control and Prevention (CDC; Viral Special Pathogens Branch: 404-639-1115) should be contacted to assist with case investigation, diagnosis, treatment, and control measures.

ISOLATION OF THE HOSPITALIZED PATIENT: In addition to standard precautions, contact and droplet precautions, including careful prevention of needlestick injuries and management of clinical specimens, are indicated for patients with CCHF for the duration for their illness. Airborne isolation may be required in certain circumstances when patients undergo procedures that stimulate coughing and promote generation of aerosols. Standard precautions should be followed with RVF and HFRS.

CONTROL MEASURES:

Care of Exposed People. People having direct contact with blood or other secretions from patients with CCHF should be observed closely for 21 days with daily monitoring for fever. Immediate therapy with intravenous ribavirin should be considered at the first sign of disease.

Environmental.

Hemorrhagic Fever With Renal Syndrome. Monitoring of laboratory rat colonies and urban rodent control may be effective for ratborne HFRS.

Crimean-Congo Hemorrhagic Fever. Arachnicides for tick control generally have limited benefit but should be used in stockyard settings. Personal protective measures (eg, physical tick removal and protective clothing with permethrin sprays) may be effective for people at-risk (farmers, veterinarians, abattoir workers).

Rift Valley Fever. Regular immunization of domestic animals should have an effect on limiting or preventing RVF outbreaks and protecting humans but is not performed routinely. Personal protective clothing (with permethrin sprays) and insect repellants may be effective for people at risk (farmers, veterinarians, abattoir workers). Mosquito control measures are difficult to implement.

Immunoprophylaxis. No vaccines currently are approved for use in humans against HFs caused by bunyaviruses.

Public Health Reporting. Because of the risk of health care-associated transmission of CCHF and diagnostic confusion with other viral hemorrhagic fevers, state health departments and the CDC should be contacted about any suspected diagnosis of viral hemorrhagic fever and the management plan for the patient. CCHF is reportable in the United States according to guidelines of the US Council of State and Territorial Epidemiologists.

Hemorrhagic Fevers Caused by Filoviruses: Ebola and Marburg

CLINICAL MANIFESTATIONS: Data on Ebola and Marburg virus infections primarily are derived from adult populations. More is known about Ebola virus disease than Marburg virus disease, although the same principles apply generally to all filoviruses that cause human disease. Asymptomatic cases of human filovirus infections have been reported, and symptomatic disease ranges from mild to severe disease; case fatality rates for severely affected people range from 25% to 90% (approximately 70% in the 2014 outbreak). After a typical incubation period of 8 to 10 days (range, 2–21 days), disease in children and adults begins with nonspecific signs and symptoms including fever, headache, myalgia, abdominal pain, and weakness followed several days later by vomiting, diarrhea, and unexplainedbleeding or bruising. Respiratory symptoms are more common in children, and central nervous system manifestations are less common in children than in adults. A fleeting maculopapular rash on the torso or face after approximately 4 to 5 days of illness may occur. Conjunctival injection or subconjunctival hemorrhage may be present. Hepatic dysfunction, with elevations in aspartate transaminase (AST) markedly higher than alanine transaminase (ALT), and metabolic derangements, including hypokalemia, hyponatremia, hypocalcemia, and hypomagnesemia, are common. In the most severe cases, microvascular instability ensues around the end of the first week of disease. Although hemostasis is impaired, hemorrhagic manifestations develop in a minority of patients. In the 2001 Uganda Sudan Ebola virus outbreak, all children with laboratory-confirmed Ebola virus disease were febrile, and only 16% had hemorrhage. The most common hemorrhagic manifestations consist of bleeding from the gastrointestinal tract, sometimes with oozing from the mucus membranes or venipuncture sites in the late stages. Central nervous system manifestations and renal failure are frequent in end-stage disease. In fatal cases, death typically occurs around 10 to 12 days after symptom onset, usually resulting from viral- or bacterial-induced septic shock and multi-organ system failure. Approximately 30% of pregnant women with Ebola virus disease present with spontaneous abortion and vaginal bleeding. Maternal mortality approaches 90% when infection occurs during the third trimester. All neonates born to mothers with active Ebola virus disease to date have died. The exact cause of the neonatal deaths is unknown, but high viral loads of Ebola virus have been documented in amniotic fluid, placental tissue, and fetal tissues of stillborn neonates.

ETIOLOGY: The *Filoviridae* (from the Latin *filo* meaning thread, referring to their filamentous shape) are single-stranded, negative-sense RNA viruses. Four of the 5 species of virus in the *Ebolavirus* genus and both of the known species of virus in the *Marburgvirus* genus are associated with human disease. All of the known human pathogenic filoviruses are endemic only in sub-Saharan Africa.

EPIDEMIOLOGY: Fruit bats are believed to be the animal reservoir for Ebolaviruses. Human infection is believed to occur from inadvertent exposure to infected bat excreta or saliva following entry into roosting areas in caves, mines, and forests. Nonhuman primates, especially gorillas and chimpanzees, and other wild animals also may become infected from bat contact and serve as intermediate hosts that transmit filoviruses to humans through contact with their blood and bodily fluids, usually associated with hunting and butchering (see Control Measures, Environmental). For unclear reasons, filovirus outbreaks tend to occur after prolonged dry seasons.

Molecular epidemiologic evidence shows that most outbreaks result from a single point introduction (or very few) into humans from wild animals, followed by human-to-human transmission, almost invariably fueled by health care-associated transmission in areas with inadequate infection control equipment and resources. Although filoviruses are the most transmissible of all hemorrhagic fever viruses, secondary attack rates in households still generally are only 15% to 20% in African communities, and are lower if proper universal and contact precautions are maintained. Human-to-human transmission usually occurs through oral, mucous membrane, or nonintact skin exposure to bodily fluids of a symptomatic person with filovirus disease, most often in the context of providing care to a sick family or community member (community transmission) or patient (health care-associated transmission). Funeral rituals that entail the touching of the corpse also have been implicated, as has transmission through breastfeeding from infected mothers (see Control Measures, Breastfeeding). Infection through fomites cannot be excluded. Health care-associated transmission is highly unlikely if rigorous infection control practices are in place in health care facilities (see Isolation of the Hospitalized Patient). Ebola is not spread through the air, by water, or in general by food (with the exception of bush meat; see Control Measures, Environmental). Respiratory spread of virus does not occur.

Children may be less likely to become infected from intrafamilial spread than adults when a primary case occurs in a household, possibly secondary to the fact that they are not typically primary caregivers of sick individuals and are less likely to take part in funeral rituals that involve touching and washing of the deceased person's body. Underreporting of Ebola cases in children also is possible. In 2 outbreaks in which large numbers of children were affected, school-aged children and adolescents had increased survival rates compared with children younger than 5 years and adults.

The degree of viremia appears to correlate with the clinical state. People are most infectious late in the course of severe disease, especially when copious vomiting, diarrhea, and/or bleeding are present. Transmission during the incubation period, when the person is asymptomatic, is not believed to occur. Virus may persist in a few immunologically protected sites for several weeks after clinical recovery, including in testicles/semen, human milk, and the chambers of the eye (resulting in transient uveitis and other ocular problems). Because of the risk of sexual transmission, abstinence or use of condoms is recommended for 3 months after recovery.

The 2014 West Africa Ebola outbreak is the largest since the virus was first identified in 1976 and the first in that region of the continent. A simultaneous outbreak of Ebola occurred in the Democratic Republic of the Congo (formerly Zaire), but this outbreak was caused by a different species than the species causing the outbreak in West Africa. Updated information on identification and current management of people traveling from areas of transmission or with contact with a person with Ebola virus infection can be found on the Centers for Disease Control and Prevention (CDC) Web site (**www.cdc. gov/vhf/ebola/**) and the AAP Web site (for pediatricians: **www.aap.org/en-us/ advocacy-and-policy/aap-health-initiatives/Children-and-Disasters/ Pages/Ebola.aspx** and for parents or caregivers: **www.healthychildren.org/ English/health-issues/conditions/infections/Pages/Ebola.aspx** and **www. cdc.gov/vhf/ebola/pdf/how-talk-children-about-ebola.pdf**).

The **incubation period** typically is 8 to 10 days (range, 2–21 days).

DIAGNOSTIC TESTS: The diagnosis of Ebola virus infection should be considered in a person who develops a fever within 21 days of travel to an endemic area (particularly Sierra Leone, Liberia, and Guinea in the 2014 outbreak). Because initial clinical manifestations are difficult to distinguish from those of more common febrile diseases, prompt laboratory testing is imperative in a suspected case. Filovirus disease can be diagnosed by testing of blood by reverse transcriptase-polymerase chain reaction (RT-PCR) assay, enzyme-linked immunosorbent assay (ELISA) for viral antigens or immunoglobulin (Ig) M, and cell culture, with the latter being attempted only under biosafety level-4 conditions. Viral RNA generally is detectable by RT-PCR assay within 3 to 10 days after the onset of symptoms. Postmortem diagnosis can be made via immunohistochemistry testing of skin, liver, or spleen. Testing generally is not performed in routine clinical laboratories. Local or state public health department officials must be contacted and can facilitate testing at a regional certified laboratory or at the CDC.

Malaria, measles, typhoid fever, Lassa fever, and dengue should be included in the differential diagnosis of a symptomatic person returning from Africa within 21 days.

TREATMENT: People suspected of having Ebola or Marburg virus infection immediately should be placed in isolation and public health officials should be notified. Management of patients with filovirus disease primarily is supportive, including oral or intravenous fluids with electrolyte repletion, vasopressors, blood products, total parenteral nutrition, and antimalarial and antibiotic medications when coinfections are suspected or confirmed (**www.cdc.gov/vhf/ebola/treatment/index.html**). Volume losses can be enormous (10 L/day in adults), and some centers report better results with repletion using lactated Ringer solution rather than normal saline solution in management of adult patients in the United States. When antibiotic agents are used to treat sepsis, the medications should have coverage for intestinal microbiota based on limited evidence of translocation of gut bacteria into the blood of patients with filovirus disease. Nonsteroidal anti-inflammatory drugs (NSAIDs), aspirin, and intramuscular injections should be avoided because of the risk of bleeding.

There currently are no specific therapies approved by the US Food and Drug Administration (FDA) for filovirus infection, although a number of experimental approaches show promise in animal models. Expanded-access programs for monoclonal antibodies, small inhibitory RNAs, antisense compounds, nucleoside analogues, and convalescent plasma have been employed on a limited scale to date in humans; the effect of these therapies on the course of human disease is unclear. Although active in other hemorrhagic fever virus infections, ribavirin has no efficacy against filoviruses and should not be used. Corticosteroids should not be administered except for replacement in suspected or confirmed adrenal insufficiency or refractory septic shock.

ISOLATION OF THE HOSPITALIZED PATIENT: Standard, contact, and droplet precautions are recommended for management of hospitalized patients with known or suspected Ebola virus disease. Although not required, it may be prudent to place the patient in a negative-pressure room when available, despite the lack of evidence for natural aerosol transmission between humans, because of the large amount of fluid losses and copious vomiting that may lead to temporary aerosolization of the virus. Access to the patient should be limited to a small number of designated staff and family members with specific instructions and training on filovirus infection control and on the use of personal protective equipment. Although experience suggests that standard universal and contact protections usually are protective, viral hemorrhagic fever precautions consisting of at least 2 pairs of gloves, fit-tested N95 or particulate respirator, impermeable or fluid-resistant gown, face shield, protective apron, and shoe covers or rubber boots are recommended when filovirus infection is confirmed or suspected. No skin should be showing, and a buddy system should be employed for donning and doffing the personal protective equipment. All health care workers should be knowledgeable with and proficient in the donning and doffing of personnel protective equipment prior to participating in management of a patient. Particulate respirators are recommended when aerosol-generating procedures, such as endotracheal intubation, are performed. Current guidance from the CDC on personal protective equipment can be found on the CDC Web site (**www.cdc.gov/vhf/ ebola/hcp/index.html**).

CONTROL MEASURES

Contact Tracing. Monitoring and movement of people with potential Ebola virus exposure currently is based on the degree of possible risk. Categories include high risk, some risk, low risk, and no identifiable risk. Full descriptions of recommended management for people in these categories can be found on the CDC Web site (**www.cdc.gov/vhf/ebola/ exposure/monitoring-and-movement-of-persons-with-exposure.html**). Asymptomatic people at high, some, or low risk should have active monitoring consisting of, at a minimum, daily reporting of measured temperatures and symptoms consistent with Ebola (including severe headache, fatigue, muscle pain, weakness, diarrhea, vomiting, abdominal pain, or unexplained hemorrhage) by the individual to the public health authority. People being actively monitored should measure their temperature twice daily, monitor themselves for symptoms, report as directed to the public health authority, and immediately notify the public health authority if they develop fever or other symptoms. Restrictions on movement apply to asymptomatic people in the high-risk category and may be considered by public health authorities for asymptomatic people with some risk as well. Restrictions on movement are not recommended for asymptomatic people with low or no identifiable risk. Despite lack of evidence for transmission during the incubation period, it usually is recommended that exposed people avoid close contact or activities with household members that might result in exposure to bodily fluids, such as sharing of utensils, kissing, and sexual intercourse. Hospitalization of asymptomatic contacts is not warranted, but people who develop fever or other manifestations of filovirus disease should be isolated immediately until the diagnosis can be ruled out.

Immunoprophylaxis. Although there are currently no FDA-approved vaccines, a number of experimental vaccines and other compounds have been shown to be efficacious in nonhuman primate models, including when given as postexposure prophylaxis. Several Ebola virus vaccine candidates are presently in Phase I trials in humans.

Breastfeeding. Although Ebola virus has been detected in human milk, it is not known whether Ebola virus can be transmitted from mothers to their infants through breastfeeding. However, given what is known about transmission of Ebola virus, regardless of breastfeeding status, infants whose mothers are infected with Ebola virus already are at high risk of acquiring Ebola virus infection through close contact with the mother and are at high risk of death overall. Therefore, when safe replacements to breastfeeding and infant care exist, mothers with probable or confirmed Ebola virus infection should not have close contact with their infants (including breastfeeding). In resource-limited settings, however, because nonbreastfed infants are at increased risk of death from starvation and other infectious diseases, such as diarrheal and respiratory diseases, these risks must be carefully weighed against the risk of Ebola virus infection. There is not enough evidence to provide guidance on when it is safe to resume breastfeeding after a mother's recovery, unless her milk can be demonstrated to be Ebola virus-free by laboratory testing. In the 1 case in which human milk was tested, Ebola virus was identified in the milk of a lactating woman 7 and 15 days after disease onset.

Travelers. Nonessential travel to areas affected by the 2014 Ebola outbreak is not recommended. Travelers to an area affected by an Ebola outbreak should practice careful hygiene (eg, wash hands with soap and water or a 9:1 water to bleach solution, use an alcohol-based hand sanitizer, avoid contact with blood and body fluids). Travelers should not handle items that may have come in contact with an infected person's blood or body fluids, such as clothes, bedding, needles, and medical equipment. Funeral or burial rituals that require handling the body of someone who has died from Ebola should be avoided. Given the current countries affected by the 2014 Ebola outbreak, travelers should avoid hospitals where Ebola patients are being treated in areas of Africa with endemic disease; the United States embassy or consulate often is able to provide advice on facilities that should be avoided. Following return to the United States, travelers should monitor their health closely for 21 days and seek medical care immediately if they develop symptoms of Ebola (see see Control Measures, Environmental). State laws mandating confinement or quarantine may apply. Current travel information for countries affected by Ebola can be found on the CDC Web site (**www.cdc.gov/vhf/ebola/travelers/index.html**)·

Environmental. Avoiding contact with bats, primarily by avoiding entry into caves and mines in areas with endemic disease, is a key prevention measure for filoviruses. People also should avoid exposure to fresh blood, bodily fluids, or meat of wild animals, especially nonhuman primates but also bats, porcupines, duikers (a type of antelope), and other mammals, in areas with endemic filovirus disease.

Public Health Reporting. Because of the risk of health care-associated transmission, state/local health departments and the CDC should be contacted for specific advice about confirmation and management of suspected cases. In the United States, Ebola and Marburg hemorrhagic fevers are reportable by guidelines of the Council of State and Territorial Epidemiologists. If a filoviral hemorrhagic fever is suspected, the state/local health department or CDC Emergency Operations Center (770-488-7100) should be contacted to assist with case investigation, diagnosis, management, and control measures.

Hepatitis A

CLINICAL MANIFESTATIONS: Hepatitis A characteristically is an acute, self-limited illness associated with fever, malaise, jaundice, anorexia, and nausea. Symptomatic hepatitis A virus (HAV) infection occurs in approximately 30% of infected children younger than 6 years; few of these children will have jaundice. Among older children and adults, infection usually is symptomatic and typically lasts several weeks, with jaundice occurring in 70% or more. Signs and symptoms typically last less than 2 months, although 10% to 15% of symptomatic people have prolonged or relapsing disease lasting as long as 6 months. Fulminant hepatitis is rare but is more common in people with underlying liver disease. Chronic infection does not occur.

ETIOLOGY: HAV is an RNA virus classified as a member of the *Picornavirus* family, genus *Hepatovirus*.

EPIDEMIOLOGY: The most common mode of transmission is person to person, resulting from fecal contamination and oral ingestion (ie, the fecal-oral route). In resource-limited countries where infection is endemic, most people are infected during the first decade of life. In the United States, hepatitis A was one of the most frequently reported vaccine-preventable diseases in the prevaccine era, but incidence of disease attributable to HAV has declined significantly since hepatitis A vaccine was licensed in 1995. These declining rates have been accompanied by a shift in age-specific rates. Historically, the highest rates occurred among children 5 to 14 years of age, and the lowest rates occurred among adults older than 40 years. Beginning in the late 1990s, national age-specific rates declined more rapidly among children than among adults; as a result, in recent years, rates have been similar among all age groups. In addition, the previously observed unequal geographic distribution of hepatitis A incidence in the United States, with the highest rates of disease occurring in a limited number of states and communities, disappeared after introduction of targeted immunization in 1999. Rates in the United States were 1.0/100 000 in 2007, which was the year hepatitis A vaccine was recommended for routine use in all US children 12 through 23 months of age, and declined to 0.4/100 000 in 2011. The 1398 HAV cases in 2011 represented the lowest number ever recorded; in 2012, there were 1562 cases, and in 2013, there were 1781 cases. Seroprevalence of antibodies to HAV (anti-HAV) was 38% in children 6 to 19 years of age in 2007–2010. White and non-Hispanic children had the lowest rates, consistent with relatively low rates of hepatitis A vaccination coverage in these groups. An increasing proportion of adults in the United States are susceptible to hepatitis A because of reduced exposure to HAV earlier in life. There have been significant decreases in anti-HAV seroprevalence in older adults (40 years and older). The overwhelming majority of HAV cases are in adults 20 years and older. The mean age of people hospitalized for HAV infection has increased significantly between 2002 and 2011 (mean age, 37.6 years in 2002–2003, compared with 45.5 years in 2010–2011).

Among cases of hepatitis A reported to the Centers for Disease Control and Prevention (CDC), recognized risk factors include close personal contact with a person infected with HAV, international travel, household or personal contact with a child who attends a child care center, household or personal contact with a newly arriving international adoptee, a recognized foodborne outbreak, men who have sex with men, and use of illegal drugs. In approximately two thirds of reported cases, the source cannot be determined. Fecal-oral spread from people with asymptomatic infections, particularly young children, likely accounts for many of these cases with an unknown source. Transmission by blood transfusion or from mother to newborn infant (ie, vertical transmission) seldom occurs.

Before availability of vaccine, most HAV infection and illness occurred in the context of community-wide epidemics, in which infection primarily was transmitted in households and extended-family settings. However, community-wide epidemics have not been observed in recent years. Common-source foodborne outbreaks occur; waterborne outbreaks are rare. Waterborne outbreaks usually are associated with sewage-contaminated or inadequately treated water. Health care-associated transmission is unusual, but very rarely outbreaks have occurred in neonatal intensive care units from neonates infected through transfused blood who subsequently transmitted HAV to other neonates and staff.

In child care centers, recognized symptomatic (icteric) illness occurs primarily among adult contacts of children. Most infected children younger than 6 years are asymptomatic or have nonspecific manifestations. Hence, spread of HAV infection within and outside a child care center often occurs before recognition of the index case(s). Outbreaks have occurred most commonly in large child care centers and specifically in facilities that enroll children in diapers.

Patients infected with HAV are most infectious during the 1 to 2 weeks before onset of jaundice or elevation of liver enzymes, when concentration of virus in the stool is highest. The risk of transmission subsequently diminishes and is minimal by 1 week after onset of jaundice. However, HAV can be detected in stool for longer periods, especially in neonates and young children.

The **incubation period** is 15 to 50 days, with an average of 28 days.

DIAGNOSTIC TESTS: Serologic tests for HAV-specific total (ie, immunoglobulin [Ig] G and IgM) anti-HAV are available commercially. The presence of serum IgM anti-HAV indicates current or recent infection, although false-positive results may occur. IgM anti-HAV is detectable in up to 20% of vaccinees when measured 2 weeks after hepatitis A immunization. In most infected people, serum IgM anti-HAV becomes detectable 5 to 10 days before onset of symptoms and declines to undetectable concentrations within 6 months after infection. People who test positive for IgM anti-HAV more than 1 year after infection have been reported. IgG anti-HAV is detectable shortly after appearance of IgM. A positive total anti-HAV (ie, IgM and IgG) test result with a negative IgM anti-HAV test result indicates immunity from past infection or vaccination. PCR assays for hepatitis A are available.

TREATMENT: Supportive.

ISOLATION OF THE HOSPITALIZED PATIENT: In general, hospitalization is not required for patients with uncomplicated acute hepatitis A. When hospitalization is necessary, contact precautions are recommended in addition to standard precautions for diapered and incontinent patients for at least 1 week after onset of symptoms.

Table 3.13. Recommendations for Preexposure Immunoprophylaxis of Hepatitis A Virus (HAV) for Travelers to Countries With High or Intermediate Hepatitis A Endemicity[a]

Age	Recommended Prophylaxis	Notes
Younger than 12 mo	IGIM	0.02 mL/kg[b] protects for up to 3 mo. For trips of 3 mo or longer, 0.06 mL/kg[b] should be given at departure and every 5 mo if exposure to HAV continues.
12 mo through 40 y	HepA vaccine[c]	
41 y or older	HepA vaccine, with or without IGIM[c]	If departure is in less than 2 wk, older adults, immunocompromised people, and people with chronic liver disease or other chronic medical conditions can receive IGIM with the initial dose of HepA vaccine to ensure optimal protection.

IGIM indicates Immune Globulin Intramuscular; HepA, hepatitis A vaccine.

[a]All people 12 months of age or older at high risk of HAV disease should be immunized routinely (see People at Increased Risk, p 396).

[b]IGIM should be administered deep into a large muscle mass. Ordinarily, no more than 5 mL should be administered in one site in an adult or large child; lesser amounts (maximum 3 mL in one site) should be given to small children and infants.

[c]People who have a contraindication to HepA vaccine should receive IGIM.

CONTROL MEASURES[1,2,3]:

General Measures. The major methods of prevention of HAV infections are improved sanitation (eg, in food preparation and of water sources) and personal hygiene (eg, hand hygiene after diaper changes in child care settings), immunization with hepatitis A vaccine, and administration of Immune Globulin (IG).

Schools, Child Care, and Work. Children and adults with acute HAV infection who work as food handlers or attend or work in child care settings should be excluded for 1 week after onset of the illness.

Immune Globulin. Immune Globulin Intramuscular (IGIM), when given within 2 weeks after exposure to HAV, is more than 85% effective in preventing symptomatic infection. When administered for preexposure prophylaxis, 1 dose of 0.02 mL/kg confers protection against hepatitis A for up to 3 months, and a dose of 0.06 mL/kg protects for 3 to 5 months. Recommended preexposure and postexposure IGIM doses and duration of protection are given in Tables 3.13 and 3.14 (p 394). HAV vaccine is preferred for preexposure protection

[1]Centers for Disease Control and Prevention. Prevention of hepatitis A through active or passive immunization: recommendations of the Advisory Committee on Immunization Practices (ACIP). *MMWR Recomm Rep.* 2006;55(RR-7):1–23

[2]Centers for Disease Control and Prevention. Prevention after exposure and in international travelers. *MMWR Morb Mortal Wkly Rep.* 2007;56(41):1080–1084

[3]Centers for Disease Control and Prevention. Use of vaccine in close contacts of international adoptees. *MMWR Morb Mortal Wkly Rep.* 2009;58(36):1006–1007

in all populations unless contraindicated and should be administered at least 2 weeks before expected exposure. Vaccine may be used for postexposure prophylaxis for most people 1 through 40 years of age (see Postexposure Prophylaxis, p 398).

Hepatitis A Vaccine. Two inactivated hepatitis A (HepA) vaccines, Havrix (GlaxoSmithKline, Research Triangle Park, NC) and Vaqta (Merck & Co Inc, Whitehouse Station, NJ), are available in the United States. The vaccines are prepared from cell culture-adapted HAV, which is propagated in human fibroblasts, purified from cell lysates, formalin inactivated, and adsorbed to an aluminum hydroxide adjuvant. Both HepA vaccines are formulated without a preservative.

Administration, Dosages, and Schedules (see Table 3.15, p 395). HepA vaccines are licensed for people 12 months and older and have pediatric and adult formulations that are administered in a 2-dose schedule. The adult formulations are recommended for people 19 years and older. Recommended doses and schedules for these different products and formulations are given in Table 3.15, p 395. A combination HepA/hepatitis B vaccine (Twinrix) is licensed in the United States for people 18 years and older and can be administered in a 3-dose schedule or an accelerated 4-dose schedule (see Table 3.15, p 395). All HepA-containing vaccines are administered intramuscularly.

Immunogenicity. Available HepA vaccines are highly immunogenic when given in their respective recommended schedules and doses. At least 95% of healthy children, adolescents, and adults have protective antibody concentrations when measured 1 month after receipt of the first dose of either single-antigen vaccine. One month after a second dose, more than 99% of healthy children, adolescents, and adults have protective antibody concentrations.

Available data on the immunogenicity of HepA vaccine in young children indicate high rates of seroconversion, but antibody concentrations are lower in infants with

Table 3.14. Recommendations for Postexposure Immunoprophylaxis of Hepatitis A Virus (HAV)

Time Since Exposure	Age of Patient	Recommended Prophylaxis
2 wk or less	Younger than 12 mo	IGIM, 0.02 mL/kg[a]
	12 mo through 40 y	HepA vaccine[b]
	41 y or older	IGIM, 0.02 mL/kg,[a] but HepA vaccine[b] can be used if IGIM is unavailable[a]
	People of any age who are immunocompromised, have chronic liver disease, or contraindication to vaccination	IGIM, 0.02 mL/kg[a]
More than 2 wk	Younger than 12 mo	No prophylaxis
	12 mo or older	No prophylaxis, but HepA vaccine may be indicated for ongoing exposure[b]

IGIM indicates Immune Globulin Intramuscular; HepA, hepatitis A vaccine.

[a]IGIM should be administered deep into a large muscle mass. Ordinarily, no more than 5 mL should be administered in one site in an adult or large child; lesser amounts (maximum 3 mL in one site) should be given to small children and infants.

[b]Dosage and schedule of hepatitis A vaccine as recommended according to age in Table 3.15. Only monovalent hepatitis A vaccine (Havrix or Vaqta) should be used for postexposure prophylaxis.

passively acquired maternal anti-HAV in comparison with vaccine recipients lacking anti-HAV. By 12 months of age, passively acquired maternal anti-HAV antibody no longer is detectable in most infants. HepA vaccine is highly immunogenic for children who begin immunization at 12 months or older, regardless of maternal anti-HAV status.

Efficacy. In double-blind, controlled, randomized trials, the protective efficacy in preventing clinical HAV infection was 94% to 100%.

Duration of Protection. The need for additional booster doses beyond the 2-dose primary immunization series has not been determined, because long-term efficacy of HepA vaccines has not been established. Detectable antibody persists after a 2-dose series for at least 17 years in adults and 15 years in children. Kinetic models of antibody decline indicate that protective levels of anti-HAV could be present for 25 years or longer in adults and 14 to 20 years in children.

Vaccine in Immunocompromised Patients. The immune response in immunocompromised people, including people with human immunodeficiency virus, may be suboptimal.

Vaccine Interchangeability. The 2 single-antigen HepA vaccines licensed by the US Food and Drug Administration (FDA), when given as recommended, seem to be similarly effective. Studies among adults have found no difference in the immunogenicity of a vaccine series that mixed the 2 currently available vaccines, compared with using the same vaccine throughout the licensed schedule. Therefore, although completion of the immunization regimen with the same product is preferable, immunization with either product is acceptable.

Administration With Other Vaccines. Data indicate that HepA vaccine may be administered simultaneously with other vaccines. Vaccines should be given in a separate

Table 3.15. Recommended Doses and Schedules for Inactivated Hepatitis A Virus (HepA) Vaccines[a]

Age	Vaccine	Hepatitis A Antigen Dose	Volume per Dose, mL	No. of Doses	Schedule
12 mo through 18 y	Havrix	720 ELU	0.5	2	Initial and 6–12 mo later
12 mo through 18 y	Vaqta	25 U[b]	0.5	2	Initial and 6–18 mo later
19 y or older	Havrix	1440 ELU	1.0	2	Initial and 6–12 mo later
19 y or older	Vaqta	50 U[b]	1.0	2	Initial and 6–18 mo later
18 y or older	Twinrix[c]	720 ELU	1.0	3 or 4	Initial, 1 mo, and 6 mo later **OR** Initial, 7 days, and 21–30 days, followed by a dose at 12 mo

ELU indicates enzyme-linked immunosorbent assay units.

[a]Havrix and Twinrix are manufactured by GlaxoSmithKline Biologicals (Research Triangle Park, NC); Vaqta is manufactured and distributed by Merck & Co Inc (Whitehouse Station, NJ).

[b]Antigen units (each unit is equivalent to approximately 1 µg of viral protein).

[c]A combination of hepatitis B (Engerix-B, 20 µg) and hepatitis A (Havrix, 720 ELU) vaccine (Twinrix) is licensed for use in people 18 years and older in 3-dose and 4-dose schedules.

syringe and at a separate injection site (see Simultaneous Administration of Multiple Vaccines, p 35).

Adverse Events. Adverse reactions are mild and include local pain and, less commonly, induration at the injection site. No serious adverse events attributed definitively to HepA vaccine have been reported. The vaccine can be administered either in the thigh or the arm, because the site of injection does not affect the incidence of local reactions.

Precautions and Contraindications to Immunization. The vaccine should not be administered to people with hypersensitivity to any of the vaccine components. Safety data in pregnant women are not available, but the risk to the fetus is considered to be low or nonexistent, because the vaccine contains inactivated, purified virus particles. In pregnant women, the risk associated with vaccination should be weighed against the risk of HAV infection. Because HepA vaccine is inactivated, no special precautions need to be taken when vaccinating immunocompromised people.

Preimmunization Serologic Testing. Preimmunization testing for anti-HAV generally is not recommended for children because of their expected low prevalence of infection. Testing may be cost-effective for people who have a high likelihood of immunity from previous infection, including people whose childhood was spent in a country with high endemicity, people with a history of jaundice potentially caused by HAV, and people older than 50 years.

Postimmunization Serologic Testing. Postimmunization testing for anti-HAV is not indicated because of the high seroconversion rates in adults and children. In addition, some commercially available anti-HAV tests may not detect low but protective concentrations of antibody among immunized people.

RECOMMENDATIONS FOR IMMUNOPROPHYLAXIS:

Preexposure Prophylaxis Against HAV Infection (see Tables 3.13, p 393, and 3.15, p 395). Immunization with HepA vaccine is recommended routinely for children 12 through 23 months of age, for people who are at increased risk of infection, for people who are at increased risk of severe manifestations of hepatitis A if infected, and for any person who wants to obtain immunity.

Children Who Routinely Should Be Immunized or Considered for Immunization. All children in the United States should receive HepA vaccine at 12 through 23 months of age, as recommended in the routine childhood immunization schedule **(http://redbook.solutions. aap.org/SS/Immunization_Schedules.aspx)**. Table 3.15 (p 395) shows HepA-containing vaccines licensed by the US Food and Drug Administration (FDA), their doses, and schedules. Children who are not immunized or have not completed the series by 2 years of age can be immunized at subsequent visits.

People at Increased Risk of HAV Infection or its Consequences Who Routinely Should Be Immunized.
- **People traveling internationally.**[1] All susceptible people traveling to or working in countries that have high or intermediate hepatitis A endemicity should be immunized or receive IGIM before departure (see Table 3.13, p 393). Travelers to Western Europe, Scandinavia, Australia, Canada, Japan, and New Zealand (ie, countries in which endemicity is low) are at no greater risk of HAV infection than are people living in or traveling to the United States. HepA vaccine at the age-appropriate dose is preferred

---

[1]Centers for Disease Control and Prevention. Update: prevention of hepatitis A after exposure to hepatitis A virus and in international travelers. Updated recommendations of the Advisory Committee on Immunization Practices (ACIP). *MMWR Morb Mortal Wkly Rep.* 2007;56(41):1080–1084

to IGIM. The first dose of HepA vaccine should be administered as soon as travel is considered.

- One dose of single-antigen vaccine administered at any time before departure can provide adequate protection for most healthy people. However, no data are available for other populations or other hepatitis A vaccine formulations (eg, the combination HepA-hepatitis B vaccine).

- Older adults, immunocompromised people, and people with chronic liver disease or other chronic medical conditions who are traveling to an area with endemic infection in 2 weeks or less should receive the initial dose of vaccine and simultaneously can receive IGIM (0.02 mL/kg) at a separate anatomic site. The vaccine series then should be completed according to the licensed schedule.

- Travelers who elect not to receive vaccine, are younger than 12 months, or are allergic to a vaccine component should receive a single dose of IGIM (0.02 mL/kg), which provides effective protection for up to 3 months.

- **Close contacts of newly arriving international adoptees.**[1,2] Data from a study conducted at 3 adoption clinics in the United States indicate that 1% to 6% of newly arrived international adoptees have acute HAV infection. The risk of HAV infection among close personal contacts of international adoptees is estimated at 106 (range, 90–819) per 100 000 household contacts of international adoptees within the first 60 days of their arrival in the United States. Therefore, HepA vaccine should be administered to all previously unvaccinated people who anticipate close personal contact (eg, household contact or regular babysitting) with an international adoptee from a country with high or intermediate endemicity during the first 60 days following arrival of the adoptee in the United States. The first dose of the 2-dose HepA vaccine series should be administered as soon as adoption is planned, ideally 2 or more weeks before the arrival of the adoptee.

- **Men who have sex with men.** Outbreaks of hepatitis A among men who have sex with men have been reported often, including in urban areas in the United States, Canada, and Australia. Therefore, men (adolescents and adults) who have sex with men should be immunized. Preimmunization serologic testing may be cost-effective for older people in this group.

- **Users of injection and noninjection drugs.** Periodic outbreaks among injection and noninjection drug users have been reported in many parts of the United States and in Europe. Adolescents and adults who use illegal drugs should be immunized. Preimmunization serologic testing may be cost-effective for older people in this group.

- **Patients with clotting-factor disorders.** Reported outbreaks of hepatitis A in patients with hemophilia receiving solvent-detergent–treated factor VIII and factor IX concentrates were identified during the 1990s, primarily in Europe, although 1 case was reported in the United States. Therefore, susceptible patients with chronic clotting disorders who receive clotting-factor concentrates should be immunized. Preimmunization testing for anti-HAV may be cost-effective for older people in this group.

- **People at risk of occupational exposure (eg, handlers of nonhuman primates and people working with HAV in a research laboratory setting).**

[1]Centers for Disease Control and Prevention. Updated recommendations from the Advisory Committee on Immunization Practices (ACIP) for use of hepatitis A vaccine in close contacts of newly arriving international adoptees. *MMWR Morb Mortal Wkly Rep.* 2009;58(36):1006–1007

[2]American Academy of Pediatrics, Committee on Infectious Diseases. Recommendations for administering hepatitis A vaccine to contacts of international adoptees. *Pediatrics.* 2011;128(4):803–804

Outbreaks of hepatitis A have been reported among people working with nonhuman primates. These infected primates were born in the wild and were not primates that had been born and raised in captivity. People working with HAV-infected primates or with HAV in a research laboratory setting should be immunized.

- **People with chronic liver disease.** Because people with chronic liver disease are at increased risk of fulminant hepatitis A, susceptible patients with chronic liver disease should be immunized. Susceptible people who are awaiting or have received liver transplants should be immunized.

Postexposure Prophylaxis (see Table 3.14, p 394).[1] A randomized clinical trial conducted among people 2 through 40 years of age comparing postexposure efficacy of IGIM and HAV vaccine found that the efficacy of a single dose of HAV vaccine was similar to that of IGIM in preventing symptomatic infection when administered within 14 days after exposure.

People who have been exposed to HAV and previously have not received HepA vaccine should receive a single dose of single-antigen HepA vaccine or IGIM as soon as possible (see Table 3.14, p 394, for prophylaxis guidance and dosages). The efficacy of IGIM or vaccine for postexposure prophylaxis when administered more than 2 weeks after exposure has not been established. No data are available for people older than 40 years or people with underlying medical conditions.

For healthy people 12 months through 40 years of age, HepA vaccine at the age-appropriate dose is preferred to IGIM because of vaccine advantages, including long-term protection and ease of administration.

- For people older than 40 years, IGIM is preferred because of the absence of data regarding vaccine performance in this age group and the increased risk of severe manifestations of hepatitis A with increasing age. However, HepA vaccine can be used if IGIM is unavailable.
- IGIM should be used for children younger than 12 months, immunocompromised people, people with chronic liver disease, and people for whom HepA vaccine is contraindicated.
- People who are given IGIM and for whom HepA vaccine also is recommended for other reasons should receive a dose of vaccine simultaneously with IGIM at a different site. For people who receive HepA vaccine, the second dose should be given according to the licensed schedule to complete the series.
- **Household and sexual contacts.** All previously unimmunized people with close personal contact with a person with serologically confirmed HAV infection, such as household and sexual contacts, should receive HepA vaccine or IGIM within 2 weeks after the most recent exposure (Table 3.14, p 394). Serologic testing of contacts is not recommended, because testing adds unnecessary cost and may delay administration of postexposure prophylaxis.
- **Newborn infants of HAV-infected mothers.** Perinatal transmission of HAV is rare. Some experts advise giving IGIM (0.02 mL/kg) to an infant if the mother's symptoms began between 2 weeks before and 1 week after delivery. Efficacy in this circumstance has not been established. Severe disease in healthy infants is rare.
- **Child care center staff, employees, and children and their household contacts.** Outbreaks of HAV infection at child care centers have been recognized since the

---

[1]Centers for Disease Control and Prevention. Update: prevention of hepatitis A after exposure to hepatitis A virus and in international travelers. Updated recommendations of the Advisory Committee on Immunization Practices (ACIP). *MMWR Morb Mortal Wkly Rep.* 2007;56(41):1080–1084

1970s, but their frequency has decreased as HAV immunization rates in children have increased and as hepatitis A incidence among children has declined. Because infections in children usually are mild or asymptomatic, outbreaks often are identified only when adult contacts (eg, parents) become ill. Serologic testing to confirm HAV infection in suspected cases is indicated.

Routine immunization of staff at child care centers is not recommended. HepA vaccine or IGIM (Table 3.14, p 394) should be administered to all previously unimmunized staff members and attendees of child care centers or homes if (1) one or more cases of hepatitis A are recognized in children or staff members; or (2) cases are recognized in 2 or more households of center attendees. In centers that provide care only to children who do not wear diapers, vaccine or IGIM need be given only to classroom contacts of an index-case patient. When an outbreak occurs (ie, hepatitis A cases in 2 or more families), HepA vaccine or IGIM also should be considered for members of households that have children (center attendees) in diapers.

Children and adults with hepatitis A should be excluded from the center until 1 week after onset of illness, until the postexposure prophylaxis program has been completed in the center, or until directed by the health department. Although precise data concerning the onset of protection after postexposure prophylaxis are not available, allowing prophylaxis recipients to return to the child care center setting immediately after receipt of the vaccine or IGIM dose seems reasonable.

- **Schools.** Schoolroom exposure generally does not pose an appreciable risk of infection, and postexposure prophylaxis is not indicated when a single case occurs and the source of infection is outside the school. However, HepA vaccine or IGIM could be used for unimmunized people who have close contact with the index patient if transmission within the school setting is documented.

- **Hospitals.** Usually, health care-associated HAV in hospital personnel has occurred through spread from patients with acute HAV infection in whom the diagnosis was not recognized. Careful hygienic practices should be emphasized when a patient with jaundice or known or suspected hepatitis A is admitted to the hospital. When outbreaks occur, HepA vaccine or IGIM is recommended for people in close contact with infected patients (Table 3.14, p 394). Routine preexposure use of HAV vaccine for hospital personnel is not recommended.

- **Exposure to an infected food handler.** If a food handler is diagnosed with hepatitis A, HepA vaccine or IGIM should be provided to other food handlers at the same establishment (Table 3.14, p 394). Food handlers with acute HAV infection should be excluded for 1 week after onset of illness. Because common-source transmission to patrons is unlikely, postexposure prophylaxis with HepA vaccine or IGIM typically is not indicated but may be considered if the food handler directly handled food during the time when the food handler likely was infectious and had diarrhea or poor hygiene practices and if prophylaxis can be provided within 2 weeks of exposure. Routine HepA immunization of food handlers is not recommended.

- **Common-source exposure.** Postexposure prophylaxis usually is not recommended, because these outbreaks commonly are recognized too late for prophylaxis to be effective in preventing HAV infection in exposed people. HepA vaccine or IGIM can be considered if it can be administered to exposed people within 2 weeks of an exposure to the HAV-contaminated water or food.

Hepatitis B

CLINICAL MANIFESTATIONS: People acutely infected with hepatitis B virus (HBV) may be asymptomatic or symptomatic. The likelihood of developing symptoms of acute hepatitis is age dependent: less than 1% of infants younger than 1 year, 5% to 15% of children 1 through 5 years of age, and 30% to 50% of people older than 5 years are symptomatic, although few data are available for adults older than 30 years. The spectrum of signs and symptoms is varied and includes subacute illness with nonspecific symptoms (eg, anorexia, nausea, or malaise), clinical hepatitis with jaundice, or fulminant hepatitis. Extrahepatic manifestations, such as arthralgia, arthritis, macular rashes, thrombocytopenia, polyarteritis nodosa, glomerulonephritis, or papular acrodermatitis (Gianotti-Crosti syndrome), can occur early in the course of illness and may precede jaundice. Acute HBV infection cannot be distinguished from other forms of acute viral hepatitis on the basis of clinical signs and symptoms or nonspecific laboratory findings.

Chronic HBV infection is defined as presence of any one of the following: hepatitis B surface antigen (HBsAg), HBV DNA, or hepatitis B e antigen (HBeAg) in serum for at least 6 months. Chronic HBV infection is likely in the presence of HBsAg, nucleic acid, HBV DNA, or HBeAg in serum from a person who tests negative for antibody of the immunoglobulin (Ig) M subclass to hepatitis B core antigen (IgM anti-HBc).

Age at the time of infection is the primary determinant of risk of progressing to chronic infection. Up to 90% of infants infected perinatally or in the first year of life will develop chronic HBV infection. Between 25% and 50% of children infected between 1 and 5 years of age become chronically infected, whereas 5% to 10% of infected older children and adults develop chronic HBV infection. Patients who become HBV infected while immunosuppressed or with an underlying chronic illness (eg, end-stage renal disease) have an increased risk of developing chronic infection. In the absence of treatment, up to 25% of infants and children who acquire chronic HBV infection will die prematurely from HBV-related hepatocellular carcinoma or cirrhosis. Risk factors for developing hepatocellular carcinoma include long duration of infection, male gender, elevation of serum alanine aminotransferase (ALT), HBeAg positivity, degree of histologic injury of the liver, replicative state of the virus (HBV DNA levels), presence of cirrhosis, and concomitant infection with hepatitis C virus (HCV) or human immunodeficiency virus (HIV).

The clinical course of untreated chronic HBV infection varies according to the population studied, reflecting differences in age at acquisition, rate of loss of HBeAg, and possibly HBV genotype. Most children have asymptomatic infection. Perinatally infected children usually have normal ALT concentrations and minimal or mild liver histologic abnormalities, with detectable HBeAg and high HBV DNA concentrations (≥20 000 IU/mL) for years to decades after initial infection ("immune tolerant phase"). Children with chronic HBV may exhibit growth impairment. Chronic HBV infection acquired during later childhood or adolescence usually is accompanied by more active liver disease and increased serum aminotransferase concentrations. Patients with detectable HBeAg *(HBeAg-positive chronic hepatitis B)* usually have high concentrations of HBV DNA and HBsAg in serum and are more likely to transmit infection. Because HBV-associated liver injury is thought to be immune mediated, in people coinfected with HIV and HBV, the return of immune competence with antiretroviral treatment of HIV infection may lead to a reactivation of HBV-related liver inflammation and damage. Over time (years to decades), HBeAg becomes undetectable in many chronically infected people. This transition often is accompanied by development of antibody to HBeAg (anti-HBe) and decreases in serum HBV DNA and serum aminotransferase concentrations and may be preceded by a temporary exacerbation of liver disease. These patients have *inactive chronic infection* but still may have exacerbations of hepatitis. Serologic reversion (reappearance of HBeAg) is more common if loss of HBeAg is not accompanied by development of anti-HBe; reversion with loss of anti-HBe also can occur.

Some patients who lose HBeAg may continue to have ongoing histologic evidence of liver damage and moderate to high concentrations of HBV DNA *(HBeAg-negative chronic hepatitis B)*. Patients with histologic evidence of chronic HBV infection, regardless of HBeAg status, remain at higher risk of death attributable to liver failure compared with HBV-infected people with no histologic evidence of liver inflammation and fibrosis. Other factors that may adversely influence the natural history of chronic infection include male gender, high HBV DNA level, elevation of serum aminotransferase concentrations, HBeAg positivity, race, alcohol use, and coinfection with HCV, hepatitis D virus (HDV), or HIV.

Resolved hepatitis B is defined as clearance of HBsAg, normalization of serum aminotransferase concentrations, and development of antibody to HBsAg (anti-HBs). Chronically infected adults clear HBsAg and develop anti-HBs at the rate of 1% to 2% annually; during childhood, the annual clearance rate is less than 1%. Reactivation of resolved chronic infection is possible if these patients become immunosuppressed and also is well reported among HBsAg-positive patients receiving anti-tumor necrosis factor agents or disease-modifying antirheumatic drugs (12% of patients).

ETIOLOGY: HBV is a DNA-containing, 42-nm-diameter hepadnavirus. Important components of the viral particle include an outer lipoprotein envelope containing HBsAg and an inner nucleocapsid consisting of hepatitis B core antigen (anti-HBc). Viral polymerase activity can be detected in preparations of plasma containing HBV.

EPIDEMIOLOGY: HBV is transmitted through infected blood or body fluids. Although HBsAg has been detected in multiple body fluids including human milk, saliva, and tears, only blood, serum, semen, vaginal secretions, and cerebrospinal, synovial, pleural, pericardial, peritoneal, and amniotic fluids are considered the most potentially infectious. People with chronic HBV infection are the primary reservoirs for infection. Common modes of transmission include percutaneous and permucosal exposure to infectious body fluids; sharing or using nonsterilized needles, syringes, or glucose monitoring equipment or devices; sexual contact with an infected person; perinatal exposure to an infected mother; and household exposure to a person with chronic HBV infection. The risk of HBV acquisition when a susceptible child bites a child who has chronic HBV infection is unknown. A theoretical risk exists if HBsAg-positive blood enters the oral cavity of the biter, but transmission by this route has not been reported. Transmission by transfusion of contaminated blood or blood products is rare in the United States because of routine screening of blood donors and viral inactivation of certain blood products before administration (see Blood Safety, p 112).

Perinatal transmission of HBV is highly efficient and usually occurs from blood exposures during labor and delivery. In utero transmission accounts for less than 2% of all vertically transmitted HBV infections in most studies. Without postexposure prophylaxis, the risk of an infant acquiring HBV from an infected mother as a result of perinatal exposure is 70% to 90% for infants born to mothers who are HBsAg and HBeAg positive; the risk is 5% to 20% for infants born to HBsAg-positive but HBeAg-negative mothers.

Person-to-person spread of HBV can occur in settings involving interpersonal contact over extended periods, such as in a household with a person with chronic HBV infection. In regions of the world with a high prevalence of chronic HBV infection, transmission between children in household settings may account for a substantial amount of transmission. The precise mechanisms of transmission from child to child are unknown; however, frequent interpersonal contact of nonintact skin or mucous membranes with blood-containing secretions, open skin lesions, or blood-containing saliva are potential means of transmission. Transmission from sharing inanimate objects, such as razors or toothbrushes, also may occur. HBV can survive in the environment for 7 or more days but is inactivated by commonly used disinfectants, including household bleach diluted 1:10 with water. HBV is not transmitted by the fecal-oral route.

Transmission among children born in the United States is unusual because of high coverage with hepatitis B (HepB) vaccine starting at birth. The risk of HBV transmission is higher in children who have not completed a vaccine series, children undergoing hemodialysis, institutionalized children with developmental disabilities, and children emigrating from countries with endemic HBV (eg, Southeast Asia, China, Africa). Person-to-person transmission has been reported in child care settings, but risk of transmission in child care facilities in the United States has become negligible as a result of high infant hepatitis B immunization rates.

Acute HBV infection is reported most commonly among adults 30 through 49 years of age in the United States. Since 1990, the incidence of acute HBV infection has declined in all age categories, with a 98% decline in children younger than 19 years and a 93% decline in young adults 20 through 29 years of age, with most of the decline among people 20 through 24 years of age. Among patients with acute hepatitis B interviewed in 2010, groups constituting the largest proportion of acute hepatitis B cases included users of injection drugs, people with multiple heterosexual partners, men who have sex with men, and people who reported surgery during the 6 weeks to 6 months before onset of symptoms. Others at increased risk include people with occupational exposure to blood or body fluids, staff of institutions and nonresidential child care programs for children with developmental disabilities, patients undergoing hemodialysis, and sexual or household contacts of people with an acute or chronic infection. Approximately 68% of infected people who were interviewed in 2010 did not have a readily identifiable risk characteristic. HBV infection in adolescents and adults is associated with other sexually transmitted infections, including syphilis and HIV. Investigations have indicated an increased risk of HBV infection among adults with diabetes mellitus. Outbreaks in nonhospital health care settings, including assisted-living facilities and nursing homes, highlight the increased risk among people with diabetes mellitus undergoing assisted blood glucose monitoring.[1]

The prevalence of HBV infection and patterns of transmission vary markedly throughout the world (see Table 3.16, p 403). Approximately 45% of people worldwide live in regions of high HBV endemicity, where the prevalence of chronic HBV infection is 8% or greater. Historically in these regions, most new infections occurred as a result

---

[1]Centers for Disease Control and Prevention. Use of hepatitis B vaccination for adults with diabetes mellitus: recommendations of the Advisory Committee on Immunization Practices (ACIP). *MMWR Morb Mortal Wkly Rep.* 2011;60(50):1709–1711

Table 3.16. Estimated International HBsAg Prevalence[a]

Region	Estimated HBsAg Prevalence[b]
North America	0.1%
Mexico and Central America	0.3%
South America	0.7%
Western Europe	0.7%
Australia and New Zealand	0.9%
Caribbean (except Haiti)	1.0%
Eastern Europe and North Asia	2.8%
South Asia	2.8%
Middle East	3.2%
Haiti	5.6%
East Asia	7.4%
Southeast Asia	9.1%
Africa	9.3%
Pacific Islands	12.0%

HBsAg indicates hepatitis B surface antigen.

[a]Centers for Disease Control and Prevention. A comprehensive immunization strategy to eliminate transmission of hepatitis B virus infection in the United States. Recommendations of the Advisory Committee on Immunization Practices (ACIP). Part II: immunization of adults. *MMWR Recomm Rep.* 2006;55(RR-16):1–33

[b]Level of HBV endemicity defined as high (≥8%), intermediate (2%–7%), and low (<2%).

of perinatal or early childhood infections. In regions of intermediate HBV endemicity, where the prevalence of HBV infection is 2% to 7%, multiple modes of transmission (ie, perinatal, household, sexual, injection drug use, and health care-associated) contribute to the burden of infection. In countries of low endemicity, where chronic HBV infection prevalence is less than 2% (including the United States) and where routine immunization has been adopted, new infections increasingly are among unimmunized age groups. Many people born in countries with high endemicity live in the United States. Infant immunization programs in some of these countries have, in recent years, reduced greatly the seroprevalence of HBsAg, but many other countries with endemic HBV have yet to implement widespread routine childhood hepatitis B immunization programs. The **incubation period** for acute infection is 45 to 160 days, with an average of 90 days.

DIAGNOSTIC TESTS: Serologic antigen tests are available commercially to detect HBsAg and HBeAg. Serologic assays also are available for detection of anti-HBs, anti-HBc (total), IgM anti-HBc, and anti-HBe (see Table 3.17, p 404, and Fig 3.4, p 405). In addition, nucleic acid amplification testing, gene-amplification techniques (eg, polymerase chain reaction assay, branched DNA methods), and hybridization assays are available to detect and quantify HBV DNA. Tests to quantify HBsAg and HBeAg currently are being developed but are not yet commercially available. HBsAg is detectable during acute infection. If HBV infection is self-limited, HBsAg disappears in most patients within a few weeks to several months after infection, followed by appearance of anti-HBs. The time between

Table 3.17. Diagnostic Tests for Hepatitis B Virus (HBV) Antigens and Antibodies

Factors to Be Tested	HBV Antigen or Antibody	Use
HBsAg	Hepatitis B surface antigen	Detection of acutely or chronically infected people; antigen used in hepatitis B vaccine; can be detected for up to a month after a dose of hepatitis B vaccine
Anti-HBs	Antibody to HBsAg	Identification of people who have resolved infections with HBV; determination of immunity after immunization
HBeAg	Hepatitis B e antigen	Identification of infected people at increased risk of transmitting HBV
Anti-HBe	Antibody to HBeAg	Identification of infected people with lower risk of transmitting HBV
Anti-HBc (total)	Antibody to HBcAg[a]	Identification of people with acute, resolved, or chronic HBV infection (not present after immunization); passively transferred maternal anti-HBc is detectable for as long as 24 months among infants born to HBsAg-positive women
IgM anti-HBc	IgM antibody to HBcAg	Identification of people with acute or recent HBV infections (including HBsAg-negative people during the "window" phase of infection; unreliable for detecting perinatal HBV infection)

HBcAg indicates hepatitis B core antigen; IgM, immunoglobulin M.
[a] No test is available commercially to measure HBcAg.

disappearance of HBsAg and appearance of anti-HBs is termed the *window period* of infection. During the window period, the only marker of acute infection is IgM anti-HBc, which is highly specific for establishing the diagnosis of acute infection. However, IgM anti-HBc usually is not present in infants infected perinatally. People with chronic HBV infection have circulating HBsAg and circulating total anti-HBc (Fig 3.5, p 405); on rare occasions, anti-HBs also is present. Both anti-HBs and total anti-HBc are present in people with resolved infection, whereas anti-HBs alone is present in people immunized with hepatitis B vaccine. Transient HBsAg antigenemia can occur following receipt of HepB vaccine, with HBsAg being detected as early as 24 hours after and up to 2 to 3 weeks following administration of the vaccine. The presence of HBeAg in serum correlates with higher concentrations of HBV and greater infectivity. Tests for HBeAg and HBV DNA are useful in selection of candidates to receive antiviral therapy and to monitor response to therapy.

TREATMENT: No specific therapy for *acute* HBV infection is available, and acute HBV infection usually does not warrant referral to a hepatitis specialist. However, acute HBV infection may be difficult to distinguish from reactivation of HBV, so if reactivation is a possibility, referral to a hepatitis specialist would be warranted. Hepatitis B Immune Globulin (HBIG) and corticosteroids are not effective treatment for acute or chronic disease.

FIG 3.4. TYPICAL SEROLOGIC COURSE OF ACUTE HEPATITIS B VIRUS INFECTION WITH RECOVERY.

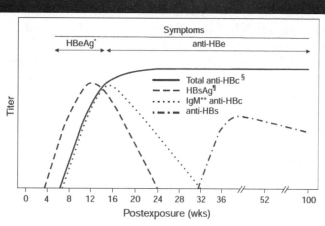

* Hepatitis B e antigen.
† Antibody to HBeAg.
§ Antibody to hepatitis B core antigen.
¶ Hepatitis B surface antigen.
** Immunoglobulin M.
†† Antibody to HBsAg.

From Centers for Disease Control and Prevention. Recommendations for identification and public health management of persons with chronic hepatitis B virus infection. *MMWR Recomm Rep.* 2008;57(RR-8):1–20

FIG 3.5. TYPICAL SEROLOGIC COURSE OF ACUTE HEPATITIS B VIRUS (HBV) INFECTION WITH PROGRESSION TO CHRONIC HBV INFECTION

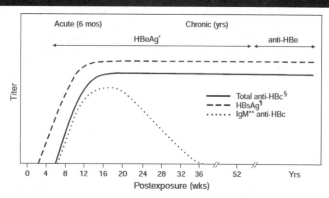

* Hepatitis B e antigen.
† Antibody to HBeAg.
§ Antibody to hepatitis B core antigen.
¶ Hepatitis B surface antigen.
** Immunoglobulin M.

From Centers for Disease Control and Prevention. Recommendations for identification and public health management of persons with chronic hepatitis B virus infection. *MMWR Recomm Rep.* 2008;57(RR-8):1–20

Children and adolescents who have chronic HBV infection are at risk of developing serious liver disease, including primary hepatocellular carcinoma (HCC), with advancing age, and therefore should receive hepatitis A vaccine. Although the peak incidence of primary HCC attributable to HBV infection is in the fifth decade of life, HCC occurs in children as young as 6 years who become infected perinatally or in early childhood. Several algorithms have been published describing the initial evaluation, monitoring, and criteria for treatment. Children with chronic HBV infection should be screened periodically for hepatic complications using serum aminotransferase tests, alpha-fetoprotein concentration, and abdominal ultrasonography. Definitive recommendations on the frequency and indications for specific tests are not yet available because of lack of data on their reliability in predicting sequelae. Patients with serum ALT concentrations persistently exceeding the upper limit of normal and patients with an increased serum alpha-fetoprotein concentration or abnormal findings on abdominal ultrasonography should be referred to a specialist in management of chronic HBV infection for further management and treatment.

The goal of treatment in chronic HBV infection is to prevent progression to cirrhosis, hepatic failure, and HCC. Current indications for treatment of chronic HBV infection include evidence of ongoing HBV viral replication, as indicated by the presence for longer than 6 months of serum HBV DNA greater than 20 000 IU/mL without HBeAg positivity, greater than 2000 IU/mL with HBeAg positivity, and elevated serum ALT concentrations for longer than 6 months or evidence of chronic hepatitis on liver biopsy. Children without necroinflammatory liver disease and children with immunotolerant chronic HBV infection (ie, normal ALT concentrations despite presence of HBV DNA) usually do not warrant antiviral therapy. Treatment response is measured by biochemical, virologic, and histologic response. An important consideration in the choice of treatment is to avoid selection of antiviral-resistant mutations.

The US Food and Drug Administration (FDA) has approved 3 nucleoside analogues (eg, entecavir, lamivudine, and telbivudine), 2 nucleotide analogues (tenofovir and adefovir), and 2 interferon-alfa drugs (interferon alfa-2b and pegylated interferon alfa-2a) for treatment of chronic HBV infection in adults. Tenofovir, entecavir, and pegylated interferon alfa-2a are preferred in adults as first-line therapy because of the lower likelihood of developing antiviral resistance mutations over long-term therapy. Of these, FDA licensure in the pediatric population is as follows: interferon, ≥1 year of age; lamivudine, ≥3 months of age; adefovir, ≥12 years of age; telbivudine, ≥16 years of age; and entecavir, ≥16 years of age. Pediatric trials of telbivudine, tenofovir, pegylated interferon, and entecavir currently are underway. Specific therapy guidelines for HIV- and HBV-coinfected children can be accessed online (**http://aidsinfo.nih.gov/guidelines**). Developments in antiviral therapies of HBV may be found on the American Association for the Study of Liver Diseases Web site (**www.aasld.org**).

The optimal agent(s) and duration of therapy for chronic HBV infection in children remain unclear. There are few large randomized controlled trials of antiviral therapies for chronic hepatitis B in childhood. Studies indicate that approximately 17% to 58% of children with increased serum aminotransferase concentrations who are treated with interferon alfa-2b for 6 months lose HBeAg, compared with approximately 8% to 17% of untreated controls. Response to interferon-alfa is better for children from Western countries (20%–58%) as compared with Asian countries (17%). Children from Asian countries with HBV infection are more likely to: (1) have acquired infection perinatally; (2) have a prolonged immune tolerant phase of infection; and (3) be infected with HBV genotype C. All 3 of these factors are associated with lower response rates to interferon-alfa, which is less effective for chronic infections acquired during early childhood, especially if serum aminotransferase concentrations are normal. Children with chronic HBV infection who were treated with lamivudine had higher rates of virologic response (loss of detectable HBV DNA and loss of HBeAg) after 1 year of treatment than did children who received placebo (23% vs 13%). Resistance to lamivudine can develop while on treatment and may occur early. The optimal duration of lamivudine therapy is not known, but a minimum of 1 year is required. For those who have not yet seroreverted but do not have resistant virus, therapy beyond 1 year may be beneficial (ie, continued seroreversions). However, the high rates of lamivudine resistance (~70% after 3 years of therapy) have decreased enthusiasm for the use of this drug. Combination therapy with lamivudine and interferon-alfa has been studied with mixed results, as compared with monotherapy with interferon-alfa. Children coinfected with HIV and HBV should receive the lamivudine dose approved for treatment of HIV. Consultation with health care professionals with expertise in treating chronic hepatitis B in children is recommended.

ISOLATION OF THE HOSPITALIZED PATIENT: Standard precautions are indicated for patients with acute or chronic HBV infection. For infants born to HBsAg-positive mothers, no special care in addition to standard precautions is needed, other than removal of maternal blood by a gloved attendant.

CONTROL MEASURES:

Strategy for Prevention of HBV Infection. The primary goal of hepatitis B-prevention programs is to eliminate transmission of HBV, thereby decreasing rates of chronic HBV infection and HBV-related chronic liver disease. A secondary goal is prevention of acute HBV infection. In the United States over the past 2 decades, a comprehensive immunization strategy to eliminate HBV transmission has been implemented progressively and now includes the following 4 components[1,2]: (1) universal immunization of infants beginning at birth; (2) prevention of perinatal HBV infection through routine screening of all pregnant women and appropriate immunoprophylaxis of infants born to HBsAg-positive women and infants born to women with unknown HBsAg status; (3) routine immunization of children and adolescents who previously have not been immunized; and (4) immunization of previously unimmunized adults at increased risk of infection.

Hepatitis B Immunoprophylaxis. Two types of products are available for immunoprophylaxis. HBIG provides short-term protection (3–6 months) and is indicated only in specific postexposure circumstances (see Care of Exposed People, p 419). HepB vaccine is used for preexposure and postexposure protection and provides long-term protection. Preexposure immunization with HepB vaccine is the most effective means to prevent HBV transmission. Accordingly, HepB immunization is recommended for all infants, children, and adolescents through 18 years of age. Infants should receive HepB vaccine as part of the routine childhood immunization schedule. All children 11 through

[1]Centers for Disease Control and Prevention. A comprehensive immunization strategy to eliminate transmission of hepatitis B virus infection in the United States: recommendations of the Advisory Committee on Immunization Practices (ACIP). Part I: immunization of infants, children, and adolescents. *MMWR Recomm Rep.* 2005;54(RR-16):1–31

[2]Centers for Disease Control and Prevention. A comprehensive immunization strategy to eliminate transmission of hepatitis B virus infection in the United States: recommendations of the Advisory Committee on Immunization Practices (ACIP). Part II: immunization of adults. *MMWR Recomm Rep.* 2006;55(RR-16):1–33

12 years of age should have their immunization records reviewed and should complete the HepB vaccine series if they have not received the vaccine or did not complete the immunization series.

Postexposure immunoprophylaxis either with HepB vaccine and HBIG or with HepB vaccine alone effectively prevents most infections after exposure to HBV. For infants, use of both HepB vaccine plus HBIG appears to provide greater protection than HepB vaccine alone. Effectiveness of postexposure immunoprophylaxis is related directly to the time elapsed between exposure and administration. Immunoprophylaxis of perinatal infection is most effective if given within 12 hours of birth; data are limited on effectiveness when administered between 25 hours and 7 days of life. Serologic testing of all pregnant women for HBsAg during each pregnancy is essential for identifying women whose infants will require postexposure immunoprophylaxis beginning at birth (see Care of Exposed People, p 419).

Hepatitis B Immune Globulin.[1] HBIG is prepared from hyperimmunized donors whose plasma is known to contain a high concentration of anti-HBs. Plasma donors are required to have negative serologic and nucleic acid test results for HIV and HCV. Additionally, the processes used to manufacture HBIG products are demonstrated to inactivate HBV, HIV, and HCV. Standard Immune Globulin is not effective for postexposure prophylaxis against HBV infection, because concentrations of anti-HBs are too low.

Hepatitis B Vaccine. Highly effective and safe HepB vaccines produced by recombinant DNA technology are licensed in the United States in single-antigen formulations and as components of combination vaccines. Plasma-derived hepatitis B vaccines no longer are available in the United States but may be used successfully in a few countries. Recombinant vaccines contain 10 to 40 µg of HBsAg protein/mL, and a completed vaccine series results in production of anti-HBs of at least 10 mIU/mL in most recipients, which provides long-term protection. Single-dose (including pediatric) formulations contain no thimerosal as a preservative. Although the concentration of recombinant HBsAg protein differs among vaccine products, rates of seroprotection are equivalent when given to immunocompetent infants, children, adolescents, or young adults in the doses recommended (see Table 3.18, p 409).

HepB vaccine can be given concurrently with other vaccines (see Simultaneous Administration of Multiple Vaccines, p 35).

Vaccine Interchangeability. In general, the various brands of age-appropriate HepB vaccines are interchangeable within an immunization series. The immune response using 1 or 2 doses of a vaccine produced by one manufacturer followed by 1 or more subsequent doses from a different manufacturer is comparable to a full course of immunization with a single product. However, until additional data supporting interchangeability of acellular pertussis-containing HepB combination vaccines are available, vaccines from the same manufacturer should be used, whenever feasible, for at least the first 3 doses in the pertussis series (see Pertussis, p 608). In addition, a 2-dose schedule of the adult formulation of Recombivax HB (Merck & Co, Whitehouse Station, NJ) is licensed for adolescents 11 through 15 years of age (see Table 3.18, p 409).

Routes of Administration. Vaccine is administered intramuscularly in the anterolateral thigh for infants or deltoid area for children and adults (see Vaccine Administration, p 26).

---

[1] Dosages recommended for postexposure prophylaxis are for products licensed in the United States. Because concentration of anti-HBs in other products may vary, different dosages may be recommended in other countries.

Table 3.18. Recommended Dosages of Hepatitis B Vaccines

Patients	Vaccine[a]		Combination Vaccines		
	Recombivax HB[b] Dose, μg (mL)	Engerix-B[c] Dose, μg (mL)	Comvax[d] Dose, μg (mL)	Pediarix[e] Dose, μg/mL	Twinrix Dose, μg (mL)[f]
Infants of HBsAg-negative mothers and children and adolescents younger than 20 y	5 (0.5)	10 (0.5)	5 μg HBsAg (0.5)	10 μg HBsAg (0.5)	No applicable
Infants of HBsAg-positive mothers (HBIG [0.5 mL] also is recommended)	5 (0.5)	10 (0.5)	5 μg HBsAg (0.5)	10 μg HBsAg (0.5)	Not applicable
Adolescents 11–15 y of age[b]	10 (1)	Not applicable	Not applicable	Not applicable	Not applicable
Adults 20 y or older	10 (1)	20 (1)	Not applicable	Not applicable	20 (1)
Adults undergoing dialysis and other immunosuppressed adults	40 (1)[g]	40 (2)[h]	Not applicable	Not applicable	Not applicable

HBsAg indicates hepatitis B surface antigen; HBIG, Hepatitis B Immune Globulin.

[a] Both vaccines are administered in a 3-dose schedule at 0, 1, and 6 months; 4 doses may be administered if a birth dose is given and a combination vaccine is used (at 2, 4, and 6 months) to complete the series. Only single-antigen hepatitis B vaccine can be used for the birth dose. Single-antigen or combination vaccine containing hepatitis B vaccine may be used to complete the series.

[b] Available from Merck & Co Inc. (Whitehouse Station, NJ). A 2-dose schedule, administered at 0 months and then 4 to 6 months later, is licensed for adolescents 11 through 15 years of age using the adult formulation of Recombivax HB (10 μg [Merck & Co Inc.]).

[c] Available from GlaxoSmithKline Biologicals (Research Triangle Park, NC). The US Food and Drug Administration also has licensed this vaccine for use in an optional 4-dose schedule at 0, 1, 2, and 12 months for all age groups. A 0-, 12-, and 24-months schedule is licensed for children 5 through 16 years of age for whom an extended administration schedule is appropriate based on risk of exposure.

[d] Available from Merck & Co Inc. A combination of hepatitis B (Recombivax, 5 μg) and Haemophilus influenzae type b (PRP-OMP) vaccine is approved for use at 2, 4, and 12 through 15 months of age (Comvax). This vaccine should not be administered at birth, before 6 weeks of age, or after 71 months of age. For additional information, see Haemophilus influenzae infections (p 368).

[e] A combination of diphtheria and tetanus toxoids and acellular pertussis (DTaP), inactivated poliovirus (IPV), and hepatitis B (Engerix-B 10 μg) is approved for use at 2, 4, and 6 months of age (Pediarix [GlaxoSmithKline]). This vaccine should not be administered at birth, before 6 weeks of age, or at 7 years of age or older. For additional information, see Pertussis (p 608).

[f] A combination of hepatitis B (Engerix-B, 20 μg) and hepatitis A (Havrix, 720 enzyme-linked immunosorbent assay units [ELU]) vaccine; Twinrix is licensed for use in people 18 years of age and older in a 3-dose schedule at 0, 1, and 6 months. Alternately, a 4-dose schedule at days 0, 7, and 21 to 30 followed by a booster dose at 12 months may be used.

[g] Special formulation for adult dialysis patients given at 0, 1, and 6 months.

[h] Two 1-mL doses given in 1 or 2 injections in a 4-dose schedule at 0, 1, 2, and 6 months of age.

Administration in the buttocks has been associated with decreased immunogenicity; intradermal vaccination has been associated with mixed results and is not an approved route of administration. Administration in the buttocks or by the intradermal route is not recommended at any age.

Efficacy and Duration of Protection. HepB vaccines licensed in the United States have a 90% to 95% efficacy for preventing HBV infection and clinical HBV disease among susceptible children and adults. Long-term studies of immunocompetent adults and children indicate that immune memory remains intact for up to 2 decades and protects against symptomatic acute and chronic HBV infection, even though anti-HBs concentrations may become low or undetectable over time. Breakthrough infections (detected by presence of anti-HBc or HBV DNA) have occurred in a limited number of immunized people, but these infections typically are transient and asymptomatic. Chronic HBV infection in immunized people has been documented in dialysis patients whose anti-HBs concentrations fell below 10 mIU/mL and rarely among people who did not respond to vaccination (eg, adults and infants born to HBsAg-positive mothers).

Booster Doses. For children and adults with normal immune status, routine booster doses of HepB vaccine are not recommended. For hemodialysis patients, children with cystic fibrosis liver disease, and other immunocompromised people at continued risk of infection, the need for booster doses should be assessed by annual anti-HBs testing, and a booster dose should be given when the anti-HBs concentration is less than 10 mIU/mL. For other immunocompromised people (eg, HIV-infected people, hematopoietic stem cell transplant recipients, and people receiving chemotherapy), the need for booster doses has not been determined. Annual anti-HBs testing and booster doses when anti-HBs levels decline to less than10 mIU/mL should be considered for immunocompromised people with an ongoing risk for exposure.

Adverse Reactions. Adverse effects most commonly reported in adults and children are pain at the injection site, reported by 3% to 29% of recipients, and a temperature greater than 37.7°C (99.8°F), reported by 1% to 6% of recipients. Anaphylaxis is uncommon, occurring in approximately 1 in 600 000 recipients, according to vaccine adverse events passive reporting surveillance systems. Large, controlled epidemiologic studies and review by the Institute of Medicine[1] (see Institute of Medicine Reviews of Adverse Events After Immunization, p 44) found no evidence of an association between HepB vaccine and sudden infant death syndrome, type 1 diabetes mellitus, seizures, encephalitis, or autoimmune (eg, vasculitis) or demyelinating disease, including multiple sclerosis.

Immunization During Pregnancy or Lactation. No adverse effect on the developing fetus has been observed when pregnant women have been immunized. Because HBV infection may result in severe disease in the mother and chronic infection in the newborn infant, pregnancy is not a contraindication to immunization. Lactation is not a contraindication to immunization.

Serologic Testing. Susceptibility testing before immunization is not indicated routinely for children or adolescents. Testing for past or current infection may be considered for people in risk groups with high rates of HBV infection, including people born in countries with intermediate and high HBV endemicity (even if immunized), users of

---

[1]Institute of Medicine. *Adverse Effects of Vaccines: Evidence and Causality.* Washington, DC: National Academies Press; 2011

injection drugs, men who have sex with men, and household and sexual contacts of HBsAg-positive people, provided testing does not delay or impede immunization efforts. A substantial proportion of people with chronic HBV infection are unaware of their infection.

Routine postimmunization testing for anti-HBs is not necessary after routine vaccination of healthy people but is recommended 1 to 2 months after the third vaccine dose for the following specific groups: (1) hemodialysis patients; (2) people with HIV infection; (3) people at occupational risk of exposure from percutaneous injuries or mucosal or nonintact skin exposures (certain health care and public safety workers); (4) other immunocompromised patients (eg, hematopoietic stem-cell transplant recipients or people receiving chemotherapy); and (5) sexual partners of HBsAg-positive people. Testing of infants born to HBsAg-positive mothers should be deferred until at least 6 months after the last vaccine dose; these infants should have postimmunization testing for HBsAg and anti-HBs performed at 9 to 18 months of age, generally at the next well-child visit after completion of the vaccine series (see Prevention of Perinatal HBV Infection, p 419). If seronegative at 9 months, repeat the test at 6 months after last dose of HepB vaccine.

Management of Nonresponders. Vaccine recipients who do not develop a serum anti-HBs response (10 mIU/mL or greater) after a primary vaccine series should be tested for HBsAg to rule out the possibility of a chronic infection as an explanation of failure to respond to the vaccine. If the HBsAg test result is negative, an additional 3-dose series should be administered. Fewer than 5% of immunocompetent infants, children, and young adults receiving 6 doses of HepB vaccine administered by the appropriate schedule in the deltoid muscle fail to develop detectable antibody. People who remain anti-HBs negative 1 to 2 months after a reimmunization series are unlikely to respond to additional doses of vaccine and should be considered nonimmune if they are exposed to HBV in the future (Tables 3.19, p 412, and 3.20, p 413).

Altered Doses and Schedules. Larger vaccine doses are required to induce protective anti-HBs concentrations in adult hemodialysis patients and immunocompromised adults, including HIV-seropositive people (see Table 3.18, p 409). Humoral immune response to HepB vaccine also may be reduced in children and adolescents who are receiving hemodialysis or are immunocompromised. However, few data exist concerning the response to higher doses of vaccine in children and adolescents, and no specific recommendations can be made for these age groups. For unvaccinated people with progressive chronic renal failure, and possibly cardiac or other transplant recipients, HepB vaccine should be administered as early as possible in the disease course to provide protection and potentially improve responses to vaccination.

Preexposure Universal Immunization of Infants, Children, and Adolescents. Hepatitis B immunization is recommended for all infants, children, and adolescents through 18 years of age. Delivery hospitals should develop policies and procedures that ensure administration of a birth dose as part of the routine care of all medically stable infants weighing 2000 g or more at birth, unless under rare circumstances a physician orders deferred immunization. If vaccination is deferred, a report of the negative serologic status of the mother must be placed in the infant's medical record. The HepB vaccine series (3 or 4 doses; see discussion about birth dose in next paragraph) for infants born to HBsAg-negative mothers should be completed by 6 to 18 months of age. All children and adolescents who have not been immunized against HBV should begin the series during any visit.

Table 3.19. Recommendations for Hepatitis B Virus (HBV) Prophylaxis After Occupational Percutaneous or Mucosal Exposure to Blood or Body Fluids[a]

Exposed Person	HBsAg Positive	Treatment When Source Is		
		HBsAg Negative	Unknown or Not Tested	
Unimmunized	Administer HBIG[b] (1 dose) and initiate HBV series	Initiate HBV series	Initiate HBV vaccine series	
Previously immunized				
Known responder	No treatment	No treatment	No treatment	
Known nonresponder		No treatment	If known high-risk source, treat as if source were HBsAg positive	
After 3 doses:	HBIG: 1 dose and initiate reimmunization[c]			
After 6 doses	HBIG: 2 doses separated by 1 month			
Response unknown	Test exposed person for anti-HBs[d]	No treatment	Test exposed person for anti-HBs[d]	
	If adequate, no treatment		• If adequate, no treatment	
	If inadequate, HBIG × 1 and vaccine booster		• If inadequate, vaccine booster dose[e]	

HBsAg indicates hepatitis B surface antigen; HBIG, Hepatitis B Immune Globulin; anti-HBs, antibody to HBsAg.

[a] Centers for Disease Control and Prevention. Immunization of health-care personnel: recommendations of the Advisory Committee on Immunization Practices (ACIP). *MMWR Recomm Rep.* 2011;60(RR-7):1–45

[b] Dose of HBIG, 0.06 mL/kg, intramuscularly.

[c] The option of giving 1 dose of HBIG (0.06 mL/kg) and reinitiating the vaccine series is preferred for nonresponders who have not completed a second 3-dose vaccine series. For people who previously completed a second vaccine series but failed to respond, 2 doses of HBIG (0.06 mL/kg) are preferred, 1 dose as soon as possible after exposure and the second 1 month later.

[d] Adequate anti-HBs is ≥10 mIU/mL.

[e] The person should be evaluated for antibody response after the vaccine booster dose. For people who receive HBIG, anti-HBs testing should be performed when passively acquired antibody from HBIG no longer is detectable (eg, 4–6 months); for people who did not receive HBIG, anti-HBs testing should be performed 1 to 2 months after the vaccine booster dose. If anti-HBs is inadequate (less than 10 mIU/mL) after the vaccine booster dose, 2 additional doses should be administered to complete a 3-dose reimmunization series, followed by postimmunization testing for anti-HBs and HBsAg.

High seroconversion rates and protective concentrations of anti-HBs (10 mIU/mL or greater) are achieved when HepB vaccine is administered in any of the various recommended schedules, including schedules begun soon after birth in term infants. Only single-antigen HepB vaccine can be used for doses given between birth and 6 weeks of age. Single-antigen or combination vaccine may be used to complete the series; 4 doses of vaccine may be administered if a birth dose is given and a combination vaccine containing a hepatitis B component is used to complete the series.[1] For guidelines for minimum scheduling time between vaccine doses for infants, see Table 1.8 (p 32). The schedule should be chosen to facilitate a high rate of adherence to the primary vaccine series. For immunization of older children and adolescents, doses may be given in a schedule of 0, 1, and 6 months; a schedule of 0, 1, and 4 months; or a schedule of 0, 2, and 4 months (although shorter intervals between first and last doses result in lower immunogenicity). For older children and adolescents, spacing at 0,

[1] Centers for Disease Control and Prevention. General recommendations on immunization. Recommendations of the Advisory Committee on Immunization Practices (ACIP). *MMWR Recomm Rep.* 2011;60(RR-2):1–64

Table 3.20. Guidelines for Postexposure Prophylaxis[a] of People With Nonoccupational Exposures[b] to Blood or Body Fluids That Contain Blood, by Exposure Type and Vaccination Status

Exposure	Treatment	
	Unvaccinated Person[c]	Previously Vaccinated Person[d]
HBsAg-positive source		
Percutaneous (eg, bite or needlestick) or mucosal exposure to HBsAg-positive blood or body fluids	Administer hepatitis B vaccine series and hepatitis B immune globulin (HBIG)	Administer hepatitis B vaccine booster dose
Sexual or needle-sharing contact of an HBsAg-positive person	Administer hepatitis B vaccine series and HBIG	Administer hepatitis B vaccine booster dose
Victim of sexual assault/abuse by a perpetrator who is HBsAg positive	Administer hepatitis B vaccine series and HBIG	Administer hepatitis B vaccine booster dose
Source with unknown HBsAg status		
Victim of sexual assault/abuse by a perpetrator with unknown HBsAg status	Administer hepatitis B vaccine series	No treatment
Percutaneous (eg, bite or needlestick) or mucosal exposure to potentially infectious blood or body fluids from a source with unknown HBsAg status	Administer hepatitis B vaccine series	No treatment
Sex or needle-sharing contact of person with unknown HBsAg status	Administer hepatitis B vaccine series	No treatment

HBsAg indicates hepatitis B surface antigen.

[a] When indicated, immunoprophylaxis should be initiated as soon as possible, preferably within 24 hours. Studies are limited on the maximum interval after exposure during which postexposure prophylaxis is effective, but the interval is unlikely to exceed 7 days for percutaneous exposures or 14 days for sexual exposures. The hepatitis B vaccine series should be completed.

[b] These guidelines apply to nonoccupational exposures. Guidelines for occupational exposures can be found in Table 3.19.

[c] A person who is in the process of being vaccinated but who has not completed the vaccine series should complete the series and receive treatment as indicated.

[d] A person who has written documentation of a complete hepatitis B vaccine series and who did not receive postvaccination testing.

Recommendations of the Advisory Committee on Immunization Practices (ACIP). Part II: immunization of adults. *MMWR Recomm Rep.* 2006;55(RR-16):30–31

12, and 24 months results in equivalent immunogenicity and can be used when an extended administration schedule is acceptable on the basis of low risk of exposure. A 2-dose schedule for one vaccine using the adult formulation is licensed for people 11 through 15 years of age; the schedule is 0 and then 4 to 6 months later (see Table 3.18, p 409).

The recommended schedule for routine hepatitis B immunization of infants born to HBsAg-negative mothers is provided in the annual immunization schedule **(http://redbook.solutions.aap.org/SS/Immunization_Schedules.aspx)**. Age-specific vaccine dosages are provided in Table 3.18 (p 409). Combination products containing HepB vaccine may be given in the United States, provided they are licensed by the FDA for the child's current age and administration of the other vaccine component(s) also is indicated. Children and adolescents who previously have not received HepB vaccine should be immunized routinely at any age with the age-appropriate doses and schedule. Selection of a vaccine schedule should consider the need to achieve completion of the vaccine series. In all settings, immunization should be initiated, even though completion of the vaccine series might not be ensured.

Preexposure Immunization of Adults.[1]
- Hepatitis B immunization is recommended as a 3-dose series for all unimmunized adults at risk of HBV infection (see Table 3.21) and for all adults seeking protection from HBV infection. Acknowledgment of a specific risk factor is not a requirement for immunization.
- In settings where a high proportion of adults are likely to have risk factors for HBV infection, all unimmunized adults should be assumed to be at risk and should receive hepatitis B immunization. These settings include: (1) sexually transmitted infection treatment facilities; (2) HIV testing and treatment facilities; (3) facilities providing drug abuse treatment and prevention services; (4) health care settings targeting services to injection drug users; (5) correctional facilities; (6) health care settings serving men who have sex with men; (7) chronic hemodialysis facilities and end-stage renal disease programs; and (8) institutions and nonresidential care facilities for people with developmental disabilities.
- HepB vaccine should be administered to unimmunized adults with diabetes mellitus who are 19 through 59 years of age.[2] HepB vaccine may be administered at the discretion of the treating clinician to unimmunized adults with diabetes mellitus who are 60 years or older.
- Standing orders should be implemented to identify and immunize eligible adults in primary care and specialty medical settings. If ascertainment of risk for HBV infection is a barrier to immunization in these settings, health care professionals may use alternative immunization strategies, such as offering hepatitis B vaccine to all unimmunized adults in age groups with highest risk of infection (eg, younger than 49 years).

Lapsed Immunizations. For infants, children, adolescents, and adults with lapsed immunizations (ie, the interval between doses is longer than that in one of the recommended schedules), the vaccine series should be completed without repeating doses, as long as

---

[1]Centers for Disease Control and Prevention. A comprehensive immunization strategy to eliminate transmission of hepatitis B virus infection in the United States: recommendations of the Advisory Committee on Immunization Practices (ACIP). Part II: immunization of adults. *MMWR Recomm Rep.* 2006;55(RR-16):1–33

[2]Centers for Disease Control and Prevention. Use of hepatitis B vaccination for adults with diabetes mellitus: recommendations of the Advisory Committee on Immunization Practices (ACIP). *MMWR Morb Mortal Wkly Rep.* 2011;60(50):1709–1711

Table 3.21. Adults Recommended to Receive Hepatitis B Virus (HBV) Vaccine[a]

People at Risk of Infection by Sexual Exposure
- Sex partners of hepatitis B surface antigen (HBsAg)-positive people
- Sexually active people who are not in a long-term, mutually monogamous relationship (eg, people with more than 1 sex partner during the previous 6 months)
- People seeking evaluation or treatment for a sexually transmitted infection
- Men who have sex with men

People at Risk of Infection by Percutaneous or Mucosal Exposure to Blood
- Current or recent injection-drug users
- Household contacts of HBsAg-positive people
- Residents and staff of facilities for people with developmental disabilities
- Health-care and public safety workers with reasonably anticipated risk of exposure to blood or blood-contaminated body fluids
- People with end-stage renal disease, including predialysis, hemodialysis, peritoneal dialysis, and home dialysis patients
- People with diabetes mellitus 19 through 59 years of age; people with diabetes mellitus 60 years of age and older may be immunized at the discretion of their physician

Others
- International travelers to regions with high or intermediate levels (HBsAg prevalence of 2% or greater) of endemic HBV infection (see Table 3.16, p 403)
- People with chronic liver disease
- People with human immunodeficiency (HIV) infection
- All other people seeking protection from HBV infection

[a]Centers for Disease Control and Prevention. A comprehensive immunization strategy to eliminate transmission of hepatitis B virus infection in the United States: recommendations of the Advisory Committee on Immunization Practices (ACIP). Part II: immunization of adults. *MMWR Recomm Rep.* 2006;55(RR-16):1-33

minimum dosing intervals between the remaining doses necessary to complete the series are heeded (see Lapsed Immunizations, p 37).

SPECIAL CONSIDERATIONS:

Infants Weighing <2000 g at Birth. Studies demonstrate that decreased seroconversion rates might occur among preterm infants with a birth weight of less than 2000 g after administration of hepatitis B vaccine at birth. However, by the chronologic age of 1 month, all medically stable preterm infants (see Immunization in Preterm and Low Birth Weight Infants, p 68), regardless of initial birth weight or gestational age, are as likely to respond to hepatitis B immunization as are term and larger infants.

All infants weighing <2000 g who are born to an HBsAg-positive mother should receive immunoprophylaxis with HepB vaccine and HBIG within 12 hours after birth; the birth dose of HepB vaccine should not be counted toward completion of the HepB vaccine series, and 3 additional doses of HepB vaccine should be administered beginning when the infant is 1 month of age (see Table 3.22, p 416). Only monovalent HepB vaccines should be used from birth through 6 weeks of age.

If maternal HBsAg status is unknown at birth, the infant weighing less than 2000 g should receive HepB vaccine within 12 hours of birth. The mother's HBsAg status should be determined as quickly as possible. If the infant's birth weight is less than 2000 g and

Table 3.22. Hepatitis B Virus (HBV) Immunoprophylaxis Scheme by Infant Birth Weight[a]

Maternal Status	Infant Birth Weight 2000 g or More	Infant Birth Weight Less Than 2000 g
HBsAg positive	Hepatitis B vaccine 1 HBIG (within 12 h of birth)	Hepatitis B vaccine 1 HBIG (within 12 h of birth)
	Continue vaccine series beginning at 1–2 mo of age according to recommended schedule for infants born to HBsAg-positive mothers (see Table 3.23)	Continue vaccine series beginning at 1–2 mo of age according to recommended schedule for infants born to HBsAg-positive mothers (ie, administer 3 additional hepatitis B vaccine doses with single-antigen vaccine at ages 1, 2–3, and 6 months, OR hepatitis B-containing combination vaccine at ages 2, 4, and 6 months (Pediarix) or 2, 4 , and 12–15 months (Comvax) (see Table 3.23)
		Immunize with 4 vaccine doses; do not count birth dose as part of the 3-dose vaccine series
	Check anti-HBs and HBsAg after completion of vaccine series[b]	Check anti-HBs and HBsAg after completion of vaccine series[b]
	HBsAg-negative infants with anti-HBs levels 10 mIU/mL or greater are protected and need no further medical management	HBsAg-negative infants with anti-HBs levels 10 mIU/mL or greater are protected and need no further medical management
	HBsAg-negative infants with anti-HBs levels less than 10 mIU/mL should be reimmunized with a second 3-dose series and retested	HBsAg-negative infants with anti-HBs levels less than 10 mIU/mL should be reimmunized with a second 3-dose series and retested
	Infants who are HBsAg positive should receive appropriate follow-up, including medical evaluation for chronic liver disease	Infants who are HBsAg positive should receive appropriate follow-up, including medical evaluation for chronic liver disease
HBsAg status unknown	Test mother for HBsAg immediately after admission for delivery	Test mother for HBsAg immediately after admission for delivery
	Hepatitis B vaccine (within 12h of birth)	Hepatitis B vaccine (within 12h of birth)
	Administer HBIG (within 7 days) if mother tests HBsAg positive; if mother's HBsAg status remains unknown, some experts would administer HBIG (within 7 days)	Administer HBIG within 12 hours of birth if mother tests HBsAg positive or if mother's HBsAg result is not available/unknown within 12 h of birth

Table 3.22. Hepatitis B Virus (HBV) Immunoprophylaxis Scheme by Infant Birth Weight,[a] continued

Maternal Status	Infant Birth Weight 2000 g or More	Infant Birth Weight Less Than 2000 g
	Continue the 3-dose vaccine series beginning at 1–2 mo of age according to recommended schedule based on mother's HBsAg result (see Table 3.23)	Continue vaccine series beginning at 1–2 mo of age according to recommended schedule based on mother's HBsAg result (ie, administer 3 additional hepatitis B vaccine doses with single-antigen vaccine at ages 1, 2–3, and 6 months, OR hepatitis B-containing combination vaccine at ages 2, 4, and 6 months (Pediarix) or 2, 4 and 12–15 months (Comvax) (see Table 3.23)
		Immunize with 4 vaccine doses; do not count birth dose as part of the 3-dose vaccine series
HBsAg negative	HBV vaccine at birth[c]	Delay first dose of hepatitis B vaccine until 1 mo of age or hospital discharge, whichever is first
	Continue vaccine series beginning at 1–2 mo of age (see Table 3.23)	Continue the 3-dose vaccine series beginning at 2 mo of age (see Table 3.23)
	Follow-up anti-HBs and HBsAg testing not needed	Follow-up anti-HBs and HBsAg testing not needed

HBsAg indicates hepatitis B surface antigen; HBIG, hepatitis B Immune Globulin; anti-HBs, antibody to HBsAg.
[a] Extremes of gestational age and birth weight no longer are a consideration for timing of hepatitis B vaccine doses.
[b] Test at 9 to 18 months of age, generally at the next well-child visit after completion of the primary series. Use testing method that allows determination of a protective concentration of anti-HBs (10 mIU/mL or greater).
[c] The first dose may be delayed until after hospital discharge in rare circumstances for an infant who weighs 2000 g or greater and whose mother is HBsAg negative, but only if a physician's order to withhold the birth dose and a copy of the mother's original HBsAg-negative laboratory report are documented in the infant's medical record.

the maternal HBsAg status cannot be determined within 12 hours of life, HBIG should be given, because the less reliable immune response in preterm infants weighing less than 2000 g precludes the option of the 7-day waiting period acceptable for term and larger preterm infants. Only monovalent HepB vaccine should be used from birth through 6 weeks of age.

All infants of HBsAg-negative mothers with a birth weight of less than 2000 g should receive the first dose of HepB vaccine series starting at 1 month of chronologic age or at hospital discharge if before 1 month of chronologic age. Infants born to HBsAg-negative mothers do not need to have postimmunization serologic testing for anti-HBs. Table 3.22 provides a summary of the recommendations for immunization of infants on the basis of maternal hepatitis B status and infant birth weight. For information on use of combination vaccines containing HepB vaccine as a component to complete the series, see Table 3.23 (p 418).

Table 3.23. Hepatitis B Vaccine Schedules for Infants by Maternal Hepatitis B Surface Antigen (HBsAg) Status[a,b]

Maternal HBsAg Status	Single-Antigen Vaccine		Single-Antigen + Combination	
	Dose	Age	Dose	Age
Positive	1[c]	Birth (12 h or less)	1[c] Birth (12 h or less) (Combination vaccine should not be used for birth dose)	
	HBIG[d]	Birth (12 h or less)	HBIG[d]	Birth (12 h or less)
	2	1 through 2 mo	2	2 mo
	3[e]	6 mo	3	4 mo
			4[e]	6 mo (Pediarix) or 12 through 15 mo (Comvax)
Unknown[f]	1[c]	Birth (12 h or less)	1[c] Birth (12 h or less) (Combination vaccine should not be used for birth dose)	
	2	1 through 2 mo	2	2 mo
	3[e]	6 mo	3	4 mo
			4[e]	6 mo (Pediarix) or 12 through 15 mo (Comvax)
Negative	1[c,g]	Birth (before discharge)	1[c,g] Birth (before discharge) (Combination vaccine should not be used for birth dose)	
	2	1 through 2 mo	2	2 mo
	3[e]	6 through 18 mo	3	4 mo
			4[e]	6 mo (Pediarix) or 12 through 15 mo (Comvax)

HBIG indicates Hepatitis B Immune Globulin.

[a] Centers for Disease Control and Prevention. A comprehensive immunization strategy to eliminate transmission of hepatitis B virus infection in the United States: recommendations of the Advisory Committee on Immunization Practices (ACIP). Part 1: immunization of infants, children, and adolescents. *MMWR Recomm Rep.* 2005;54(RR-16):1–31.

[b] See Table 3.22 for vaccine schedules for preterm infants weighing less than 2000 g.

[c] Recombivax HB or Engerix-B should be used for the birth dose. Comvax and Pediarix should not be administered at birth or before 6 weeks of age.

[d] HBIG (0.5 mL) administered intramuscularly in a separate site from vaccine.

[e] The final dose in the vaccine series should not be administered before 24 weeks (164 days) of age.

[f] Mothers should have blood drawn and tested for HBsAg as soon as possible after admission for delivery; if the mother is found to be HBsAg positive, the infant should receive HBIG as soon as possible but no later than 7 days of age.

[g] On a case-by-case basis and only in rare circumstances, the first dose may be delayed until after hospital discharge for an infant who weighs 2000 g or more and whose mother is HBsAg negative, but only if a physician's order to withhold the birth dose and a copy of the mother's original HBsAg-negative laboratory report are documented in the infant's medical record.

Considerations for High-Risk Groups:

Health Care Personnel and Others With Occupational Exposure to Blood. The risk of HBV exposure to a health care professional depends on the tasks the person performs. Health care personnel who have the potential for contact with blood or other potentially infectious body fluids should be immunized. Because the risks of occupational HBV infection often are highest during the training period, immunization should be initiated as early as possible before or during training and before contact with blood, followed by postimmunization testing for anti-HBs for health care personnel with high risk of exposure. Health care personnel with anti-HBs less than 10 mIU/mL should be reimmunized (3 additional doses) and retested for anti-HBs within 1 to 2 months of the sixth dose.

Patients Undergoing Hemodialysis. Immunization is recommended for susceptible patients undergoing hemodialysis. Immunization early in the course of renal disease is encouraged, because response is better than in advanced disease. Specific dosage recommendations have not been made for children undergoing hemodialysis. Some experts recommend increased doses of HepB vaccine for children receiving hemodialysis to increase immunogenicity.

People Born in Countries Where the Prevalence of Chronic HBV Infection Is 2% or Greater. Foreign-born people (including immigrants, refugees, asylum seekers, and internationally adopted children) from countries where the prevalence of chronic HBV infection is 2% or greater (see Table 3.16, p 403) should be screened for HBsAg regardless of immunization status. Previously unimmunized family members and other household contacts should be immunized if a household member is found to be HBsAg positive. In addition, positive HBsAg test results are nationally notifiable (see Appendix IV, p 992). People with positive HBsAg tests should be reported to the local or state health department and referred for medical management to reduce their risk of complications from chronic HBV infection and to reduce the risk of transmission.

Inmates in Juvenile Detention and Other Correctional Facilities. Unimmunized or underimmunized people in juvenile and adult correctional facilities should be immunized. If the length of stay is not sufficient to complete the immunization series, the series should be initiated, and follow-up mechanisms with a health care facility should be established to ensure completion of the series (see Hepatitis and Youth in Correctional Settings, p 189).

International Travelers. People traveling to areas where the prevalence of chronic HBV infection is 2% or greater (see Table 3.16, p 403) should be immunized. Immunization should begin at least 4 to 6 months before travel so that a 3-dose regimen can be completed (see Preexposure Universal Immunization, p 411). If immunization is initiated fewer than 4 months before departure, the alternative 4-dose schedule of 0, 1, 2, and 12 months, licensed for one vaccine (see Table 3.18, p 409), might provide protection if the first 3 doses can be administered before travel. Individual clinicians may choose to use an accelerated schedule (eg, doses at days 0, 7, and 21) for travelers who will depart before an approved immunization schedule can be completed. People who receive immunization on an accelerated schedule that is not FDA licensed also should receive a dose at 12 months after initiation of the series to promote long-term immunity.

Care of Exposed People (Postexposure Immunoprophylaxis) (Also See Table 3.24, p 420).

Prevention of Perinatal HBV Infection. Transmission of perinatal HBV infection can be prevented in approximately 95% of infants born to HBsAg-positive mothers by early active and passive immunoprophylaxis of the infant (ie, immunization and HBIG administration within 12 hours of birth). Immunization subsequently should be completed during the first 6 months of life. HepB vaccination alone, initiated at or shortly after birth, also is highly effective for preventing perinatal HBV infections. However, women with HBV DNA greater than 10^6 to 10^8 IU/mL or who are HBeAg positive have an increased risk of perinatal transmission even if appropriate active and passive vaccination is given to the newborn infant (~15%–30% risk of transmission versus less than 5% risk of transmission for women with lower HBV DNA or who are HBeAg negative). Tenofovir and telbivudine are the only nucleoside analogues that are not pregnancy category C drugs; these are category B drugs, and in small pilot studies, treatment of pregnant women in

Table 3.24. Guide to Postexposure Immunoprophylaxis of Unimmunized People to Prevent Hepatitis B Virus (HBV) Infection

Type of Exposure	Immunoprophylaxis[a]
Household contact of HBsAg-positive person	Administer hepatitis B vaccine series
Discrete exposure to an HBsAg-positive source[b]:	
• Percutaneous (eg, bite, needlestick, nonintact skin) or mucosal exposure to HBsAg-positive blood or body fluids	Administer hepatitis B vaccine + HBIG; complete vaccine series
• Sexual contact or needle sharing with an HBsAg-positive person	Administer hepatitis B vaccine + HBIG; complete vaccine series
• Victim of sexual assault/abuse by a perpetrator who is HBsAg positive	Administer hepatitis B vaccine + HBIG; complete vaccine series
Discrete exposure to a source with unknown HBsAg status:	
• Percutaneous (eg, bite, needlestick) or mucosal exposure to blood or body fluids with unknown HBsAg status	Administer hepatitis B vaccine series
• Victim of sexual assault/abuse by a perpetrator with unknown HBsAg status	Administer hepatitis B vaccine series
Susceptible child biting someone with chronic HBV infection	Initiate or complete the hepatitis B vaccine series Do not give HBIG (assumes no oral mucosal disease when the amount of blood transferred from a child with chronic HBV infection is small)

HBsAg indicates hepatitis B surface antigen; HBIG, Hepatitis B Immune Globulin.

[a] Immunoprophylaxis should be administered as soon as possible, preferably within 24 hours after exposure. Studies are limited on the maximum interval after exposure during which postexposure prophylaxis is effective, but the interval is unlikely to exceed 7 days for percutaneous exposures and 14 days for sexual exposures.

[b] If person previously was immunized with hepatitis B vaccine series, administer hepatitis B vaccine booster dose (see Table 3.19).

the third trimester with either of these drugs or lamivudine has been effective in preventing transmission to offspring of high-risk women. A recent small open-label study from China demonstrated that telbivudine (600 mg, orally, daily) given in the second and third trimester of pregnancy completely eliminated perinatal transmission of HBV in women who were both HBeAg and HBsAg positive compared with a 9% transmission rate in a control group of women who did not receive the drug. All infants in both groups received HBV vaccine and HBIG within 6 hours of delivery.

Serologic Screening of Pregnant Women. Prenatal HBsAg testing of all pregnant women, regardless of HepB vaccination history, is recommended to identify newborn infants who require immediate postexposure prophylaxis. All pregnant women should be tested during an early prenatal visit with every pregnancy. Testing should be repeated at the time of admission to the hospital for delivery for HBsAg-negative women who are at high risk of HBV infection or who have had clinical HBV infection. Women who are HBsAg positive should be reported to local health departments for appropriate case management to ensure follow-up of their infants and immunization of sexual and household contacts. In populations where HBsAg testing of pregnant women is not feasible (eg, in remote areas without access to a laboratory), all infants should receive HepB vaccine within 12 hours of birth, should receive the second dose by 2 months of age, and should receive the third dose at 6 months of age. Pregnant women and their contacts who are HBsAg-positive should be referred for medical management to reduce their risk of chronic liver disease.

Management of Infants Born to HBsAg-Positive Women. Infants born to HBsAg-positive mothers, including infants weighing less than 2000 g, should receive the initial dose of HepB vaccine within 12 hours of birth (see Table 3.18, p 409, for appropriate dosages), and HBIG (0.5 mL) should be given concurrently but at a different anatomic site. The effectiveness of HBIG diminishes the longer after exposure that it is initiated. The interval of effectiveness is unlikely to exceed 7 days. Subsequent doses of vaccine should be given as recommended in Table 3.22 (p 416) and Table 3.23 (p 418). For infants who weigh less than 2000 g at birth, the initial vaccine dose should not be counted in the required 3-dose schedule (a total of 4 doses of HepB vaccine should be administered), and the subsequent 3 doses should be given in accordance with the schedule for immunization of infants weighing <2000 g (see Immunization in Preterm and Low Birth Weight Infants, p 68).

Infants born to HBsAg-positive women should be tested for anti-HBs and HBsAg at 9 to 18 months of age (generally at the next well-child visit after completion of the immunization series). Testing should not be performed before 9 months of age to maximize the likelihood of detecting late onset of HBV infections. Testing for HBsAg will identify infants who become infected chronically despite immunization (because of intrauterine infection or vaccine failure) and will aid in their long-term medical management. Testing for IgM anti-HBc is unreliable for infants. Infants with anti-HBs concentrations less than 10 mIU/mL and who are HBsAg negative should receive 3 additional doses of vaccine (see Table 3.22, p 416) followed by testing for anti-HBs and HBsAg 1 to 2 months after the sixth dose.

Term Infants (Weighing ≥2000 g at Birth) Born to Mothers Not Tested During Pregnancy for HBsAg. Pregnant women whose HBsAg status is unknown at delivery should undergo blood testing as soon as possible to determine their HBsAg status. While awaiting results, the infant should receive the first HepB vaccine dose within 12 hours of birth, as recommended for infants born to HBsAg-positive mothers (see Table 3.18, p 409). Because HepB vaccine, when given at birth, is highly effective for preventing perinatal infection in term infants, the possible added value and the cost of HBIG do not warrant its immediate use in term infants when the mother's HBsAg status is not known. If the woman is found to be HBsAg positive, term infants should receive HBIG (0.5 mL) as soon as possible, but within 7 days of birth, and should complete the HepB immunization series as recommended (see Tables 3.18, p 409, and 3.20, p 413). If the mother is found to be HBsAg negative, HepB immunization in the dose and schedule recommended for term infants born to HBsAg-negative mothers should be completed (see Table 3.18, p 409). If the mother's HBsAg status remains unknown, some experts would administer HBIG within 7 days of birth and complete the HepB immunization series as recommended for infants born to mothers who are HBsAg positive (Table 3.22, p 416).

Infants Weighing Less Than 2000 g Born to Mothers Not Tested During Pregnancy for HBsAg. Maternal HBsAg status should be determined as soon as possible. Infants weighing less than 2000 g born to mothers whose HBsAg status is unknown should receive HepB vaccine within the first 12 hours of life. Because of the potentially decreased immunogenicity of the HepB vaccine in infants weighing less than 2000 g at birth, these infants should receive HBIG (0.5 mL) if the mother's HBsAg status cannot be determined within the initial 12 hours of birth. In these infants, the initial vaccine dose should not be counted toward the 3 doses of HepB vaccine required to complete the immunization series. The subsequent 3 doses (for a total of 4 doses) are given in accordance with recommendations for immunization of infants with a birth weight less than 2000 g, according to the HBsAg status of the mother (see Table 3.22, p 416). Follow-up HBsAg and anti-HBs testing on completion of the immunization series is recommended for all infants weighing less than 2000 g born to HBsAg-positive mothers (see Management of Infants Born to HBsAg-Positive Women, p 421).

Breastfeeding. Breastfeeding of the infant by an HBsAg-positive mother poses no additional risk of acquisition of HBV infection by the infant with appropriate administration of hepatitis B vaccine and HBIG (see Human Milk, p 125).

Household Contacts and Sexual Partners of HBsAg-Positive People. Household and sexual contacts of HBsAg-positive people (acute or chronic HBV infection) identified through prenatal screening, blood donor screening, or diagnostic or other serologic testing should be screened for HBV infection with anti-HBc or anti-HBs and HBsAg. Unvaccinated and uninfected people should be immunized. The first dose of vaccine should be given after the serologic tests are obtained while waiting on the results. People with chronic HBV should be referred for medical evaluation to prevent complications of the infection.

Prophylaxis with HBIG for other unimmunized household contacts of HBsAg-positive people is not indicated unless they have a discrete, identifiable exposure to the index patient (see next paragraph).

Postexposure Prophylaxis for People With Discrete Identifiable Exposures to Blood or Body Fluids. Management of people with a discrete, identifiable percutaneous (eg, needlestick, laceration, bite or nonintact skin), mucosal (eg, ocular or mucous membrane), or sexual exposure to blood or body fluids includes consideration of whether the HBsAg status of the person who was the source of exposure is known and the hepatitis B immunization and response status of the exposed person (also see Table 3.20, p 413). Immunization is recommended for any person who was exposed but not previously immunized. If possible, a blood specimen from the person who was the source of the exposure should be tested for HBsAg, and appropriate prophylaxis should be administered according to the hepatitis B immunization status and anti-HBs response status (if known) of the exposed person (see Table 3.20, p 413, and Injuries From Discarded Needles in the Community, p 201). Detailed guidelines for management of health care personnel and other people exposed to blood that is or might be HBsAg positive is provided in Table 3.19 and the recommendations of the Advisory Committee on Immunization Practices of the Centers for Disease Control and Prevention.[1]

HBsAg-Positive Source. If the source is HBsAg positive, unimmunized people should receive both HBIG and hepatitis B vaccine as soon as possible after exposure, preferably within 24 hours (see Table 3.19, p 412). The vaccine series should be completed using an age-appropriate dose and schedule. People who are in the process of being immunized but who have not completed the vaccine series should receive the appropriate dose of HBIG and should complete the vaccine series. Children and adolescents who have written documentation of a complete hepatitis B vaccine series and who did not receive postimmunization testing should receive a single vaccine booster dose with postimmunization testing 1 to 2 months later (Table 3.19, p 412).

[1] Centers for Disease Control and Prevention. Immunization of health-care personnel: recommendations of the Advisory Committee on Immunization Practices (ACIP). *MMWR Recomm Rep.* 2011;60(RR-7):1–45

Source With Unknown HBsAg Status. If the HBsAg status of the source is unknown, unimmunized people should begin the hepatitis B vaccine series with the first dose initiated as soon as possible after exposure, preferably within 24 hours (see Table 3.19, p 412). The vaccine series should be completed using an age-appropriate dose and schedule. Children and adolescents with written documentation of a complete hepatitis B vaccine series require no further treatment (Table 3.19, p 412).

Victims of Sexual Assault or Abuse. For unimmunized victims of sexual assault or abuse, active postexposure prophylaxis (ie, vaccine alone) should be initiated, with the first dose of HepB vaccine given as part of the initial clinical evaluation. If the offender is known to be HBsAg positive, HBIG also should be administered. The vaccine series should be completed using an age-appropriate dose and schedule. (For discussion of management of previously immunized people, see Postexposure Prophylaxis for People With Discrete Identifiable Exposures to Blood or Body Fluids, p 422.)

Child Care. All children, including children who attend child care, should receive HepB vaccine as part of their routine immunization. Immunization not only will decrease the potential for HBV transmission after human bites but also will allay anxiety about transmission from attendees who may be HBsAg positive.

Children who are HBsAg positive and who have no behavioral or medical risk factors, such as unusually aggressive behavior (eg, frequent biting), generalized dermatitis, or a bleeding problem, should be admitted to child care without restrictions. Under these circumstances, the risk of HBV transmission in child care settings is negligible, and routine screening for HBsAg is not warranted. Admission of HBsAg-positive children with behavioral or medical risk factors should be assessed on an individual basis by the child's physician.

Effectiveness of Hepatitis B Prevention Programs. Routine hepatitis B immunization programs have resulted in significant decreases in the prevalence of chronic HBV infection among children in populations with a high incidence of HBV infection. There is an association between higher coverage with HepB vaccine and larger decreases in HBsAg prevalence. The incidence of acute HBV infection among US children younger than 19 years decreased by 98% between 1990 and 2010.

Although the long-term sequelae of chronic HBV infection usually are not recognized until adolescence and adulthood, cirrhosis and HCC occur in children. In Taiwan, the average annual incidence of HCC among children 6 to 14 years of age decreased significantly within 10 years of routine infant hepatitis B immunization. Worldwide, routine infant immunization programs and introduction of immunization schedules starting within the first 24 hours of life are expected to decrease significantly the incidence of death from cirrhosis and HCC attributable to HBV infection over the next 30 to 50 years.

The Centers for Disease Control and Prevention Division of Viral Hepatitis maintains a Web site (**www.cdc.gov/hepatitis**) with information on hepatitis for health care professionals and the public.

Hepatitis C

CLINICAL MANIFESTATIONS: Signs and symptoms of hepatitis C virus (HCV) infection are indistinguishable from those of hepatitis A or hepatitis B virus infections. Acute disease tends to be mild and insidious in onset, and most infections are asymptomatic. Jaundice occurs in fewer than 20% of patients, and abnormalities in serum aminotransferase concentrations generally are less pronounced than abnormalities in patients with hepatitis B virus infection. Persistent infection with HCV occurs in up to 80% of infected children, even in the absence of biochemical evidence of liver disease. Most children with chronic infection are asymptomatic. Although chronic hepatitis develops in approximately 70% to 80% of infected adults, limited data indicate that chronic hepatitis and cirrhosis occur less commonly in children, in part because of the usually indolent nature of infection in pediatric patients. Liver failure secondary to HCV infection is the leading indication for liver transplantation among adults in the United States.

ETIOLOGY: HCV is a small, single-stranded RNA virus and is a member of the *Flavivirus* family. At least 6 HCV genotypes exist with multiple subtypes.

EPIDEMIOLOGY: The incidence of acute symptomatic HCV infection in the United States was 0.2 per 100 000 in 2005; after asymptomatic infection and underreporting were considered, approximately 20 000 new cases were estimated to have occurred. For all age groups, the incidence of HCV infection has markedly decreased in the United States since the 1990s and has remained low since 2006. However, there was a 45% increase in reported cases of acute HCV in the United States in 2011 compared with 2004–2010. This increase was mostly seen in white, nonurban young people with a history of using injection drugs and opioid agonists such as oxycodone (**www.cdc.gov/ hepatitis/statistics/2011surveillance/commentary.htm**). A substantial burden of disease still exists in the United States because of the propensity of HCV to establish chronic infection and the high incidence of acute HCV infection through the 1980s. The prevalence of HCV infection in the general population of the United States is estimated at 1.3%, equating to an estimated 3.2 million people in the United States who have chronic HCV infection. Seroprevalence varies among populations according to risk factors. The pediatric prevalence of HCV corresponding to NHANES 1999–2002 was approximately 0.1%, although the numbers of HCV infections in the younger age groups were too small for reliable estimates. Worldwide, the prevalence of chronic HCV infection is highest in Africa, especially Egypt.

HCV primarily is spread by parenteral exposure to blood of HCV-infected people. The most common risk factors for adults to acquire infection are injection drug use, multiple sexual partners, or receipt of blood products before 1992. The most common route of infection for children is maternal-fetal transmission. The current risk of HCV infection after blood transfusion in the United States is estimated to be 1 per 2 million units transfused because of exclusion of high-risk donors and of HCV-positive units after antibody testing as well as screening of pools of blood units by nucleic acid amplification test (NAAT; see Blood Safety, p 112). All intravenous and intramuscular Immune Globulin products available commercially in the United States undergo an inactivation procedure for HCV or are documented to be HCV RNA negative before release.

Approximately 60% of chronic HCV cases reported to public health authorities are in acknowledged injection drug users who have shared needles or injection paraphernalia and, to a lesser extent, in people who received transfusions before 1992, when routine screening of donor blood for HCV began; almost all infected people are outside the pediatric age range. Data from recent multicenter, population-based cohort studies indicate that approximately one third of young injection drug users 18 to 30 years of age are infected with HCV. People with sporadic percutaneous exposures, such as health care professionals (approximately 1% of cases), may be infected. Approximately half of the

18 000 people with hemophilia who received transfusions before adoption of heat treatment of clotting factors in 1987 are HCV seropositive. Also, more recently appreciated has been the number of infections acquired in the health care setting, especially nonhospital clinics where infection control and needle and intravenous hygienic procedures have not been practiced strictly. Prevalence is high among people with frequent but smaller direct percutaneous exposures, such as patients receiving hemodialysis (10%–20%).

Sexual transmission of HCV between heterosexual partners has not been demonstrated in prospective studies. Intravenous drug users often have a greater number of sex partners, so the role of sexual transmission is not fully understood. Sexual transmission of HCV among people coinfected with HIV has been described between HIV-infected men who have sex with men or HIV-infected heterosexual women.

Transmission among family contacts is uncommon but can occur from direct or inapparent percutaneous or mucosal exposure to blood.

Seroprevalence among pregnant women in the United States has been estimated at 1% to 2%. The risk of perinatal transmission averages 5% to 6%, and transmission occurs only from women who are HCV RNA positive at the time of delivery. Maternal coinfection with HIV has been associated with increased risk of perinatal transmission of HCV, with transmission rates between 10% and 20%; transmission depends in part on the concentration of HCV RNA in the mother's blood. Serum antibody to HCV (anti-HCV) and HCV RNA have been detected in colostrum, but the risk of HCV transmission is similar in breastfed and formula-fed infants.

All people with HCV RNA in their blood are considered to be infectious.

The **incubation period** for HCV disease averages 6 to 7 weeks, with a range of 2 weeks to 6 months. The time from exposure to development of viremia generally is 1 to 2 weeks.

DIAGNOSTIC TESTS[1]: The 2 types of tests available for laboratory diagnosis of HCV infections are immunoglobulin (Ig) G antibody enzyme immunoassays for HCV and NAATs to detect HCV RNA. Assays for IgM to detect early or acute infection are not available. Third-generation enzyme immunoassays are at least 97% sensitive and more than 99% specific. In June 2010, the US Food and Drug Administration (FDA) approved for use in people 15 years and older the OraQuick rapid blood test, which uses a test strip that produces a blue line within 20 minutes if anti-HCV antibodies are present. False-negative results early in the course of acute infection can result from any of the HCV serologic tests because of the prolonged interval between exposure and onset of illness and seroconversion. Within 15 weeks after exposure and within 5 to 6 weeks after onset of hepatitis, 80% of patients will have positive test results for serum anti-HCV antibody. Among infants born to anti-HCV–positive mothers, passively acquired maternal antibody may persist for up to 18 months.

FDA-licensed diagnostic NAATs for qualitative detection of HCV RNA are available. HCV RNA can be detected in serum or plasma within 1 to 2 weeks after exposure to the virus and weeks before onset of liver enzyme abnormalities or appearance of anti-HCV. Assays for detection of HCV RNA are used commonly in clinical practice to identify anti-HCV–positive patients who are viremic, for identifying infection in infants early in life (ie, perinatal transmission) when maternal antibody interferes with ability to detect antibody

---

[1]Centers for Disease Control and Prevention. Testing for HCV Infection: an update of guidance for clinicians and laboratorians. *MMWR Morb Mortal Wkly Rep.* 2013;62(18):362–365

produced by the infant, and for monitoring patients receiving antiviral therapy. However, false-positive and false-negative results of NAATs can occur from improper handling, storage, and contamination of test specimens. Viral RNA may be detected intermittently in acute infection (ie, in the first 6 or 12 months following infection); thus, a single negative assay result is not conclusive if performed during this acute infection period. Highly sensitive quantitative assays for measuring the concentration of HCV RNA have largely replaced qualitative assays. The clinical value of these quantitative assays appears to be primarily as a prognostic indicator for patients undergoing or about to undergo antiviral therapy.

TREATMENT: Patients diagnosed with HCV infection should be referred to a pediatric hepatitis specialist for clinical monitoring and consideration of antiviral treatment. Therapy is aimed at inhibiting HCV replication, eradicating infection, and improving the natural history of disease. Therapies are expensive and can have significant adverse reactions. Response to treatment varies depending on the genotype with which the person is infected. Genotype 1 is the most common genotype in North America. Genotypes 1 and 4 respond less well than genotypes 2 and 3 to antiviral therapy. Currently, the only FDA-approved treatment for HCV treatment in children 3 to 17 years of age consists of a combination of peginterferon and ribavirin. Using this regimen, sustained virologic response (SVR, defined as undetectable HCV RNA concentrations 6 or more months after treatment cessation) rates range from 38% to 50% for genotypes 1 and 4 and 80% to 100% for genotypes 2 and 3.

The few studies of peginterferon and ribavirin combination therapy in children suggest that children have fewer adverse events compared with adults; however, all treatment regimens are associated with adverse events. Major adverse effects of combination therapy in pediatric patients include influenza-like symptoms, hematologic abnormalities, neuropsychiatric symptoms, thyroid abnormalities, ocular abnormalities including ischemic retinopathy and uveitis, and growth disturbances. Of 107 patients 3 to 17 years of age in a clinical trial of pegylated interferon-alfa-2b plus ribavirin, severely inhibited growth velocity (<3rd percentile) was observed in 70% of the subjects during treatment. Of subjects experiencing severely inhibited growth, 20% had continued inhibited growth velocity (<3rd percentile) 6 months after treatment. Education of patients, their family members, and caregivers about adverse effects and their prospective management is an integral aspect of treatment with peginterferon and ribavirin.

Recently, tremendous progress has occurred in the treatment of HCV infection in adults with the introduction of several new direct-acting antiviral agents (DAAs) and several more in clinical trials. These drugs include protease inhibitors, polymerase inhibitors, and inhibitors of the nonstructural NS5A enzyme replication complex of HCV. Telaprevir and boceprevir, the first wave of protease inhibitors, were approved by the FDA in 2011 and were associated with significant improvements in SVR in combination with peginterferon and ribavirin for patients with genotype 1 compared with the use of just peginterferon and ribavirin (range, 65%–75% versus 25%–40%). Simeprevir is a second-wave protease inhibitor that received FDA approval in 2013 and provides the added benefit of once-daily dosing with similar or better efficacy versus the multiple daily doses needed for the first-wave agents. The first NS5B polymerase inhibitor (sofosbuvir) was licensed by the FDA in 2013 and was associated with even greater improvements in SVR when combined with peginterferon and ribavirin for genotypes 1 (~90%) and 4 (96%). Although these response rates have been impressive for genotype 1, the use with peginterferon and ribavirin remains a challenge for many patients because of the significant adverse effects associated with both drugs. As a result, one recently completed study and other studies in progress are combining different DAAs in interferon- and ribavirin-free protocols. As an example, sofosbuvir, when combined with once a day daclatasvir (a nonstructural NS5A enzyme replication complex inhibitor) to treat patients either previously treated or untreated with chronic HCV without peginterferon and with and without ribavirin demonstrated response rates of 94% to 98% for genotype 1. Cure rates were also >90% for other genotypes. Ledipasvir is an HCV NS5A inhibitor that was licensed in combination with sofosbuvir in 2014; in phase II and phase III trials in fixed dose combination with sofosbuvir, treatment for 8 to 12 weeks results in SVR rates greater than 90% with no serious adverse effects and relatively few significant drug-drug interactions. Another treatment regimen approved in 2014 consists of 4 drugs with 3 distinct mechanisms of action: the protease inhibitor paritaprevir, boosted with ritonavir; the NS5A inhibitor ombitasvir, and the nonnucleoside polymerase inhibitor dasabuvir. Collectively, this regimen is known as Viekira Pak (AbbVie Inc, North Chicago, IL) and is licensed for the treatment of HCV genotype 1 adult patients. Sustained virologic response rates are comparable to the other recently approved treatment advances for hepatitis C.

Together, these data offer hope for a future cure without significant adverse effects for a large population of adult and, ultimately, pediatric patients with HCV infection. At the current time, however, the DAAs have not been adequately studied in children to recommend their clinical use. In addition, adults with HCV genotype 1 and evidence of rapid virologic response within the first 4 to 8 weeks of treatment may be successfully treatment with shorter durations of DAAs plus standard of care therapy.

Management of Chronic HCV Infection. All patients with chronic HCV infection should be immunized against hepatitis A and hepatitis B because of the very high rate of severe hepatitis in patients with chronic liver disease from HCV infection who become coinfected with hepatitis A or B virus. With advancing age, chronic HCV infection increases the risk of chronic hepatitis and its complications, including cirrhosis and primary hepatocellular carcinoma (HCC). Factors associated with more severe disease include older age at acquisition, HIV coinfection, excessive alcohol consumption, and male gender. Among children, progression of liver disease appears to be accelerated when comorbid conditions, including childhood cancer, iron overload, or thalassemia are present. Pediatricians need to be alert to concomitant infections, alcohol abuse, and concomitant use of drugs, such as acetaminophen and some antiretroviral agents (such as stavudine), in patients with HCV infection. Children with chronic infection should be followed closely, including sequential monitoring of serum aminotransferase concentrations, because of the potential for chronic liver disease. Definitive recommendations on frequency of screening of hepatic enzymes have not been established. The need for screening for HCC in HCV-positive children has not been determined; however, the North American Society of Pediatric Gastroenterology, Hepatology and Nutrition recently published guidelines for children with HCV infection.[1] Evidence-based, consensus recommendations from the Infectious Diseases Society of America, the American Association for the Study of Liver Diseases, and the International Antiviral Society-USA for screening, treatment, and management of patients with HCV can be found online (**www.HCVguidelines.org**).

---

[1] Mack CL, Gonzalez-Peralta RP, Gupta N, et al; North American Society for Pediatric Gastroenterology, Hepatology, and Nutrition. NASPGHAN practice guidelines: diagnosis and management of hepatitis C infection in infants, children, and adolescents. *J Pediatr Gastroenterol Nutr.* 2012;54(6):838–855

ISOLATION OF THE HOSPITALIZED PATIENT: Standard precautions are recommended.

CONTROL MEASURES:

Care of Exposed People.

Immunoprophylaxis. On the basis of lack of clinical efficacy in humans and data from studies using animals, use of Immune Globulin for postexposure prophylaxis against HCV infection is not recommended. Potential donors of immune globulin are screened for antibody to HCV and excluded from donation if positive, so Immune Globulin preparations are devoid of anti-HCV antibody.

Breastfeeding. Mothers infected with HCV should be advised that transmission of HCV by breastfeeding has not been documented. According to guidelines of the American Academy of Pediatrics and the Centers for Disease Control and Prevention (CDC), maternal HCV infection is not a contraindication to breastfeeding. Mothers who are HCV positive and choose to breastfeed should consider abstaining if their nipples are cracked or bleeding.

Child Care. Exclusion of children with HCV infection from out-of-home child care is not indicated.

Serologic Testing for HCV Infection.

People Who Have Risk Factors for HCV Infection.

HCV testing (Table 3.25) is recommended for anyone at increased risk for HCV infection, including[1,2,3]:

- People born from 1945 through 1965;
- People who have ever injected illegal drugs, including those who injected only once many years ago;
- Recipients of clotting factor concentrates made before 1987;
- Recipients of blood transfusions or solid organ transplants before July 1992;
- Patients who have ever received long-term hemodialysis treatment;
- People with known exposures to HCV, such as
  - health care workers after needlesticks involving HCV-positive blood;
  - recipients of blood or organs from a donor who later tested HCV-positive;
- All people with HIV infection;
- Patients with signs or symptoms of liver disease (eg, abnormal liver enzyme tests);
- Children born to HCV-positive mothers (to avoid detecting maternal antibody, these children should not be tested before age 18 months).

Pregnant Women. Routine serologic testing of pregnant women for HCV infection is not recommended.

Children Born to Women With HCV Infection. Children born to women previously identified to be HCV infected should be tested for HCV infection, because 5% to 6% of these children will acquire the infection. Transmission depends in part on the concentration of HCV RNA in the mother's blood, and if the mother does not have detectable HCV RNA at the time of delivery, then the likelihood of transmission to the infant is very low. The

---

[1]Centers for Disease Control and Prevention. Recommendations for the identification of chronic hepatitis C virus infection among persons born during 1945–1965. *MMWR Recomm Rep.* 2012;61(RR–4):1–32

[2]Centers for Disease Control and Prevention. Guidelines for prevention and treatment of opportunistic infections in HIV-infected adults and adolescents: recommendations from CDC, the National Institutes of Health, and the HIV Medicine Association of the Infectious Diseases Society of America. *MMWR Recomm Rep.* 2009;58(RR–4):1–207

[3]**http://aidsinfo.nih.gov/guidelines**

Table 3.25. People for Whom Screening for HCV Infection Is Indicated

Group	Screening[a]
People who have injected illicit drugs in the recent and remote past, including those who injected only once and do not consider themselves to be drug users	Antibody
People with conditions associated with a high prevalence of HCV infection, including: People with HIV infection People who have ever been on hemodialysis People with unexplained abnormal aminotransferase concentrations	Antibody or RNA
Recipients of transfusions or organ transplants before July 1992, including: People who were notified that they had received blood from a donor who later tested positive for HCV infection People who received a transfusion of blood or blood products People who received an organ transplant	Antibody or RNA
Children born to HCV-infected mothers	Antibody after 18 mo of age, RNA for younger ages
Health care, emergency medical, and public safety workers after a needlestick injury or mucosal exposure to HCV-positive blood	Antibody or RNA
Current sexual partners of HCV-infected people	Antibody
Children with chronically elevated serum aminotransferase concentrations	Antibody
Children from a region with a high prevalence of HCV infection	Antibody

Adapted from reference Mack CL, Gonzalez-Peralta RP, Gupta N, et al; North American Society for Pediatric Gastroenterology, Hepatology, and Nutrition. NASPGHAN practice guidelines: diagnosis and management of hepatitis C infection in infants, children, and adolescents. *J Pediatr Gastroenterol Nutr.* 2012;54(6):838–855.

HCV indicates hepatitis C virus; HIV, human immunodeficiency virus.

[a] All of the positive anti-HCV antibody tests should be followed up with a HCV RNA test to determine active infection.

duration of passively acquired maternal antibody in infants can be as long as 18 months. Therefore, testing for anti-HCV should not be performed until after 18 months of age. If earlier diagnosis is desired, an NAAT to detect HCV RNA may be performed at or after the infant's first well-child visit at 1 to 2 months of age.

Adoptees. Routine serologic testing of adoptees, either domestic or international, is not recommended. See Medical Evaluation for Infectious Diseases for Internationally Adopted, Refugee, and Immigrant Children (p 194) for specific situations when serologic testing is warranted.

Counseling of Patients With HCV Infection. All people with HCV infection should be considered infectious, should be informed of the possibility of transmission to others, and should refrain from donating blood, organs, tissues, or semen and from sharing toothbrushes and razors.

Infected people should be counseled to avoid hepatotoxic agents, including medications, and should be informed of the risks of excessive alcohol ingestion. All patients with chronic HCV infection should be immunized against hepatitis A and hepatitis B.

Changes in sexual practices of infected people with a long-term partner are not recommended; however, they should be informed of the possible risks and use of precautions to prevent transmission. People with multiple sexual partners should be advised to decrease the number of partners and to use condoms to prevent transmission. No data exist to support counseling a woman against pregnancy.

The CDC Division of Viral Hepatitis maintains a Web site (**www.cdc.gov/ hepatitis/HCV**) with information on hepatitis for health care professionals and the public, including specific information for people who have received blood transfusions before 1992. Information also can be obtained from the National Institutes of Health Web site (**www2.niddk.nih.gov/Research/ScientificAreas/ DigestiveDiseases/Liver/VHID.htm**).

Evidence-based, consensus recommendations from the Infectious Diseases Society of America, the American Association for the Study of Liver Diseases, and the International Antiviral Society-USA for screening, treatment, and management of patients with HCV can be found online (**www.HCVguidelines.org**).

Hepatitis D

CLINICAL MANIFESTATIONS: Hepatitis D virus (HDV) causes infection only in people with acute or chronic hepatitis B virus (HBV) infection. HDV requires HBV as a helper virus for replication and cannot produce infection in the absence of HBV. The importance of HDV infection lies in its ability to convert an asymptomatic or mild chronic HBV infection into fulminant or more severe or rapidly progressive disease. Acute coinfection with HBV and HDV usually causes an acute illness indistinguishable from acute HBV infection alone, except that the likelihood of fulminant hepatitis can be as high as 5%.

ETIOLOGY: HDV measures 36 to 43 nm in diameter and consists of an RNA genome and a delta protein antigen, both of which are coated with hepatitis B surface antigen (HBsAg).

EPIDEMIOLOGY: HDV infection is present worldwide, in all age groups, and an estimated 18 million people are infected with the virus. Over the past 20 years, HDV prevalence has decreased significantly in Western and Southern Europe because of long-standing hepatitis B vaccination programs, although HDV remains a significant health problem in resource-limited countries. At least 8 genotypes of HDV have been described, each with a typical geographic pattern, with genotype I being the predominant type in Europe and North America. HDV can cause an infection at the same time as the initial HBV infection (coinfection), or it can infect a person already chronically infected with HBV (superinfection). Acquisition of HDV is by parenteral, percutaneous, or mucous membrane inoculation. HDV can be acquired from blood or blood products, through injection drug use, or by sexual contact, but only if HBV also is present. Transmission from mother to newborn infant is uncommon. Intrafamilial spread can occur among people with chronic HBV infection. High-prevalence areas include parts of Eastern Europe, South America, Africa, Central Asia (particularly Pakistan), and the Middle East. In the United States, HDV infection is found most commonly in people who abuse injection drugs, people with hemophilia, and people who have emigrated from areas with endemic HDV infection.

The **incubation period** for HDV superinfection is approximately 2 to 8 weeks. When HBV and HDV viruses infect simultaneously, the incubation period is similar to that of HBV (45–160 days; average, 90 days).

DIAGNOSTIC TESTS: People with chronic HBV infection are at risk of HDV coinfection. Accordingly, their care should be supervised by an expert in hepatitis treatment, and consideration should be given to testing for anti-HDV immunoglobulin (Ig) G antibodies using a commercially available test if they have increased transaminase concentrations, particularly if they recently came from a country with high prevalence of HDV. Anti-HDV may not be present until several weeks after onset of illness, and acute and convalescent sera may be required to confirm the diagnosis. In a person with anti-HDV, the absence of IgM hepatitis B core antibody (anti-HBc), which is indicative of chronic HBV infection, suggests that the person has both chronic HBV infection and superinfection with HDV. Presence of anti-HDV IgG antibodies does not prove active infection, and thus, HDV RNA testing should be performed for diagnostic and therapeutic considerations. Patients with circulating HDV RNA should be staged for severity of liver disease, have surveillance for development of hepatocellular carcinoma, and be considered for treatment. Presence of anti-HDV IgM is of lesser utility, because it is present in both acute and chronic HDV infections.

TREATMENT: HDV has proven difficult to treat. However, data suggest pegylated interferon-alfa may result in up to 40% of patients having a sustained response to treatment. Clinical trials suggest at least a year of therapy may be associated with sustained responses, and longer courses may be warranted if the patient is able to tolerate therapy. Further study of pegylated interferon monotherapy or as combination therapy with a direct acting antiviral agent needs to be performed before treatment of HDV can be advised routinely.

ISOLATION OF THE HOSPITALIZED PATIENT: Standard precautions are recommended.

CONTROL MEASURES: The same control and preventive measures used for HBV infection are indicated. Because HDV cannot be transmitted in the absence of HBV infection, HBV immunization protects against HDV infection. People with chronic HBV infection should take extreme care to avoid exposure to HDV.

Hepatitis E

CLINICAL MANIFESTATIONS: Hepatitis E virus (HEV) infection causes an acute illness with symptoms including jaundice, malaise, anorexia, fever, abdominal pain, and arthralgia. Disease is more common among adults than among children and is more severe in pregnant women, in whom mortality rates can reach 10% to 25% during the third trimester. Chronic HEV infection is rare and has been reported only in recipients of solid organ transplants and people with severe immunodeficiency.

ETIOLOGY: Hepatitis E virus (HEV) is a spherical, nonenveloped, positive-sense RNA virus. HEV is classified in the genus *Hepevirus* of the family *Hepeviridae*. There are 4 major recognized genotypes with a single known serotype.

EPIDEMIOLOGY: HEV is the most common cause of viral hepatitis in the world. Globally, an estimated 20 million HEV infections occur annually, resulting in 3.4 million cases of acute hepatitis and 70 000 deaths. In developing countries, ingestion of fecally contaminated water is the most common route of HEV transmission, and large waterborne outbreaks occur frequently. Sporadic HEV infection has been reported throughout the world and is common in Africa and the Indian subcontinent. Unlike the other agents of viral hepatitis, certain HEV genotypes (genotypes 3 and 4) also have zoonotic hosts, such as swine, and can be transmitted by eating undercooked pork. HEV genotypes 1 and 2 exclusively infect humans. Person-to-person transmission appears to be much less efficient than with hepatitis A virus but occurs in sporadic and outbreak settings. Mother-to-infant transmission of HEV occurs frequently and accounts for a significant proportion of fetal loss and perinatal mortality. Hepatitis E also is transmitted through blood product transfusion. Transfusion-transmitted hepatitis E occurs primarily in countries with endemic disease and is reported rarely in areas without endemic infection. In the United States, serologic studies have demonstrated that approximately 20% of the population has immunoglobulin (Ig) G against HEV. However, symptomatic HEV infection in the United States is uncommon and generally occurs in people who acquire HEV genotype 1 infection after traveling to countries with endemic HEV. Nonetheless, a number of people without a travel history have been diagnosed with acute HEV, and evidence for the infection should be sought in cases of acute hepatitis without an etiology. Acute HEV may masquerade as drug-induced liver injury.

DIAGNOSTIC TESTS: Testing for IgM and IgG anti-HEV is available through some research and commercial reference laboratories. Because anti-HEV assays are not approved by the US Food and Drug Administration and their performance characteristics are not well defined, results should be interpreted with caution, particularly in cases lacking a discrete onset of illness associated with jaundice or with no recent history of travel to a country with endemic infection. Definitive diagnosis may be made by demonstrating viral RNA in serum or stool by means of reverse transcriptase-polymerase chain reaction assay, which is available only in research settings (eg, with prior approval through the Centers for Disease Control and Prevention). Because virus circulates in the body for a relatively short period, the inability to detect HEV in serum or stool does not eliminate the possibility that the person was infected with HEV.

TREATMENT: Supportive. However preliminary reports suggest that ribavirin may be effective for the treatment of chronic hepatitis E.

ISOLATION OF THE HOSPITALIZED PATIENT: In addition to standard precautions, contact precautions are recommended for diapered and incontinent patients for the duration of illness.

CONTROL MEASURES: Provision of safe water is the most effective prevention measure. A recombinant HEV vaccine evaluated in a phase III clinical trial was demonstrated to be effective in preventing disease and is approved for use by the Chinese Food and Drug Administration.

Herpes Simplex

CLINICAL MANIFESTATIONS:

Neonatal. In newborn infants, herpes simplex virus (HSV) infection can manifest as the following: (1) disseminated disease involving multiple organs, most prominently liver and lungs, and in 60% to 75% of cases also involving the central nervous system (CNS); (2) localized CNS disease, with or without skin involvement (CNS disease); or (3) disease localized to the skin, eyes, and/or mouth (SEM disease). Approximately 25% of cases of neonatal HSV manifest as disseminated disease, 30% of cases manifest as CNS disease, and 45% of cases manifest as SEM disease. More than 80% of neonates with SEM disease have skin vesicles; those without have infection limited to the eyes and/or oral mucosa. Approximately two thirds of neonates with disseminated or CNS disease have skin lesions, but these lesions may not be present at the time of onset of symptoms. In the absence of skin lesions, the diagnosis of neonatal HSV infection is challenging. Disseminated infection should be considered in neonates with sepsis syndrome, negative bacteriologic culture results, severe liver dysfunction, or consumptive coagulopathy. HSV also should be considered as a causative agent in neonates with fever, a vesicular rash, or abnormal cerebrospinal fluid (CSF) findings, especially in the presence of seizures or during a time of year when enteroviruses are not circulating in the community. Although asymptomatic HSV infection is common in older children, it rarely, if ever, occurs in neonates.

Neonatal herpetic infections often are severe, with attendant high mortality and morbidity rates, even when antiviral therapy is administered. Recurrent skin lesions are common in surviving infants, occurring in approximately 50% of survivors often within 1 to 2 weeks of completing the initial treatment course of parenteral acyclovir.

Initial signs of HSV infection can occur anytime between birth and approximately 6 weeks of age, although almost all infected infants develop clinical disease within the first month of life. Infants with disseminated disease and SEM disease have an earlier age of onset, typically presenting between the first and second weeks of life; infants with CNS disease usually present with illness between the second and third weeks of life.

Children Beyond the Neonatal Period and Adolescents. Most primary HSV childhood infections beyond the neonatal period are asymptomatic. Gingivostomatitis, which is the most common clinical manifestation of HSV during childhood, is caused by HSV type 1 (HSV-1) and is characterized by fever, irritability, tender submandibular adenopathy, and an ulcerative enanthem involving the gingiva and mucous membranes of the mouth, often with perioral vesicular lesions.

Genital herpes, which is the most common manifestation of primary HSV infection in adolescents and adults, is characterized by vesicular or ulcerative lesions of the male or female genital organs, perineum, or both. Until recent years, genital herpes most often was caused by HSV type 2 (HSV-2), but HSV-1 now accounts for more than half of all cases of genital herpes in the United States. Most cases of primary genital herpes infection in males and females are asymptomatic and are not recognized by the infected person or diagnosed by a health care professional.

Eczema herpeticum can develop in patients with atopic dermatitis who are infected with HSV. Examination may reveal skin with punched-out erosions, hemorrhagic crusts, and/or vesicular lesions.

In immunocompromised patients, severe local lesions and, less commonly, disseminated HSV infection with generalized vesicular skin lesions and visceral involvement can occur.

After primary infection, HSV persists for life in a latent form. The site of latency for virus causing herpes labialis is the trigeminal ganglion, and the usual site of latency for genital herpes is the sacral dorsal root ganglia, although any of the sensory ganglia can be involved depending on the site of primary infection. Reactivation of latent virus most commonly is asymptomatic. When symptomatic, recurrent HSV-1 herpes labialis manifests as single or grouped vesicles in the perioral region, usually on the vermilion border of the lips (typically called "cold sores" or "fever blisters"). Symptomatic recurrent genital herpes manifests as vesicular lesions on the penis, scrotum, vulva, cervix, buttocks, perianal areas, thighs, or back. Among immunocompromised patients, genital HSV-2 recurrences are more frequent and of longer duration. Recurrences may be heralded by a prodrome of burning or itching at the site of an incipient recurrence, identification of which can be useful in instituting antiviral therapy early.

Conjunctivitis and keratitis can result from primary or recurrent HSV infection. Herpetic whitlow consists of single or multiple vesicular lesions on the distal parts of fingers. HSV infection can be a precipitating factor in erythema multiforme, and recurrent erythema multiforme often is caused by symptomatic or asymptomatic HSV recurrences. Wrestlers can develop herpes gladiatorum if they become infected with HSV.

HSV encephalitis (HSE) occurs in children beyond the neonatal period or in adolescents and adults and can result from primary or recurrent HSV-1 infection. One fifth of HSE cases occur in the pediatric age group. Symptoms and signs usually include fever, alterations in the state of consciousness, personality changes, seizures, and focal neurologic findings. Encephalitis commonly has an acute onset with a fulminant course, leading to coma and death in untreated patients. HSE usually involves the temporal lobe; thus, temporal lobe abnormalities on imaging studies or electroencephalography in the context of a consistent clinical picture should increase the suspicion of HSE. Magnetic resonance imaging is the most sensitive neuroradiologic imaging modality to demonstrate involvement of the temporal lobe. CSF pleocytosis with a predominance of lymphocytes is typical. Historically, erythrocytes in the CSF were considered suggestive of HSE, but with earlier diagnosis (prior to full manifestations of a hemorrhagic encephalitis), this laboratory finding is rare today.

HSV infection also can cause aseptic meningitis with nonspecific clinical manifestations that usually are mild and self-limited. Such episodes of meningitis usually are associated with genital HSV-2 infection. A number of unusual CNS manifestations of HSV have been described, including Bell palsy, atypical pain syndromes, trigeminal neuralgia, ascending myelitis, transverse myelitis, postinfectious encephalomyelitis, and recurrent (Mollaret) meningitis.

ETIOLOGY: HSVs are enveloped, double-stranded, DNA viruses. More than 100 herpesviruses have been identified across species; at least 9, including HSV, infect humans. Two distinct HSV types exist: HSV-1 and HSV-2. Infections with HSV-1 usually involve the face and skin above the waist; however, an increasing number of genital herpes cases are attributable to HSV-1. Infections with HSV-2 usually involve the genitalia and skin below the waist in sexually active adolescents and adults. However, either type of virus can be found in either area, and both HSV-1 and HSV-2 cause herpes disease in neonates. As with all human herpesviruses, HSV-1 and HSV-2 establish latency following primary infection, with periodic reactivation to cause recurrent symptomatic disease or asymptomatic viral shedding.

EPIDEMIOLOGY: HSV infections are ubiquitous and can be transmitted from people who are symptomatic or asymptomatic with primary or recurrent infections.
Neonatal. The incidence of neonatal HSV infection is estimated to range from 1 in 3000 to 1 in 20 000 live births. HSV is transmitted to a neonate most often during birth through an infected maternal genital tract but can be caused by an ascending infection through ruptured or apparently intact amniotic membranes. Intrauterine infections causing congenital malformations have been implicated in rare cases. Other less common sources of neonatal infection include postnatal transmission from a parent or other caregiver, most often from a nongenital infection (eg, mouth or hands).

The risk of HSV transmission to a neonate born to a mother who acquires primary genital infection near the time of delivery is estimated to be 25% to 60%. In contrast, the risk to a neonate born to a mother shedding HSV as a result of reactivation of infection acquired during the first half of pregnancy or earlier is less than 2%. Distinguishing between primary and recurrent HSV infections in women by history or physical examination alone may be impossible, because primary and recurrent genital infections may be asymptomatic or associated with nonspecific findings (eg, vaginal discharge, genital pain, or shallow ulcers). History of maternal genital HSV infection is not helpful in diagnosing neonatal HSV disease, because more than three quarters of infants who contract HSV infection are born to women with no history or clinical findings suggestive of genital HSV infection during or preceding pregnancy and who, therefore, are unaware of their infection. **Children Beyond the Neonatal Period and Adolescents.** Twenty-six percent of US children have serologic evidence of HSV-1 infection by 7 years of age. Patients with primary gingivostomatitis or genital herpes usually shed virus for at least 1 week and occasionally for several weeks. Patients with symptomatic recurrences shed virus for a shorter period, typically 3 to 4 days. Intermittent asymptomatic reactivation of oral and genital herpes is common and likely occurs throughout the remainder of a person's life. The greatest concentration of virus is shed during symptomatic primary infections and the lowest concentration of virus is shed during asymptomatic reactivation.

Infections with HSV-1 usually result from direct contact with virus shed from visible or microscopic orolabial lesions or in infected oral secretions. Infections with HSV-2 usually result from direct contact with virus shed from visible or microscopic genital lesions or in genital secretions during sexual activity. Genital HSV infections increase the risk of acquisition of HIV. Genital infections caused by HSV-1 in children can result from autoinoculation of virus from the mouth. Sexual abuse always should be considered in prepubertal children with genital HSV-2 infections. Therefore, genital HSV isolates from children should be typed to differentiate between HSV-1 and HSV-2.

The incidence of HSV-2 infection correlates with the number of sexual partners and with acquisition of other sexually transmitted infections. After primary genital infection, which often is asymptomatic, some people experience frequent clinical recurrences, and others have no clinically apparent recurrences. Genital HSV-2 infection is more likely to recur than is genital HSV-1 infection.

Inoculation of abraded skin occurs from direct contact with HSV shed from oral, genital, or other skin sites. This contact can result in herpes gladiatorum among wrestlers, herpes rugbiaforum among rugby players, or herpetic whitlow of the fingers in any exposed person.

The **incubation period** for HSV infection occurring beyond the neonatal period ranges from 2 days to 2 weeks.

DIAGNOSTIC TESTS: HSV grows readily in cell culture. Special transport media are available that allow transport to local or regional laboratories for culture. Cytopathogenic effects typical of HSV infection usually are observed 1 to 3 days after inoculation. Methods of culture confirmation include fluorescent antibody staining, enzyme immunoassays (EIAs), and monolayer culture with typing. Cultures that remain negative by day 5 likely will continue to remain negative. Polymerase chain reaction (PCR) assay often can detect HSV DNA in CSF from neonates with CNS infection (neonatal HSV CNS disease) and from older children and adults with HSE and is the diagnostic method of choice for CNS HSV involvement. PCR assay of CSF can yield negative results in cases of HSE, however, especially early in the disease course. In difficult cases in which repeated CSF PCR assay results are negative, histologic examination and viral culture of a brain tissue biopsy specimen is the most definitive method of confirming the diagnosis of HSE. Detection of intrathecal antibody against HSV also can assist in the diagnosis. Viral cultures of CSF from a patient with HSE usually are negative.

For diagnosis of neonatal HSV infection, the following specimens should be obtained: (1) swab specimens from the mouth, nasopharynx, conjunctivae, and anus ("surface cultures") for HSV culture and, if desired, for HSV PCR assay; (2) specimens of skin vesicles for HSV culture and, if desired, for PCR assay; (3) CSF sample for HSV PCR assay; (4) whole blood sample for HSV PCR assay; and (5) whole blood sample for measuring alanine aminotransferase (ALT). The performance of PCR assay on skin and mucosal specimens from neonates has not been studied; if used, surface or skin PCR assays should be performed in addition to (and not instead of) the gold-standard surface culture. Positive cultures obtained from any of the surface sites more than 12 to 24 hours after birth indicate viral replication and are, therefore, suggestive of infant infection rather than merely contamination after intrapartum exposure. As with any PCR assay, false-negative and false-positive results can occur. Whole blood PCR assay may be of benefit in diagnosis of neonatal HSV disease, but its use should not supplant the standard work-up of such patients (which includes surface cultures and CSF PCR assay). Any of the 3 manifestations of neonatal HSV disease (disseminated, CNS, SEM) can have viremia associated with it, so a positive whole blood PCR assay should not be used to determine extent of disease and thus duration of treatment; likewise, no data exist to support use of serial blood PCR assay to monitor response to therapy. Rapid diagnostic techniques also are available, such as direct fluorescent antibody (DFA) staining of vesicle scrapings or EIA detection of HSV antigens. These techniques are as specific but slightly less sensitive than culture. Typing HSV strains differentiates between HSV-1 and HSV-2 isolates. Radiographs and clinical manifestations can suggest HSV pneumonitis, and elevated transaminase values can suggest HSV hepatitis; both occur commonly in neonatal HSV disseminated disease. Histologic examination of lesions for presence of multinucleated giant cells and eosinophilic intranuclear inclusions typical of HSV (eg, with Tzanck test) has low sensitivity and should not be performed.

HSV PCR assay and cell culture are the preferred tests for detecting HSV in genital ulcers or other mucocutaneous lesions consistent with genital herpes. The sensitivity of viral culture is low, especially for recurrent lesions, and declines rapidly as lesions begin to heal. PCR assays for HSV DNA are more sensitive and increasingly are used in many settings. Failure to detect HSV in genital lesions by culture or PCR assay does not indicate an absence of HSV infection, because viral shedding is intermittent.

Both type-specific and type-common antibodies to HSV develop during the first several weeks after infection and persist indefinitely. The median time to seroconversion is 21 days with the Focus type-specific ELISA assay, and more than 95% of people seroconvert by 12 weeks following infection. Although type-specific HSV-2 antibody usually indicates previous anogenital infection, the presence of HSV-1 antibody does not distinguish anogenital from orolabial infection reliably, because a substantial proportion of initial genital infections are caused by HSV-1 in some populations. Type-specific serologic tests can be useful in confirming a clinical diagnosis of genital herpes caused by HSV-2. Additionally, these serologic tests can be used to evaluate recurrent or atypical genital tract symptoms with negative HSV culture or PCR evaluations and to manage sexual partners of people with genital herpes. There is growing evidence that type-specific antibody avidity testing may prove useful for evaluating risk of neonatal infection. The presence of low-avidity HSV-2 immunoglobulin (Ig) G in serum of near-term pregnant women has been correlated with an elevated risk of neonatal infection. Serologic testing is not useful in neonates.

Several glycoprotein G (gG)-based type-specific assays have been approved by the US Food and Drug Administration (FDA), including at least 1 that can be used as a point-of-care test. The sensitivities and specificities of these tests for detection of HSV-2 IgG antibody vary from 90% to 100%; false-negative results may occur, especially early after infection, and false-positive results can occur, especially in patients with low likelihood of HSV infection. Therefore, repeat testing or a confirmatory test (eg, an immunoblot assay if the initial test was an EIA) may be indicated in some settings.

TREATMENT: For recommended antiviral dosages and duration of therapy with systemically administered acyclovir, valacyclovir, and famciclovir for different HSV infections, see Non-HIV Antiviral Drugs (p 919). Valacyclovir is an L-valyl ester of acyclovir that is metabolized to acyclovir after oral administration, resulting in higher serum concentrations than are achieved with oral acyclovir and similar serum concentrations as are achieved with intravenous administration of acyclovir. Famciclovir is converted rapidly to penciclovir after oral administration. Table 3.26 shows drugs for treatment of HSV by type of infection. Valacyclovir has been approved by the FDA for use in children with chickenpox. Instructions for preparing a compounded liquid formulation of valacyclovir with a 28-day shelf-life are provided in the drug's package insert.

Neonatal. Parenteral acyclovir is the treatment for neonatal HSV infections. Parenteral acyclovir should be administered to all neonates with HSV disease, regardless of manifestations and clinical findings. The dosage of acyclovir is 60 mg/kg per day in 3 divided doses (20 mg/kg/dose), given intravenously for 14 days in SEM disease and for a minimum of 21 days in CNS disease or disseminated disease. The best outcomes in terms of

Table 3.26. Recommended Therapy for Herpes Simplex Virus Infections[a]

Infection	Drug[b]
Neonatal	Parenteral acyclovir
Keratoconjunctivitis	Trifluridine[c]
	OR
	Iododeoxyuridine
	OR
	Topical ganciclovir
Genital	Acyclovir
	OR
	Famciclovir
	OR
	Valacyclovir
Mucocutaneous (immunocompromised or primary gingivostomatitis)	Acyclovir
	OR
	Famciclovir
	OR
	Valacyclovir
Acyclovir-resistant (severe infections, immunocompromised)	Parenteral foscarnet
Encephalitis	Parenteral acyclovir

[a] See text and Table 4.9 (p 919) for details.
[b] Famciclovir and valacyclovir are approved by the US Food and Drug Administration for treatment of adults.
[c] Treatment of herpes simplex virus ocular infection should involve an ophthalmologist.

morbidity and mortality are observed among infants with SEM disease. Although most neonates treated for HSV CNS disease survive, most survivors suffer substantial neurologic sequelae. Approximately 30% of neonates with disseminated disease die despite antiviral therapy. Approximately 50% of infants surviving neonatal HSV experience cutaneous recurrences, with the first skin recurrence often occurring within 1 to 2 weeks of stopping parenteral acyclovir treatment. All infants with neonatal HSV disease regardless of disease classification should have an ophthalmologic examination and neuroimaging to establish baseline brain anatomy; magnetic resonance imaging is the most sensitive neuroradiologic imaging modality but also may require sedation, so computed tomography or ultrasonography of the head are acceptable alternatives. All infants with CNS involvement should have a repeat lumbar puncture performed near the end of therapy to document that the CSF is negative for HSV DNA on PCR assay; in the unlikely event that the PCR result remains positive near the end of a 21-day treatment course, intravenous acyclovir should be administered for another week, with repeat CSF PCR assay performed near the end of the extended treatment period and another week of parenteral therapy if it remains positive. Consultation with an infectious diseases specialist is warranted in these cases.

Oral acyclovir suppressive therapy for the 6 months following treatment of acute neonatal HSV disease improves neurodevelopmental outcomes in infants with HSV CNS disease and prevents skin recurrences in infants with any disease classification of neonatal HSV. Infants surviving neonatal HSV infections of any classification of infection (disseminated, CNS, or SEM) should receive oral acyclovir suppression at 300 mg/m^2/dose, administered 3 times daily for 6 months; the dose should be adjusted each month to account for growth. Absolute neutrophil counts should be assessed at 2 and 4 weeks after initiating suppressive therapy and then monthly during the treatment period. Longer durations or higher doses of antiviral suppression do not further improve neurodevelopmental outcomes. Valacyclovir has not been studied for longer than 5 days in young infants, so it should not be used routinely for antiviral suppression in this age group.

Infants with ocular involvement attributable to HSV infection should receive a topical ophthalmic drug (1% trifluridine, 0.1% iododeoxyuridine, or 0.15% ganciclovir) as well as parenteral antiviral therapy. An ophthalmologist should be involved in the management and treatment of acute neonatal ocular HSV disease.

Genital Infection.

Primary. Many patients with first-episode genital herpes initially have mild clinical manifestations but may go on to develop severe or prolonged symptoms with viral reactivation. Therefore, most patients with initial genital herpes should receive antiviral therapy. In adults, acyclovir and valacyclovir decrease the duration of symptoms and viral shedding in primary genital herpes. Oral acyclovir therapy (400 mg, orally, 3 times/day for 10 days; or 200 mg, orally, 5 times/day for 10 days), initiated within 6 days of onset of disease, shortens the duration of illness and viral shedding by 3 to 5 days. Valacyclovir and famciclovir do not seem to be more effective than acyclovir but offer the advantage of less frequent dosing (famciclovir, 250 mg, orally, 3 times/day for 10 days; valacyclovir, 1 g, orally, 2 times/day for 10 days). Intravenous acyclovir is indicated for patients with a severe or complicated primary infection that requires hospitalization (5–10 mg/kg, intravenously, every 8 hours for 2–7 days or until clinical improvement is observed, followed by oral antiviral therapy to complete at least 10 days of total therapy). Treatment of primary herpetic lesions does not affect the subsequent frequency or severity of recurrences.

Recurrent. Antiviral therapy for recurrent genital herpes can be administered either episodically to ameliorate or shorten the duration of lesions or continuously as suppressive therapy to decrease the frequency of recurrences. Many patients benefit from antiviral therapy; therefore, options for treatment should be discussed with all patients. Many people prefer suppressive therapy, which has the additional advantage of decreasing the risk of genital HSV-2 transmission to susceptible partners.

In adults with frequent genital HSV recurrences, daily oral acyclovir suppressive therapy is effective for decreasing the frequency of symptomatic recurrences and improving quality of life. After approximately 1 year of continuous daily therapy, acyclovir should be discontinued, and the recurrence rate should be assessed. If frequent recurrences are observed, additional suppressive therapy should be considered. Acyclovir appears to be safe for adults receiving the drug for more than 15 years, but longer-term effects are unknown. Data also support suppressive therapy in adults with valacyclovir or famciclovir.

Oral acyclovir therapy initiated within 1 day of lesion onset or during the prodrome that precedes some outbreaks shortens the mean clinical course by approximately 1 day. If episodic therapy is used, a prescription for the medication should be provided with instructions to initiate treatment immediately when symptoms begin. Valacyclovir and famciclovir also are licensed and efficacious for treatment of adults with recurrent genital herpes. Available data do not indicate an increased risk of major birth defects in comparison with the general population in women treated with acyclovir during the first trimester. Acyclovir or valacyclovir may be administered orally to pregnant women with first-episode genital herpes or severe recurrent herpes, and acyclovir should be given intravenously to pregnant women with severe HSV infection. Counseling and education of infected adolescents/ adults and their sexual partners, especially on the potential for recurrent episodes and how to reduce transmission to partners, is a critical part of management. Pregnant women or women of childbearing age with genital herpes should be encouraged to inform their health care professionals and those who will care for the newborn infant.

Mucocutaneous.

Immunocompromised Hosts. Intravenous acyclovir is effective for treatment of mucocutaneous HSV infections. Acyclovir-resistant strains of HSV have been isolated from immunocompromised people receiving prolonged treatment with acyclovir. Under these circumstances, progressive disease may be observed despite acyclovir therapy. Foscarnet is the drug of choice for disease caused by acyclovir-resistant HSV isolates.

Immunocompetent Hosts. Limited data are available on effects of acyclovir on the course of primary or recurrent nongenital mucocutaneous HSV infections in immunocompetent hosts. Therapeutic benefit has been noted in a limited number of children with primary gingivostomatitis treated with oral acyclovir. Slight therapeutic benefit of oral acyclovir therapy has been demonstrated among adults with recurrent herpes labialis. When used as treatment for HSV orolabial disease, a dose of 80 mg/kg per day, in 4 divided doses, should be used, with a maximum of 3200 mg/day. Famciclovir or valacyclovir also can be considered. Topical acyclovir is ineffective. A topical formulation of penciclovir (Denavir [Prestium Pharma, Newtown, PA]) and a topical alcohol, docosanol (Abreva [GlaxoSmithKline, Research Triangle Park, NC]), have only limited activity for therapy of herpes labialis and are not recommended.

In a controlled study of a small number of adults with recurrent herpes labialis (6 or more episodes per year), prophylactic acyclovir at a dosage of 400 mg, twice a day, was effective for decreasing the frequency of recurrent episodes. Although no studies of prophylactic therapy have been performed in children, those with frequent recurrences may benefit from continuous oral acyclovir therapy, with reevaluation being performed after 6 months to 1 year of continuous therapy; a dose of 30 mg/kg per day, in 3 divided doses, with a maximum 1000 mg/day is reasonable to begin as suppressive therapy in children. Valacyclovir has been approved for suppression of genital herpes in immunocompetent adults.

Other HSV Infections.

Central Nervous System. Patients with HSE should be treated for 21 days with intravenous acyclovir. Patients who are comatose or semicomatose at initiation of therapy have a poorer outcome. For people with Bell palsy, the combination of acyclovir and prednisone may be considered.

Ocular. Treatment of eye lesions should be undertaken in consultation with an ophthalmologist. Several topical drugs, such as 1% trifluridine, 0.1% iododeoxyuridine, and 0.15% ganciclovir, have proven efficacy for superficial keratitis. Topical corticosteroids, by themselves, are contraindicated in suspected HSV conjunctivitis; however, ophthalmologists may choose to use corticosteroids in conjunction with antiviral drugs to treat locally invasive infections. For children with recurrent ocular lesions, oral suppressive therapy with acyclovir (800 mg/day, in 2 divided doses, for patients 12 years or older) may be of benefit.

ISOLATION OF THE HOSPITALIZED PATIENT: In addition to standard precautions, the following recommendations should be followed.

Neonates With HSV Infection. Neonates with HSV infection should be hospitalized and managed with contact precautions if mucocutaneous lesions are present.

Neonates Exposed to HSV During Delivery. Infants born to women with active HSV lesions should be managed with contact precautions during the incubation period. Some experts believe that contact precautions are unnecessary if exposed infants were born by cesarean delivery, provided membranes were ruptured for less than 4 hours. The risk of HSV infection in infants born to mothers with a history of recurrent genital herpes who have no genital lesions at delivery is low, and special precautions are not necessary. Specific management options for neonates born to women with active genital HSV lesions are detailed in the Prevention of Neonatal Infection section.

Women in Labor and Postpartum Women With HSV Infection. Women with active HSV lesions should be managed with contact precautions during labor, delivery, and the postpartum period. These women should be instructed about the importance of careful hand hygiene before and after caring for their infants. The mother may wear a clean covering gown to help avoid contact of the infant with lesions or infectious secretions. A mother with herpes labialis or stomatitis should wear a disposable surgical mask when touching her newborn infant until the lesions have crusted and dried. She should not kiss or nuzzle her newborn until lesions have cleared. Herpetic lesions on other skin sites should be covered.

Breastfeeding is acceptable if no lesions are present on the breasts and if active lesions elsewhere on the mother are covered (see Human Milk, p 125).

Children With Mucocutaneous HSV Infection. Contact precautions are recommended for patients with severe mucocutaneous HSV infection. Patients with localized recurrent lesions should be managed with standard precautions.

Patients With HSV Infection of the CNS. Standard precautions are recommended for patients with infection limited to the CNS.

CONTROL MEASURES:

Prevention of Neonatal Infection.

During Pregnancy. During prenatal evaluations, all pregnant women should be asked about past or current signs and symptoms consistent with genital herpes infection in themselves and their sexual partners. However, the absence of previous signs and symptoms of genital herpes infections has poor sensitivity in determining the risk of genital HSV infection in a pregnant woman. The American College of Obstetricians and Gynecologists (ACOG) recommends that women with active recurrent genital herpes should be offered suppressive antiviral therapy at or beyond 36 weeks of gestation. Cases of neonatal HSV disease have occurred among infants born to women who received antiviral prophylaxis during the latter weeks of pregnancy.

Care of Newborn Infants Whose Mothers Have Active Genital Lesions at Delivery. The risk of transmitting HSV to the newborn infant during delivery is influenced directly by the mother's classification of HSV infection (Table 3.27); women with primary genital HSV infections who are shedding HSV at delivery are 10 to 30 times more likely to transmit the virus to their newborn infants, compared with women with a recurrent infection. With the commercial availability of serologic tests that can reliably distinguish type-specific HSV antibodies, the means to further refine management of asymptomatic neonates delivered to women with active genital HSV lesions now is possible. The American Academy of Pediatrics recently published an algorithm (Fig 3.6 and 3.7) addressing management of asymptomatic neonates following vaginal or cesarean delivery to women with active

Table 3.27. Maternal Infection Classification by Genital HSV Viral Type and Maternal Serologic Test Results[a]

Classification of Maternal Infection	PCR/Culture From Genital Lesion	Maternal HSV-1 and HSV-2 IgG Antibody Status
Documented first-episode primary infection	Positive, either virus	Both negative
Documented first-episode nonprimary infection	Positive for HSV-1	Positive for HSV-2 **AND** negative for HSV-1
	Positive for HSV-2	Positive for HSV-1 **AND** negative for HSV-2
Assumed first-episode (primary or nonprimary) infection	Positive for HSV-1 **OR** HSV-2	Not available
	Negative **OR** not available[b]	Negative for HSV-1 and/or HSV-2, **OR** not available
Recurrent infection	Positive for HSV-1	Positive for HSV-1
	Positive for HSV-2	Positive for HSV-2

HSV indicates herpes simplex virus; PCR, polymerase chain reaction (assay); IgG, immunoglobulin G.

[a] To be used for women without a clinical history of genital herpes.

[b] When a genital lesion is strongly suspicious for HSV, clinical judgment should supersede the virologic test results for the conservative purposes of this neonatal management algorithm. Conversely, if, in retrospect, the genital lesion was not likely to be caused by HSV and the PCR assay result/culture is negative, departure from the evaluation and management in this conservative algorithm may be warranted.

FIG 3.6. ALGORITHM FOR THE EVALUATION OF ASYMPTOMATIC NEONATES FOLLOWING VAGINAL OR CESAREAN DELIVERY TO WOMEN WITH ACTIVE GENITAL HERPES LESIONS.

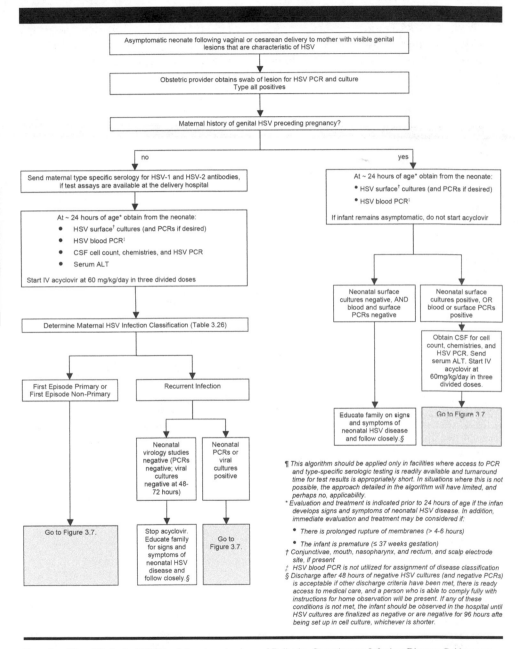

Reproduced from Kimberlin DW, Baley J; American Academy of Pediatrics, Committee on Infectious Diseases. Guidance on management of asymptomatic neonates born to women with active genital herpes lesions. *Pediatrics.* 2013;131(2):e635–e646

FIG 3.7. ALGORITHM FOR THE TREATMENT OF ASYMPTOMATIC NEONATES FOLLOWING VAGINAL OR CESAREAN DELIVERY TO WOMEN WITH ACTIVE GENITAL HERPES LESIONS.

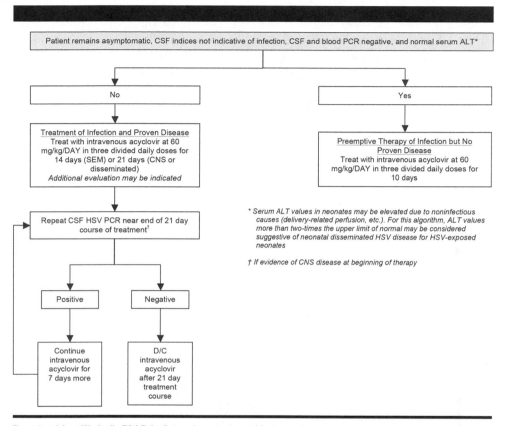

Reproduced from Kimberlin DW, Baley J; American Academy of Pediatrics, Committee on Infectious Diseases. Guidance on management of asymptomatic neonates born to women with active genital herpes lesions. *Pediatrics.* 2013;131(2):e635–e646

genital HSV lesions.[1] It is intended to outline one approach to the management of these neonates and may not be feasible in settings with limited access to PCR assays for HSV DNA or to the newer type-specific serologic tests. If, at any point during the evaluation outlined in the algorithm, an infant develops symptoms that could possibly indicate neonatal HSV disease (eg, fever, hypothermia, lethargy, irritability, vesicular rash, seizures, etc), a full diagnostic evaluation should be undertaken and intravenous acyclovir therapy should be initiated. In applying this algorithm, obstetric providers and pediatricians likely will need to work closely with their diagnostic laboratories to ensure that serologic and virologic testing is available and turnaround times are acceptable. In situations where this is not possible, the approach detailed in the algorithm will have limited, and perhaps no, applicability.

---

[1]Kimberlin DW, Baley J; American Academy of Pediatrics, Committee on Infectious Diseases. Guidance on management of asymptomatic neonates born to women with active genital herpes lesions. *Pediatrics.* 2013;131(2):e635–e646

Care of Newborn Infants Whose Mothers Have a History of Genital Herpes But No Active Genital Lesions at Delivery. An infant whose mother has known, recurrent genital infection but no genital lesions at delivery should be observed for signs of infection (eg, vesicular lesions of the skin, respiratory distress, seizures, or signs of sepsis) but should not have specimens for surface cultures for HSV obtained at 12 to 24 hours of life and should not receive empiric parenteral acyclovir. Education of parents and caregivers about the signs and symptoms of neonatal HSV infection during the first 6 weeks of life is prudent.

Infected Health Care Professionals. Transmission of HSV in hospital nurseries from infected health care professionals to newborn infants rarely has been documented. The risk of transmission to infants by health care professionals who have herpes labialis or who are asymptomatic oral shedders of virus is low. Compromising patient care by excluding health care professionals with cold sores who are essential for the operation of the hospital nursery must be weighed against the potential risk of newborn infants becoming infected. Health care professionals with cold sores who have contact with infants should cover and not touch their lesions and should comply with hand hygiene policies. Transmission of HSV infection from health care professionals with genital lesions is not likely as long as they comply with hand hygiene policies. Health care professionals with an active herpetic whitlow should not have responsibility for direct care of neonates or immunocompromised patients and should wear gloves and use hand hygiene during direct care of other patients.

Infected Household, Family, and Other Close Contacts of Newborn Infants. Intrafamilial transmission of HSV to newborn infants occurs rarely. Household members with herpetic skin lesions (eg, herpes labialis or herpetic whitlow) should be counseled about the risk of transmission and should avoid contact of their lesions with newborn infants by taking the same measures as recommended for infected health care professionals, as well as avoiding kissing and nuzzling the infant while they have active lip lesions or touching the infant while they have a herpetic whitlow. Cases of HSV transmission to the genitalia of male neonates have been reported following ritual circumcision (metzitzah b'peh) involving mouth suction of the site by the performer of the circumcision.

Care of People With Extensive Dermatitis. Patients with dermatitis are at risk of developing eczema herpeticum. If these patients are hospitalized, special care should be taken to avoid their exposure to HSV. These patients should not be kissed by people with cold sores or touched by people with herpetic whitlow.

Care of Children With Mucocutaneous Infections Who Attend Child Care or School. Oral HSV infections are common among children who attend child care or school. Most of these infections are asymptomatic, with shedding of virus in saliva occurring in the absence of clinical disease. Only children with HSV gingivostomatitis (ie, primary infection) who do not have control of oral secretions should be excluded from child care. Exclusion of children with cold sores (ie, recurrent infection) from child care or school is not indicated.

Children with uncovered lesions on exposed surfaces pose a small potential risk to contacts. If children are certified by a physician to have recurrent HSV infection, covering the active lesions with clothing, a bandage, or an appropriate dressing when they attend child care or school is sufficient. Additional control measures include avoiding the sharing of respiratory secretions through contact with objects and washing and sanitizing mouthed toys, bottle nipples, and utensils that have come in contact with saliva.

HSV Infections Among Wrestlers and Rugby Players. HSV-1 has been transmitted during athletic competition involving close physical contact and frequent skin abrasions, such as wrestling (herpes gladiatorum) and rugby (herpes rugbiaforum or scrum pox). Competitors often do not recognize or may deny possible infection. Transmission of these infections can be limited or prevented by the following: (1) examination of wrestlers and rugby players for vesicular or ulcerative lesions on exposed areas of their bodies and around their mouths or eyes before practice or competition by a person familiar with the appearance of mucocutaneous infections (including HSV, herpes zoster, and impetigo); (2) exclusion of athletes with these conditions from competition or practice until healing (fully crusted lesions) occurs or a physician's written statement declaring their condition noninfectious is obtained; and (3) cleaning wrestling mats with a freshly prepared solution of household bleach (one quarter cup of bleach in 1 gallon of water) applied for a minimum contact time of 15 seconds at least daily and, preferably, between matches. Consideration of suppressive antiviral therapy should be limited to athletes with a history of recurrent herpes gladiatorum or herpes labialis to reduce the risk of reactivation during wrestling season. Hydration of wrestlers on suppressive antiviral therapy should be ensured to minimize the likelihood of nephrotoxicity from acyclovir or valacyclovir. Despite these precautions, HSV spread during wrestling and other sports involving close personal contact still can occur through contact with asymptomatic infected people.

Histoplasmosis

CLINICAL MANIFESTATIONS: *Histoplasma capsulatum* causes symptoms in fewer than 5% of infected people. Clinical manifestations are classified according to site (pulmonary or disseminated), duration (acute, subacute, or chronic), and pattern (primary or reactivation) of infection. Most symptomatic patients have acute pulmonary histoplasmosis, a self-limited illness characterized by fever, chills, nonproductive cough, and malaise. The typical radiographic finding in mild infections is an area of focal pneumonitis associated with hilar or mediastinal adenopathy; high inoculum exposure may result in diffuse interstitial or reticulonodular pulmonary infiltrates. Most patients recover without treatment 2 to 3 weeks after onset of symptoms. Exposure to a large inoculum of conidia can cause severe pulmonary infection associated with high fevers, hypoxemia, diffuse reticulonodular infiltrates, and acute respiratory distress syndrome (ARDS). Mediastinal involvement, usually a complication of pulmonary histoplasmosis, includes mediastinal lymphadenitis, which can cause airway encroachment in young children. Inflammatory syndromes (pericarditis and rheumatologic syndromes) also can develop; erythema nodosum can occur in adolescents and adults. Primary cutaneous infections after trauma are rare. Chronic cavitary pulmonary histoplasmosis is extremely rare in children.

Disseminated histoplasmosis can be either self-limited or progressive. Progressive disseminated histoplasmosis (PDH) may occur in otherwise healthy infants and children younger than 2 years of age or in older children with primary or acquired cellular immune dysfunction. PDH can be a rapidly progressive illness following acute infection or can be a more chronic, slowly progressive disease. PDH in adults occurs most often in people with underlying immune deficiency (eg, human immunodeficiency virus/acquired immunodeficiency syndrome, solid organ transplant, hematologic malignancy, biologic response modifiers including tumor necrosis factor antagonists) or in people older than 65 years. Early manifestations of PDH in children include prolonged fever, failure to thrive, and hepatosplenomegaly; if untreated, malnutrition, diffuse adenopathy, pneumonitis, mucosal ulceration, pancytopenia, disseminated intravascular coagulopathy, and gastrointestinal tract bleeding can ensue. Central nervous system involvement is common. Chronic PDH generally occurs in adults with immune suppression and is characterized by prolonger fever, night sweats, weight loss, and fatigue; signs include hepatosplenomegaly, mucosal ulcerations, adrenal insufficiency, and pancytopenia. Clinicians should be alert to the risk of disseminated endemic mycoses in patients receiving tumor necrosis factor-alpha antagonists and disease-modifying antirheumatic drugs.

ETIOLOGY: *Histoplasma capsulatum* var *capsulatum* is a thermally dimorphic, endemic fungus that grows in the environment as a microconidia-bearing mold but converts to its yeast phase at 37°C. *H capsulatum* var *duboisii* is the cause of African histoplasmosis and is found only in central and western Africa.

EPIDEMIOLOGY: *H capsulatum* is encountered in most parts of the world (including Africa, the Americas, Asia, and Europe) and is highly endemic in the central United States, particularly the Mississippi, Ohio, and Missouri River valleys. Infection is acquired following inhalation of conidia that are aerosolized by disturbance of soil or abandoned structures contaminated with bat guano or bird droppings. The inoculum size, strain virulence, and immune status of the host affect the severity of the ensuing illness. Infections occur sporadically, in outbreaks when weather conditions (dry and windy) predispose to spread of conidia, or in point-source epidemics after exposure to activities that disturb contaminated sites. In regions with endemic disease, recreational and occupational activities, such as playing in hollow trees, caving, construction, excavation, demolition, farming, and cleaning of contaminated buildings, have been associated with outbreaks. Person-to-person transmission does not occur. Prior infection confers partial immunity; reinfection can occur but requires a larger inoculum.

The **incubation period** is variable but usually is 1 to 3 weeks.

DIAGNOSTIC TESTS: Culture is the definitive method of diagnosis. *H capsulatum* organisms from bone marrow, blood, sputum, and tissue specimens grow on standard mycologic media in 1 to 6 weeks. The lysis-centrifugation method is preferred for blood cultures. A DNA probe for *H capsulatum* permits rapid identification of cultured isolates.

Demonstration of typical intracellular yeast forms by examination with Gomori methenamine silver or other stains of tissue, blood, bone marrow, or bronchoalveolar lavage specimens strongly supports the diagnosis of histoplasmosis when clinical, epidemiologic, and other laboratory studies are compatible.

Detection of *H capsulatum* antigen in serum, urine, bronchoalveolar lavage fluid, or cerebrospinal fluid using a quantitative immunoassay is possible with a rapid, commercially available diagnostic test. Antigen detection in blood and urine specimens is most sensitive for severe, acute pulmonary infections and for progressive disseminated infections. Results often are transiently positive early in the course of acute, self-limited pulmonary infections. A negative test result does not exclude infection. If the result initially is positive, the antigen test also is useful for monitoring treatment response and, thereafter, promptly identifying relapse or reexposure to *H capsulatum* conidia. Cross-reactions occur in patients with blastomycosis, coccidioidomycosis, paracoccidioidomycosis, and penicilliosis; clinical and epidemiologic distinctions aid in differentiating these entities.

Serologic testing is available and is most useful in patients with subacute or chronic pulmonary disease. A fourfold increase in either yeast-phase or mycelial-phase complement fixation titers or a single titer of ≥1:32 in either test is strong presumptive evidence of active or recent infection in patients exposed to or residing within regions of endemicity. Cross-reacting antibodies can result from *Aspergillus* species, *Blastomyces dermatitidis,* and *Coccidioides* species infections. The immunodiffusion test is more specific than the complement fixation test, but the complement fixation test is more sensitive.

TREATMENT: Immunocompetent children with uncomplicated or mild-to-moderate acute pulmonary histoplasmosis may not require antifungal therapy, because infection usually is self-limited. However, if the patient does not improve within 4 weeks, itraconazole should be given for 6 to 12 weeks.

For severe or disseminated infections, a lipid formulation of amphotericin B followed by itraconazole is recommended (see Table 4.6, p 907). Itraconazole is preferred over other azoles by most experts; when used in adults, itraconazole is more effective, has fewer adverse effects, and is less likely to induce resistance than is fluconazole. Although safety and efficacy of itraconazole for use in children have not been established, anecdotal experience has found it to be well tolerated and effective. Serum trough concentrations of itraconazole should be ≥ 1 but <10 $\mu g/mL$. Concentrations should be checked after 2 weeks of therapy to ensure adequate drug exposure.

For severe, acute pulmonary infections, treatment with a lipid formulation of amphotericin B is recommended for 1 to 2 weeks. After clinical improvement occurs, itraconazole is recommended for an additional 12 weeks. Methylprednisolone during the first 1 to 2 weeks of therapy may be considered if severe respiratory complications develop.

All patients with chronic pulmonary histoplasmosis (eg, progressive cavitation of the lungs) should be treated. Mild to moderate cases should be treated with itraconazole for 1 to 2 years. Severe cases should be treated initially with a lipid formulation amphotericin B followed by itraconazole for the same duration.

Mediastinal and inflammatory manifestations of infection generally do not need to be treated with antifungal agents. However, mediastinal adenitis that causes obstruction of a bronchus, the esophagus, or another mediastinal structure may improve with a brief course of corticosteroids. In these instances, itraconazole should be used concurrently and continued for 6 to 12 weeks thereafter. Dense fibrosis of mediastinal structures without an associated granulomatous inflammatory component does not respond to antifungal therapy, and surgical intervention may be necessary for severe cases. Pericarditis and rheumatologic syndromes may respond to treatment with nonsteroidal anti-inflammatory agents (indomethacin).

For treatment of moderately severe to severe progressive disseminated histoplasmosis (PDH) in an infant or child, a lipid formulation of amphotericin B is the drug of choice and usually is given for a minimum of 2 weeks. When the child has demonstrated substantial clinical improvement and a decline in the serum concentration of *Histoplasma* antigen, oral itraconazole is administered for 12 weeks. Prolonged therapy for up to 12 months may be required for patients with severe disease, primary immunodeficiency syndromes, acquired immunodeficiency that cannot be reversed, or patients who experience relapse despite appropriate therapy. For those with mild to moderate PDH, itraconazole for 12 months is recommended for treatment. After completion of treatment for PDH, urine antigen concentrations should be monitored for 6 months. Stable, low, and decreasing concentrations that are unaccompanied by signs of active infection may not necessarily require prolongation or resumption of treatment.

ISOLATION OF THE HOSPITALIZED PATIENT: Standard precautions are recommended.

CONTROL MEASURES: In outbreaks, investigation for a common source of infection is indicated. Exposure to soil and dust from areas with significant accumulations of bird and bat droppings should be avoided, especially by immunocompromised individuals, including those receiving tumor necrosis factor inhibitors or disease-modifying antirheumatic drugs. If exposure is unavoidable, it should be minimized through use of appropriate respiratory protection (eg, N95 respirator), gloves, and disposable clothing. Areas suspected of being contaminated with *Histoplasma* species should be remediated. Old or abandoned structures likely to have been contaminated with bird or bat droppings should be saturated with water in an effort to reduce the aerosolization of spores during demolition. Guidelines for preventing histoplasmosis have been designed for health and safety professionals, environmental consultants, and people supervising workers involved in activities in which contaminated materials are disturbed. Additional information about the guidelines is available from the National Institute for Occupational Safety and Health (NIOSH; publication No. 2005–109, available from Publications Dissemination, 4676 Columbia Parkway, Cincinnati, OH 45226-1998; telephone 800-356-4674) and the NIOSH Web site (**www.cdc.gov/niosh/docs/2005-109/pdfs/2005-109.pdf**).

Hookworm Infections
(*Ancylostoma duodenale* and *Necator americanus*)

CLINICAL MANIFESTATIONS: Patients with hookworm infection often are asymptomatic; however, chronic hookworm infection is a common cause of moderate and severe hypochromic, microcytic anemia in people living in tropical developing countries, and heavy infection can cause hypoproteinemia with edema. Chronic hookworm infection in children may lead to physical growth delay, deficits in cognition, and developmental delay. After contact with contaminated soil, initial skin penetration of larvae, often involving the feet, can cause a stinging or burning sensation followed by pruritus and a papulovesicular rash that may persist for 1 to 2 weeks. Pneumonitis associated with migrating larvae (Löffler-like syndrome) is uncommon and usually mild, except in heavy infections. Colicky abdominal pain, nausea, diarrhea, and marked eosinophilia can develop 4 to 6 weeks after exposure. Blood loss secondary to hookworm infection develops 10 to 12 weeks after initial infection, and symptoms related to serious iron-deficiency anemia can develop in long-standing moderate or heavy hookworm infections. Pharyngeal itching, hoarseness, nausea, and vomiting can develop shortly after oral ingestion of infectious *Ancylostoma duodenale* larvae.

ETIOLOGY: *Necator americanus* is the major cause of hookworm infection worldwide, although *A duodenale* also is an important hookworm in some regions. Mixed infections also can occur. Both are roundworms (nematodes) with similar life cycles.

EPIDEMIOLOGY: Humans are the only reservoir. Hookworms are prominent in rural, tropical, and subtropical areas where soil contamination with human feces is common. Although the prevalence of both hookworm species is equal in many areas, *A duodenale* is the predominant species in the Mediterranean region, northern Asia, and selected foci of South America. *N americanus* is predominant in the Western hemisphere, sub-Saharan Africa, Southeast Asia, and a number of Pacific islands. Larvae and eggs survive in loose, sandy, moist, shady, well-aerated, warm soil (optimal temperature 23°C–33°C [73°F–91°F]). Hookworm eggs from stool hatch in soil in 1 to 2 days as rhabditiform larvae. These larvae develop into infective filariform larvae in soil within 5 to 7 days and can persist for 3 to 4 weeks. Percutaneous infection occurs after exposure to infectious larvae. *A duodenale* transmission can occur by oral ingestion and possibly through human milk. Untreated infected patients can harbor worms for 5 years or longer.

The time from exposure to development of noncutaneous symptoms is 4 to 12 weeks.

DIAGNOSTIC TESTS: Microscopic demonstration of hookworm eggs in feces is diagnostic. Adult worms or larvae rarely are seen. Approximately 5 to 8 weeks are required after infection for eggs to appear in feces. A direct stool smear with saline solution or potassium iodide saturated with iodine is adequate for diagnosis of heavy hookworm infection; light infections require concentration techniques. Quantification techniques (eg, Kato-Katz, Beaver direct smear, or Stoll egg-counting techniques) to determine the clinical significance of infection and the response to treatment may be available from state or reference laboratories.

TREATMENT: Albendazole, mebendazole, and pyrantel pamoate all are effective treatments (see Drugs for Parasitic Infections, p 927). Although data suggest that these drugs are safe in children younger than 2 years, the risks and benefits of therapy should be considered before administration. In 1-year-old children, the World Health Organization recommends reducing the albendazole dose to half of that given to older children and adults. Albendazole is not approved by the US Food and Drug Administration for hookworm infection. Reexamination of stool specimens 2 weeks after therapy to determine whether worms have been eliminated is helpful for assessing response to therapy. Retreatment is indicated for persistent infection. Nutritional supplementation, including iron, is important when severe anemia is present. Severely affected children also may require blood transfusion.

ISOLATION OF THE HOSPITALIZED PATIENT: Only standard precautions are recommended, because there is no direct person-to-person transmission.

CONTROL MEASURES: Sanitary disposal of feces to prevent contamination of soil is necessary in areas with endemic infection. Treatment of all known infected people and screening of high-risk groups (ie, children and agricultural workers) in areas with endemic infection can help decrease environmental contamination. Wearing shoes protects against hookworm infection if no other parts of the body are in contact with contaminated soil; children playing in contaminated soil would still be at risk if other body surfaces are in contact with the soil. Despite relatively rapid reinfection, periodic deworming treatments targeting preschool-aged and school-aged children have been advocated to prevent morbidity associated with heavy intestinal helminth infections.

Human Herpesvirus 6 (Including Roseola) and 7

CLINICAL MANIFESTATIONS: Clinical manifestations of primary infection with human herpesvirus 6 (HHV-6) include roseola (exanthem subitum) in approximately 20% of infected children, with the other 80% having undifferentiated febrile illness without rash or localizing signs. HHV-6 infection often is accompanied by cervical and characteristic postoccipital lymphadenopathy, gastrointestinal tract or respiratory tract signs, and inflamed tympanic membranes. Fever usually is high (temperature >39.5°C [103.0°F]) and persists for 3 to 7 days. Approximately 20% of all emergency department visits for febrile children 6 through 12 months of age are attributable to HHV-6. Roseola is distinguished by the erythematous maculopapular rash that appears once fever resolves and can last hours to days. Febrile seizures, sometimes leading to status epilepticus, are the most common complication and reason for hospitalization among children with primary HHV-6 infection. Approximately 10% to 15% of children with primary HHV-6 illnesses develop febrile seizures, predominantly between the ages of 6 and 18 months. Other neurologic manifestations that may accompany primary infection include a bulging fontanelle and encephalopathy or encephalitis. Hepatitis has been reported as a rare manifestation. Approximately 5% of mononucleosis cases are attributable to HHV-6. Congenital HHV-6 infection, which occurs in approximately 1% of newborn infants, has not been linked to any clinical disease.

The clinical manifestations occurring with human herpesvirus 7 (HHV-7) infection are less clear. Most primary infections with HHV-7 presumably are asymptomatic or mild and not distinctive. Some initial infections can present as typical roseola and may account for second or recurrent cases of roseola. Febrile illnesses associated with seizures also have been documented to occur during primary HHV-7 infection. Some investigators suggest that the association of HHV-7 with these clinical manifestations results from the ability of HHV-7 to reactivate latent HHV-6.

Following primary infection, HHV-6 and HHV-7 remain in latent state and may reactivate. The clinical circumstances and manifestations of reactivation in healthy people are unclear. Illness associated with HHV-6 reactivation has been described primarily among recipients of solid organ and hematopoietic stem cell transplants. Among the clinical findings associated with HHV-6 reactivation in these patients are fever, rash, hepatitis, bone marrow suppression, graft rejection, pneumonia, and encephalitis. A few cases of central nervous system symptoms have been reported in association with HHV-7 reactivation in immunocompromised hosts, but clinical findings generally have been reported less frequently with HHV-7 than with HHV-6 reactivation.

ETIOLOGY: HHV-6 and HHV-7 are lymphotropic agents that are closely related members of the *Herpesviridae* family, subfamily *Betaherpesvirinae*. Among the human herpesviruses, HHV-6 and HHV-7 are most closely related to cytomegalovirus. As with all human herpesviruses, HHV-6 and HHV-7 establish lifelong infection after initial exposure. There are 2 species of HHV-6, HIIV-6A and HHV-6B. Essentially all postnatally acquired primary infections in children are caused by HHV-6B, except infections in some parts of Africa. Among congenital HHV-6 infections, however, as many as one third may be caused by HHV-6A.

EPIDEMIOLOGY: HHV-6 and HHV-7 cause ubiquitous infections in children worldwide. Humans are the only known natural host. Nearly all children acquire HHV-6 infection within the first 2 years of life, probably resulting from asymptomatic shedding of infectious virus in secretions of a healthy family member or other close contact. During the acute phase of primary infection, HHV-6 and HHV-7 can be isolated from peripheral blood mononuclear cells and from saliva of some children. Viral DNA subsequently may be detected throughout life by the polymerase chain reaction (PCR) assay in multiple body sites. Although both HHV-6 and HHV-7 may be detected in blood mononuclear cells, salivary glands, lung, and skin, only HHV-6 is found in brain and only HHV-7 is found in mammary glands. Virus-specific maternal antibody, which is present uniformly in the sera of infants at birth, provides transient partial protection. As maternal antibody concentration decreases during the first year of life, the infection rate increases rapidly, peaking between 6 and 24 months of age. Essentially all children are seropositive for HHV-6 before 4 years of age. Infections occur throughout the year without a seasonal pattern. Secondary cases rarely are identified. Occasional outbreaks of roseola have been reported.

Congenital infection with HHV-6 occurs in approximately 1% of newborn infants, as determined by the presence of HHV-6 DNA in cord blood. Most congenital infections appear to result from the germline passage of maternal or paternal chromosomally integrated HHV-6, a unique mechanism of transmission of human viral congenital infection. Transplacental HHV-6 infection also may occur from reinfection or reactivation of maternal HHV-6 infection or from reactivated maternal chromosomally integrated HHV-6. HHV-6 has not been identified in human milk.

HHV-7 infection usually occurs later in childhood HHV-6 infection. By adulthood, the seroprevalence of HHV-7 is approximately 85%. Infectious HHV-7 is present in more than 75% of saliva specimens obtained from healthy adults. Contact with infected respiratory tract secretions of healthy contacts is the probable mode of transmission of HHV-7 to young children. HHV-7 has been detected in human milk, peripheral blood mononuclear cells, cervical secretions, and other body sites. Congenital HHV-7 infection has not been demonstrated by the examination of large numbers of cord blood samples for HHV-7 DNA.

The mean **incubation period** for HHV-6 is 9 to 10 days. For HHV-7, the incubation period is not known.

DIAGNOSTIC TESTS: Multiple assays for detection of HHV-6 and HHV-7 have been developed, but few are available commercially, and many do not differentiate between new, past, and reactivated infection. Moreover, because laboratory diagnosis of HHV-6 or HHV-7 usually does not influence clinical management (infections among the severely immunocompromised may be an exception), these tests have limited utility in clinical practice.

Serologic tests include immunofluorescent antibody, neutralization, immunoblot, and enzyme immunoassays (EIAs). A fourfold increase in serum antibody concentration alone does not necessarily indicate new infection, because an increase in titer also may occur with reactivation and in association with other infections, especially other beta-herpesvirus infections. However, seroconversion from negative to positive in paired sera is evidence of recent primary infection. Detection of specific immunoglobulin (Ig) M antibody also is not reliable for diagnosing new infection, because IgM antibodies to HHV-6 and HHV-7 are not always detectable in children with primary infection yet may be present in asymptomatic previously infected people. These antibody assays do not differentiate HHV-6A from HHV-6B infections. In addition, the diagnosis of primary HHV-7 infection in children with previous HHV-6 infection is confounded by concurrent rise in HHV-6 antibody titer from antigenic cross-reactivity or from reactivation of HHV-6 by a new HHV-7 infection. Detection of low-avidity HHV-6 or HHV-7 antibody with subsequent maturation to high-avidity antibody has been used in such situations to identify recent primary infection. Isolation of HHV-6 or HHV-7 in conjunction with seroconversion or, in the infant with maternal antibodies, a fourfold titer rise confirms primary infection.

Reference laboratories offer diagnostic testing for HHV-6 and HHV-7 infections by detection of viral DNA in blood and cerebrospinal fluid (CSF) specimens. However, detection of HHV-6 DNA or HHV-7 DNA in peripheral blood mononuclear cells, other body fluids, and tissues generally does not differentiate between new infection and persistence of virus from past infection. DNA detection by PCR assay in plasma and sera has been used to diagnose acute primary infection, but these assays are not sensitive in young children or specific in children with chromosomally integrated HHV-6 infection. Chromosomal integration of HHV-6 is supported by consistently positive PCR test results for HHV-6 DNA in blood, tissue, or other fluids with high viral loads ($\geq$1 copy of HHV-6 DNA per cell) and is confirmed by detection of HHV-6 DNA in hair follicles.

TREATMENT: Supportive. Anecdotal reports suggest that use of ganciclovir (and therefore valganciclovir) or foscarnet may be beneficial for immunocompromised patients with serious HHV-6 disease, but resistance may occur.

ISOLATION OF THE HOSPITALIZED PATIENT: Standard precautions are recommended.

CONTROL MEASURES: None.

Human Herpesvirus 8

CLINICAL MANIFESTATIONS: Human herpesvirus (HHV-8) is the etiologic agent associated with Kaposi sarcoma (KS), primary effusion lymphoma, and multicentric Castleman disease (MCD). More recently, a syndrome termed "the Kaposi sarcoma herpesvirus-associated inflammatory cytokine syndrome (KICS)," which presents as a systemic inflammatory illness, has been described in adults with HHV-8 infection in the United States. HHV-8 is one of the triggers of hemophagocytic lymphohistiocytosis. In regions with endemic HHV-8, a primary infection syndrome in immunocompetent children has been described, which consists of fever and a maculopapular rash, often accompanied by upper respiratory tract signs. Primary infection among immunocompromised people and men who have sex with men tends to have more severe manifestations that include pancytopenia, fever, rash, lymphadenopathy, splenomegaly, diarrhea, arthralgia, disseminated disease, and KS. In parts of Africa, among children with and without human immunodeficiency virus (HIV) infection, KS is a frequent, aggressive malignancy. In the United States, KS is rare in children but occurs commonly in severely immunocompromised HIV patients. Among organ transplant recipients and other immunosuppressed patients, KS is an important cause of cancer-related deaths. Primary effusion lymphoma is rare among children. MCD has been described in immunosuppressed and immunocompetent children, but the proportion of cases attributable to infection with HHV-8 is unknown.

ETIOLOGY: HHV-8 is a member of the family *Herpesviridae,* the *Gammaherpesvirinae* subfamily, and the *Rhadinovirus* genus and is related closely to herpesvirus saimiri of monkeys and Epstein-Barr virus.

EPIDEMIOLOGY: In areas of Africa, the Amazon basin, Mediterranean, and Middle East with endemic HHV-8, seroprevalence ranges from approximately 30% to 80%. Low rates of seroprevalence, generally less than 5%, have been reported in the United States, Northern and Central Europe, and most areas of Asia. Higher rates, however, occur in specific geographic regions, among adolescents and adults with or at high risk of acquiring HIV infection, injection drug users, and internationally adopted children coming from some Eastern European countries.

Acquisition of HHV-8 in areas with endemic infection frequently occurs before puberty, likely by oral inoculation of saliva of close contacts, especially secretions of mothers and siblings. Virus is shed frequently in saliva of infected people and becomes latent for life in peripheral blood mononuclear cells, primarily CD19+ B lymphocytes, and lymphoid tissue. In areas where infection is not endemic, sexual transmission appears to be the major route of infection, especially among men who have sex with men. Studies from areas with endemic infection have suggested transmission may occur by blood transfusion, but in the United States such evidence is lacking. Transplantation of infected donor organs has been documented to result in HHV-8 infection in the recipient. HHV-8 DNA has been detected in blood drawn at birth from infants born to HHV-8 seropositive mothers, but vertical transmission seems to be rare. Viral DNA has been detected in human milk, but transmission via human milk is yet to be proven.

The **incubation period** of HHV-8 is unknown.

DIAGNOSTIC TESTS: Nucleic acid amplification testing and serologic assays for HHV-8 are available, and new assays with greater clinical utility are being developed. Polymerase chain reaction (PCR) tests may be used on peripheral blood and tissue biopsy specimens of patients with HHV-8–associated disease, such as KS. Detection of HHV-8 in peripheral blood specimens by PCR assay has been used to support the diagnosis of KS and to identify exacerbations of HHV-8-associated diseases, primarily MCD and KICS. However, HHV-8 DNA detection in the peripheral blood does not differentiate between latent and active replicating infection.

Currently available serologic assays measuring antibodies to HHV-8 include immunofluorescence assay (IFA), enzyme immunoassays (EIAs), and Western blot assays using recombinant HHV-8 proteins. These serologic assays can detect both latent and lytic infection, but each has challenges with accuracy or convenience, therefore limiting use in the diagnosis and management of acute clinical disease.

TREATMENT: No antiviral treatment is approved for HHV-8 disease. Several antiviral agents have in vitro activity against HHV-8. Ganciclovir has been shown to inhibit HHV-8 replication in the only randomized trial of an antiviral drug for this infection. Case reports document an effect of ganciclovir, ganciclovir combined with zidovudine, cidofovir, and foscarnet. Valacyclovir and famciclovir more modestly reduce HHV-8 replication. Retrospective cohort studies suggest that antiretroviral therapy (particularly zidovudine and nelfinavir) may inhibit HHV-8 replication in HIV infected patients. Antiviral therapy may play a more significant role in the treatment of diseases associated with active HHV-8 replication, specifically MCD and KICS. HHV-8 associated malignancies can be treated with radiation and cancer chemotherapies.

ISOLATION OF THE HOSPITALIZED PATIENT: Standard precautions are recommended.

CONTROL MEASURES: None.

Human Immunodeficiency Virus Infection[1]

CLINICAL MANIFESTATIONS: Human immunodeficiency virus (HIV) infection results in a wide array of clinical manifestations and varied natural history. HIV type 1 (HIV-1) is much more common in the United States than is HIV type 2 (HIV-2). Unless otherwise specified, this chapter addresses HIV-1 infection.

Acquired immunodeficiency syndrome (AIDS) is the name given to an advanced stage of HIV infection. The Centers for Disease Control and Prevention (CDC) uses a case

---

[1]For a complete listing of current policy statements from the American Academy of Pediatrics regarding human immunodeficiency virus and acquired immunodeficiency syndrome, see **http://aappolicy.aappublications. org/**.

Table 3.28. 1993 Revised Case Definition of AIDS-Defining Conditions for Adults and Adolescents 13 Years of Age and Older[a]

- Candidiasis of bronchi, trachea, or lungs
- Candidiasis, esophageal
- Cervical cancer, invasive
- Coccidioidomycosis, disseminated or extrapulmonary
- Cryptococcosis, extrapulmonary
- Cryptosporidiosis, chronic intestinal (greater than 1 mo duration)
- Cystoisosporiasis (isosporiasis), chronic intestinal (greater than 1 mo duration)
- Cytomegalovirus disease (other than liver, spleen, or nodes)
- Cytomegalovirus retinitis (with loss of vision)
- Encephalopathy, HIV related
- Herpes simplex: chronic ulcer(s) (greater than 1 mo duration) or bronchitis, pneumonitis, or esophagitis
- Histoplasmosis, disseminated or extrapulmonary
- Kaposi sarcoma
- Lymphoma, Burkitt (or equivalent term)
- Lymphoma, immunoblastic (or equivalent term)
- Lymphoma, primary or brain
- *Mycobacterium avium* complex or *Mycobacterium kansasii* infection, disseminated or extrapulmonary
- *Mycobacterium tuberculosis* infection, any site, pulmonary or extrapulmonary
- *Mycobacterium,* other species or unidentified species infection, disseminated or extrapulmonary
- *Pneumocystis jirovecii* pneumonia
- Pneumonia, recurrent
- Progressive multifocal leukoencephalopathy
- *Salmonella* septicemia, recurrent
- Toxoplasmosis of brain
- Wasting syndrome attributable to HIV
- CD4+ T-lymphocyte count less than 200/μL (0.20×10^9/L) or CD4+ T-lymphocyte percentage less than 15%

AIDS indicates acquired immunodeficiency syndrome; HIV, human immunodeficiency virus.

[a]Modified from Centers for Disease Control and Prevention. 1993 revised classification system for HIV infection and expanded surveillance case definition for AIDS among adolescents and adults. *MMWR Recomm Rep.* 1992;41(RR-17):1–19.

definition that comprises AIDS-defining conditions for surveillance (Table 3.28). The CDC classifies all HIV-infected children younger than 13 years according to clinical stage of disease (Table 3.29, p 455) and immunologic status (Table 3.30, p 457).[1,2] For purposes of surveillance of HIV disease, the CDC has updated the immunologic classification system[3];

[1]Centers for Disease Control and Prevention. 1993 revised classification system for HIV infection and expanded surveillance case definition for AIDS among adolescents and adults. *MMWR Recomm Rep.* 1992;41(RR-17):1–19

[2]Centers for Disease Control and Prevention. 1994 revised classification system for human immunodeficiency virus infection in children less than 13 years of age. Official authorized addenda: human immunodeficiency virus infection codes and official guidelines for coding and reporting ICD-9-CM. *MMWR Recomm Rep.* 1994;43(RR-12):1–19

[3]Centers for Disease Control and Prevention. Revised surveillance case definition for HIV infection—United States, 2014. *MMWR Recomm Rep.* 2014;63(RR-3):1–10

Table 3.29. Clinical Categories for Children Younger Than 13 Years With Human Immunodeficiency Virus (HIV) Infection[a]

Category N: Not Symptomatic

Children who have no signs or symptoms considered to be the result of HIV infection or have only 1 of the conditions listed in Category A.

Category A: Mildly Symptomatic

- Children with 2 or more of the conditions listed but none of the conditions listed in categories B and C.
- Lymphadenopathy (≥0.5 cm at more than 2 sites; bilateral at 1 site)
- Hepatomegaly
- Splenomegaly
- Dermatitis
- Parotitis
- Recurrent or persistent upper respiratory tract infection, sinusitis, or otitis media

Category B: Moderately Symptomatic

- Children who have symptomatic conditions other than those listed for category A or C that are attributed to HIV infection.
- Anemia (hemoglobin <8 g/dL [<80 g/L], neutropenia (white blood cell count <1000/μL [<1.0 × 10^9/L]), and/or thrombocytopenia (platelet count <100 × 10^3/μL [<100 × 10^9/L]) persisting for ≥30 days
- Bacterial meningitis, pneumonia, or sepsis (single episode)
- Candidiasis, oropharyngeal (thrush), persisting (>2 mo) in children older than 6 mo of age
- Cardiomyopathy
- Cytomegalovirus infection, with onset before 1 mo of age
- Diarrhea, recurrent or chronic
- Hepatitis
- Herpes simplex virus (HSV) stomatitis, recurrent (>2 episodes within 1 year)
- HSV bronchitis, pneumonitis, or esophagitis with onset before 1 mo of age
- Herpes zoster (shingles) involving at least 2 distinct episodes or more than 1 dermatome
- Leiomyosarcoma
- Lymphoid interstitial pneumonia or pulmonary lymphoid hyperplasia complex
- Nephropathy
- Nocardiosis
- Persistent fever (lasting >1 mo)
- Toxoplasmosis, onset before 1 mo of age
- Varicella, disseminated (complicated chickenpox)

continued

Table 3.29. Clinical Categories for Children Younger Than 13 Years With Human Immunodeficiency Virus (HIV) Infection,[a] continued

Category C: Severely Symptomatic

- Serious bacterial infections, multiple or recurrent (ie, any combination of at least 2 culture-confirmed infections within a 2-y period), of the following types: septicemia, pneumonia, meningitis, bone or joint infection, or abscess of an internal organ or body cavity (excluding otitis media, superficial skin or mucosal abscesses, and indwelling catheter-related infections)
- Candidiasis, esophageal or pulmonary (bronchi, trachea, lungs)
- Coccidioidomycosis, disseminated (at site other than or in addition to lungs or cervical or hilar lymph nodes)
- Cryptococcosis, extrapulmonary
- Cryptosporidiosis or cystoisosporiasis with diarrhea persisting >1 mo
- Cytomegalovirus disease with onset of symptoms after 1 mo of age (at a site other than liver, spleen, or lymph nodes)
- Encephalopathy (at least 1 of the following progressive findings present for at least 2 mo in the absence of a concurrent illness other than HIV infection that could explain the findings): (1) failure to attain or loss of developmental milestones or loss of intellectual ability, verified by standard developmental scale or neuropsychologic tests; (2) impaired brain growth or acquired microcephaly demonstrated by head circumference measurements or brain atrophy demonstrated by computed tomography or magnetic resonance imaging (serial imaging required for children younger than 2 y of age); (3) acquired symmetric motor deficit manifested by 2 or more of the following: paresis, pathologic reflexes, ataxia, or gait disturbance
- HSV infection causing a mucocutaneous ulcer that persists for greater than 1 mo or bronchitis, pneumonitis, or esophagitis for any duration affecting a child older than 1 mo of age
- Histoplasmosis, disseminated (at a site other than or in addition to lungs or cervical or hilar lymph nodes)

- Kaposi sarcoma
- Lymphoma, primary, in brain
- Lymphoma, small, noncleaved cell (Burkitt), or immunoblastic; or large-cell lymphoma of B-lymphocyte or unknown immunologic phenotype
- *Mycobacterium tuberculosis*, disseminated or extrapulmonary
- *Mycobacterium*, other species or unidentified species infection, disseminated (at a site other than or in addition to lungs, skin, or cervical or hilar lymph nodes)
- *Pneumocystis jiroveci* pneumonia
- Progressive multifocal leukoencephalopathy
- *Salmonella* (nontyphoid) septicemia, recurrent
- Toxoplasmosis of the brain with onset at after 1 mo of age
- Wasting syndrome in the absence of a concurrent illness other than HIV infection that could explain the following findings: (1) persistent weight loss >10% of baseline; (2) downward crossing of at least 2 of the following percentile lines on the weight-for-age chart (eg, 95th, 75th, 50th, 25th, 5th) in a child 1 y of age or older; OR (3) <5th percentile on weight-for-height chart on 2 consecutive measurements, ≥30 days apart; PLUS
  - (1) chronic diarrhea (ie, at least 2 loose stools per day for >30 days); OR
  - (2) documented fever (for >30 days, intermittent or constant)

[a]Modified from Centers for Disease Control and Prevention. 1994 revised classification system for human immunodeficiency virus infection in children less than 13 years of age. Official authorized addenda: human immunodeficiency virus infection codes and official guidelines for coding and reporting ICD-9-CM. *MMWR Recomm Rep.* 1994;43(RR-12):1–19.

Table 3.30. HIV Infection Stage, Based on Age-Specific CD4+ T-Lymphocyte Count or CD4+ T-Lymphocyte Percentage of Total Lymphocytes[a]

| | Age on Date of CD4 T-Lymphocyte Test | | | | | |
| | <1 y | | 1 Through 5 y | | 6 y Through Adult | |
State[a]	Cells/µL	%	Cells/µL	%	Cells/µL	%
1	≥1500	≥30	≥1000	≥26	≥500	≥26[b]
2	750–1499	20–29	500–999	14–25	200–499	14–25
3	<750	<20	<500	<14	<200	<14

[a]The stage is based primarily on the CD4+ T-lymphocyte count; it is based on the CD4+ T-lymphocyte percentage only if the count is missing. There are 3 situations in which the stage is not based on this table: (1) if the criteria for stage 0 are met, the stage is 0 regardless of criteria for other stages (CD4+ T-lymphocyte test results and opportunistic illness diagnoses); (2) if the criteria for stage 0 are not met and a stage-3-defining opportunistic illness has been diagnosed, then the stage is 3 regardless of CD4+ T-lymphocyte test results; and (3) if the criteria for stage 0 are not met and information on the above criteria for other stages is missing, then the stage is U (unknown).

[b]The change in the upper CD4+ T-lymphocyte percentage threshold from 29% (as in the case definition of 2008) to 26% (as in the revision above) is contingent on data being published that support it, to corroborate unpublished analyses of surveillance data.

however, some clinical guidelines continue to make use of the 1994 CDC immunologic classification. This pediatric classification system emphasizes the importance of the CD4+ T-lymphocyte count and percentage as critical immunologic parameters and as markers of prognosis. Data regarding plasma HIV-1 RNA concentration (viral load) are not included in this classification.

With timely diagnostic testing and appropriate treatment, clinical manifestations of HIV-1 infection and occurrence of AIDS-defining illnesses now are rare among children in the United States and other industrialized countries. Early clinical manifestations of pediatric HIV infection include unexplained fevers, generalized lymphadenopathy, hepatomegaly, splenomegaly, failure to thrive, persistent or recurrent oral and diaper candidiasis, recurrent diarrhea, parotitis, hepatitis, central nervous system (CNS) disease (eg, hyperreflexia, hypertonia, floppiness, developmental delay), lymphoid interstitial pneumonia, recurrent invasive bacterial infections, and other opportunistic infections (OIs) (eg, viral and fungal).[1]

In the era of combination antiretroviral therapy (cART), there has been a substantial decrease in frequency of all OIs. The frequency of different OIs in the pre-cART era varied by age, pathogen, previous infection history, and immunologic status. In the pre-cART era, the most common OIs observed among children in the United States were infections caused by invasive encapsulated bacteria, *Pneumocystis jirovecii*, varicella-zoster virus, cytomegalovirus (CMV), *Herpes simplex* virus, *Mycobacterium avium* complex (MAC), and *Candida* species. Less commonly observed opportunistic pathogens included Epstein-Barr virus (EBV), *Mycobacterium tuberculosis*, *Cryptosporidium* species, *Cystoisospora* (formerly *Isospora*) species, other enteric pathogens, *Aspergillus* species, and *Toxoplasma gondii*.

Immune reconstitution inflammatory syndrome (IRIS) is a paradoxical clinical deterioration often seen in severely immunosuppressed people that occurs shortly after the

---

[1]Panel on Opportunistic Infections in HIV-Exposed and HIV-Infected Children. Guidelines for the Prevention and Treatment of Opportunistic Infections in HIV-Exposed and HIV-Infected Children. Department of Health and Human Services. Available at: **http://aidsinfo.nih.gov/contentfiles/lvguidelines/oi_guidelines_pediatrics.pdf.**

initiation of cART. Local and/or systemic symptoms develop secondary to an inflammatory response as cell-mediated immunity is restored. Underlying infection with mycobacteria (including *Mycobacterium tuberculosis)*, herpesviruses, and fungi (including *Cryptococcal* species) predispose to IRIS.

Malignant neoplasms in children with HIV-1 infection are relatively uncommon, but leiomyosarcomas and non-Hodgkin B-cell lymphomas of the Burkitt type (including some that occur in the CNS) occur more commonly in children with HIV infection than in immunocompetent children. Kaposi sarcoma is rare in children in the United States but has been documented in HIV-infected children who have emigrated from sub-Saharan African countries. The incidence of malignant neoplasms in HIV-infected children has decreased during the cART era.

The incidence of HIV encephalopathy is high among untreated HIV-infected infants and young children. In the United States, pediatric HIV encephalopathy has decreased substantially in the cART era, although other neurologic signs and symptoms have been appreciated, such as myelopathy or peripheral neuropathies, sometimes associated with antiretroviral therapy.

The prognosis for survival is poor for untreated infants who acquired HIV infection through mother-to-child transmission and who have high viral loads (ie, >100 000 copies/mL) and severe suppression of CD4+ T-lymphocyte counts (see Table 3.30, p 457). In these children, AIDS-defining conditions developing during the first 6 months of life, including *P jirovecii* pneumonia (PCP), progressive neurologic disease, and severe wasting, are predictors of a poor outcome. When cART regimens are begun early, prognosis and survival rates improve dramatically. Although deaths attributable to OIs have declined, non–AIDS-defining infections and multiorgan failure remain major causes of death. In the United States, mortality in a longitudinal cohort of HIV-infected children whose age at enrollment ranged from birth to 21 years declined from 7.2/100 person years in 1993 to 0.8/100 person years in 2006. The HIV mortality rate in 2006 was equivalent to that of the general US pediatric population <5 years of age (0.8/100) in 2011.[1]

Although B-lymphocyte counts remain normal or are somewhat increased, humoral immune dysfunction may precede or accompany cellular dysfunction. Polyclonal B-lymphocyte hyperactivation occurs as part of a spectrum of chronic immune activation, leading to production of immunoglobulins that are not directed against specific pathogens encountered by the child. With advancing immunosuppression, recall antibody responses, including responses to vaccine-associated antigens, are slow and diminish in magnitude. A small proportion (less than 10%) of patients will develop panhypogammaglobulinemia. In the absence of treatment with cART, such patients have a particularly poor prognosis.

ETIOLOGY: As noted previously, 2 types of HIV cause disease in humans: HIV-1 and HIV-2. These viruses are cytopathic lentiviruses belonging to the family *Retroviridae*, and they are related closely to the simian immunodeficiency viruses (SIVs), agents found in a variety of nonhuman primate species in sub-Saharan Africa. HIV-1 species infecting humans have evolved from SIVs found in chimpanzees and gorillas, whereas HIV-2 evolved from an SIV in sooty mangabeys. Three distinct genetic groups of HIV-1 exist worldwide: M (major), O (outlier), and N (new). Group M viruses are the most prevalent worldwide and comprise 8 genetic subtypes, or clades, known as A through H, which

[1]UNICEF, Under-Five Mortality. Available at: **www.childinfo.org/mortality_ufmrcountrydata.php**

each have distinct geographic distribution. The HIV-1 genome is 10 kb in length and has both conserved and highly variable domains. Three principal genes (*gag, pol,* and *env*) encode the major structural and enzymatic proteins, and 6 accessory genes regulate gene expression and aid in assembly and release of infectious virions. The envelope glycoprotein interacts with the CD4+ receptor and with 1 of 2 major coreceptors (CCR5 or CXCR4) on the host cell membrane. HIV-1 is a single-stranded RNA virus that requires the activity of a viral enzyme, reverse transcriptase, to convert to double-stranded DNA. A double-stranded DNA copy of the viral genome then randomly integrates into the host cell genome, where it persists as a provirus.

HIV-2, the second AIDS-causing virus, predominantly is found in West Africa, with the highest rates of infection in Guinea-Bissau. The prevalence of HIV-2 in the United States is extremely low. HIV-2 is thought to have a milder disease course with a longer time to development of AIDS than HIV-1. Nonnucleoside reverse transcriptase inhibitors (NNRTIs) and at least 1 fusion inhibitor (enfuvirtide) are not effective against HIV-2, whereas nucleoside reverse transcriptase inhibitors (NRTIs) and protease inhibitors have varying efficacy against HIV-2. CDC guidelines state that HIV-2 serologic testing should be performed in patients who: (1) are from countries of high prevalence, mainly in Western Africa; (2) share needles or have sex partners known to be infected with HIV-2 or from areas with endemic infection; (3) received transfusions or nonsterile medical care in areas with endemic infection; or (4) are children of women with risk factors for HIV-2 infection. The identification of HIV-2 represents a diagnostic challenge. HIV immunoassays (IAs) currently approved by the US Food and Drug Administration (FDA) detect HIV-1 and HIV-2 antibodies, but an HIV-1 Western blot might report a negative or indeterminate result or, in >60% of cases, misclassify the HIV-2 virus as HIV-1 (eg, detection of only p24 and gp160 bands). FDA-approved HIV-1/HIV-2 antibody differentiation assays can be used in lieu of the Western Blot to identify antibodies and distinguish HIV-1 from HIV-2. Therefore, it is especially important to notify the laboratory when ordering serologic tests for a patient in whom HIV-2 infection is a possibility. Nucleic acid amplification tests approved by the FDA for detection and quantitation of viral load are specific to HIV-1; these do not detect HIV-2. No nucleic acid amplification tests are approved by the FDA for HIV-2 viral load. Clinicians wishing to obtain assistance from the CDC laboratory to make an HIV-2 diagnosis should request a referral to the CDC laboratory from their local or state health department laboratory.

EPIDEMIOLOGY: Humans are the only known reservoir for HIV-1 and HIV-2. Latent virus persists in peripheral blood mononuclear cells and in cells of the brain, bone marrow, and genital tract even when plasma viral load is undetectable. Only blood, semen, cervicovaginal secretions, and human milk have been implicated epidemiologically in transmission of infection.

Established modes of HIV transmission include: (1) sexual contact (vaginal, anal, or orogenital); (2) percutaneous blood exposure (from contaminated needles or other sharp instruments); (3) mucous membrane exposure to contaminated blood or other body fluids; (4) mother-to-child transmission in utero, around the time of labor and delivery, and postnatally through breastfeeding; and (5) transfusion with contaminated blood products. Cases of probable HIV transmission from an HIV-infected caregiver to an infant through feeding blood-tinged premasticated food have been reported in the United States. As a result of highly effective screening methods, transfusion of blood, blood components, and clotting factors virtually has been eliminated as a cause of HIV transmission in the United

States since 1985. In the United States, transmission of HIV has not been documented with normal activities in households; transmission has been documented after contact of nonintact skin with blood-containing body fluids. Moreover, transmission of HIV has not been documented in schools or child care settings in the United States.

In the United States, children younger than 13 years accounted for 0.05% and 0.8% of all estimated AIDS diagnoses in 2011 and cumulative AIDS diagnoses through 2011, respectively. Children younger than 13 years accounted for 0.3% of all estimated HIV diagnoses in the United States in 2011. Since the mid-1990s, the number of reported pediatric AIDS cases has decreased significantly, primarily because of prevention of mother-to-child transmission of HIV. This decrease in rate of mother-to-child transmission of HIV in the United States was attributable to the development and implementation of antenatal HIV testing programs and other interventions to prevent transmission: antiretroviral (ARV) prophylaxis during the antepartum, intrapartum, and postnatal periods; cesarean delivery before labor and before rupture of membranes; and complete avoidance of breastfeeding. Combination ARV regimens during pregnancy have been associated with lower rates of mother-to-child transmission than zidovudine monotherapy taken antenatally. Currently in the United States, most HIV-infected pregnant women receive 3-drug combination ARV regimens either for treatment of their own HIV infection or, if criteria for treatment are not yet met, for prevention of mother-to-child transmission of HIV (in which case the drugs may be stopped after delivery). The CDC estimates perinatally transmitted HIV cases in the United States have decreased from a peak of 1650 in 1991 to 57 in 2010.

The risk of infection for an infant born to an HIV-seropositive mother who did not receive interventions to prevent transmission is estimated to range from 22.6%[1] to 25.5%[2] in the United States. Most mother-to-child transmission occurs during the intrapartum period, with fewer transmission events occurring in utero and postnatally through breastfeeding. Risk factors for mother-to-child transmission of HIV can be categorized as follows: (1) the amount of virus to which the child is exposed (especially related to the maternal viral load; a higher maternal viral load is associated with a lower maternal CD4+ T-lymphocyte count and with more advanced maternal clinical disease or with recent seroconversion); (2) the duration of exposure (eg, duration of ruptured membranes or of breastfeeding, vaginal versus cesarean delivery before labor and before rupture of membranes); and (3) factors that facilitate the transfer of virus from mother to child (eg, maternal breast pathologic lesions, infant oral candidiasis). In addition to these factors, characteristics of the virus and the child's susceptibility to infection are important. Of note, although maternal viral load is a critical determinant affecting the likelihood of mother-to-child transmission of HIV, transmissions have been observed across the entire range of maternal viral loads. The risk of mother-to-child transmission increases with each hour increase in the duration of rupture of membranes, and the duration of ruptured membranes should be considered when evaluating the need for obstetric interventions. Cesarean delivery performed before onset of labor and before rupture of membranes has been shown to reduce mother-to-child intrapartum transmission. Current US

[1]Connor EM, Sperling RS, Gelbar R, et al. Reduction of maternal infant transmission of human immunodeficiency virus with zidovudine treatment. Pediatric AIDS Clinical Trials Group Protocol 076 Study Group. *N Engl J Med*. 1994;331(18):1173–1180

[2]Sperling RS, Shapiro DE, McSherry GD, et al. Safety of the maternal–infant zidovudine regimen utilized in the Pediatric AIDS Clinical Trials Group 076 Study. *AIDS*. 1998;12(14):1805–1813

guidelines recommend cesarean delivery at 38 weeks' gestation, before onset of labor and before rupture of membranes, for HIV-infected women with a viral load >1000 copies/mL (irrespective of use of ARVs during pregnancy) and for women with unknown viral load near the time of delivery[1,2] (**http://aidsinfo.nih.gov/Guidelines**). Cesarean delivery for women with an undetectable viral load is not routinely recommended.

Postnatal transmission to neonates and young infants occurs mainly through breast-feeding. Worldwide, an estimated one third to one half of cases of mother-to-child transmission of HIV occur as a result of breastfeeding. HIV genomes have been detected in cell-associated and cell-free fractions of human milk. In the United States, HIV-infected mothers are advised not to breastfeed, because safe alternatives to human milk are available readily. Because human milk cell-associated HIV can be detected even in women receiving cART and perinatal transmission still occurs among a small percentage of cART-receiving virologically suppressed women, replacement (formula) feeding continues to be recommended for US mothers receiving cART. In resource-limited locations, women whose HIV infection status is unknown are encouraged to breastfeed their infants exclusively for the first 6 months of life, because the morbidity associated with formula feeding is unacceptably high. In addition, these women should be offered HIV testing. The World Health Organization recommended in 2010 that HIV-infected mothers exclusively breastfeed their infants for the first 6 months of life. The introduction of complementary foods should occur after 6 months of life, and breastfeeding should continue through 12 months of life. Breastfeeding should be replaced only when a nutritionally adequate and safe diet can be maintained without human milk. In areas where ARVs are available, infants should receive daily nevirapine prophylaxis until 1 week after human milk consumption stops, and mothers should receive ARV (consisting of an effective cART regimen) for the first 6 months of their infants' lives. For infants known to be HIV-infected, mothers are encouraged to breastfeed exclusively for the first 6 months of life, and after the introduction of complementary foods should continue to breastfeed up to 2 years of age, as per recommendations for the general population.

Although the rate of acquisition of HIV infection among infants has decreased significantly in the United States, the rate of new HIV infections during adolescence and young adulthood continues to increase. HIV infection in adolescents occurs disproportionately among youth of minority race or ethnicity. Transmission of HIV to adolescents is attributable primarily to sexual exposure and secondarily to illicit intravenous drug use. It is estimated that, in 2011, males accounted for approximately 77% and 86% of adolescents 13 to 19 years of age and 20 to 24 years of age, respectively, diagnosed with HIV infection. Young men who have sex with men (MSM) particularly are at high risk of acquiring HIV infection, and the rates of HIV infection in young MSM continue to increase. In the United States and 6 dependent areas in 2011, an estimated 77% and 91% of diagnoses of HIV infections among all adolescents and young adults 13 to 24 years of

---

[1]Panel on Treatment of HIV-Infected Pregnant Women and Prevention of Perinatal Transmission. Recommendations for Use of Antiretroviral Drugs in Pregnant HIV-1-Infected Women for Maternal Health and Interventions to Reduce Perinatal HIV Transmission in the United States. Washington, DC: US Department of Health and Human Services; 2014. Available at **http://aidsinfo.nih.gov/contentfiles/lvguidelines/PerinatalGL.pdf**

[2]American College of Obstetricians and Gynecologists, Committee on Obstetric Practice. *Scheduled Cesarean Delivery and the Prevention of Vertical Transmission of HIV Infection.* ACOG Committee Opinion No. 234. Washington, DC: American College of Obstetricians and Gynecologists; 2000

age and among male adolescent and young adults 13 to 24 years of age, respectively, were attributed to male-to-male sexual contact.[1] In contrast, 92% of diagnoses of HIV infection in 2011 among young adolescent and adult women 13 to 24 years of age were attributed to heterosexual contact. In 2010, there were an estimated 39035 adolescents and young adults living with a diagnosis of HIV infection in the United States and 6 dependent areas.[2] Of these, 63% were black/African American, 19% were Hispanic/Latino, and 15% were non-Hispanic white. Rates of HIV infection among adolescents are particularly high in the Southeastern and Northeastern United States. Most HIV-infected adolescents and young adults are asymptomatic and, without testing, remain unaware of their infection. Youth 13 to 24 years of age represent 26% of new HIV infections annually, and 60% are unaware they are infected.[3]

INCUBATION PERIOD: The usual age of onset of symptoms is approximately 12 to 18 months of age for untreated infants in the United States who acquire HIV infection through mother-to-child transmission. However, some HIV-infected infants become ill in the first few months of life, whereas others remain relatively asymptomatic for more than 5 years and, rarely, until early adolescence. Without therapy, a bimodal distribution of symptomatic infection has been described: 15% to 20% of untreated HIV-infected children die before 4 years of age, with a median age at death of 11 months (rapid progressors), and 80% to 85% of untreated HIV-infected children have delayed onset of milder symptoms and survive beyond 5 years of age (slower progressors).

Following HIV acquisition in adolescents and adults, primary seroconversion syndrome can occur 7 to 14 days following viral acquisition and can last for 5 to 7 days. Only a minority of patients are ill enough to seek medical care with primary seroconversion syndrome, although more may recall a prior viral illness when queried about it later.

DIAGNOSTIC TESTS[4]: Laboratory diagnosis of HIV-1 infection during infancy is based on detection of the virus or viral nucleic acid (Table 3.31, p 463). Because infants born to HIV-infected mothers acquire maternal antibodies passively, antibody assays are not informative for diagnosis of infection in children younger than 24 months unless assay results are negative. In children 24 months and older, HIV antibody assays can be used for diagnosis. Historically, 18 months was considered the age at which a positive antibody assay could accurately distinguish between presence of maternal and infant antibodies. However, using medical record data for a cohort of HIV-uninfected infants born from 2000 to 2007, it was demonstrated that clearance of maternal HIV antibodies occurred later than previously reported.[5] Despite a median age of seroreversion of 13.9 months,

[1]Centers for Disease Control and Prevention. HIV Surveillance in Adolescents and Young Adults (through 2011) (CDC Slide set). Available at: **www.cdc.gov/hiv/library/slideSets/index.html**

[2]Centers for Disease Control and Prevention. Table 15B: Rates of HIV infection among adults and adolescents, by area of residence, 2011—United States and 6 dependent areas. In: HIV Surveillance Report. Atlanta, GA: Centers for Disease Control and Prevention; 2011. Available at: **www.cdc.gov/hiv/pdf/statistics_2011_ HIV_Surveillance_Report_vol_23.pdf#Page=54**

[3]Centers for Disease Control and Prevention. Vital Signs: HIV infection, testing, and risk behaviors among youths—United States. *MMWR Morb Mortal Wkly Rep.* 2012;61(47):971–976

[4]Read JS; American Academy of Pediatrics, Committee on Pediatric AIDS. Diagnosis of HIV-1 infection in children younger than 18 months in the United States, *Pediatrics.* 2007;120(6):e1547–e1562 (Reaffirmed April 2010). Available at: **http://pediatrics.aappublications.org/cgi/content/full/120/6/e1547**

[5]Gutierrez M, Ludwig DA, Khan SS, et al. Has highly active antiretroviral therapy increased the time to seroconversion in HIV exposed but uninfected children? *Clin Infect Dis.* 2012;55(9):1255–1261

Table 3.31. Laboratory Diagnosis of HIV Infection[a]

Test	Comment
HIV DNA PCR	Preferred test to diagnose HIV-1 subtype B infection in infants and children younger than 18 mo; highly sensitive and specific by 2 wk of age and available; performed on peripheral blood mononuclear cells. False-negative results can occur in non-B subtype HIV-1 infections.
HIV p24 Ag	Less sensitive, false-positive results during first month of life, variable results; not recommended.
ICD p24 Ag	Negative test result does not rule out infection; not recommended.
HIV culture	Expensive, not easily available, requires up to 4 wk for results; not recommended.
HIV RNA PCR	Preferred test to identify non-B subtype HIV-1 infections. Similar sensitivity and specificity to HIV DNA PCR in infants and children younger than 18 mo, but DNA PCR is generally preferred because of greater clinical experience with that assay.

HIV indicates human immunodeficiency virus; PCR, polymerase chain reaction; Ag, antigen; and ICD, immune complex dissociated.

[a] Read JS; American Academy of Pediatrics, Committee on Pediatric AIDS. Diagnosis of HIV-1 infection in children younger than 18 months in the United States, *Pediatrics.* 2007;120(6):e1547–e1562 (Reaffirmed April 2010). Available at: **http://pediatrics.aappublications.org/cgi/content/full/120/6/e1547**

14% of infants remained seropositive after 18 months, 4.3% after 21 months, and 1.2% after 24 months.

In the United States, the preferred test for diagnosis of HIV infection in infants is the HIV DNA polymerase chain reaction (PCR) assay. The DNA PCR assay can detect 1 to 10 DNA copies of proviral DNA in peripheral blood mononuclear cells. Approximately 30% to 40% of HIV-infected infants will have a positive HIV DNA PCR assay result in samples obtained before 48 hours of age. A positive result by 48 hours of age suggests in utero transmission. Approximately 93% of infected infants have detectable HIV DNA by 2 weeks of age, and approximately 95% of HIV-infected infants have a positive HIV DNA PCR assay result by 1 month of age. A single HIV DNA PCR assay has a sensitivity of 95% and a specificity of 97% for samples collected from infected children 1 to 36 months of age.

HIV isolation by culture is less sensitive, less available, and more expensive than the DNA PCR assay. Definitive results may take up to 28 days. This test no longer is recommended for routine diagnosis.

Detection of the p24 antigen (including immune complex dissociated) is less sensitive than the HIV DNA PCR assay or culture. False-positive test results occur in samples obtained from infants younger than 1 month. This test generally should not be used, although newer assays have been reported to have sensitivities similar to HIV DNA PCR assays.

Plasma HIV RNA assays also have been used to diagnose HIV infection. However, a false-negative test result may occur in neonates receiving ARVs as prophylaxis. Although use of ART can reduce plasma viral loads to undetectable levels, results of DNA PCR assay, which detects cell-associated integrated HIV DNA, remain positive even among individuals with undetectable plasma viral loads.

In the absence of therapy, plasma viral loads among infants who acquired HIV infection through mother-to-child transmission increase rapidly to very high levels (typically from several hundred thousand to more than 1 million copies/mL) after birth, decreasing only slowly to a "set point" by approximately 2 years of age. This is in contrast to infection in adults, in whom viral load generally does not reach the high levels that are seen in newly infected infants and for whom the "set point" occurs approximately 6 months after acquisition of infection. An HIV RNA assay result with only low-level viral copy number in an HIV-exposed infant may indicate a false-positive result, reinforcing the importance of repeating any positive assay result to confirm the diagnosis of HIV infection in infancy. Like HIV DNA PCR assays, the sensitivity of HIV RNA assays for diagnosing infections in the first week of life is low (25%–40%), because transmission usually occurs around the time of delivery. The RNA assays approved by the FDA provide quantitative results as a predictor of disease progression rather than for routine diagnosis of HIV infection in infants. RNA assays also are useful in monitoring changes in viral load during the course of ART.

Diagnostic testing with HIV DNA or RNA assays is recommended at 14 to 21 days of age, and if results are negative, again at 1 to 2 months of age and at 4 to 6 months of age. An infant is considered infected if 2 samples from 2 different time points test positive by DNA or RNA PCR assay.[1]

Viral diagnostic testing in the first 2 days of life is recommended by some experts to allow for early identification of infants with presumed in utero infection. If testing is performed shortly after birth, umbilical cord blood should not be used because of possible contamination with maternal blood. Obtaining the sample as early as 14 days of age may facilitate decisions about initiating ARV therapy. HIV-infected infants should be transitioned from neonatal ARV prophylaxis to cART treatment. In nonbreastfed children younger than 18 months with negative HIV virologic test results, *presumptive* exclusion of HIV infection is based on:

- Two negative HIV DNA or RNA virologic test results, from separate specimens, both of which were obtained at 2 weeks of age or older and one of which was obtained at 4 weeks of age or older; **OR**
- One negative HIV DNA or RNA virologic test result from a specimen obtained at 8 weeks of age or older; **OR**
- One negative HIV antibody test result obtained at 6 months of age or older; **AND**
- No other laboratory or clinical evidence of HIV infection (ie, no subsequent positive results from virologic tests if tests were performed and no AIDS-defining condition for which there is no other underlying condition of immunosuppression).

In nonbreastfed children younger than 18 months of age with negative HIV virologic test results, *definitive* exclusion of HIV is based on:

- At least 2 negative HIV DNA or RNA virologic test results, from separate specimens, both of which were obtained at 1 month of age or older and one of which was obtained at 4 months of age or older; **OR**
- At least 2 negative HIV antibody test results from separate specimens obtained at 6 months of age or older; **AND**
- No other laboratory or clinical evidence of HIV infection (ie, no subsequent positive results from virologic tests if tests were performed and no AIDS-defining condition for which there is no other underlying condition of immunosuppression).

---

[1]Centers for Disease Control and Prevention. Revised surveillance case definitions for HIV infection among adults, adolescents, and children aged <18 months and for HIV infection and AIDS among children aged 18 months to <13 years—United States, 2008. *MMWR Recomm Rep.* 2008;57(RR-10):1–12

In children with 2 negative HIV DNA PCR test results, many clinicians will confirm the absence of antibody (ie, loss of passively acquired natural antibody) to HIV on testing at 12 through 24 months of age ("seroreversion"). In addition, some clinicians have a slightly more stringent requirement that the 2 separate antibody-negative blood samples obtained after 6 months of age be drawn at least 1 month apart for a child to be considered HIV uninfected.

Immunoassays (IAs) are used widely as the initial test for serum HIV antibody or for p24 antigen and HIV antibody. These tests are highly sensitive and specific. Repeated IA testing of initially reactive specimens is common practice and is followed by additional testing to establish the diagnosis of HIV. A positive HIV antibody test result (reactive IA followed by positive Western blot or HIV-1/HIV-2 antibody differentiation assay) in a child 18 months or older almost always indicates infection, although passively acquired maternal antibody rarely can persist beyond 18 months of age. HIV antibody tests can be performed on samples of blood or oral fluid; antigen/antibody tests can be performed only on serum or plasma. Rapid tests for HIV antibodies have been approved for use in the United States; these tests are used widely throughout the world, particularly to screen mothers of undocumented serostatus in maternity settings. As with laboratory IAs, additional testing is required after a reactive rapid test. Results from rapid tests are available within 20 minutes; however, IA results and follow-up testing might take 2 days or longer.

Infants who acquire HIV infection through mother-to-child transmission commonly have high viral set-points with progressive cellular immune dysfunction and immunosuppression resulting from a decrease in the total number of circulating CD4+ T lymphocytes. Sometimes, T-lymphocyte counts do not decrease until late in the course of infection. Changes in cell populations frequently result in a decrease in the normal CD4+ to CD8+ T-lymphocyte ratio of 1.0 or greater. This nonspecific finding, although characteristic of HIV-1 infection, also occurs with other acute viral infections, including infections caused by CMV and EBV, and tuberculosis. The risk of OIs correlates with the CD4+ T-lymphocyte percentage and count. The normal values for peripheral CD4+ T-lymphocyte counts are age related, and the lower limits of normal are provided in Table 3.30 (p 457).

Adolescents and HIV Testing. The American Academy of Pediatrics (AAP) recommends that routine screening be offered to all adolescents at least once by 16 through 18 years of age in health care settings. Use of any licensed HIV antibody test is appropriate. For any positive test result, referral to an HIV specialist is appropriate to confirm diagnosis and initiate management. Adolescents with behaviors that increase risk of HIV acquisition (eg, multiple sex partners, illicit drug use) should be tested annually.

Consent for Diagnostic Testing. CDC recommends that diagnostic HIV testing and opt-out HIV screening be part of routine clinical care in all health care settings for patients 13 through 64 years of age, thus preserving the patient's option to decline HIV testing and allowing a provider-patient relationship conducive to optimal clinical and preventive care. Patients or people responsible for the patient's care should be notified orally that testing is planned, advised of the indication for testing and the implications of positive and negative test results, and offered an opportunity to ask questions and to decline testing. With such notification, the patient's general consent for medical care is considered sufficient for diagnostic HIV testing. Although parental involvement in an adolescent's health care may be desirable, it typically is not required when the adolescent consents to HIV testing. However, laws concerning consent and confidentiality for HIV care differ among states. Public health statutes and legal precedents allow for evaluation and treatment of minors for sexually transmitted infections without parental knowledge or consent, but not every state has explicitly defined HIV infection as a condition for which testing or treatment may proceed without parental consent. Health care professionals should endeavor to respect an adolescent's request for privacy. HIV screening should be discussed with all adolescents and encouraged for adolescents who are sexually active. Periodic HIV antibody testing should be performed for adolescents who remain at risk of HIV infection. Providing information regarding HIV infection, diagnostic testing, transmission including secondary transmission, and implications of infection is an essential component of the anticipatory guidance provided to all adolescents as part of primary care.

Access to clinical care, preventive counseling, and support services is essential for people with positive HIV test results.

TREATMENT: Because HIV treatment options and recommendations change with time and vary with occurrence of ARV drug resistance and adverse event profile, consultation with an expert in pediatric HIV infection is recommended in the care of HIV-infected infants, children, and adolescents. Current treatment recommendations for HIV-infected children are available online (**http://aidsinfo.nih.gov**). Whenever possible, enrollment of HIV-infected children in clinical trials should be encouraged. Information about trials for adolescents and children can be obtained by contacting the AIDS Clinical Trials Information Service.[1]

cART is indicated for most HIV-infected children. The principal objectives of therapy are to suppress viral replication maximally, to restore and preserve immune function, to reduce HIV-associated morbidity and mortality, to minimize drug toxicity, to maintain normal growth and development, and to improve quality of life. Initiation of cART depends on the age of the child and on a combination of virologic, immunologic, and clinical criteria.[2] Data from both observational studies and clinical trials indicate that very early initiation of therapy reduces morbidity and mortality compared with starting treatment when clinically symptomatic or immune suppressed. Effective administration of early therapy will maintain the viral load at low or undetectable concentrations and will reduce viral mutation and evolution.

Initiation of cART is recommended as follows[3]: (1) HIV-infected infants ≤12 months of age should receive cART irrespective of clinical symptoms, immune status, or viral load; (2) children from 1 to 3 years of age should receive cART: if they (a) have AIDS or significant HIV-related symptoms (CDC clinical categories C and B [except for the following category B condition: single episode of serious bacterial infection]), regardless of CD4+ T-lymphocyte counts or plasma viral load values; (b) have a CD4+ T-lymphocyte percentage <25% or CD4+ T-lymphocyte count <1000 cells/mm³, regardless of symptoms or viral load; or (c) are asymptomatic or mildly symptomatic (CDC clinical category A or N or the following category B condition: single episode of serious bacterial infection) and

---

[1]See Appendix I, Directory of Resources, p 975: AIDS Clinical Trials Information Service (available at **http://aidsinfo.nih.gov**).

[2]Panel on Antiretroviral Therapy and Medical Management of HIV-Infected Children. *Guidelines for the Use of Antiretroviral Agents in Pediatric HIV Infection.* August 11, 2011:1–268. Available at: **http://aidsinfo.nih.gov/ContentFiles/PediatricGuidelines.pdf**

[3]Centers for Disease Control and Prevention. Revised surveillance case definitions for HIV infection among adults, adolescents, and children aged <18 months and for HIV infection and AIDS among children aged 18 months to <13 years—United States, 2008. *MMWR Recomm Rep.* 2008;57(RR-10):1–12

have a CD4+ T-lymphocyte percentage ≥25% and a viral load of ≥100 000 copies/mL; (3) children 3 to 5 years of age should receive cART if they (a) have AIDS or significant HIV-related symptoms (CDC clinical categories C and B [except for the following category B condition: single episode of serious bacterial infection]); (b) have a CD4+ T-lymphocyte count ≤750 cells/mm³ or CD4 + T-lymphocyte percentage <25%; or (c) are asymptomatic or mildly symptomatic (CDC clinical category A or N or the following category B condition: single episode of serious bacterial infection) and have a CD4+ T-lymphocyte count >750 cells/mm³ and a viral load ≥100 000 copies/mL; (4) children ≥5 years of age should receive cART if they: (a) have AIDS or significant HIV-related symptoms (CDC clinical categories C and B [except for the following B condition: single episode of serious bacterial infection]); or (b) have a CD4 + T-lymphocyte count <500 cells/mm³. Starting cART should be considered[1] for HIV-infected children from 1 to 3 years of age who are asymptomatic or have mild symptoms (clinical category N or A, or the following clinical category B condition: single episode of serious bacterial infection) and have a CD4+ T-lymphocyte percentage ≥25% and a viral load <100 000 copies/mL. Initiation of cART also should be considered for HIV-infected children ≥5 years of age who are asymptomatic or have mild symptoms (clinical category N or A, or the following clinical category B condition: single episode of serious bacterial infection) and have a CD4+ T-lymphocyte count >500 cells/mm³ and a viral load <100 000 copies/mL. The child and the child's primary caregiver must be able to adhere to the prescribed regimen.

Initiation of treatment of adolescents[2] generally follows guidelines for adults, for whom initiation of treatment is strongly recommended: if an AIDS-defining illness is present or if the CD4+ T-lymphocyte count is <500 cells/mm³; or regardless of CD4+ T-lymphocyte count in patients with HIV-associated nephropathy or with hepatitis B virus infection when treatment of hepatitis B virus is recommended. cART should be considered for patients with CD4+ T-lymphocyte counts >500 cells/mm³. Dosages of ARVs can be prescribed according to age, weight, body surface area, or Tanner staging of puberty. Adolescents in early puberty (Tanner stages I and II) should be prescribed doses based on pediatric schedules, and adolescents in late puberty (Tanner stage III, IV, and V) should be prescribed doses based on adult schedules. In general, cART with at least 3 active drugs is recommended for all HIV-infected individuals requiring ARV therapy. Drug regimens most often include 2 NRTIs plus either a protease inhibitor or an NNRTI (**http://aidsinfo.nih.gov**). ARV resistance testing (viral genotyping) is recommended before starting treatment. Suppression of virus to undetectable levels is the desired goal. A change in ARV therapy should be considered if there is evidence of disease progression (virologic, immunologic, or clinical), toxicity of or intolerance to drugs, initial presence or development of drug resistance, or availability of data suggesting the possibility of a superior regimen.

---

[1]Guidelines for prevention and treatment of opportunistic infections in HIV-exposed and HIV-infected children. Recommendations from the National Institutes of Health, Centers for Disease Control and Prevention, the HIV Medicine Association of the Infectious Diseases Society of America, the Pediatric Infectious Diseases Society, and the American Academy of Pediatrics. *Pediatr Infect Dis J.* 2013;32(Suppl 2):i-KK4. Available at: **http://aidsinfo. nih.gov/guidelines/html/5/pediatric-oi-prevention-and-treatment-guidelines/0**

[2]Panel on Opportunistic Infections in HIV-Infected Adults and Adolescents. Guidelines for the prevention and treatment of opportunistic infections in HIV-infected adults and adolescents: recommendations from the Centers for Disease Control and Prevention, the National Institutes of Health, and the HIV Medicine Association of the Infectious Diseases Society of America. Washington, DC: US Department of Health and Human Services; 2013. Available at: **http://aidsinfo.nih.gov/contentfiles/lvguidelines/adult_oi.pdf**

Immune Globulin Intravenous (IGIV) therapy has been used in combination with cART for HIV-infected children with hypogammaglobulinemia (IgG <400 mg/dL [4.0 g/L]) and can be considered for HIV-infected children who have recurrent, serious bacterial infections, such as bacteremia, meningitis, or pneumonia. Trimethoprim-sulfamethoxazole prophylaxis may provide comparable protection. Typically, neither form of prophylaxis is necessary for patients receiving effective cART.

Early diagnosis, prophylaxis, and aggressive treatment of OIs may prolong survival.[1,2] This particularly is true for PCP, which accounts for approximately one third of pediatric AIDS diagnoses overall and may occur early in the first year of life. Prophylaxis is not recommended for infants who meet criteria for presumptive or definitive HIV-uninfected status. Thus, for infants with negative HIV diagnostic test results at 2 and 4 weeks of age (eg, no positive test results or clinical symptoms and who, therefore, are presumptively not infected with HIV), PCP prophylaxis would not need to be initiated. Because mortality rates are high, PCP chemoprophylaxis should be given to all HIV-exposed infants with indeterminate HIV infection status starting at 4 to 6 weeks of age but can be stopped if the child subsequently meets criteria for presumptive or definitive absence of HIV infection. All infants with HIV infection should receive PCP prophylaxis through 1 year of age regardless of immune status. The need for PCP prophylaxis for HIV-infected children 1 year and older is determined by the degree of immunosuppression from CD4+ T-lymphocyte percentage and count (see *Pneumocystis jirovecii* Infections, p 638).

Guidelines for prevention and treatment of OIs in children, adolescents, and adults provide indications for administration of drugs for infection with MAC, CMV, *T gondii*, and other organisms.[1,2] Successful suppression of HIV replication in the blood to undetectable levels by cART has resulted in relatively normal CD4+ and CD8+ T-lymphocyte counts, leading to a dramatic decrease in the occurrence of most OIs. Limited data on the safety of discontinuing prophylaxis in HIV-infected children receiving cART are available; however, prophylaxis should not be discontinued in HIV-infected infants younger than 1 year irrespective of the viral or immunologic response. For older children, many experts consider discontinuing PCP prophylaxis on the basis of CD4+ T-lymphocyte count[2] for those who have received at least 6 months of effective cART: (1) for children 1 through 5 years of age, CD4+ T-lymphocyte percentage of at least 15% or CD4+ T-lymphocyte absolute count of at least 500 cells/µL for more than 3 consecutive months; and (2) for children 6 years or older, CD4+ T-lymphocyte percentage of at least 15% or the CD4+ T-lymphocyte absolute count of at least 200 cells/µL for more than 3 consecutive months. Subsequently, the CD4+ T-lymphocyte absolute count or percentage should be reevaluated at least every 3 months. Prophylaxis should be reinstituted if the original criteria for prophylaxis are reached again.

---

[1]Guidelines for prevention and treatment of opportunistic infections in HIV-exposed and HIV-infected children. Recommendations from the National Institutes of Health, Centers for Disease Control and Prevention, the HIV Medicine Association of the Infectious Diseases Society of America, the Pediatric Infectious Diseases Society, and the American Academy of Pediatrics. *Pediatr Infect Dis J.* 2013;32(Suppl 2):i-KK4. Available at: **http:// aidsinfo.nih.gov/ guidelines/ html/ 5/ pediatric-oi-prevention-and-treatment-guidelines/ 0**

[2]Panel on Opportunistic Infections in HIV-Infected Adults and Adolescents. Guidelines for the Prevention and Treatment of Opportunistic Infections in HIV-Infected Adults and Adolescents: Recommendations from the Centers for Disease Control and Prevention, the National Institutes of Health, and the HIV Medicine Association of the Infectious Diseases Society of America. Washington, DC: US Department of Health and Human Services; 2013. Available at: **http:// aidsinfo.nih.gov/ contentfiles/ lvguidelines/ adult_oi.pdf**

Immunization Recommendations (also see Immunization in Special Clinical Circumstances, p 68, and Table 1.15, p 75). All recommended childhood immunizations should be given to HIV-exposed infants. If HIV infection is confirmed, guidelines for the HIV-infected child should be followed. Children with HIV infection should be immunized as soon as is age appropriate with inactivated vaccines. Inactivated influenza vaccine (IIV) should be given annually according to the most current recommendations. Additionally, live-virus vaccines (measles-mumps-rubella [MMR] and varicella) can be given to asymptomatic HIV-infected children and adolescents without severe immunosuppression (ie, CD4 + T-lymphocyte percentage greater than 15% for at least 6 months in children 1 through 5 years of age and CD4+ T-lymphocyte percentage greater than 15% and a CD4+ T-lymphocyte count greater than 200 lymphocytes/mm^3 for a 6-month period in those 6 years and older). Severely immunocompromised HIV-infected infants, children, adolescents, and young adults should not receive measles virus-containing vaccine, because vaccine-related pneumonia has been reported. The quadrivalent measles-mumps-rubella-varicella (MMRV) vaccine should not be administered to any HIV-infected infants, regardless of degree of immunosuppression, because of lack of safety data in this population. Rotavirus vaccine may be given to HIV-exposed and HIV-infected infants irrespective of CD4+ T-lymphocyte percentage or count. All HIV-infected children should receive a dose of 23-valent polysaccharide pneumococcal vaccine after 24 months of age, with a minimal interval of 8 weeks since the last conjugate pneumococcal vaccine. Although HIV infection is not an indication for pneumococcal vaccine, people at increased risk of meningococcal disease who have HIV infection and are 2 years or older should receive a 2-dose primary series of the quadrivalent meningococcal vaccine at least 8 weeks apart. Adolescents 11 through 18 years of age who are HIV infected should receive all inactivated vaccines recommended for this age group, including the 3-dose series of human papillomavirus vaccine. The suggested schedule for administration of these vaccines is provided in the recommended childhood and adolescent immunization schedule **(http://redbook.solutions.aap.org/SS/ Immunization_Schedules.aspx).**

Children Who Are HIV Uninfected Residing in the Household of an HIV-Infected Person. Members of households in which an adult or child has HIV infection can receive MMR vaccine, because these vaccine viruses are not transmitted person to person. To decrease the risk of transmission of influenza to patients with symptomatic HIV infection, all household members 6 months or older should receive yearly influenza immunization (see Influenza, p 476). Immunization with varicella vaccine of siblings and susceptible adult caregivers of patients with HIV infection is encouraged to prevent acquisition of wild-type varicella-zoster virus infection, which can cause severe disease in immunocompromised hosts. Transmission of varicella vaccine virus from an immunocompetent host to a household contact is very uncommon.

Postexposure Passive Immunization of HIV-Infected Children.

Measles (see Measles, p 535). All HIV-infected children exposed to measles should receive Immune Globulin Intramuscular (IGIM), with the dose depending on the level of immune suppression. Asymptomatic mildly or moderately immune compromised HIV-infected patients should receive intramuscular IGIM at a dose of 0.5 mL/kg (maximum 15 mL), regardless of immunization status. Severely immunocompromised HIV-infected patients should receive IGIV at a dose of 400 mg/kg. Children who have received IGIV within 2 weeks of exposure do not require additional passive immunization.

Tetanus. HIV-infected children with severe immune suppression who sustain wounds classified as tetanus prone (see Tetanus, p 773, and Table 3.75, p 775) should receive Tetanus Immune Globulin regardless of immunization status, as recommended in the general HIV-uninfected pediatric population.

Varicella. HIV-infected children without a history of previous chickenpox or who lack evidence of immunity to varicella, including detectable varicella-zoster virus-specific immune response (either antibody or cell-mediated immune response or both) or children who have not received 2 doses of varicella vaccine should receive Varicella-Zoster Immune Globulin, if available, ideally within 96 hours but potentially beneficial up to 10 days, after close contact with a person who has chickenpox or shingles (see Varicella-Zoster Infections, p 846). Although many experts limit this recommendation to severely immune compromised children (ie, CDC immunologic category 3),[1] especially if also categorized as CDC Clinical Category C and experiencing a high plasma RNA viral load, other experts elect to extend the recommendation to include children who previously have been immunized with varicella vaccine and are moderately or severely immune compromised (ie, CDC immunologic category 2 or 3). An alternative to Varicella-Zoster Immune Globulin for passive immunization is IGIV, 400 mg/kg, administered once within 10 days after exposure. Children who have received IGIV within 2 weeks of exposure do not require additional passive immunization.

ISOLATION OF THE HOSPITALIZED PATIENT: Standard precautions should be followed by all health care professionals regardless of suspected or confirmed status of the patient. The risk to health care professionals of acquiring HIV infection from a patient is minimal, even after accidental exposure from a needlestick injury (see Epidemiology, p 459). Nevertheless, every effort should be made to avoid direct exposures to blood and other body fluids, especially those that could contain HIV. Guidelines for use of occupational postexposure prophylaxis have been published by the CDC and should be started as soon as possible after the exposure but within 72 hours for maximal effectiveness (**http://aidsinfo.nih.gov/contentfiles/HealthCareOccupExpoGL.pdf**).

CONTROL MEASURES:

Interruption of Mother-to-Child Transmission of HIV. Development and implementation of efficacious interventions to prevent mother-to-child transmission of HIV has resulted in a marked decrease in cases of mother-to-child transmission of HIV infection in the United States. Following are the recommendations of the US Public Health Service, AAP, and American College of Obstetricians and Gynecologists for the prevention of mother-to-child transmission of HIV.[2,3,4]

---

[1]Centers for Disease Control and Prevention. 1994 revised classification system for human immunodeficiency virus infection in children less than 13 years of age. Official authorized addenda: human immunodeficiency virus infection codes and official guidelines for coding and reporting ICD-9-CM. *MMWR Recomm Rep.* 1994;43(RR-12):1–19

[2]For complete listing of current policy statements from the American Academy of Pediatrics regarding human immunodeficiency virus and acquired immunodeficiency syndrome, see **http://aappolicy.aappublications.org/**.

[3]American Academy of Pediatrics, American College of Obstetricians and Gynecologists. Human immunodeficiency virus screening. Joint statement of the American Academy of Pediatrics and the American College of Obstetricians and Gynecologists. *Pediatrics.* 1999;104(1 Pt 1):128 (Reaffirmed May 2012)

[4]American Academy of Pediatrics, Committee on Pediatric AIDS. HIV testing and prophylaxis to prevent mother-to-child transmission in the United States. *Pediatrics.* 2008;122(5):1127–1134 (Reaffirmed June 2011)

The AAP and CDC recommend an opt-out approach for HIV testing of all pregnant women in all health care settings in the United States[1,2]: routine HIV screening for every pregnant woman after she is notified that testing will be performed unless she declines. For women in labor with undocumented HIV infection status during the current pregnancy, immediate maternal HIV testing with opt-out consent, using a rapid HIV antibody test, is recommended. In many states, routinely offering HIV testing during pregnancy is mandated by law. Education about HIV infection and testing should be part of a comprehensive program of health care for all women during their childbearing years.

Four effective interventions to prevent mother-to-child transmission of HIV are utilized in the United States: antiretroviral prophylaxis, as indicated (viral load >1000 copies/mL), cesarean delivery before labor (at 38 weeks' completed gestation) and before rupture of membranes, complete avoidance of breastfeeding, and complete avoidance of premastication. It is important to diagnose HIV infection early in pregnancy to allow antenatal implementation of interventions to prevent transmission (ARV prophylaxis and cesarean delivery before labor and before rupture of membranes). In resource-limited countries where complete avoidance of breastfeeding (replacement feeding) often is not safe, exclusive breastfeeding is associated with a lower risk of postnatal HIV transmission or infant morbidity/mortality than are mixed breastfeeding and formula feeding. Both maternal and infant ARV prophylaxis during breastfeeding are effective in reducing mother-to-child transmission of HIV.

Maternal ARV Therapy and Perinatal HIV Prophylaxis. HIV-infected pregnant women should use cART regimens, both for treatment of the mother's HIV infection and for prevention of mother-to-child transmission of HIV. Virologic suppression is the goal both during pregnancy and following delivery for mothers presenting for care. Detailed recommendations for use of ARVs in HIV-infected pregnant women can be found online (**http://aidsinfo.nih.gov**). Ideally, women initiating such a regimen during pregnancy should be tested for the presence of ARV resistance. However, initiation of ARV prophylaxis should not be delayed, especially if these decisions are being made late in pregnancy. Most women in industrialized nations are treated with potent combinations of 3 ARVs started after the first trimester (unless treatment is required for maternal health reasons, in which case the benefit of starting during the first trimester outweighs potential risk to the infant) and continuing to delivery. Oral zidovudine may be used as part of that therapy, because it was the drug used in the first successful clinical trial of ARV prophylaxis during the prepartum, intrapartum, and postpartum periods for prevention of mother-to-child transmission of HIV. This intervention decreased mother-to-child transmission of HIV by two thirds (see Table 3.32, p 472). HIV-infected women with HIV RNA ≥400 copies/mL (or unknown HIV RNA) near delivery should be administered intravenous (IV) zidovudine during labor, regardless of antepartum regimen or mode of delivery. On the basis of pharmacokinetic data, in women with HIV RNA ≥400 copies/mL near delivery for whom zidovudine is recommended, IV would be preferred to oral administration in the United States; in situations where IV administration is not possible, oral administration can be considered (Table 3.32, p 472). A pregnant woman already receiving treatment that does not include zidovudine need not have her ARV regimen changed if her viral

---

[1]Centers for Disease Control and Prevention. 1993 revised classification system for HIV infection and expanded surveillance case definition for AIDS among adolescents and adults. *MMWR Recomm Rep.* 1992;41(RR-17):1–19

[2]Centers for Disease Control and Prevention. Revised recommendations for HIV testing of adults, adolescents, and pregnant women in health-care settings. *MMWR Recomm Rep.* 2006;55(RR-14):1–18

Table 3.32. Zidovudine Regimen for Decreasing the Rate of Mother-to-Child Transmission of HIV[a,b]

Period of Time	Route	Dosage
During pregnancy, initiate anytime after week 14 of gestation and continue throughout pregnancy[c]	Oral	200 mg, 3 times per day, or 300 mg, 2 times per day
During labor and delivery[d]	Intravenous	2 mg/kg during the first hour, then 1 mg/kg per hour until delivery
For the newborn infant ≥35 weeks' gestation, as soon as possible after birth[b,e]	Oral	4 mg/kg, twice daily, for the first 6 weeks of life[f]
For the newborn infant ≥30 to <35 weeks' gestation, as soon as possible after birth[b,e]	Oral	2 mg/kg, twice daily for 14 days then increase to 3 mg/kg, twice daily, to complete a total of 6 weeks of treatment[f]
	Intravenous	1.5 mg/kg, twice daily (maximum of 6 weeks). When able to tolerate oral medications, the twice-daily dose is 2 mg/kg until 14 days of life and then 3 mg/kg to complete 6 weeks of treatment[f]
For the newborn infant <30 weeks' gestation, as soon as possible after birth[b,e]	Oral	2 mg/kg, twice daily for 28 days, then increase to 3 mg/kg, twice daily, to complete a total of 6 weeks of treatment[f]
	Intravenous	1.5 mg/kg, twice daily (maximum of 6 weeks). When able to tolerate oral medications, the twice-daily dose is 2 mg/kg until 28 days of life and then 3 mg/kg to complete a total of 6 weeks of treatment[f]

IV indicates Intravenous; PO, oral.

[a] Modified from Panel on Treatment of HIV-Infected Pregnant Women and Prevention of Perinatal Transmission: Recommendations for Use of Antiretroviral Drugs in Pregnant HIV-1-Infected Women for Maternal Health and Interventions to Reduce Perinatal HIV Transmission in the United States. Washington, DC: US Department of Health and Human Services; 2014. Available at: **http://aidsinfo.nih.gov/contentfiles/PerinatalGL.pdf.** Information about other antiretroviral drugs for decreasing the rate of perinatal transmission of HIV can be found online (**http://aidsinfo.nih.gov).**

[b] For infants whose mothers received no antepartum antiretroviral prophylaxis, nevirapine in the following birth weight-based doses' should be given as soon after delivery as possible, in addition to zidovudine. Weight-based dosing: birth weight 1.5-2 kg: 8 mg total for each dose; birth weight: >2 kg: 12 mg total for each dose. The first dose should be given as soon as possible after delivery up to 48 hours of life. The second dose should be given 48 hours after the first dose. The third dose should be given 96 hours after the second dose.

[c] Most women in industrialized nations are treated with potent combinations of 3 antiretroviral agents (antiretroviral therapy [ART]) started after the first trimester (unless treatment is required for maternal health reasons, in which case the benefit of starting during the first trimester outweighs potential risk to the infant) and continuing to delivery. Oral zidovudine may be used as part of that therapy.

[d] IV zidovudine no longer is required for HIV-infected women receiving combination antiretroviral regimens who have HIV RNA <400 copies/mL near delivery. HIV-infected women with HIV RNA ≥400 copies/mL (or unknown HIV RNA) near delivery should be administered IV zidovudine during labor, regardless of antepartum regimen or mode of delivery. On the basis of pharmacokinetic data, in women with HIV RNA ≥400 copies/mL near delivery for whom zidovudine is recommended, IV would be preferred to oral administration in the United States; in situations where IV administration is not possible, oral administration can be considered.

[e] The effectiveness of antiretroviral agents for prevention of mother-to-child transmission of HIV decreases with delay in initiation after birth. Initiation of postexposure prophylaxis after the first 48 hours of life is not likely to be effective in preventing transmission.

[f] In the United Kingdom and many other European countries, a 4-week neonatal chemoprophylaxis regimen is recommended for infants born to mothers who have received antenatal combination ARV drug regimens. This approach also can be considered in cases in which adherence to or toxicity from the 6-week zidovudine prophylaxis regimen is a concern.

load is suppressed. Regardless of the mother's ARV regimen, after birth, the infant should receive 6 weeks of oral zidovudine. As noted previously, observational studies suggest that use of cART regimens during pregnancy is associated with a lower risk of mother-to-child transmission of HIV than zidovudine monotherapy alone.

Note that efavirenz is classified as a class D teratogen by the FDA and should not normally be included in maternal regimens begun during the first trimester. However, because the risk of neural tube defects is restricted to the first 5 to 6 weeks of pregnancy and because unnecessary ARV drug changes occurring during pregnancy may lead to loss of viral control, efavirenz can be continued in pregnant women presenting after the first 6 weeks of pregnancy who are on an efavirenz-containing regimen with successful virologic suppression.

Health care professionals who treat HIV-infected pregnant women and their infants should report instances of prenatal exposure to ARVs (either alone or in combination) to the Antiretroviral Pregnancy Registry (1-800-258-4263 or **www.apregistry.com**). Long-term follow-up is recommended for all infants exposed to ARVs in utero or postnatally.

Intrapartum management of HIV-infected women and the immediate postnatal care of their newborn infants is multifaceted. The woman's regular HIV medical subspecialist and the delivering physician should be contacted to discuss the impending delivery and to review the patient's current and postpartum ARV regimen. For women in labor with undocumented HIV infection status, a rapid HIV test should be performed as soon as possible. For an HIV-infected woman, her routine oral ARVs should be continued on schedule (with the exception of stavudine [d4T, Zerit], which should not be coadministered with zidovudine). Any procedures that compromise the integrity of fetal skin during labor and delivery (eg, fetal electrodes) or that increase the occurrence of maternal bleeding (eg, instrumented vaginal delivery, episiotomy, vaginal tears) should be avoided when possible. As noted previously, prolonged rupture of membranes is associated with an increased risk of mother-to-child transmission of HIV, whereas cesarean delivery before labor and before rupture of membranes reduces the risk of mother-to-child transmission and is recommended at 38 weeks' gestation for women with plasma viral loads >1000 copies/mL and women with unknown plasma viral loads around the time of delivery (**http://aidsinfo.nih.gov/Guidelines**).

The newborn infant should be bathed and cleaned of maternal secretions (especially bloody secretions) as soon as possible after birth. Newborn infants should begin ARV prophylaxis as soon as possible after birth, preferably within 12 hours. In the United States, neonatal prophylaxis generally consists of zidovudine for 6 weeks. Among infants whose mothers did not receive any ARVs before onset of labor, neonatal postexposure prophylaxis with a 2- or 3-drug ARV regimen results in a lower rate of mother-to-child transmission of HIV than zidovudine alone. A 2-drug regimen of zidovudine for 6 weeks with 3 doses of nevirapine during the first week of life (as soon as possible after birth, 48 hours after first dose, and 96 hours after second dose) is as effective but less toxic than a 3-drug regimen of zidovudine, lamivudine, and nelfinavir. Therefore, current recommendations for infants of HIV-infected women who did not receive any ARVs before onset of labor are for administration of this 2-drug neonatal prophylaxis regimen (Table 3.32, p 472). Detailed guidance is available regarding infant ARV prophylaxis regimens.[1]

---

[1]Panel on Treatment of HIV-Infected Pregnant Women and Prevention of Perinatal Transmission. Recommendations for Use of Antiretroviral Drugs in Pregnant HIV-1-Infected Women for Maternal Health and Interventions to Reduce Perinatal HIV Transmission in the United States. Washington, DC: US Department of Health and Human Services; 2014. Available at: **http://aidsinfo.nih.gov/contentfiles/PerinatalGL.pdf**

Both mother and infant should have prescriptions for the HIV drugs when they leave the hospital, and the infant should have an appointment for a postnatal visit at 2 to 4 weeks of age to monitor medication adherence and to screen the infant for anemia attributable to zidovudine.

For a newborn infant whose mother's HIV infection status is unknown, the newborn infant's physician should perform rapid HIV antibody testing on the mother or the infant, with appropriate consent as required by state and local law. Test results should be reported to the physician as soon as possible to allow effective ARV prophylaxis to be administered to the infant, ideally within 12 hours. In some states, rapid testing of the neonate is required by law if the mother has refused to be tested.

The newborn infant's physician should be informed of the mother's HIV infection status so that appropriate care and follow-up of the infant can be accomplished. An HIV-infected mother and her infant should be referred to a facility that provides HIV-related services for both women and children.

Breastfeeding (also see Human Milk, p 125). Transmission of HIV by breastfeeding accounts for one third to one half of perinatal HIV transmission worldwide and is more likely among mothers who acquire HIV infection late in pregnancy or during the postpartum period. The rate of late postnatal HIV transmission (after 4 weeks of age) in sub-Saharan African countries is approximately 9 transmissions per 100 child-years of breastfeeding (0.7% transmission/month of breastfeeding) and is relatively constant. Late postnatal transmission is associated with reduced maternal CD4+ T-lymphocyte count, high plasma and human milk viral load, mastitis/breast abscess, and infant oral lesions (eg, oral thrush). Clinical trials in resource-limited settings have demonstrated efficacy of ARV treatment of HIV-infected women while breastfeeding and of ARV prophylaxis to breastfeeding children of HIV-infected women. However, because such prophylaxis cannot be assumed to be completely protective against mother-to-child transmission of HIV, in countries where safe alternative sources of infant feeding readily are available, affordable, and culturally accepted, such as the United States, HIV-infected women should be counseled not to breastfeed their infants or donate to human milk banks. Similarly, women in industrialized countries who are receiving cART for their own health, even if they have undetectable HIV viral loads, also should be counseled not to breastfeed because of the continued possibility of HIV transmission.

In general, women who are known to be HIV uninfected should be encouraged to breastfeed. However, women who are HIV uninfected but who are known to have HIV-infected sex partners or bisexual partners or are active injection drug users should be counseled about the potential risk of acquiring HIV infection themselves and of then transmitting HIV through human milk. Such women should be counseled to use condoms and to undergo frequent HIV testing (eg, monthly to every 3 months) during the breastfeeding period to detect potential maternal HIV seroconversion. In addition, in the case of condom breakage during sexual intercourse with the HIV-infected discordant partner, women should be counseled to undergo immediate HIV testing and initiation of HIV postexposure prophylaxis within 72 hours of the condom breakage.

Premastication. Probable transmission of HIV by caregivers who premasticated food for infants has been described in 3 cases in the United States. In 2 of the cases, the caregivers had bleeding gums or sores in their mouths during the time they premasticated the food. Phylogenetic testing was conducted and documented matches of the viral strains in 2 of the caregiver-infant dyads. It is hypothesized that the transmission was via bloodborne virus in the saliva rather than via salivary virus. The CDC recommends that in the United States, where safe alternative methods of feeding are available, HIV-infected caregivers should be asked about whether they practice premastication and counseled not to premasticate food for infants.

HIV in the Athletic Setting. Athletes and staff of athletic programs can be exposed to blood during certain athletic activities. Recommendations have been developed by the AAP for prevention of transmission of HIV and other bloodborne pathogens in the athletic setting (see School Health, Infections Spread by Blood and Body Fluids, p 158).

Sexual Abuse. In cases of proven or suspected sexual abuse, the child should be tested serologically as soon as possible and then periodically for 6 months (eg, at 2–6 weeks, 3 months, and 6 months after last known sexual contact) (see Sexual Victimization and STIs, p 185). Serologic evaluation for HIV infection of the perpetrator should be attempted soon after the incident but may not be able to be performed until indictment has occurred. Counseling of the child and family needs to be provided (see Sexually Transmitted Infections, p 177).

Prevention of HIV Transmission Through Adult Behaviors (Sexual Activity). Abstinence from sexual activity is the only certain way to prevent sexual transmission of HIV. Safer sex practices, including use of condoms for all sexual encounters (vaginal, anal, and oral sex) can reduce HIV transmission significantly by reducing exposure to body fluids containing HIV. Suppressing HIV viral load to undetectable levels in the blood with cART regimens has resulted in decreases in transmission in discordant couples by as much as 96%.[1] In MSM, continuous preexposure prophylaxis with ARV therapy (tenofovir and emtricitabine) was associated with reduction in HIV acquisition by 44% in the uninfected partner in a discordant couple. The efficacy of preexposure prophylaxis is higher with improved medication adherence. Preexposure prophylaxis also is effective in heterosexual couples and injecting drug users.[2,3] Because data on efficacy and long-term safety of preexposure ARV prophylaxis in MSM are limited, preexposure prophylaxis should be performed using guidelines provided by the CDC (**www.cdc.gov/hiv/prep/pdf/PREPfactsheet.pdf**). ARV-based vaginal microbicides (1% tenofovir gel) have reduced HIV acquisition in uninfected women by 39%. Data from Africa also provide evidence that medical male circumcision can reduce HIV acquisition in uninfected heterosexual males by 38% to 66% over 24 months.

Postexposure Prophylaxis for Possible Sexual or Other Nonoccupational Exposure to HIV.[4] Decisions to provide ARVs after possible nonoccupational (ie, community) exposure to HIV must balance the potential benefits and risks. Decisions regarding the need for ARV prophylaxis in such instances are predicated on the probability that the source is infected or contaminated with HIV, the likelihood of transmission by the particular exposure, and the

---

[1]Cohen MS, McCauley M, Gamble TR. HIV treatment as prevention and HPTN 052. *Curr Opin HIV AIDS.* 2012;7(2):99–105

[2]Thigpen MC, Kebaabetswe PM, Paxton LA, et al. Antiretroviral preexposure prophylaxis for heterosexual HIV transmission in Botswana. *N Engl J Med.* 2012;367(5):423–434

[3]Choopanya K, Martin M, Suntharasamai P, et al. Antiretroviral prophylaxis for HIV infection among injecting drug users in Bangkok, Thailand: a randomised, double-blind, placebo-controlled phase 3 trial. *Lancet.* 2013;381(9883):2083–2090

[4]US Department of Health and Human Services. Antiretroviral postexposure prophylaxis after sexual, injection-drug use, or other nonoccupational exposure to HIV in the United States: recommendations from the US Department of Health and Human Services. *MMWR Recomm Rep.* 2005;54(RR-2):1–20

interval between exposure and initiation of therapy, balanced against expected adverse effects associated with the regimen.

The risk of transmission of HIV from a puncture wound attributable to a needle found in the community is likely lower than 0.3%,[1] the estimated probability of HIV transmission associated with a puncture wound involving a known HIV-contaminated needle in a health care setting. The actual risks of HIV infection in an infant or child after a needlestick injury or sexual abuse are unknown. To date, there are no confirmed transmissions of HIV from accidental nonoccupational needlestick injuries (needles found in the community). The estimated risk of HIV transmission per episode of receptive penile-anal sexual exposure is 50 per 10 000 exposures, whereas the estimated risk per episode of receptive vaginal exposure is 10 per 10 000 exposures.

All ARVs are associated with adverse effects. In HIV-infected adults receiving cART regimens for treatment of HIV, an estimated 24% to 36% discontinue the drugs because of adverse effects. Adverse effects also are reported by a significant proportion of adults without HIV infection receiving ARV postexposure prophylaxis. Use of daily nevirapine for postexposure prophylaxis is not recommended because of the high incidence of severe (and rarely fatal) adverse effects in adults with normal CD4+ T-lymphocyte counts. Such adverse effects have not been reported with single-dose intrapartum/infant nevirapine used for prevention of mother-to-child transmission of HIV.

ARVs generally should not be used if the risk of transmission is low (eg, trivial needlestick injury with a drug needle from an unknown nonoccupational source) or if care is sought more than 72 hours after the reported exposure.[2] The benefits of postexposure prophylaxis are greatest when risk of infection is high, intervention is prompt, and adherence is likely. Consultation with an experienced pediatric HIV health care professional is essential.

Transition of Adolescents to Adult HIV Health Care Settings. In industrialized countries, it increasingly has become likely that HIV-infected children will survive (and thrive) well into adolescence and young adulthood. Therefore, pediatric and adult HIV programs may benefit from establishment of transition programs to introduce adolescents to the adult health care setting. Successful transition requires careful proactive planning by caregivers in both pediatric and adult venues and a multifaceted, deliberate attention to the medical, psychosocial, life-skills, educational, and family-centered needs of the patient.

The transition period is a convenient time to stress repeatedly the need for adherence to the cART regimen. Compliance is of paramount importance to virologic success. It also is an ideal time to reemphasize topics of contraception, prevention of sexually transmitted infections, and safer sex practices.

Influenza

CLINICAL MANIFESTATIONS: Influenza typically begins with sudden onset of fever, often accompanied by chills or rigors, headache, malaise, diffuse myalgia, and nonproductive cough. Subsequently, respiratory tract signs, including sore throat, nasal congestion,

---

[1]Bell TA, Hagan HC. Management of children with hypodermic needle injuries. *Pediatr Inf Dis J.* 1995;14(3):254–255

[2]Havens PL; American Academy of Pediatrics, Committee on Pediatric AIDS. Postexposure prophylaxis in children and adolescents for nonoccupational exposure to human immunodeficiency virus. *Pediatrics.* 2003;111(6):1475–1489 (Reaffirmed October 2008)

rhinitis, and cough, become more prominent. Conjunctival injection, abdominal pain, nausea, vomiting, and diarrhea less commonly are associated with influenza illness. In some children, influenza can appear as an upper respiratory tract infection or as a febrile illness with few respiratory tract symptoms. Influenza is an important cause of otitis media. Acute myositis characterized by calf tenderness and refusal to walk has been described. In infants, influenza can produce a sepsis-like picture and occasionally can cause croup, bronchiolitis, or pneumonia. Although the large majority of children with influenza recover fully after 3 to 7 days, previously healthy children can have severe symptoms and complications. In the 2013–2014 influenza season, approximately 43% of all children hospitalized with influenza had no known underlying conditions. Neurologic complications associated with influenza range from febrile seizures to severe encephalopathy and encephalitis with status epilepticus, with resulting neurologic sequelae or death. Reye syndrome, which now is a very rare condition, has been associated with influenza infection and the use of aspirin therapy during the illness. Children with influenza or suspected influenza should not be given aspirin. Death from influenza-associated myocarditis has been reported. Invasive secondary infections or coinfections with group A streptococcus, *Staphylococcus aureus* (including methicillin-resistant *S aureus* [MRSA]), *Streptococcus pneumoniae*, or other bacterial pathogens can result in severe disease and death.

ETIOLOGY: Influenza viruses are orthomyxoviruses of 3 genera or types (A, B, and C). Epidemic disease is caused by influenza virus types A and B, and both influenza A and B virus antigens are included in influenza vaccines. Type C influenza viruses cause sporadic mild influenza-like illness in children and antigens are not included in influenza vaccines. The virus type or subtype may have an effect on the number of hospitalizations and deaths that season. For example, seasons with influenza A (H3N2) as the predominant circulating strain have had 2.7 times higher average mortality rates than other seasons. The 2009 influenza A (H1N1) pandemic combined both exceptional pediatric virulence and lack of immunity, which resulted in nearly 4 times as many pediatric deaths as usually recorded.

Influenza A viruses are subclassified into subtypes by 2 surface antigens, hemagglutinin (HA) and neuraminidase (NA). Examples of these include H1N1 and H3N2 viruses. Specific antibodies to these various antigens, especially to hemagglutinin, are important determinants of immunity. Minor antigenic variation within the same influenza B type or influenza A subtypes is called *antigenic drift*. Antigenic drift occurs continuously and results in new strains of influenza A and B viruses, leading to seasonal epidemics. On the basis of ongoing global surveillance data, there have been only 5 times since 1986 that the vaccine strains in the influenza vaccine have not changed from the previous season. *Antigenic shifts* are major changes in influenza A viruses that result in new subtypes that contain a new HA alone or with a new NA. Antigenic shift occurs only with influenza A viruses and can lead a to pandemic if the new strain can infect humans and be transmitted efficiently from person to person in a sustained manner in the setting of little or no preexisting immunity.

From April 2009 to August 2010, the World Health Organization declared such a pandemic caused by influenza A (H1N1) virus. There now have been 4 influenza pandemics caused by antigenic shift in the 20th and 21st centuries. The 2009 pandemic was associated with 2 waves of substantial activity in the United States, occurring in the spring and fall of 2009 and extending well into winter 2010. During this time, more than 99% of virus isolates characterized were the 2009 pandemic influenza A (H1N1) virus. As with previous antigenic shifts, the 2009 pandemic influenza A (H1N1) viral strain has replaced the previously circulating seasonal influenza A (H1N1) strain.

Humans of all ages occasionally are infected with influenza A viruses of swine or avian origin. Human infections with swine viruses have manifested as typical influenza-like illness, and confirmation of infection caused by an influenza virus of swine origin has been discovered retrospectively during routine typing of human influenza isolates. For example, influenza A (H3N2v) viruses with the matrix (M) gene from the 2009 H1N1 pandemic virus first were detected in people in 2011 and were responsible for a multistate outbreak in summer 2012. Most cases were associated with exposure to swine at agricultural fairs, and no sustained human-to-human transmission was observed. Similarly, human infections with avian influenza viruses are uncommon but may result in a spectrum of disease including mild respiratory symptoms and conjunctivitis to severe lower respiratory tract disease, acute respiratory distress syndrome (ARDS), and death. Most notable among avian influenza viruses are A (H5N1) and A (H7N9), both of which have been associated with severe disease and high case-fatality rates. Influenza A (H5N1) viruses emerged as human infections in 1997 and have since caused human disease in Asia, Africa, Europe, and the Middle East, areas where these viruses are present in domestic or wild birds. Influenza A (H7N9) infections were first detected in 2013 and have been associated with sporadic disease in China. Infection with a novel influenza A virus is a nationally reportable disease and should be reported to the Centers for Disease Control and Prevention (CDC) through state health departments.

EPIDEMIOLOGY: Influenza is spread from person to person, primarily by respiratory tract droplets created by coughing or sneezing. Contact with respiratory tract droplet-contaminated surfaces followed by autoinoculation is another mode of transmission. During community outbreaks of influenza, the highest incidence occurs among school-aged children. Secondary spread to adults and other children within a family is common. Incidence and disease severity depend, in part, on immunity developed as a result of previous experience (by natural disease) or recent influenza immunization with the circulating strain or a related strain. Influenza A viruses, including 2 subtypes (H1N1 and H3N2), and influenza B viruses circulate worldwide, but the prevalence of each can vary among communities and within a single community over the course of an influenza season. Antigenic drift in the circulating strain(s) is associated with seasonal epidemics. In temperate climates, seasonal epidemics usually occur during winter months. Peak influenza activity in the United States can occur anytime from November to May but most commonly occurs between January and March. Community outbreaks can last 4 to 8 weeks or longer. Circulation of 2 or 3 influenza virus strains in a community may be associated with a prolonged influenza season of 3 months or more and bimodal peaks in activity. Influenza is highly contagious, especially among semi-enclosed institutionalized populations and other ongoing, closed-group gatherings, such as school and preschool/child care classrooms. Patients may be infectious 24 hours before onset of symptoms. Viral shedding in nasal secretions usually peaks during the first 3 days of illness and ceases within 7 days but can be prolonged in young children and immunodeficient patients for 10 days or even longer. Viral shedding is correlated directly with degree of fever.

Incidence of influenza in healthy children generally is 10% to 40% each year, but illness rates as low as 3% also have been reported, depending on the circulating strain. Tens of thousands of children visit clinics and emergency departments because of influenza illness each season. Influenza and its complications have been reported to result in a 10%

to 30% increase in the number of courses of antimicrobial agents prescribed to children during the influenza season. Although bacterial coinfections with a variety of pathogens, including MRSA, have been reported, medical care encounters for children with influenza are an important cause of inappropriate antimicrobial use.

Hospitalization rates among children younger than 2 years are similar to hospitalization rates among people 65 years and older. Rates vary among studies (190–480 per 100 000 population) because of differences in methodology and severity of influenza seasons. However, children younger than 24 months consistently are at a substantially higher risk of hospitalization than older children. Antecedent influenza infection sometimes is associated with development of pneumococcal or staphylococcal pneumonia in children. Methicillin-resistant staphylococcal community-acquired pneumonia, with a rapid clinical progression and a high fatality rate, has been reported in previously healthy children and adults with concomitant influenza infection. Rates of hospitalization and morbidity attributable to complications, such as bronchitis and pneumonia, are even greater in children with high-risk conditions, including asthma, diabetes mellitus, hemodynamically significant cardiac disease, immunosuppression, and neurologic and neurodevelopmental disorders. Influenza virus infection in neonates also has been associated with considerable morbidity, including a sepsis-like syndrome, apnea, and lower respiratory tract disease.

Fatal outcomes, including sudden death, have been reported in both chronically ill and previously healthy children. Since influenza-related pediatric deaths became nationally notifiable in 2004, the number of deaths among children reported annually in nonpandemic seasons has ranged from 46 (2005–2006 season) to 171 (2012–2013 season); during the 2009–2010 season, the number of pediatric deaths in the United States was 288. During the entire influenza A (H1N1) pandemic period lasting from April 2009 to August 2010, a total of 344 laboratory-confirmed, influenza-associated pediatric deaths were reported. Both influenza A and B viruses have been associated with deaths in children, most of which have occurred in children younger than 5 years. Almost half of children who die do not have a high-risk condition as defined by the Advisory Committee on Immunization Practices (ACIP). All influenza-associated pediatric deaths are nationally notifiable and should be reported to the CDC through state health departments.

The **incubation period** usually is 1 to 4 days, with a mean of 2 days.

Influenza Pandemics. A pandemic is defined by emergence and global spread of a new influenza A virus subtype to which the population has little or no immunity and that spreads rapidly from person to person. Pandemics, therefore, can lead to substantially increased morbidity and mortality rates compared with seasonal influenza. During the 20th century, there were 3 influenza pandemics, in 1918 (H1N1), 1957 (H2N2), and 1968 (H3N2). The pandemic in 1918 killed at least 20 million people in the United States and perhaps as many as 50 million people worldwide. The 2009 influenza A (H1N1) pandemic was the first in the 21st century, lasting from April 2009 to August 2010; there were 18 449 deaths among laboratory-confirmed influenza cases. However, this is believed to represent only a fraction of the true number of deaths. On the basis of a modeling study from the CDC, it is estimated that the 2009 influenza A (H1N1) pandemic was associated with between 151 700 and 575 400 deaths worldwide. Public health authorities have developed plans for pandemic preparedness and response to a pandemic in the United States. Pediatric health care professionals should be familiar with national, state, and institutional pandemic plans, including recommendations for vaccine and antiviral drug use, health care surge capacity, and personal protective strategies that can be communicated to patients and families. Up-to-date information on pandemic influenza can be found at **www.pandemicflu.gov.**

DIAGNOSTIC TESTS: Specimens for viral culture, reverse transcriptase-polymerase chain reaction (RT-PCR), rapid influenza molecular assays, or rapid diagnostic tests should be obtained, if possible, during the first 72 hours of illness, because the quantity of virus shed decreases rapidly as illness progresses beyond that point. Specimens of nasopharyngeal secretions obtained by swab, aspirate, or wash should be placed in appropriate transport media for culture. After inoculation into eggs or cell culture, influenza virus usually can be isolated within 2 to 6 days. Rapid diagnostic tests for identification of influenza A and B antigens in respiratory tract specimens are available commercially, although their reported sensitivity (44%–97%) and specificity (76%–100%) compared with viral culture, RT-PCR, and rapid influenza molecular assays are variable and differ by test and specimen type. Additionally, many rapid diagnostic antigen tests cannot distinguish between influenza subtypes, a feature that can be critical during seasons with strains that differ in antiviral susceptibility and/or relative virulence. Results of rapid diagnostic tests should be interpreted in the context of clinical findings and local community influenza activity. Careful clinical judgment must be exercised, because the prevalence of circulating influenza viruses influences the positive and negative predictive values of these influenza screening tests. False-positive results are more likely to occur during periods of low influenza activity; false-negative results are more likely to occur during periods of peak influenza activity. Decisions on treatment and infection control can be made on the basis of positive rapid diagnostic test results. Positive results are helpful, because they may reduce additional testing to identify the cause of the child's influenza-like illness. Treatment should not be withheld in high-risk patients awaiting RT-PCR test results. Serologic diagnosis can be established retrospectively by a fourfold or greater increase in antibody titer in serum specimens obtained during the acute and convalescent stages of illness, as determined by hemagglutination inhibition testing, complement fixation testing, neutralization testing, or enzyme immunoassay (EIA). However, serologic testing rarely is useful in patient management, because 2 serum samples collected 10 to 14 days apart are required. Rapid influenza molecular assays are becoming more widely available. RT-PCR, viral culture tests, and rapid influenza molecular assays offer potential for high sensitivity as well as specificity and are recommended as the tests of choice.

TREATMENT: In the United States, 2 classes of antiviral medications currently are approved for treatment or prophylaxis of influenza infections: neuraminidase inhibitors (oseltamivir and zanamivir) and adamantanes (amantadine and rimantadine). Guidance for use of these 4 antiviral agents is summarized in Table 3.33. Oseltamivir, an oral drug, remains the antiviral drug of choice. Zanamivir, an inhaled drug, is an acceptable alternative but is more difficult to administer, especially to young children. The US Food and Drug Administration (FDA) licensed oseltamivir for people as young as 2 weeks of age in 2012. Given preliminary pharmacokinetic data and limited safety data, oseltamivir can be used to treat influenza in both term and preterm infants from birth, because benefits of therapy are likely to outweigh possible risks of treatment.

Widespread resistance to adamantanes has been documented among H3N2 and H1N1 influenza viruses since 2005 (influenza B viruses intrinsically are not susceptible to adamantanes). Since January 2006, neuraminidase inhibitors (oseltamivir, zanamivir) have been the only recommended influenza antiviral drugs against influenza viruses. The 2009 pandemic

Table 3.33. Antiviral Drugs for Influenza[a]

Drug (Trade Name)	Virus	Administration	Treatment Indications	Chemoprophylaxis Indications	Adverse Effects
Oseltamivir (Tamiflu)	A and B	Oral	Birth or older[b]	3 mo or older	Nausea, vomiting
Zanamivir (Relenza)	A and B	Inhalation	7 y or older	5 y or older	Bronchospasm
Amantadine[c] (Symmetrel)	A	Oral	1 y or older	1 y or older	Central nervous system, anxiety, gastrointestinal
Rimantadine[c] (Flumadine)	A	Oral	13 y or older	1 y or older	Central nervous system, anxiety, gastrointestinal

[a] For current recommendations about treatment and chemoprophylaxis of influenza, including specific dosing information, see **www.cdc.gov/flu/professionals/antivirals/index.htm** or **www.aapredbook.org/flu**.

[b] Approved by the FDA for children as young as 2 wk of age. Given preliminary pharmacokinetic data and limited safety data, oseltamivir can be used to treat influenza in both term and preterm infants from birth because benefits of therapy are likely to outweigh possible risks of treatment.

[c] High levels of resistance to amantadine and rimantadine persist, and these drugs should not be used unless resistance patterns change significantly. Antiviral susceptibilities of viral strains are reported weekly at **www.cdc.gov/flu/weekly/fluactivitysurv.htm.**

influenza A (H1N1) virus largely is susceptible to neuraminidase inhibitors (oseltamivir and zanamivir) and resistant to adamantanes (amantadine and rimantadine). Resistance to oseltamivir has been documented to be around 1% at most for any of the tested influenza viral samples during the past few years. These resistance patterns among circulating influenza A virus strains simplify antiviral treatment, as 2009 influenza A (H1N1), influenza A (H3N2), and influenza B all have been susceptible to neuraminidase inhibitors and resistant to adamantanes. Enhanced surveillance for influenza antiviral resistance is ongoing at the CDC in collaboration with local and state health departments. Each year, options for treatment or chemoprophylaxis of influenza in the United States will depend on influenza strain resistance patterns. Recommendations for influenza chemoprophylaxis and treatment can be found online (**www.cdc.gov/flu/professionals/antivirals/index.htm** or **www.aapredbook.org/flu**).

Therapy for influenza virus infection should be offered to any hospitalized child who has severe, complicated, or progressive respiratory illness that may be influenza related, regardless of influenza-immunization status or whether onset of illness has been greater than 48 hours before admission. Outpatient therapy should be offered for influenza infection of any severity in children at high risk of complications of influenza infection, such as children younger than 2 years. Treatment may be considered for any otherwise healthy child with influenza infection for whom a decrease in duration of clinical symptoms is believed to be warranted by his or her pediatrician. The greatest impact on outcome will occur if treatment can be initiated within 48 hours of illness onset but treatment still should be considered if later in the course of illness, especially for hospitalized patients. Antiviral treatment also should be considered for symptomatic siblings of children younger than 6 months or with underlying medical conditions that predispose them to complications of influenza. Children with severe influenza should be evaluated carefully for possible coinfection with bacterial pathogens (eg, *S aureus*) that might require antimicrobial therapy. Clinicians who want to have influenza isolates tested for susceptibility should contact their state health department.

If antiviral therapy is prescribed, treatment should be started as soon after illness onset as possible and should not be delayed while waiting for a definitive influenza test result, because early therapy provides the best outcomes.[1] The duration of treatment is 5 days for the neuraminidase inhibitors (oseltamivir and zanamivir). Recommended dosages for drugs approved for treatment and prophylaxis of influenza are provided in Table 4.9 (p 919). Patients with any degree of renal insufficiency should be monitored for adverse events. Only zanamivir, which is administered by inhalation, does not require adjustment for people with severe renal insufficiency.

The most common adverse effects of oseltamivir are nausea and vomiting. Postmarketing reports, mostly from Japan, have noted self-injury and delirium with use of oseltamivir among pediatric patients, but other data suggest that these occurrences may have been related to influenza disease itself rather than antiviral therapy. Nevertheless, cautioning parents and patients regarding abnormal behavior is advised. Zanamivir use has been associated with bronchospasm in some people and is not recommended for use in patients with underlying airway disease.

Control of fever with acetaminophen or another appropriate nonsalicylate-containing antipyretic agent may be important in young children, because fever and other symptoms of influenza could exacerbate underlying chronic conditions. Children and adolescents with influenza should not receive aspirin or any salicylate-containing products because of the potential risk of developing Reye syndrome.

ISOLATION OF THE HOSPITALIZED PATIENT: In addition to standard precautions, droplet precautions are recommended for children hospitalized with influenza or an influenza-like illness for the duration of illness. Respiratory tract secretions should be considered infectious, and strict hand hygiene procedures should be used.

CONTROL MEASURES:

Influenza Vaccine. The influenza virus strains selected for inclusion in the seasonal vaccine may change yearly in anticipation of the predominant influenza strains expected to circulate in the United States in the upcoming influenza season. During the past 28 years, there have been only 5 times that the vaccine strains in the influenza vaccine have not changed from the previous year.

There are 2 forms of the vaccine, inactivated influenza vaccine (IIV), administered intramuscularly or intradermally, and live-attenuated influenza vaccine (LAIV), administered intranasally. In the past, IIV and LAIV contained the same 3 virus strains (A [H3N2], A [H1N1], and B [1 of 2 lineages]), which were selected annually on the basis of influenza circulation in the southern hemisphere. In the 2013–2014 season, quadrivalent vaccines that contained both antigenically distinct lineages (ie, Victoria or Yamagata) of influenza B viruses, in addition to A(H3N2) and A(H1N1), were introduced. The trivalent LAIV formulation has been replaced by a quadrivalent LAIV formulation (LAIV4).

---

[1] Centers for Disease Control and Prevention. Antiviral agents for the treatment and chemoprophylaxis of influenza: recommendations of the Advisory Committee on Immunization Practices (ACIP). *MMWR Recomm Rep.* 2011;60(RR-01):1–24

IIVs now are available in both trivalent (IIV3) and quadrivalent (IIV4) formulations. There is no preference from the American Academy of Pediatrics for vaccine formulation or individual vaccine as long as the vaccine is licensed for the appropriate age group.

IIVs contain no live virus. Those distributed in the United States are either subvirion vaccines, prepared by disrupting the lipid-containing membrane of the virus, or purified surface-antigen vaccines. IIVs are administered via intramuscular (IM) or intradermal (ID) injection. The IM formulation is licensed for administration to those 6 months and older and is available in both trivalent (IIV3) and quadrivalent (IIV4) formulations. IIV4 is likely to offer broader protection than IIV3, especially if the circulating B strain is not included in the IIV3. Some IM vaccines are licensed for use in different age groups of children.

An ID formulation of IIV3 is licensed for use in people 18 through 64 years of age. This method of delivery involves a microinjection with a needle 90% shorter than needles used for intramuscular administration. There is no preference for IM or ID immunization with IIV3 in people 18 years or older. Therefore, pediatricians may choose to use either the IM or ID product in their young adult patients as well as for any adults they may be vaccinating (ie, as part of a cocooning strategy). IIV4 is not currently available as an ID formulation.

During the 2 influenza seasons spanning 2010–2012, there were increased reports of febrile seizures in the United States in young children who received IIV and the 13-valent pneumococcal conjugate vaccine (PCV13) concomitantly, but this has not been observed in more recent seasons. Simultaneous administration of IIV and PCV13 continues to be recommended when both vaccines are indicated. Receipt of recommended childhood vaccines during a single visit has important benefits of protecting children against many infectious diseases; minimizing the number of visits that parents, caregivers, and children must make; and preventing febrile seizures by protecting children against influenza and pneumococcal infections, both of which can cause fever. Additional information can be found online (**www.cdc.gov/vaccinesafety/concerns/FebrileSeizures.html**).

A high-dose inactivated influenza vaccine is available for adults 65 years and older (**www.cdc.gov/flu/protect/vaccine/qa_fluzone.htm**).

LAIV4 is a quadrivalent live-attenuated influenza virus vaccine administered by intra-nasal spray. It is licensed by the FDA for healthy people 2 through 49 years of age. The 4 vaccine strains are attenuated, cold adapted, temperature sensitive viruses that replicate in the cooler temperature of the upper respiratory tract and stimulate both an immuno-globulin (Ig) A and IgG antibody response.

Two IIVs manufactured using new technologies that do not use eggs are available for people 18 years or older: cell culture-based inactivated influenza vaccine (ccIIV3) and recombinant influenza vaccine (RIV3). ccIIV3 is indicated for people 18 years or older and is administered as an IM injection. ccIIV3 has comparable immunogenicity to US-licensed IIV3 comparator vaccines. Contraindications are similar to those for other IIVs. RIV3 is indicated for people 18 through 49 years of age and is administered as an IM injection. Both of these manufacturing methods would probably permit a more rapid scale up of vaccine production when needed, such as during a pandemic.

Immunogenicity in Children. Children 9 years and older require only 1 dose of influenza vaccine annually, regardless of their influenza immunization history. Children 6 months through 8 years of age who previously have **not** been immunized against influenza require 2 doses of IIV or LAIV administered at least 4 weeks apart to produce a satisfactory

Table 3.34. Schedule for Inactivated Influenza Vaccine (IIV) Dosage by Age[a]

Age	Dose, mL[b]	No. of Doses	Route[c]
6 through 35 mo	0.25	1–2[d]	Intramuscular
3 through 8 y	0.5	1–2[d]	Intramuscular
9 y or older	0.5	1	Intramuscular
18 y or older (Intradermal)	0.1	1	Intradermal
18 y or older (Non-egg-based)	0.5	1	Intramuscular

[a]Manufacturers include Sanofi Pasteur (Fluzone and Fluzone Quadrivalent, split-virus vaccines licensed for people 6 months or older, and Fluzone Intradermal, split virus vaccine licensed for people 18 years and older), Novartis Vaccines (Fluvirin, purified surface antigen, licensed for people 4 years or older, and Flucelvax, purified surface antigen, licensed for people 18 years and older), bioCSL (Afluria, split-virus vaccine licensed for people 9 years or older), GlaxoSmithKline Biologicals (Fluarix and Fluarix Quadrivalent, split-virus vaccines licensed for people 3 years of age or older), ID Biomedical Corporation of Quebec (FluLaval and FluLaval Quadrivalent, split-virus vaccines licensed for people 3 years or older), and Protein Sciences (Flublok, recombinant vaccine licensed for people 18 years or older). Age indication for Afluria during the 2014–2015 season, per package insert, is 5 years or older; however, the Advisory Committee on Immunization Practices and American Academy of Pediatrics recommend Afluria not be used in children 6 months through 8 years of age because of increased reports of febrile reactions noted in this age group. If no other age-appropriate, licensed inactivated seasonal influenza vaccine is available for a child 5 through 8 years of age who has a medical condition that increases the child's risk of influenza complications, Afluria can be used; however, providers should discuss with parents or caregivers the benefits and risks of influenza immunization with Afluria before administering this vaccine.

[b]From: American Academy of Pediatrics, Committee on Infectious Diseases. Recommendations for prevention and control of influenza in children, 2014–2015. *Pediatrics.* 2014;134(5):e1503–e1519. Dosages are those recommended in recent years. Physicians should refer to the product circular each year to ensure that the appropriate dosage is given.

[c]For adults and older children, the recommended site of immunization is the deltoid muscle. For infants and young children, the preferred site is the anterolateral aspect of the thigh.

[d]Two doses administered at least 4 weeks apart are recommended for children younger than 9 years who are receiving inactivated trivalent influenza vaccine for the first time.

antibody response (see Table 3.34 and Table 3.35, p 485). Significant protection against disease is achieved 1 to 2 weeks after the second dose. In subsequent years, children 6 months through 8 years of age may require 1 or 2 doses, depending on the child's age at the time of the first administered dose, his or her vaccine history, and the makeup of the current year's vaccine. A dosing algorithm for children 6 months through 8 years of age is prepared each year and can be found in the annual policy statement on influenza from the American Academy of Pediatrics (AAP) published in September in *Pediatrics* and available at *Red Book* Online (**http://redbook.solutions.aap.org/redbook.aspx**).[1]

For children requiring 2 doses, vaccination should not be delayed to obtain a specific product for either dose. Any available, age-appropriate trivalent or quadrivalent vaccine can be used; IIV and LAIV are considered interchangeable. A child who receives only 1 of the 2 doses as a quadrivalent formulation is likely to be less primed against the additional B virus.

Vaccine Efficacy and Effectiveness. The efficacy (ie, prevention of illness among vaccine recipients in controlled trials) and effectiveness (ie, prevention of illness in populations receiving vaccine) of influenza vaccines depend primarily on the age and immunocompetence of vaccine recipients, the degree of similarity between the viruses in the vaccine and those in circulation, and the outcome being measured. Protection against virologically

[1]American Academy of Pediatrics, Committee on Infectious Diseases. Recommendations for prevention and control of influenza in children, 2014–2015. *Pediatrics.* 2014;134(5):e1503–e1519

Table 3.35. Schedule for Live-Attenuated Influenza Vaccine (LAIV)[a]

Age	Dose, mL[b]	No. of Doses	Route
2 through 8 y	0.2	1–2[c]	Intranasal
9 y through 49 y	0.2	1	Intranasal

[a]Manufacturer: MedImmune Vaccines, Inc (FluMist Quadrivalent).
[b]From: American Academy of Pediatrics, Committee on Infectious Diseases. Recommendations for prevention and control of influenza in children, 2014–2015. *Pediatrics.* 2014;134(5):e1503–e1519. Dosage is the one recommended in recent years. Physicians should refer to the product circular each year to ensure that the appropriate dosage is given.
[c]Two doses administered at least 4 weeks apart are recommended for children younger than 9 years who are receiving LAIV for the first time.

confirmed influenza illness after immunization with IIV in healthy children older than 2 years ranges from 50% to 95% depending on the closeness of vaccine strain match to the circulating wild strain. Efficacy of LAIV was 86% to 96% against virologically confirmed influenza A (H3N2) virus infection in a large clinical pediatric trial during 1 year. Efficacy of IIV in children 6 through 23 months of age appears to be lower than in older children, although data are limited. Two randomized controlled trials have shown that, among young children, LAIV has a 32% to 55% greater relative efficacy in preventing laboratory-confirmed influenza compared with IIV. Observational data presented in October 2014 from the US Flu Vaccine Effectiveness Network and 2 additional studies conducted during the 2013–2014 influenza season unexpectedly showed that LAIV was not effective against the 2009 influenza A (H1N1) virus when compared with IIV in children 2 through 8 years of age. Specifically, children 2 through 8 years immunized with LAIV were not protected against 2009 influenza A (H1N1). Additional experience over multiple influenza seasons will help to determine optimal utilization of these 2 vaccines in children. The effectiveness of influenza immunization on acute respiratory tract illness is less evident in pediatric than in adult populations because of the frequency of upper respiratory tract infections and influenza-like illness caused by other viral agents in young children. Antibody titers for all seasonal influenza vaccines wane up to 50% of their original levels 6 to 12 months after immunization. An annual dose is critical to maintain protection in all populations.

Coadministration With Other Vaccines. IIV can be administered simultaneously with other live and inactivated vaccines. Although information on how concurrent administration of LAIV with other vaccines affects the safety or efficacy of either LAIV or the simultaneously administered vaccine has not been well studied, inactivated or live vaccines can be administered simultaneously with LAIV. After administration of a live vaccine, at least 4 weeks should pass before another live vaccine is administered.

Recommendations for Influenza Immunization.[1,2] All people 6 months and older should receive influenza vaccine annually. Influenza immunization should begin in September or as soon as the vaccine becomes available and continue into May or for as long as vaccine is

[1]Centers for Disease Control and Prevention. Prevention and control of seasonal influenza with vaccines: recommendations of the Advisory Committee on Immunization Practices (ACIP)—United States, 2014–2015 influenza season. *MMWR Recomm Rep.* 2014;63(32):691–697 (for updates, see **www.cdc.gov/flu**)

[2]American Academy of Pediatrics, Committee on Infectious Diseases. Recommendations for prevention and control of influenza in children, 2014–2015. *Pediatrics.* 2014;134(5):e1503–e1519

available. LAIV should be considered for *healthy* children 2 through 8 years of age who have no contraindications or precautions to the intranasal vaccine. This is based on a GRADE analysis performed by the CDC, which concluded that there is an increased relative efficacy of LAIV as compared with IIV against laboratory-confirmed influenza among younger children. If LAIV is not readily available, IIV should be used; vaccination should not be delayed to obtain LAIV. Particular focus should be on the administration of IIV for all children and adolescents with underlying medical conditions associated with an elevated risk of complications from influenza, including the following:

- Asthma or other chronic pulmonary diseases, such as cystic fibrosis
- Hemodynamically significant cardiac disease
- Immunosuppressive disorders or therapy (see Special Considerations, p 488)
- Human immunodeficiency virus (HIV) infection (see Human Immunodeficiency Virus Infection, p 453)
- Sickle cell anemia and other hemoglobinopathies
- Diseases that necessitate long-term aspirin therapy, including juvenile idiopathic arthritis or Kawasaki disease
- Chronic renal dysfunction
- Chronic metabolic disease, including diabetes mellitus
- Any condition that can compromise respiratory function or handling of secretions or can increase the risk of aspiration, such as neurodevelopmental disorders, spinal cord injuries, seizure disorders, or neuromuscular abnormalities.

LAIV Indications. LAIV is indicated for healthy, nonpregnant people 2 through 49 years of age. IIV is preferred for close contacts of severely immunosuppressed people (ie, people requiring care in a protective environment).

People should not receive LAIV if they received other live vaccines within the last 4 weeks, have a moderate to severe febrile illness, are receiving salicylates, have a known or suspected immune deficiency disease or are receiving immunosuppressive or immunomodulatory therapies, are pregnant or considering pregnancy, have the diagnosis of asthma, have a history of egg allergy, or have a condition that can compromise respiratory function or handling of secretions or can increase the risk for aspiration (eg, neurodevelopmental disorders, spinal cord injuries, seizure disorders, or neuromuscular abnormalities).

IIV is preferred over LAIV for children with chronic underlying medical conditions, including metabolic disease, diabetes mellitus, other chronic disorders of the pulmonary or cardiovascular systems, renal dysfunction, or hemoglobinopathies. The safety of LAIV in these populations has not been established.

Special Considerations, LAIV. Clinicians and immunization programs should screen for possible reactive airway disease when considering use of LAIV for children 2 through 4 years of age and avoid use in children with asthma or a recent wheezing episode. Health care professionals should consult the patient's medical record, when available, to identify children 2 through 4 years of age with asthma or recurrent wheezing that might indicate asthma. Some children 2 through 4 years of age have a history of wheezing with respiratory tract illnesses but have not been diagnosed with asthma. Therefore, to identify children who might be at higher risk of asthma and possibly at increased risk of wheezing after receiving LAIV, people administering LAIV also should ask parents/guardians of children 2 through 4 years of age: "In the past 12 months, has a health care professional ever told you that your child had wheezing or asthma?" LAIV is not recommended for children whose parent or guardian answers yes to this question or for children who have had a wheezing episode or asthma diagnosis noted in his or her medical record within the past 12 months. Precaution also should be taken when considering LAIV administration to people with minor acute illness, such as a mild upper respiratory tract infection, with or without fever. Although the vaccine most likely can be given in this case, LAIV should not be administered if nasal congestion will impede delivery of the vaccine to the nasopharyngeal mucosa until the congestion-inducing illness is resolved.

Children taking an influenza antiviral medication should not receive LAIV until 48 hours after stopping the influenza antiviral therapy. If a child recently received LAIV but has an influenza illness for which antiviral agents are appropriate, the antiviral agents should be given. Reimmunization may be indicated because of the potential effects of antiviral medications on LAIV replication and immunogenicity.

Special Considerations, IIV. In children receiving immunosuppressive chemotherapy, influenza immunization may result in a less robust response than in immunocompetent children. The optimal time to immunize children with malignant neoplasms who must undergo chemotherapy is more than 3 weeks after chemotherapy has been discontinued, when the peripheral granulocyte and lymphocyte counts are greater than $1000/\mu L$ $(1.0 \times 10^9/L)$. Children who no longer are receiving chemotherapy generally have high rates of seroconversion. IIV is the influenza vaccine of choice for any child living with a family member or household contact who is immunocompromised severely (ie, in a protected environment). The preference of IIV over LAIV for such people is because of the theoretical risk of transmission of LAIV vaccine strain to an immunocompromised contact of an LAIV-immunized child. As a precautionary measure, people recently immunized with LAIV should restrict contact with severely immunocompromised patients for 7 days after immunization, even though there have been no reports of LAIV transmission between these 2 groups. In the theoretical scenario in which symptomatic LAIV infection develops in an immunocompromised host, oseltamivir or zanamivir could be prescribed because LAIV strains are susceptible to these antiviral medications.

Children with hemodynamically unstable cardiac disease constitute a large group potentially at high risk of complications of influenza. The immune response to and safety of IIV in these children are comparable to immune response and safety in healthy children.

Corticosteroids administered for brief periods or every other day seem to have a minimal effect on antibody response to influenza vaccine. Prolonged administration of high doses of corticosteroids (ie, a dose of prednisone of either 2 mg/kg or greater or a total of 20 mg/day or greater or an equivalent) may impair antibody response. Influenza immunization can be deferred temporarily during the time of receipt of high-dose corticosteroids, provided deferral does not compromise the likelihood of immunization before the start of influenza season (see Vaccine Administration, p 26).

Pregnancy. Women, including adolescents, who will be pregnant or considering pregnancy during influenza season should receive IIV, because pregnancy increases the risk of complications and hospitalization from influenza. Because intramuscular IIV is not a live-virus vaccine and rarely is associated with major systemic reactions, influenza vaccine is considered safe during any stage of pregnancy. LAIV is contraindicated during pregnancy. Studies have shown that infants born to women who received influenza vaccine have better influenza-related health outcomes. However, data suggest that only about half of pregnant women receive seasonal influenza vaccine, even though both pregnant women and their infants are at higher risk of complications, indicating that opportunities to improve neonatal and infant health through vaccination of pregnant women remain. In addition, data from some studies suggest that influenza vaccination in pregnancy may decrease the risk of preterm birth as well as giving birth to infants who are small for gestational age.

Close Contacts of High-Risk Patients. Immunization of people who are in close contact with children with high-risk conditions or with any child younger than 60 months (5 years) is an important means of protection for these children. In addition, immunization of pregnant women may benefit their unborn infants, because transplacentally acquired antibodies and human milk may protect infants from infection with influenza virus. Special outreach efforts for annual influenza immunization are recommended for the following people:

- Close contacts of infants younger than 6 months (see Recommendations for Influenza Immunization, p 485), because this high-risk group cannot be protected directly by immunization
- Household contacts and out-of-home care providers of children younger than 5 years and at-risk children of all ages (healthy contacts 2 through 49 years of age can receive either IIV or LAIV)
- Health care personnel (HCP) or health care volunteers
- Any woman who is pregnant or considering pregnancy (IIV only), is in the postpartum period, or is breastfeeding during the influenza season
- Close contacts of immunosuppressed people
- Children and adolescents of American Indian or Alaska Native heritage
- Children who are members of households with high-risk adults (ie, adults with underlying medical conditions that predispose them to severe influenza infection or adults 50 years or older), any children 6 through 59 months of age, and children with HIV infection

Health Care Personnel. The AAP recommends a mandatory annual immunization program for HCP, because they frequently come into contact with patients at high risk of influenza illness in their clinical settings.[1] Influenza vaccination of HCP has been shown to reduce both morbidity and mortality among patients. In the 2013–2014 influenza season, 36% of HCP reported having an influenza vaccination requirement at their institution. Since 2010, coverage among HCP who reported having such a requirement has ranged from 94% to 98% each year. Influenza vaccination coverage among HCP was not nearly as high in settings where vaccination was promoted but not required (65%–77%) and even lower in settings where there was neither a requirement nor promotion (48%–57%). Higher coverage rates have been associated with offering vaccination on-site, over multiple days, and at no cost. A mandate is necessary to achieve herd immunity, reach *Healthy People 2020* objectives, and sufficiently protect people who come in contact with HCP. Influenza causes significant morbidity and mortality for both patients and HCP. A mandate is expected to cut costs and increase efficiency in health care settings. There has been widespread support and success by medical organizations and hospitals that have implemented mandatory influenza immunization for HCP.

---

[1]Bernstein HH; Starke JR; and the American Academy of Pediatrics, Committee on Infectious Diseases. Policy statement: recommendation for mandatory influenza immunization of all health care personnel. *Pediatrics.* 2010;126(4):809–815 (Reaffirmed February 2014)

Breastfeeding. Breastfeeding is not a contraindication for immunization with either IIV or LAIV. Special effort should be made to vaccinate all women who are breastfeeding during the influenza season.

Timing of Vaccine Administration. Influenza vaccine should be administered as soon as available each year, preferably before the start of influenza season, at the time specified in the annual recommendations of the ACIP (**www.cdc.gov/flu/**). Providers should continue to offer vaccine until the vaccine expiration date (June 30, marking the end of the influenza season), because influenza is unpredictable. Protective immune responses persist throughout the influenza season, which can have >1 disease peak and may extend into March or later. Although the peak of influenza activity in the United States tends to occur in January through March, influenza activity can occur in early fall (ie, October and November) or late spring (eg, influenza circulated through the end of May during the 2013–2014 season). This approach also provides ample opportunity to administer a second dose of vaccine when indicated. The recommended vaccine dose and schedule for different age groups are given in Tables 3.34 (p 484) and 3.35 (p 485).

Annual influenza immunization is recommended, because immunity can decrease during the year after immunization and because in most years, at least one of the vaccine antigens is changed to match ongoing antigenic changes in circulating strains. The AAP and CDC recommend vaccine administration at any visit to the medical home during influenza season when it is not contraindicated. Strategies to make seasonal influenza vaccine easily accessible for all children include alerts to families that vaccine is available (eg, e-mails, texts, and patient portals); creating walk-in influenza clinics; extending hours beyond routine times during peak vaccination periods; administering influenza vaccine during both well and sick visits; considering how to immunize parents, adult caregivers, and siblings at the same time in the same office setting as children; and working with other institutions (eg, schools, child care programs, and religious organizations) or alternative care sites, such as emergency departments, to expand venues for administering vaccine. If a child or adult receives influenza vaccine outside of his or her medical home, such as at a pharmacy, retail-based clinic, or another practice, a system of patient record transfer is beneficial to ensuring maintenance of accurate immunization records.

Reactions, Adverse Effects, and Contraindications. Although most IIV and LAIV vaccines are produced in eggs and contain measurable amounts of egg protein, recent data have shown that IIV administered in a single, age-appropriate dose is well tolerated by most recipients with a history of egg allergy. More conservative approaches in children with a history of egg allergy, such as skin testing or a 2-step graded challenge, no longer are recommended. No data have been published on the safety of administering LAIV to egg-allergic recipients.

Fig 3.8 outlines an approach for administration of IIV to children with presumed egg allergy. As a precaution, clinicians should determine whether the presumed egg allergy is based on a mild (ie, hives alone) or severe reaction (ie, anaphylaxis involving cardiovascular changes, respiratory and/or gastrointestinal tract symptoms, or reactions that required the use of epinephrine). Pediatricians should consult with an allergist for children with a history of severe reaction. Most vaccine administration to people with egg allergy can happen without the need for referral. Data indicate that approximately 1% of children have immunoglobulin E (IgE)-mediated sensitivity to egg, and of those, a rare minority has a severe allergy.

FIG 3.8. PRECAUTIONS FOR ADMINISTERING IIV TO PRESUMED EGG-ALLERGIC CHILDREN.[a]

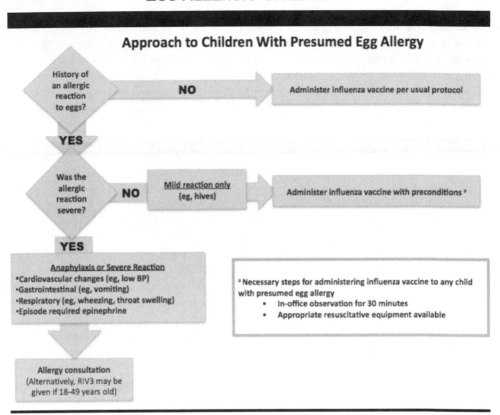

Approach to Children With Presumed Egg Allergy

History of an allergic reaction to eggs? — **NO** → Administer influenza vaccine per usual protocol

YES

Was the allergic reaction severe? — **NO** — Mild reaction only (eg, hives) → Administer influenza vaccine with preconditions [a]

YES

Anaphylaxis or Severe Reaction
- Cardiovascular changes (eg, low BP)
- Gastrointestinal (eg, vomiting)
- Respiratory (eg, wheezing, throat swelling)
- Episode required epinephrine

[a] Necessary steps for administering influenza vaccine to any child with presumed egg allergy
- In-office observation for 30 minutes
- Appropriate resuscitative equipment available

Allergy consultation (Alternatively, RIV3 may be given if 18-49 years old)

[a] American Academy of Pediatrics, Committee on Infectious Diseases. Recommendations for prevention and control of influenza in children, 2014–2015. *Pediatrics.* 2014;134(5):e1503–e1519

Standard immunization practice should include the ability to respond to acute hypersensitivity reactions. Therefore, influenza vaccine should be given to children with mild egg allergy with the following preconditions (Fig 3.8):
- Appropriate resuscitative equipment must be readily available.[1]
- The vaccine recipient should be observed in the office for 30 minutes after immunization (the usual observation time for receiving immunotherapy).

Providers may consider use of ccIIV3 or RIV3 vaccines produced via non–egg-based technologies for adults with egg allergy in settings in which these vaccines are available and otherwise age appropriate. Because there is no known safe threshold for ovalbumin content in vaccines, ccIIV3, which does contain trace amounts of ovalbumin, should be administered according to the guidance for other IIVs (Fig 3.8). In contrast, RIV3, which contains no ovalbumin, may be administered to people with egg allergy of any severity

---

[1] American Academy of Pediatrics, Committee on Pediatric Emergency Medicine. Preparation for emergencies in the offices of pediatricians and pediatric primary care providers. *Pediatrics.* 2007;120(1):200–212 (Reaffirmed June 2011)

who are 18 years or older and do not have other contraindications. However, vaccination of individuals with mild egg allergy should not be delayed if RIV3 or ccIIV3 are not available. Instead, any licensed, age-appropriate IIV should be used.

Although a very slight increase in the number of cases of Guillain-Barré syndrome (GBS) was reported during the "swine flu" vaccine program of 1976, obtaining strong epidemiologic evidence for a possible limited increase in risk of a rare condition with multiple causes is difficult. GBS has an annual background incidence of 10 to 20 cases per 1 million adults, and during the 1976 swine influenza vaccine program, 1 case of GBS was reported per 100 000 people immunized. The risk of influenza vaccine-associated GBS was higher among people 25 years or older than among people younger than 25 years. If there is an association between seasonal influenza vaccine and GBS, the risk is rare, at no more than 1 to 2 cases per million doses. Whether influenza immunization specifically might increase the risk of recurrence of GBS is unknown. The decision not to immunize should be thoughtfully balanced against the potential morbidity and mortality associated with influenza for that individual.

Immunization of children who have asthma or cystic fibrosis with available IIV is not associated with a detectable increase in adverse events or exacerbations. IIV immunization for individuals with HIV infection is considered safe. HIV-infected children should receive annual influenza vaccination according to the HIV-specific recommended immunization schedule.

Inactivated Influenza Vaccine. IIVs contain only inactivated subvirion or surface antigen particles and, therefore, cannot produce active influenza infection. The most common adverse events after IIV3 administration are local injection site pain and tenderness. Fever may occur within 24 hours after immunization in approximately 10% to 35% of children younger than 2 years but rarely in older children and adults. Mild systemic symptoms, such as nausea, lethargy, headache, muscle aches, and chills, may occur after administration of IIV3.

In children, the most common injection site adverse reactions associated with IIV4 administration are pain, redness, and swelling. The most common systemic adverse events are drowsiness, irritability, loss of appetite, fatigue, muscle aches, headache, arthralgia, and gastrointestinal tract symptoms. These events are reported with comparable frequency among participants receiving the licensed comparator trivalent vaccines.

The most common adverse events after administration of the ID formulation of IIV3 are redness, induration, swelling, pain, and itching, which occur at the site of administration; although all adverse events occur at a slightly higher rate with the IM formulation of IIV3, the rate of pain is similar between ID and IM. Headache, myalgia, and malaise may occur and tend to occur at the same rate as that with the IM formulation of IIV3. The most common solicited adverse reactions after ccIIV3 administration are injection site pain, erythema at the injection site, headache, fatigue, myalgia, and malaise. The most frequently reported adverse events for RIV3 are pain, headache, myalgia, and fatigue.

Live-Attenuated Influenza Vaccine. The most commonly reported reactions in children are runny nose or nasal congestion, headache, decreased activity or lethargy, and sore throat. LAIV4 should not be administered to people with notable nasal congestion that would impede vaccine delivery.

LAIV should not be administered to people with asthma or children younger than 5 years with recurrent wheezing. The risk of wheezing caused by LAIV among children 2 through 4 years of age with a history of asthma or wheezing is not well defined. The safety of LAIV in people with a history of high-risk medical conditions associated with an elevated risk of complications from influenza has not been established. In post-licensure surveillance of LAIV over 7 seasons, the Vaccine Adverse Event Reporting System (VAERS), jointly sponsored by the FDA and CDC, did not identify any new or unexpected safety concerns, even though there were reports of use of LAIV in people with a contraindication or precaution. The use of LAIV in young children with chronic medical conditions, including asthma, has been implemented outside of the United States, but the vaccine is not licensed for these indications in the United States.

LAIV shedding can occur after immunization, although the amount of detectable virus is less than occurs during natural influenza infection. The proposed explanation for the low incidence of transmission is that the vaccine virus is shed for a shorter duration and in a much smaller quantity than are wild-type strains. Further evaluation of transmission of LAIV is being conducted.

Chemoprophylaxis: An Adjunct Method of Protecting Children Against Influenza.
Chemoprophylaxis should not be considered a substitute for immunization. Influenza vaccine always should be offered if not contraindicated, even after influenza virus has begun circulating in the community. Antiviral medications currently licensed are important adjuncts to influenza immunization for control and prevention of influenza disease. Because of high rates of resistance of 2009 pandemic influenza A (H1N1), influenza A (H3N2), and influenza B strains to amantadine or rimantadine, only oseltamivir or zanamivir currently are recommended. However, recommendations for use of these drugs for chemoprophylaxis may vary by location and season, depending on susceptibility patterns. Pediatricians should inform recipients of antiviral chemoprophylaxis that the risk of influenza is lowered but still remains while taking medication, and susceptibility to influenza returns when medication is discontinued. Oseltamivir use is not a contraindication to immunization with IIV (unlike LAIV). For current recommendations about chemoprophylaxis against influenza, see **www.cdc.gov/flu/professionals/antivirals/index. htm** or **www.aapredbook.org/flu/**.

Indications for Chemoprophylaxis. Although immunization is the preferred approach to prevention of infection, chemoprophylaxis during an influenza outbreak, as defined by the CDC, is recommended:
- For children at high risk of complications from influenza for whom influenza vaccine is contraindicated
- For children at high risk during the 2 weeks after IIV immunization
- For family members or HCP who are unimmunized and are likely to have ongoing, close exposure to:
  - unimmunized children at high risk; or
  - unimmunized infants and toddlers who are younger than 24 months
- For control of influenza outbreaks for unimmunized staff and children in a closed institutional setting with children at high risk (eg, extended-care facilities)
- As a supplement to immunization among children at high risk, including children who are immunocompromised and may not respond to vaccine
- As postexposure prophylaxis for family members and close contacts of an infected person if those people are at high risk of complications from influenza

- For children at high risk and their family members and close contacts, as well as HCP, when circulating strains of influenza virus in the community are not matched with seasonal influenza vaccine strains, on the basis of current data from the CDC and local health departments

These recommendations apply to routine circumstances, but it should be noted that guidance may change on the basis of updated recommendations from the CDC in concert with antiviral availability, local resources, clinical judgment, recommendations from local or public health authorities, risk of influenza complications, type and duration of exposure contact, and change in epidemiology or severity of influenza. Chemoprophylaxis is not recommended for infants younger than 3 months, unless the situation is judged critical, because of limited safety and efficacy data in this age group.

Chemoprophylaxis does not interfere with the immune response to IIV; however, people immunized with LAIV should not receive antiviral prophylaxis for 14 days after receipt of LAIV because of the potential effects of antiviral medications on LAIV replication and immunogenicity.

Information about influenza surveillance is available through the CDC Voice Information System (influenza update, 888-232-3228) or through **www.cdc.gov/flu/**.

Isosporiasis (now designated as Cystoisosporiasis)

CLINICAL MANIFESTATIONS: Watery diarrhea is the most common symptom of cystoisosporiasis, and can be profuse and protracted, even in immunocompetent people. Manifestations are similar to those caused by other enteric protozoa (eg, *Cryptosporidium* and *Cyclospora* species) and can include abdominal pain, cramping, anorexia, nausea, vomiting, weight loss, and low-grade fever. Eosinophilia also can occur. The proportion of infected people who are asymptomatic is unknown. Severity of infection ranges from self-limiting in immunocompetent hosts to debilitating and life threatening in immunocompromised patients, particularly people infected with human immunodeficiency virus (HIV). Infections of the biliary tract and reactive arthritis also have been reported.

ETIOLOGY: *Cystoisospora belli* (formerly *Isospora belli*) is a coccidian protozoan; oocysts (rather than cysts) are passed in stools.

EPIDEMIOLOGY: Infection occurs predominantly in tropical and subtropical regions of the world and can cause traveler's diarrhea. Infection results from ingestion of sporulated oocysts (eg, in contaminated food or water). Humans are the only known host for *C belli* and shed noninfective oocysts in feces. These oocysts must mature (sporulate) outside the host in the environment to become infective. Under favorable conditions, sporulation can be completed in 1 to 2 days and perhaps more quickly in some settings. Oocysts probably are resistant to most disinfectants and can remain viable for prolonged periods in a cool, moist environment.

The **incubation period** is uncertain but has ranged from 7 to 12 days in reported cases associated with accidental laboratory exposures.

DIAGNOSTIC TESTS: Identification of oocysts in feces or in duodenal aspirates or finding developmental stages of the parasite in biopsy specimens (eg, of the small intestine) is diagnostic. Oocysts in stool are elongate and ellipsoidal (length, 25 to 30 μm). Oocysts can be shed in low numbers, even by people with profuse diarrhea. This constraint underscores the utility of repeated stool examinations, sensitive recovery methods (eg, concentration methods), and detection methods that highlight the organism (eg, oocysts stain bright red with modified acid-fast techniques and autofluoresce when viewed by ultraviolet fluorescent microscopy).

TREATMENT: Trimethoprim-sulfamethoxazole, typically for 7 to 10 days, is the drug of choice (see Drugs for Parasitic Infections, p 927). Immunocompromised patients may need higher doses and a longer duration of therapy. Pyrimethamine (plus leucovorin, to prevent myelosuppression) is an alternative treatment for people who cannot tolerate trimethoprim-sulfamethoxazole. Ciprofloxacin is less effective than trimethoprim-sulfamethoxazole. Nitazoxanide also has been reported to be effective, but data are limited. In adolescents and adults, maintenance therapy is recommended to prevent recurrent disease for people infected with HIV with CD4+ T-lymphocyte counts of <200 mm^3. In adults, a CD4+ T-lymphocyte count >200 cells/µL for at least 6 months is recommended to discontinue secondary prophylaxis. In children, a reasonable time to discontinue secondary prophylaxis would be after sustained improvement in CD4+ T-lymphocyte count or CD4+ T-lymphocyte percentage from CDC immunologic category 3 to 1 or 2.

ISOLATION OF THE HOSPITALIZED PATIENT: In addition to standard precautions, contact precautions are recommended for diapered and incontinent people.

CONTROL MEASURES: Preventive measures include avoiding fecal exposure (eg, food, water, skin, and fomites contaminated with stool), practicing hand and personal hygiene, and thorough washing of fruits and vegetables before eating.

Kawasaki Disease

CLINICAL MANIFESTATIONS: Kawasaki disease is a self-limited vasculitis characterized by fever and mucocutaneous signs that is recognized across the globe. If untreated, approximately 20% of children will develop coronary artery abnormalities, including aneurysms. The illness is characterized by fever and the following clinical features: (1) bilateral bulbar conjunctival injection with limbic sparing and without exudate; (2) erythematous mouth and pharynx, strawberry tongue, and red, cracked lips; (3) a polymorphous, generalized, erythematous rash that can be morbilliform, maculopapular, or scarlatiniform or may resemble erythema multiforme; (4) changes in the peripheral extremities consisting of induration of the hands and feet with erythematous palms and soles, often with later periungual desquamation; and (5) acute, nonsuppurative, usually unilateral, cervical lymphadenopathy with at least one node 1.5 cm in diameter. Kawasaki disease diagnosis may be delayed in patients who come to attention because of fever and unilateral cervical lymphadenitis, which mistakenly is thought to be bacterial lymphadenitis; a distinguishing feature is that in Kawasaki disease, lymphadenitis is unlikely to be necrotizing/suppurative on imaging studies. For diagnosis of classic Kawasaki disease, patients should have fever for at least 5 days (or fever until the date of treatment if given before the fifth day of illness) and at least 4 of the above 5 features without alternative explanation for the findings. The presence of a concurrent or preceding viral upper respiratory infection does not exclude the diagnosis of Kawasaki disease. The epidemiologic case definition also allows diagnosis of incomplete Kawasaki disease when a patient has fewer than 4 principal clinical criteria in the presence of fever and coronary artery abnormalities. Irritability, abdominal pain, diarrhea, and vomiting are common associated features. Other findings include urethritis with sterile pyuria (70% of cases), mild anterior uveitis (80%), mild elevation of hepatic transaminase levels (50%), arthritis or arthralgia (10%–20%), meningismus with cerebrospinal fluid pleocytosis (40%), pericardial effusion of at least 1 mm (less than 5%), gallbladder hydrops (less than 10%), and myocarditis manifested by congestive heart failure (less than 5%). A persistent resting tachycardia and the presence of an S3 gallop often are appreciated. Fine desquamation in the groin area can occur in the acute phase of disease (Fink sign).[1] Inflammation or ulceration may be observed at the inoculation scar of previous bacille Calmette-Guérin immunization. Rarely, Kawasaki disease can present with what appears to be "septic shock" with need for intensive care; these children often have significant thrombocytopenia at admission. Group A streptococcal or *Staphylococcus aureus* toxic shock syndrome should be excluded in such cases.

The diagnosis of incomplete Kawasaki disease should be considered in febrile patients when fever plus 2 or 3 of the characteristic features are present. If patients have purulent conjunctivitis, exudative pharyngitis, or splenomegaly, they are highly unlikely to have Kawasaki disease. The proportion of children with Kawasaki disease with incomplete manifestations is higher among patients younger than 12 months. Infants with Kawasaki disease have a higher risk of developing coronary artery aneurysms than do older children, making diagnosis and timely treatment especially important in this age group. Laboratory findings in incomplete cases are similar to findings in classic cases. Therefore, although laboratory findings in Kawasaki disease are nonspecific, they may prove useful in increasing or decreasing the likelihood of incomplete Kawasaki disease. Incomplete Kawasaki disease should be considered in any child with unexplained fever for 5 days or longer in association with 2 or more of the principal features of this illness and supportive laboratory data (eg, erythrocyte sedimentation rate [ESR] ≥40 mm/hour or C-reactive protein [CRP] concentration ≥3 mg/dL). Kawasaki disease also should be considered in any infant younger than 6 months with prolonged fever and no other explanation for the fever and in infants with shock-like syndrome in whom an inciting infection is not confirmed. If coronary artery aneurysm, ectasia, or dilation is evident (z score ≥2.5), a presumptive diagnosis of Kawasaki disease should be made. A normal early echocardiographic study is typical and does not exclude the diagnosis but may be useful in evaluation of patients with suspected incomplete Kawasaki disease. In one study, 80% of Kawasaki disease patients who ultimately developed coronary artery disease had abnormalities (z score ≥2.5) on their admission echocardiogram. The majority of these patients were evaluated before day 10 of fever. Fig 3.9 is the American Heart Association algorithm for diagnosis and treatment of suspected incomplete Kawasaki disease.

The average duration of fever in untreated Kawasaki disease is 10 days; however, fever can last 2 weeks or longer. After fever resolves, patients can remain anorectic and/or irritable with decreased energy for 2 to 3 weeks. During this phase, desquamation of fingers and toes, and fine desquamation of other areas may occur. Recurrent disease develops in approximately 2% of patients months to years later.

Coronary artery abnormalities are serious sequelae of Kawasaki disease and may occur in 20% to 25% of untreated children. Increased risk of developing coronary artery abnormalities is associated with male gender; age younger than 12 months or older than 8 years;

---

[1]For further information on the diagnosis of this disease, see Newburger JW, Takahashi M, Gerber MA, et al. Diagnosis, treatment and long-term management of Kawasaki disease: a statement for health professionals from the Committee on Rheumatic Fever, Endocarditis and Kawasaki Disease, Council on Cardiovascular Disease in the Young, American Heart Association. *Circulation.* 2004;110(17):2747–2771 (also in *Pediatrics.* 2004;114[6]:1708–1733).

FIG 3.9. EVALUATION OF SUSPECTED INCOMPLETE KAWASAKI DISEASE (KD).[a]

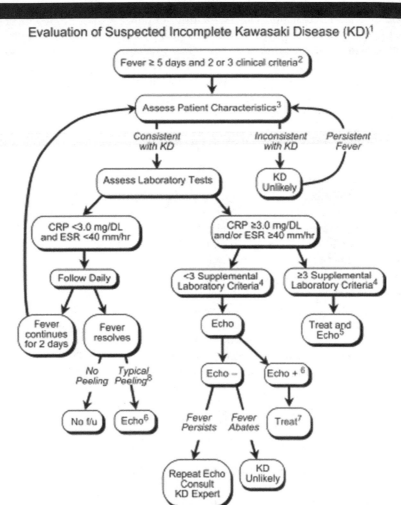

Evaluation of suspected incomplete Kawasaki disease. (1) In the absence of gold standard for diagnosis, this algorithm cannot be evidence based but rather represents the informed opinion of the expert committee. Consultation with an expert should be sought anytime assistance is needed. (2) Infants ≤6 months old on day ≥7 of fever without other explanation should undergo laboratory testing and, if evidence of systemic inflammation is found, an echocardiogram, even if the infants have no clinical criteria. (3) Patient characteristics suggesting Kawasaki disease are provided in text. Characteristics suggesting disease other than Kawasaki disease include exudative conjunctivitis, exudative pharyngitis, discrete intraoral lesions, bullous or vesicular rash, or generalized adenopathy. Consider alternative diagnoses. (4) Supplemental laboratory criteria include albumin ≤3.0 g/dL, anemia for age, elevation of alanine aminotransferase, platelets after 7 d ≥450 000/mm³, white blood cell count ≥15 000/mm³, and urine ≥10 white blood cells/high-power field. (5) Can treat before performing echocardiogram. (6) Echocardiogram is considered positive for purposes of this algorithm if any of 3 conditions are met: z score of LAD or RCA ≥2.5, coronary arteries meet Japanese Ministry of Health criteria for aneurysms, or ≥3 other suggestive features exist, including perivascular brightness, lack of tapering, decreased LV function, mitral regurgitation, pericardial effusion, or z scores in LAD or RCA of 2–2.5. (7) If the echocardiogram is positive, treatment should be given to children within 10 d of fever onset and those beyond day 10 with clinical and laboratory signs (CRP, ESR) of ongoing inflammation. (8) Typical peeling begins under nail bed of fingers and then toes.
[a] Reprinted from Newburger JW, Takahashi M, Gerber MA, et al. Diagnosis, treatment and long-term management of Kawasaki disease: a statement for health professionals from the Committee on Rheumatic Fever, Endocarditis and Kawasaki Disease, Council on Cardiovascular Disease in the Young, American Heart Association. *Pediatrics.* 2004;114(6):1708–1733.

fever for more than 10 days; high baseline relative neutrophil and band count (>80%); white blood cell count >15 000/mm³; low hemoglobin concentration (<10 g/dL); hypoalbuminemia, hyponatremia, or thrombocytopenia at presentation; fever persisting or occurring after Immune Globulin Intravenous (IGIV) administration; and persistence of elevated CRP concentration for more than 30 days or recurrent CRP elevations. Aneurysms of the coronary arteries have been demonstrated by echocardiography as early as 4 to 7 days after onset of illness but more typically occur between 1 and 4 weeks after onset of illness; onset later than 6 weeks is extremely uncommon. Giant coronary artery aneurysms (internal diameter ≥8 mm) are highly predictive of long-term complications. Aneurysms occurring in other medium-sized arteries (eg, iliac, femoral, renal, and axillary vessels) are uncommon and generally do not occur in the absence of significant coronary abnormalities. In addition to coronary artery disease, carditis can involve the pericardium, myocardium, or endocardium, and mitral or aortic regurgitation or both can develop. Carditis generally resolves when fever resolves.

In children with mild coronary artery dilation or ectasia, coronary artery dimensions often return to baseline within 6 to 8 weeks after onset of disease. Approximately 50% of coronary aneurysms (but a small proportion of giant aneurysms) regress to normal luminal size within 1 to 2 years, although this process can be accompanied by development of coronary stenosis. In addition, regression of aneurysm(s) may result in a poorly compliant, fibrotic vessel wall.

The current case-fatality rate for Kawasaki disease in the United States and Japan is less than 0.2%. The principal cause of death is myocardial infarction resulting from coronary artery occlusion attributable to thrombosis or progressive stenosis. Rarely, a large coronary artery aneurysm may rupture during the acute phase. The relative risk of mortality is highest within 6 weeks of onset of acute symptoms of Kawasaki disease, but myocardial infarction and sudden death can occur months to years after the acute episode. There is no current evidence that the vasculitis of Kawasaki disease predisposes to premature atherosclerotic coronary artery disease, although this seems plausible.

ETIOLOGY: The etiology is unknown. Epidemiologic and clinical features strongly suggest an infectious cause or trigger. Studies also suggest genetic susceptibility.

EPIDEMIOLOGY: Peak age of occurrence in the United States is between 18 and 24 months. Fifty percent of patients are younger than 2 years, and 80% are younger than 5 years; children older than 8 years less commonly develop the disease, but rare cases may occur even in adults. In children younger than 6 months, the diagnosis often is delayed, because the symptom complex of Kawasaki disease is incomplete and individual features can be subtle. The prevalence of coronary artery abnormalities is higher when diagnosis and treatment are delayed beyond the 10th day of illness. The male-to-female ratio is approximately 1.5:1. In the United States, 4000 to 5500 cases are estimated to occur each year; the incidence is highest in children of Asian ancestry. Kawasaki disease first was described in Japan, where a pattern of endemic occurrence with superimposed epidemic outbreaks was recognized. A similar pattern of disease occurrence with occasional community-wide epidemics has been recognized in North America. More cases, including clusters, occur during winter and spring. No evidence indicates person-to-person or common-source spread, although the incidence is somewhat higher in siblings of children with the disease.

The **incubation period** is unknown.

DIAGNOSTIC TESTS: No specific diagnostic test is available. The diagnosis is established by fulfillment of the clinical criteria (see Clinical Manifestations, p 493) after consideration of other possible illnesses, such as staphylococcal or streptococcal toxin-mediated disease; drug reactions (eg, Stevens-Johnson syndrome); measles, adenovirus, Epstein-Barr virus, parvovirus B19, or enterovirus infections; rickettsial exanthems; leptospirosis; systemic-onset juvenile idiopathic arthritis; and reactive arthritis. The identification of a respiratory virus by molecular testing does not necessarily exclude the diagnosis of Kawasaki disease in infants and children that otherwise meet diagnostic criteria. A greatly increased ESR and/or serum CRP concentration during the first 2 weeks of illness and an increased platelet count ($>450\,000/mm^3$) on days 10 to 21 of illness are almost universal laboratory features. ESR and platelet count usually are normal within 6 to 8 weeks; CRP concentration returns to normal much sooner.

TREATMENT: Management during the acute phase is directed at decreasing inflammation of the myocardium and coronary artery wall and providing supportive care. Therapy should be initiated as soon as the diagnosis is established or strongly suspected. Once the acute phase has subsided, therapy is directed at prevention of coronary artery thrombosis. Specific recommendations for therapy include IGIV and aspirin therapy.

Immune Globulin Intravenous. Therapy with high-dose IGIV and aspirin initiated within 10 days of the onset of fever substantially decreases the risk of development of coronary artery dilatation and aneurysms in children with normal echocardiograms at admission, compared with treatment with aspirin alone, and results in more rapid resolution of fever and other clinical and laboratory indicators of acute inflammation. Therapy with IGIV should be initiated as soon as possible; efficacy when initiated later than the 10th day of illness or after detection of aneurysms has not been fully evaluated. However, therapy with IGIV and aspirin should be provided for patients in whom the diagnosis is made more than 10 days after the onset of fever who have manifestations of continuing inflammation (eg, fever and/or elevated ESR or CRP concentration) or of evolving coronary artery disease. Despite prompt treatment with IGIV and aspirin, approximately 4% of patients develop coronary artery aneurysms if treatment is initiated before the onset of coronary artery abnormalities.

Dose. A single dose of 2 g/kg of IGIV, given over 10 to 12 hours, has been proven to reduce the risk of coronary artery aneurysms from 17% to 4% in children with normal echocardiograms at admission. Patients in whom acute Kawasaki disease is diagnosed should receive IGIV regardless of whether they have coronary artery abnormalities detected. Hemolysis requiring transfusion has occurred after IGIV treatment in children with Kawasaki disease because of isoagglutinins in the products. The risk of hemolysis is increased in patients receiving high/repeated IGIV doses (usually ≥ 2 g/kg) and those with blood groups A, B, or AB. When significant hemolysis occurs, it usually happens within 5 to 10 days of infusion. Disseminated intravascular coagulopathy and renal dysfunction attributable to hemoglobinuria have been reported in adult patients after IGIV-mediated hemolysis. Hemoglobin concentrations should be monitored after high/repeated-dose IGIV infusions in at-risk children. Additional confirmatory testing should be performed if signs or symptoms of hemolysis are observed. Adequate cross-matching is necessary if transfusion is indicated, because donor A, B, or AB red blood cells also may be hemolyzed after transfusion. Other complications, such as infusion reactions (fever, chills, hypotension) can occur, and IGIV-induced aseptic meningitis is seen as an uncommon complication. ESR becomes elevated as a result of the IGIV infusion and, thus, is not useful to monitor disease activity after infusion of IGIV.

Retreatment. Many patients have fever in the 24 hours after completing the IGIV infusion. Persistent or recrudescent fever present 36 or more hours after the end of the IGIV infusion is used to define IGIV-resistant cases. Up to 15% of Kawasaki patients are resistant to the standard single dose of 2 g/kg of IGIV. In these situations, the diagnosis of Kawasaki disease should be reevaluated. If Kawasaki disease still is considered to be most likely, retreatment with IGIV (2 g/kg) and continued high-dose aspirin therapy generally is given. For the limited number of patients (2%–4%) who are refractory to 2 doses of IGIV, infliximab (5 mg/kg, intravenously, over 2 hours) or intravenous methylprednisolone (usually 30 mg/kg/day for 3 days) or a third IGIV dose may be considered in attempt to reduce inflammation and improve coronary artery outcomes. Lack of comparative data on use of these modalities precludes definitive recommendations. The benefit and potential risks of initial systemic corticosteroids in treatment of Kawasaki disease are under investigation; recent publications from Japan suggest that IGIV plus systemic corticosteroid (methylprednisolone 2 mg/kg, orally, until CRP concentration has been normal for 2 weeks) may be useful in treating children at high risk of coronary artery disease.

Aspirin. Aspirin is used for its anti-inflammatory and antithrombotic activity, although aspirin alone does not decrease the risk of coronary artery abnormalities. Aspirin is administered in doses of 80 to 100 mg/kg per day in 4 divided doses once the diagnosis is made. Children with acute Kawasaki disease have decreased aspirin absorption and increased clearance and rarely achieve therapeutic serum concentrations, although low serum albumin concentrations result in high concentrations of free salicylate. It generally is not necessary to monitor salicylate concentrations. High-dose aspirin therapy usually is given until the patient has been afebrile for 48 to 72 hours. Low-dose aspirin (3 to 5 mg/kg/day, in a single daily dose) then is given until a follow-up echocardiogram at 6 to 8 weeks after onset of illness is normal, or is continued indefinitely for children in whom coronary artery abnormalities are present. Because of the theoretical risk of Reye syndrome in patients with influenza or varicella receiving salicylates, parents of children receiving aspirin should be instructed to contact their child's physician promptly if the child develops symptoms of or is exposed to either of these diseases. In general, ibuprofen should be avoided in children with coronary aneurysms taking aspirin for its antiplatelet effects, because ibuprofen antagonizes the platelet inhibition that is induced by aspirin. The child and all household contacts older than 6 months should receive influenza vaccine according to seasonal recommendations. If a child with Kawasaki disease is still receiving aspirin, the inactivated injectable influenza vaccine (not live-attenuated vaccine) should be used. Household contacts older than 2 years may receive either live-attenuated or inactivated injectable vaccine, unless contraindications exist.

Cardiac Care.[1] An echocardiogram should be obtained at the time of diagnosis and repeated at 2 weeks and 6 to 8 weeks after diagnosis. Children at higher risk—for example, children with persistent or recrudescent fever after initial IGIV or baseline coronary abnormalities—may require more frequent echocardiograms to guide the need for

[1]Newburger JW, Takahashi M, Gerber MA, et al. Diagnosis, treatment and long-term management of Kawasaki disease: a statement for health professionals from the Committee on Rheumatic Fever, Endocarditis and Kawasaki Disease, Council on Cardiovascular Disease in the Young, American Heart Association. *Circulation.* 2004;110(17):2747–2771 (also in *Pediatrics.* 2004;114[6]:1708–1733)

additional therapies. Children also should be assessed during this time for arrhythmias, congestive heart failure, and valvular regurgitation. The care of patients with significant cardiac abnormalities should involve a pediatric cardiologist experienced in management of patients with Kawasaki disease and in assessing echocardiographic studies of coronary arteries in children. Long-term management of Kawasaki disease should be based on the extent of coronary artery involvement. In patients with persistent moderately large coronary artery aneurysms that are not large enough to warrant anticoagulation, prolonged low-dose aspirin and clopidogrel (1 mg/kg/day) are recommended in combination. Development of giant coronary artery aneurysms (diameter 8 mm or larger) usually requires addition of anticoagulant therapy, such as warfarin or low-molecular weight heparin, to prevent thrombosis. Anticoagulation also is sometimes warranted in young infants with coronary artery aneurysms measuring less than 8 mm in diameter but for whom the size is equivalent to giant aneurysms when body surface area is considered. Recommendations regarding criteria for systemic anticoagulation and the use of antiplatelet agents are evolving, and patients should be managed by pediatric cardiologists aware of the latest guidance.

Subsequent Immunization. Measles- and varicella-containing vaccines should be deferred for 11 months after receipt of high-dose IGIV for treatment of Kawasaki disease because of possible interference with the immune response. If the child's risk of exposure to measles or varicella within this period is high, the child should be immunized and then reimmunized at least 11 months after administration of IGIV (see Table 1.10, p 39). Live-attenuated varicella-containing vaccines should be avoided during aspirin therapy because of a theoretical concern of Reye syndrome. If the child is receiving low-dose aspirin therapy and the risk of exposure is high, or if aspirin therapy is prolonged beyond 11 months, benefits and theoretical risk of Reye syndrome should be discussed; usually, varicella vaccine is given. The schedule for administration of inactivated childhood vaccines should not be interrupted.

ISOLATION OF THE HOSPITALIZED PATIENT: Standard precautions are indicated.

CONTROL MEASURES: None.

Kingella kingae Infections

CLINICAL MANIFESTATIONS: The most common infections attributable to *Kingella kingae* are pyogenic arthritis, osteomyelitis, and bacteremia. The vast majority of *K kingae* infections affect children, predominantly between 6 and 48 months of age, with most cases occurring in those younger than 2 years. *K kingae* is the most common cause of skeletal infections in children younger than 3 years in some geographic locations. *K kingae* pyogenic arthritis generally is monoarticular and most commonly involves the knee, hip, or ankle. *K kingae* osteomyelitis most often involves the femur or tibia and also has an unusual predilection for small bones, including the small bones of the foot. The clinical manifestations of *K kingae* pyogenic arthritis and osteomyelitis are similar to manifestations of skeletal infection due to other bacterial pathogens in immunocompetent children, although a subacute course may be more common. A case of Brodie abscess of bone attributable to *K kingae* has been reported. Bacteremia can occur in previously healthy children and in children with preexisting chronic medical problems. Children with *K kingae* bacteremia present with fever and frequently have concurrent findings of respiratory or gastrointestinal tract disease. Other infections caused by *K kingae* include diskitis, endocarditis (*K kingae* belongs to the HACEK group of organisms), meningitis, and pneumonia.

ETIOLOGY: *K kingae* is a gram-negative organism that belongs to the *Neisseriaceae* family. It is a fastidious, facultative anaerobic, β-hemolytic small bacillus that appears as pairs or short chains with tapered ends and that often resists decolorization, sometimes resulting in misidentification as a gram-positive organism.

EPIDEMIOLOGY: The usual habitat of *K kingae* is the human posterior pharynx. The organism more frequently colonizes young children than adults and can be transmitted among children in child care centers, occasionally causing clusters of cases. Infection may be associated with preceding or concomitant stomatitis or upper respiratory tract infection.

The **incubation period** is variable.

DIAGNOSTIC TESTS: *K kingae* can be isolated from blood, synovial fluid, bone exudate, cerebrospinal fluid, respiratory tract secretions, and other sites of infection. Organisms grow better in aerobic conditions with enhanced carbon dioxide. In patients with *K kingae* pyogenic arthritis or osteomyelitis, blood cultures often are negative. *K kingae* is difficult to isolate on routinely used solid media, and synovial fluid and bone aspirates from patients with suspected *K kingae* infection should be inoculated into Bactec, BacT/Alert, or similar blood culture systems and held for at least 7 days to maximize recovery. Conventional and real-time polymerase chain reaction methods have improved detection of *K kingae*. *K kingae* should be suspected in young children with culture-negative skeletal infections.

TREATMENT: *K kingae* is almost always highly susceptible to penicillins and cephalosporins, although in vitro susceptibility to oxacillin is relatively reduced and β-lactamase production has been reported in rare isolates. Nearly all isolates also are susceptible to aminoglycosides, macrolides, trimethoprim-sulfamethoxazole, tetracyclines, and fluoroquinolones. Between 40% and 100% of isolates are resistant to clindamycin, and virtually all isolates are resistant to trimethoprim (although most strains are susceptible to trimethoprim-sulfamethoxazole) and glycopeptide antibiotics (vancomycin and teicoplanin). Most cases of *K kingae* infection are treated with penicillin or ampicillin-sulbactam or a second-generation or third-generation cephalosporin.

ISOLATION OF THE HOSPITALIZED PATIENT: Standard precautions are recommended.

CONTROL MEASURES: None.

Legionella pneumophila Infections

CLINICAL MANIFESTATIONS: Legionellosis is associated with 2 clinically and epidemiologically distinct illnesses: Legionnaires disease and Pontiac fever. **Legionnaires' disease** varies in severity from mild to severe pneumonia characterized by fever, cough, and progressive respiratory distress. Legionnaires disease can be associated with chills, myalgia, and gastrointestinal tract, central nervous system, and renal manifestations. Respiratory failure and death can occur. **Pontiac fever** is a milder febrile illness without pneumonia that occurs in epidemics and is characterized by an abrupt onset and a self-limited, influenza-like illness.

ETIOLOGY: *Legionella* species are fastidious aerobic bacilli that stain gram negative after recovery on buffered charcoal yeast extract (BCYE) media. At least 20 different species have been implicated in human disease, but the most common species causing infections in the United States is *Legionella pneumophila*, with most isolates belonging to serogroup 1. Multiplication of *Legionella* organisms in water sources occurs optimally in temperatures between 25°C and 45°C.

EPIDEMIOLOGY: Legionnaires disease is acquired through inhalation of aerosolized water contaminated with *L pneumophila*. Person-to-person transmission has not been demonstrated. More than 80% of cases are sporadic; the sources of infection can be related to exposure to *L pneumophila*-contaminated water in the home, workplace, or hospitals or other medical facilities or to aerosol-producing devices in public places. Outbreaks have been ascribed to common-source exposure to contaminated cooling towers, evaporative condensers, potable water systems, whirlpool spas, humidifiers, and respiratory therapy equipment. Outbreaks have occurred in hospitals, hotels, and other large buildings as well as on cruise ships. Health care-associated infections can occur and often are related to contamination of the hot water supply. In patients who develop pneumonia during or after their hospitalization, Legionnaires' disease should be considered in the differential diagnosis. Legionnaires' disease occurs most commonly in people who are elderly, are immunocompromised, or have underlying lung disease. Infection in children is rare and usually is asymptomatic or mild and unrecognized. Severe disease has occurred in children with malignant neoplasms, severe combined immunodeficiency, chronic granulomatous disease, organ transplantation, end-stage renal disease, underlying pulmonary disease, and immunosuppression; in children receiving systemic corticosteroids; and as a health care-associated infection in newborn infants.

The **incubation period** for Legionnaires' disease (pneumonia) is 2 to 10 days; for Pontiac fever, the incubation period is 1 to 2 days.

DIAGNOSTIC TESTS: Recovery of *Legionella* from respiratory tract secretions, lung tissue, pleural fluid, or other normally sterile fluid specimens by using buffered charcoal yeast extract (BCYE) media provides definitive evidence of infection, but the sensitivity of culture is laboratory dependent. When a patient is suspected of having Legionnaires' disease, culture of a respiratory specimen should be conducted in addition to urine antigen testing. Detection of *Legionella* antigen in urine by commercially available immunoassays is highly specific. Such tests are sensitive for *L pneumophila* serogroup 1, but these tests rarely detect antigen in patients infected with other *L pneumophila* serogroups or other *Legionella* species. The bacterium can be demonstrated in specimens by direct immunofluorescent assay, but this test is less sensitive and the specificity is technician dependent and lower than culture or urine immunoassay. Genus-specific polymerase chain reaction-based assays have been developed that detect *Legionella* DNA in respiratory secretions as well as in blood and urine of some patients with pneumonia. For serologic diagnosis, a fourfold increase in titer of antibodies to *L pneumophila* serogroup 1, measured by indirect immunofluorescent antibody (IFA) assay, confirms a recent infection. Convalescent serum samples should be obtained 3 to 4 weeks after onset of symptoms; however, a titer increase can be delayed for 8 to 12 weeks. The positive predictive value of a single titer of 1:256 or greater is low and does not provide definitive evidence of infection. Antibodies to several gram-negative organisms, including *Pseudomonas* species, *Bacteroides fragilis*, and *Campylobacter jejuni*, can cause false-positive IFA test results.

TREATMENT: Azithromycin has replaced erythromycin as the drug of choice. Once the condition of a patient is improving, oral therapy can be substituted. Levofloxacin (or another fluoroquinolone) is the drug of choice for immunocompromised adults. Doxycycline and trimethoprim-sulfamethoxazole are alternative drugs. Tetracycline-based antimicrobial agents, including doxycycline, may cause permanent tooth discoloration for children younger than 8 years if used for repeated treatment courses. However, doxycycline binds less readily to calcium compared with older tetracyclines, and in some studies, doxycycline was not associated with visible teeth staining in younger children (see Tetracyclines, p 873). Duration of therapy is 5 to 10 days for azithromycin and 14 to 21 days for other drugs. Longer courses of therapy are recommended for patients who are immunocompromised or who have severe disease.

ISOLATION OF THE HOSPITALIZED PATIENT: Standard precautions are recommended.

CONTROL MEASURES: Monochloramine (rather than free chlorine) treatment of municipal water supplies has been associated with a decrease in health care-associated Legionnaires' disease.[1] Hospitals should maintain hot water at the highest temperature allowable by state regulations or codes, preferably 60°C (140°F) or greater, and maintain cold water temperature at less than 20°C (68°F) to minimize waterborne *Legionella* contamination. Occurrence of even a single laboratory-confirmed health care-associated case of legionellosis warrants consideration of an epidemiologic and environmental investigation. Hospitals with transplantation programs (solid organ or hematopoietic stem cell) should maintain a high index of suspicion of legionellosis, use sterile water for the filling and terminal rinsing of nebulization devices, and consider performing periodic culturing for *Legionella* species in the potable water supply of the transplant unit. Some hospitals may choose to perform periodic, routine culturing of water samples from the hospital's potable water system to detect *Legionella* species.

For emergency disinfection, superheating (to 66°C [150°F] or greater) followed by maintenance of a hot water temperature at the faucet of greater than 50°C (122°F) and/or shock chlorination or targeted use of point-of-use water filters can be used. Disinfectants that have been used for long-term decontamination of potable water supplies to prevent health care-associated cases are chlorine, monochloramine, chlorine dioxide, ultraviolet light, and copper-silver ionization.

Leishmaniasis

CLINICAL MANIFESTATIONS: The 3 main clinical syndromes are as follows:
* **Cutaneous leishmaniasis.** After inoculation by the bite of an infected female phlebotomine sand fly (approximately 2–3 mm long), parasites proliferate locally in mononuclear phagocytes, leading to an erythematous papule, which typically slowly enlarges to become a nodule and then an ulcerative lesion with raised, indurated borders. Ulcerative lesions may become dry and crusted or may develop a moist granulating base with an overlying exudate. Lesions can, however, persist as nodules or papules and may be single or multiple. Lesions commonly are on exposed areas of the body (eg, face and extremities) and may be accompanied by satellite lesions, sporotrichoid-like nodules, and regional adenopathy. Clinical manifestations of Old World and New World (American) cutaneous leishmaniasis are similar. Spontaneous resolution of lesions may

---

[1]Centers for Disease Control and Prevention. Guidelines for preventing health-care-associated pneumonia, 2003: recommendations of CDC and the Healthcare Infection Control Practices Advisory Committee (HICPAC). *MMWR Recomm Rep.* 2004;53(RR-3):1–36. Available at: **www.cdc.gov/mmwr/preview/mmwrhtml/rr5303a1.htm**

take weeks to years—depending, in part, on the *Leishmania* species/strain—and usually results in a flat, atrophic scar.

- **Mucosal leishmaniasis (espundia)** traditionally refers to a metastatic sequela of New World cutaneous infection, which results from dissemination of the parasite from the skin to the naso-oropharyngeal mucosa; this form of leishmaniasis typically is caused by species in the *Viannia* subgenus (see **Etiology**). (Mucosal involvement because of local extension of cutaneous facial lesions has a different pathophysiology.) Mucosal disease usually becomes evident clinically months to years after the original cutaneous lesions healed; however, mucosal and cutaneous lesions may be noted simultaneously, and some affected people have had subclinical cutaneous infection. Granulomatous inflammation may cause hypertrophy of the nose and lips. Untreated mucosal leishmaniasis can progress to cause ulcerative destruction of the mucosa (eg, perforation of the nasal septum) and facial disfigurement.

- **Visceral leishmaniasis (kala-azar).** After cutaneous inoculation by an infected sand fly, the parasite spreads throughout the reticuloendothelial system (eg, spleen, liver, bone marrow). The stereotypical clinical manifestations include fever, weight loss, pancytopenia (anemia, leukopenia, and thrombocytopenia), hypoalbuminemia, and hypergammaglobulinemia. Peripheral lymphadenopathy is quite common in East Africa (eg, South Sudan). Some patients in South Asia (the Indian subcontinent) develop grayish discoloration of their skin; this manifestation gave rise to the Hindi term kala-azar ("black sickness"). Untreated, advanced cases of visceral leishmaniasis almost always are fatal, either directly from the disease or from complications, such as secondary bacterial infections or hemorrhage. At the other end of the spectrum, visceral infection can be asymptomatic or oligosymptomatic. Latent visceral infection can activate years to decades postexposure in people who become immunocompromised (eg, because of coinfection with human immunodeficiency virus [HIV] or post-transplantation immunosuppression) or who receive immunomodulatory therapy (eg, with anti-tumor necrosis factor-alpha) because of other medical conditions.

ETIOLOGY: In the human host, *Leishmania* species are obligate intracellular parasites of mononuclear phagocytes. To date, approximately 20 *Leishmania* species (in the *Leishmania* and *Viannia* subgenera) are known to infect humans. Cutaneous leishmaniasis typically is caused by Old World species *Leishmania tropica*, *Leishmania major*, and *Leishmania aethiopica* and by New World species *Leishmania mexicana*, *Leishmania amazonensis*, *Leishmania (Viannia) braziliensis*, *Leishmania (V) panamensis*, *Leishmania (V) guyanensis*, and *Leishmania (V) peruviana*. Mucosal leishmaniasis typically is caused by species in the *Viannia* subgenus (especially *L [V] braziliensis* but also *L [V] panamensis* and sometimes *L [V] guyanensis*). Most cases of visceral leishmaniasis are caused by *Leishmania donovani* or *Leishmania infantum* (*Leishmania chagasi* is synonymous). *L donovani* and *L infantum* also can cause cutaneous leishmaniasis; however, people with typical cutaneous leishmaniasis caused by these organisms rarely develop visceral leishmaniasis.

EPIDEMIOLOGY: In most settings, leishmaniasis is a zoonosis, with mammalian reservoir hosts, such as rodents or dogs. However, some transmission cycles are anthroponotic: infected humans are the primary or only reservoir hosts of *L donovani* in South Asia (potentially also in East Africa) and of *L tropica*. Congenital and parenteral transmission also have been reported.

Overall, leishmaniasis is endemic in more than 90 countries in the tropics, subtropics, and southern Europe. Visceral leishmaniasis (an estimated 0.2–0.4 million new cases annually) is found in focal areas of more than 60 countries: in the Old World, in parts of Asia (particularly South, Southwest, and Central Asia), Africa (particularly East Africa), the Middle East, and southern Europe; and, in the New World, particularly in Brazil, with scattered foci elsewhere. Most (>90%) of the world's cases of visceral leishmaniasis occur in South Asia (India, Bangladesh, and Nepal), East Africa (Sudan, South Sudan, and Ethiopia), and Brazil. Cutaneous leishmaniasis is more common (an estimated total of 0.7 to 1.2 million new cases annually) and more widespread than visceral leishmaniasis. Cutaneous leishmaniasis is found in focal areas of more than 90 countries: in the Old World, in parts of the Middle East, Asia (particularly Southwest and Central Asia), Africa (particularly North and East Africa, with some cases elsewhere), and southern Europe; and, in the New World, in parts of Mexico, Central America, and South America (not in Chile or Uruguay). Occasional cases of cutaneous leishmaniasis have been acquired in Texas and Oklahoma. The geographic distribution of leishmaniasis cases identified in the United States reflects immigration and travel patterns (eg, the locations of popular tourist destinations in Latin America and of various military activities).

The incubation periods for the various forms of leishmaniasis range from weeks to years. In cutaneous leishmaniasis, the primary skin lesions typically appear within several weeks postexposure. In visceral infection, the incubation period usually ranges from approximately 2 to 6 months.

DIAGNOSTIC TESTS: Definitive diagnosis is made by detecting the parasite in infected tissue by light-microscopic examination of stained slides (eg, of aspirates, touch preparations, or histologic sections), by in vitro culture, or by molecular methods. In cutaneous and mucosal disease, tissue can be obtained by a 3-mm punch biopsy, lesion scrapings, or needle aspiration of the raised nonnecrotic edge of the lesion. In visceral leishmaniasis, although the sensitivity (diagnostic yield) is highest for splenic aspiration (approximately 95%), the procedure can be associated with life-threatening hemorrhage; bone marrow aspiration is safer and generally is preferred. Other potential sources of specimens include liver, lymph node, and, in some patients (eg, those coinfected with HIV), whole blood or buffy coat. Identification of the *Leishmania* species (eg, via isoenzyme analysis of cultured parasites or molecular approaches) may affect prognosis and influence treatment decisions. The Centers for Disease Control and Prevention (CDC) (**www.cdc.gov/ parasites/leishmaniasis**) can assist in all aspects of diagnostic testing. Serologic testing usually is not helpful in the evaluation of potential cases of cutaneous leishmaniasis but can provide supportive evidence for the diagnosis of visceral or mucosal leishmaniasis, particularly if the patient is immunocompetent.

TREATMENT: Systemic antileishmanial treatment always is indicated for patients with visceral or mucosal leishmaniasis, whereas not all patients with cutaneous leishmaniasis need to be treated or require systemic therapy. Consultation with infectious disease or tropical medicine specialists and with staff of the CDC Division of Parasitic Diseases and Malaria is recommended (telephone: 404-718-4745; e-mail: parasites@cdc.gov; CDC Emergency Operations Center [after business hours and on weekends]: 770-488-7100). The relative merits of various treatment approaches/regimens for an individual patient should be considered, taking into account that the therapeutic response may vary not only for different *Leishmania* species but also for the same species in different geographic regions (see Drugs for Parasitic Infections, p 927). In addition, special considerations apply in the United States regarding the availability of particular medications. For example, the pentavalent antimonial compound sodium stibogluconate is not commercially available but can be obtained by US-licensed physicians through the CDC Drug Service (404-639-3670), under an investigational new drug (IND) protocol, for parenteral (intravenous or intramuscular) treatment of leishmaniasis. Liposomal amphotericin B, which is administered by intravenous infusion, is approved by the Food and Drug Administration (FDA) for treatment of visceral leishmaniasis. The oral agent miltefosine is approved for treatment of cutaneous and mucosal as well as visceral leishmaniasis; the FDA-approved indications are limited to infection caused by particular *Leishmania* species and to patients who are at least 12 years of age, weigh at least 30 kg (66 pounds), and are not pregnant or breastfeeding.

ISOLATION OF THE HOSPITALIZED PATIENT: Standard precautions are recommended.

CONTROL MEASURES: The best way for travelers to prevent leishmaniasis is by protecting themselves from sand-fly bites. Vaccines and drugs for preventing infection are not available. To decrease the risk of being bitten, travelers should:

- Stay in well-screened or air-conditioned areas when feasible. Avoid outdoor activities, especially from dusk to dawn, when sand flies generally are most active.
- When outside, wear long-sleeved shirts, long pants, and socks.
- Apply insect repellent on uncovered skin and under the ends of sleeves and pant legs. Follow instructions on the label of the repellent. The most effective repellents generally are those that contain the chemical N,N-diethyl-meta-toluamide (DEET) (see Prevention of Mosquitoborne Infections, p 213).
- Spray clothing items with a pyrethroid-containing insecticide several days before travel, and allow them to dry. The insecticide should be reapplied after every 5 washings. Permethrin should never be applied to skin.
- Spray living and sleeping areas with an insecticide.
- If not sleeping in an area that is well screened or air conditioned, a bed net tucked under the mattress is recommended. If possible, a bed net that has been soaked in or sprayed with a pyrethroid-containing insecticide should be used. The insecticide will be effective for several months if the bed net is not washed. Sand flies are much smaller than mosquitoes and, therefore, can penetrate through smaller holes. Fine-mesh netting (at least 18 holes to the inch) is needed for an effective barrier against sand flies. This is particularly important if the bed net has not been treated with a pyrethroid-containing insecticide. However, sleeping under such a closely woven net in hot weather can be uncomfortable.
- Bed nets, repellents containing DEET, and permethrin should be purchased before traveling.

Leprosy

CLINICAL MANIFESTATIONS: Leprosy (Hansen disease) is a curable infection involving skin, peripheral nerves, mucosa of the upper respiratory tract, and testes. The clinical forms of leprosy reflect the cellular immune response to *Mycobacterium leprae,* and in turn the number, size, structure, and bacillary content of the lesions. The organism has unique tropism for peripheral nerves, and all forms of leprosy exhibit nerve involvement. Leprosy lesions usually do not itch or hurt. They lack sensation to heat, touch, and pain but otherwise may be difficult to distinguish from other common maladies. There may be madarosis (loss of eyelashes or eyebrows) and other ocular problems. However, the stereotypical presentations of leonine facies with nasal deformity or clawed hands with loss of digits are manifestations of late-stage untreated disease that seldom are seen today. Although the nerve injury caused by leprosy is irreversible, early diagnosis and drug therapy can prevent sequelae.

Leprosy manifests over a broad clinical and histopathologic spectrum. In the United States, the Ridley-Jopling scale is used to classify patients according to the histopathologic features of their lesions and organization of the underlying granuloma. The scale includes: (1) tuberculoid, (2) borderline tuberculoid, (3) borderline, (4) borderline lepromatous, and (5) lepromatous. A simplified scheme introduced by the World Health Organization for circumstances where pathologic examination and diagnosis is unavailable is based purely on clinical skin examination. Under this scheme, leprosy is classified by the number of skin patches seen on skin examination, classifying disease as either paucibacillary (1–5 lesions, usually tuberculoid or borderline tuberculoid) or multibacillary (>5 lesions, usually borderline, borderline lepromatous, or lepromatous). Patients in the tuberculoid spectrum have active cell-mediated immunity with low antibody responses to *M leprae* and few well-defined lesions containing few bacilli. Lepromatous spectrum cases have high antibody responses with little cell mediated immunity to *M leprae* and several somewhat-diffuse lesions usually containing numerous bacilli.

Serious consequences of leprosy occur from immune reactions and nerve involvement with resulting anesthesia, which can lead to repeated unrecognized trauma, ulcerations, fractures, and even bone resorption. Injuries can have a significant effect on life quality. Leprosy is a leading cause of permanent physical disability among communicable diseases worldwide. Eye involvement can occur, and patients should be examined by an ophthalmologist. A diagnosis of leprosy should be considered in any patient with hypoesthetic or anesthetic skin rash, or skin patches, especially those that do not respond to ordinary therapies, and among those with a history of residence in areas with endemic leprosy or contact with armadillos.

Leprosy Reactions. Acute clinical exacerbations reflect abrupt changes in the immunologic balance. They are especially common during initial years of treatment but can occur in the absence of therapy. Two major types of leprosy reactions (LRs) are seen: type 1 (reversal reaction, LR-1) predominantly is observed in borderline tuberculoid and borderline lepromatous leprosy and is the result of a sudden increase in effective cell-mediated immunity. Acute tenderness and swelling at the site of cutaneous and neural lesions with development of new lesions are major manifestations. Ulcerations can occur, but polymorphonuclear leukocytes are absent from the LR-1 lesion. Fever and systemic toxicity are uncommon. Type 2 (erythema nodosum leprosum, LR-2) occurs in borderline and lepromatous forms as a systemic inflammatory response. Tender, red dermal papules or nodules resembling erythema nodosum along with high fever, migrating polyarthralgia, painful swelling of lymph nodes and spleen, iridocyclitis, and rarely, nephritis can occur.

ETIOLOGY: Leprosy is caused by *M leprae*, an obligate intracellular bacterium that can have variable findings on Gram stain and is rod-shaped and weakly acid-fast on standard Ziehl-Nielsen staining. It is best visualized using the Fite stain.[1] *M leprae* is the only bacterium known to infect Schwann cells of peripheral nerves, and demonstration of acid-fast bacilli in peripheral nerves is pathognomonic for leprosy.

---

[1] Job CK, Chacko CJ. A modification of Fite's stain for demonstration of *M. leprae* in tissue sections. *Indian J Lepr.* 1986;58(1):17–18

EPIDEMIOLOGY: Leprosy is considered a neglected tropical disease and is most prevalent in tropical and subtropical zones. It is not highly infectious. Several human genes have been identified that are associated with susceptibility to *M leprae*, and fewer than 5% of people appear to be genetically susceptible to the infection. Accordingly, spouses of leprosy patients are not likely to develop leprosy, but biological parents, children, and siblings who are household contacts of untreated patients with leprosy are at increased risk.

Transmission is thought to be most effective through long-term close contact with an infected individual, and it likely occurs through respiratory shedding of infectious droplets by untreated cases or individuals incubating subclinical infections. The 9-banded armadillo (*Dasypus novemcinctus*) and 6-banded armadillo (*Euphractus sexcinctus*) are the only known nonhuman reservoirs of *M leprae*, and zoonotic transmission is reported in the southern United States. People with human immunodeficiency virus (HIV) infection do not appear to be at increased risk of becoming infected with *M leprae*. However, concomitant HIV infection and leprosy can lead to worsening of leprosy symptoms during HIV treatment and result in immune reconstitution inflammatory syndrome. Like many other chronic infectious diseases, onset of leprosy is associated increasingly with use of anti-inflammatory autoimmune therapies and immunologic senescence among elderly patients.

There are approximately 6500 people with leprosy living in the United States; with 3300 under active medical management. During 1994–2011, there were 2323 new cases of leprosy, with an average annual incidence rate of 0.45 cases per 1 million people. Over this period, a decline in the rate of new diagnoses from 0.52 (1994–1996) to 0.43 (2009–2011) per million was observed. The rate among foreign-born people decreased from 3.66 to 2.29, whereas the rate among US-born people was 0.16 in both 1994–1996 and 2009–2011.[1] Delayed diagnosis was more common among foreign-born people. The majority of leprosy cases reported in the United States occurred among residents of Texas, California, and Hawaii or among immigrants and other citizens who lived or worked in leprosy-endemic countries and likely acquired their disease while abroad. More than 65% of the world's leprosy patients reside in South and Southeast Asia—primarily India. Other areas of high endemicity include Angola, Brazil, Central African Republic, Democratic Republic of Congo, Madagascar, Mozambique, the Republic of the Marshall Islands, South Sudan, the Federated States of Micronesia, and the United Republic of Tanzania.

The **incubation period** usually is 3 to 5 years but ranges from 1 to 20 years. The average age at onset varies according to endemicity within the population. Younger patients (15 to 30 years of age) predominate in areas of high endemicity, and older average ages predominate in areas of low endemicity.

DIAGNOSTIC TESTS: There are no early diagnostic tests or methods to detect subclinical leprosy. Histopathologic examination of skin biopsy by an experienced pathologist is the best method of establishing the diagnosis and is the basis for classification of leprosy. These specimens can be sent to National Hansen's Disease (Leprosy) Programs (NHDP) [800-642-2477; **www.hrsa.gov/hansensdisease**] in formalin or embedded in paraffin. Acid-fast bacilli may be found in slit smears or biopsy specimens of skin lesions of

---

[1]Centers for Disease Control and Prevention. Incidence of Hansen's disease—United States, 1994–2011. *MMWR Recomm Rep.* 2014;63(43):969–972

patients with lepromatous forms of the disease but rarely are visualized from patients with tuberculoid and indeterminate forms of disease.

M leprae have not been cultured successfully in vitro. A polymerase chain reaction (PCR) test for *M leprae* is available to assist diagnosis after consultation with the NHDP and can be performed on the basis of clinical suspicion. Molecular tests for mutations causing drug resistance also are available, as is strain typing based on single nucleotide polymorphism (SNP) and other genomic elements.

TREATMENT: Leprosy is curable. The primary goal of therapy is prevention of permanent nerve damage, which can be accomplished by early diagnosis and treatment. Combination antimicrobial multidrug therapy can be obtained free of charge from the NHDP in the United States and from the World Health Organization in other countries. Certain criteria must be met for physicians wishing to obtain the antimicrobial therapy from the NHDP (**www.hrsa.gov/hansensdisease/diagnosis/ recommendedtreatment.html**).

It is important to treat *M leprae* infections with more than 1 antimicrobial agent to minimize development of antimicrobial-resistant organisms. Adults are treated with dapsone, rifampin, and clofazimine. Resistance to all 3 drugs has been documented but is rare. The infectivity of leprosy patients ceases within a few days of initiating standard multidrug therapy.

Treatment Regimens Recommended by the NHDP.

Multibacillary Leprosy (6 Patches or More):

1. Dapsone, 100 mg/day, orally, for 24 months. Pediatric dose: 1 mg/kg, orally, every 24 hours. Maximum dose: 100 mg/day for 24 months; **and**
2. Rifampin, 600 mg/day, orally, for 24 months. Pediatric dose: 10 mg/kg per day for 24 months; **and**
3. Clofazimine, 50 mg/day, orally, for 24 months. Clarithromycin can be used in place of clofazimine for children. Pediatric dose: 7.5 mg/kg per day, orally, for 24 months. Clofazimine is not available commercially; in the United States, it is available only as an investigational drug for treatment of leprosy and is obtained through the NHDP.

Paucibacillary Leprosy (1–5 Patches):

1. Dapsone, 100 mg/day, orally, for 12 months. Pediatric dose: 1 to 2 mg/kg, orally, every 24 hours. Maximum dose: 100 mg/day for 12 months; **and**
2. Rifampin, 600 mg/day, orally, for 12 months. Pediatric dose: 10 to 20 mg/kg per day, orally, for 12 months.

Before beginning antimicrobial therapy, patients should be tested for glucose-6-phosphate dehydrogenase deficiency, have baseline complete blood cell counts and liver function test results documented, and be evaluated for any evidence of tuberculosis infection, especially if the patient is infected with HIV. This consideration is important to avoid monotherapy of active tuberculosis with rifampin while treating active leprosy. Gastric upset and darkening of skin caused by daily clofazimine therapy also are common adverse reactions to the therapy. Skin darkening typically resolves within several months of completing therapy.

Leprosy reactions should be treated aggressively to prevent peripheral nerve damage. Treatment with prednisone, 1 mg/kg per day, orally, can be initiated. The severe type 2 reaction (erythema nodosum leprosum) occurs in patients with multibacillary leprosy. Treatment with thalidomide (100 mg/day for 4 days) is available for erythema nodosum leprosum under the Celgene S.T.E.P.S. Program (888-771-0141) and is used under strict supervision because of its teratogenicity. Thalidomide is not approved for use in children younger than 12 years. Most patients can be treated as outpatients. Rehabilitative measures, including surgery and physical therapy, may be necessary for some patients.

All patients with leprosy should be educated about signs and symptoms of neuritis and cautioned to report signs and symptoms of neuritis immediately so that corticosteroid therapy can be instituted. Patients should receive counseling because of the social and psychological effects of this disease.

Relapse of disease after completing multidrug therapy is rare (0.01%–0.14%); the presentation of new skin patches usually is attributable to a late type 1 reaction (LR-1). When it does occur, relapse usually is attributable to reactivation of drug-susceptible organisms. People with relapses of disease require another course of multidrug therapy.

Therapy for patients with leprosy should be undertaken in consultation with an expert in leprosy. The NHDP (800-642-2477) provides medications for leprosy at no charge as well as consultation on clinical and pathologic issues, and information about local Hansen disease clinics and clinicians who have experience with the disease. Prevention of disability is an important goal of treatment and care; a critical component of this is self-examination for any patient with loss of sensitivity in the foot.

ISOLATION OF THE HOSPITALIZED PATIENT: Standard precautions are indicated; isolation is not required. Many patients suffer profound anxiety because of the stigma historically associated with leprosy.

CONTROL MEASURES: Normal hospital hygienic practices are advised. Hand hygiene is recommended for all people in contact with patients. Gloves are not required or recommended because of the associated stigma. Household contacts should be examined initially, but long-term follow-up of asymptomatic contacts is not warranted. Chemoprophylaxis is not recommended.

There are no vaccines approved for use in the United States. A single bacille Calmette-Guérin (BCG) immunization is reported to be from 28% to 60% protective against leprosy, and BCG is used as an adjunct to drug therapy in Brazil. However, the effectiveness of combined drug and immunotherapy is unknown. The International Association of Leprosy Organizations (ILep) and American Leprosy Mission (ALM) are sponsoring a new antileprosy vaccine under development at the Infectious Disease Research Institute (Seattle, WA). This preparation was scheduled to enter initial trials beginning in late 2014.

Leprosy is a reportable disease in the United States. Newly diagnosed cases should be reported to state public health authorities, the Centers for Disease Control and Prevention, and the National Hansen Disease Program.

Leptospirosis

CLINICAL MANIFESTATIONS: Leptospirosis is an acute febrile disease with varied manifestations. The severity of disease ranges from asymptomatic or subclinical to self-limited systemic illness (approximately 90% of patients) to life-threatening illness with jaundice, renal failure (oliguric or nonoliguric), myocarditis, hemorrhage (particularly pulmonary), and refractory shock. Clinical presentation may be mono- or biphasic. Classically described biphasic leptospirosis has an acute septicemia phase usually lasting 1 week during which time *Leptospira* organisms are present in blood, followed by a second immune-mediated phase that does not respond to antibiotic therapy. Regardless of its severity, the acute phase is characterized by nonspecific symptoms, including fever, chills, headache, nausea, and vomiting occasionally accompanied by rash or conjunctival suffusion. Distinct clinical findings include notable conjunctival suffusion without purulent discharge (30%–99% of cases) and myalgia of the calf and lumbar regions (40%–100% of cases). Findings commonly associated with the immune-mediated phase include fever, aseptic meningitis, and uveitis; between 5% and 10% of *Leptospira*-infected patients are estimated to experience severe illness. Severe manifestations include any combination of jaundice and renal dysfunction (Weil syndrome), pulmonary hemorrhage, cardiac arrhythmias, and circulatory collapse. The estimated case-fatality rate is 5% to 15% with severe illness, although it can increase to >50% in patients with pulmonary hemorrhage syndrome. Asymptomatic or subclinical infection with seroconversion is frequent, especially in settings of endemic infection.

ETIOLOGY: Leptospirosis is caused by pathogenic spirochetes of the genus *Leptospira.* Leptospires are classified by species and subdivided into more than 250 antigenically defined serovars and grouped into serogroups on the basis of antigenic relatedness. Currently, the molecular classification divides the genus into 20 named pathogenic (n=9), intermediate (n=5) and saprophytic (nonpathogenic; n=6) genomospecies as determined by DNA-DNA hybridization and 16S ribosomal gene phylogenetic clustering.

EPIDEMIOLOGY: Leptospirosis is among the most globally important zoonoses, affecting people in resource-rich and resource-limited countries in both urban and rural contexts. It has been estimated that approximately 868 000 people annually worldwide are currently infected (range, 327 000–1 520 000), with approximately 49 200 (range, 19 000–88 900) deaths occurring each year. The reservoirs for *Leptospira* species include a wide range of wild and domestic animals, primarily rats, dogs, and livestock (cattle, pigs) that may shed organisms asymptomatically for years. *Leptospira* organisms excreted in animal urine may remain viable in moist soil or water for weeks to months in warm climates. Humans usually become infected via entry of leptospires through contact of mucosal surfaces (especially conjunctivae) or abraded skin with contaminated environmental sources. Unusually, infection may be acquired through direct contact with infected animals or their tissues, infective urine or fluids from carrier animals, or urine-contaminated soil or water. Epidemic exposure is associated with seasonal flooding and natural disasters, including hurricanes and monsoons. Populations in regions of high endemicity in the tropics likely encounter *Leptospira* organisms commonly during routine activities of daily living. People who are predisposed by occupation include abattoir and sewer workers, miners, veterinarians, farmers, and military personnel. Recreational exposures and clusters of disease have been associated with adventure travel, sporting events including triathlons, and wading, swimming, or boating in contaminated water, particularly during flooding or following heavy rainfall. Common history includes being submerged in or swallowing water during such activities. Person-to-person transmission is not convincingly described.

The **incubation period** usually is 5 to 14 days, range 2 to 30 days.

DIAGNOSTIC TESTS: Clinical features and routine laboratory findings of leptospirosis are not specific; a high index of suspicion must be maintained for the diagnosis. *Leptospira* organisms can be isolated from blood or cerebrospinal fluid specimens during the early septicemic phase (first 7–10 days) of illness and from urine specimens 14 days or more after illness onset. Specialized culture media are required but are not routinely available in most clinical laboratories. *Leptospira* organisms can be subcultured to specific *Leptospira* semi-solid medium (ie, EMJH) from blood culture bottles used in automated systems within 1 week of inoculation. However, isolation of the organism may be difficult, requiring incubation for up to 16 weeks, weekly darkfield microscopic examination, and avoidance of contamination. In addition, the sensitivity of culture for diagnosis is low. For these reasons, serum specimens always should be obtained to facilitate diagnosis. Antibodies can develop as early as 5 to 7 days after onset of illness, and can be measured by commercially available immunoassays, which are based on sonicates of the saprophyte *Leptospira biflexa*. These assays have variable sensitivity according to regional differences of the various *Leptospira* species; however, increases in antibody titer may not be detected until more than 10 days after onset, especially if antimicrobial therapy is initiated early. Further, in populations with high endemicity, background reactivity requires establishing regionally relevant diagnostic criteria and establishment of diagnostic versus background titers. Antibody increases can be transient, delayed, or absent in some patients, which may be related to antibiotic use, bacterial virulence, immunogenetics of the individual, or other unknown factors. Microscopic agglutination, the gold standard serologic test, is performed only in reference laboratories and requires seroconversion demonstrated between acute and convalescent specimens obtained at least 10 days apart. Immunohistochemical and immunofluorescent techniques can detect leptospiral antigens in infected tissues. Polymerase chain reaction (PCR) assays for detection of *Leptospira* DNA in clinical specimens have been developed but are available only in research laboratories. *Leptospira* DNA can be detected in whole blood during the first 4 days of illness and after 1 week in urine.

TREATMENT: Antimicrobial therapy should be initiated as soon as possible after symptom onset. Intravenous penicillin is the drug of choice for patients with severe infection requiring hospitalization; penicillin has been shown to be effective in shortening duration of fever as late as 7 days into the course of illness. Penicillin G decreases the duration of systemic symptoms and persistence of associated laboratory abnormalities and may prevent development of leptospiruria. As with other spirochetal infections, a Jarisch-Herxheimer reaction (an acute febrile reaction accompanied by headache, myalgia, and an aggravated clinical picture lasting less than 24 hours) can develop after initiation of penicillin therapy. Parenteral cefotaxime, ceftriaxone, and doxycycline have been demonstrated in randomized clinical trials to be equal in efficacy to penicillin G for treatment of severe leptospirosis. Severe cases also require appropriate supportive care, including fluid and electrolyte replacement. Patients with oliguric renal insufficiency and pulmonary hemorrhage syndrome require prompt dialysis and mechanical ventilation, respectively, to improve clinical outcome. For patients with mild disease, oral doxycycline has been shown to shorten the course of illness and decrease occurrence of leptospiruria; ampicillin or amoxicillin can also be used to treat mild disease. Tetracycline-based antimicrobial agents, including doxycycline, may cause permanent tooth discoloration for children younger than 8 years if used for repeated treatment courses. However, doxycycline binds less readily to calcium compared with older tetracyclines, and in some studies, doxycycline was not associated with visible teeth staining in younger children (see Tetracyclines, p 873). Azithromycin has been demonstrated in a clinical trial to be as effective as doxycycline and can be used as an alternative in patients for whom doxycycline is contraindicated.

ISOLATION OF THE HOSPITALIZED PATIENT: In addition to standard precautions, contact precautions are recommended for contact with urine.

CONTROL MEASURES:

- Immunization of livestock and dogs can prevent clinical disease attributable to infecting serovars contained within the vaccine. However, immunization may not prevent the shedding of leptospires in their urine, thus contaminating environments with which humans may come in contact.
- In areas with known endemic infection, reservoir-control programs may be useful.
- Swimmers should attempt to avoid immersion or swallowing water in potentially contaminated fresh water.
- Protective clothing, boots, and gloves should be worn by people with occupational exposure to decrease their risk.
- Doxycycline, 200 mg, administered orally once a week to adults, may provide effective prophylaxis against clinical disease and could be considered for high-risk groups (eg, triathletes) with short-term exposure, but infection may not be prevented. Indications for prophylactic doxycycline use for children have not been established.

Listeria monocytogenes Infections
(Listeriosis)

CLINICAL MANIFESTATIONS: Listeriosis is a relatively uncommon but severe invasive infection caused by *Listeria monocytogenes*. Transmission predominantly is foodborne, and illness occurs most frequently among pregnant women and their fetuses or newborn infants, older adults, and people with impaired cell-mediated immunity resulting from underlying illness or treatment (eg, organ transplant, hematologic malignancy, immunosuppression resulting from therapy with corticosteroid or anti-tumor necrosis factor agents, or acquired immunodeficiency syndrome). Pregnancy-associated infections can result in spontaneous abortion, fetal death, preterm delivery, and neonatal illness or death. In pregnant women, infections can be asymptomatic or associated with a nonspecific febrile illness with myalgia, back pain, and occasionally gastrointestinal tract symptoms. Fetal infection results from transplacental transmission following maternal bacteremia. Approximately 65% of pregnant women with *Listeria* infection experience a prodromal illness before the diagnosis of listeriosis in their newborn infant. Amnionitis during labor, brown staining of amniotic fluid, or asymptomatic perinatal infection can occur. Neonates can present with early-onset and late-onset syndromes similar to those of group B streptococcal infections. Preterm birth, pneumonia, and septicemia are common in early-onset disease (within the first week of life), with fatality rates of 14% to 56%. An erythematous rash with small, pale papules characterized histologically by granulomas, termed "granulomatosis infantisepticum," can occur in severe newborn infection. Late-onset infections occur at 8 to 30 days of life following term deliveries and usually result in meningitis with fatality rates of approximately 25%. Late onset infection may result from acquisition of the organism during passage through the birth canal or, rarely, from environmental sources. Health care-associated nursery outbreaks have been reported.

Clinical features characteristic of invasive listeriosis outside the neonatal period or pregnancy are bacteremia and meningitis with or without parenchymal brain involvement, and less commonly brain abscess or endocarditis. *L monocytogenes* also can cause rhombencephalitis (brain stem encephalitis) in otherwise healthy adolescents and young adults. Outbreaks of febrile gastroenteritis caused by food contaminated with a very large inoculum of *L monocytogenes* have been reported. The prevalence of stool carriage of *L monocytogenes* among healthy, asymptomatic adults is estimated to be 1% to 5%.

ETIOLOGY: *L monocytogenes* is a facultatively anaerobic, nonspore-forming, nonbranching, motile, gram-positive rod that multiplies intracellularly. The organism grows readily on blood agar and produces incomplete hemolysis. *L monocytogenes* serotypes 1/2a, 4b, and 1/2b cause most human cases of invasive listeriosis. Unlike most bacteria, *L monocytogenes* grows well at refrigerator temperatures (4°C–10°C).

EPIDEMIOLOGY: *L monocytogenes* causes approximately 1600 cases of invasive disease and 260 deaths annually in the United States. The saprophytic organism is distributed widely in the environment and is an important cause of illness in ruminants. Foodborne transmission causes outbreaks and sporadic infections in humans. Commonly incriminated foods include deli-style, ready-to-eat meats, particularly poultry; unpasteurized milk,[1] and soft cheeses, including Mexican-style cheese. The US incidence of listeriosis decreased substantially during the 1990s, when US regulatory agencies began enforcing rigorous screening guidelines for *L monocytogenes* in processed foods. The last large outbreak in the United States occurred in 2011, resulting in 143 hospitalizations, and was linked to contaminated cantaloupe.

The **incubation period** for invasive disease is longer for pregnancy-associated cases (2–4 weeks or occasionally longer) than for nonpregnancy-associated cases (1 to 14 days). The incubation period for self-limiting, febrile gastroenteritis following ingestion of a large inoculum is 24 hours; illness typically lasts 2 to 3 days.

DIAGNOSTIC TESTS: *L monocytogenes* can be recovered readily on blood agar from cultures of blood, cerebrospinal fluid (CSF), meconium, placental or fetal tissue specimens, amniotic fluid, and other infected tissue specimens, including joint, pleural, or peritoneal fluid. Gram stain of meconium, placental tissue, biopsy specimens of the rash of early-onset infection, or CSF from an infected patient may demonstrate the organism. The organisms can be gram-variable and can resemble diphtheroids, cocci, or diplococci. Laboratory misidentification is not uncommon, and the isolation of a "diphtheroid" from blood or cerebrospinal fluid (CSF) should always alert one to the possibility that the organism is *L monocytogenes*.

TREATMENT: No controlled trials have established the drug(s) of choice or duration of therapy for listerial infection. Combination therapy using ampicillin and a second agent is recommended for severe infections, including meningitis, encephalitis, endocarditis, and infections in neonates and immunocompromised patients. Therapy with intravenous ampicillin and an aminoglycoside, usually gentamicin, has been used traditionally. Use of an alternative second agent that is active intracellularly (eg, trimethoprim-sulfamethoxazole, quinolones, linezolid, or rifampin) is supported by clinical reports in adults. In the penicillin-allergic patient, either trimethoprim-sulfamethoxazole or a quinolone have been used successfully as monotherapy for *Listeria* meningitis and in the setting of brain abscess. If alternatives to gentamicin are used, susceptibility should be confirmed because resistance to trimethoprim-sulfamethoxazole, quinolones, linezolid, or rifampin occasionally has been reported. Treatment failures with vancomycin have been reported. Cephalosporins are not active against *L monocytogenes*. For bacteremia without associated CNS infection, 14 days of treatment is sufficient. For *L monocytogenes* meningitis, most experts recommend 21 days of treatment. Longer courses are necessary for patients with endocarditis or parenchymal brain infection (cerebritis, rhombencephalitis, brain abscess). Diagnostic imaging of the brain near the end of the anticipated duration of therapy

---

[1]American Academy of Pediatrics, Committee on Infectious Diseases and Committee on Nutrition. Consumption of raw or unpasteurized milk and milk products by pregnant women and children. *Pediatrics.* 2014;133(1):175–179

allows determination of parenchymal involvement of the brain and the need for prolonged therapy in neonates with complicated courses and immunocompromised patients.

ISOLATION OF THE HOSPITALIZED PATIENT: Standard precautions are recommended.

CONTROL MEASURES:
- Antimicrobial therapy for infection diagnosed during pregnancy may prevent fetal or perinatal infection and its consequences.
- Neonatal listeriosis complicating successive pregnancies is virtually unknown, and intrapartum antibiotic therapy is not recommended for mothers with a history of perinatal listeriosis.
- General and specific guidelines for preventing listeriosis from foodborne sources are provided in Table 3.36.

Table 3.36. Recommendations for Preventing Foodborne Listeriosis

General recommendations
Washing and handling food
- **Rinse** raw produce thoroughly under running tap water before eating, cutting, or cooking. Even if the produce will be peeled, it should still be washed first.
- **Scrub** firm produce, such as melons and cucumbers, with a clean produce brush.
- **Dry** the produce with a clean cloth or paper towel.

Keep your kitchen and environment cleaner and safer
- Wash hands, knives, countertops, and cutting boards after handling and preparing uncooked foods.
- Be aware that *Listeria monocytogenes* can grow in foods in the refrigerator. The refrigerator temperature should be 40°F or lower and the freezer temperature should be 0°F or lower.
- Clean up all spills in your refrigerator right away–especially juices from hot dog and lunch meat packages, raw meat, and raw poultry.

Cook meat and poultry thoroughly
- Thoroughly cook raw food from animal sources, such as beef, pork, or poultry to a safe internal temperature.
- Use precooked or ready-to-eat food as soon as you can. Do not store the product in the refrigerator beyond the use-by date.
- Use leftovers within 3 to 4 days.

Choose safer foods
- Do not drink raw (unpasteurized) milk[a] (**www.cdc.gov/foodsafety/rawmilk/raw-milk-index.html**), and do not eat foods that have unpasteurized milk in them.

Recommendations for people at higher risk, such as pregnant women, people with weakened immune systems, and older adults, in addition to the recommendations listed above, include:
Meats
- Do not eat hot dogs, luncheon meats, cold cuts, other deli meats (eg, bologna), or fermented or dry sausages unless they are heated to an internal temperature of 165°F or until steaming hot just before serving.
- Avoid getting fluid from hot dog and lunch meat packages on other foods, utensils, and food preparation surfaces, and wash hands after handling hot dogs, luncheon meats, and deli meats.
- Do not eat refrigerated pâté or meat spreads from a deli or meat counter or from the refrigerated section of a store. Foods that do not need refrigeration, like canned or shelf-stable pâté and meat spreads, are safe to eat. Refrigerate after opening.

continued

Table 3.36. Recommendations for Preventing Foodborne Listeriosis, continued

Cheeses
- Do not eat soft cheese such as feta, queso blanco, queso fresco, brie, Camembert, blue-veined, or panela (queso panela) unless it is labeled as made with pasteurized milk. Make sure the label says, "MADE WITH PASTEURIZED MILK."
- Be aware that cheeses made from pasteurized milk, such as Mexican-style cheese, that were likely contaminated during cheese-making have caused listeriosis.

Seafood
- Do not eat refrigerated smoked seafood, unless it is contained in a cooked dish, such as a casserole, or unless it is a canned or shelf-stable product.
- Canned and shelf-stable tuna, salmon, and other fish products are safe to eat.

Melons
- Wash hands with warm water and soap for at least 20 seconds *before* and *after* handling any whole melon.
- Scrub the surface of melons with a clean produce brush under running water and dry them with a clean cloth or paper towel before cutting. Be sure that your scrub brush is sanitized after each use.
- Promptly consume cut melon or refrigerate promptly. Keep your cut melon refrigerated for no more than 7 days.
- Discard cut melons left at room temperature for more than 4 hours.

[a]American Academy of Pediatrics, Committee on Infectious Diseases and Committee on Nutrition. Consumption of raw or unpasteurized milk and milk products by pregnant women and children. *Pediatrics.* 2014;133(1):175–179

- Trimethoprim-sulfamethoxazole, given as pneumocystis prophylaxis for those with acquired immunodeficiency syndrome, transplant recipients, or others on long-term, high-dose corticosteroids, effectively prevents listeriosis.
- Listeriosis is a nationally notifiable disease in the United States. Cases should be reported promptly to the state or local health department to facilitate early recognition and control of common-source outbreaks. Clinical isolates should be forwarded to a public health laboratory for molecular subtyping.

Lyme Disease[1,2]
(Lyme Borreliosis, *Borrelia burgdorferi* Infection)

CLINICAL MANIFESTATIONS: Clinical manifestations of Lyme disease are divided into 3 stages: early localized, early disseminated, and late disease. Early localized disease is characterized by a distinctive lesion, erythema migrans, at the site of a recent tick bite. Erythema migrans is by far the most common manifestation of Lyme disease in children. Erythema migrans begins as a red macule or papule that usually expands over days to weeks to form a large, annular, erythematous lesion that typically increases in size to 5 cm or more in diameter, sometimes with partial central clearing. The lesion is usually but not

[1]Wormser GP, Dattwyler RJ, Shapiro ED, et al. The clinical assessment, treatment, and prevention of Lyme disease, human granulocytic anaplasmosis, and babesiosis: clinical practice guidelines by the Infectious Diseases Society of America. *Clin Infect Dis.* 2006;43(9):1089–1134

[2]Lantos PM, Charini WA, Medoff G, et al. Final report of the Lyme Disease Review Panel of the Infectious Diseases Society of America. *Clin Infect Dis.* 2010;51(1):1–5

always painless, and it is not pruritic. Localized erythema migrans can vary greatly in size and shape and can be confused with cellulitis; lesions may have a purplish discoloration or central vesicular or necrotic areas. A classic "bulls-eye" appearance with concentric rings appears in a minority of cases. Factors that distinguish erythema migrans from local allergic reaction to a tick bite include larger size (>5 cm), gradual expansion, lack of pruritus, and slower onset. Constitutional symptoms, such as malaise, headache, mild neck stiffness, myalgia, and arthralgia, often accompany the rash of early localized disease. Fever may be present but is not universal and generally is mild. In early disseminated disease, multiple erythema migrans lesions may appear several weeks after an infective tick bite and consist of secondary annular, erythematous lesions similar to but usually smaller than the primary lesion. Other manifestations of early disseminated illness (which may occur with or without rash) are palsies of the cranial nerves (especially cranial nerve VII), lymphocytic meningitis, and polyradiculitis. Ophthalmic conditions (conjunctivitis, optic neuritis, keratitis, uveitis) can occur, usually in concert with other neurologic manifestations. Systemic symptoms, such as low-grade fever, arthralgia, myalgia, headache, and fatigue, also are common during the early disseminated stage. Lymphocytic meningitis can occur and often is associated with cranial neuropathy or papilledema; patients with lymphocytic meningitis typically have a more subacute onset, lower temperature, and fewer white blood cells in cerebrospinal fluid (CSF) than those with viral meningitis. Carditis, which usually manifests as various degrees of heart block, can occur in children but is relatively less common. Occasionally, people with early Lyme disease have concurrent human granulocytic anaplasmosis or babesiosis, which are transmitted by the same tick. Coinfection may present as more severe disease than Lyme monoinfection, and the presence of a high fever with Lyme disease or inadequate response to treatment should raise suspicion of concurrent anaplasmosis or babesiosis. Certain laboratory abnormalities, such as leukopenia, thrombocytopenia, anemia, or abnormal hepatic transaminase concentrations, raise concern for coinfection.

Late disease occurs in patients who are not treated at an earlier stage of illness and most commonly manifests as Lyme arthritis in children. Lyme arthritis is characterized by inflammatory arthritis that usually is pauciarticular and affects large joints, particularly knees. Although arthralgias can be present at any stage of Lyme disease, Lyme arthritis has objective evidence of joint swelling as well as white blood cells in synovial fluid specimens. Arthritis can occur without a history of earlier stages of illness (including erythema migrans). Compared with pyogenic arthritis, Lyme arthritis tends to manifest with joint swelling/effusion out of proportion to pain or disability and with lower peripheral blood neutrophilia and erythrocyte sedimentation rate (ESR). Polyneuropathy, encephalopathy, and encephalitis are extremely rare manifestations of late disease. Children who are treated with antimicrobial agents in the early stage of disease almost never develop late disease.

Lyme disease is not thought to produce a congenital infection syndrome. No causal relationship between maternal Lyme disease and abnormalities of pregnancy or congenital disease caused by *Borrelia burgdorferi* has been documented. No evidence exists that Lyme disease can be transmitted via human milk.

Some patients with demonstrated Lyme disease have persistent subjective symptoms, such as fatigue and arthralgia, after appropriate treatment, a condition known as post-treatment Lyme disease syndrome (PTLDS). Although the cause is not known, ongoing infection with *B burgdorferi* has not been demonstrated, and long-term antibiotics have not been shown to be beneficial. Patients with PTLDS usually respond to symptomatic treatment and recover gradually.

"Chronic Lyme disease" is a nonspecific term that lacks a clinical definition. It is used by a small minority of clinicians and patient advocates to refer to patients with chronic, unexplained syndromes usually characterized by pain and fatigue. Alternative diagnoses may be responsible for symptoms and should be considered. In none of these situations is there credible evidence that persistent infection with *B burgdorferi* is demonstrable, let alone causal.

ETIOLOGY: In the United States, Lyme disease is caused by the spirochete *B burgdorferi* sensu stricto. In Eurasia, *B burgdorferi*, *Borrelia afzelii*, and *Borrelia garinii* cause borreliosis.

EPIDEMIOLOGY: Lyme disease occurs primarily in 2 distinct geographic regions of the United States. More than 90% of cases occur in New England and in the eastern Mid-Atlantic States, as far south as Virginia. The disease also occurs, but with lower frequency, in the upper Midwest, especially Wisconsin and Minnesota. Transmission also occurs at a low level on the west coast, especially northern California. The occurrence of cases in the United States correlates with the distribution and frequency of infected tick vectors—*Ixodes scapularis* in the east and Midwest and *Ixodes pacificus* in the west. In Southern states, *I scapularis* ticks are rare compared with the northeast; those ticks that are present do not commonly feed on competent reservoir mammals and are less likely to bite humans because of different questing habits. Reported cases from states without known enzootic risks may have been acquired in states with endemic infection or may be misdiagnoses resulting from false-positive serologic test results or results that are misinterpreted as positive.

Most cases of early Lyme disease occur between April and October; more than 50% of cases occur during June and July. People of all ages may be affected, but incidence in the United States is highest among children 5 through 9 years of age and adults 55 through 59 years of age. A lesion similar to erythema migrans known as "southern tick-associated rash illness" or STARI has been reported in south central and southeastern states without endemic *B burgdorferi* infection.[1] The etiology and appropriate treatment of this condition remain unknown. STARI results from the bite of the lone star tick, *Amblyomma americanum*, which is abundant in southern states and is biologically incapable of transmitting *B burgdorferi*. Patients with STARI may present with constitutional symptoms in addition to erythema migrans; however, STARI has not been associated with any of the disseminated complications of Lyme disease.

The **incubation period** from tick bite to appearance of single or multiple erythema migrans lesions ranges from 1 to 32 days, with a median of 11 days. Late manifestations can occur months after the tick bite.

Lyme disease also is endemic in eastern Canada, Europe, states of the former Soviet Union, China, and Japan. The primary tick vector in Europe is *Ixodes ricinus*, and the primary tick vector in Asia is *Ixodes persulcatus*. Clinical manifestations of infection vary somewhat from manifestations seen in the United States. In particular, European Lyme disease may cause borrelial lymphocytoma and acrodermatitis chronica atrophicans and is more

---

[1] Lantos PM, Brinkerhoff RJ, Wormser GP, Clemen R. Empiric antibiotic treatment of erythema migrans-like skin lesions as a function of geography: a clinical and cost effectiveness modeling study. *Vector Borne Zoonotic Dis.* 2013;13(12):877–883

likely to produce neurologic disease, whereas arthritis is uncommon. These differences are attributable to the different genospecies of *Borrelia* responsible for European Lyme disease.

DIAGNOSTIC TESTS: The diagnosis of Lyme disease rests first and foremost on the recognition of a consistent clinical illness in people who have had plausible geographic exposure. Early localized Lyme disease is diagnosed clinically on recognition of an erythema migrans lesion. Although erythema migrans is not strictly pathognomonic for Lyme disease, it is highly distinctive and characteristic. If a patient has a small lesion (under 5 cm diameter) that resembles erythema migrans, the patient can be followed over several days to see if the lesion expands to greater than 5 cm; this will improve the specificity of a clinical diagnosis. In areas endemic for Lyme disease during the warm months of the year, it is expected that the vast majority of erythema migrans is attributable to *B burgdorferi* infection, and early initiation of treatment is appropriate.

Diagnostic testing is based on serology; during early infection, the sensitivity is low. Thus, diagnostic testing is not recommended for this stage of illness; only approximately one third of patients with solitary erythema migrans lesions are seropositive. Neither a positive nor a negative serologic test result is helpful if the lesion truly resembles erythema migrans, because the lesion is so specific for Lyme disease. Furthermore, immunoglobulin (Ig) M-based Lyme disease serologic testing carries a substantial risk of false–positive results, so positive results cannot reliably explain a lesion that looks atypical. Patients who have multiple lesions of erythema migrans also are diagnosed clinically, although the likelihood of seropositivity is higher in this situation. There is a broad differential diagnosis for all disseminated manifestations of Lyme disease. Thus, the diagnosis of disseminated Lyme disease requires a typical clinical illness, plausible geographic exposure, and a positive serologic test result.

The standard testing method for Lyme disease is a 2-tier serologic assay. The initial test is a quantitative screening for antibodies to a whole-cell sonicate or C6 antigen of *B burgdorferi*. This test is performed using an enzyme-linked immunosorbent assay (ELISA or EIA) or immunofluorescent antibody (IFA) test. It should be noted that clinical laboratories vary somewhat in their description of this test. It may be described as "Lyme ELISA," "Lyme Antibody Screen," "Total Lyme Antibody," or "Lyme IgG/IgM." Many commercial laboratories offer EIA/IFA with reflex to Western immunoblot if the first-tier assay result is positive. This is the most foolproof way of ordering the appropriate 2-tier test for Lyme disease.

The initial EIA or IFA test result may be reported as a titer, but the role of the numerical titer is solely to categorize the result as negative, equivocal, or positive. If the first-tier ELISA result is negative, then the patient is considered seronegative and no further testing is indicated. If the result is equivocal or positive, then a second-tier test is required. Although sensitive, the first-tier test is not specific and results in a rate of false-positive results that may exceed 5% in clinically compatible cases and far higher in clinically nonsuggestive cases. This is partly because the test is not well standardized and because there are antigenic components of *B burgdorferi* that are not specific to this species. In particular, other spirochetal infections, normal spirochetes from our oral flora, other acute infections, and certain autoimmune diseases may be cross-reactive. The EIA or IFA test is the important helpful first-tier test but is too nonspecific to determine, in itself, a patient's serologic status.

Serum specimens that yield positive or equivocal EIA results then should be tested by the second-tier standardized Western immunoblot. This assay tests for the presence of antibodies to specific *B burgdorferi* antigens. Three IgM antibodies (to the 23/24, 39, and 41 kDa polypeptides) and 10 IgG antibodies (to the 18, 23/24, 28, 30, 39, 41, 45, 60, 66, and 93 kDa polypeptides) are tested. The presence of at least 2 IgM bands or 5 IgG bands is considered a positive immunoblot result. Laboratory reporting practices can produce some confusion when physicians are interpreting results. It is common for clinical laboratories to report the titers of all 13 bands and describe them as positive or negative; laboratories often print positive bands in bold, which frequently leads to physicians misinterpreting the overall result as positive despite the fact that 4 or fewer IgG bands are present. The presence of 4 or fewer IgG bands is too nonspecific to meet criteria for positivity. For example, the p41 band indicates antibody to a flagellar protein and is present in 30% to 50% of healthy people. Thus, it is imperative that the physician review the interpretive criteria for the test overall rather than risking overinterpretation of what may be a negative test result.

It is also important to note that the IgM assay is only useful for patients in the first 30 days after symptom onset. The IgM immunoblot should be disregarded (or, if possible, not ordered to begin with) in patients who have had symptoms for longer than 4 to 6 weeks, because false-positive IgM assay results are common, and most untreated patients with disseminated Lyme disease will have a positive IgG result by week 6 of illness.

Immunoblot testing should not be performed if the EIA result is negative or without a prior EIA; the specificity of immunoblot testing diminishes if this test is performed alone. The EIA and Western blot should not be thought of as "screening" and "confirmatory," respectively. They are interdependent parts of an overall testing method.

Laboratory results from patients treated for syphilis or other spirochete diseases are difficult to interpret; consultation with an infectious diseases specialist is recommended. Although immunodeficiency theoretically could affect serologic testing results, reports have described patients who produced anti-*B burgdorferi* antibodies and tested positive despite various immunocompromising conditions.

A licensed, commercially available serologic test (C6) that detects antibody to a peptide of the immunodominant conserved region of the variable surface antigen (VlsE) of *B burgdorferi* appears to have improved sensitivity for patients with early Lyme disease and Lyme disease acquired in Europe. However, when used alone, its specificity is lower than that of standard 2-tier testing. In the future, the C6 EIA may replace immunoblotting in the 2-tier method.

Polymerase chain reaction (PCR) testing (using a laboratory with excellent quality-control procedures) has been used to detect *B burgdorferi* DNA in joint fluid. This test, however, is not necessary for the diagnosis of Lyme arthritis, a late disseminated manifestation in which patients are almost invariably seropositive. For patients with persistent arthritis after a standard course of therapy, PCR testing of synovial fluid or tissue may help discriminate ongoing infection from antibiotic-refractory arthritis. PCR also can detect *B burgdorferi* in skin biopsy specimens of erythema migrans lesions, although this invasive procedure is not recommended for routine clinical practice. PCR has poor sensitivity for cerebrospinal fluid and blood specimens.

Suspected central nervous system (CNS) Lyme disease can be confirmed by demonstration of intrathecal production of antibodies against *B burgdorferi*, which is indicated by cerebrospinal fluid (CSF)/serum IgG optical density ratio >1.3 in specimens collected simultaneously. This sometimes is useful in patients with very early dissemination to the CNS who have not yet developed serum antibodies. CSF antibody tests, however, can be falsely positive in a variety of other CNS inflammatory processes; in particular, the presence of CSF antibodies to *B burgdorferi* cannot confirm a diagnosis of Lyme disease if a different diagnosis is more plausible.

The widespread practice of ordering serologic tests for patients with nonspecific symptoms, such as fatigue or arthralgia, or testing for Lyme disease because of parental/patient pressure, is strongly discouraged. Almost all positive serologic test results in these patients are false-positive results. In areas with endemic infection, previous subclinical infection with seroconversion may occur, and the patient's symptoms may be merely coincidental. Patients with active Lyme disease almost always have objective signs of infection (eg, erythema migrans, facial nerve palsy, arthritis). Nonspecific symptoms commonly accompany these specific signs but almost never are the only evidence of Lyme disease.

Some patients who are treated with antimicrobial agents for early Lyme disease never develop detectable antibodies against *B burgdorferi;* they are cured and are not at risk of late disease. Development of antibodies in patients treated for early Lyme disease does not indicate lack of cure or presence of persistent infection. Ongoing infection without development of antibodies ("seronegative Lyme") has not been demonstrated. Most patients with early disseminated disease and virtually all patients with late disease have antibodies against *B burgdorferi.* Once such antibodies develop, they persist for many years. Consequently, tests for antibodies should not be repeated or used to assess the success of treatment.

A number of tests for Lyme disease have been found to be invalid on the basis of independent testing, or to be too nonspecific to exclude false-positive results. These include urine tests for *B burgdorferi*, CD57 assay, novel culture techniques, and antibody panels that differ from those recommended as part of standardized 2-tier testing. Although these tests are commercially available from some clinical laboratories, they are not appropriate diagnostic tests for Lyme disease.

TREATMENT: Consensus practice guidelines for assessment, treatment, and prevention of Lyme disease have been published by the Infectious Diseases Society of America.[1,2] Care of children should follow recommendations in Table 3.37, p 522. Antimicrobial therapy for nonspecific symptoms or for asymptomatic seropositivity is discouraged. Antimicrobial agents administered for durations not specified in Table 3.37 are not recommended. Alternative diagnostic approaches or therapies without adequate validation studies and publication in peer-reviewed scientific literature also are discouraged.

Early Localized Disease. Doxycycline is the drug of choice for children 8 years and older and, unlike amoxicillin, also treats patients with anaplasmosis (see Tetracyclines, p 873). For children younger than 8 years, amoxicillin is recommended. For patients who are allergic to penicillin, the alternative drug is cefuroxime. Erythromycin and azithromycin are less effective. Early Lyme disease should be treated orally for 14 days. Because STARI may be indistinguishable from early Lyme disease and questions remain about appropriate treatment, some physicians treat STARI with the same antibiotics orally as for Lyme disease.

[1]Wormser GP, Dattwyler RJ, Shapiro ED, et al. The clinical assessment, treatment, and prevention of Lyme disease, human granulocytic anaplasmosis, and babesiosis: clinical practice guidelines by the Infectious Diseases Society of America. *Clin Infect Dis.* 2006;43(9):1089–1134

[2]Lantos PM, Charini WA, Medoff G, et al. Final report of the Lyme Disease Review Panel of the Infectious Diseases Society of America. *Clin Infect Dis.* 2010;51(1):1–5

Table 3.37. Recommended Treatment of Lyme Disease in Children

Disease Category	Drug(s) and Dose[a]
Early localized disease[a]	
8 y or older	Doxycycline, 4 mg/kg per day, orally, divided into 2 doses (maximum 200 mg/day) for 14 days[b]
Younger than 8 y or unable to tolerate doxycycline[b]	Amoxicillin, 50 mg/kg per day, orally, divided into 3 doses (maximum 1.5 g/day) for 14 days OR Cefuroxime, 30 mg/kg per day in 2 divided doses (maximum 1000 mg/day or 1 g/day) for 14 days
Early disseminated and late disease	
Multiple erythema migrans	Same oral regimen as for early localized disease, for 14 days
Isolated facial palsy	Same oral regimen as for early localized disease, for 14 days (range 14–21 days)[c,d]
Arthritis	Same oral regimen as for early localized disease, for 28 days
Recurrent arthritis	Same oral regimen as for first-episode arthritis, for 28 days OR Preferred parenteral regimen: Ceftriaxone sodium, 50–75 mg/kg, IV, once a day (maximum 2 g/day) for 14 days (range 14–28 days) Alternative parenteral regimen: Penicillin, 200 000–400 000 U/kg per day, IV, given in divided doses every 4 h (maximum 18–24 million U/day) for 14 days (range 14–28 days) OR Cefotaxime 150–200 mg/kg per day, IV, divided into 3 or 4 doses (maximum 6 g/day) for 14 days (range 14–28 days)
Antibiotic-refractory/persistent arthritis[e]	Symptomatic therapy
Atrioventricular heart block or carditis	Oral regimen as for early disease if asymptomatic[f] or not hospitalized, for 14 days (range 14–21 days) OR Parenteral regimen initially for hospitalized patients, dosing as for recurrent arthritis, for 14 days (range 14–21 days); oral therapy can be substituted to complete the 14–21 day course
Meningitis	Ceftriaxone[g] or alternatives of cefotaxime or penicillin[g]: dosing as for recurrent arthritis, for 14 days (range 10–21 days) OR Doxycycline, 4–8 mg/kg per day, orally, divided into 2 doses (maximum 100–200 mg for 14 days (range 14–21 days)[b]

Table 3.37. Recommended Treatment of Lyme Disease in Children, continued

Disease Category	Drug(s) and Dose[a]
Encephalitis or other late neurologic disease[h]	Ceftriaxone[g] or alternatives of cefotaxime or penicillin[g]: dosing as for recurrent arthritis, for 14 days (range 14–28 days)

IV indicates intravenously.

[a]For patients who are allergic to penicillin, alternatives are cefuroxime, azithromycin, and erythromycin.

[b]Tetracycline-based antimicrobial agents, including doxycycline, may cause permanent tooth discoloration for children younger than 8 years if used for repeated treatment courses. However, doxycycline binds less readily to calcium compared with older tetracyclines, and in some studies, doxycycline was not associated with visible teeth staining in younger children (see Tetracyclines, p 873).

[c]Corticosteroids should not be given.

[d]Treatment has no effect on the resolution of facial nerve palsy; its purpose is to prevent late disease.

[e]Arthritis is not considered persistent unless objective evidence of synovitis exists at least 2 months after completion of a course of parenteral therapy or of two 28-day courses of oral therapy. Some experts administer a second course of an oral agent before using an IV-administered antimicrobial agent.

[f]Symptoms for heart block or carditis include syncope, dyspnea, or chest pain.

[g]For treatment of meningitis or encephalitis with ceftriaxone, cefotaxime or penicillin, drug should be administered IV.

[h]Other late neurologic manifestations include peripheral neuropathy or encephalopathy.

Treatment of erythema migrans almost always prevents development of later stages of Lyme disease. Erythema migrans usually resolves within several days of initiating treatment, although constitutional symptoms may take months to resolve.

Early Disseminated Disease. Early disseminated Lyme disease typically is treated for 14 days. Oral antibiotics are appropriate and effective for most manifestations of disseminated Lyme disease, including multiple erythema migrans and some cases of Lyme carditis treated as outpatients. For patients requiring hospitalization for Lyme carditis (eg, high-grade atrioventricular block), initial therapy usually is parenteral but can be completed with oral therapy. Some experts favor up to 21 days of total therapy for select cases.

Doxycycline is appropriate for treatment of facial nerve palsy without clinical manifestations of meningitis; lumbar puncture is not indicated. Tetracycline-based antimicrobial agents, including doxycycline, may cause permanent tooth discoloration for children younger than 8 years if used for repeated treatment courses. However, doxycycline binds less readily to calcium compared with older tetracyclines, and in some studies, doxycycline was not associated with visible teeth staining in younger children (see Tetracyclines, p 873). Amoxicillin has not been sufficiently studied for facial nerve palsies in young children, although amoxicillin has been used with apparent success in clinical practice. However, Lyme-associated neuropathies affect peripheral nerves, and it is possible that these complications do not require therapy that crosses the blood-brain barrier. Lumbar puncture is indicated for patients with headache, stiff neck, or other symptoms that suggest meningitis. If cerebrospinal fluid pleocytosis is found, patients should be treated with parenteral ceftriaxone or cefotaxime. European studies provide some evidence that oral doxycycline is effective for Lyme meningitis; this must be interpreted in the different genetic context of European borreliosis. Nonetheless, for a patient with Lyme meningitis and a prohibitive allergy to cephalosporins, doxycycline may be an attractive alternative to cephalosporin desensitization. Neurologic disease typically is treated for 14 days, with select cases receiving up to 21 days of therapy.

Late Disseminated Disease. Lyme arthritis requires longer treatment than earlier manifestations of the disease. Oral antibiotics are administered for 28 days. Patients who have responded incompletely can be treated with a second 28-day course of oral antibiotics.

Patients who experience worsening of their arthritis can be treated parenterally for 14 to 28 days. Approximately 10% to 15% of patients treated for Lyme arthritis will go on to have persistent synovitis that can last for months to years. This condition, termed "antibiotic-refractory Lyme arthritis," is a strongly HLA-associated phenomenon that is most likely autoimmune in nature. Patients with persistent synovitis despite repeat treatment initially should be managed with nonsteroidal anti-inflammatory drugs. More severe cases can be referred to a rheumatologist. Methotrexate has been used successfully in some cases. Arthroscopic synovectomy may be required rarely for more disabling or refractory cases.

Late neurologic disease is uncommon, especially in the United States. This disease may present with symptoms of neuropathy or encephalopathy. Parenteral therapy for 14 days, as is the case for early-onset Lyme meningitis, probably is effective for late disease, although some patients receive up to 28 days of treatment. Symptoms may persist for some time despite adequate therapy. For ocular/neurologic disease manifesting as optic neuritis, cranial neuropathy, or uveitis, concomitant systemic or topical corticosteroids or both are used frequently.

Post-Treatment Lyme Disease Syndrome and "Chronic Lyme Disease." Some patients have prolonged, persistent symptoms following standard treatment for Lyme disease. However, it is not clear that similar symptoms occur any more frequently in patients with a history of Lyme disease than in the population at large. Several double-blinded, randomized, placebo-controlled trials have found that additional antibiotics are associated with harm and are ineffective. The few benefits in antibiotic-treated patients were unsustained and statistically questionable. Administration of additional antibiotics to a patient following standard treatment for Lyme disease is strongly discouraged except when there is objective clinical evidence of reinfection, which can occur occasionally in areas of high endemicity.

"Chronic Lyme disease" is a term that has been used by a small minority of physicians to describe a wide variety of patients with chronic, predominantly subjective illnesses. Patients in whom "chronic Lyme disease" is diagnosed usually have either a "functional" syndrome, such as chronic fatigue syndrome or fibromyalgia; an alternative medical diagnosis; or simply laboratory test results that were either falsely positive or misinterpreted as positive. The term "chronic Lyme disease" has no clinical definition. Because it is not defined based on evidence of *B burgdorferi* infection, there is no role for antimicrobial agents.

Coinfection. Patients with Lyme disease may be simultaneously infected with *Babesia microti* (babesiosis), *Anaplasma phagocytophilum* (human granulocytic anaplasmosis), or both. These diagnoses should be suspected in patients with early Lyme disease who have high fevers, hematologic abnormalities, or elevated hepatic transaminase concentrations. Additionally, patients who contract Lyme disease in Europe may be coinfected with tickborne encephalitis virus. A small number of coinfections with *Borrelia miyamotoi* have been reported. Powassan virus and *Ehrlichia muris*-like agent also are transmitted by blacklegged ticks, but coinfections have not been described to date.

Pregnancy. Tetracyclines are contraindicated. Otherwise, therapy is the same as recommended for nonpregnant people.

ISOLATION OF THE HOSPITALIZED PATIENT: Standard precautions are recommended.

CONTROL MEASURES:

Ticks. See Prevention of Tickborne Infections (p 210).

Chemoprophylaxis. In areas of high endemicity (the coastal northeast), where 30% to 50% of *I scapularis* ticks harbor *B burgdorferi*, the risk of Lyme disease is no higher than 3%, even after high-risk deer tick bites. The risk is extremely low after brief attachment (eg, a flat, non-engorged deer tick is found) and is higher after engorgement, especially if a nymphal deer tick has been attached for ≥36 hours. Testing of the tick for spirochete infection has a poor predictive value and is not recommended. In areas of high risk, a single prophylactic 200-mg dose (4 mg/kg for people weighing less than 45 kg) of doxycycline can reduce the risk of acquiring Lyme disease after the bite of an *I scapularis* tick. Benefits of prophylaxis likely outweigh risks when the tick is engorged (or has been attached for at least 36 hours based on exposure history) and prophylaxis can be started within 72 hours of tick removal. Prophylaxis is discouraged for children younger than 8 years, and doxycycline is not used routinely in this age group. Amoxicillin prophylaxis has been insufficiently studied, but it would likely require a full course because of its short half-life, which in turn would increase the likelihood of toxicity. There are no data to support antibiotic prophylaxis of other tickborne illnesses, such as anaplasmosis, ehrlichiosis, babesiosis, or Rocky Mountain spotted fever.

Blood Donation. To date, no documented cases of *B burgdorferi* transmission have occurred as a result of spirochete transmission via blood transfusion. Nevertheless, because spirochetemia occurs in early Lyme disease, patients with active disease should not donate blood. Patients who have been treated for Lyme disease can be considered for blood donation.

Vaccines. A Lyme disease vaccine was licensed by the US Food and Drug Administration 1998 for people 15 to 70 years of age but was withdrawn in 2002, principally because of poor sales and unsubstantiated public concerns about adverse effects.

Lymphatic Filariasis
(Bancroftian, Malayan, and Timorian)

CLINICAL MANIFESTATIONS: Lymphatic filariasis (LF) is caused by infection with the filarial parasites, *Wuchereria bancrofti, Brugia malayi*, or *Brugia timori*. Adult worms cause lymphatic dilatation and dysfunction, which result in abnormal lymph flow and eventually may lead to lymphedema in the legs, scrotal area (for *W bancrofti* only), and arms. Recurrent secondary bacterial infections hasten progression of lymphedema to the more severe form known as elephantiasis. Although the infection occurs commonly in young children living in LF-endemic areas, chronic manifestations of infection, such as hydrocele and lymphedema, occur infrequently in people younger than 20 years. Most filarial infections remain clinically asymptomatic, but even then they commonly cause subclinical lymphatic dilatation and dysfunction. Lymphadenopathy, most frequently of the inguinal, crural, and axillary lymph nodes, is the most common clinical sign of lymphatic filariasis in children. When the adult worm dies, there is an acute inflammatory response that progresses distally (retrograde) along the affected lymphatic vessel, usually in the limbs. Accompanying systemic symptoms, such as headache or fever, generally are mild. In postpubertal males, adult *W bancrofti* organisms are found most commonly in the intrascrotal lymphatic vessels; thus, inflammation around dead or dying adult worms may present as funiculitis (inflammation of the spermatic cord), epididymitis, or orchitis. A tender granulomatous nodule may be palpable at the site of dying or dead adult worms. Chyluria can occur as a manifestation of bancroftian filariasis. Tropical pulmonary eosinophilia, characterized by cough, fever, marked eosinophilia, and high serum immunoglobulin E concentrations, is a rare manifestation of lymphatic filariasis.

ETIOLOGY: Filariasis is caused by 3 filarial nematodes: *W bancrofti, B malayi*, and *B timori*.

EPIDEMIOLOGY: The parasite is transmitted by the bite of infected species of various genera of mosquitoes, including *Culex, Aedes, Anopheles,* and *Mansonia. W bancrofti,* the most prevalent cause of lymphatic filariasis, is found in Haiti, the Dominican Republic, Guyana, northeast Brazil, sub-Saharan and North Africa, and Asia, extending from India through the Indonesian archipelago to the western Pacific islands. Humans are the only definitive host for the parasite. *B malayi* is found mostly in Southeast Asia and parts of India. *B timori* is restricted to certain islands at the eastern end of the Indonesian archipelago. Live adult worms release microfilariae into the bloodstream. Adult worms live for an average of 5 to 8 years, and reinfection is common. Therefore, microfilariae that can infect mosquitoes may remain in the patient's blood for decades; individual microfilaria have a lifespan up to 1.5 years. The adult worm is not transmissible from person to person or by blood transfusion, but microfilariae may be transmitted by transfusion.

The **incubation period** is not well established; the period from acquisition to the appearance of microfilariae in blood can be 3 to 12 months, depending on the species of parasite.

DIAGNOSTIC TESTS: Microfilariae generally can be detected microscopically on blood smears obtained at night (10 PM–4 AM), although variations in the periodicity of microfilaremia have been described depending on the parasite strain and the geographic location. Adult worms or microfilariae can be identified in tissue specimens obtained at biopsy. Serologic enzyme immunoassays are available, but interpretation of results is affected by cross-reactions of filarial antibodies with antibodies against other helminths. Assays for circulating parasite antigen of *W bancrofti* are available commercially but are not cleared by the US Food and Drug Administration. Ultrasonography can be used to visualize adult worms. Patients with lymphedema may no longer have microfilariae or filarial antibody present.

TREATMENT: The main goal of treatment of an infected person is to kill the adult worm. Diethylcarbamazine citrate (DEC), which is both microfilaricidal and active against the adult worm, is the drug of choice for lymphatic filariasis (see Drugs for Parasitic Infections, p 927). Ivermectin is effective against the microfilariae of *W bancrofti* but has no effect on the adult parasite. Albendazole has demonstrated macrofilaricidal activity. In some studies, combination therapy with single-dose DEC-albendazole or ivermectin-albendazole has been shown to be more effective than any one drug alone in suppressing microfilaremia and is the basis for the Global Programme for Elimination of Lymphatic Filariasis. Doxycycline (up to 6 weeks), a drug that targets the *Wolbachia* (intracellular rickettsial-like bacteria) endosymbiont, has been shown to be macrofilaricidal as well. Tetracycline-based antimicrobial agents, including doxycycline, may cause permanent tooth discoloration for children younger than 8 years if used for repeated treatment courses. However, doxycycline binds less readily to calcium compared with older tetracyclines, and in some studies, doxycycline was not associated with visible teeth staining in younger children (see Tetracyclines, p 873).

For early forms of lymphedema, antifilarial chemotherapy has been shown to have limited efficacy for reversing or stabilizing the lymphedema. Doxycycline, in limited studies, has been shown to decrease the severity of lymphedema. Complex decongestive physiotherapy may be effective for treating lymphedema and requires strict attention to hygiene in the affected anatomical areas. Chyluria originating in the bladder responds to fulguration; chyluria originating in the kidney usually cannot be corrected. Prompt identification and treatment of bacterial superinfections, particularly streptococcal and staphylococcal infections, and careful treatment of intertriginous and ungual fungal infections are important aspects of therapy for lymphedema.

ISOLATION OF THE HOSPITALIZED PATIENT: Standard precautions are recommended.

CONTROL MEASURES: Control measures have been instituted on the basis of annual community-wide combinations of DEC and albendazole (worldwide except Africa) or albendazole and ivermectin (in Africa) to decrease or possibly eliminate transmission. No vaccine is available for lymphatic filariasis.

Lymphocytic Choriomeningitis

CLINICAL MANIFESTATIONS: Child and adult infections are asymptomatic in approximately one third of cases. Symptomatic infection may result in a mild to severe illness, which includes fever, malaise, myalgia, retro-orbital headache, photophobia, anorexia, and nausea. Initial symptoms may last up to 1 week. A biphasic febrile course is common; after a few days without symptoms, the second phase may occur in up to half of symptomatic patients, consisting of neurologic manifestations that vary from aseptic meningitis to severe encephalitis. Transmission of lymphocytic choriomeningitis (LCM) virus through organ transplantation can result in fatal disseminated infection with multiple organ failure. In the past, LCM virus caused up to 10% to 15% of all cases of aseptic meningitis, and it was a common cause of aseptic meningitis during winter months. Arthralgia or arthritis, respiratory tract symptoms, orchitis, and leukopenia develop occasionally. Recovery without sequelae is the usual outcome. LCM virus infection should be suspected in presence of: (1) aseptic meningitis or encephalitis during the fall-winter season; (2) febrile illness, followed by brief remission, followed by onset of neurologic illness; and (3) cerebrospinal fluid (CSF) findings of lymphocytosis and hypoglycorrhachia.

Infection during pregnancy has been associated with spontaneous abortion. Congenital infection may cause severe abnormalities, including hydrocephalus, chorioretinitis, intracranial calcifications, microcephaly, and mental retardation. Congenital LCM etiology should be considered when TORCH (**t**oxoplasma, **o**ther [syphilis], **r**ubella, **c**ytomegalovirus, **h**erpes simplex) infections are suspected. Patients with immune abnormalities may experience severe or fatal illness, as observed in patients receiving organs from LCM virus-infected donors.

ETIOLOGY: LCM virus is a single-stranded RNA virus that belongs to the family *Arenaviridae* (so named because of its appearance on electron microscopy, which resembles grains of sand). Other members of this family include Lassa virus and the Tacaribe group.

EPIDEMIOLOGY: LCM is a chronic infection of common house mice, which often are infected asymptomatically and chronically shed virus in urine and other excretions. Congenital murine infection is common and results in a normal-appearing litter with chronic viremia and particularly high virus excretion. In addition, pet hamsters, laboratory mice, guinea pigs, and colonized golden hamsters can have chronic infection and can be sources of human infection. Humans are infected by aerosol or by ingestion of dust or food contaminated with the virus from the urine, feces, blood, or nasopharyngeal secretions of infected rodents. The disease is observed more frequently in young adults. Human-to-human transmission has occurred during pregnancy from infected mothers to their fetus and through solid organ transplantation from an undiagnosed, acutely LCM virus-infected organ donor. Several such clusters of cases have been described following transplantation, and 1 case was traced to a pet hamster purchased by the donor. A number of laboratory-acquired LCM virus infections have occurred, both through infected laboratory animals and contaminated tissue-culture stocks.

The **incubation period** usually is 6 to 13 days and occasionally is as long as 3 weeks.

DIAGNOSTIC TESTS: In patients with central nervous system disease, mononuclear pleocytosis often exceeding 1000 cells/μL is present in CSF. Hypoglycorrhachia may occur. LCM virus usually can be isolated from CSF obtained during the acute phase of illness and, in severe disseminated infections, also from blood, urine, and nasopharyngeal secretion specimens. Reverse transcriptase-polymerase chain reaction assays can be used on CSF. Serum specimens from the acute and convalescent phases of illness can be tested for increases in antibody titers by enzyme immunoassays. Demonstration of virus-specific immunoglobulin M antibodies in serum or CSF specimens is useful. In congenital infections, diagnosis usually is suspected at the sequela phase, and diagnosis usually is made by serologic testing. In immunosuppressed patients, the seroconversion can take several weeks. Diagnosis can be made retrospectively by immunohistochemical assay of fixed tissues obtained from necropsy.

TREATMENT: Supportive. Limited data suggest a role for ribavirin in immunosuppressed patients infected with LCM virus.

ISOLATION OF THE HOSPITALIZED PATIENT: Standard precautions are recommended.

CONTROL MEASURES: Infection can be controlled by preventing rodent infestation in animal and food storage areas. Because the virus is excreted for long periods of time by rodent hosts, attempts should be made to monitor laboratory and wholesale colonies of mice and hamsters for infection. Pet rodents or wild mice in a patient's home should be considered likely sources of infection. Although the risk of LCM virus infection from pet rodents is low, pregnant women should avoid exposure to wild or pet rodents and their aerosolized excreta. Pregnant women should avoid working in the laboratory with LCM virus. Guidelines for minimizing risk of human LCM virus infection associated with rodents are available[1] (also see Diseases Transmitted by Animals [Zoonoses], p 219).

Malaria

CLINICAL MANIFESTATIONS: The classic symptoms of malaria are high fever with chills, rigor, sweats, and headache, which may be paroxysmal. If appropriate treatment is not administered, fever and paroxysms may occur in a cyclic pattern. Depending on the infecting species, fever classically appears every other (*Plasmodium falciparum, Plasmodium vivax*, and *Plasmodium ovale*) or every third day (*Plasmodium malariae*), although in general practice this pattern is infrequently observed, especially in children. Other manifestations, particularly as the clinical disease progresses, can include nausea, vomiting, diarrhea, cough, tachypnea, arthralgia, myalgia, and abdominal and back pain. Anemia and thrombocytopenia, along with pallor and jaundice caused by hemolysis, are common in severe illness. Hepatosplenomegaly may be present. More severe disease may occur in

---

[1]Centers for Disease Control and Prevention. Update: interim guidance for minimizing risk for human lymphocytic choriomeningitis virus infection associated with pet rodents. *MMWR Morb Mortal Wkly Rep.* 2005;54(32):799–801

people without immunity acquired as a result of previous infections, young children, and people who are pregnant or immunocompromised.

Infection with *P falciparum*, 1 of the 5 *Plasmodium* species that infect humans, potentially is fatal and most commonly manifests as a febrile nonspecific illness without localizing signs. Severe disease (most commonly caused by ***P falciparum***, although recently also caused by ***P vivax*** from India, Southeast Asia and South America) may manifest as one of the following clinical syndromes, all of which are medical emergencies and may be fatal unless treated:

- **Cerebral malaria**, characterized by unarousable coma, can manifest with a range of neurologic signs and symptoms, including generalized seizures, signs of increased intracranial pressure (confusion and progression to stupor, coma), and death;
- **Hypoglycemia**, which can present with metabolic acidosis and hypotension associated with hyperparasitemia; hypoglycemia also can be a consequence of quinine or quinidine-induced hyperinsulinemia;
- **Renal failure** caused by acute tubular necrosis (rare in children younger than 8 years);
- **Respiratory failure**, without pulmonary edema;
- **Metabolic acidosis**, usually attributed to lactic acidosis, hypovolemia, liver dysfunction, and impaired renal function;
- **Severe anemia** attributable to high parasitemia and hemolysis, sequestration of infected erythrocytes to capillaries, and hemolysis of infected erythrocytes associated with hypersplenism; or
- **Vascular collapse and shock** associated with hypothermia and adrenal insufficiency. People with asplenia who become infected may be at increased risk of more severe illness and death.
- Syndromes primarily associated with ***P vivax*** and ***P ovale*** infection are as follows:
- **Anemia** attributable to acute parasitemia;
- **Hypersplenism** with danger of splenic rupture; and
- **Relapse of infection**, for as long as 3 to 5 years after the primary infection, attributable to latent hepatic stages (hypnozoites).
- Syndromes associated with ***P malariae*** infection include:
- **Chronic asymptomatic parasitemia** for as long as decades after the primary infection, and
- **Nephrotic syndrome** resulting from deposition of immune complexes in the kidney.

Plasmodium knowlesi is a nonhuman primate malaria parasite that also can infect humans. *P knowlesi* malaria has been misdiagnosed commonly as the more benign *P malariae* malaria. Disease can be characterized by very rapid replication of the parasite and hyperparasitemia resulting in severe disease. Severe disease in patients with *P knowlesi* infection should be treated aggressively, because hepatorenal failure and subsequent death have been well documented.

Congenital malaria resulting from perinatal transmission occurs infrequently. Most congenital cases have been caused by *P vivax* and *P falciparum; P malariae* and *P ovale* account for fewer than 20% of such cases. Manifestations can resemble those of neonatal sepsis, including fever and nonspecific symptoms of poor appetite, irritability, and lethargy.

ETIOLOGY: The genus *Plasmodium* includes species of intraerythrocytic parasites that infect a wide range of mammals, birds, and reptiles. The 5 species that infect humans are *P falciparum, P vivax, P ovale, P malariae,* and *P knowlesi.* Coinfection with multiple species increasingly is recognized as polymerase chain reaction technology is applied to the diagnosis of malaria.

EPIDEMIOLOGY: Malaria is endemic throughout the tropical areas of the world and is acquired from the bite of the female nocturnal-feeding *Anopheles* genus of mosquito. Half of the world's population lives in areas where transmission occurs. Worldwide, 216 million cases and 655 000 deaths were reported in 2010. Most deaths occur in young children. Infection by the malaria parasite poses substantial risks to pregnant women, especially primigravida women in areas with endemic infection, and their fetuses and may result in spontaneous abortion and stillbirth. Malaria also contributes significantly to low birth weight in countries where *P falciparum* is endemic. The risk of malaria is highest, but variable, for travelers to sub-Saharan Africa, Papua New Guinea, the Solomon Islands, and Vanuatu; the risk is intermediate on the Indian subcontinent and is low in most of Southeast Asia and Latin America. The potential for malaria transmission is ongoing in areas where malaria previously was eliminated if infected people return and the mosquito vector is still present. These conditions have resulted in recent cases in travelers to areas such as Jamaica, the Dominican Republic, and the Bahamas. Health care professionals should check an up-to-date source (**www.cdc.gov/malaria**) to determine malaria endemicity when providing pretravel malaria advice or evaluating a febrile returned traveler. Transmission is possible in more temperate climates, including areas of the United States where anopheline mosquitoes are present.

Nearly all of the approximately 1500 annual reported cases in the United States result from infection acquired abroad.[1] Rarely, mosquitoes in airplanes flying from areas with endemic malaria have been the source of cases in people working or residing near international airports. Local transmission also occurs rarely in the United States. Uncommon modes of malaria transmission are congenital, through transfusions, or through the use of contaminated needles or syringes.

P vivax and *P falciparum* are the most common species worldwide. *P vivax* malaria is prevalent on the Indian subcontinent and in Central America. *P falciparum* malaria is prevalent in Africa, Papua New Guinea, and on the island of Hispaniola (Haiti and the Dominican Republic). *P vivax* and *P falciparum* species are the most common malaria species in southern and Southeast Asia, Oceania, and South America. *P malariae*, although much less common, has a wide distribution. *P ovale* malaria occurs most often in West Africa but has been reported in other areas. Cases of human infections with *P knowlesi* reported, so far, have been from certain countries of Southeast Asia like Borneo, Malaysia, Philippines, Thailand, the Thai-Burmese border, Singapore, and Cambodia.

Relapses may occur in *P vivax* and *P ovale* malaria because of a persistent hepatic (hypnozoite) stage of infection. Recrudescence of *P falciparum* and *P malariae* infection occurs when a persistent low-concentration parasitemia causes recurrence of symptoms of the disease or when drug resistance prevents elimination of the parasite. In areas of Africa and Asia with hyperendemic infection, repeated infection in people with partial immunity results in a high prevalence of asymptomatic parasitemia.

The spread of chloroquine-resistant *P falciparum* strains throughout the world is of increasing concern. In addition, resistance to other antimalarial drugs also is occurring in many areas where the drugs are used widely. *P falciparum* resistance to

---

[1] Centers for Disease Control and Prevention. Malaria surveillance—United States, 2011. *MMWR Surveill Summ.* 2013;62(SS-05):1–17

sulfadoxine-pyrimethamine is common throughout Africa; mefloquine resistance has been documented in Burma (Myanmar), Laos, Thailand, Cambodia, China, and Vietnam; and emerging resistance to artemisinins has been observed at the Cambodia-Thailand border. Chloroquine-resistant *P vivax* has been reported in Indonesia, Papua New Guinea, the Solomon Islands, Myanmar, India, and Guyana. Malaria symptoms can develop as soon as 7 days after exposure in an area with endemic malaria to as late as several months after departure. More than 80% of cases diagnosed in the United States occur in people who have onset of symptoms after their return to the United States. Beginning in 2012, the CDC has tested samples from US patients for molecular markers associated with antimalarial drug resistance. Of the 65 *P falciparum*-positive samples, genetic polymorphisms were associated with pyrimethamine drug resistance in 53 (82%), sulfadoxine resistance in 61 (94%), chloroquine resistance in 29 (45%), mefloquine resistance in 1 (2%), and atovaquone resistance in 2 (3%); none had genetic polymorphisms associated with artemisinin resistance.[1]

DIAGNOSTIC TESTS: Definitive diagnosis relies on identification of the parasite microscopically on stained blood films. Both thick and thin blood films should be examined. The thick film allows for concentration of the blood to find parasites that may be present in small numbers, whereas the thin film is most useful for species identification and determination of the degree of parasitemia (the percentage of erythrocytes harboring parasites). If initial blood smears test negative for *Plasmodium* species but malaria remains a possibility, the smear should be repeated every 12 to 24 hours during a 72-hour period.

Confirmation and identification of the species of malaria parasites on the blood smear is important in guiding therapy. Serologic testing generally is not helpful, except in epidemiologic surveys. Polymerase chain reaction (PCR) assay is available in reference laboratories and many state health departments. In addition, species confirmation and antimalarial drug resistance testing is available free of charge at the Centers for Disease Control and Prevention (CDC) for all cases of malaria diagnosed in the United States. A US Food and Drug Administration (FDA)-approved test for antigen detection (a rapid diagnostic test) is available in the United States. It is the only antigen-detection kit available and is approved for use by hospitals and commercial laboratories. However, an evaluation by the World Health Organization (WHO) found that this product had poor sensitivity for detecting low-density *P vivax* infections. Rapid diagnostic testing is recommended to be conducted in parallel with routine microscopy to provide further information needed for patient treatment, such as the percentage of erythrocytes harboring parasites. Both positive and negative rapid diagnostic test results should be confirmed by microscopic examination, because low-level parasitemia may not be detected, false-positive results occur, and mixed infections may not be detected accurately. Also, information about the sensitivity of rapid diagnostic tests for the 2 less common species of malaria, *P ovale* and *P malariae,* is limited. More information about rapid diagnostic testing for malaria is available on the CDC Web site (**www.cdc.gov/malaria/ diagnosis_treatment/index.html**).

TREATMENT: The choice of malaria chemotherapy is based on the infecting species, possible drug resistance, and severity of disease (see Drugs for Parasitic Infections, p 927). Severe malaria is defined as any one or more of the following: parasitemia greater than 5% of red blood cells, signs of central nervous system or other end-organ involvement,

---

[1]Centers for Disease Control and Prevention. Malaria surveillance—United States, 2012. *MMWR Surveill Summ.* 2014;63(SS-12):1–22

shock, acidosis, thrombocytopenia, and/or hypoglycemia. Patients with severe malaria require intensive care and parenteral treatment with IV quinidine until the parasite density decreases to less than 1% and they are able to tolerate oral therapy. Concurrent treatment with tetracycline, doxycycline, or clindamycin should begin orally or intravenously if oral treatment is not tolerated (see Drugs for Parasitic Infections, p 927). A recent review of available literature suggests exchange transfusion for severe disease is not efficacious.

For patients with severe malaria in the United States who do not tolerate or cannot easily access quinidine, intravenous artesunate has become available through a CDC investigational new drug protocol. Clinicians may contact the physician on call through the CDC malaria hotline (770-488-7788, Monday–Friday, 9:00 AM–5:00 PM Eastern Time; or 777-488-7100 at all other times) for additional information and release of the drug.[1] For patients with *P falciparum* malaria, sequential blood smears to determine percentage of erythrocytes harboring parasites can be useful in monitoring treatment. Assistance with management of malaria is available 24 hours a day through the CDC Malaria Hotline (770-488-7788). Guidelines for the treatment of malaria are available on the CDC Web site (**www.cdc.gov/malaria/resources/pdf/treatmenttable.pdf**).

ISOLATION OF THE HOSPITALIZED PATIENT: Standard precautions are recommended.

CONTROL MEASURES: There is no licensed vaccine against malaria. Effective measures to reduce the risk of acquiring malaria include control of *Anopheles* mosquito populations, protection against mosquito bites, treatment of infected people, and chemoprophylaxis of travelers to areas with endemic infection. Measures to prevent contact with mosquitoes, especially from dusk to dawn (because of the nocturnal biting habits of most female *Anopheles* mosquitoes), through use of bed nets impregnated with insecticide, mosquito repellents (see Prevention of Mosquitoborne Infections, p 213), and protective clothing also are beneficial and should be optimized. The most current information on country-specific malaria transmission, drug resistance, and resulting recommendations for travelers can be obtained by contacting the CDC (**www.cdc.gov/malaria/** or the Malaria Hotline at 770-488-7788).

Chemoprophylaxis for Travelers to Areas With Endemic Malaria.[2] More than 80% of malaria-infected patients reported in the United States did not follow a CDC-recommended prophylaxis regimen. The appropriate chemoprophylactic regimen is determined by the traveler's risk of acquiring malaria in the area(s) to be visited and by local prevalence of drug resistance. Indications for prophylaxis for children are identical to those for adults. Pediatric dosages should be calculated on the basis of the child's current weight; children's dosages never should exceed adult dosages. Drugs used for malaria chemoprophylaxis generally are well tolerated, although adverse reactions can occur. Minor adverse reactions do not require stopping the drug. Travelers with serious adverse reactions should be advised to contact their physician.

Chemoprophylaxis should begin before arrival in the area with endemic malaria (starting at least 2 weeks before arrival for mefloquine, 1 week before arrival for

---

[1]Centers for Disease Control and Prevention. Notice to readers: new medication for severe malaria available under an investigational new drug protocol. *MMWR Morb Mortal Wkly Rep.* 2007;56(30):769–770

[2]For further information on prevention of malaria in travelers, see the biennial publication of the US Public Health Service, *Health Information for International Travel,* 2014. Atlanta, GA: US Department of Health and Human Services, Public Health Service, Centers for Disease Control and Prevention, National Center for Infectious Diseases, Division of Global Migration and Quarantine; 2014. Oxford University Press. Available at: **wwwnc.cdc.gov/travel/page/yellowbook-home-2014.**

chloroquine, and 1–2 days before arrival for doxycycline and atovaquone-proguanil), allowing time to develop blood concentrations of the drug. If there is desire to ensure tolerance of the antimalarial drug to be used for prophylaxis, then the drug should be started earlier so that there is time to assess any adverse events before departure and time to change to another effective drug if needed. For example, if there is concern about individual tolerance with mefloquine, then prophylaxis can be started 3 weeks before travel. Most adverse events will occur during the first 3 doses, and if the person does not tolerate mefloquine, then there still is time to prescribe alternative therapy before travel.

Drugs for the prevention of malaria currently available in the United States include chloroquine, mefloquine, doxycycline, atovaquone-proguanil, and primaquine.

- Chloroquine is an option for people traveling to parts of the world where chloroquine resistance has not developed. Adverse reactions that can occur include gastrointestinal tract disturbance, headache, dizziness, blurred vision, insomnia, and pruritus, but these generally are mild and do not require discontinuation of the drug.
- A fixed-dose combination of atovaquone-proguanil is approved for prevention and treatment of chloroquine-resistant *P falciparum* malaria. Atovaquone-proguanil is taken daily, starting 1 day before exposure and continuing for the duration of exposure and for 1 week after departure from the area with endemic malaria. A pediatric formulation is available in the United States but is not approved for prophylaxis in children weighing less than 11 kg. However, the CDC suggests that atovaquone-proguanil can be used in children weighing 5 kg or more, when travel cannot be avoided to areas where chloroquine-resistant *P falciparum* exists. Atovaquone-proguanil is contraindicated for pregnant women. The rare adverse effects reported by people using atovaquone-proguanil for chemoprophylaxis are abdominal pain, nausea, vomiting, mouth ulcers, and headache.
- Doxycycline is taken daily, starting 1 to 2 days before exposure, for the duration of exposure and for 4 weeks after departure from the area with endemic malaria. Travelers taking doxycycline should be advised of the need for strict adherence to daily dosing; the advisability of always taking the drug on a full stomach; and the possible adverse effects, including diarrhea, photosensitivity, and increased risk of monilial vaginitis. Use of doxycycline should be avoided for pregnant women and for children younger than 8 years (see Tetracyclines, p 873).
- Mefloquine is taken once weekly, starting at least 2 weeks before travel, continuing weekly during travel, and for 4 weeks after travel has concluded (see Drugs for Parasitic Infections, p 927). Mefloquine is not approved by the FDA for children who weigh less than 5 kg or are younger than 6 months. However, the CDC suggests that mefloquine is considered for use in children, regardless of weight or age restrictions, when travel cannot be avoided to areas where chloroquine-resistant *P falciparum* exists. Parents should be advised not to travel to countries with endemic malaria with children weighing less than 5 kg or younger than 6 weeks because of the risks associated with infection (septicemia or malaria) in young infants. The most common central nervous system abnormalities associated with mefloquine are dizziness, headache, insomnia, and disturbing dreams. Mefloquine has been associated with rare serious adverse events (including psychoses or seizures) at prophylactic doses. These reactions are more common with the higher doses used for treatment. Other adverse events that occur with prophylactic doses include gastrointestinal tract disturbances, headache, depression, and anxiety disorders. Mefloquine is contraindicated for use in travelers with a known hypersensitivity to the drug; people

with active depression or a history of depression; people with general anxiety disorders, psychosis, schizophrenia, or other major psychiatric disturbances; people with a history of seizures (not including febrile seizures); and people with a history of cardiac conduction abnormalities. Although the product labeling contains a warning about concurrent use with beta-blockers, a review of available data suggests that mefloquine may be used by people concurrently receiving beta-blockers if they have no underlying arrhythmia. Caution should be advised for travelers involved in tasks requiring fine motor coordination and spatial discrimination. Patients in whom mefloquine prophylaxis fails should be monitored closely if they are treated with quinidine or quinine sulfate, because either drug may exacerbate known adverse effects of mefloquine.

• Primaquine is recommended for prophylaxis in areas with predominantly *P vivax* malaria. Travelers must be tested for glucose-6-phosphate dehydrogenase (G6PD) deficiency and have a documented G6PD in the normal range before primaquine use. Primary primaquine prophylaxis should begin 1 to 2 days before departure to the area with risk of malaria and should be continued once a day while in the area with risk of malaria and daily for 7 days after leaving the area. The drug should not be used during pregnancy or lactation unless the breastfed child has a documented normal G6PD concentration.

Prophylaxis During Pregnancy and Lactation. Malaria during pregnancy carries significant risks of morbidity and mortality for both the mother and fetus. Malaria may increase the risk of adverse outcomes in pregnancy, including abortion, preterm birth, and stillbirth. For these reasons and because no chemoprophylactic regimen is absolutely effective, women who are pregnant or likely to become pregnant should try to avoid travel to areas where they could contract malaria. Women traveling to areas where drug-resistant *P falciparum* has not been reported may take chloroquine prophylaxis. Harmful effects on the fetus have not been demonstrated when chloroquine is given in the recommended doses for malaria prophylaxis. Pregnancy and lactation, therefore, are not contraindications for malaria prophylaxis with chloroquine.

For pregnant women who travel to areas where chloroquine-resistant *P falciparum* exists, the CDC recommends mefloquine chemoprophylaxis in all trimesters of pregnancy. Consequently, mefloquine is the drug of choice for prophylactic use for women who are pregnant or likely to become pregnant when exposure to chloroquine-resistant *P falciparum* is unavoidable. Lactating mothers of infants weighing more than 5 kg also may use atovaquone-proguanil or mefloquine for prophylaxis when exposure to chloroquine-resistant *P falciparum* is unavoidable.

Reliable Antimalarial Supply While Traveling. Travelers to malaria-endemic settings should seek medical attention immediately if they develop fever. Malaria can be treated with good results if begun early in the course of disease, but delay of appropriate treatment can have serious or even fatal consequences. Travelers who do not take an antimalarial drug for prophylaxis, who are on a less-than-effective regimen, or who may be in very remote areas can be given a reliable supply of atovaquone-proguanil or artemether-lumefantrine. If they are diagnosed with malaria while traveling, they will have a medicine that will not interact with their other medications, is of good quality, and is not depleting local resources.

Travelers taking atovaquone-proguanil as their chemoprophylactic drug regimen should not take atovaquone-proguanil for treatment and should use an alternative antimalarial regimen recommended by a travel medicine expert.

Travelers should be advised that any fever or influenza-like illness that develops within 3 months of departure from an area with endemic malaria requires immediate medical evaluation, including blood films to rule out malaria.

Prevention of Relapses. To prevent relapses of *P vivax* or *P ovale* infection after departure from areas where these species are endemic, travelers with prolonged exposure and normal G6PD concentrations should receive presumptive antirelapse therapy (terminal prophylaxis) with primaquine for 14 days. Rarely, travelers exposed to primaquine-resistant or -tolerant parasites may require high-dose primaquine. Primaquine can cause hemolysis in patients with G6PD deficiency; thus, all patients should be screened for this condition before primaquine therapy is initiated.

Personal Protective Measures. All travelers to areas where malaria is endemic should be advised to use personal protective measures, including the following: (1) using insecticide-impregnated mosquito nets while sleeping; (2) remaining in well-screened areas; (3) wearing protective clothing; and (4) using mosquito repellents. To be effective, most repellents require frequent reapplications (see Prevention of Mosquitoborne Infections, p 213).

Measles

CLINICAL MANIFESTATIONS: Measles is an acute viral disease characterized by fever, cough, coryza, and conjunctivitis, followed by a maculopapular rash beginning on the face and spreading cephalocaudally and centrifugally. During the prodromal period, a pathognomonic enanthema (Koplik spots) may be present. Complications of measles, including otitis media, bronchopneumonia, laryngotracheobronchitis (croup), and diarrhea, occur commonly in young children and immunocompromised hosts. Acute encephalitis, which often results in permanent brain damage, occurs in approximately 1 of every 1000 cases. In the postelimination era, death, predominantly resulting from respiratory and neurologic complications, has occurred in 1 to 3 of every 1000 cases reported in the United States. Case-fatality rates are increased in children younger than 5 years and in immunocompromised children, including children with leukemia, human immunodeficiency virus (HIV) infection, and severe malnutrition (including vitamin A deficiency). Sometimes the characteristic rash does not develop in immunocompromised patients.

Subacute sclerosing panencephalitis (SSPE) is a rare degenerative central nervous system disease characterized by behavioral and intellectual deterioration and seizures that occurs 7 to 11 years after wild-type measles virus infection, occurring at a rate of 4 to 11 per 100 000 measles cases, with higher rates if measles occurs before 2 years of age. Widespread measles immunization has led to the virtual disappearance of SSPE in the United States.

ETIOLOGY: Measles virus is an enveloped RNA virus with 1 serotype, classified as a member of the genus *Morbillivirus* in the *Paramyxoviridae* family.

EPIDEMIOLOGY: The only natural host of measles virus is humans. Measles is transmitted by direct contact with infectious droplets or, less commonly, by airborne spread. Measles is one of the most highly communicable of all infectious diseases. In temperate areas, the peak incidence of infection usually occurs during late winter and spring. In the prevaccine era, most cases of measles in the United States occurred in preschool- and young school-aged children, and few people remained susceptible by 20 years of age. The childhood and adolescent immunization program in the United States has resulted in a greater than

99% decrease in the reported incidence of measles and interruption of endemic disease transmission since measles vaccine first was licensed in 1963.

From 1989 to 1991, the incidence of measles in the United States increased because of low immunization rates in preschool-aged children, especially in urban areas. Following improved coverage in preschool-aged children and implementation of a routine second dose of measles-mumps-rubella (MMR) vaccine for children, the incidence of measles declined to extremely low levels (<1 case per 1 million population). In 2000, an independent panel of internationally recognized experts reviewed available data and unanimously agreed that measles no longer was endemic (defined as continuous, year-round transmission) in the United States. In the postelimination era from 2001 through 2012, a median of 60 measles cases were reported annually (range: 37–220). In 2008, 2011, and 2013, the numbers of reported cases were 140, 220, and 189, respectively; these larger numbers of cases were attributable to an increase in the number of importations and/or spread from importations. The number of measles outbreaks (defined as 3 or more cases linked in time and space) that occurred during this time period ranged from 2 to 16 per year. In the first half of 2014, 514 measles cases from 16 outbreaks were reported in 20 states. Forty-eight separate importations occurred. Among the 506 US cases for which information was known, 81% were in unvaccinated people, 12% of those infected had an unknown vaccination status (78% of those were adults), and 7% of those infected were vaccinated (including 5% with 2 or more doses). Among the unvaccinated people who became infected, 87% cited personal belief exemptions for not being immunized, 3% were unvaccinated travelers 6 months to 2 years of age, and 5% were too young to be vaccinated. This is the largest number of measles cases in the United States since 1994.

Progress continues toward global control and regional measles elimination. During 2000–2013, annual reported measles incidence declined 72% worldwide, from 146 to 40 per million population, and annual estimated measles deaths declined 75%, from 544 200 to 145 700.[1] Four of six WHO regions have established regional verification commissions; in the European and Western Pacific regions, 19 member states successfully documented the absence of endemic measles. Resuming progress toward 2015 milestones and elimination goals will require countries and their partners to raise the visibility of measles elimination, address barriers to measles vaccination, and make substantial and sustained additional investments in strengthening health systems.

Vaccine failure occurs in as many as 5% of people who have received a single dose of vaccine at 12 months or older. Although waning immunity after immunization may be a factor in some cases, most cases of measles in previously immunized children seem to occur in people in whom response to the vaccine was inadequate (ie, primary vaccine failures). This was the main reason a 2-dose vaccine schedule was recommended routinely for children and high-risk adults.

Patients are contagious from 4 days before the rash to 4 days after appearance of the rash. Immunocompromised patients who may have prolonged excretion of the virus in respiratory tract secretions can be contagious for the duration of the illness. Patients with SSPE are not contagious.

The **incubation period** generally is 8 to 12 days from exposure to onset of symptoms. In family studies, the average interval between appearance of rash in the index case

---

[1]Centers for Disease Control and Prevention. Progress toward regional measles elimination—worldwide, 2000–2013. *MMWR Morb Mortal Wkly Rep.* 2014;63(45):1034–1038

and subsequent cases is 14 days, with a range of 7 to 21 days. In SSPE, the mean incubation period of 84 cases reported between 1976 and 1983 was 10.8 years.

DIAGNOSTIC TESTS: Measles virus infection can be diagnosed by a positive serologic test result for measles immunoglobulin (Ig) M antibody, a significant increase in measles IgG antibody concentration in paired acute and convalescent serum specimens (collected at least 10 days apart) by any standard serologic assay, or isolation of measles virus or identification of measles RNA (by reverse transcriptase-polymerase chain reaction [RT-PCR] assay) from clinical specimens, such as urine, blood, or throat or nasopharyngeal secretions (the latter 2 are preferred specimens, and sampling more than 1 site may increase yield). State public health laboratories or the Centers for Disease Control and Prevention (CDC) Measles Laboratory will process these viral specimens. Isolation of measles virus is not recommended routinely, although viral isolates are important for molecular epidemiologic surveillance. The simplest method of establishing the diagnosis of measles is testing for IgM antibody on a single serum specimen obtained during the first encounter with a person suspected of having disease, and if the result is positive, it is a good measure for a presumptive case. The sensitivity of measles IgM assays varies by timing of specimen collection, immunization status of the case, and the assay. IgM capture assays often have positive results on the day of rash onset. However, up to 20% of assays for IgM may have a false-negative result in the first 72 hours after rash onset. If the result is negative for measles IgM and the patient has a generalized rash lasting more than 72 hours, a second serum specimen should be obtained, and the measles IgM test should be repeated. Measles IgM is detectable for at least 1 month after rash onset in unimmunized people but might be absent or present only transiently in people immunized with 1 or 2 vaccine doses. Therefore, a negative IgM test result should not be used to rule out the diagnosis in immunized people. In populations with high vaccine coverage, such as the United States, it is recommended that diagnostic testing for measles include both serologic and virologic testing. People with febrile rash illness who are seronegative for measles IgM (and have negative RT-PCR assay results for measles, if tested) should be tested for rubella using the same specimens. Diagnostic testing for measles should include both serologic and virologic tests. Genotyping of viral isolates allows determination of patterns of importation and transmission, and genome sequencing can be used to differentiate between wild-type and vaccine virus infection in those who have been immunized recently. All cases of suspected measles should be reported immediately to the local or state health department without waiting for results of diagnostic tests. Measles is on the list of nationally notifiable diseases that should be reported to the CDC within 24 hours.

TREATMENT: No specific antiviral therapy is available. Measles virus is susceptible in vitro to ribavirin, which has been given by the intravenous and aerosol routes to treat severely affected and immunocompromised children with measles. However, no controlled trials have been conducted, and ribavirin is not approved by the US Food and Drug Administration for treatment of measles.

Vitamin A. Vitamin A treatment of children with measles in developing countries has been associated with decreased morbidity and mortality rates. Low serum concentrations of vitamin A also have been found in children in the United States, and children with more severe measles illness have lower vitamin A concentrations. The World Health Organization currently recommends vitamin A for all children with acute measles,

regardless of their country of residence. Vitamin A for treatment of measles is administered once daily for 2 days, at the following doses:
- 200 000 IU for children 12 months or older;
- 100 000 IU for infants 6 through 11 months of age; and
- 50 000 IU for infants younger than 6 months.
- An additional (ie, a third) age-specific dose should be given 2 through 4 weeks later to
  children with clinical signs and symptoms of vitamin A deficiency.

Even in countries where measles is not usually severe, vitamin A should be given to all
children with severe measles (eg, requiring hospitalization). Parenteral and oral formulations of vitamin A are available in the United States.

ISOLATION OF THE HOSPITALIZED PATIENT: In addition to standard precautions, airborne transmission precautions are indicated for 4 days after the onset of rash in otherwise healthy children and for the duration of illness in immunocompromised patients.
Exposed susceptible patients should be placed on airborne precautions from day 5 after
first exposure until day 21 after last exposure.[1]

CONTROL MEASURES:

Evidence of Immunity to Measles.[2] Evidence of immunity to measles includes any of the
following:
1. Documentation of age-appropriate vaccination with a live measles virus-containing
   vaccine:
   - preschool-aged children: 1 dose;
   - school-aged children (grades K-12): 2 doses;
2. Laboratory evidence of immunity;
3. Laboratory confirmation of disease;
4. Born before 1957.

Care of Exposed People.

Use of Vaccine. Available data suggest that measles vaccine, if given within 72 hours of
measles exposure to susceptible individuals, will provide protection or disease modification in some cases. Measles vaccine should be considered in all exposed individuals who
are vaccine-eligible and who have not been vaccinated or have received only 1 dose of
vaccine. If the exposure does not result in infection, the vaccine should induce protection
against subsequent measles exposures. Immunization is the intervention of choice for control of measles outbreaks in schools and child care centers and for vaccine-eligible people
12 months and older.

Use of Immune Globulin. Immune Globulin (IG) can be administered either intramuscularly (IGIM) or intravenously (IGIV) within 6 days of exposure to prevent or modify
measles in people who do not have evidence of measles immunity. The recommended dose
of IGIM is 0.50 mL/kg, administered intramuscularly (the maximum dose by volume is

---

[1]Siegal JD, Rhinehart E, Jackson M, Chiarello L; Centers for Disease Control and Prevention, Healthcare
Infection Control Practices Advisory Committee. 2007 Guideline for Isolation Precautions: Preventing
Transmission of Infectious Agents in Healthcare Settings. Atlanta, GA: Centers for Disease Control and
Prevention; 2007. Available at: **www.cdc.gov/hicpac/pdf/isolation/Isolation2007.pdf**

[2]Centers for Disease Control and Prevention. Prevention of measles, rubella, congenital rubella syndrome, and
mumps, 2013 summary: recommendations of the Advisory Committee on Immunization Practices (ACIP).
MMWR Recomm Rep. 2013;62(RR-04):1–34

15 mL). IGIV is the recommended IG preparation for pregnant women without evidence of measles immunity and for severely immunocompromised hosts[2] regardless of immunologic or vaccination status, including patients with severe primary immunodeficiency; patients who have received a bone marrow transplant until at least 12 months after finishing all immunosuppressive treatment, or longer in patients who have developed graft-versus-host disease; patients on treatment for ALL within and until at least 6 months after completion of immunosuppressive chemotherapy; and people with human immunodeficiency virus (HIV) infection or acquired immunodeficiency syndrome (AIDS) who have severe immunosuppression defined as CD4+ T-lymphocyte percentage <15% (all ages) or CD4+ T-lymphocyte count <200 lymphocytes/mm^3 (older than 5 years) and those who have not received MMR vaccine since receiving effective ART. This is because these groups may be at higher risk of severe measles and complications, and people who weigh >30 kg will receive less than the recommended dose with IGIM preparations. IGIV is administered at a dose of 400 mg/kg. For patients who already are receiving IGIV at regularly scheduled intervals, the usual dose of 400 mg/kg should be adequate for measles prophylaxis after exposures occurring within 3 weeks of receiving IGIV. For people routinely receiving Immune Globulin Subcutaneous (IGSC) therapy, administration of at least 200 mg/kg body weight for 2 consecutive weeks before measles exposure should be sufficient. IG is not indicated for household or other close contacts who have received 1 dose of vaccine at 12 months or older unless they are severely immunocompromised (as defined previously).

For children who receive IG for modification or prevention of measles after exposure, measles vaccine (if not contraindicated) should be administered 6 months (if the dose was 0.5 mL/kg) after IG administration, provided the child is at least 12 months of age. Intervals vary between administration of IGIV or other biologic products and measles-containing vaccines (see Table 1.10, p 39).

HIV Infection.[1] HIV-infected children who are exposed to measles require prophylaxis on the basis of immune status and measles vaccine history. HIV-infected children who have serologic evidence of immunity or who received 2 doses of measles vaccine after initiation of ART with no or moderate immunosuppression (see Human Immunodeficiency Virus Infection, p 453) should be considered immune and will not require any additional measures to prevent measles. Severely immunocompromised patients (including HIV-infected people with CD4+ T-lymphocyte percentages <15% [all ages] or CD4+ T-lymphocyte counts >200/mm^3 [age <5 years] and those who have not received MMR vaccine since receiving combination antiretroviral therapy [cART]) who are exposed to measles should receive IGIV prophylaxis regardless of vaccination status, because they may not be protected by the vaccine. Some experts would include all HIV-infected people, regardless of immunologic status or MMR vaccine history, as needing IGIV prophylaxis. HIV-infected children who have received IGIV within 3 weeks of exposure do not require additional passive immunization.

Health Care Personnel. To decrease health care-associated infection, immunization programs should be established to ensure that all people who work or volunteer in health care facilities (including students) who may be in contact with patients with measles have presumptive evidence of immunity to measles (see Immunization in Health Care Personnel, p 95).

[1]Centers for Disease Control and Prevention. Prevention of measles, rubella, congenital rubella syndrome, and mumps, 2013 summary: recommendations of the Advisory Committee on Immunization Practices (ACIP). *MMWR Recomm Rep.* 2013;62(RR-04):1–34

Measles Vaccine Recommendations (see Table 3.38, p 541, for summary).

Use of MMR Vaccine. The only measles vaccine licensed in the United States is a live further-attenuated strain prepared in chicken embryo cell culture. Measles vaccines provided through the Expanded Programme on Immunization in resource-limited countries meet the World Health Organization standards and usually are comparable to the vaccine available in the United States. Measles vaccine is available in combination formulations, which include measles-mumps-rubella (MMR) and measles-mumps-rubella-varicella (MMRV) vaccines. Single-antigen measles vaccine no longer is available in the United States. Measles-containing vaccine in a dose of 0.5 mL is administered subcutaneously. Measles-containing vaccines can be given simultaneously with other immunizations in a separate syringe at a separate site (see Simultaneous Administration of Multiple Vaccines, p 35).

Serum measles antibodies develop in approximately 95% of children immunized at 12 months of age and 98% of children immunized at 15 months of age. Protection conferred by a single dose is durable in most people. A small proportion (5% or less) of immunized people may lose protection after several years. For measles control and elimination, 2 doses of vaccine are required. More than 99% of people who receive 2 doses (separated by at least 28 days, and the first dose administered on or after the first birthday) develop serologic evidence of measles immunity. The second dose provides protection to those failing to respond to their primary measles immunization and, therefore, is not a booster dose. Immunization is not deleterious for people who already are immune. Immunized people do not shed or transmit measles vaccine virus.

Improperly stored vaccine may fail to protect against measles. Since 1979, an improved stabilizer has been added to the vaccine that makes it more resistant to heat inactivation. For recommended storage of MMR and MMRV vaccines, see the manufacturers' package labels. MMRV vaccine must be stored frozen between −58°F and +5°F.

Age of Routine Immunization. The first dose of MMR vaccine should be given at 12 through 15 months of age. Delays in administering the first dose contributed to large outbreaks in the United States from 1989 to 1991. The second dose is recommended routinely at school entry (ie, 4 through 6 years of age) but can be given at any earlier age (eg, during an outbreak or before international travel), provided the interval between the first and second MMR doses is at least 28 days. Catch-up second dose immunization should occur for all school children (elementary, middle, high school) who have received only 1 dose, including at the adolescent visit at 11 through 12 years of age and beyond. If a child receives a dose of measles vaccine before 12 months of age, this dose is not counted toward the required number of doses, and 2 additional doses are required beginning at 12 through 15 months of age and separated by at least 28 days.

Use of MMRV Vaccine.[1,2]

• MMRV vaccine is indicated for simultaneous immunization against measles, mumps, rubella, and varicella among children 12 months through 12 years of age; MMRV vaccine is not indicated for people outside this age group. See Varicella-Zoster Infections, p 846, for recommendations for use of MMRV vaccine for the first dose.

---

[1]Centers for Disease Control and Prevention. Use of combination measles, mumps, rubella, and varicella vaccine: recommendations of the Advisory Committee on Immunization Practices (ACIP). *MMWR Recomm Rep.* 2010;59(RR-3):1–12

[2]American Academy of Pediatrics, Committee on Infectious Diseases. Prevention of varicella: update of recommendations for use of quadrivalent and monovalent varicella vaccines in children. *Pediatrics.* 2011;128(3):630–632

Table 3.38. Recommendations for Measles Immunization[a]

Category	Recommendations
Unimmunized, no history of measles (12 through 15 mo of age)	MMR vaccine is recommended at 12 through 15 mo of age; a second dose is recommended at least 28 days after the first dose and usually is given at 4 through 6 y of age
Children 6 through 11 mo of age in epidemic situations[b] or before international travel	Immunize with MMR vaccine, but this dose is not considered valid, and 2 valid doses administered on or after the first birthday are required. The first valid dose should be administered at 12 through 15 mo of age; the second valid dose is recommended at least 28 days later and usually is given at 4 through 6 y of age
Students in kindergarten, elementary, middle, and high school who have received 1 dose of measles vaccine at 12 mo of age or older	Administer the second dose
Students in college and other post-high school institutions who have received 1 dose of measles vaccine at 12 mo of age or older	Administer the second dose
History of immunization before the first birthday	Dose not considered valid; immunize (2 doses)
History of receipt of inactivated measles vaccine or unknown type of vaccine, 1963–1967	Dose not considered valid; immunize (2 doses)
Further attenuated or unknown vaccine given with IG	Dose not considered valid; immunize (2 doses)
Allergy to eggs	Immunize; no reactions likely (see text for details)
Neomycin allergy, nonanaphylactic	Immunize; no reactions likely (see text for details)
Severe hypersensitivity (anaphylaxis) to neomycin or gelatin	Avoid immunization
Tuberculosis	Immunize (see Tuberculosis, p 804); if patient has untreated tuberculosis disease, start antituberculosis therapy before immunizing
Measles exposure	Immunize or give IG, depending on circumstances (see text, p 538)
HIV infected	Immunize (2 doses) unless severely immunocompromised (see text, p 545); administration of IG if exposed to measles is based on degree of immunosuppression and measles vaccine history (see text, p 545)
Personal or family history of seizures	Immunize; advise parents of slightly increased risk of seizures
Immunoglobulin or blood recipient	Immunize at the appropriate interval (see Table 1.10, p 39)

MMR indicates measles-mumps-rubella vaccine; MMRV, measles-mumps-rubella-varicella vaccine; IG, Immune Globulin; HIV, human immunodeficiency virus.

[a]See text for details and recommendations for use of MMRV vaccine.

[b]Determined at the local level depending on outbreak epidemiology and risk of exposure for infants (see Outbreak Control, p 546).

- Children with HIV infection also should not receive MMRV vaccine because of lack of safety data of the quadrivalent vaccine in children infected with HIV.
- MMRV vaccine may be administered with other vaccines recommended at 12 through 15 months of age and before or at 4 through 6 years of age (**http://redbook. solutions.aap.org/SS/Immunization_Schedules.aspx**).
- At least 28 days should elapse between a dose of measles-containing vaccine, such as MMR vaccine, and a dose of MMRV vaccine. However, the recommended minimal interval between MMRV vaccine doses is 90 days.
- Febrile seizures occur in 7 to 9 per 10 000 children receiving the first dose of MMRV vaccine at 12 through 23 months of age and in 3 to 4 per 10 000 children receiving the first dose of MMR and varicella vaccines administered separately at the same visit at 12 through 23 months of age. Thus, 1 additional febrile seizure is expected to occur per approximately 2300 to 2600 children 12 through 23 months of age immunized with MMRV vaccine, compared with separate MMR and monovalent varicella vaccines. The period of risk for febrile seizures is from 5 to 12 days following receipt of the vaccine. Febrile seizures do not predispose to epilepsy or neurodevelopmental delays later in life and have no lasting medical consequence. The benefit of using MMRV instead of MMR and monovalent varicella vaccines separately is that the quadrivalent product results in one fewer injection. The American Academy of Pediatrics recommends that for the first dose of measles, mumps, rubella, and varicella vaccines at ages 12 through 47 months, either MMR and varicella vaccines or MMRV vaccine be used. Pediatricians should discuss risks and benefits of the vaccine choices with the parents or caregivers. For the first dose of measles, mumps, rubella, and varicella vaccines at ages 48 months and older and for dose 2 at any age (15 months through 12 years), use of MMRV vaccine generally is preferred over separate injections of MMR and varicella vaccines to minimize the number of injections.

Colleges and Other Institutions for Education Beyond High School. Colleges and other institutions should require that all entering students have documentation of evidence of measles immunity: serologic evidence of immunity, or receipt of 2 doses of measles-containing vaccines administered at least 28 days apart. Students without documentation of measles immunity should receive MMR vaccine on entry, followed by a second dose 28 days later, if not contraindicated.

Immunization During an Outbreak. During an outbreak, MMR vaccine should be offered to all people exposed or in the outbreak setting who lack evidence of measles immunity. During a community-wide outbreak affecting infants, MMR vaccine has been shown to be efficacious and may be recommended for infants 6 through 11 months of age (see Outbreak Control, p 546). However, seroconversion rates after MMR immunization are significantly lower in children immunized before the first birthday than in children immunized after the first birthday because of the presence of maternal antibody in some children. Therefore, doses received prior to the first birthday should not count toward the recommended 2-dose series. Children immunized before their first birthday should be reimmunized with MMR or MMRV vaccine at 12 through 15 months of age (at least 28 days after the initial measles immunization) and again at school entry (4 through 6 years of age).

International Travel. People traveling internationally (any location outside of the United States) should be immune to measles. Infants 6 through 11 months of age should receive 1 dose of MMR vaccine before departure, and then they should receive a second dose of measles-containing vaccine at 12 through 15 months of age (at least 28 days after the initial measles immunization) and a third dose at 4 through 6 years of age. Children 12 through 15 months of age should be given their first dose of MMR vaccine before departure and again by 4 through 6 years of age. Children 12 months of age or older who have received 1 dose and are traveling to areas where measles is endemic or epidemic should receive their second dose before departure, provided the interval between doses is 28 days or more.

International Adoptees. The US Department of State requires that internationally adopted children 10 years and older receive several vaccines, including MMR, before entry into the United States. Internationally adopted children who are younger than 10 years are exempt from Immigration and Nationality Act regulations pertaining to immunization of immigrants before arrival in the United States (see Children Who Received Immunizations Outside the United States, p 98); adoptive parents are required to sign a waiver indicating their intention to comply with US immunization recommendations after their child's arrival in the United States.

Health Care Personnel.[1] Adequate presumptive evidence of immunity to measles for people who work in health care facilities is: (1) documented administration of 2 doses of live-virus measles vaccine with the first dose administered at ≥12 months of age and the second dose at least 28 days after the first; (2) laboratory evidence of immunity or laboratory confirmation of disease; or (3) birth before 1957. Birth before 1957 is not a guarantee of measles immunity, and therefore, facilities should consider vaccinating unimmunized personnel who lack laboratory evidence of immunity who were born before 1957 with 2 doses of MMR vaccine at the appropriate interval (see Immunization in Health Care Personnel, p 95). For recommendations during an outbreak, see Outbreak Control (p 546).

Adverse Events. A temperature of 39.4°C (103°F) or higher develops in approximately 5% to 15% of vaccine recipients, usually between 6 and 12 days after receipt of MMR vaccine; fever generally lasts 1 to 2 days but may last as long as 5 days. Most people with fever otherwise are asymptomatic. Transient rashes have been reported in approximately 5% of vaccine recipients. Recipients who develop fever and/or rash are not considered contagious. Febrile seizures 5 to 12 days after immunization occur in 1 in 3000 to 4000 people immunized with MMR vaccine. Transient thrombocytopenia occurs in 1 in 22 000 to 40 000 people after administration of measles-containing vaccines, specifically MMR (see Thrombocytopenia, p 544). There is no evidence that reimmunization increases the risk of adverse events in people already immune to these diseases. Data indicate that only people who are not immune to the viruses in MMR tend to have adverse effects. Thus, events following a second dose of MMR vaccine would be expected to be substantially lower than after a first dose, because most people who received a first dose would be immune.

Rates of most local and systemic adverse events for children immunized with MMRV vaccine are comparable to rates for children immunized with MMR and varicella vaccines administered concomitantly. However, recipients of a first dose of MMRV vaccine have a greater rate of fever 102°F (38.9°C) or higher than do recipients of MMR and varicella administered concomitantly (22% vs 15%, respectively), and measles-like rash is observed in 3% of recipients of MMRV vaccine and 2% of recipients of MMR and varicella vaccines administered concomitantly.

The reported frequency of central nervous system conditions, such as encephalitis and encephalopathy, after measles immunization is less than 1 per million doses administered in the United States. Because the incidence of encephalitis or encephalopathy

[1]Centers for Disease Control and Prevention. Immunization of health-care personnel: recommendations of the Advisory Committee on Immunization Practices (ACIP). *MMWR Recomm Rep.* 2011;60(RR-07):1–45

after measles immunization in the United States is lower than the observed incidence of encephalitis of unknown cause, some or most of the rare reported severe neurologic disorders may be related temporally, rather than causally, to measles immunization. Multiple studies, as well as an Institute of Medicine Vaccine Safety Review, refute a causal relationship between autism and MMR vaccine or between inflammatory bowel disease and MMR vaccine. The original 1998 study claiming such a relationship was retracted by the publishing journal in 2010, and the lead author has had his medical license revoked in Great Britain.

Seizures. Risk of febrile seizures following receipt of MMR and MMRV vaccines at 12 through 23 months of age is discussed earlier in the chapter (see Use of MMRV Vaccine, p 540). Children with histories of seizures or children whose first-degree relatives have histories of seizures may be at a slightly increased risk of a seizure and should be immunized with separate MMR and varicella vaccines, because the benefits greatly outweigh the risks.

Subacute Sclerosing Panencephalitis. Measles vaccine, by protecting against measles, decreases significantly the possibility of developing SSPE. Vaccine-strain measles virus never has been confirmed in a case of SSPE.

Precautions and Contraindications (also see Table 1.10, p 39).

Febrile Illnesses. Children with minor illnesses, such as upper respiratory tract infections, may be immunized (see Vaccine Contraindications and Precautions, p 52). Fever is not a contraindication to immunization. However, if other manifestations suggest a more serious illness, the immunization should be deferred until the illness has resolved.

Allergic Reactions. Hypersensitivity reactions occur rarely and usually are minor, consisting of wheal-and-flare reactions or urticaria at the injection site. Reactions have been attributed to trace amounts of neomycin or gelatin or some other component in the vaccine formulation. Anaphylaxis is rare. Measles vaccine is produced in chicken embryo cell culture and does not contain significant amounts of egg white (ovalbumin) cross-reacting proteins. Children with egg allergy are at low risk of anaphylactic reactions to measles-containing vaccines (including MMR and MMRV). Skin testing of children for egg allergy is not predictive of reactions to MMR vaccine and is not recommended before administering MMR or other measles-containing vaccines. People with allergies to chickens or feathers are not at increased risk of reaction to the vaccine.

People who have had a significant hypersensitivity reaction after the first dose of measles vaccine should: (1) be tested for measles immunity, and if immune, should not be given a second dose; or (2) receive evaluation and possible skin testing before receiving a second dose. People who have had an immediate anaphylactic reaction to previous measles immunization should not be reimmunized but should be tested to determine whether they are immune.

People who have experienced anaphylactic reactions to gelatin or topically or systemically administered neomycin should receive measles vaccine only in settings where such reactions can be managed and after consultation with an allergist or immunologist. Most often, however, neomycin allergy manifests as contact dermatitis, which is not a contraindication to receiving measles vaccine.

Thrombocytopenia. Rarely, MMR vaccine can be associated with thrombocytopenia within 2 months of immunization, with a temporal clustering 2 to 3 weeks after immunization. On the basis of case reports, the risk of vaccine-associated thrombocytopenia may be higher for people who previously experienced thrombocytopenia, especially if it occurred in temporal association with earlier MMR immunization. The decision to immunize these children should be based on assessment of immunity after the first dose and the benefits of protection against measles, mumps, and rubella in comparison with the risks of recurrence of thrombocytopenia after immunization. The risk of thrombocytopenia is higher after the first dose of vaccine than after the second dose. There have been no reported cases of thrombocytopenia associated with receipt of MMR vaccine that have resulted in hemorrhagic complications or death in otherwise healthy people.

Recent Administration of IG. IG preparations interfere with the serologic response to measles vaccine for variable periods, depending on the dose of IG administered. Suggested intervals between IG or blood-product administration and measles immunization are given in Table 1.10 (p 39). If vaccine is given at intervals shorter than those indicated, as may be warranted if the risk of exposure to measles is imminent, the child should be reimmunized at or after the appropriate interval for immunization (and at least 28 days after the earlier immunization) unless serologic testing indicates that measles-specific antibodies were produced.

If IG is to be administered in preparation for international travel, administration of vaccine should precede receipt of IG by at least 2 weeks to preclude interference with replication of the vaccine virus.

Tuberculosis. Tuberculin skin testing is not a prerequisite for measles immunization. Antituberculosis therapy should be initiated before administering MMR vaccine to people with untreated tuberculosis infection or disease. Tuberculin skin testing, if otherwise indicated, can be performed on the day of immunization. Otherwise, testing should be postponed for 4 to 6 weeks, because measles immunization temporarily may suppress tuberculin skin test reactivity.

Altered Immunity. Immunocompromised patients with disorders associated with increased severity of viral infections should not be given live-virus measles vaccine (the exception is people with HIV infection, unless they have evidence of severe immunosuppression; see Immunization in Immunocompromised Children, p 74, and HIV Infection, p 539). The risk of exposure to measles for immunocompromised patients can be decreased by immunizing their close susceptible contacts. Immunized people do not shed or transmit measles vaccine virus. Management of immunodeficient and immunosuppressed patients exposed to measles can be facilitated by previous knowledge of their immune status. If possible, children should receive measles vaccine prior to initiating treatment with biological response modifiers, such as tumor necrosis factor antagonists. Susceptible patients with immunodeficiencies should receive IG after measles exposure (see Care of Exposed People, p 538).

Corticosteroids. For patients who have received high doses of corticosteroids (≥2 mg/kg of body weight or ≥20 mg/day of prednisone or its equivalent for people who weigh >10 kg) for 14 days or more and who otherwise are not immunocompromised, the recommended interval between stopping the corticosteroids and immunization is at least 1 month (see Immunocompromised Children, p 74). In general, inhaled steroids do not cause immunosuppression and are not a contraindication to measles immunization.

HIV Infection. Measles immunization (given as MMR vaccine) is recommended for all people ≥12 months of age with HIV infection who do not have evidence of measles immunity and who do not have evidence of severe immunosuppression, because measles can be severe and often is fatal in patients with HIV infection (see Human Immunodeficiency Virus Infection, p 453). Severe immunosuppression is defined as CD4+ T-lymphocyte percentage <15% (all ages) or CD4+ T-lymphocyte count <200 lymphocytes/mm^3 (older than 5 years). The first dose of MMR vaccine should be administered at age 12 through 15 months and the second dose at age 4 through 6 years, or as early as 28 days after the first dose. Children and adults with newly diagnosed HIV infections and without acceptable evidence of measles immunity should complete a 2-dose schedule with MMR vaccine as soon as possible after diagnosis, unless they have evidence of severe immunosuppression. People with perinatal HIV infection who were vaccinated against measles prior to establishment of combination antiretroviral therapy (cART) should be considered unvaccinated and should be revaccinated with 2 doses of MMR vaccine once cART has been administered for ≥6 months with CD4+ T-lymphocyte percentage ≥15% (all ages) and CD4+ T-lymphocyte count ≥200 lymphocytes/mm^3 (age >5 years) unless they have other acceptable current evidence of measles immunity. Severely immunocompromised HIV-infected infants, children, adolescents, and young adults should not receive measles virus-containing vaccine, because vaccine-related pneumonia has been reported (see Human Immunodeficiency Virus Infection, p 453). All members of the household of an HIV-infected person should receive 2 doses of MMR unless they are HIV infected and severely immunosuppressed, were born before 1957, have laboratory evidence of measles immunity, have had age-appropriate immunizations, or have a contraindication to measles vaccine. Because measles vaccine virus is not shed after immunization, HIV-infected people are not at risk of measles vaccine virus infection if household members are immunized.

Personal or Family History of Seizures. Children with a personal or family history of seizures should be immunized after parents or guardians are advised that the risk of seizures after measles immunization is increased slightly. Risk of febrile seizures following receipt of MMR and MMRV vaccine at 12 through 23 months of age is discussed earlier in the chapter (see Use of MMRV Vaccine, p 540). Children receiving anticonvulsants should continue such therapy after measles immunization.

Pregnancy. A measles-containing vaccine should not be given to women known to be pregnant. Women who are given MMR vaccine should not become pregnant for at least 28 days. This precaution is based on the theoretical risk of fetal infection, which applies to administration of any live-virus vaccine to women who might be pregnant or who might become pregnant shortly after immunization. No data from women who were inadvertently vaccinated while pregnant substantiate this theoretical risk. In the immunization of adolescents and young adults against measles, asking women if they are pregnant, excluding women who are, and explaining the theoretical risks to others are recommended precautions.

Outbreak Control. Every suspected measles case should be reported immediately to the local health department, and every effort must be made to obtain laboratory evidence that would confirm that the illness is measles (including obtaining specimens for virus detection), especially if the illness may be the first case in the community. During an outbreak, MMR vaccine should be offered to people in the outbreak setting who lack evidence of immunity. If the outbreak affects preschool-aged children with community-wide transmission, a second MMR dose should be considered for children ages 1 to 4 years who have received only 1 dose previously. When a community-wide outbreak involves infants younger than 1 year with ongoing risk for exposure, MMR vaccine can be administered to infants 6 through 11 months of age. These decisions usually are made at the local level with input from the health department and are based on the local epidemiology of the outbreak. People who have not been immunized, including those who have been exempted from measles immunization for medical, religious, or other reasons, should be excluded from school, child care, and health care settings until at least 21 days after the onset of rash in the last case of measles. Extra doses of measles vaccine administered to previously immunized people are not associated with an increased risk of reactions.

Schools and Child Care Facilities. During measles outbreaks in child care facilities, schools, and colleges and other institutions of higher education, all students, their siblings, and personnel born in 1957 or after who cannot provide documentation that they received 2 doses of measles-containing vaccine on or after their first birthday or other evidence of measles immunity should be immunized. People receiving their second dose, as well as unimmunized people receiving their first dose as part of the outbreak-control program, may be readmitted immediately to the school or child care facility.

Health Care Facilities. If an outbreak occurs in an area served by a hospital or within a hospital, all employees and volunteers who cannot provide documentation that they have received 2 doses of measles vaccine, with the first dose given on or after their first birthday, or laboratory evidence of immunity to measles should receive 2 doses of MMR vaccine. Because some health care personnel born before 1957 have acquired measles in health care facilities, immunization with 2 doses of MMR vaccine is recommended for health care personnel without serologic evidence of immunity in this age category during outbreaks. Serologic testing is not recommended during an outbreak before immunization, because rapid immunization is required to halt disease transmission. Health care personnel without evidence of immunity who have been exposed should be relieved of direct patient contact from the fifth to the 21st day after exposure, regardless of whether they received vaccine or IG after the exposure. Health care personnel who become ill should be relieved of patient contact until 4 days after rash develops.

Meningococcal Infections

CLINICAL MANIFESTATIONS: Invasive infection usually results in meningitis (~50% of cases), bacteremia (~35%–40% of cases) or both. Bacteremic pneumonia is uncommon (~9% of cases). Onset can be insidious and nonspecific but typically is abrupt, with fever, chills, malaise, myalgia, limb pain, prostration, and a rash that initially can be macular, maculopapular, petechial, or purpuric (meningococcemia). The maculopapular and petechial rash is indistinguishable from the rash caused by some viral infections. Purpura also can occur in severe sepsis caused by other bacterial pathogens. In fulminant cases, purpura, limb ischemia, coagulopathy, pulmonary edema, shock (characterized by tachycardia, tachypnea, oliguria, and poor peripheral perfusion, with confusion and hypotension), coma, and death can ensue within hours despite appropriate therapy. Signs and symptoms of meningococcal meningitis are indistinguishable from those associated with acute meningitis caused by other meningeal pathogens (eg, *Streptococcus pneumoniae).* In severe and fatal cases of meningococcal meningitis, raised intracranial pressure is a predominant presenting feature. The overall case-fatality rate for meningococcal disease is 10% to 15% and is somewhat higher in adolescents. Death is more common in those with coma, hypotension, leukopenia, and thrombocytopenia and among those who do not have meningitis. Less common manifestations of meningococcal infection include conjunctivitis, septic arthritis, and chronic meningococcemia. Rarely, occult bacteremia may be seen. Invasive infections can be complicated by arthritis, myocarditis, pericarditis, and endophthalmitis. A self-limiting postinfectious inflammatory syndrome occurs in fewer than 10% of cases 4 or more days after onset of meningococcal infection and most commonly presents as fever and arthritis or vasculitis. Iritis, scleritis, conjunctivitis, pericarditis, and polyserositis are less common manifestations of postinfectious inflammatory syndrome.

Sequelae associated with meningococcal disease occur in 11% to 19% of survivors and include hearing loss, neurologic disability, digit or limb amputations, and skin scarring. In addition, patients may also experience subtle long-term neurologic deficits, such as impaired school performance, behavioral problems, and attention deficit disorder.

ETIOLOGY: *Neisseria meningitidis* is a gram-negative diplococcus with at least 13 serogroups based on capsular type.

EPIDEMIOLOGY: Strains belonging to groups A, B, C, Y, and W are implicated most commonly in invasive disease worldwide. Serogroup A has been associated frequently with epidemics outside the United States, primarily in sub-Saharan Africa. A serogroup A meningococcal conjugate vaccine was introduced in the "meningitis belt" of sub-Saharan Africa in December 2010. This novel vaccine is highly effective and has the potential to end epidemic meningitis as a public health concern in sub-Saharan Africa. An increase in cases of serogroup W meningococcal disease has been associated with the Hajj pilgrimage in Saudi Arabia. Since 2002, serogroup W meningococcal disease has been reported in sub-Saharan African countries during epidemic seasons. More recently, serogroup W outbreaks have occurred in South America. Prolonged outbreaks of serogroup B meningococcal disease have occurred in New Zealand, France, and Oregon. More recently, several clusters of serogroup B meningococcal disease have occurred on college campuses in the United States. Serogroup X causes a substantial number of cases of meningococcal disease in parts of Africa but is rare on other continents.

The incidence of meningococcal disease varies over time and by age and location. During the past 60 years, the annual incidence of meningococcal disease in the United States has varied from ≤0.3 to 1.5 cases per 100 000 population. Incidence cycles have occurred over multiple years. Since the early 2000s, annual incidence rates have decreased, and since 2005 only an estimated 800 to 1000 US cases have been reported annually. The reasons for this decrease, which preceded introduction of meningococcal polysaccharide-protein conjugate vaccine into the immunization schedule, are not known but may be related to immunity of the population to circulating meningococcal strains and to the changes in behavioral risk factors (eg, smoking and exposure to secondhand smoke among adolescents and young adults).

Distribution of meningococcal serogroups in the United States has shifted in the past 2 decades. Serogroups B, C, and Y each account for approximately 30% of reported cases, but serogroup distribution varies by age, location, and time. Approximately three quarters of cases among adolescents and young adults are caused by serogroups C, Y, or W and potentially are preventable with available vaccines. In infants and children younger than 60 months, 60% of cases are caused by serogroup B and therefore are not preventable with vaccines licensed in the United States for those ages.

Since introduction in the United States of *Haemophilus influenzae* type b and pneumococcal polysaccharide-protein conjugate vaccines for infants, *N meningitidis* has become the leading cause of bacterial meningitis in children and remains an important cause of septicemia. Disease rates are highest in children 2 years or younger; the peak incidence occurs in infants. Other peaks occur in adolescents and young adults 16 through 21 years of age and adults older than 65 years. Historically, freshman college students who lived in dormitories and military recruits in barracks had a higher rate of disease compared with people who are the same age and who are not living in such accommodations. Close contacts of patients with meningococcal disease are at increased risk of becoming infected. Patients with persistent complement component deficiencies (eg, C5–C9, properdin, or factor H or factor D deficiencies) or anatomic or functional asplenia are at increased risk of invasive and recurrent meningococcal disease. Asymptomatic colonization of the upper respiratory tract provides the source from which the organism is spread. The highest rates of meningococcal colonization occur in older adolescents and young adults. Transmission occurs from person-to-person through droplets from the respiratory tract and requires close contact. Patients should be considered capable of transmitting the organism for up to 24 hours after initiation of effective antimicrobial treatment.

Outbreaks occur in communities and institutions, including child care centers, schools, colleges, and military recruit camps. However, most cases of meningococcal disease are sporadic, with fewer than 5% associated with outbreaks. The attack rate for household contacts is 500 to 800 times the rate for the general population. Serologic typing, multilocus sequence typing, multilocus enzyme electrophoresis, and pulsed-field gel electrophoresis of enzyme-restricted DNA fragments can be useful epidemiologic tools during a suspected outbreak to detect concordance among invasive strains.

The **incubation period** is 1 to 10 days, usually less than 4 days.

DIAGNOSTIC TESTS: Cultures of blood and cerebrospinal fluid (CSF) are indicated for patients with suspected invasive meningococcal disease. Culture of a petechial or purpuric lesion scraping, synovial fluid, and other usually sterile body fluid specimens yield the organism in some patients. A Gram stain of a petechial or purpuric scraping, CSF, and buffy coat smear of blood can be helpful. Because *N meningitidis* can be a component of the nasopharyngeal flora, isolation of *N meningitidis* from this site is not helpful diagnostically. A serogroup-specific polymerase chain reaction (PCR) test to detect *N meningitidis* from clinical specimens is used routinely in the United Kingdom and some European countries, where up to 56% of cases are confirmed by PCR testing alone. This test particularly is useful in patients who receive antimicrobial therapy before cultures are obtained. In the United States, PCR-based assays are available in some research and public health laboratories. A recently described multiplex PCR assay appears to have a sensitivity and specificity approaching 100% for detection of serogroups A, B, C, W, and Y.

Case definitions for invasive meningococcal disease are given in Table 3.39.

Table 3.39. Surveillance Case Definitions for Invasive Meningococcal Disease

Confirmed case

A clinically compatible case and isolation of *Neisseria meningitidis* from a usually sterile site, for example:
- Blood
- Cerebrospinal fluid
- Synovial fluid
- Pleural fluid
- Pericardial fluid
- Isolation from skin scraping of petechial or purpuric lesions

Probable case

A clinically compatible case with **EITHER** a positive result of antigen test or immunohistochemistry of formalin-fixed tissue **OR** a positive polymerase chain reaction test of blood or cerebrospinal fluid, without a positive sterile site culture.

Suspect
- A clinically compatible case and gram-negative diplococci in any sterile fluid, such as cerebrospinal fluid, synovial fluid, or scraping from a petechial or purpuric lesion
- Clinical purpura fulminans without a positive culture

TREATMENT: The priority in management of meningococcal disease is treatment of shock in meningococcemia and of raised intracranial pressure in severe cases of meningitis. Empirical therapy for suspected meningococcal disease should include an extended-spectrum cephalosporin, such as cefotaxime or ceftriaxone. Once the microbiologic diagnosis is established, definitive treatment with penicillin G (300 000 U/kg/day; maximum, 12 million U/day, divided every 4–6 hours), ampicillin, or an extended-spectrum cephalosporin (cefotaxime or ceftriaxone) is recommended. Some experts recommend susceptibility testing before switching to penicillin. However, susceptibility testing is not standardized, and the clinical significance of intermediate susceptibility is unknown. Resistance of *N meningitidis* to penicillin is rare in the United States. Ceftriaxone clears nasopharyngeal carriage effectively after 1 dose and allows outpatient management for completion of therapy when appropriate. For patients with a life-threatening penicillin allergy characterized by anaphylaxis, chloramphenicol is recommended, if available. If chloramphenicol is not available, meropenem can be used, although the rate of cross-reactivity in penicillin-allergic adults is 2% to 3%. For travelers from areas where penicillin resistance has been reported, cefotaxime, ceftriaxone, or chloramphenicol is recommended. Five to 7 days of antimicrobial therapy is adequate. In meningococcemia, early and rapid fluid resuscitation and early use of inotropic and ventilatory support may reduce mortality. The postinfectious inflammatory syndromes associated with meningococcal disease often respond to nonsteroidal anti-inflammatory drugs.

ISOLATION OF THE HOSPITALIZED PATIENT: In addition to standard precautions, droplet precautions are recommended until 24 hours after initiation of effective antimicrobial therapy.

CONTROL MEASURES:
Care of Exposed People.

Chemoprophylaxis. Regardless of immunization status, close contacts of all people with invasive meningococcal disease (see Table 3.40), whether endemic or in an outbreak situation, are at high risk of infection and should receive chemoprophylaxis. Currently licensed

Table 3.40. Disease Risk for Contacts of People With Meningococcal Disease

High risk: chemoprophylaxis recommended (close contacts)
- Household contact, especially children younger than 2 years
- Child care or preschool contact at any time during 7 days before onset of illness
- Direct exposure to index patient's secretions through kissing or through sharing toothbrushes or eating utensils, markers of close social contact, at any time during 7 days before onset of illness
- Mouth-to-mouth resuscitation, unprotected contact during endotracheal intubation at any time 7 days before onset of illness
- Frequently slept in same dwelling as index patient during 7 days before onset of illness
- Passengers seated directly next to the index case during airline flights lasting more than 8 hours

Low risk: chemoprophylaxis not recommended
- Casual contact: no history of direct exposure to index patient's oral secretions (eg, school or work)
- Indirect contact: only contact is with a high-risk contact, no direct contact with the index patient
- Health care personnel without direct exposure to patient's oral secretions

In outbreak or cluster
- Chemoprophylaxis for people other than people at high risk should be administered only after consultation with local public health authorities

vaccines, including a serogroup B vaccine licensed in 2014 for people 10 through 25 years of age, are not 100% effective. The decision to give chemoprophylaxis to contacts of people with meningococcal disease is based on risk of contracting invasive disease. Throat and nasopharyngeal cultures are not recommended, because these cultures are of no value in deciding who should receive chemoprophylaxis.

Chemoprophylaxis is warranted for people who have been exposed directly to a patient's oral secretions through close social contact, such as kissing or sharing of tooth-brushes or eating utensils, as well as for child care and preschool contacts during the 7 days before onset of disease in the index case. People who frequently slept in the same dwelling as the infected person within this period also should receive chemoprophylaxis. For airline travel lasting more than 8 hours, passengers who are seated directly next to an infected person should receive prophylaxis. It is emphasized that routine prophylaxis is not recommended for health care personnel (Table 3.40, p 550) unless they have had intimate exposure to respiratory tract secretions, such as occurs with unprotected mouth-to-mouth resuscitation, intubation, or suctioning before or less than 24 hours after anti-microbial therapy was initiated. Chemoprophylaxis ideally should be initiated within 24 hours after the index patient is identified; prophylaxis given more than 2 weeks after expo-sure has little value.

Antimicrobial Regimens for Prophylaxis (see Table 3.41). Rifampin, ceftriaxone, ciprofloxa-cin, and azithromycin are appropriate drugs for chemoprophylaxis in adults, but neither rifampin nor ciprofloxacin are recommended for pregnant women. The drug of choice for most children is rifampin or ciprofloxacin (Table 3.41). Rifampin alters the pharma-cokinetics of a number of medications. If antimicrobial agents other than ceftriaxone or cefotaxime (each of which will eradicate nasopharyngeal carriage) are used for treatment of invasive meningococcal disease, the child should receive chemoprophylaxis before hos-pital discharge to eradicate nasopharyngeal carriage of *N meningitidis*. Rifampin requires 4 doses over 2 days to eradicate nasopharyngeal carriage, but ceftriaxone, ciprofloxacin, and azithromycin only require a single dose.

In areas of the United States where ciprofloxacin-resistant strains of *N meningitidis* have been detected, ciprofloxacin should not be used for chemoprophylaxis.[1] Use of azithromy-cin as a single oral dose has been shown to be effective for eradication of nasopharyngeal carriage in one study and can be used where ciprofloxacin resistance has been detected.

Postexposure Immunoprophylaxis. Because secondary cases can occur several weeks or more after onset of disease in the index case, meningococcal vaccine is an adjunct to chemopro-phylaxis when an outbreak is caused by a serogroup prevented by a meningococcal vaccine. For control of meningococcal outbreaks caused by serogroups A, C, Y, and W, the preferred vaccine in adults and children 2 months and older is a meningococcal conjugate vaccine (see Table 3.42). The Centers for Disease Control and Prevention (CDC) Advisory Committee on Immunization Practices has recommended that either of the 2 new serogroup B vaccines be used in people 10 years and older who are at increased risk of meningococcal disease because of a serogroup B meningococcal disease outbreak. The same vaccine product should be used for all doses.

Meningococcal Vaccines. In the United States, 4 meningococcal vaccines are licensed for use in children and adults against serogroups A, C, Y, or W, and 2 vaccines are licensed for people 10 through 25 years of age against serogroup B.

---

[1]Centers for Disease Control and Prevention. Emergence of fluoroquinolone-resistant *Neisseria meningitidis*— Minnesota and North Dakota, 2007–2008. *MMWR Morb Mortal Wkly Rep.* 2008;57(7):173–175

Table 3.41. Recommended Chemoprophylaxis Regimens for High-Risk Contacts and People With Invasive Meningococcal Disease

Age of Infants, Children, and Adults	Dose	Duration	Efficacy, %	Cautions
Rifampin[a]				
<1 mo	5 mg/kg, orally, every 12 h	2 days		
≥1 mo	10 mg/kg (maximum 600 mg), orally, every 12 h	2 days	90–95	Can interfere with efficacy of oral contraceptives and some seizure and anticoagulant medications; can stain soft contact lenses
Ceftriaxone				
<15 y	125 mg, intramuscularly	Single dose	90–95	To decrease pain at injection site, dilute with 1% lidocaine
≥15 y	250 mg, intramuscularly	Single dose	90–95	To decrease pain at injection site, dilute with 1% lidocaine
Ciprofloxacin[a,b]				
≥1 mo	20 mg/kg (maximum 500 mg), orally	Single dose	90–95	
Azithromycin	10 mg/kg (maximum 500 mg)	Single dose	90	*Not* recommended routinely; equivalent to rifampin for eradication of *Neisseria meningitidis* from nasopharynx in one study

[a] Not recommended for use in pregnant women.
[b] Use only if fluoroquinolone resistant strains of *N meningitidis* have not been identified in the community.

- Quadrivalent (serogroups A, C, Y, and W) meningococcal polysaccharide vaccine (MPSV4) was licensed in 1981 for use in children 2 years and older, is administered **subcutaneously** as a single 0.5-mL dose, and can be given concurrently with other vaccines but at different anatomic sites.
- Three meningococcal conjugate vaccines (MenACWY-D [Menactra, Sanofi Pasteur], MenACWY-CRM [Menveo, Novartis Vaccines], and HibMenCY-TT [MenHibrix, [GlaxoSmithKline]) are licensed for use in people 9 months through 55 years of age, 2 months through 55 years of age, and 6 weeks through 18 months of age, respectively. Each meningococcal conjugate vaccine is administered **intramuscularly** as a 0.5-mL dose.
- All 3 meningococcal conjugate vaccines (MenACWY-D, MenACWY-CRM, and HibMenCY-TT) are licensed for infants but with different administration schedules. MenACWY-D is administered as a 2-dose primary series, 3 months apart, among children 9 through 23 months of age. MenACWY-CRM is licensed for infants as a 4-dose series at 2, 4, 6, and 12 months of age. HibMenCY-TT is licensed for infants as a 4-dose series at 2, 4, 6, and 12 through 15 months of age.

Table 3.42. Recommended Meningococcal Vaccines for Immunocompetent Children and Adults

Age	Vaccine	Status
2 mo through 10 y	MenACWY-D[a] (Menactra, Sanofi Pasteur, Swiftwater, PA) MenACWY-CRM[b] (Menveo, Novartis, Cambridge, MA) HibMenCY-TT[c] (MenHibrix, GlaxoSmith-Kline, Research Triangle Park, NC)	Not routinely recommended; see Table 3.43 (p 555) for recommendations for people at increased risk
10 through 25 y	rLP2086 serogroup B (Trumenba, Pfizer Inc, Philadelphia, PA) or 4CmenB serogroup B (Bexsero, Novartis Vaccines and Diagnostics, Siena, Italy)	Not routinely recommended; see text of 4th bullet (below) for recommendations for people at increased risk
11 through 21 y	MenACWY-D or MenACWY-CRM	Primary: • 11 through 12 y of age, 1 dose • 13 through 18 y of age, 1 dose if not previously immunized • 19 through 21 y of age, not routinely recommended but may be given as catch-up immunization for those who have not received a dose after their 16th birthday Booster: • 1 dose recommended for adolescents if first dose administered prior to 16th birthday
22 through 55 y	MenACWY-D or MenACWY-CRM	Not recommended routinely; see Table 3.43 (p 555) for people at increased risk
≥56 y	MPSV4, MenACWY-D, or MenACWY-CRM	Not routinely; see Table 3.43 for people at increased risk

[a] Licensed only for people 9 months through 55 years.
[b] Licensed only for people 2 months through 55 years.
[c] Licensed only for children aged 6 weeks through 18 months of age.

• In October 2014, rLP2086 serogroup B meningococcal vaccine (Pfizer, Philadelphia, PA) was approved by the FDA with a 3-dose schedule (0, 2, 6 months). The vaccine is based on lipoprotein 2086, which is a surface-exposed factor H binding protein (fHBP) expressed in more than 97% of invasive meningococcal B strains. It functions as an important meningococcal virulence factor. fHBP sequences segregate into 2 genetically and immunologically distinct subfamilies, A and B. The bivalent rLP2086 contains 2 lipidated fHBP variants (A05 and B01), 1 from each subfamily. No long-term immunogenicity data are available. In January 2015, the 4CmenB serogroup B meningococcal vaccine (Novartis Vaccines and Diagnostics, Siena, Italy) was licensed. It also has been approved for use in Australia, Canada, and Europe, and has been used in several outbreaks on US college campuses as an investigational product. The antigenic components of the 4CmenB serogroup B meningococcal vaccine are fHbp fusion protein, NadA, NHBA fusion protein, and the outer membrane vesicle that was part of the New Zealand vaccine. Immunity from this vaccine wanes by 5% to 25% after 2 years. Potential differences in immunogenicity and breadth of coverage between these 2 serogroup B vaccines are not known. Recommendations for use of these new meningococcal serogroup B vaccines are under consideration by the American Academy of Pediatrics. The Advisory Committee on Immunization Practices of the CDC recommends that people 10 years and older who are at increased risk of meningococcal disease receive this vaccine. This includes people with persistent complement component deficiencies, people with anatomic or functional asplenia, and people at increased risk because of a serogroup B meningococcal disease outbreak. The same vaccine product should be used for all doses.

   Indications for Use of Meningococcal Vaccines (Table 3.42, p 553, and Table 3.43, p 555). Considerations for possible routine use of the 2 newly licensed meningococcal serogroup B vaccines are under development at the American Academy of Pediatrics and the CDC. The remainder of this section on meningococcal vaccines, as well as Table 3.43, relates only to the MenACWY and MenCY vaccines. Routine childhood immunization with meningococcal conjugate vaccines is not recommended for children 2 months through 10 years of age because of the low proportion of infections that are preventable with vaccination; approximately 60% of disease among children aged ≤59 months is caused by serogroup B, which is not prevented with licensed vaccines approved for use in those ages. Meningococcal conjugate vaccination is recommended routinely for adolescents (Table 3.42) and for high-risk children (Table 3.43). Recommendations for use of a meningococcal conjugate vaccine are as follows[1,2,3,4] (Tables 3.42 and 3.43):

- Adolescents should be immunized routinely at the 11- through 12-year of age health care visit (see **http://redbook.solutions.aap.org/SS/Immunization_Schedules.aspx**), when immunization status and other preventive health services can be addressed (Table 3.42). A booster dose at 16 years of age is recommended for adolescents immunized at 11 through 12 years of age.
- Adolescents 13 through 18 years of age should be immunized routinely with a meningococcal conjugate vaccine if not previously immunized. Adolescents who receive the first dose at 13 through 15 years of age should receive a 1-time booster dose at 16 through 18 years of age.

[1]Centers for Disease Control and Prevention. Infant meningococcal vaccination: Advisory Committee on Immunization Practices (ACIP) recommendations and rationale. *MMWR Morb Mortal Wkly Rep.* 2013;62(3):52–54

[2]Centers for Disease Control and Prevention. Prevention and control of meningococcal disease: recommendations of the Advisory Committee on Immunization Practices (ACIP). *MMWR Recomm Rep.* 2013;62(RR-02):1–28

[3]Centers for Disease Control and Prevention. Use of MenACWY-CRM vaccine in children aged 2 through 23 months at increased risk for meningococcal disease: recommendations of the Advisory Committee on Immunization Practices, 2013. *MMWR Morb Mortal Wkly Rep.* 2014;63(24):527–530

[4]American Academy of Pediatrics, Committee on Infectious Diseases. Updated recommendations on the use of meningococcal vaccines. *Pediatrics.* 2014;134(2):400–403

Table 3.43. Recommended Immunization Schedule and Intervals for Children at Risk of Invasive Meningococcal Disease[a]

Age	Subgroup	Primary Immunization	Booster Dose[b]
2 through 18 mo[c]	Children who: • have persistent complement deficiencies • have functional or anatomic asplenia • are at risk during a community outbreak attributable to a vaccine serogroup	4 doses of HibMenCY-TT (MenHibRix) at 2, 4, 6, and 12–15 months[e]	Person remains at increased risk and first dose received at age: • **2 mo through 6 y of age:** Should receive additional dose of MenACWY 3 y after primary immunization. Boosters should be repeated every 5 y thereafter. • **≥7 y of age:** Should receive additional dose of MenACWY 5 y after primary immunization. Boosters should be repeated every 5 y thereafter.
2 through 23 mo of age, with high-risk conditions	Children who: • have persistent complement deficiencies • have functional or anatomic asplenia • travel to or are residents of countries where meningococcal disease is hyperendemic or epidemic • are at risk during a community outbreak attributable to a vaccine serogroup	4 doses of MenACWY-CRM (Menveo) at 2, 4, 6, and 12 months	
9 through 23 mo of age, with high-risk conditions	Children who: • have persistent complement deficiencies • travel to or are residents of countries where meningococcal disease is hyperendemic or epidemic • are at risk during a community outbreak attributable to a vaccine serogroup	2 doses of MenACWY (Menactra), 12 weeks apart[d]	

continued

Table 3.43. Recommended Immunization Schedule and Intervals for Children at Risk of Invasive Meningococcal Disease,[a] continued

Age	Subgroup	Primary Immunization	Booster Dose[b]
2 through 55 y with high-risk conditions and not immunized previously[e,f]	People who: • have persistent complement deficiencies • have functional or anatomic asplenia • have HIV, if another indication for immunization exists	2 doses of MenACWY, 8–12 wk apart[e]	
	People who: • travel to or are residents of countries where meningococcal disease is hyperendemic or epidemic • are at risk during a community outbreak attributable to a vaccine serogroup	1 dose of MenACWY[e]	

[a] Includes children who have persistent complement deficiencies (eg, C5-C9, properdin, or factor H or factor D) and anatomic or functional asplenia; travelers to or residents of countries in which meningococcal disease is hyperendemic or epidemic; and children who are part of a community outbreak of a vaccine-preventable serogroup.

[b] If child remains at increased risk of meningococcal disease.

[c] Infants and children who received Hib-MenCY-TT and are traveling to areas with highly endemic rates of meningococcal disease, such as the African "meningitis belt," are not protected against serogroups A and W and should receive a quadrivalent meningococcal vaccine licensed for children ≥2 months of age prior to travel.

[d] Because of high risk of invasive pneumococcal disease, children with functional or anatomic asplenia should not be immunized with MenACWY-D (Menactra) before 2 years of age to avoid interference with the immune response to the pneumococcal conjugate vaccine (PCV) series.

[e] If MenACWY-D is used, administer at least 4 weeks after completion of all PCV doses.

[f] If an infant is receiving the vaccine prior to travel, 2 doses can be administered as early as 2 months apart.

- Adolescents who receive their first dose of meningococcal conjugate vaccine at or after 16 years of age do not need a booster dose unless they have risk factors (Table 3.43).
- People at increased risk of invasive meningococcal disease should be immunized with a meningococcal conjugate vaccine beginning at 2 months of age. People at increased risk include:
  - People 2 months and older, including adults, who have a persistent complement component deficiency (C5–C9, properdin, or factor H or factor D).
  - People 2 months or older, including adults, who have anatomic or functional asplenia (see Asplenia and Functional Asplenia, p 86). Because of high risk of invasive pneumococcal disease, children with functional or anatomic asplenia should not be immunized with MenACWY-D (Menactra) before 2 years of age to avoid interference with the immune response to the pneumococcal conjugate vaccine series, which also is conjugated to diphtheria toxoid; MenACWY-CRM (Menveo) can be used before 2 years of age, however, since it is not conjugated to diphtheria toxoid.
  - Children 2 months of age or older and adults who travel to or reside in countries in which meningococcal disease is hyperendemic or epidemic. Infants and children who receive HibMenCY-TT and are traveling to areas with highly endemic rates of meningococcal disease are not protected against serogroups A and W and should receive a quadrivalent meningococcal vaccination before travel.
  - Military recruits.
  - Booster doses. Children who remain at increased risk should receive a first booster dose 3 years after the primary series if they received their primary series before their 7th birthday, then every 5 years thereafter. If the primary series was given after the 7th birthday, then the first booster dose should be 5 years later and then every 5 years thereafter (CDC Travelers' Health Hotline, 877-FYI-TRIP or **www.cdc. gov/travel**).
  - The risk of meningococcal disease in HIV-infected individuals is not well defined. People with HIV infection who are 2 years or older should receive a 2-dose primary series at least 8 weeks apart.
- People may elect to receive a meningococcal conjugate vaccine if they are 2 months of age or older.
- For control of meningococcal outbreaks caused by vaccine-preventable serogroups (A, C, Y, or W), a meningococcal conjugate vaccine containing the outbreak serogroup should be used for people 2 months through 55 years of age. HibMenCY-TT can be used in infants 6 weeks through 18 months of age who are in communities with serogroup C and Y meningococcal disease outbreaks. For outbreaks of meningococcal disease caused by serogroup B, the rLP2086 serogroup B meningococcal vaccine from Pfizer was approved in October 2014 by the FDA, and Novartis has submitted a rolling biologics license application to the FDA for its serogroup B meningococcal vaccine.

Reimmunization. Children previously immunized with a meningococcal conjugate vaccine who are at ongoing increased risk for meningococcal disease should receive booster immunizations. Children who remain at increased risk should receive a first booster dose of MenACWY-D or Men-ACWY-CRM 3 years after the primary series if they received their primary series before their 7th birthday, then every 5 years thereafter. If the primary series was given after the 7th birthday, then the first booster dose should be 5 years later and then every 5 years thereafter. Infants at increased risk who are vaccinated with HibMenCY-TT do not need to be vaccinated with MenACWY-D or MenACWY-CRM until the first booster dose (3 years after completing of the HibMenCY-TT series), unless another indication is present (eg, travel to countries in which meningococcal disease is hyperendemic or epidemic).

Adverse Events. Common adverse events after MPSV4 and the quadrivalent meningococcal conjugate vaccines include pain, erythema, and swelling at the injection site, headache, fatigue, and irritability. Syncope can occur after vaccination and is most common among adolescents and young adults. Patients, particularly adolescents, should be observed while seated or lying down for 15 minutes after vaccination to decrease the risk for injury should they faint. Adolescents should be seated or lying down during vaccination, and having vaccine recipients *sit or lie down for at least 15 minutes* after immunization could avert many syncopal episodes and secondary injuries. If syncope develops, patients should be observed until symptoms resolve.[1] Syncope following receipt of a vaccine is not a contraindication to subsequent doses.

Precautions. Controlled studies of meningococcal vaccines have not been performed in pregnant women, but pregnancy should not preclude vaccination if the vaccine is indicated.

Public Health Reporting. All confirmed, presumptive, and probable cases of invasive meningococcal disease must be reported to the appropriate health department (see Table 3.39, p 549). Timely reporting can facilitate early recognition and containment of outbreaks and serogrouping of isolates so that appropriate prevention recommendations can be implemented rapidly.

Counseling and Public Education. When a case of invasive meningococcal disease is detected, the physician should provide accurate and timely information about meningococcal disease and the risk of transmission to families and contacts of the infected person, provide or arrange for prophylaxis, and contact the local public health department. Some experts recommend that patients with invasive meningococcal disease be evaluated for a terminal complement deficiency; screening can be accomplished with inexpensive CH50 and AH50 testing. If a deficiency is detected, patients should receive a meningococcal conjugate vaccine if 2 months of age or older, and patients and parents should be counseled about the risk of recurrent invasive meningococcal disease. Public health questions, such as whether a mass immunization program is needed, should be referred to the local health department. In appropriate situations, early provision of information in collaboration with the local health department to schools or other groups at increased risk and to the media may help minimize public anxiety and unrealistic or inappropriate demands for intervention.

Human Metapneumovirus

CLINICAL MANIFESTATIONS: Since its discovery in 2001, human metapneumovirus (hMPV) has been shown to cause acute respiratory tract illness in people of all ages. hMPV is one of the leading causes of bronchiolitis in infants and also causes pneumonia, asthma exacerbations, croup, and upper respiratory tract infections (URIs) with concomitant acute otitis media in children. hMPV also is associated with acute exacerbations of chronic obstructive pulmonary disease (COPD) and pneumonia in adults. Otherwise healthy young children infected with hMPV usually have mild or moderate symptoms, but some young children have severe disease requiring hospitalization. hMPV infection in

---

[1] Centers for Disease Control and Prevention. Syncope after vaccination—United States, January 2005–July 2007. *MMWR Morb Mortal Wkly Rep.* 2008;57(17):457–460

immunosuppressed people may result in severe disease, and fatalities have been reported in hematopoietic stem cell or lung transplant recipients. Preterm birth and underlying cardiopulmonary disease likely are risk factors, but the degree of risk associated with these conditions is not defined fully. Recurrent infection occurs throughout life and, in previously healthy people, usually is mild or asymptomatic.

ETIOLOGY: hMPV is an enveloped single-stranded negative-sense RNA virus of the family *Paramyxoviridae*. Four major genotypes of virus have been identified with 2 major antigenic subgroups (designated A and B). These different subgroups cocirculate each year, in varying proportions; whether the subgroups exhibit pathogenic differences remains to be determined.

EPIDEMIOLOGY: Humans are the only source of infection. Formal transmission studies have not been reported, but spread is likely to occur by direct or close contact with contaminated secretions. Health care-associated infections have been reported.

hMPV infections usually occur annually during winter and early spring in temperate climates, coinciding with or overlapping with the latter half of the respiratory syncytial virus (RSV) season. Sporadic infection may occur throughout the year. In otherwise healthy infants, the duration of viral shedding is 1 to 2 weeks. Prolonged shedding (weeks to months) has been reported in severely immunocompromised hosts.

Serologic studies suggest that most children are infected at least once by 5 years of age. The population incidence of hospitalizations attributable to hMPV generally is thought to be lower than that attributable to RSV but comparable to that of influenza and parainfluenza 3 in children younger than 5 years. Large studies have shown that hMPV is detected in 6% to 7% of children with lower respiratory illnesses who are hospitalized or seen in the outpatient and emergency departments. Overall annual rates of hospitalization associated with hMPV infection are about 1 per 1000 children younger than 5 years, 2 per 1000 children 6 to 11 months of age, and 3 per 1000 infants younger than 6 months. Coinfection with RSV and other respiratory viruses can occur. The **incubation period** is estimated to be 3 to 5 days in most cases.

DIAGNOSTIC TESTS: hMPV can be difficult to isolate in cell culture. Reverse transcriptase-polymerase chain reaction (RT-PCR) assays are the diagnostic method of choice for hMPV. Several RT-PCR assays for hMPV are available commercially. Immunofluorescence assays using monoclonal antibodies for hMPV antigen also are available, with reported sensitivities varying from 65% to 90%. Testing of acute and convalescent serum specimens for titer rises is used in research settings to confirm initial infections.

TREATMENT: Treatment is supportive and includes hydration, careful clinical assessment of respiratory status, including measurement of oxygen saturation, use of supplemental oxygen, and if necessary, mechanical ventilation. Studies in vitro and in animal models have shown that ribavirin has activity against hMPV, but no controlled clinical data are available to assess whether it has any therapeutic benefit, and its use is not recommended.

Antimicrobial agents are not indicated in the treatment of infants hospitalized with uncomplicated hMPV bronchiolitis or pneumonia unless evidence exists for the presence of a concurrent bacterial infection.

ISOLATION OF THE HOSPITALIZED PATIENT: In addition to standard precautions, contact precautions are recommended for the duration of hMPV-associated illness. Prolonged shedding of virus in respiratory tract secretions may occur, particularly in immunocompromised people, and therefore, the duration of contact precautions should be extended in these situations.

CONTROL MEASURES: Appropriate respiratory hygiene and cough etiquette should be followed. Control of health care-associated hMPV infection depends on adherence to contact precautions. Exposure to hMPV-infected people, including other patients, staff, and family members, may not be recognized, because illness may be mild.

Preventive measures include limiting exposure to settings where contact with hMPV may occur (eg, child care centers) and emphasis on hand hygiene in all settings, including the home, especially when contacts of high-risk children have respiratory tract infections.

Microsporidia Infections
(Microsporidiosis)

CLINICAL MANIFESTATIONS: Patients with intestinal infection have watery, nonbloody diarrhea, generally without fever. Abdominal cramping can occur. Data suggest that asymptomatic infection is more common than previously thought. Symptomatic intestinal infection is most common in immunocompromised people, especially in organ transplant recipients and people who are infected with human immunodeficiency virus (HIV) with low CD4+ lymphocyte counts, in whom infection often results in chronic diarrhea. The clinical course can be complicated by malnutrition and progressive weight loss. Chronic infection in immunocompetent people is rare. Other clinical syndromes that can occur in HIV-infected and immunocompromised patients include keratoconjunctivitis, encephalitis, sinusitis, dermatitis, myositis, osteomyelitis, nephritis, hepatitis, cholangitis, peritonitis, prostatitis, urethritis, cystitis, disseminated disease, pulmonary disease, cardiac disease, and wasting syndrome.

ETIOLOGY: Microsporidia are obligate intracellular, spore-forming organisms classified as fungi. *Enterocytozoon bieneusi* and *Encephalitozoon intestinalis* are the most commonly reported pathogens in humans and are most often associated with chronic diarrhea in HIV-infected people. Multiple genera, including *Encephalitozoon, Enterocytozoon, Nosema, Pleistophora, Trachipleistophora, Anncaliia,* and *Vittaforma* and *Microsporidium,* have been implicated in human infection, as have unclassified species.

EPIDEMIOLOGY: Most microsporidian infections are transmitted by oral ingestion of spores. Microsporidium spores commonly are found in surface water, and human strains have been identified in municipal water supplies and ground water. Several studies indicate that waterborne transmission occurs. Person-to-person spread by the fecal-oral route also occurs. Spores also have been detected in other body fluids, but their role in transmission is unknown. Data suggest the possibility of zoonotic transmission.

The **incubation period** is unknown.

DIAGNOSTIC TESTS: Infection with gastrointestinal microsporidia species can be documented by identification of organisms in biopsy specimens from the small intestine. Microsporidia species spores also can be detected in formalin-fixed stool specimens or duodenal aspirates stained with a chromotrope-based stain (a modification of the trichrome stain) and examined by an experienced microscopist. Chemofluorescent agents like calcofluor, as well as Gram, acid-fast, periodic acid-Schiff, Warthin-Starry silver, and Giemsa stains, can also be used to detect organisms in tissue sections. Organisms often are not noticed, because they are small (1–4 μm), stain poorly, and evoke minimal inflammatory response. Use of stool concentration techniques does not seem to improve the ability to detect *E bieneusi* spores. Polymerase chain reaction assay also can be used for diagnosis. Identification for classification purposes and diagnostic confirmation of species requires transmission electron microscopy or molecular techniques.

TREATMENT: Restoration of immune function is critical for control of any microsporidian infection. For a limited number of patients, albendazole, fumagillin, metronidazole, atovaquone, and nitazoxanide have been reported to decrease diarrhea but without eradication of the organism. Albendazole is the drug of choice for infections caused by *E intestinalis* but is ineffective against *E bieneusi* and *Vittaforma corneae* infections, which may respond to fumagillin. However, fumagillin is associated with bone marrow toxicity, recurrence of diarrhea is common after therapy is discontinued, and the drug is not available in the United States. In patients infected with human immunodeficiency virus (HIV), antiretroviral therapy, which is associated with improvement in the CD4+ T-lymphocyte count, can modify the course of disease favorably and should be considered as a main part of the treatment plan. None of these therapies have been studied in children with microsporidia infection. Investigational topical fumagillin eye drops can be considered for keratoconjunctival infections caused by microsporidia. Oral therapy with albendazole also is recommended for keratoconjunctivitis, because systemic organisms may remain after local clearance.

ISOLATION OF THE HOSPITALIZED PATIENT: In addition to standard precautions, contact precautions are recommended for diapered and incontinent children for the duration of illness.

CONTROL MEASURES: None have been documented. In HIV-infected and other immunocompromised people, decreased exposure may result from attention to hand hygiene, drinking bottled or boiled water, and avoiding unpeeled fruits and vegetables.

Molluscum Contagiosum

CLINICAL MANIFESTATIONS: Molluscum contagiosum is a benign viral infection of the skin with no systemic manifestations. It usually is characterized by 1 to 20 discrete, 2- to 5-mm-diameter, flesh-colored to translucent, dome-shaped papules, some with central umbilication. Lesions commonly occur on the trunk, face, and extremities, but rarely are generalized. Molluscum contagiosum is a self-limited epidermal infection that usually resolves spontaneously in 6 to 12 months but may take as long as 4 years to disappear completely. An eczematous reaction encircles lesions in approximately 10% of patients. People with eczema, immunocompromising conditions, and human immunodeficiency virus infection tend to have more widespread and prolonged eruptions.

ETIOLOGY: The cause is a poxvirus, which is the sole member of the genus *Molluscipoxvirus.* DNA subtypes can be differentiated, but the specific subtype probably is insignificant in pathogenesis.

EPIDEMIOLOGY: Humans are the only known source of the virus, which is spread by direct contact, including sexual contact, or by fomites. Vertical transmission has been suggested in case reports of neonatal molluscum contagiosum infection. Lesions can be disseminated by autoinoculation. Infectivity generally is low, but occasional outbreaks have been reported, including outbreaks in child care centers. The period of communicability is unknown.

The **incubation period** seems to vary between 2 and 7 weeks but may be as long as 6 months.

DIAGNOSTIC TESTS: The diagnosis usually can be made clinically from the characteristic appearance of the lesions. Wright or Giemsa staining of cells expressed from the central core of a lesion reveals characteristic intracytoplasmic inclusions. Electron microscopic examination of these cells identifies typical poxvirus particles. If questions persist, nucleic acid testing via polymerase chain reaction is available at certain reference centers. Adolescents and young adults with genital molluscum contagiosum should have screening tests for other sexually transmitted infections.

TREATMENT: There is no consensus on management of molluscum contagiosum in children and adolescents. Genital lesions should be treated to prevent spread to sexual contacts. Treatment of nongenital lesions is mainly for cosmetic reasons. Lesions in healthy people typically are self-limited, and treatment may not be necessary. However, therapy may be warranted to: (1) alleviate discomfort, including itching; (2) reduce autoinoculation; (3) limit transmission of the virus to close contacts; (4) reduce cosmetic concerns; and (5) prevent secondary infection. Physical destruction of the lesions is the most rapid and effective means of curing molluscum contagiosum. Modalities available include curettage, cryotherapy with liquid nitrogen, electrodesiccation, and chemical agents designed to initiate a local inflammatory response (podophyllin, tretinoin, cantharidin, 25% to 50% trichloroacetic acid, liquefied phenol, silver nitrate, tincture of iodine, or potassium hydroxide). Most data available for any of these modalities are anecdotal. Randomized trials usually are limited because of small sample sizes. These options require a trained physician and can result in postprocedural pain, irritation, and scarring. Because physical destruction of the lesions is painful, appropriate local anesthesia may be required, particularly in young children. Systemic therapy with cimetidine has been tried because of its systemic immunomodulatory effects. However, available data have not supported a benefit. Data from larger randomized, vehicle-controlled, double-blind trials have failed to demonstrate efficacy of imiquimod cream, a local immune modulator, for molluscum contagiosum in children 2 to 12 years of age. Cidofovir is a cytosine nucleotide analogue with in vitro activity against molluscum contagiosum; successful intravenous treatment of immunocompromised adults with severe involvement has been reported. However, use of cidofovir should be reserved for extreme cases because of potential carcinogenicity and known toxicities (neutropenia and potentially permanent nephrotoxicity) associated with systemic administration of cidofovir. Successful treatment using topical cidofovir, in a combination vehicle, has been reported in both adult and pediatric cases, most of whom were immunocompromised. Solitary genital lesions in children usually are not acquired by sexual transmission and do not necessarily denote sexual abuse, as other modes of direct contact with the virus, including autoinoculation, may result in genital infection.

ISOLATION OF THE HOSPITALIZED PATIENT: Standard precautions are recommended.

CONTROL MEASURES: No control measures are known for isolated cases. For outbreaks, which are common in the tropics, restricting direct person-to-person contact and sharing of potentially contaminated fomites, such as towels and bedding, may decrease spread. Molluscum contagiosum should not prevent a child from attending child care or school or from swimming in public pools. No covering of lesions is necessary for child care, but when possible, lesions not covered by clothing should be covered by a watertight bandage when participating in contact sports/activities or swimming. The bandage should be changed daily or when soiled.

Moraxella catarrhalis Infections

CLINICAL MANIFESTATIONS: *Moraxella catarrhalis* commonly is implicated in acute otitis media (AOM), otitis media with effusion, and sinusitis. AOM caused by *M catarrhalis* is seen predominantly in younger infants and frequently recovered in mixed infections. Although it has been described as a pathogen in pneumonia and bacteremia in healthy children, it is more commonly reported in children with chronic lung disease or impaired host defenses, such as leukemia with neutropenia or congenital immunodeficiency. In immunocompetent patients, bacteremia usually is associated with a respiratory tract focus; in immunocompromised children, most often no focus of infection is identified. Other clinical manifestations include hypotension with or without a rash indistinguishable from that observed in meningococcemia, neonatal meningitis, and focal infections, such as preseptal cellulitis, osteomyelitis, or septic arthritis. Rare manifestations include endocarditis, shunt-associated ventriculitis, and mastoiditis.

ETIOLOGY: *M catarrhalis* is a gram-negative aerobic diplococcus. More than 95% of strains produce beta-lactamase that mediates resistance to penicillins.

EPIDEMIOLOGY: *M catarrhalis* is part of the normal flora of the upper respiratory tract of humans. Two thirds of children are colonized within the first year of life. The mode of transmission is presumed to be direct contact with contaminated respiratory tract secretions or droplet spread. Infection is most common in infants and young children, but also occurs in immunocompromised people at all ages. Duration of carriage by infected and colonized children and the period of communicability are unknown.

The incubation period is unknown.

DIAGNOSTIC TESTS: The organism can be isolated on blood or chocolate agar culture media after incubation in air or with increased carbon dioxide. On gram stain, *Moraxella* species are short and plump gram-negative rods, usually occurring in pairs or short chains. Culture of middle ear or sinus aspirates is indicated for patients with unusually severe infection, for patients with infection that fails to respond to treatment, and for immunocompromised children. *Moraxella catarrhalis* often is recovered as part of mixed infections. Polymerase chain reaction tests for *M catarrhalis* have been developed but currently are used for research purposes only.

TREATMENT: Most strains of *Moraxella* species produce beta-lactamase and are resistant to amoxicillin. When beta-lactamase–producing *M catarrhalis* is isolated from appropriately obtained specimens (middle ear fluid, sinus aspirates, or lower respiratory tract secretions), in vitro data indicate that cefotaxime and ceftriaxone are likely to be effective if parenteral antimicrobial therapy is needed. Pharmacokinetic/pharmacodynamic studies support the use of oral high dose amoxicillin-clavulanate, cefixime, azithromycin, cefdinir, cefpodoxime, trimethoprim-sulfamethoxazole, or a fluoroquinolone. Pharmacokinetic/pharmacodynamic studies suggest that cefuroxime axetil, high-dose amoxicillin, and cefaclor are likely to be ineffective.

ISOLATION OF THE HOSPITALIZED PATIENT: Standard precautions are recommended.

CONTROL MEASURES: None.

Mumps

CLINICAL MANIFESTATIONS: Mumps is a systemic disease characterized by swelling of one or more of the salivary glands, usually the parotid glands. Approximately one third of infections do not cause clinically apparent salivary gland swelling and may be asymptomatic (subclinical) or manifest primarily as respiratory tract infection. More than 50% of people with mumps have cerebrospinal fluid pleocytosis, but fewer than 10% have symptoms of viral meningitis. Orchitis is a commonly reported complication after puberty, although sterility rarely results. Rare complications include arthritis, thyroiditis, mastitis, glomerulonephritis, myocarditis, endocardial fibroelastosis, thrombocytopenia, cerebellar ataxia, transverse myelitis, encephalitis, pancreatitis, oophoritis, and permanent hearing impairment. In the absence of an immunization program, mumps typically occurs during childhood. Infection in adults is more likely to result in complications. An association between maternal mumps infection during the first trimester of pregnancy and spontaneous abortion or intrauterine fetal death has been reported in some studies but not in others. Although mumps virus can cross the placenta, no evidence exists that this results in congenital malformation.

ETIOLOGY: Mumps is an RNA virus in the *Paramyxoviridae* family. Other infectious causes of parotitis include Epstein-Barr virus, cytomegalovirus, parainfluenza virus types 1 and 3, influenza A virus, enteroviruses, lymphocytic choriomeningitis virus, human immunodeficiency virus (HIV), nontuberculous mycobacterium, gram-positive bacteria, and less often gram-negative bacteria.

EPIDEMIOLOGY: Mumps occurs worldwide, and humans are the only known natural hosts. The virus is spread by contact with infectious respiratory tract secretions and saliva. Mumps virus is the only known cause of epidemic parotitis. Historically, the peak incidence of mumps was between January and May and among children younger than 10 years. Mumps vaccine was licensed in the United States in 1967 and recommended for routine childhood immunization in 1977. After implementation of the 1-dose mumps vaccine recommendation, the incidence of mumps in the United States declined from an incidence of 50 to 251 per 100 000 in the prevaccine era to 2 per 100 000 in 1988. After implementation of the 2-dose measles-mumps-rubella (MMR) vaccine recommendation in 1989 for measles control, mumps further declined to extremely low levels, with an incidence of 0.1/100 000 by 1999. From 2000 to 2005, seasonality no longer was evident, and there were fewer than 300 reported cases per year (incidence of 0.1/100 000), representing a greater than 99% reduction in disease incidence since the prevaccine era. In early 2006, a large-scale mumps outbreak occurred in the Midwestern United States, with 6584 reported cases (incidence of 2.2/100 000). Most of the cases occurred among people 18 through 24 years of age, many of whom were college students who had received 2 doses of mumps vaccine. Another outbreak in 2009–2010 affected more than 3500 people, mainly students in grades 6 through 12 who were members of traditional observant religious communities in New York and New Jersey and who had received 2 doses of MMR vaccine. Two doses of the mumps vaccine are approximately 88% effective in preventing disease. In settings of high immunization coverage such as the United States, most mumps cases likely will occur in people who have received 2 doses. The period of maximum communicability begins several days before parotitis onset. The recommended isolation period is for 5 days after onset of parotid swelling. However, virus has been isolated from saliva from 7 days before through 8 days after onset of swelling.

The **incubation period** usually is 16 to 18 days, but cases may occur from 12 to 25 days after exposure.

DIAGNOSTIC TESTS: Despite the outbreaks in 2006 and 2009–2010, mumps remains an uncommon infection in the United States, and parotitis has other etiologies, including other infectious agents. People with parotitis without other apparent cause should undergo diagnostic testing to confirm mumps virus as the cause or to diagnose other etiologies (eg, influenza A virus, parainfluenza viruses 1 and 3, and bacterial causes). Mumps can be confirmed by isolation of mumps virus or by detection of mumps virus nucleic acid via reverse transcriptase-polymerase chain reaction (RT-PCR) assay in specimens from buccal swabs (Stenson duct exudates), throat washings, saliva, or spinal fluid; by detection of mumps-specific immunoglobulin (Ig) M antibody; or by a significant increase between acute and convalescent titers in serum mumps IgG antibody titer determined by standard quantitative or semi-quantitative serologic assay (most commonly, semi-quantitative enzyme immunoassay). With the availability of RT-PCR assays, culture rarely is performed any longer.

Confirming the diagnosis of mumps in highly immunized populations is challenging, because the IgM response may be absent or short lived; acute IgG titers already might be high, so no significant increase can be detected between acute and convalescent specimens; and mumps virus might be present in clinical specimens only during the first few days after illness onset. Emphasis should be placed on obtaining clinical specimens within 1 to 3 days after onset of parotitis. In immunized people, a negative IgM result does not rule out mumps.

TREATMENT: Supportive.

ISOLATION OF THE HOSPITALIZED PATIENT: In addition to standard precautions, droplet precautions are recommended until 5 days after onset of parotid swelling.

CONTROL MEASURES:

Evidence of Immunity to Mumps.[1] Evidence of immunity to mumps includes any of the following:

1. Documentation of age-appropriate vaccination with a live mumps virus-containing vaccine:
   * preschool-aged children: 1 dose;
   * school-aged children (grades K-12): 2 doses;
   * adults not at high risk: 1 dose;
2. Laboratory evidence of immunity;
3. Laboratory confirmation of disease;
4. Born before 1957.

School and Child Care. Children should be excluded for 5 days from onset of parotid gland swelling.

Exclusion. When determining means to control outbreaks, exclusion of unimmunized students without evidence of immunity from affected schools and schools judged by local public health authorities to be at risk of transmission should be considered. Excluded students can be readmitted immediately after immunization. Students who continue to be

---

[1]Centers for Disease Control and Prevention. Prevention of measles, rubella, congenital rubella syndrome, and mumps, 2013 summary: recommendations of the Advisory Committee on Immunization Practices (ACIP). *MMWR Recomm Rep.* 2013;62(RR-04):1–34

unimmunized should be excluded until at least 26 days after onset of parotitis in the last person with mumps in the affected school.

Care of Exposed People. Mumps vaccine has not been demonstrated to be effective in preventing infection after exposure. However, MMR vaccine (or measles-mumps-rubella-varicella vaccine [MMRV], if thought to be susceptive to varicella and 12 months through 12 years of age) still should be given after exposure, because immunization will provide protection against subsequent exposures. Immunization during the incubation period presents no increased risk of adverse events.

During an outbreak, the first dose of MMR vaccine (or MMRV, if age appropriate) should be offered to all unimmunized people 12 months and older, and a second dose of MMR vaccine (or MMRV, if age appropriate) should be offered to all students (including those in postsecondary school) and to all health care personnel born in or after 1957 who have only received 1 dose of MMR vaccine. A second dose also may be considered for preschool-aged children and other adults depending on outbreak epidemiology. Health care personnel born before 1957 without a history of 2 doses of MMR immunization should obtain a mumps antibody titer to document their immune status and, if negative, should receive 2 appropriately spaced doses of MMR vaccine.

The Centers for Disease Control and Prevention has issued guidance for consideration for the use of a third dose in specifically identified target populations along with criteria for public health departments to consider for decision making (**www.cdc.gov/vaccines/pubs/surv-manual/chpt09-mumps.html**).

Immune Globulin (IG) preparations are not effective as postexposure prophylaxis for mumps.

Mumps Vaccine. Live-attenuated mumps vaccine containing the Jeryl-Lynn strain has been licensed in the United States since 1967. Vaccine is administered by subcutaneous injection of 0.5 mL of MMR vaccine (licensed for people 12 months or older) or MMRV vaccine (licensed for children 12 months through 12 years of age). Monovalent mumps vaccine no longer is available in the United States. Postlicensure data indicate that the effectiveness of 1 dose of mumps vaccine has been approximately 78% (range, 49%–92%), and 2-dose vaccine effectiveness is 88% (range, 66%–95%). Some studies and investigations conducted during the recent mumps outbreaks indicate that vaccine-induced immunity might wane, possibly explaining the recent occurrence of mumps in the 15- through 24-year age group.

Vaccine Recommendations.

- The first dose of MMR or MMRV vaccine (see MMRV vaccine recommendations in Varicella-Zoster Infections, p 846) should be given routinely to children at 12 through 15 months of age, with a second dose of MMR or MMRV vaccine administered at 4 through 6 years of age. The second dose of MMR or MMRV vaccine may be administered before 4 years of age, provided at least 28 days have elapsed since the first dose. Administration of MMR or MMRV vaccine is not harmful if given to a person already immune to one or more of the viruses from previous infection or immunization.
- People should be immunized unless they have evidence of mumps immunity (p 567). Adequate immunization is 2 doses of mumps-containing vaccine (≥28 days apart) for school-aged children and adults at high risk (ie, health care personnel, students at post-high school educational institutions, and international travelers). A single dose of mumps-containing vaccine is considered adequate for other adults born in or after

1957. Health care personnel born before 1957 should consider receiving 1 dose of MMR vaccine unless they have laboratory evidence of immunity or disease.

- Because mumps is endemic throughout most of the world, unless they have evidence of immunity, people 12 months or older should be offered 2 doses of MMR vaccine according to vaccine policy before beginning travel. Children younger than 12 months need not be given mumps vaccine before travel, but they may receive it as MMR vaccine if measles immunization is indicated.
- If a child receives a dose of mumps vaccine before 12 months of age, this dose is not counted toward the required number of doses, and 2 additional doses are required beginning at 12 through 15 months of age and separated by at least 28 days.
- A mumps-containing vaccine may be given with other vaccines at different injection sites and with separate syringes (see Simultaneous Administration of Multiple Vaccines, p 35).

Adverse Reactions. Adverse reactions associated with the mumps component of US-licensed MMR or MMRV vaccines are rare. Orchitis, parotitis, and low-grade fever have been reported rarely after immunization. Temporally related reactions, including febrile seizures, nerve deafness, aseptic meningitis, encephalitis, rash, pruritus, and purpura, may follow immunization rarely; however, causality has not been established. Allergic reactions also are rare (see Measles, Precautions and Contraindications [p 544], and Rubella, Precautions and Contraindications [p 694]). Other reactions that occur after immunization with MMR or MMRV vaccine may be attributable to other components of the vaccines (see Measles, p 535, Adverse Events, p 543, Rubella, p 688, and Varicella-Zoster Infections, p 846).

A second dose of MMR vaccine is not associated with an increased incidence of reactions. Postlicensure data on MMRV vaccine are limited.

Precautions and Contraindications. See Measles, p 535, Rubella, p 688, and Varicella-Zoster Infections, p 846, if MMRV is used.

Febrile Illness. Children with minor illnesses with or without fever, such as upper respiratory tract infections, may be immunized (see Vaccine Contraindications and Precautions, p 52). Fever is not a contraindication to immunization. However, if other manifestations suggest a more serious illness, the child should not be immunized until recovered.

Allergies. Hypersensitivity reactions occur rarely and usually are minor, consisting of wheal-and-flare reactions or urticaria at the injection site. Reactions have been attributed to trace amounts of neomycin or gelatin or some other component in the vaccine formulation. Anaphylaxis is rare; MMR and MMRV vaccines are produced in chicken embryo cell culture and do not contain significant amounts of egg white (ovalbumin) cross-reacting proteins. Children with egg allergy are at low risk of anaphylactic reactions to MMR or MMRV vaccine. Skin testing of children for egg allergy is not predictive of reactions to MMR or MMRV vaccine and is not required before administering MMR vaccine. People with allergies to chickens or feathers are not at increased risk of reaction to the vaccine. People who have experienced anaphylactic reactions to gelatin or topically or systemically administered neomycin should receive mumps vaccine only in settings where such reactions could be managed and after consultation with an allergist or immunologist. Most often, however, neomycin allergy manifests as contact dermatitis, which is not a contraindication to receiving mumps vaccine (see Measles, p 535).

Recent Administration of IG. Although the effect of IG administration on the immune response to mumps vaccine is unknown, MMR vaccine should be given at least 2 weeks before planned administration of IG, blood transfusion, or other blood products because of the theoretical possibility that antibody will neutralize vaccine virus and interfere with successful immunization. Administration of MMR or MMRV vaccine should be delayed from 3 to 11 months following receipt of specific blood products or IG (see Table 1.10, p 39).

Altered Immunity. Patients with immunodeficiency diseases and people receiving immunosuppressive therapy or expected to receive such therapy within 4 weeks (eg, patients with leukemia, lymphoma, or generalized malignant disease), including high doses of systemically administered corticosteroids, alkylating agents, antimetabolites, or radiation, or people who otherwise are immunocompromised should not receive live-attenuated vaccines including MMR or MMRV (see Immunization in Immunocompromised Children, p 74). Exceptions are patients with HIV infection who are not severely immuncompromised (age-specific CD4+ T-lymphocyte percentages of 15% or greater), who can receive MMR but not MMRV vaccine (see Human Immunodeficiency Virus Infection, p 453). The risk of mumps exposure for patients with altered immunity can be decreased by immunizing their close susceptible (ie, household) contacts. Immunized people do not transmit mumps vaccine virus.

After cessation of immunosuppressive therapy, MMR immunization should be deferred for at least 3 months (with the exception of corticosteroid recipients [see next paragraph]). This interval is based on the assumptions that immunologic responsiveness will have been restored in 3 months and the underlying disease for which immunosuppressive therapy was given is in remission or under control. However, because the interval can vary with the intensity and type of immunosuppressive therapy, radiation therapy, underlying disease, and other factors, a definitive recommendation for an interval after cessation of immunosuppressive therapy when mumps vaccine (as MMR) can be administered safely and effectively often is not possible.

Corticosteroids. For patients who have received high doses of corticosteroids (2 mg/kg/day or greater or greater than 20 mg/day of prednisone or equivalent) for 14 days or more and who otherwise are not immunocompromised, the recommended interval is at least 1 month after corticosteroids are discontinued (see Immunization in Immunocompromised Children, p 74).

Pregnancy. Conception should be avoided for 28 days after mumps immunization because of the theoretical risk associated with live-virus vaccine. Susceptible postpubertal females should not be immunized if they are known to be pregnant. However, mumps immunization during pregnancy has not been associated with congenital malformations (see Measles, p 535, and Rubella, p 688).

Mycoplasma pneumoniae and Other *Mycoplasma* Species Infections

CLINICAL MANIFESTATIONS: *Mycoplasma pneumoniae* is a frequent cause of upper and lower respiratory tract infections in children, including pharyngitis, acute bronchitis, and pneumonia. Acute otitis media is uncommon. Bullous myringitis, once considered pathognomonic for mycoplasma, now is known to occur with other pathogens as well. Coryza, sinusitis, and croup are rare. Symptoms are variable and include cough, malaise, fever, and occasionally headache. Acute bronchitis and upper respiratory tract illness caused by *M pneumoniae* generally are mild and self-limited. Approximately 10% of infected school-aged children will develop pneumonia with cough and widespread rales on physical examination within days after onset of constitutional symptoms. Cough often initially is nonproductive but later can become productive. Cough can persist for 3 to 4 weeks and can be accompanied by wheezing. Approximately 10% of children with *M pneumoniae* infection will exhibit a rash, which most often is maculopapular. Radiographic abnormalities are variable. Bilateral diffuse infiltrates or focal abnormalities, such as consolidation, effusion, or hilar adenopathy, can occur.

Unusual manifestations include nervous system disease (eg, aseptic meningitis, encephalitis, acute disseminated encephalomyelitis, cerebellar ataxia, transverse myelitis, peripheral neuropathy) as well as myocarditis, pericarditis, arthritis, erythema nodosum, polymorphous mucocutaneous eruptions (including classic and atypical Stevens-Johnson syndrome), hemolytic anemia, thrombocytopenic purpura, and hemophagocytic syndromes. In patients with sickle cell disease, Down syndrome, immunodeficiencies, and chronic cardiorespiratory disease, severe pneumonia with pleural effusion may develop. Acute chest syndrome and pneumonia have been associated with *M pneumoniae* in patients with sickle cell disease. Infection also has been associated with exacerbations of asthma.

Several other *Mycoplasma* species colonize mucosal surfaces of humans and can produce disease in children. *Mycoplasma hominis* infection has been reported in neonates (especially at scalp electrode monitor site) and children (both immunocompetent and immunocompromised). Intra-abdominal abscesses, septic arthritis, endocarditis, pneumonia, meningoencephalitis, brain abscess, and surgical wound infections all have been reported.

ETIOLOGY: Mycoplasmas, including *M pneumoniae*, are pleomorphic bacteria that lack a cell wall. Mycoplasmas cannot be detected using light microscopy.

EPIDEMIOLOGY: Mycoplasmas are ubiquitous in animals and plants, but *M pneumoniae* causes disease only in humans. *M pneumoniae* is transmissible by respiratory droplets during close contact with a symptomatic person. Outbreaks have been described in hospitals, military bases, colleges, and summer camps. Occasionally, *M pneumoniae* causes ventilator-associated pneumonia. *M pneumoniae* is a leading cause of pneumonia in school-aged children and young adults but is an infrequent cause of community-acquired pneumonia in preschool-aged children younger than 5 years. In the United States, an estimated 2 million infections are caused by *M pneumoniae* each year; approximately 20% of hospitalized community-acquired pneumonia is suggested to be caused by *M pneumoniae*. Infections occur throughout the world, in any season, and in all geographic settings. In family studies, approximately 30% of household contacts develop pneumonia. Asymptomatic carriage after infection may occur for weeks to months. Immunity after infection is not long lasting.

The **incubation period** usually is 2 to 3 weeks (range, 1–4 weeks).

DIAGNOSTIC TESTS: When Gram stain of colonies is performed, no bacteria are noted. *M pneumoniae* can be grown in special enriched broth followed by passage to SP4 agar media or on commercially-available mixed liquid broth/agar slant media, but most clinical facilities lack the capacity to perform this culture. Isolation takes up to 21 days.

Serologic tests using immunofluorescence and enzyme immunoassays that detect *M pneumoniae*-specific immunoglobulin (Ig) M and IgG antibodies are available commercially. IgM antibodies generally are not detectable within the first 7 days after onset of symptoms. Although the presence of IgM antibodies may indicate recent *M pneumoniae* infection, false-positive test results occur, and antibodies persist in serum for several months and may not indicate current infection. IgM antibodies may not be elevated in older children and adults who have had recurrent *M pneumoniae* infection. Serologic diagnosis is best made by demonstrating a fourfold or greater increase in antibody titer between acute and convalescent serum specimens. Complement-fixation assay results should be interpreted cautiously, because the assay is both less sensitive and less specific than is immunofluorescent assay or enzyme immunoassay. IgM antibody titer peaks at approximately 3 to 6 weeks and persists for 2 to 3 months after infection. Measurement of serum cold hemagglutinin titer has limited value, because titers of ≥1:64 are present in only 50% of patients with pneumonia caused by *M pneumoniae*, and lower titers are nonspecifically present during respiratory viral infections.

Polymerase chain reaction (PCR) tests for *M pneumoniae* are available commercially and increasingly are replacing other tests, because PCR tests performed on respiratory tract specimens (nasal wash, nasopharyngeal swab, pharyngeal swab) have sensitivity and specificity between 80% and 100%, yield positive results earlier in the course of illness than serologic tests, and are rapid. Identification of *M pneumoniae* by PCR or culture in a patient with compatible clinical manifestations suggests causation; attributing a nonclassic clinical disorder to *Mycoplasma* is problematic, however, because *M pneumoniae* can colonize the respiratory tract for several weeks after acute infection, even after appropriate antimicrobial therapy. A recent study detected *M pneumoniae* DNA by PCR in 21.2% (95% CI: 17.2%–25.2%) of asymptomatic children 3 months to 16 years of age. Performance characteristics of individual institutions' PCR tests (which are not cleared by the US Food and Drug Administration), using different primer sequences and targeting different genes, are not generalizable.

The diagnosis of mycoplasma-associated central nervous system disease is challenging, both because disease may not be the result of direct invasion and because there is no reliable single test for cerebrospinal fluid to establish a diagnosis.

PCR assay of body fluids for *Mycoplasma hominis* is available at reference laboratories and may be helpful diagnostically.

TREATMENT: *Mycoplasma* infection is an infrequent cause of community-acquired pneumonia (CAP) in preschool-aged children. Evidence of benefit of antimicrobial therapy for nonhospitalized children with lower respiratory tract disease attributable to *M pneumoniae* is limited. Some data suggest benefit of appropriate antimicrobial therapy in hospitalized children. Antimicrobial therapy is not recommended for preschool-aged children with CAP, because viral pathogens are responsible for the great majority of cases. There is no evidence that treatment of other possible manifestations of *M pneumoniae* infection (eg, upper respiratory tract infection, extrapulmonary infection) with antimicrobial agents alters the course of illness. Because *Mycoplasma* organisms lack a cell wall, they inherently are resistant to beta-lactam agents. Macrolides, including azithromycin, clarithromycin, and erythromycin, are the preferred antimicrobial agents for treatment of pneumonia in school-aged children who have moderate to severe infection and those with underlying conditions, such as sickle cell disease. Fluoroquinolones and doxycycline also are effective (see Tetracyclines, p 873). Macrolide-resistant strains are increasingly common.

M hominis usually is resistant to erythromycin and azithromycin but generally is susceptible to clindamycin, tetracyclines, and fluoroquinolones.

ISOLATION OF THE HOSPITALIZED PATIENT: In addition to standard precautions, droplet precautions are recommended for the duration of symptomatic illness.

CONTROL MEASURES: Hand hygiene decreases household transmission of respiratory pathogens and should be encouraged.

Tetracycline or azithromycin prophylaxis for close contacts has been shown to limit transmission in family and institutional outbreaks. However, antimicrobial prophylaxis for asymptomatic exposed contacts is not recommended routinely, because most secondary illnesses will be mild and self-limited. Prophylaxis with a macrolide or tetracycline can be considered for people at increased risk of severe illness with *M pneumoniae*, such as children with sickle cell disease who are close contacts of a person who is acutely ill with *M pneumoniae* infection.

Nocardiosis

CLINICAL MANIFESTATIONS: Immunocompetent children typically develop cutaneous or lymphocutaneous disease with pustular or ulcerative lesions that remain localized after soil contamination of a skin injury. Invasive disease occurs most commonly in people with chronic granulomatous disease, organ transplantation, human immunodeficiency virus infection, or disease requiring long-term systemic corticosteroid therapy. Infection has occurred in adults receiving tumor necrosis factor inhibitors, especially infliximab. In immunocompromised children, infection characteristically begins in the lungs, and illness can be acute, subacute, or chronic. Pulmonary disease commonly manifests as rounded nodular infiltrates that can undergo cavitation. Hematogenous spread may occur from the lungs to the brain (single or multiple abscesses), in skin (pustules, pyoderma, abscesses, mycetoma), or occasionally in other organs. Some experts recommend neuroimaging in patients with pulmonary disease attributable to the frequency of concurrent central nervous system (CNS) disease, which initially can be asymptomatic. *Nocardia* organisms can be recovered from patients with cystic fibrosis, but their role as a lung pathogen in these patients is not clear.

ETIOLOGY: *Nocardia* are gram-positive, filamentous bacteria that belong to a group informally known as the aerobic actinomycetes. Other members of this group include: *Actinomadura madurae*, one of several species that are the causative agent of actinomycetoma; *Rhodococcus equi*; and *Gordonia bronchialis*. In the United States, nocardiosis most commonly presents as pulmonary or disseminated disease in immunocompromised individuals, or as primary cutaneous infection in immunocompetent individuals. The most prevalent species isolated from human clinical sources in the United States are from the *Nocardia asteroides* complex (*Nocardia nova, Nocardia farcinica, Nocardia cyriacigeorgica,* and *Nocardia abscessus*). Primary cutaneous infection most often is associated with *Nocardia brasiliensis,* and skin infection with this organism can be indistinguishable from sporotrichosis. To date, 46 of the 88 valid species of *Nocardia* have been isolated from clinical sources. Other less common pathogenic species include*: Nocardia brevicatena, Nocardia otitidiscaviarum, Nocardia pseudobrasiliensis, Nocardia transvalensis* complex, and *Nocardia veterana.*

EPIDEMIOLOGY: *Nocardia* species are ubiquitous environmental saprophytes, living in soil, organic matter, and water. Infections caused by *Nocardia* species typically are the result of environmental exposure through inhalation of soil or dust particles or through traumatic inoculation with a soil-contaminated object. Person-to-person and animal-to-human transmission is not known to occur.

The **incubation period** is unknown.

DIAGNOSTIC TESTS: Isolation of *Nocardia* species from primary clinical specimens can require extended incubation periods because of their slow growth. Specimens from sterile sites can be inoculated directly onto solid media such as buffered charcoal yeast extract (BCYE) agar with an incubation time of up to 2 weeks. Specimens from contaminated sites, such as tissue or sputum, should be inoculated onto selective media such as Thayer

Martin or BCYE with vancomycin with incubation of at least 3 weeks. Recovery of *Nocardia* species from tissue can be improved if the laboratory is requested to observe cultures for 3 to 4 weeks in an appropriate liquid medium at optimal growth temperature (between 25°C and 35°C for most species). Stained smears of sputum, body fluids, or pus demonstrating beaded, branching rods that stain weakly gram positive and partially acid fast by the modified Kinyoun method suggest the diagnosis. Because of the difficulty in interpretation of the acid-fast stain, utilization of positive and negative controls is suggested. Brown-Brenn tissue Gram-stain method and Grocott-Gomori methenamine silver stains are recommended to demonstrate microorganisms in tissue specimens. Serologic tests for *Nocardia* species are not useful.

Accurate identification of *Nocardia* isolates paired with antimicrobial susceptibility testing greatly increases the chances of positive patient care outcome. Because of the unstable nature of phenotypic traits in the aerobic actinomycetes and difficulty growing the organisms on commercial biochemical testing media, accurate identification is accomplished through molecular methods. For *Nocardia* species, 16S rRNA gene sequence analysis of a nearly full length (~1440 bp) sequence will allow for resolution of the isolate to the species level. *Nocardia* species are well documented to be resistant to multiple drugs. A few of the most common pathogenic *Nocardia* species have unique susceptibility patterns. Invasive infections with resistant strains can result in delayed or failed treatment and increased risk of disseminated infection or subsequent relapse. Rapid and accurate identification of *Nocardia* isolates along with antimicrobial susceptibility testing are essential tools for successful treatment of nocardiosis.

TREATMENT: Trimethoprim-sulfamethoxazole or a sulfonamide alone (eg, sulfisoxazole or sulfamethoxazole) has been the drug of choice for mild infections. Sulfonamides that are less urine soluble, such as sulfadiazine, should be avoided. A high mortality rate with sulfonamide monotherapy in immunocompromised patients and patients with severe disease, disseminated disease, or central nervous system involvement has led to use of combination therapy for the first 4 to 12 weeks based on results of antimicrobial susceptibility testing and clinical improvement. Suggested combinations include trimethoprim-sulfamethoxazole plus amikacin, meropenem or imipenem, or ceftriaxone. Immunocompetent patients with primary lymphocutaneous disease usually respond after 6 to 12 weeks of therapy. Drainage of abscesses is beneficial. Immunocompromised patients and patients with serious disease should be treated for 6 to 12 months and for at least 3 months after apparent cure because of the propensity for relapse. Patients with acquired immunodeficiency syndrome may need even longer therapy, and suppressive therapy should be considered for life. Patients with meningitis or brain abscess should be monitored with serial neuroimaging studies.

If infection does not respond to trimethoprim-sulfamethoxazole, other agents such as clarithromycin *(N nova)*, amoxicillin-clavulanate *(N brasiliensis* and *N abscessus)*, imipenem, or meropenem may be beneficial. Linezolid is highly active against all *Nocardia* species in vitro; case series including a small number of patients demonstrated that linezolid may be effective for treatment of some invasive infections. Drug susceptibility testing should guide therapy and is recommended by the Clinical and Laboratory Standards Institute for isolates from patients with invasive disease and patients who are unable to tolerate a sulfonamide as well as patients in whom sulfonamide therapy fails.

ISOLATION OF THE HOSPITALIZED PATIENT: Standard precautions are recommended.

CONTROL MEASURES: None.

Norovirus and Other Human Calicivirus Infections

CLINICAL MANIFESTATIONS: Abrupt onset of vomiting accompanied by watery diarrhea, abdominal cramps, and nausea are characteristic of norovirus gastroenteritis. Acute diarrhea without vomiting may also occur, most notably in children. Symptoms last from 24 to 60 hours. However, more prolonged courses of illness can occur, particularly among elderly people, young children, and hospitalized patients. Systemic manifestations, including fever, myalgia, malaise, anorexia, and headache, may accompany gastrointestinal tract symptoms. Since introduction of rotavirus vaccines, noroviruses have become the leading cause of gastroenteritis in the United States.

ETIOLOGY: Noroviruses are 27- to 40-nm, nonenveloped, single-stranded RNA viruses of the family *Caliciviridae.* This family is divided into at least 5 genera (*Lagovirus, Nebovirus, Vesivirus, Sapovirus,* and *Norovirus*), with noroviruses and sapoviruses often referred to as human caliciviruses (HuCVs). Noroviruses are genetically diverse and currently are divided into 6 genogroups (I–VI), of which 3 (I, II, and IV) can cause human illness. Based on the analysis of the major viral capsid protein VP1, noroviruses can be further classified into more than 25 different genotypes.

EPIDEMIOLOGY: Noroviruses are a major cause of both sporadic cases and outbreaks of gastroenteritis. Norovirus causes an estimated 1 in 15 US residents to become ill each year as well as 56 000 to 71 000 hospitalizations and 570 to 800 deaths, predominantly among young children and the elderly.[1] As a result at the success of the rotavirus vaccine, noroviruses have become the predominant agent of pediatric viral gastroenteritis in the United States.[2] The norovirus genogroup II, genotype 4 (GII.4) has been predominant worldwide during the past decade. Sapovirus infections are reported mainly among children with sporadic acute diarrhea, although they increasingly have been recognized as a cause of outbreaks. Asymptomatic norovirus excretion is common across all age groups, with the highest prevalence in children. Outbreaks with high attack rates tend to occur in closed populations, such as long-term care facilities, schools, and cruise ships. Transmission is by person-to-person spread via the fecal-oral or vomitus-oral routes, through contaminated food or water, or by touching surfaces contaminated with norovirus and then touching mucous membranes. Norovirus is recognized as the most common cause of foodborne illness and foodborne disease outbreaks in the United States.[3] Common-source outbreaks have been described after ingestion of ice, shellfish, and a variety of ready-to-eat foods, including salads, berries, and bakery products, usually contaminated by infected food handlers. Transmission via vomitus has been documented, and exposure to contaminated surfaces and aerosolized vomitus has been implicated in some outbreaks. Norovirus has been detected in raw or unpasteurized milk or milk products.[4] Viral excretion may start

[1]Centers for Disease Control and Prevention. Vital Signs: foodborne norovirus outbreaks—United States, 2009–2012. *MMWR Morb Mortal Wkly Rep.* 2014;63(22):491–495

[2]Payne DC, Vinje J, Szilagyi PG, et al. Norovirus and medically attended gastroenteritis in U.S. children. *N Engl J Med.* 201321;368(12):1121–1130

[3]Centers for Disease Control and Prevention. Surveillance for foodborne disease outbreaks—United States, 2009–2010. *MMWR Morb Mortal Wkly Rep.* 2013;62(3):41–47

[4]American Academy of Pediatrics, Committee on Infectious Diseases and Committee on Nutrition. Consumption of raw or unpasteurized milk and milk products by pregnant women and children. *Pediatrics.* 2014;133(1):175–179

before onset of symptoms, peaks several days after exposure, and may persist for 3 weeks or more. Prolonged excretion has been reported in immunocompromised hosts. Infection occurs year round but is more common during the colder months of the year.

The **incubation period** is 12 to 48 hours.

DIAGNOSTIC TESTS: A multiplex nucleic acid-based assay for the detection of gastrointestinal pathogens, which includes norovirus, is cleared by the US Food and Drug Administration (FDA), although it may not be widely available in diagnostic laboratories. An enzyme immunoassay (EIA) kit has also been cleared by the FDA for preliminary identification of norovirus as the cause of gastroenteritis outbreaks.

Most state and local public health laboratories use real-time reverse transcriptase-polymerase chain reaction (RT-PCR) for detection of viral RNA in stool. Laboratory and epidemiologic support for investigation of suspected viral gastroenteritis outbreaks is available at the Centers for Disease Control and Prevention (CDC) by request.

TREATMENT: Supportive therapy includes oral or intravenous rehydration solutions to replace and maintain fluid and electrolyte balance.

ISOLATION OF THE HOSPITALIZED PATIENT: In addition to standard precautions, contact precautions are recommended for suspected cases of acute gastroenteritis attributable to norovirus infection until 48 hours after symptom resolution.

CONTROL MEASURES: Appropriate hand hygiene is likely the single most important method to prevent norovirus infection and control transmission. Reducing any norovirus present on hands is best accomplished by thorough handwashing with running water and plain or antiseptic soap. Washing hands with soap and water after contact with a patient with norovirus infection is more effective than use of alcohol gels for reducing transmission. Several factors favor transmission of noroviruses including low infectious dose, large numbers of virus particles can be excreted, and shedding can last for several weeks after symptoms have subsided. The spread of infection can be decreased by standard measures for control of diarrhea, such as educating child care providers and food handlers about infection control, maintaining cleanliness of surfaces and food preparation areas, using appropriate disinfectants (principally sodium hypochlorite [chlorine bleach]), excluding caregivers or food handlers who are ill and for a period after recovery (eg, 24–72 hours), exercising appropriate hand hygiene, as discussed previously, and excluding infected children from group child care (see Children in Out-of-Home Child Care, p 132). If a source of transmission can be identified (eg, contaminated food or water) during an outbreak, then specific interventions to interrupt transmission can be effective. Candidate norovirus virus-like-particle vaccines are in an early stage of development. Sporadic cases are not nationally notifiable, but outbreaks should be reported to local and state public health authorities as required and to the CDC via the National Outbreak Reporting System and virus typing data to CaliciNet. Updated guidance on norovirus is available on the CDC Web site (**www.cdc. gov/mmwr/pdf/rr/rr6003.pdf**).[1] A toolkit designed to help health care professionals control and prevent norovirus gastroenteritis in health care settings is available (**www.cdc. gov/hai/pdfs/norovirus/229110-ANorovirusIntroLetter508.pdf**).

---

[1]Centers for Disease Control and Prevention. Updated norovirus outbreak management and disease prevention guidelines. *MMWR Recomm Rep.* 2011;60(3):1–15

Onchocerciasis
(River Blindness, Filariasis)

CLINICAL MANIFESTATIONS: The disease involves skin, subcutaneous tissues, lymphatic vessels, and eyes. Subcutaneous, nontender nodules that can be up to several centimeters in diameter containing male and female worms develop 6 to 12 months after initial infection. In patients in Africa, nodules tend to be found on the lower torso, pelvis, and lower extremities, whereas in patients in Central and South America, the nodules more often are located on the upper body (the head and trunk) but may occur on the extremities. After the worms mature, fertilized females produce microfilariae that migrate to the dermis and may cause a papular dermatitis. Pruritus often is highly intense, resulting in patient-inflicted excoriations over the affected areas. After a period of years, skin can become lichenified and hypo- or hyperpigmented. Microfilariae may invade ocular structures, leading to inflammation of the cornea, iris, ciliary body, retina, choroid, and optic nerve. Loss of visual acuity and blindness can result if the disease is untreated.

ETIOLOGY: *Onchocerca volvulus* is a filarial nematode.

EPIDEMIOLOGY: *O volvulus* has no significant animal reservoir. Microfilariae in human skin infect *Simulium* species flies (black flies) when they take a blood meal and then in 10 to 14 days develop into infectious larvae that are transmitted with subsequent bites. Black flies breed in fast-flowing streams and rivers (hence, the colloquial name for the disease, "river blindness"). The disease occurs primarily in equatorial Africa, but small foci are found in southern Mexico, Guatemala, northern South America, and Yemen. Prevalence is greatest among people who live near vector breeding sites. The infection is not transmissible by person-to-person contact or blood transfusion.

The **incubation period** from larval inoculation to microfilariae in the skin usually is 12 to 18 months but can be as long as 3 years.

DIAGNOSTIC TESTS: Direct examination of a 1- to 2-mg shaving or biopsy specimen of the epidermis and upper dermis (usually taken from the posterior iliac crest area) can reveal microfilariae. Microfilariae are not found in blood. Adult worms may be demonstrated in excised nodules that have been sectioned and stained. A slit-lamp examination of an involved eye may reveal motile microfilariae in the anterior chamber or "snowflake" corneal lesions. Eosinophilia is common. Specific serologic tests and polymerase chain reaction techniques for detection of microfilariae in skin are available only in research laboratories, including those of the National Institutes of Health.

TREATMENT: Ivermectin, a microfilaricidal agent, is the drug of choice for treatment of onchocerciasis. Treatment decreases dermatitis and the risk of developing severe ocular disease but does not kill the adult worms (which can live for more than a decade) and, thus, is not curative. One single oral dose of ivermectin (150 µg/kg) should be given every 6 to 12 months until asymptomatic. Adverse reactions to treatment are caused by death of microfilariae and can include rash, edema, fever, myalgia, and rarely, asthma exacerbation and hypotension. Such reactions are more common in people with higher skin loads of microfilaria and decrease with repeated treatment in the absence of reexposure. Precautions to ivermectin treatment include pregnancy (class C drug), central nervous system disorders, and high levels of circulating *Loa loa* microfilaraemia (determined by examining a Giemsa-stained thick blood smear between 10 AM and 2 PM; see

Drugs for Parasitic Infections, p 927). Treatment of patients with high levels of circulating *L loa* microfilaraemia with ivermectin sometimes can result in fatal encephalopathy. The American Academy of Pediatrics notes that ivermectin usually is compatible with breastfeeding. Because low levels of drug are found in human milk after maternal treatment, some experts recommend delaying maternal treatment until the infant is 7 days of age, but risk versus benefit should be considered. Safety and effectiveness of ivermectin in pediatric patients weighing less than 15 kg have not been established.

A 6-week course of doxycycline (100–200 mg/day) can be used to kill adult worms through depletion of the endosymbiotic rickettsia-like bacteria, which appear to be required for survival of *O volvulus*. This approach may be used as adjunctive therapy for children 8 years or older and nonpregnant adults (see Antimicrobial Agents and Related Therapy, Tetracyclines, p 873) to obviate the need for years of ivermectin treatment. Doxycycline treatment should be initiated several days after treatment with ivermectin, because there are no studies of the safety of simultaneous treatment.

Diethylcarbamazine is contraindicated, because it may cause adverse ocular reactions. Nodules also be removed surgically.

ISOLATION OF THE HOSPITALIZED PATIENT: Standard precautions are recommended.

CONTROL MEASURES: Repellents and protective clothing (long sleeves and pants) can decrease exposure to bites from black flies, which bite by day. Treatment of vector breeding sites with larvicides was effective for controlling black fly populations, particularly in West Africa. Vector control, however, largely has been supplanted by community-wide mass drug administration programs. A highly successful global initiative being led by the World Health Organization has mass distributed hundreds of millions of ivermectin treatments (donated by the drug manufacturer for this purpose) to communities with onchocerciasis. As a result of these programs, transmission largely has been eliminated from the Americas and markedly curtailed throughout Africa.

Human Papillomaviruses

CLINICAL MANIFESTATIONS: Human papillomaviruses (HPV) are a large family of viruses. Most HPV infections are inapparent clinically. However, HPVs can cause benign epithelial proliferation (warts) of the skin and mucous membranes and are associated with cancers. HPVs can be grouped into cutaneous and genital (mucosal) types. The cutaneous types cause nongenital warts including common skin warts, plantar warts, flat warts, thread-like (filiform) warts, and epidermodysplasia verruciformis. Some mucosal types (low risk) are associated with warts or papillomas of mucous membranes, including the upper respiratory tract, anogenital, oral, nasal, and conjunctival areas. Other mucosal types (high risk) are associated with cancers and precancers, including cervical, anogenital, and oropharyngeal cancers.

Common **skin warts** are dome-shaped with conical projections that give the surface a rough appearance. They usually are painless and multiple, occurring commonly on the hands and around or under the nails. When small dermal vessels become thrombosed, black dots appear in the warts.

Plantar warts on the foot are often larger than warts at other sites and may not project through much of the skin surface. They may be painful when walking and are characterized by marked hyperkeratosis, sometimes with black dots.

Flat warts ("juvenile warts") commonly are found on the face and extremities of children and adolescents. They usually are small, multiple, and flat topped; seldom exhibit papillomatosis; and rarely cause pain. Filiform warts occur on the face and neck. Cutaneous warts are benign.

Anogenital warts, also called **condylomata acuminata,** are skin-colored warts with a papular, flat or cauliflower-like surface that range in size from a few millimeters to several centimeters; these warts often occur in groups. In males, these warts may be found on the penis, scrotum, or anal or perianal area. In females, these lesions may occur on the vulva, anal or perianal areas, and less commonly, in the vagina or on the cervix. Warts usually are painless, although they may cause itching, burning, local pain, or bleeding.

Anogenital **low-grade squamous intraepithelial lesions (L-SILs)** can result from persistent infection with low-risk and high-risk HPV types, whereas **high-grade squamous intraepithelial lesions (H-SILs)** result from persistent infection with high-risk HPV types. H-SILs are considered precancers. In the cervix, these lesions are detected through routine screening with cytologic testing (Papanicolaou [Pap] test); tissue biopsy is required to make the diagnosis. In the past, cervical lesions have been called dysplasias (mild, moderate, severe) or cervical intraepithelial neoplasia (CIN grades 1, 2 or 3, with only grades 2 or 3 being considered cancer precursors). Endocervical glandular precancer, **adenocarcinoma in situ** (AIS), also may result from high-risk HPV types. **Invasive cancers** associated with HPV include those of cervix, vagina, vulva, penis, anus, and oropharynx (back of throat, base of tongue, and tonsils).

Juvenile recurrent respiratory papillomatosis is a rare condition characterized by recurring papillomas in the larynx or other areas of the upper respiratory tract. This condition is diagnosed most commonly in children between 2 and 5 years of age and manifests as a voice change (eg, hoarseness), stridor, or abnormal cry. Respiratory papillomas can cause respiratory tract obstruction in young children. Recurrent respiratory papillomatosis is divided into juvenile onset and adult onset forms based on age at presentation. Juvenile recurrent papillomatosis is defined as onset before 18 years and is believe to result from vertical transmission from mother to infant at the time of delivery.

Epidermodysplasia verruciformis is a rare, inherited disorder believed to be a consequence of a deficiency of cell-mediated immunity resulting in an abnormal susceptibility to certain HPV types and manifesting as chronic cutaneous HPV infection and frequent development of skin cancer. Lesions may resemble flat warts but often are similar to tinea versicolor, covering the torso and upper extremities. Most appear during the first decade of life, but malignant transformation, which occurs in 30% to 60% of affected people, usually is delayed until adulthood.

ETIOLOGY: HPVs are DNA viruses of the *Papillomavirus* family, which can be grouped into cutaneous and mucosal types on the basis of their tendency to infect specific epithelial tissue. In children, the most common lesions from cutaneous HPVs are hand and foot warts. Mucosal HPVs infect the genital tract and other mucosal surfaces and are grouped into low-risk and high-risk types on the basis of their epidemiologic association with cancers. Types are designated on the basis of the nucleotide sequence of specific regions of the genome. Low-risk types 6 and 11 are associated with about 90% of condylomata acuminata, recurrent respiratory papillomatosis, and conjunctival papillomas. High-risk types (currently including types 16, 18, 31, 33, 35, 39, 45, 51, 52, 56, 58, 59, 68, 69, 73, and 82) can cause low-grade cervical cell abnormalities, high-grade cervical cell abnormalities that are precursors to cancer, and anogenital cancers. High-risk HPV types are detected in 99% of cervical cancers. Type 16 is the cause of approximately 50% of cervical cancers worldwide, and types 16 and

18 together account for approximately 70% of cervical cancers. Type 16 also is the cause of most HPV-related oropharyngeal cancers. Infection with a high-risk HPV type is considered necessary for the development of cervical cancer but is not sufficient to cause cancer, because the vast majority of women who experience an HPV infection do not develop cancer.

EPIDEMIOLOGY: HPV types involved in common hand and foot warts are quite different from mucosal types. Nongenital hand and foot warts occur commonly among school-aged children; the prevalence rate is as high as 50%. These can be acquired through casual contact and facilitated through minor skin trauma. Autoinoculation can result in spread of lesions. The intense and often widespread appearance of cutaneous warts in patients with compromised cellular immunity (particularly patients who have undergone transplantation and people with human immunodeficiency virus infection) suggests that alterations in T-lymphocyte immunity may impair clearance of infection.

Genital HPV infections are transmitted primarily by skin-to-skin contact, usually through sexual intercourse; other genital contact has been associated with transmission. In US females, the highest prevalence of infection is in 20- to 24-year-olds. Most infections are subclinical and clear spontaneously within 2 years. Persistent infection with high-risk types of HPV is associated with development of cervical cancer, resulting in approximately 12 000 new cases and 4000 deaths annually in the United States. Cervical cancer is a rare outcome of infection that generally requires decades of persistent infection. HPV also is the cause of most vulvar, vaginal, penile, and anal cancers as well as a significant percentage of oropharyngeal cancers. Nearly 27 000 cases of HPV-related cancers are diagnosed annually in the United States. The risk of development of cancer precursor lesions is greater in people with HIV infection and people with cellular immune deficiencies.

Rarely, infection is transmitted to a child through the birth canal during delivery or transmitted from nongenital sites. Respiratory papillomatosis is believed to be acquired by aspiration of infectious secretions during passage through an infected birth canal. When anogenital warts are identified in a child who is beyond infancy but is prepubertal, sexual abuse must be considered (see Sexual Victimization and STIs, p 185).

The **incubation period** is estimated to range from 3 months to several years. Papillomavirus acquired by a neonate at the time of birth may never cause clinical disease or may become apparent over several years (eg, respiratory papillomatosis).

DIAGNOSTIC TESTS: Most cutaneous and anogenital warts are diagnosed through clinical inspection. Serologic testing for HPV does not inform clinical decisions and is not indicated. Respiratory papillomatosis is diagnosed using endoscopy and biopsy. Cytologic screening (Pap test) and sometimes HPV testing of cervical specimens will identify women requiring follow-up with colposcopy and biopsy. Vulvar, vaginal, penile, and anal lesions may be identified using visual inspection, sometimes using magnification, and in some cases, cytologic screening (Pap test) is used and suspicious lesions are biopsied; there is no routine screening recommended for these cancers. For all anogenital lesions, diagnosis is made on the basis of histologic findings.

Although cytologic and histologic changes can be suggestive of HPV, these findings are not diagnostic of HPV. Detection of HPV infection is based on detection of viral nucleic acid (DNA or RNA) or capsid protein. Clinical tests for high-risk HPV may be used in combination with Pap testing for cervical cancer screening in women 30 years or older and for triage of equivocal Pap test abnormalities (atypical squamous cells of undetermined significance [ASCUS]) in women 21 years or older.[1] The advantages to using these HPV tests in women 30 years or older is that the Pap screening interval can be prolonged to 5 years. These HPV tests are not recommended for use in adolescents or men.

TREATMENT[2]: There is no treatment for HPV infection. Treatment is directed toward lesions caused by HPV. Treatment of anogenital warts may differ from treatment of cutaneous nongenital warts. Treatment options for warts should be discussed with a health care professional. Regression of nongenital and genital warts occurs in approximately 30% of cases within 6 months. Most methods of treatment of cutaneous warts use chemical or physical destruction of the infected epithelium, including cryotherapy with liquid nitrogen, laser or surgical removal of warts, application of salicylic acid products, or application of topical immune-modulating agents. Daily treatment with tretinoin has been useful for widespread flat warts in children. Care must be taken to avoid a deleterious cosmetic result with therapy. Pharmacologic treatments for refractory warts, including cimetidine, have been used with varying success.

Treatments for genital warts are characterized as patient applied or provider administered. No one treatment is superior to another. Interventions include ablational/excisional treatments, antiproliferative methods, and immune-modulating therapy. Many agents used for treatment have not been tested for safety and efficacy in children, and some are contraindicated in pregnancy. Although most forms of therapy are successful for initial removal of warts, treatment may not eradicate HPV infection from the surrounding tissue. Recurrences are common and may be attributable to reactivation rather than reinfection. Follow-up visits during and after treatment for genital warts may be advantageous, because treatments can result in local symptoms or adverse effects (**www.cdc.gov/std/treatment/2010/genital-warts.htm**).

Cancer precursor lesions that are identified in the cervix (H-SIL, AIS) and elsewhere in the genital tract require excision or destruction. Overtreatment of cervical lesions can cause substantial economic, emotional, and reproductive adverse effects, including higher risk of preterm birth. Management of invasive cervical and other anogenital and orpharyngeal cancers requires a specialist and should be conducted according to existing guidance.

Respiratory papillomatosis is difficult to treat and is best managed by an experienced otolaryngologist. Local recurrence is common, and repeated surgical procedures for removal often are necessary. Extension or dissemination of respiratory papillomas from the larynx into the trachea, bronchi, or lung parenchyma is rare but can result in increased morbidity and mortality; carcinoma can occur rarely. Intralesional interferon, indole-3-carbinole, photodynamic therapy, intralesional mumps vaccine, and intralesional cidofovir have been used as investigational treatments, but the lack of adequately powered controlled trials with any of these interventions makes conclusions regarding efficacy difficult.

Oral warts can be removed through cryotherapy, electrocautery, or surgical excision.

ISOLATION OF THE HOSPITALIZED PATIENT: Standard precautions are recommended.

---

[1]American Society for Colposcopy and Cervical Pathology. *Updated Consensus Guidelines on the Management of Women with Abnormal Cervical Cancer Screening Tests and Cancer Precursors.* Frederick, MD: American Society for Colposcopy and Cervical Pathology; 2013. Available at: **www.asccp.org/Guidelines-2/Management-Guidelines-2**

[2]Centers for Disease Control and Prevention. Sexually transmitted diseases treatment guidelines—2014. *MMWR Recomm Rep.* 2015; in press

CONTROL MEASURES AND CARE OF EXPOSED PEOPLE: Suspected child sexual abuse should be reported to the appropriate local agency if anogenital warts are found in a child who is beyond infancy but is prepubertal (see Sexual Victimization and STIs, p 185). HPV vaccine is recommended beginning at 9 years of age in children with suspected child sexual abuse.

Sexual abstinence, monogamous relationships, delayed sexual debut, and minimizing the number of sex partners are modes of reducing risk of anogenital HPV infection. Consistent and correct use of latex condoms may reduce the risk of anogenital HPV infection when infected areas are covered or protected by the condom. Use of latex condoms has been associated with a decrease in the risk of genital warts and cervical cancer. The degree and duration of contagiousness in patients with a history of genital HPV infection is unknown. People with genital warts should refrain from sex with new partners while warts are present, and sex partners of people with genital warts may benefit from a clinical evaluation for anogenital warts or other sexually transmitted infections.

Although infection with HPV types 6 and 11 leading to respiratory papillomatosis is believed to be acquired during passage through the birth canal, this condition has occurred in infants born by cesarean delivery. Because the preventive value of cesarean delivery is unknown, it should not be performed solely to prevent transmission of HPV to the newborn infant.

Cervical Cancer Screening. A variety of professional organizations offer guidance on cervical cancer screening, including the American College of Obstetricians and Gynecologists (**www.acog.org**), American Cancer Society (**www.cancer.org**), and US Preventive Services Task Force (**www.ahrq.gov/clinic/uspstfix.htm**). These organizations recommend that Pap testing begin at 21 years of age for all healthy women, regardless of sexual history. Female adolescents with a recent diagnosis of HIV infection should undergo cervical Pap test screening twice in the first year after diagnosis and annually thereafter (**http://aidsinfo.nih.gov/guidelines**). Sexually active female adolescents who have had an organ transplant or are receiving long-term corticosteroid therapy also should undergo similar cervical Pap test screening. If cytologic screening has been initiated before 21 years of age, patients with abnormal Pap test results should be cared for by a physician who is knowledgeable in the management of cervical dysplasia. The American Society for Colposcopy and Cervical Pathology's 2013 Consensus Guidelines include algorithms for management of abnormal Pap test results that are specific for adolescence (**www.asccp.org/Guidelines-2/Management-Guidelines-2**).

HPV Vaccines. Three HPV vaccines are licensed by the US Food and Drug Administration (FDA) for use in the United States. A quadrivalent vaccine (HPV4 [types 6, 11, 16, and 18], Gardasil [Merck & Co Inc, Whitehouse Station, NJ]) was licensed by the FDA for use in females 9 through 26 years of age in 2006 and in males 9 through 26 years of age in 2009. In December 2014, an expanded 9-valent HPV vaccine (HPV9 [types 6, 11, 16, 18, 31, 33, 45, 52, and 58], Gardasil 9 [Merck & Co Inc, Whitehouse Station, NJ]) was licensed by the FDA for use in females ages 9 through 26 and in males ages 9 through 15. A bivalent vaccine (HPV2 [types 16 and 18], Cervarix [GlaxoSmithKline, Research Triangle Park, NC]) was licensed for use in 2009 and is indicated for females 9 through 25 years of age.

Women who have received an HPV vaccine must continue to have regular Pap tests performed. HPV vaccines do not provide protection against all HPV types associated with development of cancer.

Immunogenicity. More than 99% of healthy vaccine recipients develop HPV antibodies to vaccine HPV types 1 month after receipt of the third dose. In clinical trials of HPV4 vaccine, antibody titers in young adolescent females and males 9 through 15 years of age were higher than antibody responses in females and males 16 through 26 years of age. For HPV2 vaccine, antibody responses in young adolescent females 9 through 14 years of age were higher than antibody titers in females 15 through 25 years of age. HPV9 has been shown to be noninferior to HPV4 for anti-HPV 6, 11, 16, and 18 in boys, girls, young men, and young women.

Antibody concentrations decrease over time after the third dose but plateau by 18 to 24 months after receipt of the third dose for either vaccine. In continuing studies of vaccine recipients, antibody concentrations remain much higher than those associated with naturally acquired HPV infection. However, the clinical significance of antibody concentrations is not clear, because a serologic correlate of protection has not been established.

Efficacy. HPV4 and HPV2 vaccines have been shown to be highly effective in preventing cervical cancers related to HPV types 16 and 18 in females in clinical trials through 26 years of age. HPV4 vaccine has been shown to be highly effective in preventing genital warts related to HPV types 6 and 11 in females and males in clinical trials through 26 years of age. HPV4 vaccine also has been shown to be highly effective in preventing anal precancers in males through 26 years of age. HPV9 provides 97% protection against the additional 5 HPV types in the 9-valent product (31, 33, 45, 52, and 58), and has noninferior immunogenicity for the 4 HPV types in the 4-valent product (6, 11, 16, and 18). Vaccines currently have not been proven to have therapeutic effect on existing HPV infection or disease and offer no protection against progression of infection to disease from HPV acquired before immunization. Therefore, HPV vaccines are most effective for both males and females when given at ages 11 or 12 years, well before most are exposed to HPV through sexual contact.

Follow-up studies 8 to 10 years after HPV4 and HPV2 vaccination have shown no waning of protection. Long-term follow-up studies are being conducted to determine the duration of efficacy for all HPV vaccines.

Vaccine Recommendations.[1,2] The American Academy of Pediatrics and the Advisory Committee on Immunization Practices of the Centers for Disease Control and Prevention recommend HPV9, HPV4 (as availabilities last), or HPV2 vaccine for routine immunization of females 11 or 12 years of age, and recommend either HPV9 or HPV4 (as availabilities last) for routine immunization of males 11 or 12 years of age. The vaccination series can be started as young as 9 years of age, and in the case of sexual abuse, HPV vaccination is recommended beginning at 9 years of age.

Providers are encouraged to recommend use of this vaccine as they do all other childhood and adolescent vaccines. Current HPV vaccination rates are lower than expected when compared with other adolescent vaccines within the first few years of incorporation into the immunization schedule. Research has demonstrated that parents often are influenced by the strong recommendations of their child's pediatrician, and opportunities to prevent cervical cancer deaths are being missed by physicians focusing on the HPV vaccine as an STI vaccine rather than a cancer prevention vaccine.

---

[1] American Academy of Pediatrics, Committee on Infectious Diseases. HPV vaccine recommendations. *Pediatrics.* 2012;129(3):602–605

[2] Centers for Disease Control and Prevention. Human papillomavirus vaccination: recommendations of the Advisory Committee on Immunization Practices (ACIP). *MMWR Recomm Rep.* 2014;63(RR-5):1–30

The HPV9, HPV4 (as availabilities last), and HPV2 vaccines also are recommended for females 13 through 26 years of age not previously immunized. HPV9 and HPV4 (as availabilities last) also are recommended for males 13 through 21 years of age not previously immunized. Males 22 through 26 years of age may be immunized with HPV9 or HPV4, and both are recommended for men who have sex with men and people who are immunocompromised (including those with HIV infection) through 26 years of age. No HPV vaccines are not licensed for use in people older than 26 years of age.

Dosage and Administration. The recommended dose and administration schedule for HPV9, HPV4, and HPV2 vaccines are the same. The vaccines are given in three 0.5-mL doses, administered intramuscularly, preferably in a deltoid muscle. The second dose should be administered at least 1 to 2 months after the first dose, and the third dose should be administered at least 6 months after the first dose. The minimum interval between doses 1 and 2 is 4 weeks. The minimum interval between doses 2 and 3 is 12 weeks (and at least 24 weeks after the first dose).

- Dose(s) of vaccine received after a shorter-than-recommended interval should be repeated.
- If the vaccine schedule is interrupted, the vaccine series does not need to be restarted.
- Whenever feasible, the same HPV vaccine should be used for the entire immunization series, because no studies have addressed interchangeability of HPV vaccines. However, if the vaccine provider does not know which HPV vaccine was previously administered, then any of the vaccines maybe used to complete the series to provide protection against HPV types 16 and 18 in females. HPV2 vaccine is not licensed by the FDA for use in males and is not recommended in boys or men.
- The vaccines are available in single-dose vials and prefilled syringes and contain no antimicrobial agents or preservative.
- HPV vaccines should be stored at 2°C to 8°C (36°F–46°F) and not frozen.
- HPV vaccine can be coadministered with any live or inactivated vaccine indicated at the same visit.
- People in the recommended age groups with evidence of current HPV infection or disease, such as abnormal Pap test results, cervical lesions, anogenital warts, or a positive HPV DNA test result, should receive immunization. Existing infection with all vaccine HPV types is unlikely, and so the vaccine could provide protection against HPV types not already acquired.

Recommendations for Special Populations. HPV vaccines are not live vaccines. HPV vaccines are recommended for people in the recommended age groups who are immunocompromised as a result of infection (including HIV), disease, or medications. The immune response and vaccine efficacy in immunocompromised people might be less than that in immunocompetent people. There are ongoing evaluations on duration of efficacy and immunogenicity in immunocompromised populations, including those with HIV-infection.

Vaccine Adverse Events, Precautions, and Contraindications. Injection site discomfort or pain, redness (erythema), and edema (swelling) are the most commonly reported local adverse events. Systemic symptoms after HPV vaccine can include headache, dizziness, fever, nausea, and fatigue/malaise. Syncope (fainting) is reported in adolescents after receipt of recommended adolescent vaccines, including the HPV vaccine. HPV vaccines can be administered to people with minor acute illnesses.

- Immunization of people with moderate or severe acute illnesses should be deferred until after the patient improves.

- HPV vaccines are contraindicated in people with a history of immediate hypersensitivity to any vaccine component (HPV2, HPV4, and HPV9) and to yeast (HPV4 and HPV9). HPV2 vaccine in the prefilled syringe formulation should not be administered to latex-sensitive individuals, because the rubber stopper contains latex.
- HPV vaccines are not recommended for use during pregnancy. The health care professional should inquire about pregnancy in sexually active patients, but a pregnancy test is not required before starting the immunization series. If a vaccine recipient becomes pregnant, subsequent doses should be postponed until the postpartum period. If a dose has been administered inadvertently during pregnancy, no action is recommended. Data to date show no evidence of adverse effect of HPV9, HPV4, or HPV2 vaccine on outcomes of pregnancy. For pregnant women who receive HPV9 or HPV4, providers can call 1-800-672-6372. Pregnancy registries for HPV2 and HPV4 have been closed with concurrence from the FDA.
- Vaccine providers, particularly when vaccinating adolescents, should be encouraged to observe patients (with patients seated or lying down) for 15 minutes after vaccination to decrease the risk for injury should they faint. If syncope develops, patients should be observed until symptoms resolve.
- HPV9 and HPV4 vaccine may be administered to lactating women. The HPV2 vaccine has not been studied in lactating women.

Paracoccidioidomycosis
(South American Blastomycosis)

CLINICAL MANIFESTATIONS: Disease occurs primarily in adults, in whom the site of initial infection is the lungs. Disease is infrequent in children, in whom approximately 5% to 10% of all cases occur. Clinical patterns can include subclinical infection or progressive disease that can be either acute-subacute (juvenile type) or chronic (adult type). In both adult and juvenile forms, constitutional symptoms, such as fever, malaise, anorexia, and weight loss, are common. In the juvenile form, the initial pulmonary infection usually is asymptomatic, and manifestations are related to dissemination of infection to the reticuloendothelial system, resulting in enlarged lymph nodes and involvement of liver, spleen, and bone marrow. Skin lesions are observed regularly and are located typically on the face, neck, and trunk. Involvement of bones, joints, and mucous membranes is less common. Enlarged lymph nodes occasionally coalesce and form abscesses or fistulas. The chronic form of the illness can be localized to the lungs or can disseminate. Oral mucosal lesions are observed in half of the cases. Skin involvement is common but occurs in a smaller proportion than in patients with the acute-subacute form. Infection can be latent for years before causing illness.

ETIOLOGY: *Paracoccidioides brasiliensis* is a thermally dimorphic fungus with yeast and mycelia phases.

EPIDEMIOLOGY: The infection occurs in Latin America, from Mexico to Argentina. The natural reservoir is unknown, although soil is suspected. The mode of transmission is unknown, but most likely occurs via inhalation of contaminated soil or dust; person-to-person transmission does not occur.

The **incubation period** is highly variable, ranging from 1 month to many years.

DIAGNOSTIC TESTS: Round, multiple-budding cells with a distinguishing pilot's wheel appearance can be seen in preparations of sputum, bronchoalveolar lavage specimens, scrapings from ulcers, and material from lesions or in tissue biopsy specimens. Several procedures, including wet or KOH wet preparations, or histologic staining with hematoxylin and eosin, silver, or periodic-acid Schiff, are adequate for visualization of fungal elements. The mycelia form of *P brasiliensis* can be cultured on most enriched media, including blood agar at 37°C (98°F) and Mycosel or Sabouraud dextrose agar at 24°C (75°F). Its appearance is not distinctive, and confirmation requires conversion to the yeast phase or DNA sequence determination. A number of serologic tests are available; quantitative immunodiffusion is the preferred test. The antibody titer by immunodiffusion usually is ≥1:32 in acute infection.

TREATMENT: Amphotericin B is preferred by many experts for initial treatment of severe paracoccidioidomycosis (see Antifungal Drugs for Systemic Fungal Infections, p 905). An alternative is intravenous trimethoprim-sulfamethoxazole (8–10 mg/kg/day of the trimethoprim component, divided into 3 daily doses). Children treated initially by the intravenous route can transition to orally administered therapy after clinical improvement has been observed, usually after 3 to 6 weeks.

Oral therapy with itraconazole (5 mg/kg, twice daily; maximum dose 200 mg) is the treatment of choice for less severe or localized infection and to complete treatment when amphotericin B is used initially. Serum concentrations of itraconazole should be ≥1 but <10 μg/mL. Concentrations should be checked after 2 weeks of therapy to ensure adequate drug exposure. Prolonged therapy for 6 to 12 months is necessary to minimize the relapse rate. Children with severe disease can require a longer course. Itraconazole is associated with fewer adverse effects and a lower relapse rate (3%–5%) than ketoconazole, which is now uncommonly used for treatment. Voriconazole is as well tolerated and as effective as itraconazole in adults, but data for its use in children with paracoccidioidomycosis are not available. Trimethoprim-sulfamethoxazole orally (10 mg/kg/day of the trimethoprim component divided into 2 doses daily) is an alternative but treatment must be continued for 2 years or longer to lessen the risk of relapse, which occurs in 10% to 15% of optimally treated patients.

Serial serologic testing by quantitative immunodiffusion is useful for monitoring the response to therapy. The expected response is a progressive decline in titers after 1 to 3 months of treatment with stabilization at a low titer.

ISOLATION OF THE HOSPITALIZED PATIENT: Standard precautions are recommended.

CONTROL MEASURES: None.

Paragonimiasis

CLINICAL MANIFESTATIONS: There are 2 major forms of paragonimiasis: (1) disease principally attributable to *Paragonimus westermani, Paragonimus heterotremus, Paragonimus africanus, Paragonimus uterobilateralis,* and *Paragonimus kellicotti* causing primary pulmonary disease with or without extrapulmonary manifestations; and (2) disease attributable to other species of *Paragonimus,* most notably *Paragonimus skrjabini,* for which humans are accidental hosts and manifestations generally are extrapulmonary, resulting in a larva migrans syndrome similar to that caused by *Toxocara canis.* The former disease is especially likely to have an insidious onset and a chronic course. Pulmonary disease is associated with chronic cough and dyspnea, but most infections probably are inapparent or result in mild symptoms. Heavy infestations cause paroxysms of coughing, which often produce blood-tinged sputum that is brown because of the presence of *Paragonimus* species eggs. Hemoptysis can be severe.

Pleural effusion, pneumothorax, bronchiectasis, and pulmonary fibrosis with clubbing can develop. Extrapulmonary manifestations also may involve liver, spleen, abdominal cavity, intestinal wall, intra-abdominal lymph nodes, skin, and central nervous system, with meningoencephalitis, seizures, and space-occupying tumors attributable to invasion of the brain by adult flukes, usually occurring within a year of pulmonary infection. Symptoms tend to subside after approximately 5 years but can persist for as many as 20 years.

Extrapulmonary paragonimiasis is associated with migratory allergic subcutaneous nodules containing juvenile worms. Pleural effusion is common, as is invasion of the brain.

ETIOLOGY: In Asia, classical paragonimiasis is caused by adult flukes and eggs of *P westermani* and *P heterotremus*. In Africa, the adult flukes and eggs of *P africanus* and *P uterobilateralis* produce the disease, whereas in North America the endemic species is *P kellicotti*. In North America, disease also has been caused by *P westermani*, present in imported crab. The adult flukes of *P westermani* are up to 12 mm long and 7 mm wide and occur throughout the Asia. A triploid parthenogenetic form of *P westermani*, which is larger, produces more eggs, and elicits greater disease, has been described in Japan, Korea, Taiwan, and parts of eastern China. *P heterotremus* occurs in Southeast Asia and adjacent parts of China.

Extrapulmonary paragonimiasis (ie, visceral larva migrans) is caused by larval stages of *P skrjabini* and *P miyazakii*. The worms rarely mature in infected human tissues. *P skrjabini* occurs in China, whereas *P miyazakii* occurs in Japan. *P mexicanus* and *P ecuadoriensis* occur in Mexico, Costa Rica, Ecuador, and Peru. *P kellicotti*, a lung fluke of mink and opossums in the United States, also can cause infection in humans.

EPIDEMIOLOGY: Transmission occurs when raw or undercooked freshwater crabs or crayfish containing larvae (metacercariae) are ingested. Numerous cases have been associated with ingestion of uncooked crawfish during river raft trips in the Midwestern United States. The metacercariae excyst in the small intestine and penetrate the abdominal cavity, where they remain for a few days before migrating to the lungs. *P westermani* and *P heterotremus* mature within the lungs over 6 to 10 weeks, when they then begin egg production. Eggs escape from pulmonary capsules into the bronchi and exit from the human host in sputum or feces. Eggs hatch in freshwater within 3 weeks, giving rise to miracidia. Miracidia penetrate freshwater snails and emerge several weeks later as cercariae, which encyst within the muscles and viscera of freshwater crustaceans before maturing into infective metacercariae. A less common mode of transmission that may also occur is human infection through the ingestion of raw pork, usually from wild pigs, containing the juvenile stages of *Paragonimus* species (described as occurring in Japan).

Humans are accidental ("dead-end") hosts for *P skrjabini* and *P miyazakii* in visceral larva migrans. These flukes cannot mature in humans and, hence, do not produce eggs.

Paragonimus species also infect a variety of other mammals, such as canids, mustelids, felids, and rodents, which serve as animal reservoir hosts.

The **incubation period** is variable; egg production begins by approximately 8 weeks after ingestion of *P westermani* metacercariae.

DIAGNOSTIC TESTS: Microscopic examination of stool, sputum, pleural effusion, cerebrospinal fluid, and other tissue specimens may reveal eggs. A Western blot serologic antibody test based on *P westermani* antigen, available at the Centers for Disease Control and Prevention (CDC), is sensitive and specific; antibody concentrations detected by immunoblot decrease slowly after the infection is cured by treatment. Charcot-Leyden crystals and eosinophils in sputum are useful diagnostic elements. Chest radiographs may appear normal or resemble radiographs from patients with tuberculosis. Misdiagnosis is likely unless paragonimiasis is suspected.

TREATMENT: Praziquantel in a 2-day course is the treatment of choice (see Drugs for Parasitic Infections, p 927) and is associated with high cure rates as demonstrated by disappearance of egg production and radiographic lesions in the lungs. The drug also is effective for some extrapulmonary manifestations. An alternative drug for patients unable to take praziquantel (eg, because of previous allergic reaction) is triclabendazole, given in 1 or 2 doses. Triclabendazole is not available commercially in the United States but may be obtained from the CDC under an investigational drug protocol. For patients with central nervous system paragonimiasis, a short course of steroids may be beneficial in addition to the praziquantel to reduce the inflammatory response associated with the dying flukes.

ISOLATION OF THE HOSPITALIZED PATIENT: Standard precautions are recommended.

CONTROL MEASURES: Cooking of crabs and crayfish for several minutes until the meat has congealed and turned opaque kills metacercariae. Similarly, meat from wild pigs should be well cooked before eating (160°F[71°C]). Control of animal reservoirs is not possible.

Parainfluenza Viral Infections

CLINICAL MANIFESTATIONS: Parainfluenza viruses (PIVs) are the major cause of laryngotracheobronchitis (croup), and may cause bronchiolitis and pneumonia as well as upper respiratory tract infection.[1] PIV type 1 (PIV1) and, to a lesser extent, PIV type 2 (PIV2) are the most common pathogens associated with croup. PIV type 3 (PIV3) most commonly is associated with bronchiolitis and pneumonia in infants and young children. Infections with PIV type 4 (PIV4) are less well characterized, but studies using sensitive molecular assays suggest that they may be more common than previously appreciated. Rarely, PIVs have been isolated from patients with parotitis, aseptic meningitis, encephalitis, or Guillain-Barré syndrome. PIV infections can exacerbate symptoms of chronic lung disease and asthma in children and adults. In children with immunodeficiency and recipients of hematopoietic stem cell transplants, PIVs can cause refractory infections with persistent shedding, severe pneumonia with viral dissemination, and even fatal disease, most commonly caused by PIV3. PIV infections do not confer complete protective immunity; therefore, reinfections can occur with all serotypes and at any age, but reinfections usually cause a mild illness limited to the upper respiratory tract.

ETIOLOGY: PIVs are enveloped single-stranded negative-sense RNA viruses classified in the family *Paramyxoviridae*. Four antigenically distinct types—1, 2, 3, and 4 (with 2 subtypes, 4A and 4B)—that infect humans have been identified.

EPIDEMIOLOGY: PIVs are transmitted from person to person by direct contact and exposure to contaminated nasopharyngeal secretions through respiratory tract droplets and fomites. PIV infections can be sporadic or associated with outbreaks of acute respiratory tract disease. Seasonal patterns of infection are distinct, predictable, and cyclic in temperate regions. Different serotypes have distinct epidemiologic patterns. PIV1 tends to

---

[1] American Academy of Pediatrics, Subcommittee on Diagnosis and Management of Bronchiolitis. Clinical practice guideline: the diagnosis, management, and prevention of bronchiolitis. *Pediatrics.* 2014;134(5):e1474–e1502

produce outbreaks of respiratory tract illness, usually croup, in the autumn of every other year. A major increase in the number of cases of croup in the autumn usually indicates a PIV1 outbreak. PIV2 also can cause outbreaks of respiratory tract illness in the autumn, often in conjunction with PIV1 outbreaks, but PIV2 outbreaks tend to be less severe, irregular, and less common. PIV3 is endemic and usually is prominent during spring and summer in temperate climates but often continues into autumn, especially in years when autumn outbreaks of PIV1 or PIV2 are absent. Infections with PIV4 are recognized less commonly and can be associated with illnesses ranging from mild to severe.

The age of primary infection varies with serotype. Primary infection with all types usually occurs by 5 years of age. Infection with PIV3 more often occurs in infants and is a prominent cause of bronchiolitis and pneumonia in this age group. By 12 months of age, 50% of infants have acquired PIV3 infection. Infections between 1 and 5 years of age more commonly are associated with PIV1 and, to a lesser extent, PIV2. Age at acquisition of PIV4 infection is not as well defined. Rates of PIV-associated hospitalizations for children vary depending on clinical syndrome, PIV type, and patient age.

Immunocompetent children with primary PIV infection may shed virus for up to 1 week before onset of clinical symptoms and for 1 to 3 weeks after symptoms have disappeared, depending on serotype. Severe lower respiratory tract disease with prolonged shedding of the virus can develop in immunodeficient people. In these patients, infection may spread beyond the respiratory tract to the liver and lymph nodes.

The **incubation period** ranges from 2 to 6 days.

DIAGNOSTIC TESTS: PIVs may be isolated from nasopharyngeal secretions, usually within 4 to 7 days of culture inoculation or earlier by use of centrifugation of the specimen onto a monolayer of susceptible cells with subsequent staining for viral antigen (shell vial assay). Highly sensitive reverse transcriptase-polymerase chain reaction (RT-PCR) assays also now are available commercially for detection and differentiation of PIVs. Rapid antigen identification techniques, including immunofluorescence assays, can be used to detect the virus in nasopharyngeal secretions, but sensitivities of the tests vary. Serologic diagnosis, made retrospectively by a significant increase in antibody titer between serum specimens obtained during acute infection and convalescence, is less useful, because infection may not always be accompanied by a significant homotypic antibody response.

TREATMENT: Specific antiviral therapy is not available. Most infections are self-limited and require no treatment. Monitoring for hypoxia and hypercapnia in more severely affected children with lower respiratory tract disease may be helpful. The following treatment recommendations apply to laryngotracheobronchitis. Racemic epinephrine aerosol commonly is given to severely affected hospitalized patients with laryngotracheobronchitis to decrease airway obstruction. Parenteral, oral, and nebulized corticosteroids have been demonstrated to lessen the severity and duration of symptoms and hospitalization in patients with moderate to severe laryngotracheobronchitis. Oral steroids also are effective for outpatients with less severe croup. Management otherwise is supportive. Antimicrobial agents should be reserved for documented secondary bacterial infections. The use of ribavirin (usually inhaled) with or without concomitant administration of Immune Globulin Intravenous (IGIV) has been reported anecdotally in immunocompromised patients with severe pneumonia; however, controlled studies are lacking.

ISOLATION OF THE HOSPITALIZED PATIENT: In addition to standard precautions, contact precautions are recommended for hospitalized infants and young children for the duration of illness. In immunocompromised patients, the duration of contact precautions should be extended because of possible prolonged shedding. Hospitalized immunocompromised patients with PIV infection should be isolated to prevent spread to other patients.

CONTROL MEASURES: Appropriate respiratory hygiene and cough etiquette should be followed. Exposure to PIV-infected people, including other patients, staff, and family members, may not be recognized, because illness may be mild. Additional infection control measures should be considered in certain settings (eg, child care centers, nursing homes) when respiratory infections have been identified to limit spread.

Parasitic Diseases

Many parasitic diseases traditionally have been considered exotic and, therefore, frequently are not included in differential diagnoses of patients in the United States, Canada, and Europe. Nevertheless, a number of these organisms are endemic in industrialized countries, and overall, parasites are among the most common causes of morbidity and mortality in various and diverse geographic locations worldwide. Outside the tropics and subtropics, parasitic diseases particularly are common among tourists returning to their own countries, immigrants from areas with highly endemic infection, and immunocompromised people. Some of these infections disproportionately affect impoverished populations, such as black and Hispanic people living in the United States and aboriginal people living in Alaska and the Canadian Arctic. Selected parasitic infections, including cryptosporidiosis, giardiasis, Chagas disease, cysticercosis, and toxocariasis, may be quite common in the southern United States. Physicians and clinical laboratory personnel need to be aware of where these infections may be acquired, their clinical presentations, and methods of diagnosis and should advise people how to prevent infection. Table 3.44 (p 589) provides details on some infrequently encountered parasitic diseases.

Consultation and assistance in diagnosis and management of parasitic diseases are available from the Centers for Disease Control and Prevention (CDC), state health departments, and university departments or divisions of geographic medicine, tropical medicine, pediatric infectious diseases, international health, and public health.

Through authorized investigational new drug mechanisms, the CDC distributes several drugs that are not available commercially in the United States for treatment of parasitic diseases. To request these drugs, a physician must contact the CDC Parasitic Diseases Inquiries office (see Appendix I, Directory of Resources, p 975; 404-718-4745; e-mail: parasites@cdc.gov). Consultation with a medical officer from the CDC is required before a drug is distributed.

Important human parasitic infections are discussed in individual chapters in section 3; the diseases are arranged alphabetically, and the discussions include recommendations for drug treatment. Drugs for Parasitic Infections can be found beginning on p 927, and are compiled from recommendations on the CDC Web site. Although the recommendations for administration of these drugs given in the disease-specific chapters are similar, they may not be identical in all instances because of differences of opinion among experts. Both sources should be consulted.

Table 3.44. Parasitic Diseases Not Covered Elsewhere[a]

Disease and/ or Agent	Where Infection May Be Acquired	Definitive Host	Intermediate Host	Modes of Human Infection	Directly Communicable (Person to Person)	Diagnostic Laboratory Tests in Humans	Causative Form of Parasite	Manifestations in Humans
Angiostrongylus cantonensis (neurotropic disease)	Widespread in the tropics, particularly Pacific Islands, Southeast Asia, Central and South America, the Caribbean, and the United States	Rats	Snails and slugs	Eating improperly cooked infected mollusks or food contaminated by mollusk secretions containing larvae; prawns, fish, and land crabs that have ingested infected mollusks also may be infectious	No	Eosinophils in CSF; rarely, identification of larvae in CSF or at autopsy; serologic test	Larval worms	Eosinophilia, meningo-encephalitis
Angiostrongylus costaricensis (gastrointestinal tract disease)	Central and South America	Rodents	Snails and slugs	Eating improperly poorly cooked infected mollusks or food contaminated by mollusk secretions containing larvae	No	Gel diffusion; identification of larvae and eggs in tissue	Larval worms	Abdominal pain, eosinophilia

continued

Table 3.44. Parasitic Diseases Not Covered Elsewhere,[a] continued

Disease and/ or Agent	Where Infection May Be Acquired	Definitive Host	Intermediate Host	Modes of Human Infection	Directly Communicable (Person to Person)	Diagnostic Laboratory Tests in Humans	Causative Form of Parasite	Manifestations in Humans
Anisakiasis	Cosmopolitan, most common where eating raw fish is practiced	Marine mammal	Certain saltwater fish, squid, and octopus	Eating uncooked or inadequately treated infected marine fish	No	Identification of recovered larvae in granulomas or vomitus	Larval worms	Acute gastrointestinal tract disease
Clonorchis sinensis, Opisthorchis viverrini, Opisthorchis felineus (flukes)	East Asia, Eastern Europe, Russian Federation	Humans, cats, dogs, other mammals	Certain freshwater snails	Eating uncooked infected freshwater fish	No	Eggs in stool or duodenal fluid	Larvae and mature flukes	Abdominal pain; hepatobiliary disease Cholangiocarcinoma
Dracunculiasis (Dracunculus medinensis) (guinea worm)	Foci in Africa Global eradication nearly achieved	Humans	Crustacea (copepods)	Drinking water infested with infected copepods	No	Identification of emerging or adult worm in subcutaneous tissues	Adult female worm	Emerging roundworm; inflammatory response; systemic and local blister or ulcer in skin

Table 3.44. Parasitic Diseases Not Covered Elsewhere,[a] continued

Disease and/or Agent	Where Infection May Be Acquired	Definitive Host	Intermediate Host	Modes of Human Infection	Directly Communicable (Person to Person)	Diagnostic Laboratory Tests in Humans	Causative Form of Parasite	Manifestations in Humans
Fasciolopsiasis (*Fasciolopsis buski*)	East Asia	Humans, pigs, dogs	Certain freshwater snails, plants	Eating uncooked infected plants	No	Eggs or worm in feces or duodenal fluid	Larvae and mature worms	Diarrhea, constipation, vomiting, anorexia, edema of face and legs, ascites
Intestinal capillariasis (*Capillaria philippinensis*)	Philippines, Thailand	Humans, fish-eating birds	Fish	Ingestion of uncooked infected fish	Uncertain	Eggs and parasite in feces	Larvae and mature worms	Protein-losing enteropathy; diarrhea, malabsorption, ascites, emaciation

CSF indicates cerebrospinal fluid.

[a] For recommended drug treatment, see Drugs for Parasitic Infections (p 927).

Human Parechovirus Infections

CLINICAL MANIFESTATIONS: Human parechoviruses cause similar clinical diseases as enteroviruses, including febrile illnesses, exanthems, sepsis-like syndromes, and central nervous system manifestations, such as meningitis (often with little or no pleocytosis), encephalitis, and paralytic disease. Infections in neonates and young infants may be severe and may include sepsis, hepatitis and coagulopathy, and/or meningoencephalitis with long-term sequelae. Parechovirus infections have been associated with respiratory and gastrointestinal tract disease and a variety of other manifestations, although causation has not been established consistently.

ETIOLOGY: The parechoviruses are a genus in the picornavirus family of RNA viruses. The parechovirus genus now includes at least 16 parechovirus types. Parechoviruses 1 and 2 previously were classified as echoviruses 22 and 23, respectively.

EPIDEMIOLOGY: Human parechovirus infections have been reported worldwide. Seroepidemiologic studies suggest that parechovirus infections occur commonly during early childhood. In some studies, most school-aged children have serologic evidence of prior infection, but seroprevalence appears to vary by geographic region and specific parechovirus type. Clinical reports suggest that most severe disease occurs in infants and young children. Infections frequently are inapparent clinically. Transmission appears to occur via the fecal-oral and respiratory routes, and in utero transmission also may occur. Parechoviruses may circulate throughout the year, but infections by certain types occur more commonly during summer and fall months. Multiple parechovirus types may circulate in a community during the same time period. Community outbreaks and health care-associated transmission in neonatal and pediatric hospital units have been described. Virus is shed from the upper respiratory tract for 1 to 3 weeks and in stool for <2 weeks to 5 months. Shedding may occur in the absence of illness.

The **incubation period** for parechovirus infections has not been defined.

DIAGNOSTIC TESTS: Polymerase chain reaction (PCR) assays that detect parechoviruses, available at the Centers for Disease Control and Prevention and select reference laboratories, represent the best diagnostic modality currently available. Enterovirus PCR assays will not detect any of the human parechoviruses. Parechoviruses can be detected in stool, throat swabs, nasopharyngeal aspirates, cerebrospinal fluid, and blood. Viral culture can be used for diagnosis of parechovirus infections, but recovery in culture is less sensitive than PCR assay, requires multiple cell lines, and may take several days. The parechovirus type can be identified by genomic sequencing of the VP1 capsid region or by neutralization assay of a viral isolate, although neutralizing antisera are not available for all serotypes. Serologic assays have been developed for research but are not available commercially for diagnostic purposes.

TREATMENT: No specific therapy is available for parechovirus infections. The investigational antiviral drug pleconaril lacks significant activity against parechoviruses. Immune Globulin Intravenous (IGIV) has been used in some published case reports involving neonates with severe human parechovirus infections (HP3V1), especially myocarditis. IGIV contains neutralizing antibody titers against HP3V1 but very low neutralizing antibody titers against HP3V3.

ISOLATION OF THE HOSPITALIZED PATIENT: In addition to standard precautions, contact precautions are appropriate for infants and young children for the duration of parechovirus illness. Cohorting of infected neonates may be effective in controlling hospital nursery outbreaks.

CONTROL MEASURES: Hand hygiene is important in decreasing spread of parechoviruses within families and institutions. No vaccine for parechoviruses is available.

Parvovirus B19
(Erythema Infectiosum, Fifth Disease)

CLINICAL MANIFESTATIONS: Infection with human parvovirus B19 is recognized most often as erythema infectiosum (EI), or fifth disease, which is characterized by a distinctive rash that may be preceded by mild systemic symptoms, including fever in 15% to 30% of patients. The facial rash can be intensely red with a "slapped cheek" appearance that often is accompanied by circumoral pallor. A symmetric, macular, lace-like, and often pruritic rash also occurs on the trunk, moving peripherally to involve the arms, buttocks, and thighs. The rash can fluctuate in intensity and recur with environmental changes, such as temperature and exposure to sunlight, for weeks to months. A brief, mild, non-specific illness consisting of fever, malaise, myalgia, and headache often precedes the characteristic exanthema by approximately 7 to 10 days. Arthralgia and arthritis occur in fewer than 10% of infected children but commonly occur among adults, especially women. Knees are involved most commonly in children, but a symmetric polyarthropathy of knees, fingers, and other joints is common in adults.

Human parvovirus B19 also can cause asymptomatic infections. Other manifestations (Table 3.45) include a mild respiratory tract illness with no rash, a rash atypical for EI that may be rubelliform or petechial, papular purpuric gloves-and-socks syndrome (PPGSS; painful and pruritic papules, petechiae, and purpura of hands and feet, often with fever and an enanthem), polyarthropathy syndrome (arthralgia and arthritis in adults in the absence of other manifestations of EI), chronic erythroid hypoplasia with severe anemia in immunodeficient patients (eg, patients with human immunodeficiency virus [HIV] infection, patients receiving immune suppressive therapy), and transient aplastic crisis lasting 7 to 10 days in patients with hemolytic anemias (eg, sickle cell disease and autoimmune hemolytic anemia). For children with other conditions associated with low hemoglobin concentrations, including hemorrhage, severe anemia, and thalassemia, parvovirus B19 infection will not result in aplastic crisis but might result in prolongation of recovery

Table 3.45. Clinical Manifestations of Human Parvovirus B19 Infection

Conditions	Usual Hosts
Erythema infectiosum (fifth disease)	Immunocompetent children
Polyarthropathy syndrome	Immunocompetent adults (more common in women)
Chronic anemia/pure red cell aplasia	Immunocompromised hosts
Transient aplastic crisis	People with hemolytic anemia (ie, sickle cell anemia)
Hydrops fetalis/congenital anemia	Fetus (first 20 weeks of pregnancy)
Petechial, papular-purpuric gloves-and-socks syndrome	Immunocompetent adults

from the anemia resulting from these conditions. Patients with transient aplastic crisis may have a prodromal illness with fever, malaise, and myalgia, but rash usually is absent. In addition, human parvovirus B19 infection sometimes has been associated with decreases in numbers of platelets, lymphocytes, and neutrophils.

Human parvovirus B19 infection occurring during pregnancy can cause fetal hydrops, intrauterine growth restriction, isolated pleural and pericardial effusions, and death, but the virus is not a proven cause of congenital anomalies. The risk of fetal death is between 2% and 6% when infection occurs during pregnancy. The greatest risk appears to occur during the first half of pregnancy.

ETIOLOGY: Human parvovirus B19 is a small, nonenveloped, single-stranded DNA virus in the family *Parvoviridae*, genus *Erythrovirus*. Three distinct genotypes of the virus have been described. Parvovirus B19 replicates in human erythrocyte precursors, which accounts for some of the clinical manifestations following infection. Human parvovirus B19-associated red blood cell aplasia is related to caspase-mediated apoptosis of erythrocyte precursors.

EPIDEMIOLOGY: Parvovirus B19 is distributed worldwide and is a common cause of infection in humans, who are the only known hosts. Modes of transmission include contact with respiratory tract secretions, percutaneous exposure to blood or blood products, and vertical transmission from mother to fetus. Human parvovirus B19 infections are ubiquitous, and cases of EI can occur sporadically or in outbreaks in elementary or junior high schools during late winter and early spring. Secondary spread among susceptible household members is common, with infection occurring in approximately 50% of susceptible contacts in some studies. The transmission rate in schools is lower, but infection can be an occupational risk for school and child care personnel, with approximately 20% of susceptible contacts becoming infected. In young children, antibody seroprevalence generally is 5% to 10%. In most communities, approximately 50% of young adults and often more than 90% of elderly people are seropositive. The annual seroconversion rate in women of childbearing age has been reported to be approximately 1.5%. Timing of the presence of high-titer parvovirus B19 DNA in serum and respiratory tract secretions indicates that people with EI are infectious before rash onset and are unlikely to be infectious after onset of the rash and/or joint symptoms. In contrast, patients with aplastic crises are contagious from before the onset of symptoms through at least the week after onset. Symptoms of the PPGSS can occur in association with viremia and before development of antibody response, and affected patients should be considered infectious.

The **incubation period** from acquisition of parvovirus B19 to onset of initial symptoms (rash or symptoms of aplastic crisis) is between 4 and 14 days but can be as long as 21 days.

DIAGNOSTIC TESTS: Parvovirus B19 cannot be propagated in standard cell culture. In the immunocompetent host, detection of serum parvovirus B19-specific immunoglobulin (Ig) M antibodies is the preferred diagnostic test for parvovirus B19-associated rash illness. A positive IgM test result indicates that infection probably occurred within the previous 2 to 3 months. On the basis of immunoassay results, IgM antibodies may be detected in 90% or more of patients at the time of the EI rash and by the third day of illness in patients with transient aplastic crisis. Serum IgG antibodies appear by approximately day 2 of EI and persist for life; therefore, presence of parvovirus B19 IgG is not necessarily indicative of acute infection. These assays are available through commercial laboratories and through some state public health department and research laboratories. However, their sensitivity and specificity may vary, particularly for IgM. The optimal method for detecting transient aplastic crisis or chronic infection in the immunocompromised patient is demonstration of high titer of viral DNA by polymerase chain reaction (PCR) assays. Because parvovirus B19 DNA can be detected at low levels by PCR assay in serum for months and even years after the acute viremic phase, detection does not necessarily indicate acute infection. Low levels of parvovirus B19 DNA also can be detected by PCR in tissues (skin, heart, liver, bone marrow), independent of active disease.

TREATMENT: For most patients, only supportive care is indicated. Patients with aplastic crisis may require transfusion. For treatment of chronic infection in immunodeficient patients, Immune Globulin Intravenous (IGIV) therapy often is effective and should be considered. Some cases of parvovirus B19 infection concurrent with hydrops fetalis have been treated successfully with intrauterine blood transfusions of the fetus.

ISOLATION OF THE HOSPITALIZED PATIENT: In addition to standard precautions, droplet precautions are recommended for hospitalized children with aplastic crises, children with PPGSS, or immunosuppressed patients with chronic infection and anemia for the duration of hospitalization. For patients with transient aplastic or erythrocyte crisis, these precautions should be maintained for 7 days or until the reticulocyte count has recovered from suppression to at least 2%. Neonates who had hydrops attributable to parvovirus B19 in utero do not require isolation if the hydrops is resolved at the time of birth.

Pregnant health care workers should be informed of the potential risks to their fetus from human parvovirus B19 infections and about preventive measures that may decrease these risks (eg, attention to strict infection control procedures and not caring for immunocompromised patients with chronic parvovirus B19 infection or patients with parvovirus B19-associated aplastic crises, because patients in both groups are likely to be contagious).

CONTROL MEASURES:

- Women who are exposed to children at home or at work (eg, teachers or child care providers) are at increased risk of infection with parvovirus B19. However, because school or child care center outbreaks often indicate wider spread in the community, including inapparent infection, women are at some degree of risk of exposure from other sources at home or in the community. In view of the high prevalence of parvovirus B19 infection, the low incidence of adverse effects on the fetus, and the fact that avoidance of child care or classroom teaching can decrease but not eliminate the risk of exposure, routine exclusion of pregnant women from the workplace where EI is occurring is not recommended. Women of childbearing age who are concerned can undergo serologic testing for IgG antibody to parvovirus B19 to determine their susceptibility to infection.
- Pregnant women who discover that they have been in contact with children who were in the incubation period of EI or with children who were in aplastic crisis should have the relatively low potential risk of infection explained to them. The American College of Obstetrics and Gynecology recommends that pregnant women exposed to parvovirus B19 should have serologic testing performed to determine susceptibility and possible evidence of acute parvovirus B19 infection. Pregnant women with evidence of acute parvovirus B19 infection should be monitored closely (eg, serial ultrasonographic examinations) by their obstetric provider. In pregnant women with suspected or proven

intrauterine parvovirus B19 infection, amniotic fluid and fetal tissues should be considered infectious and contact precautions should be used in addition to standard precautions if exposure is likely.

- Children with EI may attend child care or school, because they no longer are contagious once the rash appears.
- Transmission of parvovirus B19 is likely to be decreased through use of routine infection-control practices, including hand hygiene and proper disposal of used facial tissues.
- In July 2009, the US Food and Drug Administration issued a guidance for nucleic acid amplification testing to reduce the possible risk of parvovirus B19 transmission by plasma-derived products (**www.fda.gov/biologicsbloodvaccines/ guidancecomplianceregulatoryinformation/guidances/blood/ ucm071592.htm**). The goal was to identify and prevent the use of plasma-derived products containing high levels of virus. Human parvovirus B19 viral loads in manufacturing pools should not exceed 10^4 IU/mL.

Pasteurella Infections

CLINICAL MANIFESTATIONS: The most common manifestation in children is cellulitis at the site of a bite or scratch of a cat, dog, or other animal. Cellulitis typically develops within 24 hours of the injury and includes swelling, erythema, tenderness, and serous or sanguinopurulent discharge at the site. Regional lymphadenopathy, chills, and fever can occur. The most frequent local complications are abscesses and tenosynovitis, but septic arthritis and osteomyelitis also are reported. Other less common manifestations of infection include septicemia, meningitis, ocular infections (eg, conjunctivitis, corneal ulcer, endophthalmitis), endocarditis, respiratory tract infections (eg, pneumonia, pulmonary abscesses, pleural empyema), appendicitis, hepatic abscess, peritonitis, and urinary tract infection. People with liver disease, solid organ transplant, or underlying host defense abnormalities are predisposed to bacteremia with *Pasteurella multocida*.

ETIOLOGY: Members of the genus *Pasteurella* are nonmotile, facultatively anaerobic, mostly catalase and oxidase positive, gram-negative coccobacilli that are primarily respiratory tract colonizers and pathogens in animals. The most common human pathogen is *P multocida*. Most human infections are caused by the following species or subspecies: *P multocida* subspecies *multocida* (causing more than 50% of infections), *P multocida* subspecies *septica*, *Pasteurella canis*, *Pasteurella stomatis*, and *Pasteurella dagmatis*.

EPIDEMIOLOGY: *Pasteurella* species are found in the oral flora of 70% to 90% of cats, 25% to 50% of dogs, and many other animals. Transmission can occur from the bite or scratch or licking of a previous wound by a cat or dog or, less commonly, from another animal. Infected cat bite wounds contain *Pasteurella* species more often than do dog bite wounds. Rarely, respiratory tract spread occurs from animals to humans; in a significant proportion of cases, no animal exposure can be identified. Although rare, human-to-human transmission has been documented vertically from mother to neonate, horizontally from colonized humans, and by contaminated blood products.

The **incubation period** usually is less than 24 hours.

DIAGNOSTIC TESTS: The isolation of *Pasteurella* species from skin lesion drainage or other sites of infection (eg, blood, joint fluid, cerebrospinal fluid, sputum, pleural fluid, or suppurative lymph nodes) is diagnostic. *Pasteurella* species are somewhat fastidious but may be cultured on several media generally used in clinical laboratories, including sheep blood and chocolate agars, at 35°C to 37°C without increased carbon dioxide concentration. Although they resemble several other organisms morphologically, laboratory identification to the genus level generally is not difficult; however, species and subspecies differentiation is more challenging with standard biochemical testing alone.

TREATMENT: The drug of choice is penicillin. Penicillin resistance is rare, but beta-lactamase–producing strains have been recovered, especially from adults with pulmonary disease. Other oral agents that usually are effective include ampicillin, amoxicillin, cefuroxime, cefixime, cefpodoxime, doxycycline, and fluoroquinolones. Oral and parenteral antistaphylococcal penicillins and first-generation cephalosporins including cephalexin are not as active, so these are not recommended. *Pasteurella* usually is resistant to vancomycin, clindamycin, and erythromycin. For patients who are allergic to beta-lactam agents, azithromycin or trimethoprim-sulfamethoxazole are alternative choices, but clinical experience with these agents is limited. For suspected polymicrobial infected bites, oral amoxicillin-clavulanate or, for severe infection, intravenous ampicillin-sulbactam, ticarcillin-clavulanate, or piperacillin-tazobactam can be given. The duration of therapy usually is 7 to 10 days for local infections and 10 to 14 days for more severe infections. Antimicrobial therapy should be continued for 4 to 6 weeks for bone and joint infections. Wound drainage or débridement may be necessary.

ISOLATION OF THE HOSPITALIZED PATIENT: Standard precautions are recommended.

CONTROL MEASURES: Limiting contact with wild animals and education about appropriate contact with domestic animals can help to prevent *Pasteurella* infections (see Bite Wounds, p 205). Animal bites and scratches should be irrigated, cleansed, and débrided promptly. Antimicrobial prophylaxis for selected children depending on the type of animal bite wound should be initiated according to the recommendations in Table 2.16, p 205.

Pediculosis Capitis[1]
(Head Lice)

CLINICAL MANIFESTATIONS: Itching is the most common symptom of head lice infestation, but many children are asymptomatic. Adult lice or eggs (nits) are found on the hair and are most readily apparent behind the ears and near the nape of the neck. Excoriations and crusting caused by secondary bacterial infection may occur and often are associated with regional lymphadenopathy. Head lice usually deposit their eggs on a hair shaft 4 mm or less from the scalp. Because hair grows at a rate of approximately 1 cm per month, the duration of infestation can be estimated by the distance of the nit from the scalp.

ETIOLOGY: *Pediculus humanus capitis* is the head louse. Both nymphs and adult lice feed on human blood.

EPIDEMIOLOGY: In the United States, head lice infestation is most common in children attending child care and elementary school. Head lice infestation is not a sign of poor hygiene. All socioeconomic groups are affected. In the United States, infestations are less common in black children than in children of other races. Head lice infestation is not influenced by hair length or frequency of shampooing or brushing. Head lice are not a health

---

[1]American Academy of Pediatrics, Committee on School Health and Committee on Infectious Diseases. Clinical report: head lice. *Pediatrics.* 2010;126(2):392–403

hazard, because they are not responsible for spread of any disease. Head lice are only able to crawl; therefore, transmission occurs mainly by direct head-to-head contact with hair of infested people. Transmission by contact with personal belongings, such as combs, hair brushes, and hats, is uncommon. Away from the scalp, head lice survive fewer than 2 days at room temperature, and their eggs generally become nonviable within a week and cannot hatch at a lower ambient temperature than that near the scalp.

The **incubation period** from the laying of eggs to hatching of the first nymph usually is about 8 to 9 days but can vary from 7 to 12 days, being somewhat shorter in hot climates and longer in cold climates. Lice mature to the adult stage approximately 9 to 12 days later. Adult females then may lay eggs (nits), but these will develop only if the female has mated.

DIAGNOSTIC TESTS: Identification of eggs (nits), nymphs, and lice with the naked eye is possible; diagnosis can be confirmed by using a hand lens, dermatoscope (epiluminescence microscope), or traditional microscope. Nymphal and adult lice shun light and move rapidly and conceal themselves. Wetting the hair with water, oil, or a conditioner and using a fine-tooth comb may improve the ability to diagnose infestation and shorten examination time. It is important to differentiate nits from dandruff, benign hair casts (a layer of follicular cells that may slide easily off the hair shaft), plugs of desquamated cells, external hair debris, and fungal infections of the hair. Because nits remain affixed to the hair firmly, even if dead or hatched, the mere presence of nits is not a sign of an active infestation.

TREATMENT: A number of effective pediculicidal agents are available to treat head lice infestation (see Drugs for Parasitic Infections, p 927). Costs vary by product (see Table 3.46). Safety is a major concern with pediculicides, because the infestation itself presents minimal risk to the host. Pediculicides should be used only as directed and with care. Instructions on proper use of any product should be explained carefully. Therapy can be started with over-the-counter 1% permethrin or with a pyrethrin combined with piperonyl butoxide product, both of which have good safety profiles. However, resistance to these compounds has been documented in the United States. For treatment failures not attributable to improper use of an over-the-counter pediculicide, malathion, benzyl alcohol lotion, spinosad suspension, or ivermectin lotion should be used. When lice are resistant to all topical agents, oral ivermectin may be used, although the oral formulation is not approved by the Food and Drug Administration (FDA) as a pediculicide. Drugs that

Table 3.46. Topical Pediculicides for the Treatment of Head Lice

Product	Availability	Cost Estimate[a]
Permethrin 1% lotion (Nix)	Over the counter	$
Pyrethrins + piperonyl butoxide (Rid)	Over the counter	$
Malathion 0.5% (Ovide)	Prescription	$$$$
Benzyl alcohol 5% (Ulesfia)	Prescription	$$–$$$$[b]
Spinosad 0.9% suspension (Natroba)	Prescription	$$$$
Ivermectin 0.5% lotion (Sklice)	Prescription	$$$$

[a] $, <$25; $$, $26-$99; $$$, $100-$199; $$$$, $200-$299.
[b] Cost varies by length of hair, which impacts number of units of product required.

have residual activity may kill nymphs as they emerge from eggs. Pediculicides that are not sufficiently ovicidal usually require more than one application. Ideally, retreatment should occur after the eggs that are present at the time of initial treatment have hatched but before any new eggs have been produced.

- **Permethrin (1%).** Permethrin is available without a prescription in a 1% lotion that is applied to the scalp and hair for 10 minutes after shampooing with a nonconditioning shampoo and towel drying the hair. Permethrin has a low potential for toxic effects and can be highly effective, although widespread resistance in the United States may limit overall effectiveness. Although activity of permethrin can continue for 2 weeks or more after application, some experts advise a second treatment 9 to 10 days after the first treatment, especially if hair is washed within a week after the first treatment. Product labeling recommends a second treatment 7 or more days after the first application if live lice are seen. Permethrin 1% is approved by the FDA for use on children 2 months or older.

- **Pyrethrin-based products.** Pyrethrins are natural extracts from the chrysanthemum and are available (usually formulated with the synergist piperonyl butoxide) without a prescription as shampoos or mousse preparations (both to be applied to dry hair). Pyrethrins have no residual activity and repeated application 7 to 10 days after the first application is necessary to kill newly hatched lice. Resistance to permethrin renders pyrethrin-based products ineffective. Pyrethrins are contraindicated in people who are allergic to chrysanthemums or ragweed and should only be used on children older than 2 years.

- **Malathion (0.5%).** This organophosphate pesticide that is both pediculicidal and partially ovicidal is available only by prescription as a lotion and is highly effective as formulated in the United States. The safety and effectiveness of malathion lotion have not been assessed by the FDA in children younger than 6 years. Malathion lotion is applied to dry hair, left to dry naturally, and then removed 8 to 12 hours later by washing and rinsing the hair. The product should be reapplied 7 to 9 days later only if live lice still are present at that time. The alcohol base of the lotion is flammable; therefore, the lotion or wet hair during treatment should not be exposed to lighted cigarettes, open flames, or electric heat sources such as hair dryers or curling irons. The product, if ingested, can cause severe respiratory distress. Malathion is contraindicated in children younger than 2 years because of the possibility of increased scalp permeability and absorption.

- **Benzyl alcohol lotion (5%).** Benzyl alcohol is available by prescription in a lotion formulated with mineral oil and is highly effective as a pediculicide. This agent has been evaluated by the FDA for use in children 6 months or older. When applied, sufficient amounts should be used on dry hair to saturate the scalp and entire length of the hair, and then washed off after 10 minutes. Retreatment after 7 days is recommended to kill any newly hatched lice. Benzyl alcohol use in neonates has been associated with neonatal gasping syndrome and should not be used in infants younger than 6 months.

- **Spinosad suspension (0.9%).** This product, which contains benzyl alcohol and spinosad as the active compound, was approved by the FDA in 2011 for treatment of head lice infestation in children. Enough of the suspension is used to cover dry hair completely, starting with the scalp, and is left on for 10 minutes. Spinosad is approved for topical use in children 6 months and older. Because of the benzyl alcohol, this product should not be used in infants younger than 6 months. A second treatment is applied at 7 days if live lice still are seen.

- **Ivermectin lotion (0.5%).** Ivermectin interferes with the function of invertebrate nerve and muscle cells. It is used widely as an anthelmintic agent. The 0.5% lotion was approved by the FDA in 2012 as a single-application, topical treatment of head lice in people 6 months and older. The lotion is applied to dry hair, starting with the scalp, in an amount sufficient to coat the hair and scalp thoroughly. After a 10-minute application, the lotion is rinsed off with water.
- **Oral ivermectin.** Oral ivermectin has not been evaluated by the FDA as a pediculicide. Ivermectin may be effective against head lice if sufficient concentration is present in the blood at the time a louse feeds. It has been given as a single oral dose of 200 µg/kg or 400 µg/kg, with a second dose given after 9 to 10 days. Fewer failures occur at the 400 µg/kg dose. Because it blocks essential neural transmission if it crosses the blood-brain barrier and young children may be at higher risk of this adverse drug reaction, ivermectin should not be used in children weighing less than 15 kg (33 pounds).
- **Lindane shampoo, 1%.** Because of safety concerns, a high rate of treatment failure, and availability of other treatments, **lindane shampoo should not be used in the treatment of pediculosis capitis**. Infants, children weighing less than 50 kg (110 lb), and patients with other skin conditions such as atopic dermatitis are at risk of serious neurotoxicity from lindane use. An FDA "boxed" warning is in effect for lindane shampoo.

Other off-label treatments are detailed in the clinical report on head lice published by the American Academy of Pediatrics in 2010.[1] With the recommended products available today and the limited data on effectiveness of these other treatments, including oral trimethoprim-sulfamethoxazole, it is unlikely that any would be used.

Data are lacking to determine whether suffocation of lice by application of some occlusive agents, such as petroleum jelly, olive oil, butter, or fat-containing mayonnaise, is effective as a method of treatment. Because pediculicides kill lice shortly after application, detection of living lice on scalp inspection 24 hours or more after treatment suggests incorrect use of pediculicide, hatching of lice after treatment, reinfestation, or resistance to therapy. In such situations, after excluding incorrect use, immediate retreatment with a different pediculicide followed by a second application 7 to 10 days later is recommended. Itching or mild burning of the scalp caused by inflammation of the skin in response to topical therapeutic agents can persist for many days after lice are killed and is not a reason for retreatment. Topical corticosteroid and oral antihistamine agents may be beneficial for relieving these signs and symptoms. Manual removal of nits after successful treatment with a pediculicide is helpful, because none of the pediculicides are 100% ovicidal. Fine-toothed nit combs designed for this purpose are available. Removal of nits is tedious and time consuming but may be attempted for aesthetic reasons, to decrease diagnostic confusion, or to improve therapeutic efficacy.

ISOLATION OF THE HOSPITALIZED PATIENT: In addition to standard precautions, contact precautions are recommended until the patient has been treated with an appropriate pediculicide.

CONTROL MEASURES: Household and other close contacts should be examined and treated if infested. Bedmates of infested people should be treated prophylactically at the same time as the infested household members and contacts. Prophylactic treatment of other noninfested people is not recommended. Children should not be excluded or sent

[1]American Academy of Pediatrics, Committee on School Health and Committee on Infectious Diseases. Clinical report: head lice. *Pediatrics.* 2010;126(2):392–403

home early from school because of head lice. Parents of children with infestation (ie, at least 1 live, crawling louse) should be notified and informed that their child should be treated. The presence of nits alone does not justify treatment.

"No-nit" policies requiring that children be free of nits before they return to a child care facility or school have not been effective in controlling head lice transmission and are not recommended. Egg cases farther from the scalp are easier to discover, but these tend to be empty (hatched) or nonviable and, thus, are of no consequence.

Supplemental measures generally are not required to eliminate an infestation. Head lice only rarely are transferred via fomites from shared headgear, clothing, combs, or bedding. Special handling of such items is not likely to be useful. If desired, hats, bedding, clothing, and towels worn or used by the infested person in the 2-day period just before treatment is started can be machine-washed and dried using the hot water and hot air cycles, respectively, because lice and eggs are killed by exposure for 5 minutes to temperatures greater than 53.5°C (128.3°F). Vacuuming furniture and floors can remove an infested person's hairs that might have viable nits attached. Environmental insecticide sprays increase chemical exposure of household members and have not been helpful in the control of head lice. Treatment of dogs, cats, or other pets is not indicated, because they do not play a role in transmission of human head lice.

Pediculosis Corporis
(Body Lice)

CLINICAL MANIFESTATIONS: Intense itching, particularly at night, is common with body lice infestations. Bites manifest as small erythematous macules, papules, and excoriations primarily on the trunk. In heavily bitten areas, typically around the mid-section, the skin can become thickened and discolored. Secondary bacterial infection of the skin (pyoderma) caused by scratching is common.

ETIOLOGY: *Pediculus humanus corporis* (or *humanus*) is the body louse. Nymphs and adult lice feed on human blood.

EPIDEMIOLOGY: Body lice generally are restricted to people living in crowded conditions without access to regular bathing or changes of clothing (refugees, victims of war or natural disasters, homeless people). Under these conditions, body lice can spread rapidly through direct contact or contact with contaminated clothing or bedding. Body lice live in clothes or bedding, lay their eggs on or near the seams of clothing, and move to the skin to feed. Body lice cannot survive away from a blood source for longer than approximately 5 to 7 days at room temperature. In contrast with head lice, body lice are well-recognized vectors of disease (eg, epidemic typhus, trench fever, epidemic relapsing fever, and bacillary angiomatosis).

The **incubation period** from laying eggs to hatching of the first nymph is approximately 1 to 2 weeks, depending on ambient temperature. Lice mature and are capable of reproducing 9 to 19 days after hatching, depending on whether infested clothing is removed for sleeping.

DIAGNOSTIC TESTS: Identification of eggs, nymphs, and lice with the naked eye is possible; diagnosis can be confirmed by using a hand lens, dermatoscope (epiluminescence microscope), or a traditional microscope. Adult and nymphal body lice seldom are seen on the body, because they generally are sequestered in clothing.

TREATMENT: Treatment consists of improving hygiene and regular changes of clean clothes and bedding. Infested materials can be decontaminated by washing in hot water (at least 53.5°C [128.3°F]), by machine drying at hot temperatures, by dry cleaning, or by pressing with a hot iron. Temperatures exceeding 53.5°C (128.3°F) for 5 minutes are lethal to lice and eggs. Pediculicides usually are not necessary if materials are laundered at least weekly (see Drugs for Parasitic Infections, p 927). Some people with much body hair may require full-body treatment with a pediculicide, because lice and eggs may adhere to body hair.

ISOLATION OF THE HOSPITALIZED PATIENT: In addition to standard precautions, contact precautions are recommended until the patient has been treated.

CONTROL MEASURES: The most important factor in the control of body lice infestation is the ability to change and wash clothing. Close contacts should be examined and treated appropriately; clothing and bedding should be laundered using hot water and dried using the hot cycle.

Pediculosis Pubis
(Pubic Lice, Crab Lice)

CLINICAL MANIFESTATIONS: Pruritus of the anogenital area is a common symptom in pubic lice infestations ("crabs" or "phthiriasis"). The parasite most frequently is found in the pubic region, but infestation can involve the eyelashes, eyebrows, beard, axilla, perianal area, and rarely, the scalp. A characteristic sign of heavy pubic lice infestation is the presence of bluish or slate-colored macules (maculae ceruleae) on the chest, abdomen, or thighs.

ETIOLOGY: *Pthirus pubis* is the pubic or crab louse. Nymphs and adult lice feed on human blood.

EPIDEMIOLOGY: Pubic lice infestations are more prevalent in adults and usually are transmitted through sexual contact. Transmission by contaminated items, such as towels, is uncommon. Pubic lice on the eyelashes or eyebrows of children may be evidence of sexual abuse, although other modes of transmission are possible (see Sexual Victimization and STIs, p 185). Infested people should be examined for other sexually transmitted infections (see Sexually Transmitted Infections in Adolescents and Children, p 177). Adult pubic lice can survive away from a host for up to 36 hours, and their eggs can remain viable for up to 10 days under suitable environmental conditions.

The **incubation period** from the laying of eggs to the hatching of the first nymph is approximately 6 to 10 days. Adult lice become capable of reproducing approximately 2 to 3 weeks after hatching.

DIAGNOSTIC TESTS: Identification of eggs (nits), nymphs, and lice with the naked eye is possible; the diagnosis can be confirmed by using a hand lens, microscope or dermatoscope.

TREATMENT: All areas of the body with coarse hair should be examined for evidence of pubic lice infestation. Lice and their eggs can be removed manually, or the hairs can be shaved to eliminate infestation immediately. Caution should be used when inspecting, removing or treating lice on or near the eyelashes. Pediculicides used to treat other kinds of louse infestations are effective for treatment of pubic lice (see Pediculosis Capitis, p 597; and Drugs for Parasitic Infections, p 927) although treatment is off-label for all products except pyrethrin with piperonyl butoxide and lindane shampoo. Retreatment is recommended as for head lice.

Topical pediculicides should not be used for treatment of pubic lice infestation of eyelashes; an ophthalmic-grade petrolatum ointment applied to the eyelashes 2 to 4 times daily for 8 to 10 days is effective.

ISOLATION OF THE HOSPITALIZED PATIENT: In addition to standard precautions, contact precautions are recommended until the patient has been treated with an appropriate pediculicide.

CONTROL MEASURES: All sexual contacts should be examined and treated, as needed. Patients should be advised to avoid sexual contact until they and their sex partner have been treated successfully. Bedding, towels, and clothing can be decontaminated by laundering in hot water and machine drying using a hot cycle or by dry cleaning.

Pelvic Inflammatory Disease

CLINICAL MANIFESTATIONS: Pelvic inflammatory disease (PID) comprises a spectrum of inflammatory disorders of the female upper genital tract, including any combination of endometritis, parametritis, salpingitis, oophoritis, tubo-ovarian abscess (TOA), and pelvic peritonitis. Acute PID is difficult to diagnose because of the wide variation in symptoms and signs. Symptoms of acute PID include unilateral or bilateral lower abdominal or pelvic pain, fever, vomiting, abnormal vaginal discharge, irregular vaginal bleeding, and pain with intercourse. The severity of symptoms varies widely and may range from indolent to severe. Patients occasionally present with right upper quadrant abdominal pain resulting from perihepatitis (Fitz-Hugh-Curtis syndrome). Many episodes of PID go undiagnosed and untreated because the patient and/or health care professional fails to recognize the implications of mild or nonspecific symptoms and signs. Silent PID is a term that can be applied to women with very minimal or no symptoms, and there is a growing body of evidence that this represents a large proportion of all PID cases. In subclinical PID, mild inflammation occurs within the reproductive tract at a very low level, yet damage to the fallopian tubes or surrounding structures is occurring. Clinicians need to recognize the implication of mild or nonspecific findings, particularly in a young female who might give an incomplete or inaccurate sexual history.

Examination findings vary but may include oral temperature >101°F (>38.3°C), lower abdominal tenderness with or without peritoneal signs, cervical or vaginal discharge, tenderness with lateral motion of the cervix, uterine tenderness, unilateral or bilateral adnexal tenderness, and adnexal fullness. Pyuria (presence of white blood cells [WBCs] on urine microscopy), abundant WBCs on saline microscopy of vaginal fluid, an elevated erythrocyte sedimentation rate, elevated C-reactive protein, and/or an adnexal mass demonstrated by abdominal or transvaginal ultrasonography are findings that support a diagnosis of PID.

Complications of PID include perihepatitis (Fitz-Hugh-Curtis syndrome) and tubo-ovarian abscess/complex formation. Long-term sequelae include tubal scarring that can cause infertility in 20% of females, ectopic pregnancy in 9%, and chronic pelvic pain in 18%. Factors that may increase the likelihood of infertility are delay in diagnosis or initiation of antimicrobial therapy, younger age at time of infection, chlamydial infection, and PID determined to be severe by laparoscopic examination.

ETIOLOGY: *Neisseria gonorrhoeae* and *Chlamydia trachomatis* are the pathogens most commonly isolated in PID, although the proportion of PID cases attributable to these pathogens is declining. Numerous other organisms have been isolated from upper genital tract cultures of females with PID, including anaerobes such as *Bacteroides* species and *Peptostreptococcus* species, facultative anaerobes including *Gardnerella vaginalis, Haemophilus influenzae, Streptococcus* species, *Actinomyces israeli*, enteric gram-negative bacilli, and cytomegalovirus. Genital mycoplasmas, including *Mycoplasma genitalium, Mycoplasma hominis,* and *Ureaplasma urealyticum*, also have been associated with PID. Polymicrobial infection is common. However, in more than half of cases, no organism is identified in lower genital tract specimens (ie, endocervical or vaginal specimens). More recent data suggest that *M genitalium* may play a role in the pathogenesis of PID, although there is currently no test cleared by the US Food and Drug Administration (FDA) for *M genitalium*.

EPIDEMIOLOGY: Although many of the issues pertaining to high-risk sexual behavior and acquisition of sexually transmitted infections (STIs) are common to both adolescents and adults, they often are intensified among adolescents because of both behavioral and biological predispositions. Adolescents and young women can be at higher risk of STIs and PID because of behavioral factors such as inconsistent use of barrier contraceptives, douching, greater number of current and lifetime sexual partners, and use of alcohol and other substances that may impair judgment while engaging in sexual activity. Latex condoms may reduce the risk of PID. Use of oral contraceptives have been associated with a reduced risk of PID. In addition to the protective effects, oral contraceptives seem to be associated with a decrease in the severity of inflammation. Evidence regarding the risks of PID related to use of intrauterine devices (IUDs), specifically in adolescents, is limited, but research shows that IUDs do not increase the long-term risk of PID, and the benefits of IUDs may likely outweigh the risks.

An **incubation period** for PID is undefined.

DIAGNOSTIC TESTS: Diagnostic criteria recommended by the Centers for Disease Control and Prevention (CDC) are presented in Table 3.47 (p 605). No single symptom, sign, or laboratory or imaging finding is sensitive and specific for the diagnosis of acute PID. The diagnosis of PID typically is accomplished by using a combination of clinical symptoms and signs, examination, and laboratory tests. Adnexal tenderness on bimanual examination of a patient who has been sexually active has been described as the most sensitive finding for PID. Additional criteria can be used to make the diagnosis of PID more specific (Table 3.47) in patients with no evidence of lower genital tract infection (ie, mucopurulent cervical discharge or evidence of WBCs on a microscopic evaluation of a saline preparation of vaginal fluid [ie, wet prep]). If the cervical discharge appears normal and no WBCs are observed on the wet prep of vaginal fluid, the diagnosis of PID is unlikely, and alternative causes of pain should be considered. A vaginal swab for *C trachomatis* and *N gonorrhoeae*, such as nucleic acid amplification tests, should be obtained in all patients with suspected PID. When the diagnosis of PID is in doubt, there is concern for a tubo-ovarian abscess, or the patient is not responding to conventional therapy, further diagnostic evaluation using ultrasonography and/or magnetic resonance imaging (MRI) may be helpful. Laparoscopy is the gold standard for diagnosis, allowing direct visualization of the adnexal structures as well as allowing bacteriologic specimens to be obtained directly from tubal exudate or the cul-de-sac. Endometrial biopsy may demonstrate histopathologic evidence of endometritis and may be the only sign of PID in some females. Because of their

Table 3.47. Criteria for Clinical Diagnosis of Pelvic Inflammatory Disease (PID)[a]

Minimum Criteria

Empiric treatment of PID should be initiated in sexually active young women if they are experiencing pelvic or lower abdominal pain, if one or more of the following **minimum criteria** are present, and no other cause(s) for the illness can be identified:

- Uterine tenderness
- Adnexal tenderness
- Cervical motion tenderness

Additional Criteria

These criteria may be used to enhance the specificity of the minimum criteria. Additional criteria that support a diagnosis of PID include the following:

- Oral temperature greater than 38.3°C (101°F)
- Mucopurulent cervical or vaginal discharge
- Presence of white blood cells (WBCs) on saline microscopy of vaginal secretions
- Increased erythrocyte sedimentation rate
- Increased C-reactive protein concentration
- Laboratory documentation of cervical infection with *Neisseria gonorrhoeae* or *Chlamydia trachomatis*

Most women with PID have mucopurulent cervical discharge or evidence of WBCs on a microscopic evaluation of a saline preparation of vaginal fluid. If the cervical discharge appears normal **and** no WBCs are found on the wet preparation, the diagnosis of PID is unlikely, and alternative causes of pain should be sought.

The **most specific criteria** for diagnosing PID include the following:

- Endometrial biopsy with histopathologic evidence of endometritis
- Transvaginal ultrasonography or magnetic resonance imaging techniques showing thickened, fluid-filled tubes with or without free pelvic fluid or tubo-ovarian complex, or ultrasonographic studies suggesting pelvic infection (eg, tubal hyperemia)
- Laparoscopic abnormalities consistent with PID

A diagnostic evaluation that includes some of these more extensive studies may be warranted in some cases.

[a]Adapted from the Centers for Disease Control and Prevention. Sexually transmitted diseases treatment guidelines, 2014. *MMWR Recomm Rep.* 2015; in press (see **www.cdc.gov/std/treatment**).

high cost and invasive nature, however, these procedures are not indicated for diagnosis of PID in most cases. Pregnancy must be ruled out in all patients evaluated for PID.

TREATMENT: A sexually active female with lower abdominal pain who exhibits uterine, adnexal, or cervical motion tenderness on bimanual examination should be treated for PID if no other cause is identified. To minimize risks of progressive infection and subsequent infertility, treatment should be initiated at the time of clinical diagnosis, and therapy should be completed, regardless of the results of STI testing.

Among women with mild to moderate PID, there is no difference in clinical course, recurrent PID, chronic pelvic pain, or rates of infertility between women hospitalized for PID and those treated as outpatients (Table 3.48, p 607). No evidence is available to suggest that adolescents benefit from hospitalization for treatment of PID. The decision to hospitalize adolescents with acute PID should be made on the basis of the same criteria used for older women and should be based on the judgment of the provider and whether the patient meets any of the following suggested criteria:

- surgical emergencies, such as ectopic pregnancy or appendicitis, or another serious condition cannot be excluded;
- the patient's illness is severe (eg, vomiting, severe pain, overt peritonitis, or high fever);
- the patient has a tubo-ovarian abscess;
- the patient is pregnant;
- the patient is unable to follow or tolerate an outpatient regimen; or
- the patient has failed to respond clinically to outpatient therapy.

The antimicrobial regimen chosen should provide empiric, broad-spectrum coverage directed against the most common causative agents, including *N gonorrhoeae* and *C trachomatis*, even if these pathogens are not identified in lower genital tract specimens (Table 3.48, p 607). As a result of the emergence of quinolone-resistant *N gonorrhoeae*, fluoroquinolones no longer are recommended for the treatment of PID. Although other second- and third-generation parenteral cephalosporins may be effective in the treatment of PID, cefoxitin and cefotetan are advantageous, because they are more active against anaerobic bacteria. Ceftriaxone, however, may be preferred for its greater efficacy against *N gonorrhoeae*. Empiric therapy for anaerobic pathogens should be provided for patients with tubo-ovarian abscess, severe or recurrent PID, recent pelvic surgery, or evidence of bacterial vaginosis.

Evidence is limited for alternative outpatient regimens. For people with severe cephalosporin allergy, the use of a fluoroquinolone (levofloxacin, 500 mg, once daily for 14 days, or ofloxacin, 400 mg, twice daily for 14 days) with or without metronidazole (500 mg, orally, twice daily for 14 days) can be considered, provided the community prevalence as well as individual risk for gonococcal infection are low. If a culture test for *N gonorrhoeae* is positive, antimicrobial susceptibility testing should guide therapy. If the organism is quinolone resistant or if antimicrobial susceptibility cannot be assessed, the CDC recommends the addition of azithromycin (2 g, orally, as a single dose) to the quinolone-based regimen listed above.

A critical component to the outpatient management is short-term follow-up, especially in the adolescent population. Outpatients should be reevaluated after 72 hours of therapy; hospitalization and/or further diagnostics should be considered in women without clinical improvement. Hospitalized patients may be changed to oral therapy 24 hours after demonstrating significant clinical improvement. After discharge, 14 days of therapy should be completed. A diagnosis of Fitz-Hugh-Curtis syndrome does not alter the treatment regimen. Patients with tubo-ovarian abscess should have at least 24 hours of inpatient treatment that includes anaerobic coverage; on discharge, patients should complete a 14-day course of doxycycline (100 mg, orally, twice a day) or clindamycin (450 mg, orally, 4 times a day). Evidence is insufficient to recommend the removal of IUDs in women diagnosed with acute PID. However, caution should be exercised if the IUD remains in place, and close clinical follow-up is mandatory.

ISOLATION OF THE HOSPITALIZED PATIENT: Standard precautions are recommended.

CONTROL MEASURES[1]:
- Male sexual partners of patients with PID should receive diagnostic evaluation for gonococcal and chlamydial urethritis and should be treated presumptively for both

---

[1]Centers for Disease Control and Prevention. Recommendations for partner services programs for HIV infection, syphilis, gonorrhea, and chlamydial infection. *MMWR Recomm Rep.* 2008;57(RR-9):1–63

Table 3.48. Recommended Treatment of Pelvic Inflammatory Disease (PID)[a]

Parenteral Regimen A[b]

Cefotetan, 2 g, IV, every 12 h **OR Cefoxitin,** 2 g, IV, every 6 h
PLUS

Doxycycline, 1100 mg, orally or IV, every 12 h to complete 14 days[c]

OR

Parenteral: Regimen B[d]

Clindamycin, 900 mg, IV, every 8 h
PLUS

Gentamicin: loading dose, IV or IM (2 mg/kg), followed by maintenance dose (1.5 mg/kg) every 8 h. Single daily dosing (3–5 mg/kg) can be substituted.

NOTE

Parenteral therapy may be discontinued 24 h after a patient improves clinically; continuing oral therapy should consist of doxycycline (100 mg, orally, twice a day) or clindamycin (450 mg, orally, 4 times a day) to complete a total of 14 days of therapy. Clindamycin should be used if tubo-ovarian abscess is present.

Outpatient Regimen[e]

Ceftriaxone, 250 mg, IM, once **OR Cefoxitin,** 2 g, IM, and **probenecid,** 1 g, orally,

in a single dose concurrently **OR** Other parenteral extended-spectrum **cephalosporin[f]** (eg, **ceftizoxime** or **cefotaxime**)
PLUS

Doxycycline, 100 mg, orally, twice a day for 14 days
WITH or WITHOUT

Metronidazole, 500 mg, orally, twice a day for 14 days

IV indicates intravenous; IM, intramuscular; NAAT, nucleic acid amplification test; GC, gonococcal.

[a] Additional regimens may be found in: Centers for Disease Control and Prevention. Sexually transmitted diseases treatment guidelines, 2014. *MMWR Recomm Rep.* 2015; in press (see www.cdc.gov/std/treatment).

[b] Hospitalization and parenteral treatment is recommended if patient has severe illness such as tubo-ovarian abscess, is pregnant, or is unable to tolerate or follow ambulatory regimens.

[c] Metronidazole may be added for anaerobic coverage.

[d] Alternative parenteral regimens include ampicillin-sulbactam (3 g, IV, every 6 hours) plus doxycycline (100 mg, IV or orally, every 12 hours).

[e] Patients with inadequate response to outpatient therapy after 72 hours should be reevaluated for possible misdiagnosis and may require parenteral therapy.

[f] Data to indicate whether expanded-spectrum cephalosporins (ceftizoxime, cefotaxime, ceftriaxone) can replace cefoxitin or cefotetan are limited. Many experts believe they also are effective therapy for PID, but they are less active against anaerobes.

infections if they had sexual contact with the patient during the 60 days preceding onset of symptoms in the patient. A large proportion of these males will be asymptomatic.

- The patient should abstain from sexual intercourse until she and her partner(s) have completed treatment.
- The patient and her partner(s) should be encouraged to use condoms consistently and correctly.
- The patient should be screened for other STIs, including human immunodeficiency virus (HIV).
- Unimmunized or incompletely immunized patients should complete the immunization series for human papillomavirus and hepatitis B (see **http://redbook.solutions.aap. org/SS/Immunization_Schedules.aspx**).
- Because of the high risk of reinfection, patients who test positive for *N gonorrhoeae* or *C trachomatis* should be retested 3 months after completing treatment or at their next clinical encounter within 12 months of treatment.
- Patients with *N gonorrhoeae* infection who are not treated with a parenteral cephalosporin should have a test of cure at the completion of therapy.
- The diagnosis of PID provides an opportunity to educate the adolescent about prevention of STIs, including abstinence, consistent use of barrier methods of protection, immunization, and the importance of receiving periodic screening for STIs.

Pertussis (Whooping Cough)

CLINICAL MANIFESTATIONS: Pertussis begins with mild upper respiratory tract symptoms similar to the common cold (catarrhal stage) and progresses to cough and then usually to paroxysms of cough (paroxysmal stage), characterized by inspiratory whoop and commonly followed by vomiting. Fever is absent or minimal. Symptoms wane gradually over weeks to months (convalescent stage). Cough illness in immunized children and adults can range from typical to mild and unrecognized. The duration of classic pertussis is 6 to 10 weeks. Approximately half of adolescents with pertussis cough for 10 weeks or longer. Complications among adolescents and adults include syncope, weight loss, sleep disturbance, incontinence, rib fractures, and pneumonia; among adults, complications increase with age. Pertussis is most severe when it occurs during the first 6 months of life, particularly in preterm and unimmunized infants. Disease in infants younger than 6 months can be atypical with a short catarrhal stage, followed by gagging, gasping, bradycardia, or apnea (67%) as prominent early manifestations; absence of whoop; and prolonged convalescence. Sudden unexpected death can be caused by pertussis. Complications among infants include pneumonia (23%) and pulmonary hypertension as well as complications related to severe coughing spells, such as subdural bleeding, conjunctival bleeding, and hernia; and severe coughing spells leading to hypoxia and complications such as seizures (2%), encephalopathy (less than 0.5%), apnea, and death. More than two thirds of infants with pertussis are hospitalized. Case-fatality rates are approximately 1% in infants younger than 2 months and less than 0.5% in infants 2 through 11 months of age. Previous immunization reduces morbidity and mortality in infants.

ETIOLOGY: Pertussis is caused by a fastidious, gram-negative, pleomorphic bacillus, *Bordetella pertussis.* Other causes of sporadic prolonged cough illness include *Bordetella parapertussis, Mycoplasma pneumoniae, Chlamydia trachomatis, Chlamydophila pneumoniae, Bordetella* *bronchiseptica* (the cause of kennel cough), *Bordetella holmesii* and certain respiratory tract viruses, particularly adenoviruses and respiratory syncytial viruses.

EPIDEMIOLOGY: Humans are the only known hosts of *B pertussis*. Transmission occurs by close contact with cases via aerosolized droplets. Cases occur year round, typically with a late summer-autumn peak. Neither infection nor immunization provides lifelong immunity. Lack of natural booster events and waning immunity since the most recent immunization, particularly when acellular pertussis vaccine is used for the entire immunization series, are responsible for increased cases reported in school-aged children, adolescents, and adults. Additionally, waning maternal immunity and reduced transplacental antibody in mothers who have not received Tdap vaccine during pregnancy contribute to an increase in pertussis in very young infants. More than 41 000 cases of pertussis were reported in the United States in 2012, the highest in over 50 years. As many as 80% of previously immunized household contacts of symptomatic cases are infected with pertussis because of waning vaccine-induced immunity. Symptoms in these contacts vary from asymptomatic infection to classic pertussis. Older siblings (including adolescents) and adults with mild or unrecognized atypical disease are important sources of pertussis for infants and young children. Infected people are most contagious during the catarrhal stage through the third week after onset of paroxysms. Factors affecting the length of communicability include age, immunization status or previous infection, and appropriate antimicrobial therapy.

The **incubation period** is 7 to 10 days, with a range of 5 to 21 days.

DIAGNOSTIC TESTS: Culture is considered the "gold standard" for laboratory diagnosis of pertussis; however, although culture is 100% specific, it is not optimally sensitive, because *B pertussis* is a fastidious organism. Culture requires collection of an appropriate nasopharyngeal specimen, obtained either by aspiration or with Dacron (polyethylene terephthalate) or calcium alginate swabs. Specimens must be placed into special transport media (such as Regan-Lowe) immediately and not allowed to dry while being transported promptly to the laboratory. Culture results can be negative if taken from a previously immunized person, if antimicrobial therapy has been started, if more than 2 weeks has elapsed since cough onset, or if the specimen is not handled appropriately.

Polymerase chain reaction (PCR) assay now is the most commonly used laboratory method for detection of *B pertussis* because of its improved sensitivity and more rapid turnaround time. The PCR test requires collection of an adequate nasopharyngeal specimen using a Dacron swab or nasopharyngeal wash or aspirate. Calcium alginate swabs are inhibitory to PCR and should not be used for PCR tests. The PCR test has optimal sensitivity during the first 3 weeks of cough, is unlikely to be useful if antimicrobial therapy has been given for more than 5 days, and lacks sensitivity in previously immunized people, but still is more sensitive than culture. Unacceptably high rates of false-positive results are reported from some laboratories, and pseudo-outbreaks linked to contaminated specimens also have been reported.[1] The Centers for Disease Control and Prevention (CDC) has released a "best practices" document to guide pertussis PCR assays (**www. cdc.gov/pertussis/clinical/diagnostic-testing/diagnosis-pcr-bestpractices. html**) as well as a video demonstrating optimal specimen collection. Multiple DNA target

[1]Mandal S, Tatti KM, Woods-Stout D, et al. Pertussis pseudo-outbreak linked to specimens contaminated by Bordetella pertussis DNA from clinic surfaces. *Pediatrics.* 2012;129(2):e424–e430

sequences are required to distinguish between *Bordetella* species. Direct fluorescent antibody testing no longer is recommended.

Commercial serologic tests for pertussis infection can be helpful for diagnosis, especially later in illness and in adolescents and adults. However, no commercial kit is cleared by the US Food and Drug Administration (FDA) for diagnostic use. Cutoff points for diagnostic values of immunoglobulin (Ig) G antibody to pertussis toxin (PT) have not been established by the FDA, and IgA and IgM assays lack adequate sensitivity and specificity. In the absence of recent immunization, an elevated serum IgG antibody to PT after 2 weeks of onset of cough is suggestive of recent *B pertussis* infection. An increasing titer, a single IgG anti-PT value of approximately 100 IU/mL or greater (using standard reference sera as a comparator), or a decreasing titer if obtained later in the illness are considered diagnostic.

An increased white blood cell count attributable to absolute lymphocytosis is suggestive of pertussis in infants and young children but often is absent in adolescents and adults with pertussis and can be only mildly abnormal in some young infants at the time of presentation. A markedly elevated white blood cell count is associated with a poor prognosis in young infants.

TREATMENT: Antimicrobial agents administered during the catarrhal stage may ameliorate the disease. Clinicians should begin antimicrobial therapy prior to test results if the clinical history is strongly suggestive of pertussis or the patient is at high risk of severe or complicated disease (eg, an infant). After the cough is established, antimicrobial agents have no discernible effect on the course of illness but are recommended to limit spread of organisms to others. A 5-day course of azithromycin is the appropriate first-line choice for treatment and for postexposure prophylaxis (PEP) (see Table 3.49, p 611).[1] A shorter course of azithromycin (eg, 3 days) has not been validated and is not recommended for PEP or treatment. Azithromycin should be used with caution in people with prolonged QT interval and proarrhythmic conditions. Resistance of *B pertussis* to macrolide antimicrobial agents has been reported, but rarely. Penicillins and first- and second-generation cephalosporins are not effective against *B pertussis*.

Antimicrobial agents used for infants younger than 6 months require special consideration. The FDA has not approved azithromycin or clarithromycin for use in infants younger than 6 months. An association between orally administered erythromycin and azithromycin with infantile hypertrophic pyloric stenosis (IHPS) has been reported in infants younger than 1 month. Azithromycin is the drug of choice for treatment or prophylaxis of pertussis in infants younger than 1 month in whom the risk of developing severe pertussis and life-threatening complications outweighs the potential risk of IHPS. All infants younger than 1 month (and preterm infants until a similar postconceptional age) who receive any macrolide should be monitored for development of IHPS during and for 1 month after completing the course (see Table 3.49, p 611). Cases of IHPS should be reported to MedWatch (see MedWatch, p 957).

Trimethoprim-sulfamethoxazole is an alternative for patients older than 2 months who cannot tolerate macrolides or who are infected with a macrolide-resistant strain, but studies evaluating trimethoprim-sulfamethoxazole as treatment for pertussis are limited.

---

[1] Centers for Disease Control and Prevention. Recommended antimicrobial agents for the treatment and postexposure prophylaxis of pertussis: 2005 CDC guidelines. *MMWR Recomm Rep.* 2005;54(RR-14):1–16

Table 3.49. Recommended Antimicrobial Therapy and Postexposure Prophylaxis for Pertussis in Infants, Children, Adolescents, and Adults[a]

Age	Recommended Drugs			Alternative
	Azithromycin	Erythromycin	Clarithromycin	TMP-SMX
Younger than 1 mo	10 mg/kg/day as a single dose daily for 5 days[b,c]	40 mg/kg/day in 4 divided doses for 14 days	Not recommended	Contraindicated at younger than 2 mo of age
1 through 5 mo	See above	See above	15 mg/kg per day in 2 divided doses for 7 days	2 mo of age or older: TMP, 8 mg/kg/day; SMX, 40 mg/kg/day in 2 doses for 14 days
6 mo or older and children	10 mg/kg as a single dose on day 1 (maximum 500 mg), then 5 mg/kg/day as a single dose on days 2 through 5 (maximum 250 mg/day)[b,d]	40 mg/kg/day in 4 divided doses for 7–14 days (maximum 1–2 g/day)	15 mg/kg/day in 2 divided doses for 7 days (maximum 1 g/day)	See above
Adolescents and adults	500 mg as a single dose on day 1, then 250 mg as a single dose on days 2 through 5[b,d]	2 g/day in 4 divided doses for 7–14 days	1 g/day in 2 divided doses for 7 days	TMP, 320 mg/day; SMX, 1600 mg/day in 2 divided doses for 14 days

TMP indicates trimethoprim; SMX, sulfamethoxazole.

[a] Centers for Disease Control and Prevention. Recommended antimicrobial agents for the treatment and postexposure prophylaxis of pertussis: 2005 CDC guidelines. *MMWR Recomm Rep.* 2005;54(RR-14):1–16

[b] Azithromycin should be used with caution in people with prolonged QT interval and certain proarrhythmic conditions.

[c] Preferred macrolide for this age because of risk of idiopathic hypertrophic pyloric stenosis associated with erythromycin.

[d] A 3-day course of azithromycin for PEP or treatment has not been validated and is not recommended.

Young infants are at increased risk of respiratory failure attributable to apnea or secondary bacterial pneumonia and are at risk of cardiopulmonary failure and death from severe pulmonary hypertension. Hospitalized young infants with pertussis should be managed in a setting/facility where these complications can be recognized and managed urgently. In infants with refractory pulmonary hypertension and markedly elevated lymphocyte counts, exchange transfusions or leukopheresis have been life-saving.

ISOLATION OF THE HOSPITALIZED PATIENT: In addition to standard precautions, droplet precautions are recommended for 5 days after initiation of effective therapy, or if appropriate antimicrobial therapy is not given, until 3 weeks after onset of cough.

CONTROL MEASURES:

Care of Exposed People

Household and Other Close Contacts. Close contacts who are unimmunized or under-immunized should have pertussis immunization initiated or continued using age-appropriate products according to the recommended schedule as soon as possible; this includes off-label use of tetanus toxoid, reduced-content diphtheria toxoid, and acellular pertussis vaccine (Tdap) in children 7 through 10 years of age who did not complete the diphtheria and tetanus toxoids and acellular pertussis vaccine (DTaP) series (see Table 3.50, p 613).

PEP is recommended for all household contacts of the index case and other close contacts, including children in child care, regardless of immunization status. Close contact can be considered as face-to-face exposure within 3 feet of a symptomatic person; direct contact with respiratory, nasal, or oral secretions; or sharing the same confined space in close proximity to an infected person for ≥1 hour. When considering borderline degree of exposure for a nonhousehold contact, PEP should be given if the contact lives in a household with a person at high risk of severe pertussis (eg, young infant, pregnant woman, person who has contact with infants) or is at high risk himself or herself. If 21 days have elapsed since onset of cough in the index case, PEP has limited value but should be considered for households with high-risk contacts. The agents, doses, and duration of PEP are the same as for treatment of pertussis (see Table 3.49, p 611).

People who have been in contact with an infected person should be monitored closely for respiratory tract symptoms for 21 days after last contact with the infected person. Close contacts with cough should be evaluated and treated for pertussis when appropriate.

Child Care. Pertussis immunization and chemoprophylaxis should be given as recommended for household and other close contacts. Child care providers and exposed children, especially incompletely immunized children, should be observed for respiratory tract symptoms for 21 days after last contact with the index case while infectious. Children and child care providers who are symptomatic or who have confirmed pertussis should be excluded from child care pending physician evaluation and completion of 5 days of the recommended course of antimicrobial therapy if pertussis is suspected. Untreated children and providers should be excluded until 21 days have elapsed from cough onset.

Schools. Students and staff members with pertussis should be excluded from school until they have completed 5 days of the recommended course of antimicrobial therapy. People who do not receive appropriate antimicrobial therapy should be excluded from school for 21 days after onset of symptoms. Use of PEP for large groups of students usually is not recommended, but exceptions for individuals can be considered, such as when intense, close contact simulates a household exposure or when pertussis in the exposed person would have severe medical consequences. Public health officials should be consulted for

Table 3.50. Composition and Recommended Use of Vaccines With Tetanus Toxoid, Diphtheria Toxoid, and Acellular Pertussis Components Licensed and Available in the United States[a,b]

Pharmaceutical	Manufacturer	Pertussis Antigens	Recommended Use
DTaP Vaccine for Children Younger Than 7 Years of Age			
DTaP (Infanrix)	GlaxoSmithKline Biologicals	PT, FHA, pertactin	**All 5 doses,** children 6 wk through 6 y of age
DTaP (Daptacel)	Sanofi Pasteur	PT, FHA, pertactin, fimbriae types 2 and 3	**All 5 doses,** children 6 wk through 6 y of age
DTaP-hepatitis B-IPV (Pediarix)	GlaxoSmithKline Biologicals	PT, FHA, pertactin	**First 3 doses, children 6 wk through 6 y of age; usual use** at 6- to 8-wk intervals beginning at 2 mo of age; then 2 doses of DTaP are needed to complete the 5-dose series before 7 y of age
DTaP-IPV/Hib (Pentacel)	Sanofi Pasteur	PT, FHA, pertactin, fimbriae types 2 and 3	**First 4 doses, children 6 wk through 4 y of age; usual use** at 2, 4, 6, and 15 through 18 mo of age; then 1 dose of DTaP is needed to complete the 5-dose series before 7 y of age
DTaP-IPV (Kinrix)	GlaxoSmithKline Biologicals	PT, FHA, pertactin	**Booster dose** for **fifth dose** of DTaP and **fourth dose** of IPV at 4 through 6 y of age
Tdap Vaccines for Adolescents			
Tdap (Boostrix)	GlaxoSmithKline Biologicals	PT, FHA, pertactin	**Single dose** at 11 through 12 y of age instead of Td (see text for additional recommendations)
Tdap (Adacel)	Sanofi Pasteur	PT, FHA, pertactin, fimbriae types 2 and 3	**Single dose** at 11 through 12 y of age instead of Td (see text for additional recommendations)

DTaP indicates pediatric formulation of diphtheria and tetanus toxoids and acellular pertussis vaccines; PT, pertussis toxoid; FHA, filamentous hemagglutinin; Hib, *Haemophilus influenzae* type b vaccine; IPV, inactivated poliovirus; Tdap, adolescent/adult formulation of tetanus toxoid, reduced diphtheria toxoid, and acellular pertussis vaccine; Td, tetanus and reduced diphtheria toxoids (for children 7 years of age or older and adults).

[a] DTaP recommended schedule is 2, 4, 6, and 15 through 18 months and 4 through 6 years of age. The fourth dose can be given as early as 12 months of age, provided 6 months have elapsed since the third dose was given. The fifth dose is not necessary if the fourth dose was given on or after the fourth birthday. Refer to manufacturers' product information for comprehensive product information regarding indications and use of the vaccines listed.

[b] Tripedia and TriHibit are licensed but no longer are available in the United States.

recommendations to control pertussis transmission in schools; their additional recommendations could include use of Tdap in children after their 4- to 6-year booster but before 11 years of age and institution of the DTaP series in siblings at 6 weeks of age. The immunization status of children should be reviewed, and age-appropriate vaccines should be administered, if indicated, as for household and other close contacts. Parents and teachers should be notified about possible exposures to pertussis. Exclusion of exposed people with cough illness should be considered pending evaluation by a physician.

Health Care Settings.[1] Health care facilities should maximize efforts to immunize all health care personnel (HCP) with Tdap to prevent transmission of *B pertussis*. All HCP should observe respiratory precautions when examining a patient with a cough illness.

People exposed to a patient with pertussis who did not take proper infection-control precautions should be evaluated by infection-control personnel for postexposure management and follow-up. The CDC recommends the following:

- Data on the need for PEP in Tdap-immunized HCP are inconclusive. Some immunized HCP still are at risk of *B pertussis* infection, and Tdap may not preclude the need for PEP.
- PEP is recommended for all HCP (even if immunized with Tdap) who have unprotected exposure to pertussis and are likely to expose other patients at risk of severe pertussis (eg, hospitalized neonates and pregnant women). Other HCP either should receive PEP or should be monitored daily for 21 days after exposure and treated at the onset of signs and symptoms of pertussis.
- Other people (patients, caregivers) defined as close contacts or high-risk contacts of a patient or HCP with pertussis should be given chemoprophylaxis (and immunization when indicated), as recommended for household contacts (see Table 3.49, p 611).
- HCP with symptoms of pertussis (or HCP with any respiratory illness within 21 days of exposure to pertussis who did not receive PEP) should be excluded from work for at least the first 5 days of the recommended antimicrobial therapy. HCP with symptoms of pertussis who cannot take, or who object to, antimicrobial therapy should be excluded from work for 21 days from onset of cough. Use of a respiratory mask is not sufficient protection during this time.

Immunization

Vaccine Products. Purified acellular-component pertussis vaccines replaced previously used diphtheria, tetanus, and whole-cell pertussis vaccine (DwTP or DTP) exclusively in 1997 and contain 3 or more immunogens derived from *B pertussis* organisms: inactivated pertussis toxin (toxoid), filamentous hemagglutinin, fimbrial proteins (agglutinogens) and pertactin (an outer membrane 69-kd protein; see Table 3.50 for products). Acellular pertussis vaccines are adsorbed onto aluminum salts and must be administered intramuscularly. All pertussis vaccines in the United States are combined with diphtheria and tetanus toxoids; none contains thimerosal as a preservative. DTaP products may be formulated as combination vaccines containing one or more of inactivated poliovirus vaccine, hepatitis B vaccine, and *Haemophilus influenzae* type b vaccine. Recommendations for the series of DTaP for children younger than 7 years are provided in the annual immunization schedule for children and adolescents (**http://redbook.solutions.aap.org/ SS/Immunization_Schedules.aspx**). Tdap vaccines contain reduced quantities

[1]Centers for Disease Control and Prevention. Immunization of health-care personnel. Recommendations of the Advisory Committee on Immunization Practices (ACIP). *MMWR Recomm Rep.* 2011;60(RR-07):1–45

of diphtheria toxoid and some pertussis antigens compared with DTaP. A single dose is recommended universally for people 11 years and older, including adults, in place of a decennial tetanus and diphtheria vaccine (Td). The preferred schedule is to administer Tdap at the 11- or 12- year-old preventive visit, with catch-up of older adolescents. For uses of DTaP and Tdap in special circumstances, see Recommendations for Scheduling Pertussis Immunization for Children Younger Than 7 Years in Special Circumstances (p 616) and Recommendations for Adolescent and Adult Immunization With Tdap in Special Situations (p 619).

Dose and Route. Each 0.5-mL dose of DTaP or Tdap is given intramuscularly. Use of a decreased volume of individual doses of pertussis vaccines or multiple doses of decreased-volume (fractional) doses is not recommended.

Interchangeability of Acellular Pertussis Vaccines. Insufficient data exist on the safety, immunogenicity, and efficacy of DTaP vaccines from different manufacturers when administered interchangeably for the primary series in infants. In circumstances in which the type of DTaP product(s) received previously is unknown or the previously administered product(s) is not readily available, any DTaP vaccine licensed for use in the primary series may be used. There is no need to match Tdap vaccine manufacturer with DTaP vaccine manufacturer used for earlier doses.

Recommendations for Routine Childhood Immunization With DTaP. Six doses of pertussis-containing vaccine are recommended: 4 doses of DTaP before 2 years of age, 1 dose of DTaP before school entry, and 1 dose of Tdap at 11 or 12 years of age. The first dose of DTaP may be given as early as 6 weeks of age, followed by 2 additional doses at intervals of approximately 2 months. The fourth dose of DTaP is recommended at 15 through 18 months of age, and the fifth dose of DTaP is given before school entry (kindergarten or elementary school) at 4 through 6 years of age. If the fourth dose of pertussis vaccine is delayed until after the fourth birthday, the fifth dose is not recommended.

Other recommendations are as follows:

- For the fourth dose, DTaP may be administered as early as 12 months of age if the interval between the third and fourth doses is at least 6 months.
- Simultaneous administration of DTaP and all other recommended vaccines is acceptable. Vaccines should not be mixed in the same syringe unless the specific combination is licensed by the FDA (see Simultaneous Administration of Multiple Vaccines, p 35, and *Haemophilus influenzae* Infections, p 368).
- During a pertussis outbreak in the community, public health authorities may recommend starting DTaP immunization as early as 6 weeks of age, with doses 2 and 3 in the primary series given at intervals as short as 4 weeks. Children younger than 7 years who have begun but not completed their primary immunization schedule with DTwP outside the United States should receive DTaP to complete the pertussis immunization schedule.
- DTaP is not licensed or recommended for people 7 years or older.
- Children between 7 and 10 years of age who have not completed their primary immunization schedule or have an unknown vaccine history should receive a single dose of Tdap. If they require additional tetanus and diphtheria toxoid doses, Td should be used.
- Children who have a contraindication to pertussis immunization should receive no further doses of a pertussis-containing vaccine (see Contraindications and Precautions to DTaP Immunization, p 617).

Combined Vaccines. Several pertussis-containing combination vaccines are licensed for use (see Table 3.50, p 613) and may be used when feasible and when any components are indicated and none is contraindicated.

Recommendations for Scheduling Pertussis Immunization for Children Younger Than 7 Years in Special Circumstances

- For the child whose pertussis immunization schedule is resumed after deferral or interruption of the recommended schedule, the next dose in the sequence should be given, regardless of the interval since the last dose—that is, the schedule is not restarted (see Lapsed Immunizations, p 37).
- For children who have received fewer than the recommended number of doses of pertussis vaccine but who have received the recommended number of diphtheria and tetanus toxoid (DT) vaccine doses for their age (ie, children started on DT, then given DTaP), DTaP should be given to complete the recommended pertussis immunization schedule. However, the total number of doses of diphtheria and tetanus toxoids (as DT, DTaP, or DTwP) should not exceed 6 before the seventh birthday.
- Although wild-type pertussis infection confers short-term protection against recurrent infection, the duration of protection is unknown. Age-appropriate DTaP dose(s) or a single dose of Tdap (depending on the age of the patient) should be given to complete the standard or catch-up immunization series in people who have had pertussis infection.

Medical Records. Charts of children for whom pertussis immunization has been deferred should be flagged, and the immunization status of these children should be assessed periodically to ensure that they are immunized appropriately.

Adverse Events After DTaP Immunization in Children Younger Than 7 Years

- **Local and febrile reactions.** Reactions to DTaP most commonly include redness, swelling, induration, and tenderness at the injection site as well as drowsiness; less common reactions include fretfulness, anorexia, vomiting, crying, and slight to moderate fever. These local and systemic manifestations after pertussis immunization occur within several hours of immunization and subside spontaneously within 48 hours without sequelae.
- Swelling involving the entire thigh or upper arm has been reported in 2% to 3% of vaccinees after administration of the fourth and fifth doses of a variety of acellular pertussis vaccines. Limb swelling can be accompanied by erythema, pain, and fever; it is not an infection. Although thigh swelling may interfere with walking, most children have no limitation of activity; the condition resolves spontaneously and has no sequelae. It may be helpful to inform parents preemptively of the increase in reactogenicity that has been reported after the fourth and fifth doses of DTaP vaccine. Entire limb swelling after a fourth dose of DTaP is associated with a modestly increased risk of a similar reaction or an injection-site reaction >5 cm after the fifth dose. Entire limb swelling is not a contraindication to further DTaP, Tdap, or Td immunization.
- A review by the Institute of Medicine (IOM) based on case-series reports found evidence of a rare yet causal relationship between receipt of tetanus toxoid-containing vaccines and brachial neuritis. However, the frequency of this event has not been determined. Brachial neuritis is listed in the Vaccine Injury Table.
- **Allergic reactions.** The rate of anaphylaxis to DTwP was estimated to be approximately 2 cases per 100 000 injections; the incidence of anaphylaxis after immunization with DTaP is unknown. The Institute of Medicine report titled "Adverse Effects of

Vaccines: Evidence and Causality" links tetanus-containing vaccines to anaphylaxis.[1] Severe anaphylactic reactions and resulting deaths, if any, are rare after pertussis immunization. Transient urticarial rashes that occur occasionally after pertussis immunization, unless appearing immediately (ie, within minutes), are unlikely to be anaphylactic (IgE mediated) in origin.

- **Seizures.** The incidence of seizures occurring within 48 hours of administration of DwTP was estimated to be 1 case per 1750 doses administered. Seizures have been reported substantially less often after DTaP, and a postlicensure study of children 6 to 23 months of age who received DTaP during 1997–2001 did not show an increased risk for seizures. Seizures, if associated with pertussis-containing vaccines, usually are simple febrile seizures and have not been demonstrated to result in recurrent afebrile seizures (ie, epilepsy) or other neurologic sequelae.
- **Hypotonic-hyporesponsive episode.** A hypotonic-hyporesponsive episode (HHE) (also termed "collapse" or "shock-like state") was reported to occur at a frequency of 1 per 1750 doses of DTwP administered, although reported rates varied widely. HHEs occur significantly less often after immunization with DTaP than with DTwP. A follow-up study of a group of children who experienced an HHE following DTwP immunization demonstrated no evidence of subsequent serious neurologic sequelae or intellectual impairment.
- **Temperature 40.5°C (104.8°F) or higher.** The rate of temperature 40.5°C (104.8°F) or higher after administration of DTaP is less than 0.1%.
- **Prolonged crying.** The frequency of inconsolable crying for 3 or more hours within 48 hours of receipt of DTaP is 0.2% or less. The significance of persistent crying is unknown, has been noted after receipt of immunizations other than pertussis vaccine, is not known to be associated with sequelae, and is not a contraindication to subsequent dose(s).

Evaluation of Adverse Events Temporally Associated With Pertussis Immunization. Appropriate diagnostic studies should be performed to establish the cause of serious adverse events occurring temporally after immunization, rather than assuming that they are caused by the vaccine. The CDC has established independent Clinical Immunization Safety Assessment (CISA) centers to assess people with selected adverse events and offer recommendations for management. Nonetheless, the cause of events temporally related to immunization, even when unrelated to the immunization received, cannot always be established, even after extensive diagnostic and investigative studies. Genetic testing of several cases of encephalopathy temporally associated with DTwP revealed a genetic defect in neuronal sodium channels (Dravet syndrome); fever associated with DTwP likely unmasked the genetic condition and was not the cause of encephalopathy.

The preponderance of evidence does not support a causal relationship between immunization with DTwP and sudden infant death syndrome, infantile spasms, or serious acute neurologic illness resulting in permanent neurologic injury. Active surveillance performed by the IMPACT network of Canadian pediatric centers screening more than 12 000 admissions for neurologic disorders between 1993 and 2002 found no case of encephalopathy attributable to DTaP after administration of more than 6.5 million doses. **Contraindications and Precautions to DTaP Immunization.[2]** **Anaphylaxis** after a previous dose of DTaP or to a vaccine component is a **contraindication** to further doses unless the

---

[1]Institute of Medicine. *Adverse Effects of Vaccines: Evidence and Causality.* Washington, DC: The National Academies Press; 2011

[2]Centers for Disease Control and Prevention. General recommendations on immunization: recommendations of the Advisory Committee on Immunization Practices (ACIP). *MMWR Recomm Rep.* 2011;60 (RR-02):1–60

patient has been desensitized. Children who experienced **encephalopathy** within 7 days after administration of a previous dose of diphtheria and tetanus toxoids and pertussis vaccine (DTwP, DTaP, or Tdap) not attributable to another identifiable cause should not receive additional doses of a vaccine that contains pertussis antigens.

Guillain-Barré syndrome within 6 weeks after a previous dose of tetanus toxoid-containing vaccine is a **precaution** to further doses. Moderate or severe acute illness with or without a fever is a **precaution** to (ie, a reason to defer) administration of any vaccine until the person has recovered. Children with an **evolving neurologic disorder** generally have DTaP immunization deferred temporarily to reduce confusion about reason(s) for a change in the clinical course. If deferred in the first year of life, DT should not be given, because in the United States the risk of acquiring diphtheria or tetanus by children younger than 1 year is remote. The decision to administer DTaP should be revisited frequently, and if deferral is chosen after 1 year of age, DT immunization should be completed according to the recommended schedule (see Diphtheria, p 325, and/or Tetanus, p 773).

Conditions That Are NOT Contraindications or Precautions to DTaP

Children with the following conditions should be given DTaP when indicated/on schedule:

- Preterm birth.
- A stable neurologic condition (well-controlled seizures, a history of seizure disorder, cerebral palsy).
- A family history of a seizure disorder or adverse events after receipt of a pertussis-containing vaccine in a family member.

Recommendations for Routine Adolescent Immunization With Tdap[1,2]

- Adolescents 11 years and older should receive a single dose of Tdap instead of Td for booster immunization against tetanus, diphtheria, and pertussis. The preferred age for Tdap immunizations is 11 through 12 years of age.
- Adolescents 11 years and older who received Td but not Tdap should receive a single dose of Tdap to provide protection against pertussis. Tdap can be administered regardless of time since receipt of last tetanus- or diphtheria-containing vaccine.
- Simultaneous administration of Tdap and all other recommended vaccines is recommended when feasible. Vaccines should not be mixed in the same syringe. Other indicated vaccine(s) that are not available and, therefore, cannot be given at the time of administration of Tdap can be given anytime thereafter.
- Outside of pregnancy, a second dose of Tdap is not recommended. See the following sections for special situations.

Recommendations for Scheduling Tdap in Children 7 Years and Older Who Did Not Complete Recommended DTaP Doses Before 7 Years of Age.

Children 7 through 10 years of age who have not completed their immunization schedule with DTaP before 7 years of age (see previous section) or who have an unknown vaccine history should receive a single dose of Tdap. If further dose(s) of tetanus and diphtheria toxoids are needed in a catch-up schedule, Td is used. The preferred schedule is Tdap followed by Td (if needed) at 2 months and 6 to 12 months, but a single dose of Tdap could be substituted for any dose

---

[1]Centers for Disease Control and Prevention. Updated recommendations for the use of tetanus toxoid, reduced diphtheria toxoid and acellular pertussis (Tdap) vaccine from the Advisory Committee on Immunization Practices, 2010. *MMWR Morb Mortal Wkly Rep.* 2011;60(1):13–15

[2]Centers for Disease Control and Prevention. Updated recommendations for use of tetanus toxoid, reduced diphtheria toxoid, and acellular pertussis vaccine (Tdap) in pregnant women—Advisory Committee on Immunization Practices (ACIP), 2012. *MMWR.* 2013;62(7):131–135

in the series. Children who receive Tdap at 7 through 10 years of age should not be given the standard Tdap booster at 11 or 12 years of age but should be given Td 10 years after their last Tdap/Td dose.

Recommendations for Adolescent and Adult Immunization With Tdap in Special Situations. Currently, Tdap vaccines are licensed for only a single dose. Special situations for use of Tdap, or repeated use of Tdap off label, are provided in the following sections.

Use of Tdap in Pregnancy. Providers of prenatal care should implement a Tdap immunization program for all pregnant women. Health care professionals should administer a dose of Tdap during **each** pregnancy irrespective of the mother's prior history of receiving Tdap. To maximize the maternal antibody response and passive antibody transfer to the infant, optimal timing for Tdap administration is between 27 and 36 weeks' gestation, but Tdap may be given at any time. For women not previously vaccinated with Tdap and in whom Tdap was not administered during pregnancy, Tdap should be administered immediately postpartum. Postpartum Tdap is not recommended for women who previously received Tdap at any time.

Protection of Young Infants: The Cocoon Strategy. The American Academy of Pediatrics, CDC, and American College of Obstetricians and Gynecologists recommend the cocoon strategy to protect infants from pertussis through immunization of their family members to decrease their likelihood of acquisition and subsequent transmission of *B pertussis* to young infants who have high risk of severe or fatal pertussis. Immunizing parents or other adult family contacts in the pediatric office setting could increase immunization coverage for this population.[1]

- Underimmunized children younger than 7 years should be given DTaP, and underimmunized children 7 years and older should be given Tdap (see previous discussion).
- All adolescents and adults should have received a single dose of Tdap. To ensure receipt, all adolescents and adults who have or anticipate having close contact with an infant younger than 12 months (eg, parents, siblings, grandparents, child care providers, and HCP) and who previously have not received Tdap should receive a single dose of Tdap, ideally at least 2 weeks before beginning close contact with the infant. There is no minimum interval suggested or required between Tdap and prior tetanus or diphtheria-toxoid containing vaccines.
- Cough illness in contacts of neonates should be investigated and managed aggressively, with consideration given for azithromycin prophylaxis for the neonate if pertussis contact is likely (see Control Measures).

Special Situations.

- **Wound management in people who previously received Tdap.** In the setting when tetanus prophylaxis is required following a wound in a person who previously received Tdap ≥5 years earlier or in whom Tdap history is uncertain, Tdap can be used if Td is not readily available.
- **Wound management for pregnant women.** As part of standard wound management care to prevent tetanus, if a tetanus toxoid-containing vaccine is indicated in a pregnant woman who has not received at Td-containing vaccine within 5 years, Tdap should be administered.

[1]Lessin HR; Edwards KM; American Academy of Pediatrics, Committee on Practice and Ambulatory Medicine, Committee on Infectious Diseases. Immunizing parents and other close family contacts in the pediatric office setting. *Pediatrics.* 2012;129(2):e247–e253

- **Pregnant women for whom tetanus booster is due.** If tetanus and diphtheria booster immunization is indicated during pregnancy (ie, more than 10 years since previous Td), then Tdap should be administered, preferably between weeks 27 and 36 of gestation.
- **Pregnant women with unknown or incomplete tetanus vaccination.** To ensure protection against maternal and neonatal tetanus, pregnant women who never have been immunized against tetanus should receive 3 doses of vaccines containing tetanus and reduced diphtheria toxoids during pregnancy. The recommended schedule is 0, 4 weeks, and 6 to 12 months. Tdap should replace 1 dose of Td, preferably between weeks 27 and 36 of gestation.

Health Care Professionals.[1]
- The CDC recommends a single dose of Tdap as soon as is feasible for HCP of any age who previously have not received Tdap. There is no minimum interval suggested or required between Tdap and prior receipt of any tetanus or diphtheria toxoid-containing vaccine.
- Tdap is not licensed for multiple administrations. After receipt of Tdap, HCP should receive routine decennial booster immunization against tetanus and diphtheria (Td) according to previously published guidelines.
- Hospitals and ambulatory-care facilities should provide Tdap for HCP and maximize immunization rates (eg, education about the benefits of immunization or mandatory requirement, convenient access, and provision of Tdap at no charge).

Recommendations for Adult Immunization With Tdap. The CDC recommends administration of a single dose of Tdap universally for adults of any age who previously have not received Tdap, with no minimum interval suggested or required between Tdap and prior receipt of a tetanus- or diphtheria-toxoid containing vaccine. When available, Boostrix is the preferred Tdap vaccine for adults 65 years and older; however, providers should not miss an opportunity to vaccinate and can use any available Tdap. A dose of either vaccine is considered valid.

Adverse Events After Administration of Tdap. Local adverse events after administration of Tdap in adolescents and adults are common but usually are mild. Systemic adverse events also are common but usually are mild (eg, any fever, 3%–14%; any headache, 40%–44%; tiredness, 27%–37%). Postmarketing data suggest that these events occur at approximately the same rate and severity as following receipt of Td.

Syncope can occur after immunization, is more common among adolescents and young adults, and can result in serious injury. Vaccinees should be seated and observed for 15 minutes after immunization. If syncope occurs, patients should be observed until symptoms resolve.

Contraindications, Precautions, and Deferral of Use of Tdap in Adolescents and Adults. Anaphylaxis that occurred after any component of the vaccine is a **contraindication** to Tdap (see Tetanus, p 773, for additional recommendations regarding tetanus immunization). In **latex-allergic** individuals, package inserts should be consulted regarding latex content.

History of **Guillain-Barré** syndrome within 6 weeks of a dose of a tetanus toxoid vaccine is a **precaution** to Tdap immunization. If decision is made to continue tetanus

---

[1] Centers for Disease Control and Prevention. Immunization of health-care personnel: recommendations of the Advisory Committee on Immunization Practices (ACIP) and supported by the Healthcare Infection Control Practices Advisory (HICPAC). *MMWR Recomm Rep.* 2011;60(RR-07):1–45

toxoid immunization, Tdap is preferred if indicated. A history of severe **Arthus hypersensitivity reaction** after a previous dose of a tetanus or diphtheria toxoid-containing vaccine administered less than 10 years previously should lead to **deferral** of Tdap or Td immunization for 10 years after administration of the tetanus or diphtheria toxoid-containing vaccine.

Conditions That Are NOT Contraindications or Precautions to Tdap in Adolescents and Adults. People with the following conditions should be given Tdap when indicated:

- History of an extensive or whole limb-swelling reaction after pediatric DTP/DTaP or Td immunization that was not an Arthus hypersensitivity reaction.
- Stable neurologic disorder, including well-controlled seizures, a history of seizure disorder, and cerebral palsy.
- Brachial neuritis.
- Immunosuppression, including people with human immunodeficiency virus infection. The immunogenicity of Tdap in people with immunosuppression has not been studied adequately, but there is no safety risk.

Pinworm Infection
(Enterobius vermicularis)

CLINICAL MANIFESTATIONS: Although some people are asymptomatic, pinworm infection (enterobiasis) may cause pruritus ani and, rarely, pruritus vulvae. Bacterial superinfections can result from scratching and excoriation of the area. Although pinworms have been found in the lumen of the appendix, and in some cases, these intraluminal parasites have been associated with signs of acute appendicitis, pinworms have also been observed in histologically normal appendices removed for incidental reasons. Many clinical findings, such as grinding of teeth at night, weight loss, and enuresis, have been attributed to pinworm infections, but proof of a causal relationship has not been established. Urethritis, vaginitis, salpingitis, or pelvic peritonitis may occur from aberrant migration of an adult worm from the perineum.

ETIOLOGY: *Enterobius vermicularis* is a nematode or roundworm.

EPIDEMIOLOGY: Enterobiasis occurs worldwide and commonly clusters within families. Prevalence rates are higher in preschool- and school-aged children, in primary caregivers of infected children, and in institutionalized people; up to 50% of these populations may be infected.

Egg transmission occurs by the fecal-oral route either directly or indirectly via contaminated hands or fomites such as shared toys, bedding, clothing, toilet seats, and baths. Transmission related to sexual contact has been reported in adults. Female pinworms usually die after depositing up to 10 000 fertilized eggs within 24 hours on the perianal skin. Reinfection occurs either by autoinfection, from pinworms crawling into the rectum after hatching, or by infection following ingestion of eggs from another person. A person remains infectious as long as female nematodes are discharging eggs on perianal skin. Eggs remain infective in an indoor environment usually for 2 to 3 weeks. Humans are the only known natural hosts; dogs and cats do not harbor *E vermicularis*.

The **incubation period** from ingestion of an egg until an adult gravid female migrates to the perianal region is 1 to 2 months or longer.

DIAGNOSTIC TESTS: Diagnosis is made when adult worms are visualized in the perianal region, which is best examined 2 to 3 hours after the child is asleep. No egg shedding occurs inside the intestinal lumen; thus, very few ova are present in stool, and so examination of stool specimens for ova and parasites is not recommended. Alternatively, diagnosis is made by touching the perianal skin with transparent (not translucent) adhesive tape to collect any eggs that may be present; the tape is then applied to a glass slide and examined under a low-power microscopic lens. Specimens should be obtained on 3 consecutive mornings when the patient first awakens, before washing. Eosinophilia is unusual and should not be attributed to pinworm infection. Serologic testing is not available or useful for diagnosis.

TREATMENT: Because pinworms largely are innocuous, the risk versus benefit of treatments should be weighed. Drugs of choice for treatment (see Drugs for Parasitic Infections, p 927) are pyrantel pamoate and albendazole (not approved for this use by the US Food and Drug Administration), which are given in a single dose and repeated in 2 weeks, because none of these drugs completely are effective against the egg or developing larvae stages. Pyrantel pamoate is available without prescription. For children younger than 2 years, in whom experience with these drugs is limited, risks and benefits should be considered before drug administration. Mebendazole no longer is available in the United States. Reinfection with pinworms occurs easily; prevention should be discussed when treatment is given. Infected people should bathe in the morning; bathing removes a large proportion of eggs. Frequently changing the infected person's underclothes, bedclothes, and bed sheets may decrease the egg contamination of the local environment and risk of reinfection. Specific personal hygiene measures (eg, exercising hand hygiene before eating or preparing food, keeping fingernails short, avoiding scratching of the perianal region, and avoiding nail biting) may decrease risk of autoinfection and continued transmission. Repeated infections should be treated by the same method as the first infection. All household members should be treated as a group in situations in which multiple or repeated symptomatic infections occur. Vaginitis is self-limited and does not require separate treatment.

ISOLATION OF THE HOSPITALIZED PATIENT: Standard precautions are indicated.

CONTROL MEASURES: Control is difficult in child care centers and schools, because the rate of reinfection is high. In institutions, mass and simultaneous treatment, repeated in 2 weeks, can be effective. Hand hygiene is the most effective method of prevention. Bed linens and underclothing of infected children should be handled carefully, should not be shaken (to avoid spreading ova into the air), and should be laundered promptly.

Pityriasis Versicolor
(Tinea Versicolor)

CLINICAL MANIFESTATIONS: Pityriasis versicolor (formerly tinea versicolor) is a common and benign superficial infection of the skin. It classically occurs in adolescence and involves the upper trunk and neck. Infants and children are more likely to exhibit facial involvement, particularly of the bilateral temples. The condition can occur at any age, and may involve other areas, including the scalp, genital area, and thighs. Symmetrical involvement with ovoid discrete or coalescent lesions of varying size is typical; these macules or patches vary in color, even in the same person. White, pink, tan, or brown coloration is often surmounted by faint dusty scales. The differential diagnosis includes pityriasis alba, vitiligo, seborrheic dermatitis, pityriasis rosea, progressive macular hypopigmentation, and pityriasis lichenoides.

ETIOLOGY: The cause of pityriasis versicolor is *Malassezia* species, a group of lipid-dependent yeasts that exist on healthy skin in yeast phase and cause clinical lesions only when substantial growth of hyphae occurs. Moist heat and lipid-containing sebaceous secretions encourage rapid overgrowth. Lesions fail to tan during the summer and during the winter are relatively darker, hence the term versicolor.

EPIDEMIOLOGY: Pityriasis versicolor can occur in any climate or age group but tends to favor adolescents and young adults, particularly in tropical climates. Moisture, heat, and the presence of lipids from the sebaceous glands seem to encourage hyphal overgrowth. These organisms also can cause systemic infections in neonates, particularly those receiving total parenteral nutrition with lipids, as well as folliculitis, particularly in immunocompromised individuals. Recurrence following discontinuation of therapy may approach 60% to 80%, and preventive treatments are sometimes used to decrease this rate. The **incubation period** is unknown.

DIAGNOSTIC TESTS: The presence of symmetrically distributed faintly scaling macules and patches of varying color concentrated on the upper back and chest is close to diagnostic. The "evoked scale" sign consists of stretching or scraping involved skin, which elicits a visible layer of thin scale. Involved areas fluoresce yellow-green under Wood's lamp evaluation. Potassium hydroxide wet mount prep of scraped scales reveals the classic "spaghetti and meatballs" short hyphae and clusters of yeast forms. Because this yeast is a common inhabitant of the skin, culture from the surface is nondiagnostic. Samples from pustules or sterile sites should be placed in media enriched with olive oil or another long-chain fatty acid.

TREATMENT: Multiple topical and systemic agents are efficacious, and recommendations vary substantially. The most cost-effective treatments are selenium sulfide shampoo/lotion and clotrimazole cream. However, adherence with these agents may be low because of unpleasant side effects (the shampoo has a sulfur-like odor) or duration of required therapy (most experts recommend 2–3 weeks of topical clotrimazole therapy for best results). Effective topical agents include ketoconazole, bifonazole, miconazole, econazole, oxiconazole, clotrimazole, terbinafine, and ciclopirox, as well as zinc pyrithione shampoo. Systemic therapies, including fluconazole, ketoconazole, and itraconazole, are not approved by the US Food and Drug Administration for pityriasis versicolor but are easy to use and are effective. Single doses do not appear to be as efficacious as multiple doses over several days or weeks. Fluconazole can be dosed at 300 mg weekly for 2 to 4 weeks, and ketoconazole can be used at 200 mg daily for 10 days.

Although oral agents are easier to use, they are not necessarily more effective and have possible serious side effects. Several studies have shown that topical therapy may be equivalent or superior to systemic therapy. Drug interactions can occur, and monitoring for liver toxicity must be considered in patients receiving systemic therapy, particularly if they receive multiple courses. For uncomplicated cases, most experts recommend initiating therapy with topical agents, such as ketoconazole; selenium sulfide shampoo used for 3 to 7 days for 5 to 10 minutes and then showered off; or a topical azole applied twice daily for 2 to 3 weeks. Shampoos are easier to disperse, particularly on wet skin, and may increase compliance. Systemic therapy is reserved for resistant infection or extensive involvement. Off-label regimens to decrease recurrence include use of the aforementioned shampoos/lotions on a weekly or monthly basis. The family must be counseled that return of pigment to the previously affected sites can take months.

ISOLATION OF THE HOSPITALIZED PATIENT: Standard precautions are recommended.

CONTROL MEASURES: The organism that causes pityriasis versicolor is commensal and resides on normal skin. Infected patients should be treated.

Plague

CLINICAL MANIFESTATIONS: Naturally acquired plague most commonly manifests in the **bubonic form**, with acute onset of fever and painful swollen regional lymph nodes (buboes). Buboes develop most commonly in the inguinal region but also occur in axillary or cervical areas. Less commonly, plague manifests in the **septicemic form** (hypotension, acute respiratory distress, purpuric skin lesions, intravascular coagulopathy, organ failure) or as **pneumonic plague** (cough, fever, dyspnea, and hemoptysis) and rarely as **meningeal**, **pharyngeal**, **ocular**, or **gastrointestinal plague**. Abrupt onset of fever, chills, headache, and malaise are characteristic in all cases. Occasionally, patients have symptoms of mild lymphadenitis or prominent gastrointestinal tract symptoms, which may obscure the correct diagnosis. When left untreated, plague often will progress to overwhelming sepsis with renal failure, acute respiratory distress syndrome, hemodynamic instability, diffuse intravascular coagulation, necrosis of distal extremities, and death. Plague has been referred to as the Black Death.

ETIOLOGY: Plague is caused by *Yersinia pestis*, a pleomorphic, bipolar-staining, gramnegative coccobacillus.

EPIDEMIOLOGY: Plague is a zoonotic infection primarily maintained in rodents and their fleas. Humans are incidental hosts who develop bubonic or primary septicemic manifestations typically through the bite of infected rodent fleas or through direct contact with tissues of infected animals. Secondary pneumonic plague arises from hematogenous seeding of the lungs with *Y pestis* in patients with untreated bubonic or septicemic plague. Primary pneumonic plague is acquired by inhalation of respiratory tract droplets from a human or animal with pneumonic plague. Only the pneumonic form has been shown to be transmitted from person to person, and the last known case of person-to-person transmission in the United States occurred in 1924. Rarely, humans can develop primary pneumonic plague following exposure to domestic cats with respiratory tract plague infections. Plague occurs worldwide with enzootic foci in parts of Asia, Africa, and the Americas. Most human plague cases are reported from rural, underdeveloped areas and mainly occur as isolated cases or in small, focal clusters. Since 2000, more than 95% of the approximately 22 000 cases reported to the World Health Organization have been from countries in sub-Saharan Africa. In the United States, plague is endemic in western states, with most (approximately 85%) of the 37 cases reported from 2006 through 2010 being from New Mexico, Colorado, Arizona, and California. Cases of peripatetic plague have been identified in states without endemic plague, such as Connecticut (2008) and New York (2002).

The **incubation period** is 2 to 8 days for bubonic plague and 1 to 6 days for primary pneumonic plague.

DIAGNOSTIC TESTS: *Y pestis* has a bipolar (safety-pin) appearance when stained with Wright-Giemsa or Wayson stains. A positive fluorescent antibody test result for the presence of *Y pestis* in direct smears or cultures of blood, bubo aspirate, sputum, or another clinical specimen provides presumptive evidence of *Y pestis* infection. Diagnosis of plague usually is confirmed by culture of *Y pestis* from blood, bubo aspirate, sputum, or another clinical specimen. Automated blood culture identification systems can misidentify *Y pestis*. Many clinical laboratories provide preliminary identification of *Yersinia* species, with definitive identification performed at the state or federal laboratory. Isolation of *Yersinia* species from an automated system should trigger additional evaluation to determine whether the clinical presentation is consistent with plague. A single positive serologic test result from passive hemagglutination assay or enzyme immunoassay in an unimmunized patient who previously has not had plague also provides presumptive evidence of infection. Seroconversion, defined as a fourfold difference in antibody titer between 2 serum specimens obtained at least 2 weeks apart, also confirms the diagnosis of plague. Polymerase chain reaction assay and immunohistochemical staining for rapid diagnosis of *Y pestis* are available in some reference or public health laboratories. Isolates suspected as *Y pestis* should be reported immediately to the state health department and submitted to the Division of Vector-Borne Infectious Diseases of the Centers for Disease Control and Prevention (CDC).

TREATMENT: For children, gentamicin and streptomycin administered intramuscularly or intravenously appear to be equally effective. Alternative drugs approved by the US Food and Drug Administration (FDA) include tetracycline, doxycycline, chloramphenicol, and trimethoprim-sulfamethoxazole. Trimethoprim-sulfamethoxazole should not be considered a first-line treatment option when treating bubonic plague and should not be used as monotherapy to treat pneumonic or septicemic plague, because of higher treatment failure rates. Fluoroquinolones (including ciprofloxacin) have been shown to be highly effective in animal and in vitro studies, and levofloxacin has been approved recently by the FDA for treatment of plague. The usual duration of antimicrobial treatment is 7 to 10 days or until several days after lysis of fever. Chloramphenicol is considered the treatment of choice for plague meningitis, but when chloramphenicol is unavailable, fluoroquinolones, particularly those with higher cerebrospinal fluid penetration, such as levofloxacin, should be considered as alternative therapy.

Drainage of abscessed buboes may be necessary; drainage material is infectious until effective antimicrobial therapy has been administered.

ISOLATION OF THE HOSPITALIZED PATIENT: For patients with bubonic plague, standard precautions are recommended. For patients with suspected pneumonic plague, respiratory droplet precautions should be initiated immediately and continued for 48 hours after initiation of effective antimicrobial treatment.

CONTROL MEASURES:

Care of Exposed People. All people with exposure to a known or suspected plague source, such as *Y pestis*-infected fleas or infectious tissues, in the previous 6 days should be offered antimicrobial prophylaxis or be cautioned to report fever greater than 38.3°C (101.0°F) or other illness to their physician. People with close exposure (less than 2 m) to a patient with pneumonic plague should receive antimicrobial prophylaxis, but isolation of asymptomatic people is not recommended. Pneumonic transmission typically occurs in the end stage of disease in patients with hemoptysis, thereby placing caregivers and health care professionals at high risk. For people 8 years or older, doxycycline or ciprofloxacin is recommended. For children younger than 8 years, doxycycline, tetracycline, chloramphenicol, ciprofloxacin, or trimethoprim-sulfamethoxazole are alternative drugs (see Tetracyclines, p 873, and Fluoroquinolones, p 872). Tetracycline-based antimicrobial agents, including doxycycline, may cause permanent tooth discoloration for children younger than 8 years if used for repeated treatment courses. However, doxycycline binds less readily to calcium compared with older tetracyclines, and in some studies, doxycycline was not associated with visible teeth staining in younger children. The benefits of prophylactic therapy should be weighed against the risks. Prophylaxis is given for 7 days from the time of last exposure and in the usual therapeutic doses.

Other Measures. State public health authorities should be notified immediately of any suspected cases of human plague. People living in areas with endemic plague should be informed about the importance of eliminating sources of rodent food and harborage near residences, the role of dogs and cats in bringing plague-infected rodent fleas into peridomestic environments, the need for flea control and confinement of pets, and the importance of avoiding contact with sick and dead animals. Other preventive measures include surveillance of rodent populations, use of insecticides and insect repellents, and rodent control measures by health authorities when surveillance indicates the occurrence of plague epizootics. Rodent-control measures never should be employed without prior or concurrent use of insecticides.

Vaccine. Killed whole-cell and live-attenuated vaccines have been used in humans at high risk of exposure to *Y pestis*; however, these are not currently licensed for use in the United States. New vaccines based on recombinant capsular subunit protein F1 and the low-calcium response V antigen (LcrV), either as a mixture of the 2 antigens (F1+V) or as a fusion of the 2 antigens (F1-V), are under evaluation.

Pneumococcal Infections[1,2]

CLINICAL MANIFESTATIONS: *Streptococcus pneumoniae* is a common cause of invasive bacterial infections in children, including febrile bacteremia. Pneumococci also are a common cause of acute otitis media, sinusitis, community-acquired pneumonia, pleural empyema, and conjunctivitis. *S pneumoniae* remains the most common cause of bacterial meningitis and subdural hygromas in infants and children from 2 months of age in the United States.[3] Pneumococci occasionally cause mastoiditis, periorbital cellulitis, endocarditis, osteomyelitis, pericarditis, peritonitis, pyogenic arthritis, soft tissue infection, overwhelming septicemia in patients with splenic dysfunction, and neonatal septicemia. Hemolytic-uremic syndrome can accompany complicated invasive disease (eg, pneumonia with pleural empyema).

---

[1]American Academy of Pediatrics, Committee on Infectious Diseases. Policy statement: recommendations for the prevention *Streptococcus pneumoniae* infections in infants and children: use of 13-valent pneumococcal conjugate vaccine (PCV13) and pneumococcal polysaccharide vaccine (PPSV23). *Pediatrics.* 2010;126(1):186–190

[2]Centers for Disease Control and Prevention. Prevention of pneumococcal disease among infants and children—use of 13-valent pneumococcal conjugate vaccine and 23-valent pneumococcal polysaccharide vaccine. *MMWR Recomm Rep.* 2010;59(RR-11):1–18

[3]Thigpen MC, Whitney CG, Messonnier NE, et al; Emerging Infections Programs Network. Bacterial meningitis in the United States, 1998–2007. *N Engl J Med.* 2011;364(21):2016–2025

ETIOLOGY: *S pneumoniae* organisms (pneumococci) are lancet-shaped, gram-positive catalase-negative diplococci. More than 90 pneumococcal serotypes have been identified on the basis of unique polysaccharide capsules. Before implementation of routine immunization in infants with heptavalent pneumococcal conjugate vaccine (PCV7) in 2000, serotypes 4, 6B, 9V, 14, 18C, 19F, and 23F caused most invasive childhood pneumococcal infections in the United States; these 7 types were contained in PCV7. Serotypes 6A, 6B, 9V, 14, 19A, 19F, and 23F were the most common serotypes associated with resistance to penicillin, but serotype 19A emerged as the most common cause of invasive disease and the serotype most associated with resistance in PCV7-immunized children. The 13-valent pneumococcal conjugate vaccine (PCV13) was introduced in 2010 and includes types 1, 3, 5, 6A, 7F, and 19A in addition to the serotypes in PCV7.

EPIDEMIOLOGY: Pneumococci are ubiquitous, with many people having transient colonization of the upper respiratory tract. In children, nasopharyngeal carriage rates range from 21% in industrialized countries to more than 90% in resource-limited countries. Transmission is from person to person by respiratory droplet contact. The period of communicability is unknown and may be as long as the organism is present in respiratory tract secretions but probably is less than 24 hours after effective antimicrobial therapy is begun. Among young children who acquire a new pneumococcal serotype in the nasopharynx, illness (eg, otitis media) occurs in approximately 15%, usually within a few days of acquisition. Viral upper respiratory tract infections, including influenza, can predispose to pneumococcal infection and transmission. Pneumococcal infections are most prevalent during winter months. Rates of infection are highest in infants, young children, elderly people, and black, Alaska Native, and some American Indian populations. The incidence and severity of infections are increased in people with congenital or acquired humoral immunodeficiency, human immunodeficiency virus (HIV) infection, absent or deficient splenic function (eg, sickle cell disease, congenital or surgical asplenia), diabetes mellitus, chronic liver disease, chronic renal failure or nephrotic syndrome, or abnormal innate immune responses. Children with cochlear implants have high rates of pneumococcal meningitis, as do children with congenital or acquired cerebrospinal fluid (CSF) leaks.[1] Other categories of children at presumed high risk or at moderate risk of developing invasive pneumococcal disease are outlined in Table 3.51. Since introduction of PCV7 and PCV13, racial disparities have diminished; however, rates of invasive pneumococcal disease (IPD) among some American Indian (Alaska Native and Apache) populations remain more than fivefold higher than the rate among children in the general US population.

From 1998 (before PCV7 was introduced in 2000) to 2007, the incidence of vaccine-type invasive pneumococcal infections decreased by 99%, and the incidence of all IPD decreased by 76% in children younger than 5 years. In adults 65 years and older, IPD caused by PCV7 serotypes decreased 92% compared with baseline and all serotype invasive disease by 37%. The reduction in cases in these latter groups indicates the significant indirect benefits of PCV7 immunization by interruption of transmission of pneumococci from children to adults. Further reductions in disease in children of all ages, also associated with herd protection, have been demonstrated to date for at least 3 of the additional 6 serotypes in PCV13, including serotype 19A.

---

[1] American Academy of Pediatrics, Committee on Infectious Diseases. Policy statement: cochlear implants in children: surgical site infections and prevention and treatment of acute otitis media and meningitis. *Pediatrics.* 2010;126(2):381–391

Table 3.51. Underlying Medical Conditions That Are Indications for Pneumococcal Immunization Among Children, by Risk Group[a]

Risk group	Condition
Immunocompetent children	Chronic heart disease[b]
	Chronic lung disease[c]
	Diabetes mellitus
	Cerebrospinal fluid leaks
	Cochlear implant
Children with functional or anatomic asplenia	Sickle cell disease and other hemoglobinopathies
	Chronic or acquired asplenia, or splenic dysfunction
Children with immuno-compromising conditions	HIV infection
	Chronic renal failure and nephrotic syndrome
	Diseases associated with treatment with immunosuppressive drugs or radiation therapy, including malignant neoplasms, leukemias, lymphomas, and Hodgkin disease; or solid organ transplantation
	Congenital immunodeficiency[d]

[a]Centers for Disease Control and Prevention. Licensure of a 13-valent pneumococcal conjugate vaccine (PCV13) and recommendations for use among children. Advisory Committee on Immunization Practices (ACIP). *MMWR Morb Mortal Wkly Rep.* 2010;59(9):258–261

[b]Particularly cyanotic congenital heart disease and cardiac failure.

[c]Including asthma if treated with prolonged high-dose oral corticosteroids.

[d]Includes B- (humoral) or T-lymphocyte deficiency; complement deficiencies, particularly C_1, C_2, C_3, and C_4 deficiency; and phagocytic disorders (excluding chronic granulomatous disease).

The **incubation period** varies by type of infection but can be as short as 1 to 3 days.

DIAGNOSTIC TESTS: Recovery of *S pneumoniae* from a normally sterile site (eg, blood, CSF, peritoneal fluid, middle ear fluid, joint fluid) or from a suppurative focus confirms the diagnosis. The finding of lancet-shaped gram-positive organisms and white blood cells in expectorated sputum or pleural exudate suggests pneumococcal pneumonia in older children and adults. Recovery of pneumococci by culture of an upper respiratory tract swab specimen is not sufficient to assign an etiologic diagnosis of pneumococcal disease involving the middle ear, lower respiratory tract, or sinus. Real-time polymerase chain reaction (PCR) assay using *lyt*A is investigational but may be specific and significantly more sensitive than culture of pleural fluid, CSF, and blood, particularly in patients who have received recent antimicrobial therapy. Investigational assays, such as serotype-specific urinary antigen detection and nasopharyngeal carriage as measured by quantitative lytA PCR assay, have not been validated.

Susceptibility Testing. All *S pneumoniae* isolates from normally sterile body fluids (eg, CSF, blood, middle ear fluid, pleural or joint fluid) should be tested for antimicrobial susceptibility to determine the minimum inhibitory concentration (MIC) of penicillin, cefotaxime or ceftriaxone, and clindamycin. CSF isolates also should be tested for susceptibility to vancomycin and meropenem. *Nonsusceptible* includes both *intermediate* and *resistant* isolates. Breakpoints vary depending on whether an isolate is from a nonmeningeal or meningeal site; in children with meningitis presentations, the breakpoints for meningeal isolates should be used (eg, a blood isolate in a patient with meningitis). Accordingly, current definitions by the Clinical and Laboratory Standards Institute (CLSI) for susceptibility and nonsusceptibility are provided in Table 3.52 for nonmeningeal and meningitis presentations.

For patients with meningitis caused by an organism that is nonsusceptible to penicillin, susceptibility testing of rifampin also should be performed. If the patient has a nonmeningeal infection caused by an isolate that is nonsusceptible to penicillin, cefotaxime, and ceftriaxone, susceptibility testing to other agents such as clindamycin, erythromycin, trimethoprim-sulfamethoxazole, linezolid, meropenem, and vancomycin should be performed.

Quantitative MIC testing using reliable methods, such as broth microdilution or antimicrobial gradient strips, should be performed on isolates from children with invasive infections. When quantitative testing methods are not available or for isolates from noninvasive infections, the qualitative screening test using a 1-µg oxacillin disk on an agar plate reliably identifies all penicillin-*susceptible* pneumococci using meningitis breakpoints (ie, disk-zone diameter of 20 mm or greater). Organisms with an oxacillin disk-zone size of less than 20 mm potentially are nonsusceptible for treatment of meningitis and require quantitative susceptibility testing. The oxacillin disk test is used as a screening test for resistance to beta-lactam drugs (ie, penicillins and cephalosporins).

TREATMENT: *S pneumoniae* strains that are nonsusceptible to penicillin G, cefotaxime, ceftriaxone, and other antimicrobial agents using meningitis breakpoints have been identified throughout the United States and worldwide but are uncommon using nonmeningeal breakpoints. Recommendations for treatment of pneumococcal infections are as follows.

***Bacterial Meningitis Possibly or Proven to Be Caused by* S pneumoniae.** Combination therapy with vancomycin and cefotaxime or ceftriaxone should be administered initially to all

Table 3.52. Clinical and Laboratory Standards Institute Definitions of in Vitro Susceptibility and Nonsusceptibility of Nonmeningeal and Meningeal Pneumococcal Isolates[a,b]

Drug and Isolate Location	Susceptible, µg/mL	Nonsusceptible, µg/mL	
		Intermediate	Resistant
Penicillin (oral)[c]	≤0.06	0.12–1.0	≥2.0
Penicillin (intravenous)[d]			
Nonmeningeal	≤2.0	4.0	≥8.0
Meningeal	≤0.06	None	≥0.12
Cefotaxime **OR** ceftriaxone			
Nonmeningeal	≤1.0	2.0	≥4.0
Meningeal	≤0.5	1.0	≥2.0

[a]Clinical and Laboratory Standards Institute. *Performance Standards for Antimicrobial Susceptibility Testing: 18th Informational Supplement.* CLSI Publication No. M100-S23. Wayne, PA: Clinical and Laboratory Standards Institute; 2013

[b]Centers for Disease Control and Prevention. Effects of new penicillin susceptibility breakpoints for *Streptococcus pneumoniae*—United States, 2006–2007. *MMWR Morb Mortal Wkly Rep.* 2008;57(50):1353–1355

[c]Without meningitis.

[d]Treated with intravenous penicillin.

children 1 month or older with definite or probable bacterial meningitis because of the possibility of *S pneumoniae* resistant to penicillin, cefotaxime, and ceftriaxone.

For children with serious hypersensitivity reactions to beta-lactam antimicrobial agents (ie, penicillins and cephalosporins), the combination of vancomycin and rifampin should be considered. Vancomycin should not be given alone, because bactericidal concentrations in CSF are difficult to sustain, and clinical experience to support use of vancomycin as monotherapy is minimal. Rifampin also should not be given as monotherapy, because resistance can develop during therapy. Meropenem also can be given as an alternative drug. A repeat lumbar puncture should be considered after 48 hours of therapy in the following circumstances:

- the organism is penicillin nonsusceptible by oxacillin disk or quantitative (MIC) testing, and results from cefotaxime and ceftriaxone quantitative susceptibility testing are not yet available; or
- the patient's condition has not improved or has worsened; or
- the child has received dexamethasone, which can interfere with the ability to interpret the clinical response, such as resolution of fever.

Once results of susceptibility testing are available, therapy should be modified according to the guidance in Table 3.53. Vancomycin should be discontinued and either penicillin or cefotaxime or ceftriaxone should be continued if the organism is susceptible to penicillin; if the isolate is penicillin nonsusceptible, cefotaxime or ceftriaxone should be continued.

If the organism is nonsusceptible to penicillin and cefotaxime or ceftriaxone, vancomycin should be continued. Addition of rifampin to the combination of vancomycin

Table 3.53. Antimicrobial Therapy for Infants and Children With Meningitis Caused by *Streptococcus pneumoniae* on the Basis of Susceptibility Test Results

Susceptibility Test Results	Antimicrobial Management[a]
• *Susceptible* to penicillin	**Discontinue vancomycin** **AND** Begin penicillin (and discontinue cephalosporin) **OR** Continue cefotaxime or ceftriaxone alone[b]
• *Nonsusceptible* to penicillin (*intermediate* or *resistant*) **AND** *Susceptible* to cefotaxime and ceftriaxone	**Discontinue vancomycin** **AND** Continue cefotaxime or ceftriaxone
• *Nonsusceptible* to penicillin (*intermediate* or *resistant*) **AND** *Nonsusceptible* to cefotaxime and ceftriaxone (*intermediate* or *resistant*) **AND** *Susceptible* to rifampin	Continue vancomycin and high-dose cefotaxime or ceftriaxone **AND** Rifampin may be added in selected circumstances (see text)

[a]See Table 3.54, p 631, for dosages. Some experts recommend the maximum dosages. Initial therapy of nonallergic children older than 1 month of age should be vancomycin and cefotaxime or ceftriaxone. See Bacterial Meningitis Possibly or Proven to Be Caused by *S pneumoniae*, p 629.

[b]Some physicians may choose this alternative for convenience and cost savings but only in treatment of meningitis.

and cefotaxime or ceftriaxone after 24 to 48 hours of therapy should be considered if the organism is susceptible to rifampin and (1) after 24 to 48 hours, despite therapy with vancomycin and cefotaxime or ceftriaxone, the clinical condition has worsened; (2) the subsequent culture of CSF indicates failure to eradicate or to decrease substantially the number of organisms; or (3) the organism has an unusually high cefotaxime or ceftriaxone MIC (≥4 µg/mL). Consultation with an infectious disease specialist should be considered in such circumstances.

Dexamethasone. For infants and children 6 weeks and older, adjunctive therapy with dexamethasone may be considered after weighing the potential benefits and possible risks. Some experts recommend use of corticosteroids in pneumococcal meningitis, but this issue is controversial and data are not sufficient to make a routine recommendation for children. If used, dexamethasone should be given before or concurrently with the first dose of antimicrobial agents.

Nonmeningeal Invasive Pneumococcal Infections Requiring Hospitalization. For nonmeningeal invasive infections in previously healthy children who are not critically ill, antimicrobial agents currently used to treat infections with *S pneumoniae* and other potential pathogens should be initiated at the usually recommended dosages (see Table 3.54).

For critically ill infants and children with invasive infections potentially attributable to *S pneumoniae*, vancomycin in addition to empiric antimicrobial therapy (eg, cefotaxime or ceftriaxone or others) can be considered. Such patients include those with presumed septic shock, severe pneumonia with empyema, or significant hypoxia or myopericardial involvement. If vancomycin is administered, it should be discontinued as soon as antimicrobial susceptibility test results demonstrate effective alternative agents.

If the organism has in vitro resistance to penicillin, cefotaxime, and ceftriaxone according to guidelines of the Clinical Laboratory Standards Institute, therapy should be

Table 3.54. Dosages of Intravenous Antimicrobial Agents for Invasive Pneumococcal Infections in Infants and Children[a]

Antimicrobial Agent	Meningitis		Nonmeningeal Infections	
	Dose/kg per day	Dose Interval	Dose/kg per day	Dose Interval
Penicillin G	250 000–400 000 U[b]	4–6 h	250 000–400 000 U[b]	4–6 h
Cefotaxime	225–300 mg	8 h	75–225 mg	8 h
Ceftriaxone	100 mg	12h	50–75 mg	12–24 h
Vancomycin	60 mg	6 h	40–45 mg	6–8 h
Rifampin[c]	20 mg	12 h	Not indicated	...
Chloramphenicol[d]	75–100 mg	6 h	75–100 mg	6 h
Clindamycin	Not indicated	...	25–40 mg	6–8 h
Meropenem[e]	120 mg	8 h	60 mg	8 h

[a] Doses are for children 1 month or older.
[b] Because 1 U = 0.6 µg/mL, this range is equal to 150 to 240 mg/kg per day.
[c] Indications for use are not defined completely.
[d] Drug should be considered only for patients with life-threatening allergic response after administration of beta-lactam antimicrobial agents.
[e] Drug is approved for pediatric patients 3 months and older.

modified on the basis of clinical response, susceptibility to other antimicrobial agents, and results of follow-up cultures of blood and other infected body fluids. Consultation with an infectious disease specialist should be considered.

For children with severe hypersensitivity to beta-lactam antimicrobial agents (ie, penicillins and cephalosporins), initial management should include vancomycin or clindamycin in addition to antimicrobial agents for other potential pathogens, as indicated. Vancomycin should not be continued if the organism is susceptible to other appropriate non–beta-lactam antimicrobial agents. Consultation with an infectious disease specialist should be considered.

Nonmeningeal Invasive Pneumococcal Infections in the Immunocompromised Host. The preceding recommendations for management of possible pneumococcal infections requiring hospitalization also apply to immunocompromised children. Vancomycin should be discontinued as soon as antimicrobial susceptibility test results indicate that effective alternative antimicrobial agents are available.

Dosages. The recommended dosages of intravenous antimicrobial agents for treatment of invasive pneumococcal infections are given in Table 3.54.

Acute Otitis Media.[1] According to clinical practice guidelines of the American Academy of Pediatrics (AAP) and the American Academy of Family Physicians (AAFP) on acute otitis media (AOM), amoxicillin (80–90 mg/kg/day) is recommended, except in select cases in which the option of observation without antimicrobial therapy is warranted. Optimal duration of therapy is uncertain. For younger children and children with severe disease at any age, a 10-day course is recommended; for children 6 years and older with mild or moderate disease, a duration of 5 to 7 days is appropriate.

Patients who fail to respond to initial management should be reassessed at 48 to 72 hours to confirm the diagnosis of AOM and exclude other causes of illness. If AOM is confirmed in the patient managed initially with observation, amoxicillin should be given. If the patient has failed initial antibacterial therapy, a change in antibacterial agent is indicated. Suitable alternative agents should be active against penicillin-nonsusceptible pneumococci as well as beta-lactamase–producing *Haemophilus influenzae* and *Moraxella catarrhalis.* Such agents include high-dose oral amoxicillin-clavulanate; oral cefdinir, cefpodoxime, or cefuroxime; or intramuscular ceftriaxone in a 3-day course. Amoxicillin-clavulanate should be given at 80 to 90 mg/kg per day of the amoxicillin component in the 14:1 formulation to decrease the incidence of diarrhea. Patients who continue to fail therapy with one of the aforementioned oral agents should be treated with a 3-day course of parenteral ceftriaxone. Macrolide resistance among *S pneumoniae* is high, so clarithromycin and azithromycin generally are not considered appropriate alternatives for initial therapy even in patients with a type I (immediate, anaphylactic) reaction to a beta-lactam agent. In such cases, treatment with clindamycin (if susceptibility is known) or levofloxacin is preferred. For patients with a history of non-type I allergic reaction to penicillin, agents such as cefdinir, cefuroxime, or cefpodoxime can be used orally.

Myringotomy or tympanocentesis should be considered for children failing to respond to second-line therapy and for severe cases to obtain cultures to guide therapy. For multidrug-resistant strains of *S pneumoniae,* use of levofloxacin or other agents should be considered in consultation with an expert in infectious diseases and based on the specific susceptibility profile.

Sinusitis. Antimicrobial agents effective for treatment of AOM also are likely to be effective for acute sinusitis and are recommended.

---

[1]Lieberthal AS, Carroll AE, Chonmaitree T, et al. Clinical practice guideline: diagnosis and management of acute otitis media. *Pediatrics.* 2013;131(3):e964–e999

ISOLATION OF THE HOSPITALIZED PATIENT: Standard precautions are recommended, including for patients with infections caused by drug-resistant *S pneumoniae.*

CONTROL MEASURES:

Active Immunization. Two pneumococcal vaccines are available for use in children in the United States: the 13-valent pneumococcal conjugate vaccine (PCV13) and 23-valent pneumococcal polysaccharide vaccine (PPSV23). PCV13 has replaced the 7-valent PCV7 and is licensed for use in infants and children from 6 weeks through 17 years of age and adults 50 years and older. PCV13 is composed of the 7 purified capsular polysaccharide serotypes that were in PCV7 (4, 6B, 9V, 14, 18C, 19F, and 23F) plus another 6 (1, 3, 5, 6A, 7F, and 19A) individually conjugated to a nontoxic variant of diphtheria toxin carrier protein, CRM_{197} (~34 μg). PCV13 is available in single-dose, prefilled syringes that do not contain latex or preservative but do contain 0.02% polysorbate 80, 0.125 mg of aluminum (as aluminum phosphate adjuvant), and 5 mM succinate buffer. PPSV23 is licensed for use in children 2 years and older and adults. PPSV23 is composed of 23 capsular polysaccharides in isotonic saline solution containing 0.25% phenol as preservative. Each available vaccine is recommended in a dose of 0.5 mL to be administered intramuscularly. Immunization with PPSV23 does not induce immunologic memory or boosting with subsequent doses, and no effects on nasopharyngeal carriage or indirect protection of unimmunized groups have been documented.

Routine Immunization With Pneumococcal Conjugate Vaccine. PCV13 is recommended for all infants and children 2 through 59 months of age. For infants, the vaccine should be administered at 2, 4, 6, and 12 through 15 months of age; catch-up immunization is recommended for all children 59 months of age or younger, and the schedule is the same as previously published for PCV7, with PCV13 replacing PCV7 for all doses (Table 3.55). Infants should begin the PCV13 immunization series in conjunction with other recommended vaccines at the time of the first regularly scheduled health maintenance visit after 6 weeks of age. Infants of very low birth weight (1500 g or less) should be immunized when they attain a chronologic age of 6 to 8 weeks, regardless of their gestational age at birth. PCV13 can be administered concurrently with all other age-appropriate childhood immunizations using a separate syringe and a separate injection site.

Supplemental Dose Recommendation. For fully immunized children 15 through 71 months of age who have not received at least 1 dose of PCV13 and who have an underlying medical condition (Table 3.51, p 628) that increases their risk of pneumococcal disease or complications, a single supplemental dose of PCV13 is recommended.

Immunization of Children Unimmunized or Incompletely Immunized With PCV13. For toddlers 2 through 71 months of age who have not received PCV13 or who need "catch up" immunization, the dose schedule is outlined in Table 3.55 (p 634). PCV13 is recommended for all children younger than 72 months who are at high risk or presumed high risk of acquiring invasive pneumococcal infection, as defined in Table 3.51 (p 628).

Immunization of Children 6 Through 18 Years of Age With High-Risk Conditions[1]

PPSV23-Naïve Children. For children 6 through 18 years of age who previously have not received PCV13 and who are at increased risk of IPD because of anatomic or functional asplenia (including sickle cell disease), HIV infection, cochlear implant, CSF leak, or other

---

[1]Centers for Disease Control and Prevention. Use of 13-valent pneumococcal conjugate vaccine and 23-valent pneumococcal polysaccharide vaccine among children aged 6–18 years with immunocompromising conditions: recommendations of the Advisory Committee on Immunization Practices (ACIP). *MMWR Morb Mortal Wkly Rep.* 2013;62(25):521–524

Table 3.55. Recommended Schedule for Doses of PCV13, Including Catch-up Immunizations in Previously Unimmunized and Partially Immunized Children 2 Through 71 Months of Age

Age at Examination	Immunization History	Recommended Regimen[a,b]
2 through 6 mo	0 doses	3 doses, 2 mo apart; fourth dose at 12 through 15 mo of age
	1 dose	2 doses, 2 mo apart; fourth dose at 12 through 15 mo of age
	2 doses	1 dose, 2 mo after the most recent dose; fourth dose at 12 through 15 mo of age
7 through 11 mo	0 doses	2 doses, 2 mo apart; third dose at 12 mo of age
	1 or 2 doses before age 7 mo	1 dose at age 7 through 11 mo, with another dose at 12 through 15 mo of age (≥2 mo later)
12 through 23 mo	0 doses	2 doses, ≥2 mo apart
	1 dose at <12 mo	2 doses, ≥2 mo apart
	1 dose at ≥12 mo	1 dose, ≥2 mo after the most recent dose
	2 or 3 doses at <12 mo	1 dose, ≥2 mo after the most recent dose
24 through 59 mo[c] Healthy children	Any incomplete schedule	1 dose, ≥2 mo after the most recent dose[c]
24 through 71 mo[d] Children with underlying medical conditions	Any incomplete schedule of <3 doses	2 doses, one ≥2 mo after the most recent dose and another dose ≥2 mo later
	Any incomplete schedule of 3 doses	1 dose, ≥2 mo after the most recent dose

PCV13 indicates 13-valent pneumococcal conjugate vaccine.

[a]For children immunized at younger than 12 months, the minimum interval between doses is 4 weeks. Doses administered at 12 months or older should be at least 8 weeks apart.

[b]Centers for Disease Control and Prevention. Licensure of a 13-valent pneumococcal conjugate vaccine (PCV13) and recommendations for use among children. Advisory Committee on Immunization Practices (ACIP). *MMWR Morb Mortal Wkly Rep.* 2010;59(RR-11):1–18

[c]A single dose should be administered to all healthy children 24 through 59 months of age with any incomplete schedule.

[d]Children with sickle cell disease, asplenia, chronic heart or lung disease, diabetes mellitus, cerebrospinal fluid leak, cochlear implant, human immunodeficiency virus infection, or another immunocompromising condition (see Table 3.51, p 628). PPV23 also is indicated. See Table 3.56, p 635.

immunocompromising conditions (Table 3.51, p 628), administration of a single PCV13 dose followed by a dose of PPSV23 at age ≥2 years and at least 8 weeks after the last PCV13 dose is recommended. Revaccination with PPSV23 dose is recommended 5 years after the first PPSV23 dose for children ≥2 years of age. No more than a total of 2 PPSV23 doses should be given before 65 years of age.

    Previous Vaccination With PPSV23. Children 6 through 18 years of age who previously received ≥1 dose of PPSV23 and no prior PCV13 immunizations should be given a single dose of PCV13, even if they have received PCV7 previously, at least 8 weeks after the last PPSV23 dose. If a second PPSV23 dose is indicated, it should be given at least

Table 3.56. Recommendations for Pneumococcal Immunization with PCV13 or PPSV23 Vaccine for Children at High Risk or Presumed High Risk of Pneumococcal Disease, as Defined in Table 3.51 (p 628)

Age	Previous Dose(s) of Any Pneumococcal Vaccine	Recommendations
23 mo or younger	None	PCV13, as in Table 3.53 (p 630)
24 through 71 mo	4 doses of PCV13	1 dose of PPSV23 vaccine at 24 mo of age, at least 8 wk after last dose of PCV13
		1 dose of PPSV23, 5 y after the first dose of PPV7[a]
24 through 71 mo	3 previous doses of PCV7 before 24 mo of age	1 dose of PCV13
		1 dose of PPSV23, ≥8 wk after the last dose of PCV7
		1 dose of PPSV23, 5 y after the first dose of PPSV23[a]
24 through 71 mo	<3 doses of PCV7 before 24 mo of age	2 doses of PCV13, at least 8 wk after last dose of PCV13 (if applicable)
		1 dose of PPSV23 vaccine, ≥8 wk after the last dose of PCV13
		1 dose of PPSV23 vaccine, 5 y after the first dose of PPSV23 vaccine[a]
24 through 71 mo	1 dose of PPSV23	2 doses of PCV13, 8 wk apart, beginning at 6–8 wk after last dose of PPSV23
		1 dose of PPSV23 vaccine, 5 y after the last dose of PPV23 and at least 8 wk after PCV13[a]
6 years through 18 years with immunocompromising conditions[b]	No previous doses of PCV13 or PPSV23	1 dose of PCV13 followed by 1 dose of PPSV23 at least 8 weeks later and a second dose 5 years after the first
	1 dose of PCV13	1 dose of PPSV23 and a second dose 5 years after the first (second dose is given 3 years after the first in children with sickle cell disease)
	≥1 dose of PPSV23	1 dose of PCV13 (even if PCV7 previously given) ≥8 weeks after the last PPSV23 dose. If a second PPSV23 dose is indicated, it should be given ≥5 years after the first PPSV23 dose

PCV13 indicates 13-valent pneumococcal conjugate vaccine; PPSV23, 23-valent pneumococcal polysaccharide vaccine.

[a] A second dose of PPSV23 5 years after the first dose is recommended only for children who have functional or anatomic asplenia (in those with sickle cell anemia, the second dose is given 3 years after the first), HIV infection, or other immunocompromising conditions (Table 3.51, p 628). No more than 2 doses of PPSV23 are recommended. All other children with underlying medical conditions should receive 1 dose of PPSV23.

[b] Includes anatomic or functional asplenia, HIV infection, cochlear implant, CSF leak, or other immunocompromising conditions.

5 years after the first PPSV23 dose, but no more than a total of 2 PPSV23 doses should be given before 65 years of age.

Immunization of Children 2 Through 18 Years of Age Who Are at Increased Risk of IPD With PPSV23 After PCV7 or PCV13.[1] Children 2 years or older with an underlying medical condition increasing the risk of IPD should receive PPSV23 as soon as possible after a diagnosis is made. Children who are candidates for solid organ transplantation and in cases when a splenectomy is planned for a patient older than 2 years, PPSV23 should be given at least 2 weeks before transplant or splenectomy. In candidates for solid organ transplantation, a dose of PCV13 should be given, even for those older than 6 years.

Doses of PCV13 should be completed before PPSV23 is administered, with a minimum interval of 8 weeks between the last dose of PCV13 and the first dose of PPSV23. If a child previously has received PPSV23, the child also should receive the recommended doses of PCV13. A second dose of PPSV23 is recommended 5 years after the first dose in children with sickle cell disease or functional or anatomic asplenia, HIV infection, or other immunocompromising conditions, but no more than a total of 2 PPSV23 doses should be given before 65 years of age. In children with sickle cell disease, PPSV23 is recommended routinely at 2 years of age, with a second dose at 5 years of age.

Control of Transmission of Pneumococcal Infection and Invasive Disease Among Children Attending Out-of-Home Child Care. Before routine use of PCV7, children attending out-of-home child care were twofold to threefold more likely to acquire IPD than were healthy children of the same age not enrolled in out-of-home child care. PPSV23 has not been shown to decrease nasopharyngeal carriage of pneumococci. In contrast, PCV7 and PCV13 reduce carriage of pneumococcal serotypes in the vaccine. Available data are insufficient to recommend any antimicrobial regimen for preventing or interrupting the carriage or transmission of pneumococcal infection in out-of-home child care settings. Antimicrobial chemoprophylaxis is not recommended for contacts of children with IPD, regardless of their immunization status.

General Recommendations for Use of Pneumococcal Vaccines.

- Either PPSV23 or PCV13 can be given concurrently with other childhood vaccines, with one exception. For children with functional or anatomic asplenia, the quadrivalent meningococcal conjugate vaccine conjugated to diphtheria toxoid (MenACWY-D, Menactra, Sanofi Pasteur, Swiftwater, PA) should not be administered concomitantly OR within 4 weeks of administration of PCV13 immunization, to avoid potential interference with the immune response to PCV13, which also is conjugated to diphtheria toxoid. It is for this reason that children with functional or anatomic asplenia should not be immunized with MenACWY-D before 2 years of age so that they can complete their PCV13 series; MenACWY-CRM (Menveo) can be used before 2 years of age, however, because it is not conjugated to diphtheria toxoid. Pneumococcal vaccine should be injected with a separate syringe in a separate injection site.
- When elective splenectomy is performed for any reason, immunization with PCV13 should be completed at least 2 weeks before splenectomy. Immunization also should precede initiation of immune-compromising therapy or placement of a cochlear implant by at least 2 weeks. PPSV23 can be given 8 or more weeks after PCV13 (see Immunization in Immunocompromised Children, p 74).

[1]American Academy of Pediatrics, Committee on Infectious Diseases. Immunization for *Streptococcus pneumoniae* infections in high-risk children. *Pediatrics.* 2014;134(6):1230–1233

- Generally, pneumococcal vaccines should be deferred during pregnancy, because of the absence of data when administered to a pregnant woman. Other inactivated or killed vaccines, including licensed polysaccharide vaccines, have been administered safely during pregnancy. The risk of severe pneumococcal disease in a pregnant woman who has an underlying medical condition increasing the risk of IPD should prompt immunization with PPSV23 if not previously administered within the previous 5 years.

Case Reporting. Cases of IPD in children younger than 5 years and drug-resistant infection in all ages should be reported according to state standards. Before introduction of PCV13, approximately 99% of invasive disease cases were caused by non-PCV7 serotypes. Therefore, the overwhelming majority of invasive pneumococcal disease cases occurring among unimmunized children have not represented vaccine failures. Early evidence suggests that IPD caused by PCV13 serotypes is decreasing. To differentiate PCV13 failure in an immunized child from disease caused by a serotype not included in PCV13, the isolate should be serotyped. A protocol for identifying pneumococcal serotypes using PCR is available for state public health laboratories on the CDC Web site. If the invasive isolate is a serotype included in the vaccine, an evaluation of the patient's HIV status and immunologic function should be considered, if the child had receipt of 2 or more doses of PCV13 at least 2 weeks before the onset of the invasive infection.

Adverse Reactions to Pneumococcal Vaccines. Adverse reactions after administration of polysaccharide or conjugate vaccines generally are mild to moderate. The most commonly reported adverse reactions are local reactions of injection site, pain, redness, or swelling in addition to irritability, decreased appetite, or impaired sleep. Fever may occur within the first 1 to 2 days after injections, particularly after use of conjugate vaccine. Other systemic reactions include fatigue, headache, chills, decreased appetite, and generalized muscle pain.

Passive Immunization. Intravenous administration of Immune Globulin is recommended for preventing pneumococcal infection in patients with congenital or acquired immunodeficiency diseases, including people with HIV infection who have recurrent pneumococcal infections (see Human Immunodeficiency Virus Infection, p 453).

Chemoprophylaxis. Daily antimicrobial prophylaxis is recommended for children with functional or anatomic asplenia, regardless of their immunization status, for prevention of pneumococcal disease on the basis of results of a large, multicenter study (see Asplenia and Functional Asplenia, p 86). Oral penicillin V (125 mg, twice a day, for children younger than 3 years; 250 mg, twice a day, for children 3 years and older) is recommended. The study, performed before routine use of PCV7 in the United States, demonstrated that oral penicillin V given to infants and young children with sickle cell disease decreased the incidence of pneumococcal bacteremia by 84% compared with the placebo control group. Although overall incidence of IPD is decreased after penicillin prophylaxis, cases of penicillin-resistant IPD and nasopharyngeal carriage of penicillin-resistant strains in patients with sickle cell disease have increased in recent years. Parents should be informed that penicillin prophylaxis may not be effective in preventing all cases of IPD. In children with suspected or proven penicillin allergy, erythromycin is an alternative agent for prophylaxis.[1]

---

[1] American Academy of Pediatrics, Committee on Genetics. Health supervision for children with sickle cell disease. *Pediatrics.* 2002;109(3):526–535 (Reaffirmed January 2011)

The age at which prophylaxis is discontinued is an empiric decision. Most children with sickle cell disease who have received all recommended pneumococcal vaccines for age and who had received penicillin prophylaxis for prolonged periods, who are receiving regular medical attention, and who have not had a previous severe pneumococcal infection or a surgical splenectomy may discontinue prophylactic penicillin safely at 5 years of age. However, they must be counseled to seek medical attention for all febrile events. The duration of prophylaxis for children with asplenia attributable to other causes is unknown. Some experts continue prophylaxis throughout childhood or longer.

Pneumocystis jirovecii Infections

CLINICAL MANIFESTATIONS: Symptomatic infection is extremely rare in healthy people. Disease in immunocompromised infants and children may produce a respiratory illness characterized by dyspnea, tachypnea, significant oxygen desaturation, nonproductive cough, and fever. The intensity of these signs and symptoms may vary, and in some immunocompromised children and adults, the onset may be acute and fulminant. Chest radiographs often show bilateral diffuse interstitial or alveolar disease; rarely, lobar, miliary, cavitary, and nodular lesions or even no lesions are seen. Most children with *Pneumocystis* pneumonia are significantly hypoxic. The mortality rate in immunocompromised patients ranges from 5% to 40% in treated patients and approaches 100% without therapy.

ETIOLOGY: Nomenclature for *Pneumocystis* species has evolved. Originally considered a protozoan, *Pneumocystis* now is classified as a fungus on the basis of DNA sequence analysis. Human *Pneumocystis* now is called *Pneumocystis jirovecii*, while *Pneumocystis carinii* is used for organisms infecting rats. *P carinii f* sp *hominis* or "human *P carinii*" sometimes are still used to refer to human *Pneumocystis. P jirovecii* is an atypical fungus, with several morphologic and biologic similarities to protozoa, including susceptibility to a number of antiprotozoal agents but resistance to most antifungal agents. In addition, the organism exists as 2 distinct morphologic forms: the 5- to 7-μm-diameter cysts, which contain up to 8 intracystic bodies, and the smaller, 1- to 5-μm-diameter trophozoite or trophic form.

EPIDEMIOLOGY: *Pneumocystis* species are ubiquitous in mammals worldwide, particularly rodents, and have a tropism for growth on respiratory tract epithelium. *Pneumocystis* isolates recovered from mice, rats, and ferrets differ genetically from each other and from human *P jirovecii*. Asymptomatic or mild human infection occurs early in life, with more than 85% of healthy children acquiring antibody by 20 months of age. In resource-limited countries and in times of famine, *Pneumocystis* pneumonia (PCP) can occur in epidemics, primarily affecting malnourished infants and children. Epidemics also have occurred among preterm infants. In industrialized countries, PCP occurs almost entirely in immunocompromised people with deficient cell-mediated immunity, particularly people with human immunodeficiency virus (HIV) infection, recipients of immunosuppressive therapy after solid organ transplantation or treatment for malignant neoplasm, and children with congenital immunodeficiency syndromes. Although decreasing in frequency because of effective prophylaxis and antiretroviral therapy, PCP remains one of the most common serious opportunistic infections in infants and children with perinatally acquired HIV infection and adolescents with advanced immunosuppression. Although onset of disease can occur at any age, including rare instances during the first month of life, PCP most commonly occurs in HIV-infected children in the first year of life, with peak incidence at 3 through 6 months of age. The single most important factor in susceptibility to PCP is the status of cell-mediated immunity of the host, reflected by a marked decrease in CD4+ T-lymphocyte count and percentage. The mode of transmission is unknown. Animal studies have demonstrated animal-to-animal transmission by the airborne route; evidence suggests airborne transmission among humans. Outbreaks in hospitals have been reported. Vertical transmission has been postulated. Although reactivation of latent infection with immunosuppression has been proposed as an explanation for disease after the first 2 years of life, animal models of PCP do not support the existence of latency. Studies of patients with acquired immunodeficiency syndrome (AIDS) with more than 1 episode of PCP suggest reinfection rather than relapse. In patients with cancer, the disease can occur during remission or relapse. The period of communicability is unknown.

The **incubation period** is unknown, but reports of human outbreaks of PCP in transplant recipients have demonstrated a median of 53 days from exposure to clinically apparent infection.

DIAGNOSTIC TESTS: A definitive diagnosis of PCP is made by visualization of organisms (*Pneumocystis* cysts) in lung tissue or respiratory tract secretion specimens. The most sensitive and specific diagnostic procedures involve specimen collection from open lung biopsy and, in older children, transbronchial biopsy. However, bronchoscopy with bronchoalveolar lavage, induction of sputum in older children and adolescents, and intubation with deep endotracheal aspiration are less invasive, can be diagnostic, and are sensitive in patients with HIV infection who have a large number of *Pneumocystis* organisms. Methenamine silver, toluidine blue O, calcofluor white, and fluorescein-conjugated monoclonal antibody are the most useful stains for identifying the thick-walled cysts of *P jirovecii*. Extracystic trophozoite forms are identified with Giemsa stain, modified Wright-Giemsa stain, and fluorescein-conjugated monoclonal antibody stain. The sensitivity of all microscopy-based methods depends on the skill of the laboratory technician. Polymerase chain reaction assays for detecting *P jirovecii* infection have been shown to be highly sensitive and cost effective even with noninvasive specimens, such as oral wash or expectorated sputum. Limited data suggests that serum 1,3-β-D-glucan (BG) assay may be helpful and a potential marker for *Pneumocystis* infection.

TREATMENT[1]: The drug of choice is trimethoprim-sulfamethoxazole (TMP-SMX), usually administered intravenously. Oral therapy should be reserved for patients with mild disease who do not have malabsorption or diarrhea and for patients with a favorable clinical response to initial intravenous therapy. Duration of therapy is 14 to 21 days. The rate of adverse reactions to TMP-SMX (eg, rash, neutropenia, anemia, thrombocytopenia, renal toxicity, hepatitis, nausea, vomiting, and diarrhea) is higher in HIV-infected children than in non–HIV-infected patients. It is not necessary to discontinue therapy for most mild adverse reactions. At least half of the patients with more severe reactions (excluding

---

[1]Guidelines for prevention and treatment of opportunistic infections in HIV-exposed and HIV-infected children. Recommendations from the National Institutes of Health, Centers for Disease Control and Prevention, the HIV Medicine Association of the Infectious Diseases Society of America, the Pediatric Infectious Diseases Society, and the American Academy of Pediatrics. *Pediatr Infect Dis J.* 2013;32(Suppl 2):i-KK4. Available at: **http://aidsinfo. nih.gov/guidelines/html/5/pediatric-oi-prevention-and-treatment-guidelines/0**

anaphylaxis) requiring interruption of therapy subsequently will tolerate TMP-SMX if rechallenged after the reaction resolves.

Intravenously administered pentamidine is an alternative drug for children and adults who cannot tolerate TMP-SMX or who have severe disease and have not responded to TMP-SMX after 5 to 7 days of therapy. The therapeutic efficacy of intravenous pentamidine in adults with PCP is similar to that of TMP-SMX. Pentamidine is associated with a high incidence of adverse reactions, including pancreatitis, diabetes mellitus, renal toxicity, electrolyte abnormalities, hypoglycemia, hyperglycemia, hypotension, cardiac arrhythmias, fever, and neutropenia. If a recipient of didanosine requires pentamidine, didanosine should not be administered until 1 week after pentamidine therapy has been completed because of overlapping toxicities.

Atovaquone is approved for oral treatment of mild to moderate PCP in adults who are intolerant of TMP-SMX. Experience with use of atovaquone in children is limited, although atovaquone-azithromycin appears to be as effective as TMP-SMX for preventing serious bacterial infections as well as PCP. Adverse reactions to atovaquone are limited to rash, nausea, and diarrhea. Other potentially useful drugs in adults include clindamycin with primaquine (adverse reactions are rash, nausea, and diarrhea), dapsone with trimethoprim (associated with neutropenia, anemia, thrombocytopenia, methemoglobinemia, rash, and transaminase elevation), and trimetrexate with leucovorin. Experience with the use of these combinations in children is limited.

Corticosteroids appear to be beneficial in treatment of HIV-infected adults with moderate to severe PCP (as defined by an arterial oxygen pressure [PaO_2] of less than 70 mm Hg in room air or an arterial-alveolar gradient of more than 35 mm Hg). For adolescents 13 years and older and adults, the recommended dose of oral prednisone is 80 mg/day, in 2 divided doses, for the first 5 days of therapy; 40 mg, once daily, on days 6 through 10; and 20 mg, once daily, on days 11 through 21. Studies have shown that use of corticosteroids can lead to reduced acute respiratory failure, decreased need for ventilation, and reduced mortality in children with PCP. Although no controlled studies of the use of corticosteroids in young children have been performed, most experts would recommend corticosteroids as part of therapy for children with moderate to severe PCP disease. On the basis of limited available data, a recommended regimen of oral prednisone for children younger than 13 years is 1 mg/kg/dose, twice daily, for the first 5 days of therapy; 0.5 mg/kg/dose, twice daily, on days 6 through 10; and 0.5 mg/kg, once daily, on days 11 through 21.

Coinfection with other organisms, such as cytomegalovirus or pneumococcus, has been reported in HIV-infected children. Children with dual infections may have more severe disease.

Chemoprophylaxis. Chemoprophylaxis is highly effective in preventing PCP among some high-risk groups. Prophylaxis against a first episode of PCP is indicated for many patients with significant immunosuppression, including people with HIV infection (see Human Immunodeficiency Virus Infection, p 454) and people with primary or acquired cell-mediated immunodeficiency.

In HIV-infected children, risk of PCP is associated with age-specific CD4+ T-lymphocyte cell counts and percentages that define severe immunosuppression (Immune Category 3 [see Table 3.29, p 455]). Because CD4+ T-lymphocyte cell counts and percentages can decline rapidly in HIV-infected infants, prophylaxis for PCP is recommended for all infants born to HIV-infected women with indeterminate HIV status beginning at 4 to 6 weeks of age and continuing until 12 months of age unless a diagnosis of HIV has been excluded presumptively or definitively, in which case prophylaxis should be discontinued (see Table 3.57). Children who are HIV infected or whose HIV status is indeterminate should continue prophylaxis throughout the first year of life.

For HIV-infected children 12 months or older, PCP prophylaxis should be continued or initiated in the following circumstances: Prophylaxis is recommended for all HIV-infected children 6 years or older who have CD4+ T-lymphocyte counts <200 cells/mm^3 or CD4+ T-lymphocyte percentage <15%; for children 1 through 5 years of age with CD4+ T-lymphocyte counts <500 cells/mm^3 or CD4+ T-lymphocyte percentage <15%; and for all HIV-infected infants younger than 12 months regardless of CD4+

Table 3.57. Recommendations for *Pneumocystis jirovecii* Pneumonia (PCP) Prophylaxis for Human Immunodeficiency Virus (HIV)-Exposed Infants and Children, by Age and HIV Infection Status[a]

Age and HIV Infection Status	PCP prophylaxis[b]
Birth through 4 to 6 wk of age, HIV exposed or HIV infected	No prophylaxis
4 to 6 wk through 12 mo of age HIV infected or indeterminate HIV infection presumptively or definitively excluded[c]	 Prophylaxis No prophylaxis
1 through 5 y of age, HIV infected	Prophylaxis if: CD4+ T-lymphocyte count is less than 500 cells/μL or percentage is less than 15%[d]
6 y of age or older, HIV infected	Prophylaxis if: CD4+ T-lymphocyte count is less than 200 cells/μL or percentage is less than 15%[d]

[a] Guidelines for prevention and treatment of opportunistic infections in HIV-exposed and HIV-infected children. Recommendations from the National Institutes of Health, Centers for Disease Control and Prevention, the HIV Medicine Association of the Infectious Diseases Society of America, the Pediatric Infectious Diseases Society, and the American Academy of Pediatrics. *Pediatr Infect Dis J.* 2013;32(Suppl 2):i-KK4. Available at: **http://aidsinfo.nih.gov/guidelines/html/5/pediatric-oi-prevention-and-treatment-guidelines/0**

[b] Children who have had PCP should receive lifelong ("secondary") PCP prophylaxis unless/until their CD4+ T-lymphocyte cell counts and percentages achieve and maintain designated age-specific values greater than those indicative of severe immunosuppression (Immune Category 3) for at least 6 months (see Human Immunodeficiency Virus Infection, Table 3.29, p 455).

[c] In nonbreastfeeding HIV-exposed infants with no positive virologic test results or other laboratory or clinical evidence of HIV infection, HIV presumptively can be excluded on the basis of 2 negative virologic test results, 1 performed at 2 weeks of age or older and 1 performed at 4 weeks of age or older, on 1 negative virologic test result performed at 8 weeks of age or older, or on 1 negative HIV antibody test performed at 6 months of age or older. HIV definitively can be excluded on the basis of 2 negative virologic test results, 1 performed at 4 weeks of age or older and 1 performed at 4 months of age or older, or on 2 negative HIV antibody test results from 2 separate specimens obtained at 6 months of age or older (see Human Immunodeficiency Virus Infection, p 453).

[d] Prophylaxis should be considered on a case-by-case basis for children who might otherwise be at risk of PCP, such as children with rapidly declining CD4+ T-lymphocyte cell counts or percentages or children with Clinical Category C status of HIV infection.

T-lymphocyte count or percentage (see Human Immunodeficiency Virus Infection, Table 3.29, p 455, and Table 3.57, p 641); Discontinuation of PCP prophylaxis should be considered for HIV-infected children when, after receiving combination antiretroviral therapy for ≥6 months, CD4+ T-lymphocyte percentage is ≥15% or CD4+ T-lymphocyte count is ≥200 cells/mm³ for patients 6 years or older; and CD4+ T-lymphocyte percentage is ≥15% or CD4+ T-lymphocyte count is ≥500 cells/mm³ for patients aged 1 through 5 years for >3 consecutive months.

HIV-infected children older than 1 year who are not receiving PCP prophylaxis (eg, children not previously identified as infected or children whose PCP prophylaxis was discontinued) should begin or resume prophylaxis if their CD4+ T-lymphocyte cell counts and percentages reach the targeted values for PCP prophylaxis initiation (see Table 3.57, p 641).

In patients with AIDS, prophylaxis should be initiated at the end of therapy for acute infection and should be continued until 6 months after CD4+ T-lymphocyte cell count and percentage exceed the values designated as requiring prophylaxis (see Table 3.57, p 641) or lifelong if CD4+ T-lymphocyte cells do not exceed these thresholds in response to antiretroviral therapy.

Prophylaxis for PCP is recommended for children who have received hematopoietic stem cell transplants (HSCTs)[1] or solid organ transplants; children with hematologic malignancies (eg, leukemia or lymphoma) and some nonhematologic malignancies; children with severe cell-mediated immunodeficiency, including children who received adrenocorticotropic hormone for treatment of infantile spasm; and children who otherwise are immunosuppressed and who have had a previous episode of PCP. In general, for this diverse group of immunocompromised hosts, the risk of PCP increases with duration and intensity of chemotherapy, with other immunosuppressive therapies, and with coinfection with immunosuppressive viruses (eg, cytomegalovirus) and rates of PCP for similar patients in a given locale. Consequently, the recommended duration of PCP prophylaxis will vary depending on individual circumstances. Guidelines for allogeneic HSCT recipients recommend that PCP prophylaxis be initiated at engraftment (or before engraftment, if engraftment is delayed) and administered for at least 6 months. It should be continued for more than 6 months in all children receiving ongoing or intensified immunosuppressive therapy (eg, prednisone or cyclosporin) or in children with chronic graft-versus-host disease. Guidelines for PCP prophylaxis for solid organ transplant recipients are less definitive, but some authorities suggest durations ranging from 6 months to 1 year for renal transplants and from 1 year to life for heart, lung, and liver transplants.

The recommended drug regimen for PCP prophylaxis for all immunocompromised patients is TMP-SMX, administered orally on 3 consecutive days each week (see Table 3.58). Alternatively, TMP-SMX can be administered daily, 7 days a week. For patients who cannot tolerate TMP-SMX, alternative choices include oral

---

[1]Center for International Blood and Marrow Research; National Marrow Donor program; European Blood and Marrow Transplant Group; American Society of Blood and Marrow Transplantation; Canadian Blood and Marrow Transplant Group; Infectious Diseases Society of America; Society for Healthcare Epidemiology of America; Association of Medical Microbiology and Infectious Disease Canada; Centers for Disease Control and Prevention. Guidelines for preventing infectious complications among hematopoietic cell transplant recipients: a global perspective. *Biol Blood Marrow Transplant.* 2009;15(10):1143–1238

Table 3.58. Drug Regimens for *Pneumocystis jirovecii* Pneumonia Prophylaxis for Children 4 Weeks and Older[a]

Recommended regimen:

Trimethoprim-sulfamethoxazole (trimethoprim, 150 mg/m^2 [or 5 mg/kg] per day, with sulfa-methoxazole, 750 mg/m^2 [or 25 mg/kg] per day), orally, in divided doses twice a day, 3 times per week on consecutive days (eg, Monday-Tuesday-Wednesday)

Acceptable alternative trimethoprim-sulfamethoxazole dosage schedules:

- Trimethoprim (150 mg/m^2 per day) with sulfamethoxazole (750 mg/m^2 per day), orally, **as a single daily dose,** 3 times per week on consecutive days (eg, Monday-Tuesday-Wednesday)
- Trimethoprim (150 mg/m^2 per day) with sulfamethoxazole (750 mg/m^2 per day), orally, in divided doses, twice a day, and **administered 7 days per week**
- Trimethoprim (150 mg/m^2 per day) with sulfamethoxazole (750 mg/m^2 per day), orally,
- in divided doses twice a day, and administered 3 times per week on alternate days (eg, Monday-Wednesday-Friday)

Alternative regimens if trimethoprim-sulfamethoxazole is not tolerated:

- **Dapsone (children 1 mo or older)**
- 2 mg/kg (maximum 100 mg), orally, once a day or 4 mg/kg (maximum 200 mg), orally, every week
- **Aerosolized pentamidine (children 5 y or older)**
- 300 mg, inhaled monthly via Respirgard II nebulizer
- **Atovaquone**
  - **children 1 through 3 mo of age and older than 24 mo through 12 y of age:** 30 mg/kg (maximum 1500 mg), orally, once a day
  - **children 4 through 24 mo of age:** 45 mg/kg (maximum 1500 mg), orally, once a day
  - **children older than 12 y:** 1500 mg, orally, once a day

[a]Guidelines for prevention and treatment of opportunistic infections in HIV-exposed and HIV-infected children. Recommendations from the National Institutes of Health, Centers for Disease Control and Prevention, the HIV Medicine Association of the Infectious Diseases Society of America, the Pediatric Infectious Diseases Society, and the American Academy of Pediatrics. *Pediatr Infect Dis J.* 2013;32(Suppl 2):i-KK4. Available at: **http://aidsinfo.nih.gov/guidelines/html/5/pediatric-oi-prevention-and-treatment-guidelines/0**

atovaquone or dapsone. Atovaquone is effective and safe but expensive. Dapsone is effective and inexpensive but associated with more serious adverse effects than atovaquone. Aerosolized pentamidine is recommended for children who cannot tolerate TMP-SMX, atovaquone, or dapsone and are old enough to use a Respirgard II nebulizer. Intravenous pentamidine has been used but is not generally recommended for prophylaxis. Other drug combinations with potential for prophylaxis include pyrimethamine plus dapsone plus leucovorin or pyrimethamine-sulfadoxine. Experience with these drugs in adults and children for this indication is limited. These agents should be considered only in situations in which recommended regimens are not tolerated or cannot be used for other reasons.

ISOLATION OF THE HOSPITALIZED PATIENT: Standard precautions are recommended. Some experts recommend that because of the theoretical risk for transmission, patients with PCP not share a room with other immunocompromised patients, especially patients who are not receiving chemoprophylaxis, although data are insufficient to support this recommendation as standard practice.

CONTROL MEASURES: Appropriate therapy for infected patients and prophylaxis in immunocompromised patients are the only available means of control. Detailed guidelines for children, adolescents, and adults infected with HIV have been issued by the Centers for Disease Control and Prevention and the Infectious Diseases Society of America.[1,2]

Poliovirus Infections

CLINICAL MANIFESTATIONS: Approximately 72% of poliovirus infections in susceptible children are asymptomatic. Nonspecific illness with low-grade fever and sore throat (minor illness) occurs in 24% of people who become infected. Viral meningitis, sometimes with paresthesias, occurs in 1% to 5% of patients a few days after the minor illness has resolved. Rapid onset of asymmetric acute flaccid paralysis with areflexia of the involved limb occurs in fewer than 1% of infections, and residual paralytic disease involving the motor neurons (paralytic poliomyelitis) occurs in approximately two thirds of people with acute motor neuron disease. The classical case of paralytic polio begins with a minor illness characterized by fever, sore throat, headache, nausea, constipation, and/or malaise for several days, followed by a symptom free period of 1 to 3 days. Rapid onset of paralysis then follows. However, paralysis can occur without the prodrome. Typically, paralysis is asymmetric and affects the proximal muscles more than the distal muscles. Cranial nerve involvement (bulbar poliomyelitis, often showing a tripod sign) and paralysis of respiratory tract muscles can occur. Sensation usually is intact in patients with paralytic polio. Findings in cerebrospinal fluid (CSF) are characteristic of viral meningitis, with mild pleocytosis and lymphocytic predominance. Adults who contracted paralytic poliomyelitis during childhood may develop the noninfectious postpolio syndrome 15 to 40 years later. Postpolio syndrome is characterized by slow and irreversible exacerbation of weakness, most likely occurring in those muscle groups involved during the original infection. Muscle and joint pain also are common manifestations. The prevalence and incidence of postpolio syndrome is unclear. Studies estimate the range of postpolio syndrome in poliomyelitis survivors is from 25% to 40%.

ETIOLOGY: Polioviruses are classified as members of the family *Picornaviridae*, genus *Enterovirus*, in the species enterovirus C, and include 3 serotypes. Acute paralytic disease may be caused by naturally occurring (wild) polioviruses or by circulating vaccine-derived polioviruses (cVDPVs) that have acquired virulence properties (neurovirulence and transmissibility) that are indistinguishable from naturally occurring polioviruses as a result of sustained person-to-person circulation in the absence of adequate population immunity. In addition, rare cases of vaccine-associated paralytic poliomyelitis (VAPP) occur in recipients of oral poliovirus vaccine (OPV) or their close contacts. People with primary

---

[1] Guidelines for prevention and treatment of opportunistic infections in HIV-exposed and HIV-infected children. Recommendations from the National Institutes of Health, Centers for Disease Control and Prevention, the HIV Medicine Association of the Infectious Diseases Society of America, the Pediatric Infectious Diseases Society, and the American Academy of Pediatrics. *Pediatr Infect Dis J.* 2013;32(Suppl 2):i-KK4. Available at: **http://aidsinfo.nih.gov/guidelines/html/5/pediatric-oi-prevention-and-treatment-guidelines/0**

[2] Centers for Disease Control and Prevention. Guidelines for prevention of opportunistic infections in HIV-infected adults and adolescents: recommendations from the CDC, the National Institutes of Health, and the HIV Medicine Association of the Infectious Diseases Society of America. *MMWR Recomm Rep.* 2009;58(RR-4):1-207

B-lymphocyte immunodeficiencies are at increased risk both of VAPP and of chronic infection (immunodeficiency-associated vaccine-derived polioviruses, or iVDPV) from vaccine virus. With recent progress in the World Health Organization (WHO) Global Poliomyelitis Eradication Initiative, more cases of paralytic disease are caused by vaccine-related viruses (VAPP and cVDPV) than by wild polioviruses.

EPIDEMIOLOGY: Humans are the only natural reservoir for poliovirus. Spread is by contact with feces and/or respiratory secretions. Infection is more common in infants and young children and occurs at an earlier age among children living in poor hygienic conditions. In temperate climates, poliovirus infections are most common during summer and autumn; in the tropics, the seasonal pattern is less pronounced.

The last reported case of poliomyelitis attributable to indigenously acquired, naturally occurring wild poliovirus in the United States occurred in 1979 during an outbreak among unimmunized people that resulted in 10 paralytic cases. The only identified imported case of paralytic poliomyelitis since 1986 occurred in 1993 in a child transported to the United States for medical care. Since 1986, all other cases acquired in the United States have been VAPP cases attributable to OPV vaccine. From 1980 to 1997, the average annual number of cases of VAPP reported in the United States was 8. Fewer VAPP cases were reported in 1998 and 1999, after a shift in US immunization policy in 1997 from use of OPV to a sequential inactivated poliovirus (IPV) vaccine/OPV schedule. Implementation of an all-IPV vaccine schedule in 2000 halted the occurrence of VAPP cases in the United States. In 2005, however, a healthy, unimmunized young adult from the United States acquired VAPP in Central America, most likely from an infant grandchild of the host family who recently had been immunized with OPV. In 2005, a type 1 VDPV was identified in the stool of an asymptomatic, unimmunized, immuno-deficient child in Minnesota. Subsequently, poliovirus infections in 7 other unimmunized children (35% of all children tested) within the index patient's community were documented. None of the infected children had paralysis. Phylogenetic analysis suggested that the VDPV circulated in the community for approximately 2 months before the infant's infection was detected and that the initiating OPV dose had been given (likely in another country) before the index child's birth. In 2009, a woman with longstanding common-variable immunodeficiency was diagnosed with VAPP and died of polio-associated complications. Molecular characterization of the poliovirus isolate suggested that the infection likely occurred approximately 12 years earlier, coinciding with OPV immunization of her child. Circulation of indigenous wild poliovirus strains ceased in the United States several decades ago, and the risk of contact with imported wild polioviruses has decreased in parallel with the success of the global eradication program. Of the 3 poliovirus serotypes, type 2 wild poliovirus appears to have been eradicated globally, with the last naturally occurring case detected in 1999 in India. No cases of type 3 wild poliovirus were detected during 2013, suggesting this type also is on the verge of eradication. Type 1 poliovirus now accounts for all polio cases attributable to wild poliovirus.

Communicability of poliovirus is greatest shortly before and after onset of clinical illness, when the virus is present in the throat and excreted in high concentrations in feces. Virus persists in the throat for approximately 1 to 2 weeks after onset of illness and is excreted in feces for 3 to 6 weeks. Patients potentially are contagious as long as fecal excretion persists. In recipients of OPV, virus also persists in the throat for 1 to 2 weeks and is excreted in feces for several weeks, although in rare cases excretion for more than 2 months can occur. Immunocompromised patients with significant B-lymphocyte immune deficiencies have excreted iVDPV for periods of more than 20 years.

The **incubation period** of nonparalytic poliomyelitis is 3 to 6 days. For the onset of poliomyelitis, the **incubation period** to paralysis usually is 7 to 21 days (range, 3–35 days).

DIAGNOSTIC TESTS: Poliovirus can be detected in specimens from the pharynx and feces, less commonly from urine, and rarely from CSF by isolation in cell culture or reverse transcriptase-polymerase chain reaction (RT-PCR). Two or more stool and throat swab specimens for enterovirus isolation or detection should be obtained at least 24 hours apart from patients with suspected paralytic poliomyelitis as early in the course of illness as possible, ideally within 14 days of onset of symptoms. Fecal material is most likely to yield virus in cell culture. However, poliovirus may be excreted intermittently, and a single negative test result does not rule out infection.

Because OPV no longer is available in the United States, the chance of exposure to vaccine-type polioviruses has become remote. Therefore, if a poliovirus is isolated in the United States, the isolate should be reported immediately to the state health department and sent to the Centers for Disease Control and Prevention (CDC) through the state health department for further testing. Paralytic poliomyelitis and detection of polioviruses are nationally reportable conditions in the United States. The diagnostic test of choice for confirming poliovirus disease is viral culture of stool specimens and throat swab specimens obtained as early in the course of illness as possible. Commonly used molecular tests for enteroviruses will detect poliovirus, but will not differentiate poliovirus from other enteroviruses and, therefore, are insufficient to demonstrate that poliovirus is the etiology of disease. In these situations, additional virus testing will be necessary to confirm the diagnosis of poliovirus related disease. Interpretation of acute and convalescent serologic test results can be difficult because of high levels of population immunity.

TREATMENT: Supportive.

ISOLATION OF THE HOSPITALIZED PATIENT: In addition to standard precautions, contact precautions are indicated for infants and young children for the duration of hospitalization.

CONTROL MEASURES:
Immunization of Infants and Children.

Vaccines. The 2 types of poliovirus vaccines are IPV, administered parenterally (subcutaneously or intramuscularly; Table 1.6, p 15), and live OPV, administered orally. IPV is the only poliovirus vaccine available in the United States. IPV contains the 3 types of poliovirus grown in Vero cells or human diploid cells and inactivated with formaldehyde. IPV also is available in combination with other childhood vaccines (see Table 1.9, p 37). OPV contains attenuated poliovirus types 1, 2, and 3 produced in monkey kidney cells or human diploid cells.

Immunogenicity and Efficacy. Both IPV and OPV, in their recommended schedules, are highly immunogenic and effective in preventing poliomyelitis. Administration of IPV results in seroconversion in 95% or more of vaccine recipients to each of the 3 serotypes after 2 doses and results in seroconversion in 99% to 100% of recipients after 3 doses. Immunity probably is lifelong. Following exposure to live polioviruses, most IPV-immunized children will excrete virus from stool but not from the oropharynx. Stool excretion quantities and duration are reduced compared with shedding from unimmunized people. Immunization with 3 or more doses of OPV induces excellent serum antibody responses and a variable degree of intestinal immunity against poliovirus reinfection. A 3-dose series of OPV, as formerly used in the United States, results in sustained, probably lifelong immunity. After 3 doses of OPV in tropical countries, seroconversion rates are lower than in the United States because of "tropical enteropathy," a condition describing interference by other microbes with the replication of vaccine strains at the level of the gastrointestinal tract.

Administration with Other Vaccines. Either IPV or OPV may be given concurrently with other routinely recommended childhood vaccines (see Simultaneous Administration of Multiple Vaccines, p 35). For administration of combination vaccines containing IPV (see Table 1.9, p 37) with other vaccines and interchangeability of the combined vaccine with other vaccine products, see Pertussis (p 608), Hepatitis B (p 400), *Haemophilus influenzae* (p 368), and Pneumococcal Infections (p 626).

Adverse Reactions. No serious adverse events have been associated with use of IPV. Because IPV may contain trace amounts of streptomycin, neomycin, and polymyxin B, allergic reactions are possible in recipients with hypersensitivity to one or more of these antimicrobial agents.

OPV can cause VAPP. Before exclusive use of IPV in the United States beginning in 2000, the overall risk of VAPP associated with OPV was approximately 1 case per 2.4 million doses of OPV distributed. The rate of VAPP following the first dose, including vaccine recipient and contact cases, was approximately 1 case per 750 000 doses.

Schedule.[1,2] Four doses of IPV are recommended for routine immunization of all infants and children in the United States.

- The first 2 doses of the 4-dose IPV series should be given at 2-month intervals beginning at 2 months of age (minimum age, 6 weeks), and a third dose is recommended at 6 through 18 months of age. Doses may be given at 4-week intervals when accelerated protection is indicated.
- Administration of the third dose at 6 months of age has the potential advantage of enhancing the likelihood of completion of the primary series and does not compromise seroconversion.
- A fourth and final dose in the series should be administered at 4 years or older and at a minimum interval of 6 months from the third dose.
- The final dose in the IPV series at 4 years or older should be administered regardless of the number of previous doses; a fourth dose is not necessary if the third dose was given at 4 years or older and a minimum of 6 months after the second dose.
- When IPV is given in combination with other vaccines at 2, 4, 6, and 12 through 15 months of age, it is necessary to administer a fifth and final dose of IPV at 4 years or older. The minimum interval from dose 4 to dose 5 should be at least 6 months.
- If a child misses an IPV dose at 4 through 6 years of age, the child should receive a booster dose as soon as feasible.

[1]Centers for Disease Control and Prevention. Updated recommendations of the Advisory Committee on Immunization Practices (ACIP) regarding routine poliovirus vaccination. *MMWR Morb Mortal Wkly Rep.* 2009;58(30):829–830

[2]American Academy of Pediatrics, Committee on Infectious Diseases. Poliovirus. *Pediatrics.* 2011;128(4):805–808

OPV remains the vaccine of choice for global eradication, although the Strategic Advisory Group of Experts (SAGE) on Immunization of the WHO has recommended that all countries currently using OPV introduce at least 1 dose of IPV into their routine immunization schedules by the end of 2015 in preparation for stopping all use of OPV after global certification that all wild polioviruses have been eradicated.[1] OPV no longer is licensed or available in the United States.

Children Incompletely Immunized. Children who have not received the recommended doses of poliovirus vaccines on schedule should receive sufficient doses of IPV to complete the immunization series for their age (see **http://aapredbook.aappublications.org/ site/resources/izschedules.xhtml**).

Vaccine Recommendations for Adults. Most adults residing in the United States are presumed to be immune to poliovirus from previous immunization and have only a small risk of exposure to wild poliovirus in the United States. However, immunization is recommended for adults who may be traveling to areas where polio infection occurs. Travelers to polio-affected areas should receive polio vaccination or a booster polio vaccination before travel according to CDC guidance (**wwwnc.cdc.gov/travel/yellowbook/2014/chapter-3-infectious-diseases-related-to-travel/poliomyelitis**). Countries are considered to have active wild poliovirus circulation if they have ongoing endemic circulation, active polio outbreaks, or environmental evidence of active wild poliovirus circulation. Travelers working in health care settings, refugee camps, or other humanitarian aid settings in these countries may be at particular risk.

For unimmunized adults, primary immunization with IPV is recommended. Two doses of IPV should be given at intervals of 1 to 2 months (4–8 weeks); a third dose is given 6 to 12 months after the second dose. If time does not allow 3 doses of IPV to be given according to the recommended schedule before protection is required, the following alternatives are recommended:

- If protection is not needed until 8 weeks or more, 3 doses of IPV should be administered at least 4 weeks apart (eg, at weeks 0, 4, and 8).
- If protection is not needed for 4 to 8 weeks, 2 doses of IPV should be administered at least 4 weeks apart (eg, at weeks 0 and 4).
- If protection is needed in fewer than 4 weeks, a single dose of IPV should be administered.

The remaining doses of IPV to complete the primary immunization schedule should be given subsequently at the recommended intervals if the person remains at an increased risk.

Recommendations in other circumstances are as follows:

- **Incompletely immunized adults.** Adults who previously received less than a full primary series of OPV or IPV should be given the remaining required doses of IPV regardless of the interval since the last dose and the type of vaccine that was received previously.
- **Adults who are at an increased risk of exposure to wild or vaccine-derived polioviruses and who previously completed primary immunization with OPV or IPV.** These adults can receive a single dose of IPV. Available data do not indicate the need for more than a single lifetime booster dose with IPV.

---

[1]Orenstein WA, Seib KG; American Academy of Pediatrics, Committee on Infectious Diseases. Eradicating polio: how the world's pediatricians can help stop this crippling illness forever. *Pediatrics.* 2015;135(1):196–202

Travelers also may be affected by new WHO and CDC polio vaccination recommendations for people residing for 4 or more consecutive weeks in countries with ongoing poliovirus transmission and are leaving those countries to go to polio-free countries.[1]

- All residents and long-term visitors (defined as a duration of more than 4 weeks) should receive an additional dose of OPV or IPV between 4 weeks and 12 months before international travel and have the dose documented.
- Residents and long-term visitors who currently are in those countries who must travel with fewer than 4 weeks' notice and have not been vaccinated with OPV or IPV within the previous 4 week to 12 months should receive a dose at least by the time of departure.

The list of countries affected by this new recommendation can be found online: **(www.polioradication.org/infectedcountres/PolioEmergency.aspx)**.
Precautions and Contraindications to Immunization.

Immunocompromised People. Immunocompromised patients, including people with human immunodeficiency virus (HIV) infection; combined immunodeficiency; abnormalities of immunoglobulin synthesis (ie, antibody deficiency syndromes); leukemia, lymphoma, or generalized malignant neoplasm; or people receiving immunosuppressive therapy with pharmacologic agents (see Immunization in Immunocompromised Children, p 74) or radiation therapy should receive IPV. A protective immune response to IPV in an immunocompromised patient cannot be ensured.

Household Contacts of Immunocompromised People or People With Altered Immune States, Immunosuppression Attributable to Therapy for Other Disease, or Known HIV Infection. IPV is recommended for these people, and OPV should not be used. If OPV inadvertently is introduced into a household of an immunocompromised or HIV-infected person, close contact between the patient and the OPV recipient should be minimized for approximately 4 to 6 weeks after immunization. Household members should be counseled on practices that will minimize exposure of the immunocompromised or HIV-infected person to excreted poliovirus vaccine. These practices include exercising hand hygiene after contact with the child by all and avoiding diaper changing by the immunosuppressed person.

Pregnancy. Immunization during pregnancy generally should be avoided for reasons of theoretical risk, although no convincing evidence indicates that rates of adverse reactions to IPV are increased in pregnant women or in their developing fetuses. If immediate protection against poliomyelitis is needed, IPV is recommended.

Hypersensitivity or Anaphylactic Reactions to IPV Vaccine or Antimicrobial Agents Contained in IPV. IPV is contraindicated for people who have experienced an anaphylactic reaction after a previous dose of IPV attributable to any component of the vaccine.

Breastfeeding and mild diarrhea are not contraindications to IPV or OPV administration.

Reporting of Adverse Events After Immunization. All cases of VAPP and other serious adverse events associated temporally with poliovirus vaccine should be reported (see Vaccine Adverse Event Reporting System [VAERS], p 46).

Case Reporting and Investigation. A suspected case of poliomyelitis or a nonparalytic poliovirus infection, regardless of whether the virus is suspected to be wild poliovirus or VDPV, should be considered a **public health emergency** and reported immediately to the

---

[1]Centers for Disease Control and Prevention. Interim CDC guidance for polio vaccination for travel to and from countries affected by wild poliovirus. *MMWR Morb Mortal Wkly Rep.* 2014;63(27):591–594

state health department, which then results in an immediate epidemiologic investigation. Poliomyelitis should be considered in the differential diagnosis of all cases of acute flaccid paralysis, including Guillain-Barré syndrome, transverse myelitis, and acute neurologic illness of unknown etiology associated with limb weakness in children (see Enterovirus [Nonpoliovirus], p 333).[1] If the course is compatible clinically with poliomyelitis, specimens should be obtained for virologic studies (see Diagnostic Tests, p 646). If evidence implicates wild poliovirus or a VDPV infection, an intensive investigation will be conducted, and a public health decision will be made about the need for supplementary immunizations, choice of vaccine, and other actions. Because the vast majority of people who transmit poliovirus either are clinically asymptomatic or have a minor illness, the source person who transmitted virus to the patient with paralytic polio may be very difficult to identify (eg, there may be no known contact with someone who traveled to an area with endemic or epidemic polio). Therefore, pediatricians should be guided by the clinical presentation in deciding whether a child with acute paralysis might have polio and might warrant reporting the suspected case to public health authorities. It is important to collect 2 stool specimens 24 hours apart for detection of polio.

Polyomaviruses (BK Virus and JC Virus)

CLINICAL MANIFESTATIONS: BK virus (BKV) infection and JC virus (JCV) infection in humans usually occur in childhood and seemingly result in lifelong persistence. A primary infection in immunocompetent children generally is asymptomatic. However, because of the tropism of BKV for the genitourinary tract epithelium, it may cause asymptomatic hematuria or cystitis in healthy children. BKV is more likely to cause disease in immunocompromised people, including hemorrhagic cystitis in hematopoietic stem cell transplant recipients and interstitial nephritis and ureteral stenosis in renal transplant recipients. The primary symptom of BKV-associated hemorrhagic cystitis among immunocompromised children is painful hematuria. Passage of blood clots in the urine and secondary obstructive nephropathy can occur in patients with BKV-associated hemorrhagic cystitis. BKV-associated nephropathy occurs in 3% to 8% of renal transplant recipients and less frequently in other solid organ transplant recipients. BKV-associated nephropathy should be suspected in any renal transplant recipient with allograft dysfunction. More than half of renal allograft patients with BKV-associated nephropathy may experience allograft loss.

JCV is the cause of progressive multifocal leukoencephalopathy (PML), a disease that occurs in severely immune-compromised patients, including patients with acquired immunodeficiency syndrome (AIDS), patients receiving intensive chemotherapy, and patients receiving various monoclonal antibody therapies for immune suppression (biologic response modifiers). PML, the only known disease caused by JCV, occurs in approximately 5% of untreated adults with AIDS but is rare in children with AIDS. PML is a demyelinating disease of the central nervous system. Symptoms include cognitive disturbance, hemiparesis, ataxia, cranial nerve dysfunction, and aphasia. Lytic infection of oligodendrocytes by JCV is the primary mechanism of pathogenesis for PML. In the absence of restored T-lymphocyte function, PML almost always is fatal. PML is an

---

[1]Centers for Disease Control and Prevention. Acute neurologic illness of unknown etiology in children—Colorado, August–September 2014. *MMWR Morb Mortal Wkly.* 2014;63(40):901–902

AIDS-defining illness in human immunodeficiency virus (HIV)-infected people.[1] More than 90% of adults are infected by JCV, with most infections being acquired during childhood or adolescence.

Simian virus 40 (SV40) is a polyomavirus of Asian macaque monkeys and was an unrecognized contaminant of some lots of Sabin and Salk poliovirus vaccines between 1955 and 1963. Recently, 7 additional polyomaviruses have been detected in humans. The KI polyomavirus (KIPyV) and WU polyomavirus (WUPyV) have been identified in respiratory tract secretions, primarily in association with known pathogenic viruses of the respiratory tract. The Merkel cell polyomavirus (MCPyV) has been detected in >80% of Merkel cell carcinomas, which are rare neuroendocrine tumors of the skin. Human polyomaviruses 6 and 7 (HPyV6 and HPyV7) have been detected as asymptomatic inhabitants of human skin. The trichodysplasia spinulosa-associated polyomavirus (TSPyV) has been identified in tissue from patients with trichodysplasia spinulosa, a rare follicular disease of immunocompromised patients that primarily affects the face. Human polyomavirus 9 (HPyV9) has been detected in the serum of some renal transplant recipients. The natural history, prevalence, and pathogenic potential of these recently discovered human polyomaviruses have not yet been established.

ETIOLOGY: Polyomaviruses are nonenveloped viruses with a circular double-stranded DNA genome with icosahedral symmetry of the capsid ranging 40 to 50 nm in diameter. The genome of the polyomaviruses is approximately 5 kilobase pairs in length and encodes 5 major proteins—3 for capsid proteins VP1, VP2, and VP3 and 2 for large T and small t antigens. One of the biological characteristics of polyomavirus is the maintenance of a chronic viral infection in their host with little or no symptoms. Symptomatic disease caused by commonly known human polyomavirus infections primarily occurs in immunosuppressed people.

EPIDEMIOLOGY: Humans are the only known natural hosts for BKV and JCV. The mode of transmission of BKV and JCV is uncertain, but respiratory route and oral route by water or food have been postulated for their transmission. BKV and JCV are ubiquitous in the human population, with BKV infection occurring in early childhood and JCV infection occurring primarily in adolescence and adulthood. BKV persists in the kidney, gastrointestinal tract, and leukocytes of healthy subjects, with urinary excretion occurring in 3% to 5% of healthy adults. JCV persists in the kidney and brain of healthy people. The prevalence of urinary excretion of JCV increases with age.

DIAGNOSTIC TESTS: Antibody assays commonly are used to detect the presence of specific antibodies against individual viruses, and nucleic acid-based polymerase chain reaction (PCR) assays are the most sensitive tools for rapid viral screening for polyomaviruses and quantification of viral load. Detection of BKV T-antigen by immunohistochemical analysis of renal biopsy material is the gold standard for diagnosis of BKV-associated nephropathy. Visualization of BKV particles in a renal biopsy specimen by electron

---

[1]Guidelines for prevention and treatment of opportunistic infections in HIV-exposed and HIV-infected children. Recommendations from the National Institutes of Health, Centers for Disease Control and Prevention, the HIV Medicine Association of the Infectious Diseases Society of America, the Pediatric Infectious Diseases Society, and the American Academy of Pediatrics. *Pediatr Infect Dis J.* 2013;32(Suppl 2):i–KK4. Available at: **http://aidsinfo.nih.gov/guidelines/html/5/pediatric-oi-prevention-and-treatment-guidelines/0**

microscopy is a sensitive alternative to immunohistochemical analysis. Prospective monitoring of BK viral load in plasma commonly is used after renal transplantation. Detection of BKV nucleic acid in plasma by PCR assay is associated with an increased risk of BKV-associated nephropathy, especially when BKV viral loads exceed 10 000 genomes/mL. However, detection of BKV in urine of renal transplant recipients is common and does not predict BKV disease after renal transplantation.

The diagnosis of BKV-associated hemorrhagic cystitis is made clinically when other causes of urinary tract bleeding are excluded. Among hematopoietic stem cell transplant recipients, detection of BKV in urine is common (more than 50%), but BKV-associated hemorrhagic cystitis is much less common (10%–15%). Prolonged urinary shedding of BKV and detection of BKV in plasma after hematopoietic stem cell transplantation has been associated with increased risk of developing BKV-associated hemorrhagic cystitis. Urine cytologic testing may suggest urinary shedding of BKV on the basis of presence of decoy cells, which resemble renal carcinoma cells. However, decoy cells do not have high sensitivity or specificity for BKV disease.

A confirmed diagnosis of PML requires a compatible clinical syndrome and magnetic resonance imaging or computed tomographic findings showing lesions in the brain white matter coupled with brain biopsy findings. JCV can be demonstrated by in situ hybridization, electron microscopy, or immunohistochemistry. Diagnosis of PML can be facilitated when JCV DNA is detected in cerebrospinal fluid by a nucleic acid amplification test, which may obviate the need for a brain biopsy. Early in the course of PML, false-negative PCR assay results have been reported, so repeat testing is warranted when clinical suspicion of PML is high. Measurement of JCV DNA concentrations in cerebrospinal fluid samples may be a useful marker for managing PML in patients with AIDS who are receiving combination antiretroviral therapy.

TREATMENT: Several studies evaluating treatment options (eg, cidofovir, brincidofovir, levofloxacin, leflunomide) are ongoing (**www.clinicaltrials.gov).** In patients with biopsy-confirmed BKV-associated nephropathy, reduction of immune suppression may prevent allograft loss. The role of Immune Globulin Intravenous (IGIV) in the treatment of BKV-associated nephropathy is uncertain. In renal transplant patients with BKV plasma viral loads greater than 10 000 genomes/mL, judicious reduction of immune suppression has been shown to prevent development of BKV-associated nephropathy without increasing the risk of rejection.

Most patients with BKV-hemorrhagic cystitis after hematopoietic stem cell transplantation require only supportive care, because restoration of immune function by stem cell engraftment ultimately will control BKV replication. In severe cases, surgical intervention may be required to stop bladder hemorrhage. Cidofovir has been used for treatment; however, definitive data on its efficacy and safety are not yet available.

Restoration of immune function (eg, combination antiretroviral therapy for patients with AIDS) is necessary for survival of patients with PML. Cidofovir sometimes is used for the treatment of PML but has not been shown to be effective in producing clinical improvement.

ISOLATION OF THE HOSPITALIZED PATIENT: Standard precautions are recommended.

CONTROL MEASURES: None.

Prion Diseases: Transmissible Spongiform Encephalopathies

CLINICAL MANIFESTATIONS: Transmissible spongiform encephalopathies (TSEs, or prion diseases) constitute a group of rare, rapidly progressive, universally fatal neurodegenerative diseases of humans and animals that are characterized by neuronal degeneration, spongiform change, gliosis, and accumulation of abnormal misfolded protease-resistant prion protein (protease-resistant prion protein [PrP^{res}], variably called scrapie prion protein [PrP^{sc}] or, as suggested by the World Health Organization, TSE-associated PrP [PrP^{TSE}]) that distributes diffusely throughout the brain or forms plaques of various morphology.

Human TSEs include several diseases: Creutzfeldt-Jakob disease (CJD), Gerstmann-Sträussler-Scheinker disease, fatal familial and sporadic fatal insomnia, kuru, and variant CJD (vCJD, presumably caused by the agent of bovine spongiform encephalopathy [BSE], commonly called "mad cow" disease). Classic CJD can be sporadic (approximately 85% of cases), familial (approximately 15% of cases), or iatrogenic (fewer than 1% of cases). Sporadic CJD most commonly is a disease of older adults (median age of death in the United States, 68 years) but also rarely has been described in adolescents older than 13 years and young adults. Iatrogenic CJD has been acquired through intramuscular injection of contaminated cadaveric pituitary hormones (growth hormone and human gonadotropin), dura mater allografts, corneal transplantation, and use of contaminated instrumentation at neurosurgery or during depth-electrode electroencephalographic recording. In 1996, an outbreak of vCJD linked to exposure to tissues from BSE-infected cattle was reported in the United Kingdom. Since the end of 2003, 4 presumptive cases of transfusion-transmitted vCJD have been reported: 3 clinical cases as well as 1 probable asymptomatic case in which PrP^{TSE} was detected in spleen and lymph nodes but not brain tissues. A fifth iatrogenic vCJD infection in a hemophiliac patient in the United Kingdom, also preclinical with a finding of PrP^{TSE} in spleen, was attributed to treatment with potentially vCJD-contaminated, UK-sourced fractionated plasma products. The best-known TSEs affecting animals include scrapie of sheep, BSE, and a chronic wasting disease of North American deer, elk, and moose (**www.cdc.gov/ncidod/dvrd/cwd/**). Except for vCJD, no other human TSE has been attributed to infection with an agent of animal origin.

CJD manifests as a rapidly progressive neurologic disease with escalating defects in memory, personality, and other higher cortical functions. At presentation, approximately one third of patients have cerebellar dysfunction, including ataxia and dysarthria. Iatrogenic CJD also may manifest as dementia with cerebellar signs. Myoclonus develops in at least 80% of affected patients at some point in the course of disease. Death usually occurs in weeks to months (median, 4–5 months); approximately 10% to 15% of patients with sporadic CJD survive for more than 1 year.

vCJD is distinguished from classic CJD by younger age of onset, early "psychiatric" manifestations, and other features, such as painful sensory symptoms, delayed onset of overt neurologic signs, relative absence of diagnostic electroencephalographic changes, and a more prolonged duration of illness (median, 13–14 months). In vCJD, but not in classic CJD, a high proportion of people exhibit high signal abnormalities on T2-weighted brain magnetic resonance imaging in the pulvinar region of the posterior thalamus (known as the "pulvinar sign"). In vCJD, the neuropathologic examination reveals numerous "florid" plaques (surrounded by vacuoles) and exceptionally striking accumulation of PrP^{TSE} in the brain. In addition, PrP^{TSE} is detectable in the tonsils and other lymphoid tissues of patients with vCJD.

ETIOLOGY: The infectious particle or prion responsible for human and animal prion diseases is believed to be a misfolded form of a normal ubiquitous prion protein (PrP) found on the surface of neurons and many other cells in both humans and animals. The precise protein structure and mechanism of propagation is unknown. It is generally postulated that sporadic CJD arises from a spontaneous structural change into the pathogenic form of the normal "cellular" protease-sensitive host-encoded glycoprotein (PrP^C or PrP^{sen}). Prion propagation is postulated to occur by a "recruitment" reaction (the nature of which is under investigation), in which abnormal PrP^{TSE} serves as a template or lattice for the conversion of neighboring PrP^C molecules into misfolded protein with high potential to aggregate.

EPIDEMIOLOGY: Classic CJD is rare, occurring in the United States at a rate of approximately 1 case per million people annually. The onset of disease peaks in the 60- through 74-year age group. Case-control studies of sporadic CJD have not identified any consistent environmental risk factor. No statistically significant increase in cases of sporadic CJD has been observed in people previously treated with blood, blood components, or plasma derivatives (see Blood Safety: Reducing the Risk of Transfusion-Transmitted Infections, p 112). The incidence of sporadic CJD is not increased in patients with several diseases associated with frequent exposure to blood or blood products, specifically hemophilia A and B, thalassemia, and sickle cell disease, suggesting that the risk of transfusion transmission of classic CJD, if any, is very low and appropriately regarded as theoretical. CJD has not been reported in infants born to infected mothers. Familial or genetic form of TSEs, inherited as autosomal-dominant disorder, is associated with a variety of mutations of the PrP-encoding gene (PRNP) located on chromosome 20. Familial CJD onset of disease is approximately 10 years earlier than sporadic CJD.

As of June 2014 (**www.cjd.ed.ac.uk/documents/worldfigs.pdf**), the total number of vCJD cases reported was in 177 patients in the United Kingdom, 27 in France, 5 in Spain, 4 in Ireland, 4 in the United States, 3 in the Netherlands, 2 in Portugal, 2 in Italy, 2 in Canada, and 1 each in Taiwan, Japan, and Saudi Arabia. Two of the 4 patients in the United States, 2 of the 4 in Ireland, and 1 each of the patients in France and Canada are believed to have acquired vCJD during prolonged residence in the United Kingdom. The Centers for Disease Control and Prevention (CDC) and Health Canada have concluded that one of the vCJD patient in the United States and in Canada probably were infected during their residencies as children in Saudi Arabia. Authorities suspect that the Japanese patient was infected during a short visit of 24 days to the United Kingdom in 1990, 12 years before the onset of vCJD. Most patients with vCJD were younger than 30 years, and several were adolescents. All but 3 of the primary 174 United Kingdom patients with noniatrogenic vCJD died before 60 years of age. All but 14 patients died before 50 years of age, and 151 patients (87%) died before the age of 40. The median age at death of the 173 primary vCJD cases was 27 years. The ages at death of the 3 iatrogenic vCJD transfusion transmission cases were 32, 69, and 75 years. On the basis of animal inoculation studies, comparative PrP immunoblotting, and epidemiologic investigations, almost all cases of vCJD are believed to have resulted from exposure to tissues from cattle infected with BSE. As noted, 3 clinically symptomatic patients and 1 patient with no clinical signs of the disease are believed to have been infected with vCJD through transfusion of nonleukoreduced red blood cells, and 1 hemophiliac patient, also with no clinical signs of TSE, was probably infected through injections of human plasma-derived clotting factors.

The **incubation period** for iatrogenic CJD varies by route of exposure and ranges from about 14 months to more than 30 years.

DIAGNOSTIC TESTS: The diagnosis of human prion diseases can be made with certainty only by neuropathologic examination of affected brain tissue, usually obtained at autopsy. In most patients with classic CJD, a characteristic 1-cycle to 2-cycles per second triphasic sharp-wave discharge on electroencephalographic tracing is regarded as indicative of CJD. The likelihood of finding this abnormality is enhanced when serial electroencephalographic recordings are obtained. A protein assay that detects the 14-3-3 protein in cerebrospinal fluid (CSF) has been reported to be reasonably sensitive, although not specific, as a marker for CJD. Measurement of the tau protein level in addition to the detection of 14-3-3 protein in the CSF has been reported to increase the specificity of CSF testing for CJD. Specific disease marker PrP^{TSE} was demonstrated in CSF of 80% CJD cases, but currently, testing for this marker can be performed only on an investigational basis in a few laboratories using sophisticated techniques for detecting minute amounts of the protein. No validated blood test is available, but a prototype test for vCJD that captures, enriches, and detects disease-associated prion protein from whole blood using stainless steel powder is being investigated.[1] A progressive neurologic syndrome in a person bearing a pathogenic mutation of the PRNP gene (not a normal polymorphism) is presumed to be prion disease. Because no unique nucleic acid has been detected in prions (the infectious particles) causing TSEs, genome amplification studies such as PCR are not possible. Consideration of brain biopsies for patients with possible CJD should be given when other potentially treatable diseases remain in the differential diagnosis. Complete postmortem examination of the brain is encouraged to confirm the clinical diagnosis and to detect emerging forms of CJD, such as vCJD. State-of-the-art diagnostic testing, including assays of 14-3-3 and tau proteins in CSF, PRNP gene sequencing, Western blot analysis to identify and characterize PrP^{TSE}, and histologic processing of brain tissues with expert neuropathologic consultation, are offered by the National Prion Disease Pathology Surveillance Center (telephone, 216-368-0587; **www.cjdsurveillance.com**).

TREATMENT: No treatment has been shown in humans to slow or stop the progressive neurodegeneration in prion diseases. Experimental treatments are being studied. Supportive therapy is necessary to manage dementia, spasticity, rigidity, and seizures occurring during the course of the illness. Psychological support may help families of affected people. Genetic counseling is indicated in familial disease, taking into account that penetrance has been variable in some families in which people with a PRNP mutation survived to an advanced age without neurodegenerative disease. A family support and patient advocacy group, the CJD Foundation (telephone 330-665-5590; **www.cjdfoundation.org**), offers helpful information and advice.

ISOLATION OF THE HOSPITALIZED PATIENT: Standard precautions are recommended. Available evidence indicates that even prolonged intimate contact with CJD-infected people has not resulted in transmission of disease. Tissues associated with high levels of infectivity (eg, brain, eyes, and spinal cord of affected people) and instruments in contact

[1]Jackson GS, Burk-Rafel J, Edgeworth JA, et al. Population screening for variant Creutzfeldt-Jakob disease using a novel blood test: diagnostic accuracy and feasibility study. *JAMA Neurol.* 2014:71(4):421–428

with those tissues are considered biohazards; incineration, prolonged autoclaving at high temperature and pressure after thorough cleaning, and especially exposure to a solution of 1 N or greater sodium hydroxide or a solution of 5.25% or greater sodium hypochlorite (undiluted household chlorine bleach) for 1 hour has been reported to decrease markedly or eliminate infectivity of contaminated surgical instruments.[1] Detailed CJD infection-control recommendations, distribution of infectivity in various tissues, and specific decontamination protocols are available online (**www.cdc.gov/ncidod/dvrd/ cjd/qa_cjd_infection_control.htm** and **www.who.int/csr/resources/ publications/bse/WHO_CDS_CSR_APH_2000_3/en/**). Person-to-person transmission of classic CJD by blood, milk, saliva, urine, or feces has not been reported. These body fluids should be handled using standard infection control procedures; universal blood precautions should be sufficient to prevent bloodborne transmission.

CONTROL MEASURES: Immunization against prion diseases is not available, and no protective immune response to infection has been demonstrated. Iatrogenic transmission of CJD through cadaveric pituitary hormones has been obviated by use of recombinant products. Recognition that CJD can be spread by transplantation of infected dura and corneas and that vCJD can be spread by blood transfusion has led to more stringent donor-selection criteria and improved collection protocols. Health care professionals should follow their state's prion disease reporting requirements and indicate CJD or other prion disease diagnoses appropriately on death certificates; US mortality data are used to help monitor occurrences of prion diseases. In addition, any suspected or confirmed diagnosis of a prion disease of special public health concern (eg, suspected iatrogenic disease or vCJD) should be reported promptly to the appropriate state or local health departments and to the CDC (telephone, 404-639-3091; **www.cdc.gov/ ncidod/dvrd/prions/**). Current precautionary policies of the US Food and Drug Administration to reduce the risk of transmitting CJD by human blood or blood products are available online (**www.fda.gov/downloads/BiologicsBloodVaccines/ GuidanceComplianceRegulatoryInformation/Guidances/UCM213415.pdf**). General information about BSE is available from the Food and Drug Administration (**www.fda.gov/AnimalVeterinary/ResourcesforYou/AnimalHealthLiteracy/ ucm136222.htm**), from the USDA (**www.fsis.usda.gov/wps/portal/fsis/ topics/food-safety-education/get-answers/food-safety-fact-sheets/ production-and-inspection/bovine-spongiform-encephalopathy-mad-cow- disease/bse-mad-cow-disease**), from the CDC (**www.cdc.gov/ncidod/dvrd/ bse/**), and from the World Organisation for Animal Health (**www.oie.int/en/ animal-health-in-the-world/bse-portal/**).

Q Fever (*Coxiella burnetii* Infection)

CLINICAL MANIFESTATIONS: Approximately half of acute Q fever infections result in symptoms. Acute and chronic forms of the disease exist and both can present as fever of unknown origin. Q fever in children typically is characterized by abrupt onset of fever often accompanied by chills, headache, weakness, cough, and other nonspecific systemic symptoms. Illness mainly is self-limited, although a relapsing febrile illness lasting for several months has been documented in children. Gastrointestinal tract symptoms, such

---

[1] **www.cdc.gov/ncidod/dvrd/prions**

as diarrhea, vomiting, abdominal pain, and anorexia, are reported in 50% to 80% of children. Rash also has been observed in some patients with Q fever. Q fever pneumonia usually manifests as mild cough, respiratory distress, and chest pain. Chest radiographic patterns are variable. More severe manifestations of acute Q fever are rare but include hepatitis, hemolytic-uremic syndrome, myocarditis, pericarditis, cerebellitis, encephalitis, meningitis, hemophagocytosis, lymphadenitis, acalculous cholecystitis, and rhabdomyolysis. Chronic Q fever is rare in children but can present as blood culture-negative endocarditis, chronic relapsing or multifocal osteomyelitis, or chronic hepatitis. Children who are immunocompromised or have underlying valvular heart disease may be at higher risk of chronic Q fever.

ETIOLOGY: *Coxiella burnetii*, the cause of Q fever, formerly was considered to be a *Rickettsia* organism but is a gram-negative intracellular bacterium that belongs to the order *Legionellaceae*. The infectious form of *C burnetii* is highly resistant to heat, desiccation, and disinfectant chemicals and can persist for long periods of time in the environment. *C burnetii* is classified as a category B bioterrorism agent by the Centers for Disease Control and Prevention (CDC).

EPIDEMIOLOGY: Q fever is a zoonotic infection that has been reported worldwide, including every state in the United States. *C burnetii* infection usually is asymptomatic in animals. Many different species can be infected, although cattle, sheep, and goats are the primary reservoirs for human infection. Tick vectors may be important for maintaining animal and bird reservoirs but are not thought to be important in transmission to humans. Humans most often acquire infection by inhalation of fine-particle aerosols of *C burnetii* generated from birthing fluids or other excreta of infected animals or through inhalation of dust contaminated by these materials. Infection can occur by exposure to contaminated materials, such as wool, straw, bedding, or laundry. Windborne particles containing infectious organisms can travel a half-mile or more, contributing to sporadic cases for which no apparent animal contact can be demonstrated. Unpasteurized dairy products can contain the organism.[1] Seasonal trends occur in farming areas with predictable frequency, and the disease often coincides with the livestock birthing season in spring.

The **incubation period** is 14 to 22 days, with a range from 9 to 39 days, depending on the inoculum size. Chronic Q fever can develop months or years after initial infection.

DIAGNOSTIC TESTS[2]: Serologic evidence of a fourfold increase in phase II immunoglobulin (Ig) G via immunofluorescent assay (IFA) tests between paired sera taken 3 to 6 weeks apart is the diagnostic gold standard to confirm diagnosis of acute Q fever. Polymerase chain reaction (PCR) testing on blood or serum may be useful in the first 2 weeks of symptom onset and before antibiotic administration. Although a positive PCR assay result can confirm the diagnosis, a negative PCR test result will not rule out Q fever. A single high serum phase II IgG titer (≥1:128) by IFA in the convalescent stage may be considered evidence of probable infection. Confirmation of chronic Q fever is based on an increasing phase I IgG titer (typically ≥1:1024) that often is higher than the phase II IgG titer *and* an identifiable nidus of infection (eg, endocarditis, vascular infection,

---

[1]American Academy of Pediatrics, Committee on Infectious Diseases and Committee on Nutrition. Consumption of raw or unpasteurized milk and milk products by pregnant women and children. *Pediatrics.* 2014;133(1):175–179

[2]Centers for Disease Control and Prevention. Diagnosis and management of Q fever—United States, 2013: recommendations from CDC and the Q Fever Working Group. *MMWR Recomm Rep.* 2013;62(RR-3):1–30

osteomyelitis, chronic hepatitis). Detection of *C burnetii* in tissues by immunohistochemistry or PCR assay can also confirm a diagnosis of chronic Q fever. Isolation of *C burnetii* from blood can be performed only in special laboratories because of the potential hazard to laboratory workers.

TREATMENT[2]: Acute Q fever generally is a self-limited illness, and many patients recover without antimicrobial therapy. However, early treatment is extremely effective in shortening illness duration and symptom severity and should be given to all symptomatic patients. For patients with suspected disease, immediate empiric therapy should be given, because laboratory results are often negative early in illness onset pending production of measureable antibody. Doxycycline (100 mg, orally, 2 times/day for children 8 years or older; or 4 mg/kg per day, orally, divided 2 times/day for children younger than 8 years, for 14 days) is the drug of choice for severe infections in patients of any age. Tetracycline-based antimicrobial agents, including doxycycline, may cause permanent tooth discoloration for children younger than 8 years if used for repeated treatment courses. However, doxycycline binds less readily to calcium compared with older tetracyclines, and in some studies, doxycycline was not associated with visible teeth staining in younger children (see Tetracyclines, p 873). Children younger than 8 years with mild illness, pregnant women, and patients allergic to doxycycline can be treated with trimethoprim-sulfamethoxazole.

Chronic Q fever is much more difficult to treat, and relapses can occur despite appropriate therapy, necessitating repeated courses of therapy. The recommended therapy for chronic Q fever endocarditis is a combination of doxycycline and hydroxychloroquine for a minimum of 18 months. Surgical replacement of the infected valve may be necessary in some patients.

ISOLATION OF THE HOSPITALIZED PATIENT: Standard precautions are recommended.

CONTROL MEASURES: Strict adherence to proper hygiene when handling infected parturient animals or their excreta can help decrease the risk of infection in the farm setting, as can ensuring consumption of pasteurized milk and milk products. Improved prescreening of animal herds used by research facilities may decrease the risk of infection. Special safety practices are recommended for nonpropagative laboratory procedures involving *C burnetii* and for all propagative procedures, during aerosol-generating procedures performed on infected patients, and during high-risk worker exposures in biomedical facilities that house sheep and goats. Vaccines for domestic animals and people working in high-risk occupations have been developed but are not licensed in the United States. Q fever is a nationally reportable disease, and all human cases should be reported to the state health department. Additional information about Q fever is available on the CDC Web site (**www.cdc.gov/mmwr/preview/mmwrhtml/rr6203a1.htm** or **www.cdc.gov/qfever/index.html**).

Rabies[1]

CLINICAL MANIFESTATIONS: Infection with rabies virus and other lyssaviruses characteristically produces an acute illness with rapidly progressive central nervous system manifestations, including anxiety, radicular pain, dysesthesia or pruritus, hydrophobia, and dysautonomia. Some patients may have paralysis. Illness almost invariably progresses

---

[1]For further information, see Centers for Disease Control and Prevention. Human rabies prevention: United States, 2008. Recommendations of the Advisory Committee on Immunization Practices. *MMWR Recomm Rep.* 2008;57(RR-3):1–28

to death. Three unimmunized people have recovered from clinical rabies in the United States.[1] The differential diagnosis of acute encephalitic illnesses of unknown cause or with features of Guillain-Barré syndrome should include rabies.

ETIOLOGY: Rabies virus is an RNA virus classified in the *Rhabdoviridae* family, *Lyssavirus* genus. The genus *Lyssavirus* currently contains 12 species with 2 additional putative species divided into 3 phylogroups.

EPIDEMIOLOGY: Understanding the epidemiology of rabies has been aided by viral variant identification using monoclonal antibodies and nucleotide sequencing. In the United States, human cases have decreased steadily since the 1950s, reflecting widespread immunization of dogs and the availability of effective prophylaxis after exposure to a rabid animal. From 2000 through July 2013, 31 of 43 cases of human rabies reported in the United States were acquired indigenously. Among the 31 indigenously acquired cases, all but 4 were associated with bats. Despite the large focus of rabies in raccoons in the eastern United States, only 3 human deaths have been attributed to the raccoon rabies virus variant. Historically, 2 cases of human rabies were attributable to probable aerosol exposure in laboratories, and 2 unusual cases have been attributed to possible airborne exposures in caves inhabited by millions of bats, although alternative infection routes cannot be discounted. Transmission also has occurred by transplantation of organs, corneas, and other tissues from patients dying of undiagnosed rabies. Person-to-person transmission by bite has not been documented in the United States, although the virus has been isolated from saliva of infected patients.

Wildlife rabies perpetuates throughout all of the 50 United States except Hawaii, which remains "rabies free." Wildlife, including bats, raccoons, skunks, foxes, coyotes, and bobcats, are the most important potential sources of infection for humans and domestic animals in the United States. Rabies in small rodents (squirrels, hamsters, guinea pigs, gerbils, chipmunks, rats, and mice) and lagomorphs (rabbits, pikas, and hares) is rare. Rabies may occur in woodchucks or other large rodents in areas where raccoon rabies is common. The virus is present in saliva and is transmitted by bites or, rarely, by contamination of mucosa or skin lesions by saliva or other potentially infectious material (eg, neural tissue). Worldwide, most rabies cases in humans result from dog bites in areas where canine rabies is enzootic. Most rabid dogs, cats, and ferrets shed virus for a few days before there are obvious signs of illness. No case of human rabies in the United States has been attributed to a dog, cat, or ferret that has remained healthy throughout the standard 10-day period of confinement after an exposure.

The **incubation period** in humans averages 1 to 3 months but ranges from days to years.

DIAGNOSTIC TESTS: Infection in animals can be diagnosed by demonstration of the presence of rabies virus antigen in brain tissue using a direct fluorescent antibody (DFA) test. Suspected rabid animals should be euthanized in a manner that preserves brain tissue for appropriate laboratory diagnosis. Virus can be isolated in suckling mice or in tissue culture from saliva, brain, and other specimens and can be detected by identification of viral antigens or nucleotide sequences in affected tissues. Diagnosis in suspected human cases can be made postmortem by either immunofluorescent or immunohistochemical examination of brain tissue or by detection of viral nucleotide sequences. Antemortem diagnosis can

---

[1]Centers for Disease Control and Prevention. Recovery of a patient from clinical rabies—California, 2011. *MMWR Morb Mortal Wkly Rep.* 2012;61(4):61–65

be made by DFA test on skin biopsy specimens from the nape of the neck, by isolation of the virus from saliva, by detection of antibody in serum in unvaccinated people and cerebrospinal fluid (CSF) in all people, and by detection of viral nucleotide sequences in saliva, skin, or other tissues. No single test is sufficiently sensitive because of the unique nature of rabies pathobiology. Laboratory personnel and state health or local health departments should be consulted before submission of specimens to the Centers for Disease Control and Prevention so appropriate collection and transport of materials can be arranged.

TREATMENT: There is no specific treatment. Two female adolescents fit current laboratory criteria for rabies but did not require intensive care. Once symptoms have developed, neither rabies vaccine nor Rabies Immune Globulin (RIG) improves the prognosis. Ten people have survived rabies in association with incomplete rabies vaccine schedules. Since 2004, 3 female children, all of whom had not received rabies postexposure prophylaxis, survived rabies. A combination of sedation and intensive medical intervention may be valuable adjunctive therapy.[1] Details of the management protocol used can be found at **www.mcw.edu/rabies**.

ISOLATION OF THE HOSPITALIZED PATIENT: Standard precautions (ie, gowns, gloves, goggles, and masks) are recommended for the duration of illness. If the patient has bitten another person or potentially infectious material from the patient has contaminated an open wound or mucous membrane, the involved area should be washed thoroughly with soap and water and risk assessment should be completed to determine whether postexposure prophylaxis should be administered (see Care of Exposed People, p 662).

CONTROL MEASURES: In the United States, animal rabies is common. Education of children to avoid contact with stray or wild animals is of primary importance. Inadvertent contact of family members and pets with potentially rabid animals, such as raccoons, foxes, coyotes, and skunks, may be decreased by securing garbage and pet food outdoors to decrease attraction of domestic and wild animals. Similarly, chimneys and other potential entrances for wildlife, including bats, should be identified and covered. Bats should be excluded from human living quarters. International travelers to areas with enzootic canine rabies should be warned to avoid exposure to stray dogs, and if traveling to an area with enzootic infection where immediate access to medical care and biologic agents is limited, preexposure prophylaxis is indicated.

Exposure Risk and Decisions to Administer Prophylaxis. Exposure to rabies results from a break in the skin caused by the teeth of a rabid animal or by contamination of scratches, abrasions, or mucous membranes with saliva or other potentially infectious material, such as neural tissue, from a rabid animal. The decision to immunize a potentially exposed person should be made in consultation with the local health department, which can provide information on risk of rabies in a particular area for each species of animal and in accordance with the guidance in Table 3.59. In the United States, all mammals are believed to be susceptible, but bats, raccoons, skunks, and foxes are more likely to be infected than are other animals. Coyotes, cattle, dogs, cats, ferrets, and other animals occasionally are infected. Bites of rodents (such as squirrels, mice, and rats) or lagomorphs (rabbits, hares, and pikas) rarely require prophylaxis. Additional factors must be considered when deciding whether immunoprophylaxis is indicated. An unprovoked attack may be more suggestive of a rabid animal than a bite that occurs during attempts to feed or handle an

[1]Centers for Disease Control and Prevention. Recovery of a patient from clinical rabies—California, 2011. *MMWR Morb Mortal Wkly Rep.* 2012;61(4):61–65

Table 3.59. Rabies Postexposure Prophylaxis Guide

Animal Type	Evaluation and Disposition of Animal	Postexposure Prophylaxis Recommendations
Dogs, cats, and ferrets	Healthy and available for 10 days of observation	Prophylaxis only if animal develops signs of rabies[a]
	Rabid or suspected of being rabid[b]	Immediate immunization and RIG[c]
	Unknown (escaped)	Consult public health officials for advice
Bats, skunks, raccoons, foxes, and most other carnivores; woodchucks	Regarded as rabid unless geographic area is known to be free of rabies or until animal proven negative by laboratory tests[b]	Immediate immunization and RIG[c]
Livestock, rodents, and lagomorphs (rabbits, hares, and pikas)	Consider individually	Consult public health officials; bites of squirrels, hamsters, guinea pigs, gerbils, chipmunks, rats, mice and other rodents, rabbits, hares, and pikas almost never require rabies postexposure prophylaxis

RIG indicates Rabies Immune Globulin.

[a] During the 10-day observation period, at the first sign of rabies in the biting dog, cat, or ferret, prophylaxis of the exposed person with RIG (human) and vaccine should be initiated. The animal should be euthanized immediately and tested.

[b] The animal should be euthanized and tested as soon as possible. Holding for observation is not recommended. Immunization is discontinued if immunofluorescent test result for the animal is negative.

[c] See text.

animal. Properly immunized dogs, cats, and ferrets have only a minimal chance of developing rabies. However, in rare instances, rabies has developed in properly immunized animals.

Postexposure prophylaxis for rabies is recommended for all people bitten by wild mammalian carnivores or bats or by domestic animals that are suspected to be rabid unless laboratory tests prove that the animal does not have rabies. Postexposure prophylaxis also is recommended for people who report an open wound, scratch, or mucous membrane that has been contaminated with saliva or other potentially infectious material (eg, brain tissue) from a rabid animal. The injury inflicted by a bat bite or scratch may be small and not readily evident, or the circumstances of contact with a bat may preclude accurate recall (eg, a bat in a room of a deeply sleeping or medicated person or a previously unattended child, especially an infant or toddler who cannot reliably communicate about a potential bite). Hence, postexposure prophylaxis may be indicated, following proper risk assessment, for situations in which a bat physically is present in the same room if a bite or mucous membrane exposure cannot reliably be excluded, unless prompt testing of the bat has excluded rabies virus infection. Prophylaxis should be initiated as soon as possible after bites by known or suspected rabid animals.

Risk assessment for the administration of postexposure prophylaxis is recommended for people who report a possibly infectious exposure (eg, bite, scratch, or open wound or mucous membrane contaminated with saliva or other infectious material, such as tears, CSF, or brain tissue) to a human with rabies. Rabies virus transmission after exposure to a human with rabies has not been documented convincingly in the United States, except after tissue or organ transplantation from donors who died of unsuspected rabies encephalitis. Casual contact with an infected person (eg, by touching a patient) or contact with noninfectious fluids or tissues (eg, blood or feces) alone does not constitute an exposure and is not an indication for prophylaxis (see Care of Hospital Contacts).

Handling of Animals Suspected of Having Rabies. A dog, cat, or ferret that is suspected of having rabies and has bitten a human should be captured, confined, euthanized, and tested or should be observed by a veterinarian for 10 days by order of public health authorities. If signs of rabies develop, the animal should be euthanized in a manner to allow its head to be removed and shipped under refrigeration (not frozen, which would delay testing) to a qualified laboratory for examination.

Other biting animals that may have exposed a person to rabies virus should be reported immediately to the local health department. Management of animals depends on the species, the circumstances of the bite, and the epidemiology of rabies in the area. Previous immunization of an animal may not preclude the necessity for euthanasia and testing. Because clinical manifestations of rabies in a wild animal cannot be interpreted reliably, a wild mammal suspected of having rabies should be euthanized at once, and its brain should be examined for evidence of rabies virus infection. The exposed person need not receive prophylaxis if the result of rapid examination of the brain by the direct fluorescent antibody test is negative for rabies virus infection.

Risk Assessments for Contacts of Humans With Rabies. Administration of postexposure prophylaxis to hospital contacts of patients with rabies is required only in situations in which potentially infectious material (such as saliva, CSF, or brain tissue) comes into direct contact with broken skin or mucous membranes. It is expected that in cases in which people were using appropriate protective equipment, there will likely be no risk of exposures (see Care of Exposed People).

Care of Exposed People.

Local Wound Care. The immediate objective of postexposure prophylaxis is to prevent virus from entering neural tissue. Prompt and thorough local treatment of all lesions is essential, because virus may remain localized to the area of the bite for a variable time. All wounds should be flushed thoroughly and cleaned with soap and water. Quaternary ammonium compounds (such as benzalkonium chloride) no longer are considered superior to soap. The need for tetanus prophylaxis and measures to control bacterial infection also should be considered. The wound, if possible, should not be sutured. For severe facial wounds, which often are also infected with bacteria, better cosmesis results from single sutures, widely placed, several hours after local instillation of RIG, followed by plastic surgery days later.

Prophylaxis (see Table 3.59, p 661). After wound care is completed, concurrent use of passive and active prophylaxis is optimal, with the exceptions of people who previously have received complete vaccination regimens (pre- or postexposure) with a cell culture vaccine or people who have been vaccinated with other types of rabies vaccines and have previously had a documented rabies virus-neutralizing antibody titer; these people should receive only vaccine. Prophylaxis should begin as soon as possible after exposure, ideally within 24 hours. However, a delay of several days or more may not compromise effectiveness, and prophylaxis should be initiated if reasonably indicated, regardless of the interval between exposure and initiation of therapy. In the United States, only human RIG is available for passive

Table 3.60. US Food and Drug Administration-Licensed Rabies Vaccines[a] and Rabies Immune Globulin Products

Category	Product	Manufacturer	Dose and Route of Administration
Human rabies vaccine	Human diploid cell vaccine (HDCV) (Imovax)	Sanofi Pasteur	1 mL, IM
	Purified chicken embryo cell vaccine (PCECV) (RabAvert)	Novartis Vaccines and Diagnostics	1 mL, IM
Rabies Immune Globulin	Imogam Rabies-HT	Sanofi Pasteur	20 IU/kg, infiltrate around wound[b]
	HyperRab S/D	Talecris Biotherapeutics	20 IU/kg, infiltrate around wound[b]

IM indicates intramuscular.

[a]Rabies vaccine adsorbed (RVA) is licensed in the United States but no longer is distributed in the United States.

[b]Any remaining volume should be administered intramuscularly.

immunization. Licensed cell culture rabies vaccine should be used for active immunization. Physicians can obtain expert counsel from their local or state health departments.

Active Immunization (Postexposure). Human diploid cell vaccine (HDCV) and purified chicken embryo cell vaccine (PCECV) are available for use in the United States (see Table 3.60). For a previously unvaccinated immunocompetent person, a 1.0-mL dose of vaccine is given intramuscularly in the deltoid area (the anterolateral aspect of the thigh is also acceptable for children) on the first day of postexposure prophylaxis (day 0), and repeated doses are given on days 3, 7, and 14 after the first dose, for a total of 4 doses,[1] with 1 dose of RIG given on day 0. The volume of the dose is not decreased for children. For a person with altered immunocompetence, postexposure prophylaxis should include a 5-dose vaccination regimen (ie, 1 dose of vaccine on days 0, 3, 7, 14, and 28), with 1 dose of RIG. Serologic testing to document seroconversion after administration of a rabies vaccine series usually is not necessary but occasionally has been advised for recipients who may be immunocompromised or for people with deviations from the recommended vaccination schedule. Immune response should be assessed by performing serologic testing 7 to 14 days after administration of the final dose in the series. Ideally, a vaccination series should be initiated and completed with 1 vaccine product unless serious adverse reactions occur. Clinical studies evaluating efficacy or frequency of adverse reactions when the series is completed with a second product have not been conducted.

Care should be taken to ensure that the vaccine is administered intramuscularly. Intradermal vaccine is not advised for postexposure prophylaxis in the United States, although for reasons of cost and availability, intradermal regimens are recommended by the World Health Organization and frequently are used in some countries. Because virus-neutralizing antibody responses in adults who received vaccine in the gluteal area sometimes have been less than in those who were injected in the deltoid muscle, the deltoid site always should be used except in infants and young children, in whom the anterolateral thigh is the appropriate site.

---

[1]Centers for Disease Control and Prevention. Use of a reduced (4-dose) vaccine schedule for postexposure prophylaxis to prevent human rabies: recommendations of the Advisory Committee on Immunization Practices. *MMWR Recomm Rep.* 2010;59(RR–02):1–9

- **Adverse reactions and precautions with HDCV and PCECV:** Reactions are uncommon in children. In adults, mild local reactions, such as pain, erythema, and swelling or itching at the injection site, are reported in 15% to 25%, and mild systemic reactions, such as headache, nausea, abdominal pain, muscle aches, and dizziness, are reported in 10% to 20% of recipients. Immune complex-like reactions in people receiving booster doses of HDCV have been observed, possibly because of interaction between propiolactone contained in the vaccine and human albumin. The reaction, characterized by onset 2 to 21 days after inoculation, begins with generalized urticaria and can include arthralgia, arthritis, angioedema, nausea, vomiting, fever, and malaise. The reaction is not life threatening, occurs in as many as 6% of adults receiving booster doses as part of a preexposure immunization regimen, and is rare in people receiving primary immunization with HDCV. Similar allergic reactions with primary or booster doses have been reported with PCECV. If the patient has a serious allergic reaction to HDCV, PCECV may be given according to the same schedule as HDCV, and vice-versa. If reactions following vaccine are mild, pretreatment with antihistamines just before the next vaccination can be considered. All suspected serious, systemic, para-lytic, or anaphylactic reactions to rabies vaccine should be reported immediately to the Vaccine Adverse Events Reporting System (p 46).

  Although the safety of rabies vaccine during pregnancy has not been studied specifi-cally in the United States, pregnancy should not be considered a contraindication to use of vaccine or RIG after exposure.
- **Nerve tissue vaccines:** Inactivated nerve tissue vaccines are not licensed in the United States and not recommended by the World Health Organization but still are used in some areas of the world. These preparations induce neuroparalytic reactions in 1 in 2000 to 1 in 8000 recipients. Vaccination with nerve tissue vaccine should be discontinued if meningeal or neuroparalytic reactions develop. Corticosteroids should be used only for life-threatening reactions, because they increase the risk of rabies in experimentally inoculated animals.

Passive Immunization. Human RIG should be used concomitantly with the first dose of vac-cine for postexposure prophylaxis to bridge the time between possible infection and anti-body production induced by the vaccine (see Table 3.60, p 663). If vaccine is not available immediately, RIG should be administered alone, and vaccination should be started as soon as possible. If RIG is not available immediately, vaccine should be administered and RIG administered subsequently if obtained within 7 days after initiating vaccination. If administration of both vaccine and RIG is delayed, both should be used regardless of the interval between exposure and treatment, within reason.

The recommended dose of RIG is 20 IU/kg. As much of the dose as possible should be used to infiltrate the wound(s), if present. The remainder is given intramuscularly into deltoid muscle. In cases of multiple severe wounds in which RIG is insufficient for infil-tration, dilution in saline solution to an adequate volume (twofold or threefold) has been recommended to ensure that all wound areas receive infiltrate. For children with a small muscle mass, it may be necessary to administer RIG at multiple sites. Human RIG is sup-plied in 2-mL (300 IU) and 10-mL (1500 IU) vials. Passive antibody can, in some cases, inhibit the response to rabies vaccines; therefore, the recommended dose should not be exceeded. Vaccine never should be administered in the same parts of the body or with the same syringe used to give RIG. Hypersensitivity reactions to RIG are rare.

Purified equine RIG containing rabies antibodies may be available outside the United States and generally is accompanied by a low rate of serum sickness (less than 1%). Equine RIG is administered at a dose of 40 IU/kg, and desensitization may be required.

- **Management of postexposure prophylaxis in previously immunized people:** Administration of RIG is not recommended for the following exposed people: (1) people who received postexposure prophylaxis with HDCV, RVA, or PCECV for a previous exposure; (2) people who received a 3-dose, intramuscular, preexposure regimen of HDCV, RVA, or PCECV; (3) people who received a 3-dose, intradermal, pre-exposure regimen of HDCV with the product used in the United States; and (4) people who have a documented adequate rabies virus antibody titer after previous immunization with any other rabies vaccine. These people should receive two 1.0-mL booster doses of HDCV or PCECV; the first dose is given ideally on the day of exposure, and the second dose is given 3 days later.

Preexposure Control Measures, Including Vaccination. The relatively low frequency of reactions to HDCV and PCECV has made provision of preexposure vaccination practical for people in high-risk groups, including veterinarians, animal handlers, certain laboratory workers, and people moving or traveling to areas where canine rabies is common. Others, such as spelunkers (cavers) or animal rehabilitators, who may have frequent exposures to bats and other wildlife, also should be considered for preexposure prophylaxis.

HDCV and PCECV are licensed for intramuscular administration. The preexposure prophylaxis schedule is three 1-mL intramuscular injections each, given on days 0, 7, and 21 or 28. This series of immunizations has resulted in development of rabies virus-neutralizing antibodies in all people properly immunized. Therefore, routine serologic testing for antibody after primary immunization is not indicated.

Serum antibodies usually persist for 2 years or longer after the primary series is administered intramuscularly. Preexposure booster immunization with 1.0 mL of HDCV or PCEC intramuscularly will produce an effective anamnestic response in most healthy individuals. Rabies virus-neutralizing antibody titers should be determined at 6-month intervals for people at continuous risk of infection (rabies research laboratory workers, rabies biologics production workers). Titers should be determined approximately every 2 years for people with risk of frequent exposure (rabies diagnostic laboratory workers, spelunkers/cavers, veterinarians and staff, animal-control and wildlife workers in rabies-enzootic areas, and all people who frequently handle bats or other wildlife animals). A single booster dose of vaccine should be administered only as appropriate to maintain adequate antibody concentrations. The Centers for Disease Control and Prevention currently specifies complete viral neutralization at a serum dilution of 1:5 (approximately 0.1 IU/mL or greater) by the rapid fluorescent-focus inhibition test as evidence of an adequate immune response; the World Health Organization specifies 0.5 IU/mL or greater as acceptable. Other people, such as travelers to areas where canine rabies is common, do not need serologic testing and follow-up. If they received preexposure immunization at any time prior to the time they are exposed, then they should receive booster doses of vaccine at days 0 and 3.

Public Health. A variety of approved public health measures, including vaccination of dogs, cats, and ferrets and management of stray dog population and selected wildlife, are used to control rabies in animals.[1] In regions where oral vaccination of wildlife with recombi-

---

[1]National Association of State Public Health Veterinarians Inc. Compendium of animal rabies prevention and control, 2011. *MMWR Recomm Rep.* 2011;60(RR-6):1–15

nant rabies vaccine is undertaken, the prevalence of rabies among foxes, coyotes, and raccoons may be decreased. Unvaccinated dogs, cats, ferrets, or other pets bitten by a known rabid animal should be euthanized immediately. If the owner is unwilling to allow the animal to be euthanized, the animal should be placed in strict isolation for 6 months and immunized at latest 1 month before release. If the exposed animal has been immunized within 1 to 3 years, depending on the vaccine administered and local regulations, the animal should be revaccinated and observed for 45 days.

Case Reporting. All suspected human cases of rabies should be reported promptly to public health authorities.

Rat-Bite Fever

CLINICAL MANIFESTATIONS: Rat-bite fever is caused by *Streptobacillus moniliformis* or *Spirillum minus. S moniliformis* infection (streptobacillary fever or Haverhill fever) is characterized by relapsing fever, rash, and migratory polyarthritis. There is an abrupt onset of fever, chills, muscle pain, vomiting, headache, and rarely (unlike *S minus*), lymphadenopathy. A maculopapular, purpuric, or petechial rash develops, predominantly on the peripheral extremities including the palms and soles, typically within a few days of fever onset. The bite site usually heals promptly and exhibits no or minimal inflammation. Nonsuppurative migratory polyarthritis or arthralgia follows in approximately 50% of patients. Symptoms of untreated infection resolve within 2 weeks, but fever occasionally can relapse for weeks or months. Complications include soft tissue and solid-organ abscesses, septic arthritis, pneumonia, endocarditis, myocarditis, and meningitis. The case-fatality rate is 7% to 13% in untreated patients, and fatal cases have been reported in young children. With *S minus* infection ("sodoku"), a period of initial apparent healing at the site of the bite usually is followed by fever and ulceration at the site, regional lymphangitis and lymphadenopathy, and a distinctive rash of red or purple plaques. Arthritis is rare. Infection with *S minus* is rare in the United States.

ETIOLOGY: The causes of rat-bite fever are *S moniliformis,* a microaerophilic, gram-negative, pleomorphic bacillus, and *S minus,* a small, gram-negative, spiral organism with bipolar flagellar tufts.

EPIDEMIOLOGY: Rat-bite fever is a zoonotic illness. The natural habitat of *S moniliformis* and *S minus* is the upper respiratory tract of rodents. *S moniliformis* is transmitted by bites or scratches from or exposure to oral secretions of infected rats (eg, kissing pet rodents); other rodents (eg, mice, gerbils, squirrels, weasels) and rodent-eating animals, including cats and dogs, also can transmit the infection. Haverhill fever refers to infection after ingestion of unpasteurized milk, water, or food contaminated with *S moniliformis* and may be associated with an outbreak of disease. *S minus* is transmitted by bites of rats and mice. *S moniliformis* infection accounts for most cases of rat-bite fever in the United States; *S minus* infections occur primarily in Asia.

The **incubation period** for *S moniliformis* usually is less than 7 days but can range from 3 days to 3 weeks; for *S minus,* the **incubation period** is 7 to 21 days.

DIAGNOSTIC TESTS: *S moniliformis* is a fastidious, slow-growing organism isolated from specimens of blood, synovial fluid, aspirates from abscesses, or material from the bite lesion by inoculation into bacteriologic media enriched with blood (15% rabbit blood seems optimal), serum, ascitic fluid, and 5% to 10% carbon dioxide atmosphere at 37°C. Cultures should be held up to 3 weeks if *S moniliformis* is suspected. Sodium polyanethol sulfonate (SPS), present in most blood culture media, is inhibitory to *S moniliformis;* therefore, SPS-free media should be used, and the laboratory should be alerted to hold the culture for a longer period of time. *S moniliformis* has been detected using a nucleic acid amplification-based assay. *S minus* has not been recovered on artificial media but can be visualized by darkfield microscopy in wet mounts of blood, exudate of a lesion, and lymph nodes. Blood specimens also should be viewed with Giemsa or Wright stain. *S minus* can be recovered from blood, lymph nodes, or local lesions by intraperitoneal inoculation of mice or guinea pigs.

TREATMENT: Penicillin G procaine administered intramuscularly or penicillin G administered intravenously for 7 to 10 days is the treatment for rat-bite fever caused by either agent. Initial intravenous penicillin G therapy for 5 to 7 days followed by oral penicillin V for 7 days also has been successful. Limited experience exists for ampicillin, cefuroxime, and cefotaxime. Doxycycline or streptomycin can be substituted when a patient has a serious allergy to penicillin. Patients with endocarditis should receive intravenous high-dose penicillin G for at least 4 weeks. The addition of streptomycin or gentamicin for initial therapy may be useful.

ISOLATION OF THE HOSPITALIZED PATIENT: Standard precautions are recommended.

CONTROL MEASURES: Exposed people should be observed for symptoms. Because the occurrence of *S moniliformis* after a rat bite is approximately 10%, some experts recommend postexposure administration of penicillin. Rat control is important in the control of disease. People with frequent rodent exposure should wear gloves and avoid hand-to-mouth contact during animal handling. Regular hand hygiene should be practiced.

Respiratory Syncytial Virus

CLINICAL MANIFESTATIONS: Respiratory syncytial virus (RSV) causes acute respiratory tract infections in people of all ages and is one of the most common diseases of early childhood. Most infants are infected during the first year of life, with virtually all having been infected at least once by the second birthday. Most RSV-infected infants experience upper respiratory tract symptoms, and 20% to 30% develop lower respiratory tract disease (eg, bronchiolitis and/or pneumonia) with the first infection. Signs and symptoms of bronchiolitis typically begin with rhinitis and cough, which progress to increased respiratory effort with tachypnea, wheezing, rales, crackles, intercostal and/or subcostal retractions, grunting, and nasal flaring. During the first few weeks of life, particularly among preterm infants, infection with RSV may produce minimal respiratory tract signs; lethargy, irritability, and poor feeding, sometimes accompanied by apneic episodes, may be presenting manifestations in these infants. Most previously healthy infants who develop RSV bronchiolitis do not require hospitalization, and most who are hospitalized improve with supportive care and are discharged after 2 or 3 days. Approximately 1% to 3% of all children in the first 12 months of life will be hospitalized because of RSV lower respiratory tract disease. Most RSV hospitalizations occur in the first 3 months of life. Factors that increase the risk of severe RSV lower respiratory tract illness include extreme prematurity; cyanotic or complicated congenital heart disease (CHD), especially conditions associated with pulmonary hypertension; chronic lung disease of prematurity (CLD [formerly called bronchopulmonary dysplasia]); and certain immunodeficiency states. Fewer than 100 deaths in young children are attributable to complications of RSV infection annually.

The association between RSV bronchiolitis early in life and subsequent asthma remains poorly understood. RSV bronchiolitis may be associated with short-term or long-term complications that include recurrent wheezing and abnormalities in pulmonary function. This association may reflect an underlying genetic predisposition to severe bronchiolitis and to asthma rather than a direct consequence of RSV infection.

Reinfection with RSV throughout life is common, but subsequent infections usually are less severe than primary infections. Recurrent RSV infection in older children and adults usually manifests as mild upper respiratory tract illness. Serious disease involving the lower respiratory tract may develop in older children and adults, especially in immunocompromised people, people with cardiopulmonary disease, and elderly people, particularly those with comorbidities.

ETIOLOGY: RSV is an enveloped, nonsegmented, negative strand RNA virus of the family *Paramyxoviridae*. The virus uses attachment (G) and fusion (F) surface glycoproteins for virus entry; these surface proteins lack neuraminidase and hemagglutinin activities. Only 1 serotype is known, but variations in the surface proteins (especially the attachment protein G) result in the classification of viruses in 2 major subgroups, designated A and B. Numerous genotypes have been identified in each subgroup, and strains of both subgroups often circulate concurrently in a community. The clinical and epidemiologic significance of strain variation has not been determined, but evidence suggests that antigenic differences may affect susceptibility to infection and that some strains may be more virulent than others.

EPIDEMIOLOGY: Humans are the only source of infection. RSV usually is transmitted by direct or close contact with contaminated secretions, which may occur from exposure to large-particle droplets at short distances (typically <3 to 6 feet) or from fomites. Viable RSV can persist on environmental surfaces for several hours and for 30 minutes or more on hands. Infection among health care personnel and others may occur by hand-to-eye or hand-to-nasal epithelium self-inoculation with contaminated secretions. Enforcement of infection-control policies is critical to decrease the risk of health care-associated transmission of RSV. Health care-associated spread of RSV to hematopoietic stem cell or solid organ transplant recipients or patients with cardiopulmonary abnormalities or immunocompromised conditions has been associated with severe and fatal disease in children and adults. Children with human immunodeficiency virus (HIV) infection experience extended viral shedding and sometimes prolonged illness but usually do not exhibit enhanced disease.

RSV occurs in annual epidemics during winter and early spring in temperate climates. Spread among household and child care contacts, including adults, is common. The period of viral shedding usually is 3 to 8 days but may last longer, especially in young infants and in immunosuppressed people, in whom shedding may continue for as long as 3 to 4 weeks.

The **incubation period** ranges from 2 to 8 days; 4 to 6 days is most common.

DIAGNOSTIC TESTS: Rapid diagnostic assays, including immunofluorescent and enzyme immunoassay techniques for detection of viral antigen in nasopharyngeal specimens, are available commercially for RSV and are generally reliable in infants and young children. In children, the sensitivity of these assays in comparison with culture varies between 53% and 96%, with most in the 80% to 90% range. The sensitivity may be lower in older children and is quite poor in adults, because adults typically shed low concentrations of RSV. As with all antigen detection assays, the predictive value is high during the peak season, but false-positive test results are more likely to occur when the incidence of disease is low, such as in the summer in temperate areas. Therefore, antigen detection assays should not be the only basis on which the beginning and end of monthly immunoprophylaxis is determined. In most outpatient and inpatient settings, specific viral testing has little effect on management and routine testing is not recommended.[1]

One disadvantage of targeted antigen detection relative to comprehensive virologic assessment (culture or reverse transcriptase-polymerase chain reaction [RT-PCR] assay) is that coinfections may not be detected. Up to 30% of children with RSV bronchiolitis may be coinfected with another respiratory tract pathogen, such as human metapneumovirus, rhinovirus, bocavirus, adenovirus, coronavirus, influenza virus, or parainfluenza virus. Whether children with bronchiolitis who are coinfected with more than 1 virus experience more severe disease is not clear.

Molecular diagnostic tests using RT-PCR assays are available commercially and increase RSV detection rates over viral isolation or antigen detection assays, especially in older children and adults. Many commercial tests are designed as multiplex assays to facilitate testing for multiple respiratory viruses with one test. Because of the increased sensitivity of RT-PCR testing, these tests may be preferred in many clinical settings. However, these tests should be interpreted with caution, especially when a multiplex assay identifies the presence of nucleic acid from more than 1 virus, because genetic material from some viruses (eg, rhinovirus, adenovirus, bocavirus) may persist in the airway for many weeks after cessation of shedding of infectious virus. As many as 25% of asymptomatic children test positive for respiratory viruses using RT-PCR assays in population-based studies.

RSV isolation from respiratory tract secretions in cell culture requires 1 to 5 days (shell vial techniques can produce results within 24 to 48 hours), but results and sensitivity vary among laboratories. Experienced viral laboratory personnel should be consulted for optimal methods of collection and transport of specimens, which include keeping the specimen cold but unfrozen during transport, rapid specimen processing, and stabilization in virus transport media. Conventional serologic testing of acute and convalescent serum specimens cannot be relied on to confirm infection in young infants, in whom sensitivity may be low.

TREATMENT: Primary treatment of young children hospitalized with bronchiolitis is supportive and should include hydration, careful assessment of respiratory status, measurement of oxygen saturation, suction of the upper airway, and if necessary, intubation and mechanical ventilation.[1] Clinicians may choose not to administer supplemental oxygen if the oxyhemoglobin saturation exceeds 90% in infants and children hospitalized with bronchiolitis.[1] Clinicians may choose not to use continuous pulse oximetry for children with bronchiolitis.[1] Continuous measurement of oxygen saturation may detect transient fluctuations in oxygenation that are not clinically significant, prolong oxygen use, and delay discharge. Among patients with bronchiolitis, pulse oximetry should not be used as a proxy for respiratory distress. Supplemental oxygen is recommended only when oxyhemoglobin saturation persistently falls below 90% in a previously healthy infant.[1]

---

[1]Ralston SL, Lieberthal AS, Meissner HC, et al. Clinical practice guideline: the diagnosis, management, and prevention of bronchiolitis. *Pediatrics.* 2014;134(5):e1474–e1502

Ribavirin has in vitro antiviral activity against RSV, and aerosolized ribavirin therapy has been associated with a small but statistically significant increase in oxygen saturation during the acute infection in several small studies. However, a consistent decrease in need for mechanical ventilation, decrease in length of stay in the pediatric intensive care unit, or reduction in days of hospitalization among ribavirin recipients has not been demonstrated. The aerosol route of administration, concern about potential toxic effects among exposed health care personnel, conflicting results of efficacy trials, and high cost have led to infrequent use of this drug. Ribavirin is not recommended for routine use but may be considered for use in selected patients with documented, potentially life-threatening RSV infection.

Alpha- and Beta-Adrenergic Agents. Beta-adrenergic agents are not recommended for care of first-time wheezing associated with RSV bronchiolitis. Randomized clinical trials have demonstrated that bronchodilators do not affect disease resolution, need for hospitalization, or length of stay. Bronchodilators do not improve oxygen saturation, hospital admission rates after outpatient treatment, or time to resolution of illness at home. For these reasons, a trial of albuterol no longer is included as a recommended option in the management of RSV bronchiolitis.[1] Evidence does not support the use of nebulized epinephrine in children hospitalized with bronchiolitis. Insufficient data are available to recommend routine use of epinephrine for outpatient management of children with bronchiolitis.[1]

Corticosteroid Therapy. Controlled clinical trials among children with bronchiolitis have demonstrated that corticosteroids do not reduce hospital admissions and do not reduce length of stay for inpatients. Corticosteroid treatment is not recommended for infants and children with RSV bronchiolitis. Evidence for potential benefit from combined use of corticosteroids and agents with alpha- or beta-adrenergic activity is insufficient to support a recommendation.[1]

Antimicrobial Therapy. Antimicrobial therapy is not indicated for infants with RSV bronchiolitis or pneumonia unless there is evidence of concurrent bacterial infection. Bacterial lung infections and bacteremia are uncommon in this setting. Acute otitis media (AOM) caused by RSV or bacterial superinfection may occur in infants with RSV bronchiolitis. Antimicrobial therapy for treatment of otitis media may be considered if bulging of the tympanic membrane is present.[2]

Other Therapies. Chest physiotherapy should not be used in infants and children with a diagnosis of bronchiolitis. If indicated, nasogastric or intravenous fluids may be used to maintain hydration.

Nebulized hypertonic saline (3%) appears to be safe and effective at improving the symptoms of mild to moderate bronchiolitis after 24 hours of use and in reducing hospital length of stay in settings where the duration of stay is likely to exceed 3 days. Hypertonic saline has not been shown to be effective over the short term for patients managed in the emergency room or when length of hospitalization is brief. Hypertonic saline has not been studied in intensive care settings.

High-flow nasal cannula therapy (HFNC) may be used for respiratory support in hospitalized infants with bronchiolitis. Heated, humidified flow of air is titrated to respiratory effect, typically between 2 and 12 L/minute. HFNC is initiated for difficulty with breathing and typically is not used to treat hypoxia, because the mechanism of effect is through

---

[1]Ralston SL, Lieberthal AL, Meissner HC, et al. Clinical practice guideline: the diagnosis, management, and prevention of bronchiolitis. *Pediatrics.* 2014;134(5):e1474–e1502

[2]Lieberthal AS, Carroll AE, Chonmaitree T, et al. Clinical practice guideline: the diagnosis and management of acute otitis media. *Pediatrics.* 2013;131(3):e964–e999

provision of pressure support and removal of dead-space carbon dioxide. However, oxygen may be blended with the provided gas for purposes of managing hypoxia. Utilization has been shown to decrease respiratory effort and intubation rates in hospitalized children.

Nasal continuous positive airway pressure is used in the intensive care unit for infants with marked increased work of breathing as an alternative to HFNC and improves ventilation and oxygenation in infants with severe respiratory distress. Noninvasive ventilation strategies are preferred to intubation, because there is less chance of iatrogenic error and sedation typically is not required. Intubation of infants is used only for the sickest infants who are losing the innate reserve to maintain ventilation and oxygenation despite other supportive measures.

Heliox improves ventilation in infants who have severe respiratory distress but who do not require large amounts of oxygen. Helium is blended with oxygen, and this lower-density gas improves laminar gas flow through narrowed bronchioles.

Prevention of RSV Infections. Palivizumab is a humanized mouse immunoglobulin (Ig) G1 monoclonal antibody produced by recombinant DNA technology. The antibody is directed against a conserved epitope of the A antigenic site of the fusion protein (F), which resides on the viral surface and prevents the conformational change that is necessary for fusion of the viral RSV envelope with the plasma membrane of the respiratory epithelial cell. Without fusion, the virus is unable to enter the cell and unable to replicate.

Palivizumab may be considered to reduce the risk of RSV lower respiratory tract disease in certain children at increased risk of severe disease. Palivizumab is administered intramuscularly at a dose of 15 mg/kg, once every 30 days. In some reports, palivizumab administration in a home-based program has been shown to improve compliance and to reduce exposure to microbial pathogens compared with administration in office- or clinic-based settings. A patient with a history of a severe allergic reaction following a dose of palivizumab should not receive additional doses. Palivizumab is not effective in treatment of RSV disease and is not approved or recommended for this indication.

Respiratory Syncytial Virus Immune Globulin Intravenous (RSV-IGIV), a hyperimmune, polyclonal globulin prepared from donors selected for high serum titers of RSV neutralizing antibody, previously was used for prophylaxis but no longer is available.

Cost Considerations. Results of cost-effectiveness analyses of palivizumab prophylaxis depend on several base case assumptions, including baseline RSV hospitalization rates among different groups of high-risk children, the reduction in RSV hospitalization rates among recipients of prophylaxis in different risk groups, the cost of hospitalization (amount saved by avoiding hospitalization), the threshold criteria for hospitalization of a child with bronchiolitis (which differs from country to country and even from pediatrician to pediatrician), the number of monthly doses administered, the weight of an infant who receives prophylaxis, variation in the severity of the RSV season, and the acquisition cost of palivizumab. Cost analyses conducted by independent investigators consistently demonstrate the cost of palivizumab prophylaxis far exceeds the economic benefit from a small number of hospitalizations avoided, even among infants at highest risk.

Numerous studies have documented that infants hospitalized with viral lower airway disease are more likely to experience recurrent wheezing compared with infants who do not experience severe bronchiolitis. Data suggest that avoidance of RSV infection among preterm infants from use of palivizumab may result in a slight decrease in the incidence of parent-reported wheezing episodes (not medically attended events) in the first years of life. Although the results suggesting a reduction in wheezing episodes among palivizumab recipients are statistically significant, the absolute benefit is so small as to be clinically minimal and insufficient to justify the drug cost.

Health expenditures should not be based only on cost and benefit but rather on the assessment of the benefit of the intervention relative to the expenditure. High-cost interventions may be appropriate if highly beneficial. Because the high cost of palivizumab prophylaxis is associated with minimal health benefit, this intervention cannot be considered as high-value health care for any group of infants.

Initiation and Termination of Immunoprophylaxis. During the 6 RSV seasons from July 2007 to January 2013, the median duration of the RSV season ranged from 13 to 23 weeks, with median peak activity from mid-December to early February, with the exception of Florida and Alaska. Within the 10 Health and Human Services Regions, in the few regions when the RSV season began in October, the season ended in March or early April. In regions where the RSV season began in November or December, the season ended by April or early May. Because 5 monthly doses of palivizumab at 15 mg/kg/dose will provide more than 6 months of serum palivizumab concentrations above the desired serum concentration for most infants, administration of more than 5 monthly doses is not recommended within the continental United States. Children who qualify for palivizumab prophylaxis should receive the first dose at the onset of the RSV season. For qualifying infants born during the RSV season, fewer than 5 doses will be needed to provide protection until the RSV season ends in their region (maximum of 5 doses).

A small number of sporadic RSV hospitalizations will occur before or after the main season in many areas of the United States, but the greatest benefit from prophylaxis is derived during the peak of the season and not when the incidence of RSV hospitalization is low.

Timing of Prophylaxis for Alaska Native/American Indian Infants. Hospitalization rates for all causes of bronchiolitis as high as 484 to 590/1000 infants have been described in isolated Inuit populations. Alaska Native infants in southwestern Alaska experience higher RSV hospitalization rates and a longer RSV season. On the basis of epidemiology of RSV in Alaska, particularly in remote regions where the cost of emergency air transport may alter a cost analysis, the selection of infants eligible for prophylaxis may differ from the remainder of the United States. Clinicians may wish to use RSV laboratory surveillance data generated by the state of Alaska to assist in determining onset and end of the RSV season for appropriate timing of palivizumab administration.

Limited information is available concerning the burden of RSV disease for American Indian populations. However, local assessment of the cost-benefit, as occurs for Alaska Native populations, may be prudent for certain American Indian populations. If local data support a high burden of RSV disease in select American Indian populations, selection of infants eligible for prophylaxis may differ from the remainder of the United States for infants in the first year of life.

Timing of Prophylaxis for the State of Florida. Variation in the onset and offset of the RSV season in different regions of Florida may affect the timing of palivizumab administration. Florida Department of Health data may be used to determine the appropriate timing for administration of the first dose of palivizumab for qualifying infants. Despite varying onset and offset dates of the RSV season in different regions of Florida, a maximum of 5 monthly doses of palivizumab will be adequate for qualifying infants for most RSV seasons in Florida. If the first of 5 monthly doses is administered in July, protective serum concentrations of palivizumab will be present for most infants and young children for more than 6 months (likely into February). More than 5 monthly doses are not recommended, despite the detection of a small number of cases of RSV infection outside this time window.

Eligibility Criteria for Prophylaxis of High-Risk Infants and Young Children.[1,2]

- **Infants with CLD of prematurity.**
  - ♦ Prophylaxis may be considered during the RSV season during the first year of life for preterm infants who develop CLD of prematurity defined as gestational age <32 weeks, 0 days and a requirement for >21% oxygen for at least the first 28 days after birth.
  - ♦ During the second year of life, consideration of palivizumab prophylaxis is recommended only for infants who satisfy this definition of CLD of prematurity and continue to require medical support (chronic corticosteroid therapy, diuretic therapy, or supplemental oxygen) during the 6-month period before the start of the second RSV season.
  - ♦ For infants with CLD who do not continue to require medical support in the second year of life prophylaxis is not recommended.
- **Infants with CHD.**
  - ♦ Children with hemodynamically significant CHD who are most likely to benefit from immunoprophylaxis include infants with acyanotic heart disease who are receiving medication to control congestive heart failure and will require cardiac surgical procedures and infants with moderate to severe pulmonary hypertension.
  - ♦ Decisions regarding palivizumab prophylaxis for infants with cyanotic heart defects in the first year of life may be made in consultation with a pediatric cardiologist, as the benefit of prophylaxis in infants with cyanotic heart disease is unknown.
  - ♦ These recommendations apply to qualifying infants in the first year of life who are born within 12 months of onset of the RSV season.
  - ♦ The following groups of infants with CHD are <u>not</u> at increased risk of RSV infection and generally should not receive immunoprophylaxis:
    - — Infants and children with hemodynamically insignificant heart disease (eg, secundum atrial septal defect, small ventricular septal defect, pulmonic stenosis, uncomplicated aortic stenosis, mild coarctation of the aorta, and patent ductus arteriosus)
    - — Infants with lesions adequately corrected by surgery, unless they continue to require medication for congestive heart failure
    - — Infants with mild cardiomyopathy who are not receiving medical therapy for the condition
    - — Children in the second year of life

[1]American Academy of Pediatrics, Committee on Infectious Diseases, Bronchiolitis Guideline Committee. Technical report: updated guidance for palivizumab prophylaxis among infants and young children at increased risk of hospitalization for respiratory syncytial virus infection. *Pediatrics.* 2014;134(2):e620–e638

[2]American Academy of Pediatrics, Committee on Infectious Diseases, Bronchiolitis Guideline Committee. Policy statement: updated guidance for palivizumab prophylaxis among infants and young children at increased risk of hospitalization for respiratory syncytial virus infection. *Pediatrics.* 2014;134(2):415–420

◆ Because a mean decrease in palivizumab serum concentration of 58% was observed after surgical procedures that involve cardiopulmonary bypass, for children who are receiving prophylaxis and who continue to require prophylaxis following a surgical procedure, a postoperative dose of palivizumab (15 mg/kg) should be considered after cardiac bypass or at the conclusion of extracorporeal membrane oxygenation (ECMO) for infants and children younger than 24 months.

◆ Children younger than 2 years who undergo cardiac transplantation during the RSV season may be considered for palivizumab prophylaxis.

● **Preterm infants without CLD or CHD.**

◆ Palivizumab prophylaxis may be administered to preterm infants born before 29 weeks, 0 days' gestation who are younger than 12 months at the start of the RSV season.

◆ For infants born during the RSV season, fewer than 5 monthly doses will be needed.

◆ Available data for infants born at 29 weeks, 0 days' gestation or later do not identify a gestational age cutoff for which the benefits of prophylaxis are clear. For this reason, infants born at 29 weeks, 0 days' gestation or later are not universally recommended to receive palivizumab prophylaxis. Infants 29 weeks, 0 days' gestation or later may qualify to receive prophylaxis on the basis of congenital heart disease (CHD), chronic lung disease (CLD), or another condition.

◆ Palivizumab prophylaxis is not recommended in the second year of life on the basis of a history of prematurity alone, regardless of the degree of prematurity.

◆ Some experts believe that on the basis of the data quantifying a small increase in risk of hospitalization, even for infants born earlier than 29 weeks, 0 days' gestation, palivizumab prophylaxis is not justified in the first year of life.

● **Children with anatomic pulmonary abnormalities or neuromuscular disorder.**

◆ No prospective studies or population based data are available to define the risk of RSV hospitalization in children with pulmonary abnormalities or neuromuscular disease. Infants with neuromuscular disease or a congenital anomaly that impairs the ability to clear secretions from the upper airway because of ineffective cough are known to be at risk of a prolonged hospitalization related to lower respiratory tract infection and therefore may be considered for prophylaxis during the first year of life.

● **Immunocompromised children.**

◆ No population-based data are available on the incidence of RSV hospitalization in children who undergo solid organ or hematopoietic stem cell transplantation. Severe and even fatal disease attributable to RSV is recognized in children receiving chemotherapy or who are immunocompromised because of other conditions but the efficacy of prophylaxis in this cohort is not known. Prophylaxis may be considered for children younger than 24 months who will be profoundly immunocompromised during the RSV season.

● **Children with Down syndrome.**

◆ Limited data suggest a slight increase in RSV hospitalization rates among children with Down syndrome.

◆ However, data describing more than a slight increase in hospitalization rates are insufficient to justify a recommendation for routine use of prophylaxis in children with Down syndrome unless qualifying heart disease, CLD, airway clearance issues, or prematurity (<29 weeks, 0 days' gestation) is present.

- **Children with cystic fibrosis.**
  - Routine use of palivizumab prophylaxis in patients with cystic fibrosis, including neonates diagnosed with cystic fibrosis by newborn screening, is not recommended unless other indications are present.
  - An infant with cystic fibrosis with clinical evidence of CLD and/or nutritional compromise in the first year of life may be considered for prophylaxis.
  - Continued use of palivizumab prophylaxis in the second year may be considered for infants with manifestations of severe lung disease (previous hospitalization for pulmonary exacerbation in the first year of life or abnormalities on chest radiography or chest computed tomography that persist when stable) or weight for length less than the 10th percentile.
- **Preventive measures for all high-risk infants.**
  - Infants, especially those at high risk, never should be exposed to tobacco smoke. Tobacco smoke exposure is a known risk factor for many adverse health-related outcomes, and studies have shown increased severity of RSV infection in hospitalized children exposed to secondhand smoke. In addition, smoke exposure may increase the risk of developing wheezing after RSV infection. Families with infants, especially with infants who are at increased risk of RSV disease, must control exposure to tobacco smoke.
  - In contrast to the well-documented beneficial effect of breastfeeding against many viral illnesses, existing data are conflicting regarding the specific protective effect of breastfeeding against RSV infection. Breastfeeding should be encouraged for all infants in accordance with recommendations of the American Academy of Pediatrics.
  - High-risk infants should be kept away from crowds and from situations in which exposure to infected people cannot be controlled. Participation in group child care should be restricted during the RSV season for high-risk infants whenever feasible.
  - Parents should be instructed on the importance of careful hand hygiene.
  - In addition, all infants (beginning at 6 months of age) and their contacts (beginning when the child is born) should receive influenza vaccine as well as other recommended age-appropriate immunizations.
- **Special situations.**
  - Discontinuation of palivizumab prophylaxis among children who experience breakthrough RSV hospitalization:
    - If any infant or young child receiving monthly palivizumab prophylaxis experiences a breakthrough RSV hospitalization, monthly prophylaxis should be discontinued because of the extremely low likelihood of a second RSV hospitalization in the same season (<0.5%).
  - Use of palivizumab in the second year of life:
    - Hospitalization rates attributable to RSV decline during the second RSV season for all children.
    - A second season of palivizumab prophylaxis is recommended only for preterm infants <32 weeks, 0 days' gestation who required at least 28 days of oxygen after birth and who continue to require supplemental oxygen, chronic systemic corticosteroid therapy, or diuretic therapy within 6 months of the start of the second RSV season.

- Prevention of nosocomial RSV disease:
  - No rigorous data exist to support palivizumab use in controlling outbreaks of health care-associated disease, and palivizumab use is not recommended for this purpose. Strict adherence to infection control practices is the basis for reducing nosocomial RSV disease.
  - Infants in a neonatal unit who qualify for prophylaxis because of CLD, prematurity, or CHD may receive the first dose 48 to 72 hours before discharge to home or promptly after discharge.

ISOLATION OF THE HOSPITALIZED PATIENT: In addition to standard precautions, contact precautions are recommended for the duration of RSV-associated illness among infants and young children, including patients treated with ribavirin. The effectiveness of these precautions depends on compliance and necessitates scrupulous adherence to appropriate hand hygiene practices. Patients with RSV infection should be cared for in single rooms or placed in a cohort.

CONTROL MEASURES: The control of health care-associated RSV transmission is complicated by the continuing chance of introduction through infected patients, staff, and visitors. During the peak of the RSV season, many infants and children hospitalized with respiratory tract symptoms will be infected with RSV and should be cared for with contact precautions (see Isolation of the Hospitalized Patient, discussed previously). During community outbreaks of RSV, a variety of measures have been demonstrated to reduce the risk of health care-associated transmission, including: (1) cohorting of symptomatic patients and staff; (2) excluding visitors with current or recent respiratory tract infections; (3) excluding staff with respiratory tract illness or RSV infection from caring for susceptible infants; (4) using gowns and gloves and possibly goggles or masks for protecting health care personnel; (5) emphasizing hand hygiene before and after direct contact with patients, after contact with inanimate objects in the direct vicinity of patients, and after glove removal; and (6) limiting young sibling visitation during the RSV season.

A critical aspect of RSV prevention among high-risk infants is education of parents and other caregivers about the importance of decreasing exposure to and transmission of RSV. Preventive measures include limiting, where feasible, exposure to contagious settings (eg, child care centers) and emphasis on hand hygiene in all settings, including the home, especially during periods when contacts of high-risk children have respiratory tract infections.

Rhinovirus Infections

CLINICAL MANIFESTATIONS: Rhinoviruses are the most frequent causes of the common cold, or rhinosinusitis. Rhinoviruses also can be associated with pharyngitis, otitis media, and lower respiratory tract infections (eg, bronchiolitis, pneumonia). Initial clinical manifestations include sore throat and nasal discharge that initially is watery and clear but often becomes mucopurulent and viscous after a few days and may persist for 10 to 14 days. Malaise, headache, myalgia, and low-grade fever, cough, wheezing, and sneezing may occur. In children with asthma, rhinoviruses are detected in approximately half of all acute exacerbations, even more in the autumn and spring.

ETIOLOGY: Rhinoviruses are small, nonenveloped single positive-stranded RNA viruses classified into 3 species (A, B, C) in the family *Picornaviridae*, genus *Enterovirus*. Approximately 100 serotypes have been identified by neutralization with type-specific antisera, and many additional types have been identified by molecular methods. Infection with one type confers some type-specific immunity, but immunity is of variable degree and brief duration and offers little protection against other serotypes.

EPIDEMIOLOGY: Transmission occurs predominantly by person-to-person contact, with self-inoculation by contaminated secretions on hands and/or aerosol spread. Infections occur throughout the year, but peak activity occurs during autumn and spring. Multiple serotypes circulate simultaneously, and the prevalent serotypes circulating in a given population change from season to season. By adulthood, antibodies to many different types have developed. Viral shedding in nasopharyngeal secretions is most abundant during the first 2 to 3 days of infection and usually ceases by 7 to 10 days. However, virus shedding may continue for as long as 3 weeks or more.

The **incubation period** usually is 2 to 3 days but occasionally is up to 7 days.

DIAGNOSTIC TESTS: Although used classically, cell culture now is recognized to be insensitive for many different rhinovirus strains. Polymerase chain reaction (PCR) detection methods have become the preferred way to identify rhinovirus infections and the only way to detect species C viruses, which have not been isolated successfully in cell culture. Commercial molecular diagnostic assays for rhinoviruses are available. Positive PCR assay results for rhinovirus may be detected in asymptomatic children. If characteristic symptoms are not present, this laboratory finding may indicate residual viral RNA from a previous rhinovirus infection. Serologic diagnosis of rhinovirus infection is impractical because of the large number of antigenic types and the absence of a common antigen.

TREATMENT: Treatment mainly is supportive. Antimicrobial agents are not indicated for people with symptoms caused by a rhinovirus. Antimicrobial agents do not prevent secondary bacterial infection, and their use may promote the emergence of resistant bacteria and complicate treatment for a bacterial infection (see Antimicrobial Resistance and Stewardship: Appropriate and Judicious Use of Antimicrobial Agents, p 874).

ISOLATION OF THE HOSPITALIZED PATIENT: In addition to standard precautions, droplet precautions are recommended for symptomatic hospitalized infants and children for the duration of illness. Contact precautions should be added if copious moist secretions and close contact are likely to occur (eg, young infants). In symptomatic immunocompromised patients, the duration of contact precautions should be extended because of possible prolonged shedding.

CONTROL MEASURES: Appropriate respiratory hygiene and cough etiquette should be followed. Additional infection control measures should be considered in certain settings (eg, child care centers, schools, nursing homes) when respiratory infections have been identified to limit spread.

Rickettsial Diseases

Rickettsial diseases comprise infections caused by bacterial species of the genera *Rickettsia* (endemic and epidemic typhus and spotted fever group rickettsioses), *Orientia* (scrub typhus), *Ehrlichia* (ehrlichiosis), *Anaplasma* (anaplasmosis), *Neoehrlichia*, and *Neorickettsia*.

CLINICAL MANIFESTATIONS: Rickettsial infections have many features in common, including the following:

- Fever, rash (especially in spotted fever and typhus group rickettsiae), headache, myalgia, and respiratory tract symptoms are prominent features.

- Local primary eschars occur with some rickettsial diseases, commonly with spotted fever rickettsioses, rickettsialpox, and scrub typhus.
- Systemic capillary and small vessel endothelial damage (ie, vasculitis) with increased microvascular permeability is the primary pathologic feature of most severe spotted fever and typhus group rickettsial infections.
- Rickettsial diseases can become life threatening rapidly. Risk factors for severe disease include glucose-6-phosphate dehydrogenase deficiency, male gender, and treatment with sulfonamides.

Immunity against reinfection by the same agent after natural infection usually is of long duration, except in the case of scrub typhus. Among the 4 groups of rickettsial diseases, some cross-immunity usually is conferred by infections within groups but not between groups. Reinfection of humans with *Ehrlichia* species and *Anaplasma* species has not been described.

ETIOLOGY: The rickettsiae causing human disease include: *Rickettsia* species, *Orientia tsutsugamushi*, *Ehrlichia* species, and *Anaplasma phagocytophilum*, *Neorickettsia sennetsu*, and *Neoehrlichia mikurensis*. Rickettsiae are small, coccobacillary gram-negative bacteria that are obligately intracellular pathogens and cannot be grown in cell-free media. They grow in different cellular compartments: *Orientia* and *Rickettsia* organisms in the cytoplasm and *Anaplasmataceae* organisms in different nonacidified modified phagosomes.

EPIDEMIOLOGY: Rickettsial diseases have arthropod vectors including ticks, flies, mites, and lice. The continued identification of new pathogenic rickettsial agents, such as *Rickettsia phillipi* (364D) in California in 2010 and *Rickettsia parkeri* in many states, will require ongoing research to confirm the burden of human illness. Humans are incidental hosts, except for the agent of classic epidemic typhus, for which humans are the principal reservoir and the human body louse is the vector; however, other vectors and reservoirs exist even for this disease. Rickettsial life cycles typically involve arthropod and mammalian reservoirs, and transmission occurs as a result of environmental or occupational exposure. Geographic and seasonal occurrences of rickettsial diseases are related to specific arthropod vector life cycles, activities, and distributions.

The **incubation periods** vary according to organism (see specific chapters).

DIAGNOSTIC TESTS: Group-specific antibodies are detectable in the serum of many people 7 to 14 days after onset of illness, but slower antibody responses occur commonly in some diseases. The utility of serologic diagnoses in acute illness is limited in these infections because of their short incubations; a negative serologic test result never excludes infection in the acute phase of clinical illness. Various serologic tests for detecting antirickettsial antibodies are available. The indirect immunofluorescent antibody assay is recommended in most circumstances because of its relative sensitivity and specificity; however, it cannot determine the causative agent to the species level. Treatment early in the course of illness can blunt or delay serologic responses. Polymerase chain reaction (PCR) assays can detect rickettsiae in whole blood and/or tissues collected during the acute stage of illness and before administration of antimicrobial agents; availability of these tests often is limited to reference and research laboratories. In laboratories with experienced personnel, immunohistochemical staining and PCR testing of skin biopsy specimens from patients with rash or eschar can help to diagnose rickettsial infections early in the course of disease. Weil-Felix tests are insensitive and nonspecific and no longer are recommended.

Weil-Felix tests will not detect infections caused by *Ehrlichia* species and *Anaplasma* species and are insensitive for scrub typhus. The use of tick panels is discouraged.

TREATMENT: Prompt and specific therapy is important for optimal outcome. The drug of choice for rickettsioses is doxycycline. Tetracycline-based antimicrobial agents, including doxycycline, may cause permanent tooth discoloration for children younger than 8 years if used for repeated treatment courses. However, doxycycline binds less readily to calcium compared with older tetracyclines, and in some studies, doxycycline was not associated with visible teeth staining in younger children (see Tetracyclines, p 873). The duration of treatment is 7 to 14 days. Antimicrobial treatment is most effective when individuals are treated appropriately during the first week of illness. If the disease remains untreated during the second week, therapy is less effective in preventing complications. Because confirmatory laboratory tests primarily are retrospective, treatment decisions should be made on the basis of clinical findings and epidemiologic data and should not be delayed until test results are known.

CONTROL MEASURES: Control measures primarily involve prevention of vector transmission of rickettsial agents to humans (see Prevention of Tickborne Infections, p 210).

Several rickettsial diseases, including spotted fevers, ehrlichiosis, and anaplasmosis, are nationally notifiable diseases and should be reported to state and local health departments.

For more details, the following chapters on rickettsial diseases should be consulted:
* *Ehrlichia, Anaplasma,* and Related Infections, p 329 (or **www.cdc.gov/ehrlichiosis/**).
* Rickettsialpox, p 680.
* Rocky Mountain Spotted Fever, p 682 (or **www.cdc.gov/rmsf/**).
* Endemic Typhus (Murine Typhus), p 841.
* Epidemic Typhus (Louseborne or Sylvatic Typhus), p 843.

OTHER RICKETTSIAL SPOTTED FEVER INFECTIONS: A number of other epidemiologically distinct fleaborne and tickborne spotted fever infections caused by rickettsiae have been recognized (also see **www.cdc.gov/otherspottedfever/index.html**). Many of them present with an eschar at the site of the tick bite and without rash. The causative agents of some of these infections share the same group antigen as *Rickettsia rickettsii*. These include:
* *Rickettsia africae,* the causative agent of African tick bite fever that is endemic in sub-Saharan Africa and some Caribbean Islands.
* *Rickettsia conorii* and subspecies, the causative agents of boutonneuse fever, Mediterranean spotted fever, India tick typhus, Marseilles fever, Israeli tick typhus, and Astrakhan spotted fever, that are endemic in southern Europe, Africa, the Middle East, and the Indian subcontinent.
* *Rickettsia parkeri,* a causative agent of *Amblyomma* tick infections in the Americas.
* *Rickettsia sibirica,* the causative agent of Siberian tick typhus, endemic in central Asia.
* *Rickettsia australis,* the causative agent of North Queensland tick typhus, endemic in eastern Australia.
* *Rickettsia japonica,* the causative agent of Japanese spotted fever, endemic in Japan.
* *Rickettsia honei,* the causative agent of Thai tick typhus and Flinders Island spotted fever and probably endemic throughout Southeast Asia.

- *Rickettsia slovaca*, the causative agent of tickborne lymphadenopathy (TIBOLA) and *Dermacentor*-borne necrosis-erythema-lymphadenopathy (DEBONEL), endemic in European countries; *R raoultii* infections have a similar presentation and distribution.
- *Rickettsia felis*, the causative agent of cat flea rickettsiosis that occurs worldwide; reports on the severity of illness vary widely.
- *Rickettsia aeschlimannii*, a causative agent of disease with an eschar and maculopapular rash easily confused with *R conorii* infections, reported from Africa and Europe.
- *Rickettsia heilongjiangensis*, reported from the Russian Far East and China.
- *Rickettsia helvetica*, can cause fatal perimyocarditis but generally is self-limiting; it is common in Asia.
- *R sibirica* subspecies *mongolitimonae*, reported from Europe, Africa, and Asia and causes a rickettsiosis with eschar and lymphangitis.
- *Rickettsia massiliae* is widespread in Africa and Europe; the Bar 29 type agent has been found in 3 US states and is implicated as a cause of illness in Argentina.

These infections have clinical and pathologic features that generally are milder than those of Rocky Mountain spotted fever in nonimmunocompromised people. Infection most often is confirmed using serologic assays. Demonstration of a fourfold or greater increase in specific antibodies (immunoglobulin G) in acute and convalescent serum samples taken 2 to 3 weeks apart is diagnostic of spotted fever rickettsioses; however, PCR and amplicon sequencing assays on DNA from acute whole blood or skin biopsy provide more accurate identification of the etiologic agent. These diseases are of importance among people traveling to or returning from areas where these agents are endemic and among people living in these areas. Research related to new rickettsial agents likely will shape future recommendations for clinicians, particularly because birds and reptiles appear to be a common source of exotic imported ticks that can harbor nonendemic agents.

Rickettsialpox

CLINICAL MANIFESTATIONS: Rickettsialpox is a febrile, eschar-associated illness that is characterized by generalized, relatively sparse, erythematous, papulovesicular eruptions on the trunk, face, and extremities (less often on palms and soles) or on mucous membranes of the mouth. The rash develops 1 to 4 days after onset of fever and 3 to 10 days after appearance of an eschar at the site of the bite of a house mouse mite. Regional lymph nodes in the area of the primary eschar typically become enlarged. Without specific antimicrobial therapy, systemic disease lasts approximately 7 to 10 days; manifestations include fever, headache, malaise, and myalgia. Less frequent manifestations include anorexia, vomiting, conjunctivitis, nuchal rigidity, and photophobia. The disease is mild compared with Rocky Mountain spotted fever, and no rickettsialpox-associated deaths have been described; however, disease occasionally is severe enough to warrant hospitalization.

ETIOLOGY: Rickettsialpox is caused by *Rickettsia akari*, a gram-negative intracellular bacillus, which is classified with the spotted fever group rickettsiae and related antigenically to other members of that group.

EPIDEMIOLOGY: The natural host for *R akari* in the United States is *Mus musculus*, the common house mouse. The disease is transmitted by the house mouse mite, *Liponyssoides* *sanguineus*. Disease risk is heightened in areas infested with mice and rats. The disease can occur wherever the hosts, pathogens, and humans coexist but is most frequently reported in large urban settings. In the United States, rickettsialpox has been described predominantly in northeastern metropolitan centers, especially in New York City. It also has been confirmed in many other countries, including Croatia, Ukraine, Turkey, Russia, South Korea, and Mexico. All age groups can be affected. No seasonal pattern of disease occurs. The disease is not communicable but occurs occasionally among families or people cohabiting a house mouse mite-infested dwelling.

The **incubation period** is 6 to 15 days.

DIAGNOSTIC TESTS: *R akari* can be isolated in cell culture from blood and eschar biopsy specimens during the acute stage of disease, but culture is not attempted routinely. Because antibodies to *R akari* have extensive cross-reactivity with antibodies against *Rickettsia rickettsii* (the cause of Rocky Mountain spotted fever) and other spotted fever group rickettsiae, an indirect immunofluorescent antibody assay for *R rickettsii* can be used to demonstrate a fourfold or greater change in antibody titers between acute and convalescent serum specimens taken 2 to 6 weeks apart. Use of *R akari* antigen is recommended for a more accurate serologic diagnosis but may only be available in specialized research laboratories. Direct fluorescent antibody or immunohistochemical testing of formalin-fixed, paraffin-embedded eschars or papulovesicle biopsy specimens can detect rickettsiae in the samples and are useful diagnostic techniques, but because of cross-reactivity, these assays are not able to confirm the etiologic agent. Use of polymerase chain reaction for detection of rickettsial DNA with subsequent sequence identification can confirm *R akari* infection.

TREATMENT: Doxycycline is the drug of choice in all age groups and is effective when given for 3 to 5 days. Doxycycline will shorten the course of disease; symptoms typically resolve within 12 to 48 hours after initiation of therapy. Relapse is rare. Tetracycline-based antimicrobial agents, including doxycycline, may cause permanent tooth discoloration for children younger than 8 years if used for repeated treatment courses. However, doxycycline binds less readily to calcium compared with older tetracyclines, and in some studies, doxycycline was not associated with visible teeth staining in younger children (see Tetracyclines, p 873). There are limited data describing the utility of other antimicrobials, including azithromycin and fluoroquinolones. Chloramphenicol is an alternative drug but carries a risk of serious adverse events and is not available as an oral formulation in the United States. Use of chloramphenicol should be considered only in rare cases, such as severe doxycycline allergies or during pregnancy. Untreated rickettsialpox usually will resolve within 2 to 3 weeks.

ISOLATION OF THE HOSPITALIZED PATIENT: Person-to-person spread of rickettsialpox has not been reported. Standard precautions are recommended.

CONTROL MEASURES: Application of residual acaricides can be used in heavily mite-infested environments to eliminate the vector. Rodent-control measures are important in limiting or eliminating spread of rickettsialpox; however, they should be conducted only in conjunction with acaricide application to ensure vector control. No specific management of exposed people is necessary.

Rocky Mountain Spotted Fever

CLINICAL MANIFESTATIONS: Rocky Mountain spotted fever (RMSF) is a systemic, small-vessel vasculitis that often involves a characteristic rash. Fever, myalgia, severe headache (less common in young children), photophobia, nausea, vomiting, and anorexia are typical presenting symptoms. Abdominal pain and diarrhea often are present and can obscure the diagnosis. The rash usually begins within the first 6 days of symptoms as erythematous macules or maculopapules. The rash usually appears first on the wrists and ankles, often spreading within hours proximally to the trunk and distally to the palms and soles. Although early development of a rash is a useful diagnostic sign, the rash can be atypical or absent in up to 20% of cases. It may be difficult to visualize in patients with dark skin. A petechial rash typically is a late finding and indicates progression to severe disease. Lack of a typical rash is a risk factor for misdiagnosis and poor outcome. Hepatomegaly and splenomegaly occur in 33% of patients. Meningeal signs with a positive Kernig and Brudzinski sign may occur. Thrombocytopenia, hyponatremia (serum sodium concentrations less than 130 mg/dL are observed in 20%), and elevated liver transaminase concentrations develop in many cases, are frequently mild in the early stages of disease, and worsen as disease progresses. White blood cell count typically is normal, but leukopenia and anemia can occur. If not treated, the illness can last as long as 3 weeks and can be severe, with prominent central nervous system, cardiac, pulmonary, gastrointestinal tract, and renal involvement; disseminated intravascular coagulation; and shock leading to death. RMSF can progress rapidly, even in previously healthy people. Delay in appropriate antimicrobial treatment past the fifth day of symptoms is associated with severe disease and poor outcomes. Case-fatality rates of untreated RMSF range from 20% to 80%, with a median time to death of 8 days. Significant long-term sequelae are common in patients with severe RMSF, including neurologic (paraparesis; hearing loss; peripheral neuropathy; bladder and bowel incontinence; and cerebellar, vestibular, and motor dysfunction) and nonneurologic (disability from limb or digit amputation) sequelae. Patients treated early in the course of symptoms may have a mild illness, with fever resolving in the first 48 hours of treatment.

ETIOLOGY: *Rickettsia rickettsii*, an obligate, intracellular, gram-negative bacillus and a member of the spotted fever group of rickettsiae, is the causative agent. The primary targets of infection in mammalian hosts are endothelial cells lining the small blood vessels of all major tissues and organs. Increased permeability leads to a diffuse small vessel vasculitis.

EPIDEMIOLOGY: The pathogen is transmitted to humans by the bite of a tick of the *Ixodidae* family (hard ticks). Ticks and their small mammal hosts serve as reservoirs of the pathogen in nature. Other wild animals and dogs have been found with antibodies to *R rickettsii*, but their role as natural reservoirs is not clear. People with occupational or recreational exposure to the tick vector (eg, pet owners, animal handlers, and people who spend more time outdoors) are at increased risk of acquiring the organism. People of all ages can be infected. The period of highest incidence in the United States is from April to September, although RMSF can occur year round in certain areas with endemic disease. Laboratory-acquired infection occasionally has resulted from accidental inoculation and aerosol contamination. Transmission has occurred on rare occasions by blood transfusion. Mortality is highest in males, people older than 50 years, children 5 to 9 years of age, and people with no recognized tick bite or attachment. In approximately half of pediatric RMSF cases, there is no recall of a recent tick bite. Delay in disease recognition and initiation of antirickettsial therapy after the fifth day of symptoms increase the risk of death. Factors contributing to delayed diagnosis include absence of rash or difficulty in its recognition, especially in individuals with darker complexions; initial presentation before the fourth day of illness; and onset of illness during months of low incidence.

RMSF is widespread in the United States, with a reported annual incidence that has increased eightfold from 1.8 cases per million people in 2000 to 14.3 cases per million in 2012, or about 4500 cases per year. Despite its name, RMSF is not common in the Rocky Mountain area. Most cases are reported in the south Atlantic, southeastern, and south central states, although most states in the contiguous United States record cases each year. The principal recognized vectors of *R rickettsii* are *Dermacentor variabilis* (the American dog tick) in the eastern and central United States and *Dermacentor andersoni* (the Rocky Mountain wood tick) in the western United States. Another common tick throughout the world that feeds on dogs, *Rhipicephalus sanguineus* (the brown dog tick) has been confirmed as a vector of *R rickettsii* in Arizona and Mexico and may play a role in other regions. Transmission parallels the tick season in a given geographic area. RMSF also occurs in Canada, Mexico, Central America, and South America.

The **incubation period** is approximately 1 week (range, 2–14 days).

DIAGNOSTIC TESTS: RMSF may be diagnosed by the detection of *R rickettsii* DNA in acute whole blood and serum specimens by polymerase chain reaction (PCR) assay. The specimen should preferably be obtained within the first week of symptoms and before (or within 24 hours of) doxycycline administration, and a negative result does not rule out RMSF infection. Diagnosis also may be confirmed by the detection of rickettsial DNA in biopsy or autopsy specimens by PCR assay or immunohistochemical (IHC) visualization of rickettsiae in tissues. The gold standard for serologic diagnosis of RMSF is the indirect fluorescent antibody (IFA) test. A negative serologic test result from the acute phase does not rule out a diagnosis of RMSF in any case. Both immunoglobulin (Ig) G and IgM antibodies begin to increase around day 7 to 10 after onset of symptoms; therefore, an elevated acute titer may represent past exposure rather than acute infection. Low-level elevated antibody titers can be an incidental finding in a significant proportion of the general population in some regions. IgM antibodies may remain elevated for months and are not highly specific for acute RMSF. A fourfold or greater rise in antigen-specific IgG between acute and convalescent sera obtained 2 to 6 weeks apart confirms the diagnosis. Cross-reactivity may be observed between antibodies to other spotted fever group rickettsiae. Testing of acute and convalescent sera by enzyme immunoassays or dot blot immunoassay tests can also be used for assessing antibody presence but are less useful for quantifying changes in titer. *R rickettsii* may also be isolated from acute blood specimens by animal passage or through tissue culture, but this can be hazardous, and culture is restricted to specialized procedures (not routine blood culture) at reference laboratories with at minimum Biosafety level 3 containment facilities. Cell culture cultivation of the organism must be confirmed by molecular methods.

TREATMENT: Doxycycline is the treatment of choice for RMSF in patients of any age and should be started as soon as RMSF is suspected. Use of antibiotics other than doxycycline increases the risk of mortality. The doxycycline dose for RMSF is 4 mg/kg per day, divided every 12 hours, intravenously or orally (maximum 100 mg/dose). Treatment is most effective if started in the first few days of symptoms, and treatment started after the fifth day of symptoms is less likely to prevent death or other adverse outcomes. Therefore, physicians always should treat empirically even when suspicion of the disease is low and should not postpone treatment while awaiting laboratory confirmation or classic symptoms, such as petechiae, to appear. Tetracycline-based antimicrobial agents, including doxycycline, may cause permanent tooth discoloration for children younger than 8 years if used for repeated treatment courses. However, doxycycline binds less readily to calcium compared with older tetracyclines, and in some studies, doxycycline was not associated with visible teeth staining in younger children (see Tetracyclines, p 873). Chloramphenicol sometimes is listed as an alternative treatment; however, its use is associated with a higher risk of fatal outcome. In addition, chloramphenicol carries a risk of serious adverse events and is not available as an oral formulation in the United States. Use of chloramphenicol should be considered only in rare cases, such as severe doxycycline allergies or during pregnancy. If the mother's life is in danger, doxycycline may be considered and the theoretical risk to the fetus should be discussed with the patient. These exceptions should be considered on a case-by-case basis, and the risks and benefits should be discussed with the patient. Antimicrobial treatment should be continued until the patient has been afebrile for at least 3 days and has demonstrated clinical improvement; the usual duration of therapy is 7 to 10 days.

ISOLATION OF THE HOSPITALIZED PATIENT: Standard precautions are recommended.

CONTROL MEASURES: Control of ticks in their natural habitat is difficult. Avoidance of tick-infested areas (eg, grassy areas, areas that border wooded regions) is the best preventive measure. If a tick-infested area is entered, people should wear protective clothing and apply tick or insect repellents to clothes and exposed body parts for added protection. All pets should be treated for ticks according to veterinary guidelines, and untreated animals should be excluded to prevent the yard and home from becoming a suitable habitat for ticks. Adults should be taught to inspect themselves, their children (bodies and clothing), and pets thoroughly for ticks after spending time outdoors during the tick season and to remove ticks promptly and properly (see Prevention of Tickborne Infections, p 210).

Prophylactic antimicrobial agents have no role in preventing RMSF, even in children with a documented tick bite who have not developed symptoms. Patients should not be tested or treated for RMSF until at least 1 symptom of illness is present. No licensed *R rickettsii* vaccine is available in the United States. Additional information is available on the Centers for Disease Control and Prevention's Web site (**www.cdc.gov/rmsf/**).

Rotavirus Infections

CLINICAL MANIFESTATIONS: Infection begins with acute onset of fever and vomiting followed 24 to 48 hours later by watery diarrhea. Symptoms generally persist for 3 to 8 days. In moderate to severe cases, dehydration, electrolyte abnormalities, and acidosis may occur. In certain immunocompromised children, including children with congenital cellular immunodeficiencies or severe combined immunodeficiency (SCID) and children who are hematopoietic stem cell or solid organ transplant recipients, persistent infection and diarrhea can develop.

ETIOLOGY: Rotaviruses are segmented, double-stranded RNA viruses belonging to the family *Reoviridae*, with at least 7 distinct antigenic groups (A through G). Group A viruses are the major causes of rotavirus diarrhea worldwide. Serotyping is based on the 2 surface proteins, VP7 glycoprotein (G) and VP4 protease-cleaved hemagglutinin (P). Prior to introduction of the rotavirus vaccine, G types 1 through 4 and 9 and P types 1A[8] and 1B[4] were most common in the United States.

EPIDEMIOLOGY: The epidemiology of rotavirus disease in the United States has changed following the introduction of the rotavirus vaccine. Prior to widespread use of the rotavirus vaccine, rotavirus was the most common cause of gastroenteritis in young children, the most common cause of health care-associated diarrhea in young children, and an important cause of acute gastroenteritis in children attending child care.

Rotavirus is present in high titer in stools of infected patients several days before and several days after onset of clinical disease. Transmission is by the fecal-oral route. Rotavirus can be found on toys and hard surfaces in child care centers, indicating that fomites may serve as a mechanism of transmission. Respiratory transmission likely plays a minor role in disease transmission. Spread within families and an institution is common. Rarely, common-source outbreaks from contaminated water or food have been reported.

In temperate climates, rotavirus disease is most prevalent during the cooler months. Before licensure of rotavirus vaccines in North America in 2006 and 2008, the annual rotavirus epidemic usually started during the autumn in Mexico and the southwest United States and moved eastward, reaching the northeast United States and Maritime Provinces by spring. The seasonal pattern of disease is less pronounced in tropical climates, with rotavirus infection being more common during the cooler, drier months.

The epidemiology of rotavirus disease in the United States has changed dramatically since rotavirus vaccines became available in 2006. A biennial pattern has emerged, with small, short seasons beginning in late winter/early spring (eg, 2009, 2011, and 2013) alternating with years with extremely low circulation (eg, 2008, 2010, 2012). The overall burden of rotavirus disease has declined dramatically. Beginning in 2008, annual hospitalizations for rotavirus disease among US children younger than 5 years declined by approximately 75%, with an estimated 40 000 to 50 000 fewer rotavirus hospitalizations nationally each year. In case-control evaluations in the United States, the vaccines (full series) have been found to be approximately 85% to 90% effective against rotavirus disease resulting in hospitalization. The vaccines also are highly effective against rotavirus disease resulting in emergency department care, and substantial reductions in emergency department visits for rotavirus disease have occurred in the years since vaccine was introduced. Substantial reductions in office visits for gastroenteritis attributable to rotavirus also have been observed during this time period.

The **incubation period** ranges from 1 to 3 days.

DIAGNOSTIC TESTS: It is not possible to diagnose rotavirus infection by clinical presentation or nonspecific laboratory tests. Enzyme immunoassays (EIAs), immunochromotography, and latex agglutination assays for group A rotavirus antigen detection in stool are available commercially. EIAs are used most widely because of their high sensitivity and specificity. Rotavirus also can be identified in stool by electron microscopy, by electrophoresis and silver staining, by standard or real-time reverse transcriptase-polymerase chain reaction (RT-PCR) assay for detection of viral genomic RNA, and by viral culture.

TREATMENT: No specific antiviral therapy is available. Oral or parenteral fluids and electrolytes are given to prevent or correct dehydration. Orally administered Human Immune Globulin, administered as an investigational therapy in immunocompromised patients with prolonged infection, has decreased viral shedding and shortened the duration of diarrhea.

ISOLATION OF THE HOSPITALIZED PATIENT: In addition to standard precautions, contact precautions are indicated for diapered or incontinent children for the duration of illness.

CONTROL MEASURES: Breastfeeding is associated with milder rotavirus disease and should be encouraged.

Child Care. General measures for interrupting enteric transmission in child care centers are available (see Children in Out-of-Home Child Care, p 132). Surfaces should be washed with soap and water. Few commercially available cleaning products have confirmed virucidal activity against rotavirus. A 70% ethanol solution, a bleach solution, or other disinfectants will inactivate rotavirus and may help prevent disease transmission resulting from contact with environmental surfaces. If using bleach, a freshly made solution of 1 part household bleach to 2 parts water (providing approximately 20 000 parts per million of free chlorine) to disinfect nonporous surfaces is suggested.

Vaccines. Two rotavirus vaccines are licensed for use among infants in the United States. In February 2006, a live, oral human-bovine reassortant pentavalent rotavirus (RV5 [RotaTeq, Merck & Co Inc, Whitehouse Station, NJ]) vaccine was licensed as a 3-dose series for use among infants in the United States. In April 2008, a live, oral human attenuated monovalent rotavirus (RV1 [Rotarix, GlaxoSmithKline, Research Triangle Park, NC]) vaccine was licensed as a 2-dose series for infants in the United States. The products differ in composition and schedule of administration. The American Academy of Pediatrics and the Centers for Disease Control and Prevention do not express a preference for either vaccine.

In 2010, porcine circovirus or porcine circovirus DNA was detected in both rotavirus vaccines. There is no evidence that this virus is a safety risk or causes illness in humans.

Postmarketing data from the United States, Australia, Mexico, and Brazil indicate that there is a small risk of intussusception from the currently licensed rotavirus vaccines. In the United States, the data currently available suggest the attributable risk is between approximately 1 excess intussusception case per 30 000 vaccinated infants to 1 excess case per 100 000 vaccinated infants. The risk appears to be primarily during the first week following the first or second dose; data from Australia suggest some risk may extend up to 21 days following the first dose. In the United States, as well as other parts of the world, the benefits of rotavirus vaccination in preventing severe rotavirus disease outweigh the risk of intussusception. Parents should be informed of the risk, the early signs and symptoms of intussusception, and the need for prompt care if these develop. The level of risk observed in these postmarketing studies is substantially lower than the risk of intussusception after immunization with RotaShield, the previously licensed rotavirus vaccine. Intussusception following rotavirus infection usually occurs within a week after the first or second vaccine dose. These preliminary surveillance data do not require any change in rotavirus vaccine recommendations. The benefits of rotavirus immunization include prevention of hospitalization for severe rotavirus disease in the United States and of death in other parts of the world. Currently, the benefits of these vaccines, which are known, far outweigh the rare potential risks. Postmarketing strain surveillance in the United States and other countries has revealed that RV5 vaccine reassortant strains have been detected occasionally in stool samples of children with diarrhea. In some of the reports, the reassortant virus seemed to cause diarrheal illness.

Table 3.61. Recommended Schedule for Administration of Rotavirus Vaccine

Recommendation	RV5 (RotaTeq[a])	RV1 (Rotarix[b])
Number of doses in series	3	2
Recommended ages for doses	2, 4, and 6 months of age	2 and 4 months of age
Minimum age for first dose	6 weeks of age	6 weeks of age
Maximum age for first dose	14 weeks, 6 days of age	14 weeks, 6 days of age
Minimum interval between doses	4 weeks	4 weeks
Maximum age for last dose	8 months, 0 days of age	8 months, 0 days of age

[a]Merck & Co Inc, Whitehouse Station, NJ.
[b]GlaxoSmithKline, Research Triangle Park, NC.

Following are recommendations for use of the currently licensed rotavirus vaccines[1,2] (see Table 3.61):

- Infants in the United States routinely should be immunized with 3 doses of RV5 vaccine administered orally at 2, 4, and 6 months of age or 2 doses of RV1 vaccine administered orally at 2 and 4 months of age.
- The first dose of rotavirus vaccine should be administered from 6 weeks through 14 weeks, 6 days of age (the maximum age for the first dose is 14 weeks, 6 days).
- Immunization should not be initiated for infants 15 weeks, 0 days of age or older. For infants to whom the first dose of rotavirus vaccine is inadvertently administered at 15 weeks, 0 days of age or older, the remainder of the rotavirus immunization series should be completed according to the schedule.
- The minimum interval between doses of rotavirus vaccine is 4 weeks.
- All doses of rotavirus vaccine should be administered by 8 months, 0 days of age.
- The rotavirus vaccine series should be completed with the same product whenever possible. However, immunization should not be deferred if the product used for previous doses is not available or is unknown. In this situation, the health care professional should continue or complete the series with the product available.
- If any dose in the series was RV5 vaccine or the product is unknown for any dose in the series, a total of 3 doses of rotavirus vaccine should be given.
- Rotavirus vaccine can be administered concurrently with other childhood vaccines.
- Infants with transient, mild illness with or without low-grade fever may receive rotavirus vaccine.
- Preterm infants may be immunized if the infant is at least 6 weeks of postnatal age and is clinically stable. Preterm infants should be immunized on the same schedule and with the same precautions as recommended for full-term infants. The first dose of vaccine should be given at the time of discharge or after the infant has been discharged from the nursery.

---

[1]American Academy of Pediatrics, Committee on Infectious Diseases. Prevention of rotavirus disease: updated guidelines for use of rotavirus vaccine. *Pediatrics.* 2009;123(5):1412–1420

[2]Centers for Disease Control and Prevention. Prevention of rotavirus gastroenteritis among infants and children. Recommendations of the Advisory Committee on Immunization Practices (ACIP). *MMWR Recomm Rep.* 2009;58(RR-2):1–25

- Infants living in households with immunocompromised people can and should be immunized. Infants living in households with pregnant women also should be immunized. Rotavirus vaccine should not be administered to infants who have a history of a severe allergic reaction (eg, anaphylaxis) after a previous dose of rotavirus vaccine or to a vaccine component. The tip caps of the prefilled oral applicators of the RV1 vaccine may contain natural rubber latex, so infants with a severe (anaphylactic) allergy to latex should not receive RV1; the RV1 vial stoppers are not made with natural rubber latex. The RV5 vaccine dosing tube is latex free.
- SCID and history of intussusception are contraindications for use of both rotavirus vaccines. Gastroenteritis, including severe diarrhea and prolonged shedding of vaccine virus, has been reported in infants who were administered live, oral rotavirus vaccines and later identified as having SCID.
- Precautions for administration of rotavirus vaccine include manifestations of altered immunocompetence (other than SCID, which is a contraindication); moderate to severe illness, including gastroenteritis; preexisting chronic intestinal tract disease; and spina bifida or bladder exstrophy (because of risk of latex allergy because the tip caps of the prefilled oral applicators of the RV1 vaccine may contain natural rubber latex).
- Rotavirus vaccine may be administered at any time before, concurrent with, or after administration of any blood product, including antibody-containing blood products.
- Breastfeeding infants should be immunized according to the same schedule as non-breastfed infants.
- If an infant regurgitates, spits out, or vomits during or after vaccine administration, the vaccine dose should not be repeated.
- If a recently immunized infant is hospitalized for any reason, no precautions other than standard precautions need to be taken to prevent spread of vaccine virus in the hospital setting.
- Infants who have had rotavirus gastroenteritis before receiving the full series of rotavirus immunization should begin or complete the schedule following the standard age and interval recommendations.
- Because of concern for shedding of vaccine strain in the stool, administration of rotavirus vaccine is not recommended for infants who remain hospitalized in the neonatal intensive care unit after immunization.

Rubella

CLINICAL MANIFESTATIONS:
Postnatal Rubella. Many cases of postnatal rubella are subclinical. Clinical disease usually is mild and characterized by a generalized erythematous maculopapular rash, lymphadenopathy, and slight fever. The rash starts on the face, becomes generalized in 24 hours, and lasts a median of 3 days. Lymphadenopathy, which may precede rash, often involves posterior auricular or suboccipital lymph nodes, can be generalized, and lasts between 5 and 8 days. Conjunctivitis and palatal enanthema have been noted. Transient polyarthralgia and polyarthritis rarely occur in children but are common in adolescents and adults, especially females. Encephalitis (1 in 6000 cases) and thrombocytopenia (1 in 3000 cases) are complications.
Congenital Rubella Syndrome. Maternal rubella during pregnancy can result in miscarriage, fetal death, or a constellation of congenital anomalies (congenital rubella syndrome

[CRS]). The most commonly described anomalies/manifestations associated with CRS are ophthalmologic (cataracts, pigmentary retinopathy, microphthalmos, and congenital glaucoma), cardiac (patent ductus arteriosus, peripheral pulmonary artery stenosis), auditory (sensorineural hearing impairment), or neurologic (behavioral disorders, meningoencephalitis, microcephaly, and mental retardation). Neonatal manifestations of CRS include growth restriction, interstitial pneumonitis, radiolucent bone disease, hepatosplenomegaly, thrombocytopenia, and dermal erythropoiesis (so-called "blueberry muffin" lesions). Mild forms of the disease can be associated with few or no obvious clinical manifestations at birth. Congenital defects occur in up to 85% if maternal infection occurs during the first 12 weeks of gestation, 50% if infection occurs during the first 13 to 16 weeks of gestation, and 25% if infection occurs during the end of the second trimester. Natural rubella infection in pregnancy is one of the few known causes of autism.

ETIOLOGY: Rubella virus is an enveloped, positive-stranded RNA virus classified as a *Rubivirus* in the *Togaviridae* family.

EPIDEMIOLOGY: Humans are the only source of infection. Postnatal rubella is transmitted primarily through direct or droplet contact from nasopharyngeal secretions. The peak incidence of infection is during late winter and early spring. Approximately 25% to 50% of infections are asymptomatic. Immunity from wild-type or vaccine virus usually is prolonged, but reinfection on rare occasions has been demonstrated and rarely has resulted in CRS. Although volunteer studies have demonstrated rubella virus in nasopharyngeal secretions from 7 days before to a maximum of 14 days after onset of rash, the period of maximal communicability extends from a few days before to 7 days after onset of rash. A small number of infants with congenital rubella continue to shed virus in nasopharyngeal secretions and urine for 1 year or more and can transmit infection to susceptible contacts. Rubella virus has been recovered in high titer from lens aspirates in children with congenital cataracts for several years.

Before widespread use of rubella vaccine, rubella was an epidemic disease, occurring in 6- to 9-year cycles, with most cases occurring in children. In the postvaccine era, most cases in the mid-1970s and 1980s occurred in young unimmunized adults in outbreaks on college campuses and in occupational settings. More recent outbreaks have occurred in people born outside the United States or among underimmunized populations. The incidence of rubella in the United States has decreased by more than 99% from the prevaccine era.

The United States was determined no longer to have endemic rubella in 2004, and from 2004 through 2012, 79 cases of rubella and 6 cases of CRS, including 3 cases in 2012, were reported in the United States; all of the cases were import associated or from unknown sources.[1] A national serologic survey from 1999-2004 indicated that among children and adolescents 6 through 19 years of age, seroprevalence was approximately 95%. However, approximately 10% of adults 20 through 49 years of age lacked antibodies to rubella, although 92% of women were seropositive. In addition, epidemiologic studies of rubella and CRS in the United States have identified that seronegativity is higher among people born outside the United States or from areas with poor vaccine coverage. The risk of CRS is highest in infants of women born outside the United States, because these women are more likely to be susceptible to rubella.

---

[1]Centers for Disease Control and Prevention. Three cases of congenital rubella syndrome in the postelimination era—Maryland, Alabama, and Illinois, 2012. *MMWR Morb Mortal Wkly Rep.* 2013;62(12):226–229

In 2003, the Pan American Health Organization (PAHO) adopted a resolution calling for elimination of rubella and CRS in the Americas by the year 2010. All countries with endemic rubella in the Americas implemented the recommended PAHO strategy by the end of 2008. The strategy consists of achieving high levels of measles-rubella vaccination coverage in the routine immunization program and in the supplemental vaccination campaigns to rapidly reduce the number of people in the country susceptible to acute infection. This is accomplished while simultaneously strengthening epidemiologic surveillance to monitor impact. The last confirmed endemic case in the Americas was diagnosed in Argentina in February 2009. In September 2010, the PAHO announced that the region of the Americas had achieved the rubella and CRS elimination goals on the basis of surveillance data, but documentation of elimination is ongoing.

The **incubation period** for postnatally acquired rubella ranges from 14 to 21 days, usually 16 to 18 days.

DIAGNOSTIC TESTS: Detection of rubella-specific immunoglobulin (Ig) M antibody usually indicates recent postnatal infection or congenital infection in a newborn infant, but both false-negative and false-positive results occur. Most postnatal cases are IgM-positive by 5 days after symptom onset, and most congenital cases are IgM-positive at birth to 3 months of age. For diagnosis of postnatally acquired rubella, a fourfold or greater increase in antibody titer between acute and convalescent periods or seroconversion between acute and convalescent IgG serum titers also indicate infection. Congenital infection also can be confirmed by stable or increasing serum concentrations of rubella-specific IgG over the first 7 to 11 months of life. The hemagglutination-inhibition rubella antibody test, which previously was the most commonly used method of serologic screening for rubella infection, generally has been supplanted by a number of equally or more sensitive assays for determining rubella immunity, including enzyme immunoassays and latex agglutination tests. Diagnosis of congenital rubella infection in children older than 1 year is difficult; serologic testing usually is not diagnostic, and viral isolation, although confirmatory, is possible in only a small proportion of congenitally infected children of this age.

A false-positive IgM test result may be caused by a number of factors including rheumatoid factor, parvovirus IgM, and heterophile antibodies. The presence of high-avidity IgG or lack of increase in IgG titers can be useful in identifying false-positive rubella IgM results. Low-avidity IgG is associated with recent primary rubella infection, whereas high-avidity IgG is associated with past infection or reinfection. The avidity assay is not a routine test and should be performed at reference laboratories like the Centers for Disease Control and Prevention (CDC).

Rubella virus can be isolated most consistently from throat or nasal specimens (and less consistently, urine) by inoculation of appropriate cell culture. Detection of rubella virus RNA by real time reverse-transcriptase polymerase chain reaction from a throat/nasal swab or urine sample with subsequent genotyping of strains may be valuable for diagnosis and molecular epidemiology. Most postnatal cases are positive virologically on the day of symptom onset, and most congenital cases are positive virologically at birth. Laboratory personnel should be notified that rubella is suspected, because specialized testing is required to detect the virus. Blood, urine, and cataract specimens also may yield virus, particularly in infants with congenital infection. With the successful elimination of indigenous rubella and CRS in the United States, molecular typing of viral isolates is critical in defining a source in outbreak scenarios as well as for sporadic cases.

TREATMENT: Supportive.

ISOLATION OF THE HOSPITALIZED PATIENT: In addition to standard precautions, for postnatal rubella, droplet precautions are recommended for 7 days after onset of the rash. Contact isolation is indicated for children with proven or suspected congenital rubella until they are at least 1 year of age, unless 2 cultures of clinical specimens obtained 1 month apart after 3 months of age are negative for rubella virus.

CONTROL MEASURES:

School and Child Care. Children with postnatal rubella should be excluded from school or child care for 7 days after onset of the rash. During an outbreak, children without evidence of immunity should be immunized or excluded for 21 days after onset of rash of the last case in the outbreak. Children with rubella may return to school or child care 7 days after rash onset. Children with CRS should be considered contagious until they are at least 1 year of age, unless 2 cultures of clinical specimens obtained 1 month apart are negative for rubella virus after 3 months of age. Infection-control precautions should be considered in children up to 3 years of age who are hospitalized for congenital cataract extraction. In child care settings, hand hygiene is essential for reducing transmission from the urine of children with CRS. Caregivers of these infants should be made aware of the potential hazard of the infants to susceptible pregnant contacts.

Surveillance for Congenital Infections. Accurate diagnosis and reporting of CRS are extremely important in assessing control of rubella. All birth defects in which rubella infection is suspected etiologically should be investigated thoroughly and reported to the CDC through local or state health departments.

Care of Exposed People. Evidence of rubella immunity consists of documented receipt of at least 1 dose of rubella-containing vaccine on or after the first birthday or serologic evidence of immunity. People born prior to 1957 can be considered immune. Documented evidence of rubella immunity is especially important for women who could become pregnant. Prenatal serologic screening for rubella immunity should be undertaken for all pregnant women. Women who have rubella-specific antibody concentrations above the standard positive cutoff value for the assay can be considered to have adequate evidence of rubella immunity. Those without antibody concentrations above the standard positive cutoff or those with equivocal test results should receive rubella vaccine during the immediate postpartum period before discharge. Vaccinated women of childbearing age who have received 1 or 2 doses of rubella-containing vaccine and have rubella serum IgG concentrations that are not clearly positive should be administered 1 additional dose of measles-mumps-rubella (MMR) vaccine (maximum of 3 doses) and do not need to be retested thereafter for serologic evidence of rubella immunity.

When a pregnant woman is exposed to rubella, a blood specimen should be obtained as soon as possible and tested for rubella antibody (IgG and IgM). An aliquot of frozen serum should be stored for possible repeated testing at a later time. The presence of rubella-specific IgG antibody in a properly performed test at the time of exposure indicates that the person most likely is immune. If antibody is not detectable, a second blood specimen should be obtained 2 to 3 weeks later and tested concurrently with the first specimen. If the second test result is negative, another blood specimen should be obtained 6 weeks after the exposure and also tested concurrently with the first specimen; a negative test result in both the second and third specimens indicates that infection has not occurred, and a positive test result in the second or third specimen but not the first (seroconversion) indicates recent infection.

Immune Globulin. Immune Globulin (IG) does not prevent rubella infection after exposure and is not recommended for that purpose. Although administration of IG after exposure to rubella will not prevent infection or viremia, it may modify or suppress symptoms and create an unwarranted sense of security. Therefore, IG is not recommended for routine postexposure prophylaxis of rubella in early pregnancy or any other circumstance. Infants with CRS have been born to women who received IG shortly after exposure. Administration of IG should be considered only if a pregnant woman who has been exposed to rubella will not consider termination of pregnancy under any circumstance. Administration of IG eliminates the value of IgG antibody testing to detect maternal infection. IgM antibody can be used to detect maternal infection after exposure, even after receipt of IG.

Vaccine. Although live-virus rubella vaccine administered after exposure has not been demonstrated to prevent illness, vaccine theoretically could prevent illness if administered within 3 days of exposure. Immunization of exposed nonpregnant people may be indicated, because if the exposure did not result in infection, immunization will protect these people in the future. Immunization of a person who is incubating natural rubella or who already is immune is not associated with an increased risk of adverse effects.

Rubella Vaccine.[1] The live-virus rubella vaccine distributed in the United States is the RA 27/3 strain grown in human diploid cell cultures. The RA 27/3 rubella vaccine was developed by Dr. Stanley Plotkin, to whom the 2015 *Red Book* is dedicated (p xvii). Vaccine is administered by subcutaneous injection as a combined vaccine containing MMR or measles-mumps-rubella-varicella (MMRV). Single-antigen rubella vaccine no longer is available in the United States. Vaccine can be given simultaneously with other vaccines (see Simultaneous Administration of Multiple Vaccines, p 35). Serum antibody to rubella is induced in more than 95% of recipients after a single dose at 12 months or older. Clinical efficacy and challenge studies have demonstrated that 1 dose confers long-term immunity against clinical and asymptomatic infection in more than 90% of immunized people. However, both symptomatic (rare) and asymptomatic reinfection has occurred.

Because of the 2-dose recommendations for measles- and mumps-containing vaccine (as MMR) and varicella vaccine (as MMRV), 2 doses of rubella vaccine are administered routinely. This provides an added safeguard against primary vaccine failures.

Vaccine Recommendations. At least 1 dose of live-attenuated rubella-containing vaccine is recommended for people 12 months or older. In the United States, rubella vaccine is recommended to be administered in combination with measles and mumps vaccines (MMR) or in combination with measles, mumps and varicella (MMRV), when a child is 12 through 15 months of age, with a second dose of MMR or MMRV at school entry at 4 through 6 years of age or sooner, according to recommendations for routine measles, mumps, rubella, and varicella immunization. People who have not received the dose at school entry should receive their second dose as soon as possible but optimally no later than 11 through 12 years of age (see Measles, p 535).

Special emphasis must continue to be placed on the immunization of at-risk postpubertal males and females, especially college students, military recruits, recent immigrants, health care professionals, teachers, and child care providers. People who were born in 1957 or after and who have not received at least 1 dose of vaccine or who have no serologic evidence of immunity to rubella are considered susceptible and should be

[1]Centers for Disease Control and Prevention. Prevention of Measles, Rubella, Congenital Rubella Syndrome, and Mumps, 2013 Summary: Recommendations of the Advisory Committee on Immunization Practices (ACIP). *MMWR Recomm Rep.* 2013;62(RR-4):1–34

immunized with MMR vaccine. Clinical diagnosis of infection is unreliable and should not be accepted as evidence of immunity.

Specific recommendations are as follows:

- Postpubertal females without documentation of presumptive evidence of rubella immunity should be immunized unless they are pregnant. Postpubertal females should be advised not to become pregnant for 28 days after receiving a rubella-containing vaccine (see Precautions and Contraindications, p 694, for further discussion). Routine serologic testing of nonpregnant postpubertal women before immunization is unnecessary and is a potential impediment to protection against rubella, because it requires 2 visits.
- During annual health care examinations, premarital and family planning visits, and visits to sexually transmitted infection clinics, postpubertal females should be assessed for rubella susceptibility and, if deemed susceptible, should be immunized with MMR vaccine.
- Routine prenatal screening for rubella immunity should be undertaken. If a woman is found to be susceptible, rubella vaccine should be administered during the immediate postpartum period before discharge.
- People who have rubella-specific antibody concentrations above the standard positive cutoff value for the assay can be considered to have adequate evidence of rubella immunity. Except for women of childbearing age, people who have an equivocal serologic test result should be considered susceptible to rubella unless they have documented receipt of 1 dose of rubella-containing vaccine or subsequent serologic test results indicate rubella immunity. Vaccinated women of childbearing age who have received 1 or 2 doses of rubella-containing vaccine and have rubella serum IgG concentrations that are not clearly positive should receive 1 additional dose of MMR vaccine (maximum of 3 doses) and do not need to be retested thereafter for serologic evidence of rubella immunity.
- Breastfeeding is not a contraindication to postpartum immunization of the mother (for additional information, see Human Milk, p 125).
- All susceptible health care personnel who may be exposed to patients with rubella or who take care of pregnant women, as well as people who work in educational institutions or provide child care, should be immunized to prevent infection for themselves and to prevent transmission of rubella to pregnant patients.[1]

Adverse Reactions.

- Of susceptible children who receive MMR or MMRV vaccines, fever develops in 5% to 15% from 6 to 12 days after immunization. Rash occurs in approximately 5% of immunized people. Mild lymphadenopathy occurs commonly. Febrile seizures occur slightly more frequently among children 12 through 23 months of age after administration of MMRV vaccine compared with MMR and varicella given as separate injections during the same visit (see Measles, p 535).
- Joint pain, usually in small peripheral joints, has been reported in approximately 0.5% of young children following vaccination with a rubella-containing vaccine. Arthralgia and transient arthritis tend to be more common in susceptible postpubertal females, occurring in approximately 25% and 10%, respectively, of vaccine recipients. Joint involvement usually begins 7 to 21 days after immunization and generally is transient. The incidence of joint manifestations after immunization is lower than after natural infection at the corresponding age.

---

[1]Centers for Disease Control and Prevention. Immunization of health-care personnel: recommendations of the Advisory Committee on Immunization Practices (ACIP). *MMWR Recomm Rep.* 2011;60(RR-7):1–45

- Transient paresthesia and pain in the arms and legs also have been reported, although rarely.
- Central nervous system manifestations have been reported, but no causal relationship with rubella vaccine has been established.
- Other reactions that occur after immunization with MMR or MMRV are associated with the measles, mumps, and varicella components of the vaccine (see Measles, p 535, Mumps, p 564, and Varicella-Zoster Infections, p 846).

Precautions and Contraindications.

- **Pregnancy.** Rubella vaccine should not be administered to pregnant women. If vaccine is administered inadvertently or if pregnancy occurs within 28 days of immunization, the patient should be counseled on the theoretical risks to the fetus. The maximal theoretical risk for occurrence of congenital rubella is estimated to be 1.3% on the basis of data accumulated by the CDC from more than 200 susceptible women who received the current rubella vaccine (the RA27/3 strain) from 1 to 2 weeks before to 4 to 6 weeks after conception. Of the offspring, 2% had subclinical infection, but none had congenital defects; 98% were not infected. Other more substantial data from Latin America as a result of the extremely large mass rubella vaccination campaigns conducted in the 2000s support this US experience. In view of these observations, receipt of rubella vaccine during pregnancy is not an indication for termination of pregnancy.
- **Children of pregnant women.** Immunizing susceptible children whose mothers or other household contacts are pregnant does not cause a risk. Most immunized people intermittently shed small amounts of virus from the pharynx 7 to 28 days after immunization, but no evidence of transmission of the vaccine virus from immunized children has been found.
- **Febrile illness.** Children with minor illnesses, such as upper respiratory tract infection, may be immunized (see Vaccine Safety, p 43). Fever is not a contraindication to immunization. However, if other manifestations suggest a more serious illness, the child should not be immunized until recovery has occurred.
- **Recent administration of IG.** IG preparations interfere with immune response to measles vaccine, and theoretically may interfere with the serologic response to rubella vaccine (see p 38). If rubella vaccine is indicated postpartum for a woman who has received anti-Rho (D) IG or blood products, suggested intervals are the same as used between IG administration and measles immunization (see Table 1.10, p 39).
- **Altered immunity.** Immunocompromised patients with disorders associated with increased severity of viral infections should not receive live-virus rubella vaccine (see Immunization in Immunocompromised Children, p 74). Exceptions are patients with human immunodeficiency virus infection who are not severely immunocompromised; these patients may be immunized against rubella with MMR vaccine (see Human Immunodeficiency Virus Infection, p 453). If possible, children receiving biologic response modifiers, such as anti-tumor necrosis factor-alpha (see Biologic Response Modifiers Used to Decrease Inflammation, p 83), should be immunized prior to initiating treatment.
- **Household contacts of immunocompromised people.** The risk of rubella exposure for patients with altered immunity is decreased by immunizing susceptible contacts. Although small amounts of vaccine virus may be isolated from the pharynx, no evidence of transmission of rubella vaccine virus from immunized children to immunocompromised contacts has been found. Precautions and contraindications

appropriate for the measles, mumps, and varicella components of MMR or MMRV vaccines also should be reviewed before administration (see Measles, p 535, Mumps, p 564, and Varicella-Zoster Infections, p 846).

Corticosteroids. For patients who have received high doses of corticosteroids (2 mg/kg or greater or more than 20 mg/day) for 14 days or more and who otherwise are not immunocompromised, the recommended interval between stopping the steroids and immunization is at least 1 month (see Immunization in Immunocompromised Children, p 74) after steroids have been discontinued.

Tuberculosis. Tuberculin skin testing is not a prerequisite for MMR immunization. Antituberculosis therapy should be initiated before administering MMR vaccine to people with untreated tuberculosis infection or disease. Tuberculin skin testing, if otherwise indicated, can be performed on the day of immunization with MMR vaccine. Otherwise, tuberculin skin testing should be postponed for 4 to 6 weeks, because measles immunization temporarily may suppress tuberculin skin test reactivity.

Salmonella Infections

CLINICAL MANIFESTATIONS: Nontyphoidal *Salmonella* organisms cause a spectrum of illness ranging from asymptomatic gastrointestinal tract carriage to gastroenteritis, bacteremia, and focal infections, including meningitis, brain abscess, and osteomyelitis. The most common illness associated with nontyphoidal *Salmonella* infection is gastroenteritis, in which diarrhea, abdominal cramps, and fever are common manifestations. The site of infection usually is the distal small intestine as well as the colon. Sustained or intermittent bacteremia can occur, and focal infections are recognized in as many as 10% of patients with nontyphoidal *Salmonella* bacteremia. In the United States, the incidence of invasive *Salmonella* infection is highest among infants. Certain *Salmonella* serovars (eg, Dublin, Typhi, Choleraesuis), although rare, are more likely to result in invasive infection than gastroenteritis. However, in recent years in sub-Saharan Africa, systematic blood culture-based surveillance to assess the magnitude of the burden of invasive bacterial infections such as caused by *Streptococcus pneumoniae*, *Haemophilus influenzae* type b, and group A *Neisseria meningitidis* serendipitously revealed the profound importance of invasive disease caused by certain serovars of nontyphoidal *Salmonella*. Notably, these highly lethal African nontyphoidal *Salmonella* organisms are distinct genetically from their serovar counterparts causing pediatric disease in industrialized countries and exhibit a very high lethality (approx 20% case fatality rate); two thirds of patients present without gastroenteritis or a history of antecedent diarrhea.

Salmonella enterica serovars Typhi, Paratyphi A, Paratyphi B, and Paratyphi C can cause a protracted bacteremic illness referred to, respectively, as typhoid and paratyphoid fever and collectively as enteric fevers. In older children, the onset of enteric fever typically is gradual, with manifestations such as fever, constitutional symptoms (eg, headache, malaise, anorexia, and lethargy), abdominal discomfort and tenderness, hepatomegaly, splenomegaly, dactylitis, rose spots, and change in mental status. In infants and toddlers, invasive infection with enteric fever serovars can manifest as a mild, nondescript febrile illness accompanied by self-limited bacteremia, or invasive infection can occur in association with more severe clinical symptoms and signs, sustained bacteremia, and meningitis. Either diarrhea (resembling pea soup) or constipation can be early features. Relative bradycardia (pulse rate slower than would be expected for a given body temperature) has been considered a common feature of typhoid fever in adults but in children is neither a discriminating feature in the assessment of a febrile child from an area where enteric fever is endemic nor a feature of the disease per se.

ETIOLOGY: *Salmonella* organisms are gram-negative bacilli that belong to the family *Enterobacteriaceae*. More than 2500 *Salmonella* serovars have been described; most serovars causing human disease are classified within O serogroups A through E. *Salmonella* serotype Typhi is classified in O serogroup D, along with many other common serovars Enteritidis and Dublin. In 2011, the most commonly reported human isolates in the United States were *Salmonella* serovars Enteritidis, Typhimurium, Newport, Javiana, and I 4,[5],12:i:-; these 5 serovars generally account for nearly half of all *Salmonella* infections in the United States **(www.cdc.gov/ncezid/dfwed/PDFs/salmonella-annual-report-2011-508c.pdf)**.

The relative prevalence of other serovars varies by country. Approximately 75% to 95% of the serovars associated with invasive pediatric disease in sub-Saharan Africa are *S* Typhimurium (mostly of an unusual variant, multilocus sequence type 313, that is distinct genomically), a monophasic variant of ST 313 that does not express phase 2 flagella, or *S* Enteritidis. The current *Salmonella* nomenclature is shown in Table 3.62.

EPIDEMIOLOGY: Every year, nontyphoidal *Salmonella* organisms are among of the most common causes of laboratory-confirmed cases of enteric disease. The principal reservoirs for nontyphoidal *Salmonella* organisms include birds, mammals, reptiles, and amphibians. However, it is believed that some of the African serotypes associated with invasive human disease have a human rather than animal reservoir. The major food vehicles of transmission to humans in industrialized countries include food of animal origin, such as poultry, beef, eggs, and dairy products. Multiple other food vehicles (eg, fruits, vegetables, peanut butter, frozen pot pies, powdered infant formula, cereal, and bakery products) have been implicated in outbreaks in the United States and Europe, presumably when the food was contaminated by contact with an infected animal product or a human carrier. Other modes of transmission include ingestion of contaminated water or contact with infected animals, mainly poultry (eg, chicks, chickens, ducks), reptiles or amphibians (eg, pet turtles, iguanas, lizards, snakes, frogs, toads, newts, salamanders), and rodents (eg, hamsters, mice) or other mammals (eg, hedgehogs). Reptiles and amphibians that live in tanks or aquariums can contaminate the water with germs, which can spread to people. Small turtles with a shell length of less than 4 inches are a well-known source of human *Salmonella*

Table 3.62. Nomenclature for *Salmonella* Organisms

Complete Name[a]	Serotype[b]	Antigenic Formula
S enterica[a] subspecies *enterica* serovar Typhi	Typhi	9,12,[Vi]:d:-
S enterica subspecies *enterica* serovar Typhimurium	Typhimurium	[1],4,[5],12:i:1,2
S enterica subspecies *enterica* serovar Newport	Newport	6,8,[20]:e,h:1,2
S enterica subspecies *enterica* serovar Paratyphi A	Paratyphi A	[1],2,12:a:[1,5]
S enterica subspecies *enterica* serovar Enteritidis	Enteritidis	[1],9,12:g,m:-

[a]Species and subspecies are determined by biochemical reactions. Serotype is determined based on antigenic make-up. In the current taxonomy, only 2 species are recognized, *Salmonella enterica* and *Salmonella bongori*. *S enterica* has 6 subspecies, of which subspecies I (*enterica*) contains the overwhelming majority of all *Salmonella* pathogens that affect humans, other mammals, and birds.

[b]Many *Salmonella* pathogens that previously were considered species (and, therefore, were written italicized with a small case first letter) now are considered serotypes (also called serovars). Serotypes are now written nonitalicized with a capital first letter (eg, Typhi, Typhimurium, Enteritidis). The serotype of *Salmonella* is determined by its O (somatic) and H (flagellar) antigens and whether Vi is expressed.

infections. Because of this risk, the Food and Drug Administration (FDA) has banned the interstate sale and distribution of these turtles since 1975. Animal-derived pet foods and treats have also been linked to *Salmonella* infections, especially among young children.

Unlike nontyphoidal *Salmonella* serovars, the enteric fever serovars (*Salmonella* serovars Typhi, Paratyphi A, Paratyphi B [*sensu stricto*]) are restricted to human hosts, in whom they cause clinical and subclinical infections. Chronic human carriers (mostly involving chronic infection of the gall bladder but occasionally involving infection of the urinary tract) constitute the reservoir in areas with endemic infection. Infection with enteric fever serovars implies ingestion of a food or water vehicle contaminated by a chronic carrier or person with acute infection. Although typhoid fever (300–400 cases annually) and paratyphoid fever (approx 150 cases annually) are uncommon in the United States, these infections are highly endemic in many resource-limited countries, particularly in Asia. Consequently, most typhoid fever and paratyphoid fever infections in residents of the United States usually are acquired during international travel.

Age-specific incidences for nontyphoidal *Salmonella* infection are highest in children younger than 4 years. In the United States, rates of invasive infections and mortality are higher in infants, elderly people, and people with hemoglobinopathies (including sickle cell disease) and immunocompromising conditions (eg, malignant neoplasms, human immunodeficiency virus [HIV]) infection). Most reported cases are sporadic, but widespread outbreaks, including health care-associated and institutional outbreaks, have been reported. The incidence of foodborne cases of nontyphoidal *Salmonella* gastroenteritis has diminished little in recent years.

Every year, nontyphoidal *Salmonella* organisms are one of the most common causes of laboratory-confirmed cases of enteric disease reported by the Foodborne Diseases Active Surveillance Network (FoodNet [**www.foodsafety.gov** and **www.cdc.gov/foodnet**]).

A risk of transmission of infection to others persists for as long as an infected person excretes nontyphoidal *Salmonella* organisms. Twelve weeks after infection with the most common nontyphoidal *Salmonella* serovars, approximately 45% of children younger than 5 years excrete organisms, compared with 5% of older children and adults; antimicrobial therapy can prolong excretion. Approximately 1% of adults continue to excrete nontyphoidal *Salmonella* organisms for more than 1 year.

The **incubation period** for nontyphoidal *Salmonella* gastroenteritis usually is 12 to 36 hours (range, 6–72 hours). For enteric fever, the **incubation period** usually is 7 to 14 days (range, 3–60 days).

DIAGNOSTIC TESTS: Isolation of *Salmonella* organisms from cultures of stool, blood, urine, bile (including duodenal fluid containing bile), and material from foci of infection is diagnostic. Gastroenteritis is diagnosed by stool culture. Diagnostic tests to detect *Salmonella* antigens by enzyme immunoassay, latex agglutination, and monoclonal antibodies have been developed, as have commercial immunoassays that detect antibodies to antigens of enteric fever serovars. Gene-based polymerase chain reaction diagnostic tests also are available in research laboratories. Multiplex polymerase chain reaction (PCR) platforms for detection of multiple viral, parasitic, and bacterial pathogens, including *Salmonella*, have been licensed for diagnostic use.

If enteric fever is suspected, blood, bone marrow, or bile culture is diagnostic, because organisms often are absent from stool. The sensitivity of blood culture and bone marrow culture in children with enteric fever is approximately 60% and 90%, respectively. The combination of a single blood culture plus culture of bile (collected from a bile-stained duodenal string) is 90% sensitive in detecting *Salmonella* serovar Typhi infection in children with clinical enteric fever.

TREATMENT:

- Antimicrobial therapy usually is not indicated for patients with either asymptomatic infection or uncomplicated (noninvasive) gastroenteritis caused by nontyphoidal *Salmonella* serovars, because therapy does not shorten the duration of diarrheal disease and can prolong duration of fecal excretion. Although of unproven benefit, antimicrobial therapy is recommended for gastroenteritis caused by nontyphoidal *Salmonella* serovars in people at increased risk of invasive disease, including infants younger than 3 months and people with chronic gastrointestinal tract disease, malignant neoplasms, hemoglobinopathies, HIV infection, or other immunosuppressive illnesses or therapies.

- If antimicrobial therapy is initiated in patients with gastroenteritis, amoxicillin or trimethoprim-sulfamethoxazole is recommended for susceptible strains. Resistance to these antimicrobial agents is becoming more common, especially in resource-limited countries. Resistance patterns for United States isolates can be found on the CDC Web site (**www.cdc.gov/narms/reports/index.html**). In areas where ampicillin and trimethoprim-sulfamethoxazole resistance is common, a fluoroquinolone or azithromycin usually is effective. For patients with localized invasive disease (eg, osteomyelitis, abscess, meningitis) or bacteremia in people infected with HIV, empiric therapy with ceftriaxone is recommended. Once antimicrobial susceptibility test results are available, ampicillin or ceftriaxone for susceptible strains is recommended.

- For invasive, nonfocal infections such as bacteremia or septicemia caused by nontyphoidal *Salmonella* or for enteric fever caused by *Salmonella* serovars Typhi, Paratyphi A, and Paratyphi B, 14 days of therapy is recommended, although shorter courses (7–10 days) have been effective. Therapy with a fluoroquinolone or azithromycin orally can be considered in patients with uncomplicated infections for nontyphoidal *Salmonella*. For enteric fever caused by *Salmonella* serovar Typhi, therapy should be administererd parenterally for 14 days, either entirely in the hospital or, if adequately improved, with the final 4 days with home IV therapy. For localized invasive disease (eg, osteomyelitis, meningitis), at least 4 to 6 weeks of therapy is recommended. Drugs of choice, route of administration, and duration of therapy are based on susceptibility of the organism (if known), knowledge of the antimicrobial susceptibility patterns of prevalent strains, site of infection, host, and clinical response. Multidrug-resistant isolates of *Salmonella* serovars Typhi and Paratyphi A (exhibiting R factor-encoded resistance to ampicillin, chloramphenicol, and trimethoprim/sulfamethoxazole) and strains with decreased susceptibility to fluoroquinolones are common in South and Southeast Asia and are found increasingly in travelers to areas with endemic infection. Invasive salmonellosis attributable to strains with decreased fluoroquinolone susceptibility is associated with greater risk for treatment failure. *Salmonella* serovars Typhi and Paratyphi A and nontyphoidal *Salmonella* isolates with ciprofloxacin resistance or that produce extended-spectrum beta-lactamases occasionally are reported. Empiric treatment of enteric fever with ceftriaxone or fluoroquinolone is recommended, but once antimicrobial susceptibility results are known, therapy should be changed as necessary. Azithromycin is an effective alternative for people with uncomplicated infections. Relapse of nontyphoidal *Salmonella* infection can occur, particularly in immunocompromised patients, who may require longer duration of treatment and retreatment. Aminoglycosides are not recommended for treatment of invasive *Salmonella* infections.

- For enteric fever caused by *Salmonella* servar Typhi acquired from overseas travel, culture should be performed on stool samples from all people who traveled with the index case(s), and if results are positive, people should be treated with antibiotics (eg, ciprofloxacin) and monitored for development of any symptoms. Asymptomatic people in the United States who had contact with the index case(s) do not require culture of stool samples.
- The propensity to become a chronic *Salmonella* serovar Typhi carrier (excretion longer than 1 year) following acute typhoid infection correlates with prevalence of cholelithiasis, increases with age, and is greater in females than males. Chronic carriage in children is uncommon. The chronic carrier state may be eradicated by 4 weeks of oral therapy with ciprofloxacin or norfloxacin, antimicrobial agents that are highly concentrated in bile. High-dose parenteral ampicillin also can be used if 4 weeks of oral fluoroquinolone therapy is not well tolerated (see Fluoroquinolones, p 872). Cholecystectomy may be indicated in some adults if antimicrobial therapy alone fails.
- Corticosteroids may be beneficial in patients with severe enteric fever, which is characterized by delirium, obtundation, stupor, coma, or shock. These drugs should be reserved for critically ill patients in whom relief of manifestations of toxemia may be life saving. The usual regimen is high-dose dexamethasone given intravenously at an initial dose of 3 mg/kg, followed by 1 mg/kg, every 6 hours, for a total course of 48 hours.

ISOLATION OF THE HOSPITALIZED PATIENT: In addition to standard precautions, contact precautions should be used for diapered and incontinent children for the duration of illness. In children with typhoid fever, precautions should be continued until culture results for 3 consecutive stool specimens obtained at least 48 hours after cessation of antimicrobial therapy are negative.

CONTROL MEASURES: Important measures include proper food hygiene practices; treated water supplies; proper hand hygiene; adequate sanitation to dispose of human fecal waste; exclusion of infected people from handling food or providing health care; education on the risk of *Salmonella* infections from animal contact; prohibiting the sale of pet turtles; limiting exposure of children younger than 5 years and immunocompromised children to reptiles, amphibians, poultry in backyard flocks, and rodents at home and in public settings (see Diseases Transmitted by Animals [Zoonoses], p 219); reporting cases to appropriate health authorities; and investigating outbreaks. Eggs and other foods of animal origin should be cooked thoroughly. People should not eat raw eggs or foods containing raw eggs or consume unpasteurized milk or raw milk products.[1] Notification of public health authorities and determination of serovar are of primary importance in detection and investigation of outbreaks.

Child Care. Outbreaks of *Salmonella* illness in child care centers are rare. Specific strategies for controlling infection in out-of-home child care include adherence to hygiene practices, including meticulous hand hygiene and limiting exposure to certain animals. Animals at higher risk of causing salmonellosis, including reptiles, amphibians, and poultry, are not recommended in schools, child care settings, hospitals, or nursing homes (see Children in Out-of-Home Child Care, p 132).

When nontyphoidal *Salmonella* serovars are identified in a symptomatic child care attendee or staff member with enterocolitis, older children and staff members do not

---

[1]American Academy of Pediatrics, Committee on Infectious Diseases and Committee on Nutrition. Consumption of raw or unpasteurized milk and milk products by pregnant women and children. *Pediatrics.* 2014;133(1):175–179

need to be excluded unless they are symptomatic. Stool cultures are not required for asymptomatic contacts. Likewise, children or staff members with nontyphoidal *Salmonella* enterocolitis do not require negative culture results from stool samples, and children can return to child care facilities once the diarrhea has resolved (see Children in Out-of-Home Child Care, p 132). Antimicrobial therapy is not recommended for people with asymptomatic nontyphoidal *Salmonella* infection or uncomplicated diarrhea or for people who are contacts of an infected person.

When *Salmonella* serovar Typhi infection is identified in a child care staff member, local or state health departments may be consulted regarding regulations for length of exclusion and testing, which may vary by jurisdiction. Because infections with *Salmonella* serotypes Typhi or Paratyphi are transmitted easily and can be severe, exclusion of an infected child is warranted until results of 3 stool samples obtained at least 48 hours after cessation of antimicrobial therapy have negative culture results for *Salmonella* serotypes Typhi or *Paratyphi* (see Children in Out-of-Home Child Care, p 132).

Typhoid Vaccine. Resistance to infection with *Salmonella* serovar Typhi is enhanced by typhoid immunization, but currently licensed vaccines do not provide complete protection. Two typhoid vaccines are licensed for use in the United States (see Table 3.63).

The demonstrated efficacy of the 2 vaccines licensed by the US Food and Drug Administration ranges from 50% to 80%, but the duration of protection differs notably between the vaccines. Vaccine is selected on the basis of age of the child, need for booster doses, and possible contraindications (see Precautions and Contraindications, p 701) and reactions (see Adverse Events, p 701).

Indications. In the United States, immunization is recommended only for the following people:

- **Travelers to areas where risk of exposure to *Salmonella* serovar Typhi is recognized.** Risk is greatest for travelers to the Indian subcontinent, South and Southeast Asia, Latin America including the Caribbean, the Middle East, and Africa, who may have prolonged exposure to contaminated food and drink. Such travelers need to be cautioned that typhoid vaccine is not a substitute for careful selection of food and drink (see **www.cdc.gov/travel**).
- **People with intimate exposure to a documented typhoid fever carrier,** as occurs with continued household contact.
- **Laboratory workers with frequent contact with *Salmonella* serovar Typhi.**
- **People living outside the United States in areas with endemic typhoid infection.**

Table 3.63. Commercially Available Typhoid Vaccines in the United States

Typhoid Vaccine	Type	Route	Minimum Age of Receipt, y	No. of Doses[a]	Booster Frequency, y	Adverse Effects Incidence
Ty21a	Live-attenuated	Oral	6	4	5	Less than 5%
ViCPS	Polysaccharide	Intramuscular	2	1	2	Less than 7%

ViCPS indicates Vi capsular polysaccharide vaccine.

[a]Primary immunization. For further information on dosage, schedules, and adverse events, see text.

Dosages. For primary immunization, the following dosage is recommended for each vaccine:

- **Typhoid vaccine live oral Ty21a (Vivotif).** Children (6 years and older) and adults should take 1 enteric-coated capsule every other day for a total of 4 capsules. Each capsule should be taken with cool liquid, no warmer than 37°C (98°F), approximately 1 hour before a meal. The capsules should be kept refrigerated, and all 4 doses must be taken to achieve maximal efficacy. Immunization should be completed at least 1 week before possible exposure.
- **Typhoid Vi polysaccharide vaccine (Typhim Vi).** Primary immunization of people 2 years and older with Vi capsular polysaccharide (ViCPS) vaccine consists of one 0.5-mL (25-μg) dose administered intramuscularly. Vaccine should be given at least 2 weeks before possible exposure.
- **Protection against *Salmonella* serovars Paratyphi A and Paratyphi B.** Neither Ty21a nor ViCPS vaccine provides reliable protection against *Salmonella* serotype Paratyphi A. Results of 2 field trials suggest that Ty21a may provide partial cross-protection against *Salmonella* serovar Paratyphi B.

Booster Doses. In circumstances of continued or repeated exposure to *Salmonella* serovar Typhi, periodic reimmunization is recommended to maintain immunity.

Continued efficacy for 7 years after immunization with the oral Ty21a vaccine has been demonstrated; however, the manufacturer of oral Ty21a vaccine recommends reimmunization (completing the entire 4-dose series) every 5 years if continued or renewed exposure to *Salmonella* serovar Typhi is expected. Oral Ty21a (which does not express Vi antigen) and ViCPS (which protects by stimulating serum IgG Vi antibody) vaccines mediate protection by distinct mechanisms.

ViCPS vaccine is a T-independent antigen that does not elicit immunologic memory to allow boosting of serum Vi antibody titers following an initial immunization. The manufacturer of ViCPS vaccine recommends reimmunization every 2 years if continued or renewed exposure is expected.

No data have been reported concerning use of one vaccine administered after primary immunization with the other.

Adverse Events. The oral Ty21a vaccine produces mild adverse reactions that may include abdominal pain, nausea, diarrhea, vomiting, fever, headache, and rash or urticaria. Reported adverse reactions to ViCPS vaccine also are minimal and include fever, headache, malaise, myalgia, and local reaction of tenderness and pain, erythema, or induration of 1 cm or greater.

Precautions and Contraindications. No data are available regarding efficacy of typhoid vaccines in children younger than 2 years. A contraindication to administration of parenteral ViCPS vaccine is a history of hypersensitivity to any component of the vaccine. No safety data have been reported for typhoid vaccines in pregnant women. The oral Ty21a vaccine is a live-attenuated vaccine and should not be administered to immunocompromised people, including people known to be infected with HIV, to have a phagocytic cell defect, or to have chronic granulomatous disease[1]; the parenteral ViCPS vaccine may be an alternative, although the expected immune response may not be obtained. The oral Ty21a vaccine requires replication in the gut for effectiveness; it should not be administered during gastrointestinal tract illness. Adequate immune response is achieved when

[1]Rubin LG, Levin MJ, Ljungman P, et al. 2013 IDSA clinical practice guideline for vaccination of the immunocompromised host. *Clin Infect Dis.* 2014;58(3):e44–e100

administered simultaneously with either mefloquine or chloroquine; however, if mefloquine is administered, immunization with Ty21a should be delayed for 24 hours. Also, the antimalarial agent proguanil should not be administered simultaneously with oral Ty21a vaccine but, rather, should be administered 10 or more days after the fourth dose of oral Ty21a vaccine. Atovaquone also can interfere with oral Ty21a immunogenicity. Antimicrobial agents should be avoided for 3 days before the first dose of oral Ty21a vaccine and 7 days after the fourth dose of Ty21a vaccine.

Scabies

CLINICAL MANIFESTATIONS: Scabies is characterized by an intensely pruritic, erythematous, papular eruption caused by burrowing of adult female mites in upper layers of the epidermis, creating serpiginous burrows. Itching is most intense at night. In older children and adults, the sites of predilection are interdigital folds, flexor aspects of wrists, extensor surfaces of elbows, anterior axillary folds, waistline, thighs, navel, genitalia, areolae, abdomen, intergluteal cleft, and buttocks. In children younger than 2 years, the eruption generally is vesicular and often occurs in areas usually spared in older children and adults, such as the scalp, face, neck, palms, and soles. The eruption is caused by a hypersensitivity reaction to the proteins of the parasite.

Characteristic scabietic burrows appear as gray or white, tortuous, thread-like lines. Excoriations are common, and most burrows are obliterated by scratching before a patient seeks medical attention. Occasionally, 2- to 5-mm red-brown nodules are present, particularly on covered parts of the body, such as the genitalia, groin, and axilla. These scabies nodules are a granulomatous response to dead mite antigens and feces; the nodules can persist for weeks and even months after effective treatment. Cutaneous secondary bacterial infection can occur and usually is caused by *Streptococcus pyogenes* or *Staphylococcus aureus* (including methicillin-resistant *S aureus* [MRSA]). Studies have demonstrated a correlation between poststreptococcal glomerulonephritis and scabies.

Crusted (Norwegian) scabies is an uncommon clinical syndrome characterized by a large number of mites and widespread, crusted, hyperkeratotic lesions. Crusted scabies usually occurs in people with debilitating conditions, people with developmental disabilities, or people who are immunocompromised. Crusted scabies also can occur in otherwise healthy children after long-term use of topical corticosteroid therapy.

Postscabetic pustulosis is a reactive phenomenon that may follow successful treatment of primary infestation with scabies. Affected infants and young children manifest episodic crops of sterile, pruritic papules and pustules predominantly in an acral distribution, but lesions may extend to a lesser degree onto the torso.

ETIOLOGY: The mite *Sarcoptes scabiei* subspecies *hominis* is the cause of scabies. The adult female burrows in the stratum corneum of the skin and lays eggs. Larvae emerge from the eggs in 2 to 4 days and molt to nymphs and then to adults, which mate and produce new eggs. The entire cycle takes approximately 10 to 17 days. *S scabiei* subspecies *canis*, acquired from dogs (with clinical mange), can cause a self-limited and mild infestation in humans usually involving the area in direct contact with the infested animal that will resolve without specific treatment.

EPIDEMIOLOGY: Humans are the source of infestation. Transmission usually occurs through prolonged close, personal contact. Because of the large number of mites in exfoliating scales, even minimal contact with a patient with crusted scabies may result in transmission; transmission from a patient with crusted scabies also can occur through contamination of items such as clothing, bedding, and furniture. Infestation acquired from dogs and other animals is uncommon, and these mites do not replicate in humans. Scabies of human origin can be transmitted as long as the patient remains infested and untreated, including during the interval before symptoms develop. Scabies is endemic in many countries and occurs worldwide in cycles thought to be 15 to 30 years long. Scabies affects people from all socioeconomic levels without regard to age, gender, or standards of personal hygiene. Scabies in adults often is acquired sexually.

The **incubation period** in people without previous exposure usually is 4 to 6 weeks. People who previously were infested are sensitized and develop symptoms 1 to 4 days after repeated exposure to the mite; however, these reinfestations usually are milder than the original episode.

DIAGNOSTIC TESTS: Diagnosis of scabies typically is made by clinical examination. Diagnosis can be confirmed by identification of the mite or mite eggs or scybala (feces) from scrapings of papules or intact burrows, preferably from the terminal portion where the mite generally is found. Mineral oil, microscope immersion oil, or water applied to skin facilitates collection of scrapings. A broad-blade scalpel is used to scrape the burrow. Scrapings and oil can be placed on a slide under a glass coverslip and examined microscopically under low power. Adult female mites average 330 to 450 μm in length. Skin scrapings provide definitive evidence of infection but have low sensitivity. Handheld dermoscopy (epiluminescence microscopy) has been used to identify in vivo the pigmented mite parts or air bubbles corresponding to infesting mites within the stratum corneum.

TREATMENT: Topical permethrin 5% cream or off-label use of oral ivermectin both are effective agents for treatment of scabies (see Drugs for Parasitic Infections, p 927). Most experts recommend starting with topical 5% permethrin cream as the drug of choice, particularly for infants, young children (not approved for children younger than 2 months), and pregnant or nursing women. Permethrin cream should be removed by bathing after 8 to 14 hours. Children and adults with infestation should apply lotion or cream containing this scabicide over their entire body below the head. Because scabies can affect the face, scalp, and neck in infants and young children, treatment of the entire head, neck, and body in this age group is required. Special attention should be given to trimming fingernails and ensuring application of medication to these areas. A Cochrane review found that oral ivermectin is effective for treating scabies but less effective than topical permethrin. Because ivermectin is not ovicidal, it is given as 2 doses, 1 week apart. Ivermectin is not approved for treatment of scabies by the US Food and Drug Administration. The safety of ivermectin in children weighing less than 15 kg (33 lb) has not been determined. Ivermectin is not recommended for women who are pregnant or who are lactating and intend to breastfeed.

Alternative drugs include 10% crotamiton cream or lotion, or unapproved 5% to 10% precipitated sulfur compounded into petrolatum. Because scabietic lesions are the result of a hypersensitivity reaction to the mite, itching may not subside for several weeks despite successful treatment. The use of oral antihistamines and topical corticosteroids can help relieve this itching. Topical or systemic antimicrobial therapy is indicated for secondary bacterial infections of the excoriated lesions.

Because of safety concerns and availability of other treatments, lindane lotion should not be used as a first-line agent in the treatment of scabies. It is approved by the US Food and Drug Administration for second-line therapy in patients who cannot tolerate or have failed other approved therapies. Infants, children weighing less than 50 kg (110 lb), and patients with other skin conditions, such as atopic dermatitis, are at particular risk of serious neurotoxicity from lindane. Lindane is contraindicated in preterm infants, patients with crusted scabies or other skin conditions that could increase absorption of the drug, and patients with seizure disorders.

ISOLATION OF THE HOSPITALIZED PATIENT: In addition to standard precautions, contact precautions are recommended until the patient has been treated with an appropriate scabicide.

CONTROL MEASURES:
- Prophylactic therapy is recommended for household members, particularly for household members who have had prolonged direct skin-to-skin contact. Manifestations of scabies infestation can appear as late as 2 months after exposure, during which time patients can transmit scabies. All household members should be treated at the same time to prevent reinfestation. Bedding and clothing worn next to the skin during the 3 days before initiation of therapy should be laundered in a washer with hot water and dried using a hot cycle. Mites do not survive more than 3 days without skin contact. Clothing that cannot be laundered should be removed from the patient and stored for several days to a week to avoid reinfestation.
- Children should be allowed to return to child care or school after treatment has been completed.
- Epidemics and localized outbreaks may require stringent and consistent measures to treat contacts. Caregivers who have had prolonged skin-to-skin contact with patients with infestation may benefit from prophylactic treatment.
- Environmental disinfestation is unnecessary and unwarranted. Thorough vacuuming of environmental surfaces is recommended after use of a room by a patient with crusted scabies.
- People with crusted scabies and their close contacts must be treated promptly and aggressively to avoid outbreaks.

Schistosomiasis

CLINICAL MANIFESTATIONS: Infections are established by skin penetration of infecting larvae (cercariae, shed by fresh water snails), which may be accompanied by a transient, pruritic, papular rash (cercarial dermatitis). After penetration, the parasites enter the bloodstream, migrate through the lungs, and eventually mature into adult worms that reside in the venous plexus that drains the intestines or, in the case of *Schistosoma haematobium*, the urogenital tract. Four to 8 weeks after exposure, an acute serum sickness-like illness (Katayama syndrome) can develop that manifests as fever, malaise, cough, rash, abdominal pain, hepatosplenomegaly, diarrhea, nausea, lymphadenopathy, and eosinophilia. The severity of symptoms associated with infection is related to the worm burden. People with low to moderate worm burdens may have only subclinical disease or relatively mild manifestations, such as growth stunting or anemia. Higher worm burdens are associated with a range of symptoms caused primarily by inflammation and fibrosis triggered by the immune response to eggs produced by adult worms. Severe forms of intestinal schistosomiasis (*Schistosoma mansoni* and *Schistosoma japonicum* infections) can result in hepatosplenomegaly, abdominal pain, bloody diarrhea, portal hypertension, ascites, esophageal varices, and hematemesis. Urogenital schistosomiasis (*S haematobium* infections) can result in the bladder becoming inflamed and fibrotic. Urinary tract symptoms and signs include dysuria, urgency, terminal microscopic and gross hematuria, secondary urinary tract infections, hydronephrosis, and nonspecific pelvic pain. *S haematobium* is associated with lesions of the lower genital tract (vulva, vagina, and cervix) in women, prostatitis and hematospermia in men, and certain forms of bladder cancer. Other organ systems can be involved—for example, eggs can embolize in the lungs, causing pulmonary hypertension. Less commonly, eggs can lodge in the central nervous system, causing severe neurologic complications.

Cercarial dermatitis (swimmer's itch) often is caused by larvae of schistosome parasites of birds or other wildlife. These larvae can penetrate human skin but eventually die in the dermis and do not cause systemic disease. Skin manifestations include pruritus at the penetration site a few hours after water exposure, followed in 5 to 14 days by an intermittent pruritic, sometimes papular, eruption. In previously sensitized people, more intense papular eruptions may occur for 7 to 10 days after exposure.

ETIOLOGY: The trematodes (flukes) *S mansoni*, *S japonicum*, *Schistosoma mekongi*, and *Schistosoma intercalatum* cause intestinal schistosomiasis, and *S haematobium* causes urogenital disease. All species have similar life cycles. Swimmer's itch typically is caused by various schistosome species that are parasitic only for birds and wild mammals.

EPIDEMIOLOGY: Persistence of schistosomiasis depends on the presence of an appropriate snail as an intermediate host. Eggs excreted in stool (*S mansoni*, *S japonicum*, *S mekongi*, and *S intercalatum*) or urine *(S haematobium)* into fresh water hatch into motile miracidia, which infect snails. After development and asexual replication in snails, cercariae emerge and penetrate the skin of humans in contact with water. Children commonly are first infected when they accompany their mothers to lakes, ponds, and other open fresh water sources. School-aged children typically are the most heavily infected people in the community because of prolonged wading and swimming in infected waters. They are also important in maintaining transmission through behaviors such as uncontrolled defecation and urination. Communicability lasts as long as infected snails are in the environment or live eggs are excreted in the urine and feces of humans into fresh water sources with appropriate snails. In the case of *S japonicum*, animals play an important zoonotic role (as a source of eggs) in maintaining the life cycle. Infection is not transmissible by person-to-person contact or blood transfusion.

The distribution of schistosomiasis is focal and limited by the presence of appropriate snail vectors, infected human reservoirs, and fresh water sources. *S mansoni* occurs throughout tropical Africa, in parts of several Caribbean islands, and in areas of Venezuela, Brazil, Suriname, and the Arabian Peninsula. *S japonicum* is found in China, the Philippines, and Indonesia. *S haematobium* occurs in Africa and the Middle East. *S mekongi* is found in Cambodia and Laos. *S intercalatum* is found in West and Central Africa. Adult worms of *S mansoni* can live as long as 30 years in the human host. Thus, schistosomiasis can be diagnosed in patients many years after they have left an area with endemic infection. Immunity is incomplete, and reinfection occurs commonly. Swimmer's itch can occur in all regions of the world after exposure to fresh water, brackish water, or salt water.

The **incubation period** is variable but is approximately 4 to 6 weeks for *S japonicum*, 6 to 8 weeks for *S mansoni*, and 10 to 12 weeks for *S haematobium*.

DIAGNOSTIC TESTS: Eosinophilia is common and may be intense in Katayama syndrome (acute schistosomiasis). Infection with *S mansoni* and other species (except *S haematobium*) is determined by microscopic examination of stool specimens to detect characteristic eggs, but results may be negative if performed too early in the course of infection. In light infections, several stool specimens examined by a concentration technique may be needed before eggs are found, or eggs may be seen in a biopsy of the rectal mucosa. *S haematobium* is diagnosed by examining urine for eggs. Egg excretion in urine often peaks between noon and 3 PM. Biopsy of the bladder mucosa may be used to diagnose this infection. Urine reagent dipsticks commonly will be positive for hematuria. Serologic tests, available through the Centers for Disease Control and Prevention and some commercial laboratories, may be helpful for detecting light infections; however, results of these antibody-based tests remain positive for many years and are not useful in differentiating ongoing infection from past infection or reinfection.

Swimmer's itch can be difficult to differentiate from other causes of dermatitis. A skin biopsy may demonstrate larvae, but their absence does not exclude the diagnosis.

TREATMENT: The drug of choice for schistosomiasis caused by any species is praziquantel (see Drugs for Parasitic Infections, p 927). The alternative drug for *S mansoni* is oxamniquine, although this drug is not available in the United States; it is used in some areas of Brazil. Praziquantel does not kill developing worms; therapy given within 4 to 8 weeks of exposure should be repeated 1 to 2 months later to improve the rate of parasitologic cure. Swimmer's itch is a self-limited disease that may require symptomatic treatment of the rash. More intense reactions may require a course of oral corticosteroids.

ISOLATION OF THE HOSPITALIZED PATIENT: Standard precautions are recommended. Schistosomiasis cannot be transmitted from person to person or by the fecal-oral route.

CONTROL MEASURES: Elimination of the intermediate snail host is difficult to achieve in most areas. Thus, mass or selective treatment of infected populations, sanitary disposal of human waste, and education about the source of infection are key elements of current control measures. Travelers to areas with endemic infection should be advised to avoid any contact with freshwater streams, rivers, ponds, or lakes. Swimming and wading should only occur in chlorinated pools. Sea water does not transmit human schistosomiasis.

Shigella Infections

CLINICAL MANIFESTATIONS: *Shigella* species primarily infect the large intestine, causing clinical manifestations that range from watery or loose stools with minimal or no constitutional symptoms to more severe symptoms, including high fever, abdominal cramps or tenderness, tenesmus, and mucoid stools with or without blood. *Shigella dysenteriae* serotype 1 often causes a more severe illness than other shigellae with a higher risk of complications, including septicemia, pseudomembranous colitis, toxic megacolon, intestinal perforation, hemolysis, and hemolytic-uremic syndrome (HUS). Infection attributable to *S dysenteriae* type 1 has become rare in industrialized countries. Generalized seizures have been reported among young children with shigellosis attributable to any serotype; although the pathophysiology and incidence are poorly understood, such seizures usually are self-limited and usually are associated with high fever or electrolyte abnormalities. Septicemia is rare during the course of illness and is caused either by *Shigella* organisms or by other gut flora that gain access to the bloodstream through intestinal mucosa damaged during shigellosis. Septicemia occurs most often in neonates, malnourished children, and people with *S dysenteriae* serotype 1 infection. Reactive arthritis with possible extraarticular manifestations is a rare complication that can develop weeks or months after shigellosis, especially in patients expressing HLA-B27.

ETIOLOGY: *Shigella* species are facultative aerobic, gram-negative bacilli in the family *Enterobacteriaceae*. Four species (with more than 40 serotypes) have been identified. Among *Shigella* isolates reported in the United States in 2012, approximately 81% were *Shigella sonnei*, 17% were *Shigella flexneri*, 1% were *Shigella boydii*, and less than 1% were other species (**www. cdc.gov/narms/reports/index.html**). In resource-limited countries, especially in Africa and Asia, *S flexneri* predominates, and *S dysenteriae* often causes outbreaks. Shiga toxin is produced by *S dysenteriae* serotype 1, which enhances virulence at the colonic mucosa and can cause small blood vessel and renal damage, leading to HUS.

EPIDEMIOLOGY: Humans are the natural host for *Shigella* organisms, although other primates can be infected. The primary mode of transmission is fecal-oral, although transmission also can occur via contact with a contaminated inanimate object, ingestion of contaminated food or water, or sexual contact. Houseflies also may be vectors through physical transport of infected feces. Ingestion of as few as 10 organisms, depending on the species, is sufficient for infection to occur. Prolonged organism survival in water (up to 6 months) and food (up to 30 days) can occur with *Shigella*. Children 5 years or younger in child care settings and their caregivers, people living in crowded conditions, and men who have sex with men are at increased risk of infection. Infections attributable to *S flexneri*, *S boydii*, and *S dysenteriae* are more common in older children and adults than are infections attributable to *S sonnei* in the United States; nonetheless, more than 25% of cases caused by each species are reported among children younger than 5 years. Travel to resource-limited countries with inadequate sanitation can place travelers at risk of infection. Even without antimicrobial therapy, the carrier state usually ceases within 1 to 4 weeks after onset of illness; long-term carriage is uncommon and does not correlate with underlying intestinal dysfunction.

The **incubation period** varies from 1 to 7 days, typically 1 to 3 days.

DIAGNOSTIC TESTS: Isolation of *Shigella* organisms from feces or rectal swab specimens containing feces is diagnostic; sensitivity is improved by testing stool as soon as possible after it is passed. The presence of fecal lactoferrin (or fecal leukocytes) demonstrated on a methylene-blue stained stool smear is fairly sensitive for the diagnosis of colitis but is not specific for shigellosis. Although bacteremia is rare, blood should be cultured in severely ill, immunocompromised, or malnourished children. Multiplex polymerase chain reaction (PCR) platforms for detection of multiple bacterial, viral, and parasitic pathogens including *Shigella* are commercially available, but no rapid diagnostic tests have been licensed. Other tests for bacterial detection, including qualitative and quantitative PCR assays, are available in research laboratories and some clinical laboratories.

TREATMENT:
- Although severe dehydration is rare with shigellosis, correction of fluid and electrolyte losses, preferably by oral rehydration solutions, is the mainstay of treatment.
- Most clinical infections with *S sonnei* are self-limited (48 to 72 hours), and mild episodes do not require antimicrobial therapy. Available evidence suggests that antimicrobial therapy is somewhat effective in shortening duration of diarrhea and hastening eradication of organisms from feces. Treatment is recommended for patients with severe disease or with underlying immunosuppressive conditions; in these patients, empiric

therapy should be given while awaiting culture and susceptibility results. Antimicrobial susceptibility testing of clinical isolates is indicated, because resistance to antimicrobial agents is common and susceptibility data can guide appropriate therapy. Plasmid-mediated resistance has been identified in all *Shigella* species. In 2012 in the United States, approximately 25% of *Shigella* species were resistant to ampicillin, 43% were resistant to trimethoprim-sulfamethoxazole, 4% were resistant to azithromycin, 2% were resistant to ciprofloxacin, and 1.1% were resistant to ceftriaxone (**www.cdc.gov/ narms/reports/index.html**).

- Azithromycin susceptibility testing is not performed widely for *Shigella* species, but evidence suggests that *Shigella* strains with decreased susceptibility to azithromycin are circulating in the United States. Ciprofloxacin and ceftriaxone resistance is increasing around the world.
- For cases in which treatment is required and susceptibilities are unknown or an ampicillin- and trimethoprim-sulfamethoxazole–resistant strain is isolated, parenteral ceftriaxone for 2 to 5 days, a fluoroquinolone (eg, ciprofloxacin) for 3 days, or azithromycin for 3 days should be administered. Oral cephalosporins (eg, cefixime) have been used successfully in treating shigellosis in adults. Fluoroquinolones are not approved by the US Food and Drug Administration for use in people younger than 18 years with shigellosis, although fluoroquinolones have been shown to be beneficial (see Fluoroquinolones, p 872). For susceptible strains, ampicillin or trimethoprim-sulfamethoxazole for 5 days is effective; amoxicillin is not effective because of its rapid absorption from the gastrointestinal tract. The oral route of therapy is recommended except for seriously ill patients.
- Antidiarrheal compounds that inhibit intestinal peristalsis are contraindicated, because they can prolong the clinical and bacteriologic course of disease and can increase the rate of complications.
- Nutritional supplementation, including vitamin A (200 000 IU) and zinc (10 or 20 mg elemental Zn, orally daily for 10–14 days), can be given to hasten clinical resolution in geographic areas where children are at risk of malnutrition.

ISOLATION OF THE HOSPITALIZED PATIENT: In addition to standard precautions, contact precautions are indicated for the duration of illness.

CONTROL MEASURES:

Child Care Centers. General measures for interrupting enteric transmission in child care centers are recommended (see Children in Out-of-Home Child Care, p 132). Meticulous hand hygiene is the single most important measure to decrease transmission. Waterless hand sanitizers may be effective as an adjunct to washing hands with soap and in circumstances where access to soap or clean water is limited. Eliminating access to shared water-play areas and contaminated diapers also can decrease infection rates. Child care staff members should follow all standard infection control recommendations, specifically enhancing hand hygiene and ensuring that those who change diapers are not responsible for food preparation.

When *Shigella* infection is identified in a child care attendee or staff member, stool specimens from symptomatic attendees and staff members should be cultured. The local health department should be notified to evaluate and manage potential outbreaks. Ill children and staff should not be permitted to return to the child care facility until 24 or more hours after diarrhea has ceased. State regulations may require one or more stool cultures to be negative for *Shigella* species before returning to care.

Institutional Outbreaks. The outbreaks that are most difficult to control are those that involve children not yet or only recently toilet-trained, adults who are unable to care for themselves (mentally disabled people or skilled nursing facility residents), or an inadequate supply of chlorinated water. A cohort system, combined with appropriate antimicrobial therapy, and a strong emphasis on hand hygiene should be considered until stool cultures no longer yield *Shigella* species. In residential institutions, ill people and newly admitted patients should be housed in separate areas.

General Control Measures. Strict attention to hand hygiene is essential to limit spread. Other important control measures include improved sanitation, appropriately chlorinating the water supply, proper cooking and storage of food, excluding infected people as food handlers, and measures to decrease contamination of food and surfaces by houseflies. People should refrain from recreational water venues (eg, swimming pools, water parks) while they have diarrhea, and those who are incontinent should continue to avoid recreational water activities for 1 additional week after symptoms resolve. Breastfeeding provides some protection for infants. Case reporting to appropriate health authorities (eg, hospital infection control personnel and public health departments) is essential.

Smallpox (Variola)

The last naturally occurring case of smallpox occurred in Somalia in 1977, followed by 2 cases in 1978 after a photographer was infected during a laboratory exposure and later transmitted smallpox to her mother in the United Kingdom. In 1980, the World Health Assembly declared that smallpox (variola virus) had been eradicated successfully worldwide. The United States discontinued routine childhood immunization against smallpox in 1972 and routine immunization of health care professionals in 1976. Immunization of US military personnel continued until 1990. Following eradication, 2 World Health Organization reference laboratories were authorized to maintain stocks of variola virus. As a result of terrorism events on September 11, 2001, and concern that the virus and the expertise to use it as a weapon of bioterrorism may have been misappropriated, the smallpox immunization policy was revisited. In 2002, the United States resumed immunization of military personnel deployed to certain areas of the world and in 2003 initiated a civilian smallpox immunization program for first responders to facilitate preparedness and response to a possible smallpox bioterrorism event.

CLINICAL MANIFESTATIONS: People infected with variola major strains develop a severe prodromal illness characterized by high fever (102°F–104°F [38.9°C–40.0°C]) and constitutional symptoms, including malaise, severe headache, backache, abdominal pain, and prostration, lasting for 2 to 5 days. Infected children may suffer from vomiting and seizures during this prodromal period. Most patients with smallpox are severely ill and bedridden during the febrile prodrome. The prodromal period is followed by development of lesions on mucosa of the mouth or pharynx, which may not be noticed by the patient. This stage occurs less than 24 hours before onset of rash, which usually is the first recognized manifestation of infectiousness. With onset of oral lesions, the patient becomes infectious and remains so until all skin crust lesions have separated. The rash typically begins on the face and rapidly progresses to involve the forearms, trunk, and legs, with the greatest concentration of lesions on the face and distal extremities. The majority of patients will have lesions on the palms and soles. With rash onset, fever decreases but does not resolve. Lesions begin as macules that progress to papules, followed by firm vesicles and then deep-seated, hard pustules described as "pearls of pus." Each stage lasts 1 to 2 days. By the sixth or seventh day of rash, lesions may begin to umbilicate or become confluent. Lesions increase in size for approximately 8 to 10 days, after which they begin to crust. Once all the crusts have separated, 3 to 4 weeks after the onset of rash, the patient no longer is infectious. Variola minor strains cause a disease that is indistinguishable clinically from variola major, except that it causes less severe systemic symptoms, more rapid rash evolution, reduced scarring, and fewer fatalities.

Varicella (chickenpox) is the condition most likely to be mistaken for smallpox. Generally, children with varicella do not have a febrile prodrome, but adults may have a brief, mild prodrome. Although the 2 diseases are confused easily in the first few days of the rash, smallpox lesions develop into pustules that are firm and deeply embedded in the dermis, whereas varicella lesions develop into superficial vesicles. Because varicella erupts in crops of lesions that evolve quickly, lesions on any one part of the body will be in different stages of evolution (papules, vesicles, and crusts), whereas all smallpox lesions on any one part of the body are in the same stage of development. The rash distribution of the 2 diseases differs; varicella most commonly affects the face and trunk, with relative sparing of the extremities, and lesions on the palms or soles are rare.

Variola major in unimmunized people is associated with case-fatality rates of $\leq 30\%$ during epidemics of smallpox. The mortality rate is highest in pregnant women, children younger than 1 year, and adults older than 30 years. The potential for modern supportive therapy to improve outcome is not known.

In addition to the typical presentation of smallpox (90% of cases or greater), there are 2 uncommon forms of variola major: hemorrhagic (characterized either by a hemorrhagic diathesis prior to onset of the typical smallpox rash [early hemorrhagic smallpox] or by hemorrhage into skin lesions and disseminated intravascular coagulation [late hemorrhagic smallpox]) and malignant or flat type (in which the skin lesions do not progress to the pustular stage but remain flat and soft). Each variant occurs in approximately 5% of cases and is associated with a 95% to 100% mortality rate.

ETIOLOGY: Variola is a member of the *Poxviridae* family (genus *Orthopoxvirus*). Other members of this genus that can infect humans include monkeypox virus, cowpox virus, and vaccinia virus. In 2003, an outbreak of monkeypox linked to prairie dogs exposed to rodents imported from Ghana occurred in the United States. Cowpox virus was used by Benjamin Jesty in 1774 and by Edward Jenner in 1796 as material for the first smallpox vaccine. Later, cowpox virus was replaced with vaccinia virus.

EPIDEMIOLOGY: Humans are the only natural reservoir for variola virus (smallpox). Smallpox is spread most commonly in droplets from the oropharynx of infected people, although rare transmission from aerosol spread has been reported. Infection from direct contact with lesion material or indirectly via fomites, such as clothing and bedding, also has been reported. Because most patients with smallpox are extremely ill and bedridden, spread generally is limited to household contacts, hospital workers, and other health care professionals. Secondary household attack rates for smallpox were considerably lower than for measles and similar to or lower than rates for varicella.

The **incubation period** is 7 to 17 days (mean, 12 days).

DIAGNOSTIC TESTS: Variola virus can be detected in vesicular or pustular fluid by a number of different methods, including electron microscopy, immunohistochemistry, culture, or polymerase chain reaction (PCR) assay. Only PCR assay can diagnose infection with variola virus definitively; all other methods simply screen for orthopoxviruses. Screening is available through state health departments, and final variola-specific laboratory confirmation is available only at the Centers for Disease Control and Prevention (CDC). Diagnostic work-up includes exclusion of varicella-zoster virus or other common conditions that cause a vesicular/pustular rash illness. Caution is required when collecting specimens from patients in whom a diagnosis of smallpox is considered. Detail guidelines for safe collection of specimens in patients with possible smallpox can be found on the CDC Web site (**http://emergency.cdc.gov/agent/smallpox/response-plan/files/guide-d.pdf**).

TREATMENT: There is no known effective antiviral therapy available to treat smallpox. Infected patients should receive supportive care. Cidofovir, a nucleotide analogue of cytosine, has demonstrated antiviral activity against certain orthopoxviruses in vitro and in animal models. Its effectiveness in treatment of variola in humans is unknown. Investigational agents, such as brincidofovir (CMX001, which is the lipophilic derivative of cidofovir), are being evaluated in animal models. Vaccinia Immune Globulin (VIG) is reserved for certain complications of immunization and has no role in treatment of smallpox. Physicians at civilian medical facilities may request VIG by calling the CDC Smallpox Vaccine Adverse Events Clinical Information Line at 1-800-232-4636. Physicians at military medical facilities may request VIG by calling the US Army Medical Research Institute of Infectious Diseases (USAMRIID) at 301-619-2257 or 1-888-872-7443 (1-888-USA-RIID). Tecovirimat (ST-246, an investigational agent active against orthopoxviruses) and brincidofovir have been used for the treatment of disseminated vaccinia.

ISOLATION OF THE HOSPITALIZED PATIENT: On admission, a patient suspected of having smallpox should be placed in a private, airborne infection isolation room equipped with negative-pressure ventilation with high-efficiency particulate air filtration. Standard, contact, and airborne precautions should be implemented immediately, and hospital infection control personnel and the state (and/or local) health department should be alerted at once. After evaluation by the state or local health department, if smallpox laboratory diagnostics are considered necessary, the CDC Emergency Operations Center should be consulted at 770-488-7100.

CONTROL MEASURES:

Care of Exposed People. Cases of febrile rash illness for which smallpox is considered in the differential diagnosis should be reported immediately to local or state health departments.

Use of Vaccine. Postexposure immunization (within 3–4 days of exposure) provides some protection against disease and significant protection against a fatal outcome. Except for severely immunocompromised people, who are not expected to benefit from live vaccinia vaccine, any person with a significant exposure to a patient with proven smallpox during the infectious stage of illness requires immunization as soon after exposure as possible but within 4 days of first exposure ("ring vaccination"). Because infected people are not contagious until the rash (and/or oral lesions) appears, people exposed only during the prodromal period are not at risk.

Preexposure Immunization.

Smallpox Vaccine. The only smallpox vaccine licensed in the United States is ACAM2000 (Sanofi Pasteur Biologics Co, Cambridge, MA), a live-virus vaccine.[1] The lyophilized vaccine does not contain variola virus but a related virus called vaccinia

---

[1]Centers for Disease Control and Prevention. Notice to readers: newly licensed smallpox vaccine to replace old smallpox vaccine. *MMWR Morb Mortal Wkly Rep.* 2008;57(8):207–208

virus, different from the cowpox virus initially used for immunization by Jesty and Jenner. Vaccinia vaccines are highly effective in preventing smallpox, with protection waning after 5 to 10 years following 1 dose; protection after reimmunization has lasted longer. However, substantial protection against death from smallpox persisted in the past for more than 30 years after immunization during infancy during a time of worldwide small-pox virus circulation and routine smallpox immunization practices. The manufacturer recommends that people at very high risk, such as those handling variola virus, be vac-cinated every 3 years. The vaccine generally is not available and can only be adminis-tered by specially trained providers. In the absence of a smallpox outbreak, preexposure smallpox immunization is not recommended for children. Smallpox vaccine had been recommended for adults participating in smallpox response teams and for people working with orthopoxviruses, and smallpox vaccine continues to be administered to eligible mili-tary personnel preparing to deploy to certain regions in the world. Inadvertent transmis-sion of the vaccine virus may occur from vaccine recipients to their household contacts. Children who are immunocompromised or have atopic skin disease are at increased risk of serious complications following contact transmission, including progressive vaccinia and eczema vaccinatum. Smallpox reimmunization recommendations can be found on the CDC Web site (**http://emergency.cdc.gov/agent/smallpox/revaxmemo. asp**). Information about vaccine administration contraindications to preexposure smallpox immunization and adverse events[1] can be found in the vaccine package insert and medication guide (**www.fda.gov/BiologicsBloodVaccines/Vaccines/ ApprovedProducts/ucm180810.htm** or **www.bt.cdc.gov/agent/smallpox/ index.asp**). An investigational attenuated vaccinia vaccine (Imvamune) is part of the national strategic stockpile, intended for use in patients with moderate immunocompro-mised or atopic skin disease.

Sporotrichosis

CLINICAL MANIFESTATIONS: There are 3 cutaneous patterns described for sporotri-chosis. The classic lymphocutaneous process with multiple nodules most commonly is seen in adults. Inoculation occurs at a site of minor trauma, causing a painless papule that enlarges slowly to become a nodular lesion that can develop a violaceous hue or can ulcerate. Secondary lesions follow the same evolution and develop along the lymphatic distribution proximal to the initial lesion. A localized cutaneous form of sporotrichosis, also called fixed cutaneous form, is most commonly seen in children and presents as a solitary crusted papule or papuloulcerative or nodular lesion in which lymphatic spread is not observed. The extremities and face are the most common sites of infection. A dis-seminated cutaneous form with multiple lesions is rare, usually occurring in immunocom-promised children.

Extracutaneous sporotrichosis is uncommon, with cases occurring primarily in immunocompromised patients or, in adults, those who are alcoholic or have chronic obstructive pulmonary disease. Osteoarticular infection results from hematogenous spread or local inoculation. The most commonly affected joints are the knee, elbow, wrist, and ankle. Pulmonary sporotrichosis clinically resembles tuberculosis and occurs after

---

[1] Centers for Disease Control and Prevention. Surveillance guidelines for smallpox vaccine (vaccinia) adverse reactions. *MMWR Recomm Rep.* 2006;55(RR-1):1–16

inhalation or aspiration of aerosolized conidia. Disseminated disease generally occurs after hematogenous spread from primary skin or lung infection. Disseminated sporotrichosis can involve multiple foci (eg, eyes, pericardium, genitourinary tract, central nervous system) and occurs predominantly in immunocompromised patients. Pulmonary and disseminated forms of sporotrichosis are uncommon in children.

ETIOLOGY: *Sporothrix schenckii* is a thermally dimorphic fungus that grows as a mold or mycelial form at room temperature and as a yeast at 35°C to 37°C and in host tissues. *S schenckii* is a complex of at least 6 species. The related species *Sporothrix brasiliensis*, *Sporothrix globosa*, and *Sporothrix mexicana* also cause human infection.

EPIDEMIOLOGY: *S schenckii* is a ubiquitous organism that has worldwide distribution but is most common in tropical and subtropical regions of Central and South America and parts of North America and Japan. The fungus is isolated from soil and plant material, including hay, straw, sphagnum moss, and decaying vegetation. Thorny plants, such as roses and Christmas trees, commonly are implicated, because pricks from their thorns or needles inoculate the organism from the soil or moss around the bush or tree. People engaging in gardening or farming are at risk of infection. Inhalation of conidia can lead to pulmonary disease. Zoonotic spread from infected cats or scratches from digging animals, such as armadillos, has led to cutaneous disease.

The **incubation period** is 7 to 30 days after cutaneous inoculation but can be as long as 3 months.

DIAGNOSTIC TESTS: Culture of *Sporothrix* species from a tissue, wound drainage, or sputum specimen is diagnostic. Culture of *Sporothrix* species from a blood specimen is definite evidence for the disseminated form of infection associated with immunodeficiency. Histopathologic examination of tissue may not be helpful, because the organism seldom is abundant. Special fungal stains to visualize the oval or cigar-shaped organism are required. Serologic testing and polymerase chain reaction assay show promise for accurate and specific diagnosis but are available only in research laboratories.

TREATMENT[1]**:** Sporotrichosis usually does not resolve without treatment. Itraconazole (5 mg/kg, twice daily; maximum dose 200 mg) is the drug of choice for children with lymphocutaneous and localized cutaneous disease. The duration of therapy is 2 to 4 weeks after all lesions have resolved, usually for a total duration of 3 to 6 months. Serum trough concentrations of itraconazole should be ≥1 but <10 µg/mL. Concentrations should be checked after 2 weeks of therapy to ensure adequate drug exposure. Saturated solution of potassium iodide (1 drop, 3 times daily, increasing as tolerated to a maximum of 1 drop/kg of body weight or 40 to 50 drops, 3 times daily, whichever is lowest) is an alternative therapy. Oral fluconazole, 12 mg/kg daily, should be used only if the patient cannot tolerate other agents.

Amphotericin B is recommended as the initial therapy for visceral or disseminated sporotrichosis in children (see Recommended Doses of Parenteral and Oral Antifungal Drugs, p 909). After clinical response to amphotericin B therapy is documented, itraconazole can be substituted and should be continued for at least 12 months. Itraconazole may be required for lifelong therapy in children with human immunodeficiency virus infection.

---

[1]Kauffman CA, Bustamante B, Chapman SW, Pappas PG; Infectious Diseases Society of America. Clinical practice guidelines for the management of sporotrichosis: 2007 update by the Infectious Diseases Society of America. *Clin Infect Dis.* 2007;45(10):1255–1265

Pulmonary and disseminated infections respond less well than cutaneous infection, despite prolonged therapy. Surgical débridement or excision may be necessary to resolve cavitary pulmonary disease.

ISOLATION OF THE HOSPITALIZED PATIENT: Standard precautions are indicated.

CONTROL MEASURES: Use of protective gloves and clothing for occupational and vocational activities that could lead to exposure to *S schenckii* can decrease risk of disease.

Staphylococcal Food Poisoning

CLINICAL MANIFESTATIONS: Staphylococcal foodborne illness is characterized by abrupt and sometimes violent onset of severe nausea, abdominal cramps, vomiting, and prostration, often accompanied by diarrhea. Low-grade fever or mild hypothermia can occur. The illness typically lasts 1 to 2 days, but symptoms are intense and can require hospitalization. The short incubation period, brevity of illness, and usual lack of fever help distinguish staphylococcal from other types of food poisoning except that of the vomiting syndrome caused by *Bacillus cereus*. Chemical food poisoning usually has a shorter incubation period, and *Clostridium perfringens* food poisoning usually has a longer incubation period. Patients with foodborne *Salmonella* or *Shigella* infection are more likely to have fever and a longer incubation period (see Appendix VII, Clinical Syndromes Associated With Foodborne Diseases, p 1008).

ETIOLOGY: Enterotoxins produced by strains of *Staphylococcus aureus* and, rarely, *Staphylococcus epidermidis* and *Staphylococcus intermedius* elicit the symptoms of staphylococcal food poisoning.

EPIDEMIOLOGY: Illness is caused by ingestion of food containing heat-stable staphylococcal enterotoxins. The most commonly implicated foods are sliced meats, pastries, custards, and other milk-based products that have been inadequately heated or refrigerated. Pork products, especially ham, are implicated commonly in outbreaks in the United States. Sometimes these foods have been contaminated by direct contact with the hands of food handlers, or the organism may originate from purulent discharge from an infected finger, abscess, or nasopharyngeal secretions. When contaminated foods remain at room temperature for several hours, the toxin-producing staphylococcal organisms multiply, producing increasing quantities of heat-stable toxins. Less commonly, enterotoxins can be of bovine origin and can contaminate milk or milk products, especially cheeses.[1]

The **incubation period** ranges from 30 minutes to 8 hours after ingestion, typically 2 to 4 hours.

DIAGNOSTIC TESTS: In most cases, given the short duration of illness and rapid recovery with supportive care, diagnostic testing to confirm the diagnosis is not necessary. Recovery of large numbers of staphylococci from stool or vomitus and detection of enterotoxin by commercially available kits support the diagnosis. In an outbreak, demonstration of either enterotoxin or $\geq 10^5$ colony-forming units/g in an epidemiologically implicated food confirms the diagnosis. Identification by pulsed-field gel electrophoresis of the same subtype of *S aureus* from the stool or vomitus of 2 or more ill people also confirms the diagnosis. Local public health authorities should be notified to help determine the source of the outbreak.

---

[1] American Academy of Pediatrics, Committee on Infectious Diseases and Committee on Nutrition. Consumption of raw or unpasteurized milk and milk products by pregnant women and children. *Pediatrics.* 2014;133(1):175–179

TREATMENT: Treatment is supportive. Antimicrobial agents are not indicated.

ISOLATION OF THE HOSPITALIZED PATIENT: Staphylococcal food poisoning is not spread from person to person. Standard precautions are recommended.

CONTROL MEASURES: People with boils, abscesses, and other purulent lesions of the hands, face, or nose should be excluded from food preparation and handling until lesions resolve. Strict hand hygiene before food handling should be enforced. Information on recommended safe food handling practices, including time and temperature requirements during cooking, storage, and reheating, can be found online (**www.foodsafety.gov**).

Staphylococcal Infections

CLINICAL MANIFESTATIONS:

Staphylococcus aureus. *Staphylococcus aureus* causes a variety of localized and invasive suppurative infections and 3 toxin-mediated syndromes: toxic shock syndrome, scalded skin syndrome, and food poisoning (see Staphylococcal Food Poisoning, p 714). Localized infections include cellulitis, skin and soft tissue abscesses, pustulosis, impetigo (bullous and nonbullous), paronychia, mastitis, ecthyma, erythroderma, hordeola, furuncles, carbuncles, peritonsillar abscesses (Quinsy), omphalitis, parotitis, lymphadenitis, and wound infections. *S aureus* also causes invasive infections with bacteremia associated with foreign bodies, including intravascular catheters or grafts, peritoneal catheters, cerebrospinal fluid shunts, spinal instrumentation or intramedullary rods, pressure equalization tubes, pacemakers and other intracardiac devices, and prosthetic joints. Bacteremia can be complicated by septicemia; osteomyelitis; arthritis; endocarditis; pneumonia; pleural empyema; pericarditis; soft tissue, muscle, or visceral abscesses; septic thrombophlebitis of small and large vessels; and other foci of infection. Primary *S aureus* pneumonia also can occur after aspiration of organisms from the upper respiratory tract and typically is associated with mechanical ventilation or viral infections in the community (eg, influenza). Meningitis may be seen in preterm infants but otherwise is rare unless accompanied by an intradermal foreign body (eg, ventriculoperitoneal shunt) or a congenital or acquired defect in the dura. *S aureus* infections can be fulminant. They commonly are associated with metastatic foci and abscess formation, which often require drainage, foreign body removal, and prolonged antimicrobial therapy to achieve cure. Certain chronic diseases, such as diabetes mellitus, malignancy, prematurity, immunodeficiency, nutritional disorders, surgery, and transplantation, increase the risk for severe *S aureus* infections.

    Staphylococcal toxic shock syndrome (TSS), a toxin-mediated disease, usually is caused by strains producing TSS toxin-1 or possibly other related staphylococcal enterotoxins. TSS toxin-1 acts as a superantigen that stimulates production of tumor necrosis factor and other mediators that cause capillary leak, leading to hypotension and multiorgan failure. Staphylococcal TSS is characterized by acute onset of fever, generalized erythroderma, rapid-onset hypotension, and signs of multisystem organ involvement, including profuse watery diarrhea, vomiting, conjunctival injection, and severe myalgia (see Table 3.64). Although approximately 50% of reported cases of staphylococcal TSS occur in menstruating females using tampons, nonmenstrual TSS cases occur after childbirth or abortion, after surgical procedures, and in association with cutaneous lesions. TSS also can occur in males and females without a readily identifiable focus of infection. Prevailing clones (eg, USA300) of community-associated methicillin-resistant *S aureus*

Table 3.64. *Staphylococcus aureus* Toxic Shock Syndrome: Clinical Case Definition[a]

Clinical Findings

- Fever: temperature 38.9°C (102.0°F) or greater
- Rash: diffuse macular erythroderma
- Desquamation: 1–2 wk after onset, particularly on palms, soles, fingers, and toes
- Hypotension: systolic pressure 90 mm Hg or less for adults; lower than fifth percentile for age for children younger than 16 years; orthostatic drop in diastolic pressure of 15 mm Hg or greater from lying to sitting; orthostatic syncope or orthostatic dizziness
- Multisystem organ involvement: 3 or more of the following:
  1. Gastrointestinal tract: vomiting or diarrhea at onset of illness
  2. Muscular: severe myalgia or creatinine phosphokinase concentration greater than twice the upper limit of normal
  3. Mucous membrane: vaginal, oropharyngeal, or conjunctival hyperemia
  4. Renal: serum urea nitrogen or serum creatinine concentration greater than twice the upper limit of normal or urinary sediment with 5 white blood cells/high-power field or greater in the absence of urinary tract infection
  5. Hepatic: total bilirubin, aspartate transaminase, or alanine transaminase concentration greater than twice the upper limit of normal
  6. Hematologic: platelet count 100 000/mm³ or less
  7. Central nervous system: disorientation or alterations in consciousness without focal neurologic signs when fever and hypotension are absent

Laboratory Criteria

- *Negative* results on the following tests, if obtained:
  1. Blood, throat, or cerebrospinal fluid cultures; blood culture may be positive for *S aureus*
  2. Serologic tests for Rocky Mountain spotted fever, leptospirosis, or measles

Case Classification

- *Probable:* a case that meets the laboratory criteria and in which 4 of 5 clinical findings are present
- *Confirmed:* a case that meets laboratory criteria and all 5 of the clinical findings, including desquamation, unless the patient dies before desquamation occurs.

[a]Adapted from Wharton M, Chorba TL, Vogt RL, Morse DL, Buehler JW. Case definitions for public health surveillance. *MMWR Recomm Rep.* 1990;39(RR-13):1–43.

(MRSA) rarely produce TSS toxin. People with TSS, especially menses-associated illness, are at risk of a recurrent episode.

Staphylococcal scalded skin syndrome (SSSS) is a toxin-mediated disease caused by circulation of exfoliative toxins A and B. The manifestations of SSSS are age related and include Ritter disease (generalized exfoliation) in the neonate, a tender scarlatiniform eruption and localized bullous impetigo in older children, or a combination of these with thick white/brown flaky desquamation of the entire skin, especially on the face and neck, in older infants and toddlers. The hallmark of SSSS is the toxin-mediated cleavage of the stratum granulosum layer of the epidermis (ie, Nikolsky sign). Healing occurs without scarring. Bacteremia is rare, but dehydration and superinfection can occur with extensive exfoliation.

Coagulase-Negative Staphylococci. Most coagulase-negative staphylococci (CoNS) isolates from patient specimens represent contamination of culture material (see Diagnostic Tests, p 720). Of the isolates that do not represent contamination, most come from infections associated with health care, such as patients with obvious disruptions of host defenses caused by surgery, medical device insertion, immunosuppression, or developmental maturity (eg, very low birth weight infants). CoNS are the most common cause of late-onset bacteremia and septicemia among preterm infants, typically infants weighing less than 1500 g at birth, and of episodes of health care-associated bacteremia in all age groups. CoNS are responsible for bacteremia in children with intravascular catheters or those with vascular grafts or intracardiac patches, prosthetic cardiac valves, or pacemaker wires. Infection also may occur associated with other indwelling foreign bodies, including cerebrospinal fluid shunts, peritoneal catheters, or prosthetic joints. Mediastinitis after open-heart surgery, endophthalmitis after intraocular trauma, and omphalitis and scalp abscesses in preterm neonates have been described. CoNS also can enter the bloodstream from the respiratory tract of mechanically ventilated preterm infants or from the gastrointestinal tract of infants with necrotizing enterocolitis. Some species of CoNS are associated with urinary tract infection, including *Staphylococcus saprophyticus* in adolescent females and young adult women, often after sexual intercourse, and *Staphylococcus epidermidis* and *Staphylococcus haemolyticus* in hospitalized patients with urinary tract catheters. In general, CoNS infections have an indolent clinical course in children with intact immune function, even in children who are immunocompromised.

ETIOLOGY: Staphylococci are catalase-positive, gram-positive cocci that appear microscopically as grape-like clusters. There are 32 species that are related closely on the basis of DNA base composition, but only 17 species are indigenous to humans. *S aureus* is the only species that produces coagulase, although not all *S aureus* produce coagulase. Of the 16 CoNS species, *S epidermidis, S haemolyticus, S saprophyticus, Staphylococcus schleiferi,* and *Staphylococcus lugdunensis* most often are associated with human infections. Staphylococci are ubiquitous and can survive extreme conditions of drying, heat, and low-oxygen and high-salt environments. *S aureus* has many surface proteins, including the microbial surface components recognizing adhesive matrix molecule (MSCRAMM) receptors, which allow the organism to bind to tissues and foreign bodies coated with fibronectin, fibrinogen, and collagen. This permits a low inoculum of organisms to adhere to sutures, catheters, prosthetic valves, and other devices. Many CoNS produce an exopolysaccharide slime biofilm that makes these organisms, as they bind to medical devices (eg, catheters), relatively inaccessible to host defenses and antimicrobial agents.

EPIDEMIOLOGY:

Staphylococcus aureus. *S aureus,* which is second only to CoNS as a cause of health care-associated bacteremia, is one of the most common causes of health care-associated pneumonia in children and is responsible for most health care-associated surgical site infections. *S aureus* colonizes the skin and mucous membranes of 30% to 50% of healthy adults and children. The anterior nares, throat, axilla, perineum, vagina, or rectum are usual sites of colonization. Rates of carriage of more than 50% occur in children with desquamating skin disorders or burns and in people with frequent needle use (eg, diabetes mellitus, hemodialysis, illicit drug use, allergy shots).

S aureus-mediated TSS was recognized in 1978, and many early cases were associated with tampon use. Although changes in tampon composition and use have resulted in a decreased proportion of cases associated with menses, menstrual and nonmenstrual cases of TSS continue to occur and are reported with similar frequency. Risk factors for

TSS include absence of antibody to TSS toxin-1 and focal *S aureus* infection with a TSS toxin-1–producing strain. TSS toxin-1 producing strains can be part of normal flora of the anterior nares or vagina, and colonization at these sites is believed to result in protective antibody in more than 90% of adults. Health care-associated TSS can occur and most often follows surgical procedures. In postoperative cases, the organism generally originates from the patient's own flora.

Transmission of S aureus. *S aureus* is transmitted most often by direct contact in community settings and indirectly from patient to patient via transiently colonized hands of health care professionals in health care settings. Health care professionals and family members who are colonized with *S aureus* in the nares or on skin also can serve as a reservoir for transmission. Contaminated environmental surfaces and objects also can play a role in transmission of *S aureus*, although their contribution for spread probably is minor. Although not transmitted by the droplet route routinely, *S aureus* can be dispersed into the air over short distances. Dissemination of *S aureus* from people with nasal carriage, including infants, is related to density of colonization, and increased dissemination occurs during viral upper respiratory tract infections. Additional risk factors for health care-associated acquisition of *S aureus* include illness requiring care in neonatal or pediatric intensive care or burn units; surgical procedures; prolonged hospitalization; local epidemic of *S aureus* infection; and the presence of indwelling catheters or prosthetic devices.

Staphylococcus aureus *Colonization and Disease.* Nasal, skin, vaginal, and rectal carriage are the primary reservoirs for *S aureus*. Although domestic animals can be colonized, data suggest that colonization is acquired from humans. Adults who carry MRSA in the nose preoperatively are more likely to develop surgical site infections after general, cardiac, orthopedic, or solid organ transplant surgery than are patients who are not carriers. Heavy cutaneous colonization at an insertion site is the single most important predictor of intravenous catheter-related infections for short-term percutaneously inserted catheters. For hemodialysis patients with *S aureus* skin colonization, the incidence of central line-associated bloodstream infection is sixfold higher than for patients without skin colonization. After head trauma, adults who are nasal carriers of *S aureus* are more likely to develop *S aureus* pneumonia than are noncolonized patients.

Health Care-Associated MRSA. MRSA has been endemic in most US hospitals since the 1980s, recently accounting for more than 60% of health care-associated *S aureus* infections in intensive care units reported to the Centers for Disease Control and Prevention (CDC). Health care-associated MRSA strains are resistant to beta-lactamase–resistant (BLR) beta-lactam antimicrobial agents and cephalosporins (except the fifth-generation cephalosporin, ceftaroline), as well as to antimicrobial agents of several other classes (multidrug resistance). Methicillin-susceptible *S aureus* (MSSA) strains can be heterogeneous for methicillin resistance (see Diagnostic Tests, p 720).

Risk factors for nasal carriage of health care-associated MRSA include hospitalization within the previous year, recent (within the previous 60 days) antimicrobial use, prolonged hospital stay, frequent contact with a health care environment, presence of an intravascular or peritoneal catheter or tracheal tube, increased number of surgical procedures, or frequent contact with a person with one or more of the preceding risk factors. A discharged patient known to have had colonization with MRSA should be assumed to have continued colonization when rehospitalized, because carriage can persist for years.

MRSA, both health care- and community-associated strains, and methicillin-resistant CoNS are responsible for a large portion of infections acquired in health care settings. A review of 25 pediatric hospitals demonstrated a 10-fold increase in MRSA infections since 1999 without change in the frequency of MSSA infections. Health care-associated MRSA strains are difficult to treat, because they usually are multidrug resistant and predictably are susceptible only to vancomycin, linezolid, and agents not approved by the US Food and Drug Administration (FDA) for use in children.

Community-Associated MRSA. Unique clones of MRSA are responsible for community-associated infections in healthy children and adults without typical risk factors for health care-associated MRSA infections. The most frequent manifestation of community-associated MRSA infections is skin and soft tissue infection, but invasive disease also occurs. Antimicrobial susceptibility patterns of these strains differ from those of health care-associated MRSA strains. Although community-associated MRSA are resistant to all beta-lactam antimicrobial agents except ceftaroline, they typically are susceptible to multiple other antimicrobial agents, including trimethoprim-sulfamethoxazole, gentamicin, and doxycycline; clindamycin susceptibility is variable. A review of prescribing patterns among 25 pediatric hospitals has demonstrated clindamycin to be the most commonly prescribed antimicrobial agent for non–life-threatening MRSA infections. However, attention to local resistance rates of *S aureus* to clindamycin is imperative, because community-associated MRSA and MSSA isolates with intrinsic or inducible resistance to clindamycin exceeding 20% have been reported by some institutions. Community-associated MRSA infections have occurred in settings where there is crowding; frequent skin-to-skin contact; body piercing; sharing of personal items, such as towels and clothing; and poor personal hygiene, such as occurs among athletic teams, in correctional facilities, and in military training facilities. However, most community-associated MRSA infections occur in people without direct links to those settings, including healthy full-term neonates. Transmission of community-associated MRSA from an infected classmate or teammate has been described in child care centers and among sports teams, respectively. Although community-associated MRSA arose from the community, in many health care settings, these clones are overtaking health care-associated MRSA strains as a cause of health care-associated MRSA infections, making usefulness of the epidemiologic terms "health care-associated" and "community-associated" of less value.

Vancomycin-Intermediately Susceptible S aureus. Strains of MRSA with intermediate susceptibility to vancomycin (minimum inhibitory concentration [MIC], 4–8 µg/mL) have been isolated from people (historically, dialysis patients) who had received multiple courses of vancomycin for a MRSA infection. Strains of MRSA can be heterogeneous for vancomycin resistance (see Diagnostic Tests, p 720). Extensive vancomycin use allows vancomycin-intermediately susceptible *S aureus* (VISA) strains to develop. These strains may emerge during therapy. Control measures recommended by the CDC have included using proper methods to detect VISA, using appropriate infection-control measures, and adopting measures to ensure appropriate vancomycin use. Although rare, outbreaks of VISA and heteroresistant VISA have been reported in France, Spain, and Japan. Communicability persists as long as lesions or the carrier state are present.

Vancomycin-Resistant S aureus. In 2002, 2 isolates of vancomycin-resistant *S aureus* (VRSA [MIC, 16 µg/mL or greater]) were identified in adults from 2 different states. As of May 2014, VRSA had been isolated in 13 adults from 4 states (**www.cdc.gov/HAI/ settings/lab/vrsa_lab_search_containment.html**). Each of these adults with

VRSA infections had underlying medical conditions, a history of MRSA infections, and prolonged exposure to vancomycin. No spread of VRSA beyond case patients has been documented. A concern is that most automated antimicrobial susceptibility testing methods commonly used in the United States were unable to detect vancomycin resistance in these isolates.

Coagulase-Negative Staphylococci. CoNS are common inhabitants of the skin and mucous membranes. Virtually all infants have colonization at multiple sites by 2 to 4 days of age. The most frequently isolated CoNS organism is *S epidermidis*. Different species colonize specific areas of the body. *S haemolyticus* is found on areas of skin with numerous apocrine glands. The frequency of health care-associated CoNS infections increased steadily until 2000, when these infections seem to have plateaued. Infants and children in intensive care units, including neonatal intensive care units, have the highest incidence of CoNS bloodstream infections. CoNS can be introduced at the time of medical device placement, through mucous membrane or skin breaks, through loss of bowel wall integrity (eg, necrotizing enterocolitis in very low birth weight neonates), or during catheter manipulation. Less often, health care professionals with environmental CoNS colonization on hands transmit the organism. The roles of the environment or fomites in CoNS transmission are not known.

Most CoNS strains are methicillin resistant and account for health care-associated infections associated with indwelling foreign bodies and in the neonatal population. Methicillin-resistant strains are resistant to all beta-lactam drugs, including cephalosporins (except ceftaroline), and usually several other drug classes. Once these strains become endemic in a hospital, eradication is difficult, even when strict infection-prevention practices are followed.

The **incubation period** is variable for staphylococcal disease. A long delay can occur between acquisition of the organism and onset of disease. For toxin-mediated SSSS, the **incubation period** usually is 1 to 10 days; for postoperative TSS, it can be as short as 12 hours. Menstrual-related cases can develop at any time during menses.

DIAGNOSTIC TESTS: Gram-stained smears of material from skin lesions or pyogenic foci showing gram-positive cocci in clusters can provide presumptive evidence of infection. Isolation of organisms from culture of otherwise sterile body fluid is the method for definitive diagnosis. Newer molecular assays have recently been approved by the FDA for direct detection of *S aureus* from blood culture bottles. Nonamplified molecular assays, such as peptide nucleic acid fluorescent in situ hybridization (PNA-FISH) and nucleic acid amplification tests, such as BD GenOhm Staph SR (BD Molecular diagnostics) and Xpert MRSA/SA BC (Cepheid), are approved for detection and identification of *S aureus*, including MRSA, in positive blood cultures.

S aureus almost never is a contaminant when isolated from a blood culture. CoNS isolated from a single blood culture commonly are dismissed as "contaminants." In a very preterm neonate, an immunocompromised person, or a patient with an indwelling catheter or prosthetic device, repeated isolation of the same strain of CoNS (by antimicrobial susceptibility results or molecular techniques) from blood cultures or another normally sterile body fluid suggests true infection, but genotyping more strongly supports the diagnosis. For central line-associated bloodstream infection, quantitative blood cultures from the catheter will have 5 to 10 times more organisms than cultures from a peripheral blood vessel. Criteria that suggest CoNS as pathogens rather than contaminants include the following:

- 2 or more positive blood cultures from different collection sites;
- a single positive culture from blood and another sterile site (eg, cerebrospinal fluid, joint) with identical antimicrobial susceptibility patterns for each isolate;
- growth in a continuously monitored blood culture system within 15 hours of incubation;
- clinical findings of infection;
- an intravascular catheter that has been in place for 3 days or more; and
- similar or identical genotypes among all isolates.

S aureus-mediated TSS is a clinical diagnosis (Table 3.64, p 716). S aureus grows in culture of blood specimens from fewer than 5% of patients with TSS. Specimens for culture should be obtained from an identified focal site of infection, because these sites usually will yield the organism. Because approximately one third of isolates of S aureus from nonmenstrual cases produce toxins other than TSS toxin-1, and TSS toxin-1-producing organisms can be present as normal flora, TSS-1 production by an isolate is not useful diagnostically.

Quantitative antimicrobial susceptibility testing should be performed for all staphylococci, including CoNS, isolated from normally sterile sites. Health care-associated MRSA heterogeneous or heterotypic strains appear susceptible by disk testing. However, when a parent strain is cultured on methicillin-containing media, resistant subpopulations are apparent. When these resistant subpopulations are cultured on methicillin-free media, they can continue as stable resistant mutants or revert to susceptible strains (heterogeneous resistance). Cells expressing heteroresistance grow more slowly than the oxacillin-susceptible cells and can be missed at growth conditions above 35°C (95°F).

A large proportion of community-associated S aureus strains are methicillin resistant, and a high percentage (more than 90% in some centers) of health care-associated S aureus from children are methicillin and multidrug resistant. More than 90% of health care-associated CoNS strains are methicillin-resistant. Because of the high rates of community-associated MRSA infections in the United States, clindamycin has become an often-used drug for treatment of non–life-threatening presumed S aureus infections. Routine antimicrobial susceptibility testing of S aureus strains historically did not include a method to detect strains susceptible to clindamycin that rapidly become clindamycin-resistant when exposed to this agent. This clindamycin-inducible resistance can be detected by the D zone test. When a MRSA isolate is determined to be erythromycin resistant and clindamycin susceptible by routine methods, the D zone test is performed. Many automated platforms for susceptibility testing now include testing for inducible clindamycin resistance. MRSA isolates that demonstrate clindamycin-inducible resistance will be reported by the laboratory as clindamycin resistant, and the patient should not be treated with clindamycin. All S aureus strains with an MIC to vancomycin of 4 µg/mL or greater should be confirmed and further characterized. Early detection of VISA is critical to trigger aggressive infection-control measures (see Table 3.65). Such isolates are unlikely to be effectively treated with vancomycin.

Guidelines for laboratory detection of VISA and VRSA are available at **www.cdc. gov/ncidod/dhqp/ar_visavrsa_lab.html**. S aureus and CoNS strain genotyping has become a necessary adjunct for determining whether several isolates from one

Table 3.65. Recommendations for Detecting and Preventing Spread of *Staphylococcus aureus* With Decreased Susceptibility to Vancomycin

Definitions:
- **Vancomycin-susceptible** *S aureus*
  MIC 2 µg/mL or less
- **Vancomycin-intermediately susceptible** *S aureus* **(VISA)**
  MIC 4 through 8 µg/mL
  Not transferable to susceptible strains
- **Vancomycin-resistant** *S aureus* **(VRSA)**
  MIC 16 µg/mL or greater
  Potentially transferable to susceptible strains
- **Confirmation of VISA and VRSA**
  Possible VISA and VRSA isolates should be retested using vancomycin screen plates or a
  validated MIC method.
  VISA and VRSA isolates should be reported to the local health department or CDC.

Infection control[a]:
- Isolate patient in a private room.
- Minimize numbers of people caring for VISA/VRSA patients.
- Implement appropriate infection-control precautions:
  - Use contact precautions (gown and gloves).
  - Wear mask/eye protection or face shield if performing procedures (eg, wound manipulations, suctioning) likely to generate splash or splatter of VISA/VRSA contaminated materials (eg, blood, body fluids, secretions).
  - Perform hand hygiene using appropriate agent (eg, hand washing with soap and water or alcohol-based hand sanitizer).
  - Dedicate nondisposable items for patient use.
  - Monitor and strictly enforce compliance with contact precautions and other measures.
- Educate and inform health care professionals about the need for contact isolation.
- Consult with state health department and CDC before discharging and/or transferring the patient, and notify receiving institution or unit of presence of VISA and of appropriate precautions.

MIC indicates minimum inhibitory concentration; CDC, Centers for Disease Control and Prevention.
[a] For information regarding control of spread of VISA and vancomycin-resistant *S aureus*, e-mail SEARCH@cdc.gov or visit
www.cdc.gov/ncidod/dhqp

patient or from different patients are the same. Typing, in conjunction with epidemiologic information, can facilitate identification of the source, extent, and mechanism of transmission in an outbreak. Antimicrobial susceptibility testing is the most readily available method for typing by a phenotypic characteristic. A number of molecular typing methods are available for *S aureus*. Choice of method should consider purpose of typing and available resources. The primary method used currently by the CDC is pulsed-field gel electrophoresis.

TREATMENT:

Skin and Soft Tissue Infection. Skin and soft tissue infections, such as diffuse impetigo or cellulitis attributable to MSSA, can be treated with oral penicillinase-resistant beta-lactam drugs, such as a first- or second-generation cephalosporin. However, the continued increase in prevalence of community-associated MRSA throughout the United States may limit the utility of beta lactams as empiric first-line agents. For the penicillin-allergic patient and in cases in which MRSA is considered, trimethoprim-sulfamethoxazole, doxycycline in children 8 years and older, or clindamycin can be used if the isolate is susceptible. Trimethoprim-sulfamethoxazole should not be used as a single agent in the initial treatment of cellulitis. Topical mupirocin is recommended for localized impetigo. Tetracycline-based antimicrobial agents, including doxycycline, may cause permanent tooth discoloration for children younger than 8 years if used for repeated treatment courses. However, doxycycline binds less readily to calcium compared with older tetracyclines, and in some studies, doxycycline was not associated with visible teeth staining in younger children (see Tetracyclines, p 873).

The most frequent manifestation of community-associated MRSA infection is skin and soft tissue infection. Fig 3.10 shows the initial management of skin and soft tissue infections suspected to be caused by community-associated MRSA.

For patients with complicated skin and soft tissue infection with abscess, drainage/débridement and systemic antibiotic therapy are warranted; therapy should be focused on the pathogen identified.

Invasive Staphylococcal Infections. Empiric therapy for serious suspected staphylococcal infection is vancomycin plus a semisynthetic beta lactam (eg, oxacillin). Clindamycin is bacteriostatic and should not be used for initial treatment of endovascular infection. Serious MSSA infections require intravenous therapy with a beta-lactamase–resistant (BLR) beta-lactam antimicrobial agent, such as nafcillin or oxacillin, because most *S aureus* strains produce beta-lactamase enzymes and are resistant to penicillin and ampicillin (see Table 3.66, p 725). Vancomycin is not recommended for treatment of serious MSSA infections, because outcomes are inferior compared with cases in which antistaphylococcal beta lactams are used and to minimize emergence of vancomycin resistance. First- or second-generation cephalosporins (eg, cefazolin) or vancomycin are less effective than nafcillin or oxacillin for treatment of MSSA endocarditis or meningitis.

A patient with MSSA infection (and no evidence of endocarditis or central nervous system [CNS] infection) who has a nonserious allergy to penicillin can be treated with a first- or second-generation cephalosporin or with clindamycin, if the *S aureus* strain is susceptible.

Intravenous vancomycin is recommended for treatment of serious infections caused by staphylococcal strains resistant to BLR beta-lactam antimicrobial agents (eg, MRSA and all CoNS). For empiric therapy of life-threatening *S aureus* infections, initial therapy should include vancomycin and a BLR beta-lactam antimicrobial agent (eg, nafcillin, oxacillin). For hospital-acquired CoNS infections, vancomycin is the drug of choice. Subsequent therapy should be determined by antimicrobial susceptibility results.

Guidelines for management of serious skin/soft tissue infection, complicated pneumonia/empyema, CNS infection, osteomyelitis, and endocarditis caused by MRSA are available (**www.idsociety.org/IDSA_Practice_Guidelines/**).

Vancomycin Treatment Failure and VISA Infection. VISA infection is rare in children. For seriously ill patients with a history of recurrent MRSA infections or for patients failing vancomycin therapy in whom VISA strains are a consideration, initial therapy could include linezolid or trimethoprim-sulfamethoxazole, with or without gentamicin. If antimicrobial susceptibility results document multidrug resistance, alternative agents, such as quinupristin-dalfopristin, daptomycin (not approved for pneumonia), ceftaroline, or tigecycline, could be considered.

FIG 3.10. ALGORITHM FOR INITIAL MANAGEMENT OF SKIN AND SOFT TISSUE INFECTIONS CAUSED BY COMMUNITY-ASSOCIATED *STAPHYLOCOCCUS AUREUS*

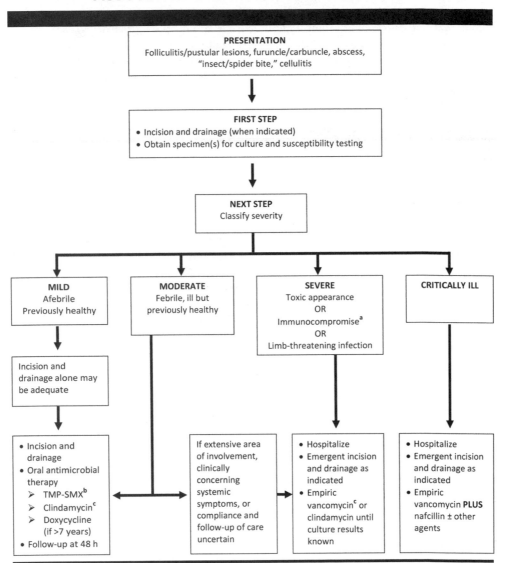

[a] Immunocompromise: any chronic illness except asthma or eczema.

[b] TMP-SMX = trimethoprim-sulfamethoxazole, if group A streptococcus unlikely.

[c] Consider prevalence of clindamycin-susceptible methicillin-susceptible *S aureus* and "D" test-negative community-associated methicillin-resistant *S aureus* strains in the community.

Table 3.66. Parenteral Antimicrobial Agent(s) for Treatment of Bacteremia and Other Serious *Staphylococcus aureus* Infections

Susceptibility	Antimicrobial Agents	Comments
I. Initial empiric therapy (organism of unknown susceptibility)		
Drugs of choice:	Vancomycin (15 mg/kg, every 6 h) + nafcillin or oxacillin	For life-threatening infections (ie, septicemia, endocarditis, CNS infection); linezolid could be substituted for vancomycin if the patient has received several recent courses of vancomycin
	Vancomycin (15 mg/kg, every 6–8 h)	For non–life-threatening infection without signs of sepsis (eg, skin infection, cellulitis, osteomyelitis, pyarthrosis) when rates of MRSA colonization and infection in the community are substantial
	Clindamycin	For non–life-threatening infection without signs of sepsis when rates of MRSA colonization and infection in the community are substantial and prevalence of clindamycin resistance is low
II. Methicillin-susceptible, penicillin-resistant *S aureus* (MSSA)		
Drugs of choice:	Nafcillin or oxacillin[a] Cefazolin	
Alternatives:	Clindamycin	Only for patients with a serious penicillin allergy and clindamycin-susceptible strain
	Vancomycin	Only for patients with a serious penicillin and cephalosporin allergy
	Ampicillin + sulbactam	For patients with polymicrobial infections caused by susceptible isolates.
III. Methicillin-resistant *S aureus* (MRSA; oxacillin MIC, 4 µg/mL or greater)		
A. Health care-associated (multidrug resistant)		
Drugs of choice:	Vancomycin ± gentamicin[a]	
Alternatives: susceptibility testing results available before alternative drugs are used	Trimethoprim-sulfamethoxazole Linezolid[b] Quinupristin-dalfopristin[b]	

continued

Table 3.66. Parenteral Antimicrobial Agent(s) for Treatment of Bacteremia and Other Serious *Staphylococcus aureus* Infections, continued

Susceptibility	Antimicrobial Agents	Comments
B. Community-associated (not multidrug resistant)		
Drugs of choice:	Vancomycin ± gentamicin[a]	For life-threatening infections or endovascular infections including those complicated by venous thrombosis.
	Clindamycin (if strain susceptible)	For pneumonia, septic arthritis, osteomyelitis, skin or soft tissue infections
	Trimethoprim-sulfamethoxazole	For skin or soft tissue infections
Alternative:	Vancomycin	For serious infections
	Linezolid	For serious infections caused by clindamycin resistant isolates in patients with renal dysfunction or those intolerant of vancomycin.
IV. Vancomycin-intermediately susceptible *S aureus* (MIC, 4 to 16 µg/mL)[b]		
Drugs of choice:	Optimal therapy is not known	Dependent on in vitro susceptibility test results
	Linezolid[b]	
	Ceftaroline	
	Daptomycin[c]	
	Quinupristin-dalfopristin[b]	
	Tigecycline	
Alternatives:	Vancomycin + linezolid ± gentamicin	
	Vancomycin + trimethoprim-sulfamethoxazole[a]	

CNS indicates central nervous system; MIC, minimum inhibitory concentration.

[a]Gentamicin should be considered for addition to the therapeutic regimen for endocarditis without prosthetic devices or CNS infection; gentamicin and rifampin should be added for endocarditis of a prosthetic device or infections with a vancomycin-intermediate *S aureus* strain. Addition of rifampin is recommended for other device related infections (spinal instrumentation, prosthetic joint). Some experts recommend achieving vancomycin trough concentrations between 15–20 µg/mL for serious MRSA infections until the patient has improved and blood cultures are sterile. Consultation with an infectious diseases specialist should be considered to determine which agent to use and duration of use.

[b]Linezolid, ceftaroline, quinupristin-dalfopristin, and tigecycline are agents with activity in vitro and efficacy in adults with multidrug-resistant, gram-positive organisms, including *S aureus*. Because experience with these agents in children is limited, consultation with an infectious diseases specialist should be considered before use.

[c]Daptomycin is active in vitro against multidrug-resistant, gram-positive organisms, including *S aureus*, but has not been evaluated in children. Daptomycin is approved by the US Food and Drug Administration only for treatment of complicated skin and skin structure infections and for *S aureus* bloodstream infections. Daptomycin is ineffective for treatment of pneumonia and is not indicated in patients 18 years and older.

Duration of Therapy for Invasive Infections. Duration of therapy for serious MSSA or MRSA infections depends on the site and severity of infection but usually is 4 weeks or more for endocarditis, osteomyelitis, necrotizing pneumonia, or disseminated infection, assuming a documented clinical and microbiologic response. The duration of bacteremia for patients with staphylococcal infection typically can be 3 to 4 days for MSSA and 7 to 9 days for MRSA. In assessing whether modification of therapy is necessary, clinicians should consider whether the patient is clinically improving, should identify and drain sequestered foci of infection, and for MRSA strains, should consider the vancomycin MIC and the achievable vancomycin trough concentrations.

Completion of the course with an oral drug can be considered if adherence can be ensured and endocarditis or CNS infection is not a consideration. For endocarditis and CNS infection, parenteral therapy is recommended for the entire treatment. Drainage of abscesses and removal of foreign bodies are desirable and almost always are required for medical treatment to be effective. In some cases, multiple débridement procedures are necessary for children with MRSA osteoarticular infection.

Duration of therapy for central line-associated bloodstream infections is controversial and depends on consideration of a number of factors, including the organism (*S aureus* vs CoNS), the type and location of the catheter, the site of infection (exit site vs tunnel vs line), the feasibility of using an alternative vascular access site at a later date, and the presence or absence of a catheter-related thrombus. Infections are more difficult to treat when associated with a thrombus, thrombophlebitis, or intra-atrial thrombus. Data detailing outcomes of treatment of serious MRSA infections in adults does not support the addition of gentamicin or rifampin to vancomycin because of an increase in adverse effects and lack of greater efficacy of the combination versus monotherapy, but the addition of rifampin can be considered in the setting of a foreign body associated infection. If a central line can be removed, there is no demonstrable thrombus, and bacteremia resolves promptly, a 5-day course of therapy seems appropriate for CoNS infections in the immunocompetent host.

A longer course is suggested if the patient is immunocompromised or the organism is *S aureus;* experts differ on recommended duration, but many suggest a minimum of 14 days provided there is no evidence of a metastatic focus. If the patient needs a new central line, waiting 48 to 72 hours after bacteremia apparently has resolved before insertion is optimal. If a tunneled catheter is needed for ongoing care, in situ treatment of the infection can be attempted. If the patient responds to antimicrobial therapy with immediate resolution of the *S aureus* bacteremia, treatment should be continued for 10 to 14 days parenterally. Antimicrobial lock therapy of tunneled central lines may result in a higher rate of catheter salvage in adults with CoNS infections, but experience with this approach is limited in children. If blood cultures remain positive for more than 2 days for *S aureus* or 3 to 5 days for CoNS or if the clinical illness fails to improve, the central line should be removed, parenteral therapy should be continued, and the patient should be evaluated for metastatic foci of infection. Vegetations or a thrombus in the heart or great vessels always should be considered when a central line becomes infected and should be suspected more strongly if blood cultures remain positive for more than 2 days or if there are other clinical manifestations associated with endocarditis. Transesophageal echocardiography, if feasible, is the most sensitive technique for identifying vegetations, but transthoracic echocardiography generally is adequate for children younger than 10 years and those weighing >60 kg.

Management of S aureus *Toxin-Mediated Diseases.* As summarized in Table 3.67, the first priority in management of *S aureus* TSS is aggressive fluid management as well as management of respiratory or cardiac failure, if present. Initial antimicrobial therapy should include a parentally administered beta-lactam antistaphylococcal antimicrobial agent and a protein synthesis-inhibiting drug, such as clindamycin, at maximum dosages. Vancomycin should be substituted for BLR penicillins or cephalosporins in regions where community-associated MRSA infections are common (see Table 3.66, p 725). Once the organism is identified and susceptibilities are known, therapy for *S aureus* should be modified, but an active antimicrobial agent should be continued for 10 to 14 days. Administration of antimicrobial agents can be changed to the oral route once the patient is tolerating oral alimentation. The total duration of therapy is based on the usual duration of established foci of infection (eg, pneumonia, osteomyelitis). Aggressive drainage and irrigation of accessible sites of purulent infection should be performed as soon as possible. All foreign bodies, including those recently inserted during surgery, should be removed if possible. Immune Globulin Intravenous (IGIV) can be considered in patients with severe staphylococcal TSS unresponsive to other therapeutic measures, because IGIV may neutralize circulating toxin. The optimal IGIV regimen is unknown, but 150 to 400 mg/kg per day for 5 days or a single dose of 1 to 2 g/kg has been used. SSSS in infants should be treated with a parenteral BLR beta-lactam antimicrobial agent or, if MRSA is a consideration, vancomycin can be used. Transition to an oral agent can be considered in nonneonates who have demonstrated excellent clinical and microbiologic response to parenteral therapy.

ISOLATION OF THE HOSPITALIZED PATIENT: Standard precautions are recommended for many patients infected or colonized with MSSA, including patients with TSS. Contact precautions also should be used for patients with abscesses or draining wounds that cannot be covered, regardless of staphylococcal strain, and should be maintained until draining ceases or can be contained by a dressing. Patients infected or colonized with MRSA should be managed with contact precautions for the duration of hospitalization and subsequent hospitalizations, because MRSA carriage can persist for years. For MSSA or MRSA pneumonia, droplet precautions are recommended for the first 24 hours of

Table 3.67. Management of Staphylococcal Toxic Shock Syndrome

- Fluid management to maintain adequate venous return and cardiac filling pressures to prevent end-organ damage
- Anticipatory management of multisystem organ failure
- Parenteral antimicrobial therapy at maximum doses
  - ◆ Kill organism with bactericidal cell wall inhibitor (eg, beta-lactamase–resistant antistaphylococcal antimicrobial agent)
  - ◆ Reduce enzyme or toxin production with protein synthesis inhibitor (eg, clindamycin)
- Immune Globulin Intravenous may be considered for infection refractory to several hours of aggressive therapy or in the presence of an undrainable focus or persistent oliguria with pulmonary edema

antimicrobial therapy. Droplet precautions should be maintained throughout the illness for MSSA or MRSA tracheitis with a tracheostomy tube in place.

To prevent transmission of VISA and VRSA, the CDC has issued specific infection-control recommendations that should be followed (see Table 3.65, p 722). For CoNS, standard precautions are recommended. For known epidemic MRSA strains, contact precautions should be used.

CONTROL MEASURES:

Coagulase-Negative Staphylococci. Prevention and control of CoNS infections have focused on prevention of intraoperative contamination by skin flora and on sterile insertion of intravascular and intraperitoneal catheters and other prosthetic devices. Catheter-related bloodstream infections can be markedly reduced with a "bundled" preventive approach. Prophylactic administration of an antimicrobial agent intraoperatively lowers the incidence of infection after cardiac surgery and implantation of synthetic vascular grafts and prosthetic devices and often has been used at the time of cerebrospinal fluid shunt placement.

Staphylococcus aureus. Measures to prevent and control *S aureus* infections can be considered separately for people and for health care facilities.

Individual Patient. Community-associated *S aureus* infections in immunocompetent hosts usually cannot be prevented, because the organism is ubiquitous and there is no vaccine. However, strategies focusing on hand hygiene and wound care have been effective at limiting transmission of *S aureus* and preventing spread of infections in community settings. Specific strategies include appropriate wound care, minimizing skin trauma and keeping abrasions and cuts covered, optimizing hand hygiene and personal hygiene practices (eg, shower after activities involving skin-to-skin contact), avoiding sharing of personal items (eg, towels, razors, clothing), cleaning shared equipment between uses, and regular cleaning of frequently touched environmental surfaces. For patients who experience recurrent *S aureus* infections or who are predisposed to *S aureus* infections because of disorders of neutrophil function, chronic skin conditions, or obesity, a variety of techniques have been used to prevent infection, including scrupulous attention to skin hygiene and to use of clothing and bed linens that minimize sweating, but none have been shown to be effective in preventing recurrent infections with community-associated MRSA. Applying mupirocin to the nares and bathing using chlorhexidine for 5 consecutive days for all family members have been associated with decreased recurrences. Use of bleach in the bath water 2 to 3 times a week (1/4–1/2 cup of bleach per full bath)[1] has been advocated for decreased recurrences; a recent randomized controlled trial of bleach baths plus hygiene education over a 3-month period were found to be associated with approximately a 20% decrease in recurrent medically attended skin and soft tissue infection recurrences compared with hygiene education alone when used for 3 months, but this was not a significant reduction ($P = .15$).[2] Studies in adults have reported success with 7-day course of the combination of oral rifampin and doxycycline plus nasal mupirocin.

---

[1]Stevens DL, Bisno AL, Chambers HF, et al. Practice guidelines for the diagnosis and management of skin and soft tissue infections: 2014 update by the Infectious Diseases Society of America. *Clin Infect Dis.* 2014;59(2):e10–e52

[2]Kaplan SK, Forbes A, Hammerman WA. Randomized trial of "bleach baths" plus routine hygienic measures vs routine hygienic measures alone for prevention of recurrent infections. *Clin Infect Dis.* 2014;58(5):679–682

Measures to prevent health care-associated *S aureus* infections in individual patients include strict adherence to recommended infection-control precautions and appropriate intraoperative antimicrobial prophylaxis, and in some circumstances, use of antimicrobial regimens to attempt to eradicate nasal carriage in certain patients can be considered.

Child Care or School Settings. Children with *S aureus* colonization or infection should not be excluded routinely from child care or school settings. Children with draining or open abrasions or wounds should have these covered with a clean, dry dressing. Routine hand hygiene should be emphasized for personnel and children in these facilities.

General Measures. Published recommendations of the CDC Healthcare Infection Control Practices Advisory Committee (HICPAC)[1] for prevention of health care-associated pneumonia should be effective for decreasing the incidence of *S aureus* pneumonia. Careful preparation of the skin before surgery, including cleansing of skin before placement of intravascular catheters using barrier methods, will decrease the incidence of *S aureus* wound and catheter-related infections. Meticulous surgical technique with minimal trauma to tissues, maintenance of good oxygenation, and minimal hematoma and dead space formation will minimize risk of surgical site infection. Appropriate hand hygiene, including before and after use of gloves, by health care professionals and strict adherence to contact precautions are of paramount importance.

Intraoperative Antimicrobial Prophylaxis. The benefits of systemic antimicrobial prophylaxis do not justify the potential risks associated with antimicrobial use in most clean surgical procedures, because the risk of overall infection (most commonly caused by *S aureus*) is only 1% to 2%. Some exceptions apply, such as a person undergoing organ transplantation, neurosurgery, or insertion of a major prosthetic device, such as a ventriculo-peritoneal shunt or a heart valve, or a known MRSA carrier undergoing a major surgical procedure. If antimicrobial prophylaxis is used, the agent is administered 30 to 60 minutes before the operation (60–120 minutes for vancomycin), and a total duration of therapy of less than 24 hours is recommended. Staphylococci are the most common pathogens causing surgical site infections, and cefazolin is the most commonly recommended drug.

Eradication of Nasal Carriage. Preprocedure detection and eradication of nasal carriage using mupirocin twice a day for 5 to 7 days before surgery can decrease the incidence of *S aureus* surgical site infections (SSIs) in some colonized adult patients after cardiothoracic, general, or neurosurgical procedures. The combination of preoperative chlorhexidine baths with intranasal mupirocin has been demonstrated to be beneficial in reducing deep SSIs in adult MRSA carriers, but data are limited in children. Use of intermittent or continuous intranasal mupirocin for eradication of nasal carriage also has been shown to decrease the incidence of invasive *S aureus* infections in adult patients undergoing long-term hemodialysis or ambulatory peritoneal dialysis. However, eradication of nasal carriage of *S aureus* is difficult, and mupirocin-resistant strains can emerge with repeated or widespread use. Treatment is not recommended for routine use, but recent recommendations support use in certain cardiac and orthopedic surgery patients. If mupirocin is used, surveillance for mupirocin resistance is recommended.

---

[1]Centers for Disease Control and Prevention. Guidelines for preventing health-care-associated pneumonia, 2003: recommendations of CDC and the Healthcare Infection Control Practices Advisory Committee. *MMWR Recomm Rep.* 2004;53(RR-3):1–36

Institutions. Measures to control spread of *S aureus* within health care facilities involve use and careful monitoring of HICPAC guidelines.[1,2] Strategies for controlling spread of MRSA also are found in recommendations for controlling spread of multidrug-resistant organisms (**www.cdc.gov/drugresistance/index.html**). These include general recommendations for all settings and focus on administrative issues; engagement, education, and training of personnel; judicious use of antimicrobial agents; monitoring of prevalence trends over time; use of standard precautions for all patients; and use of contact precautions when appropriate. When rates of endemicity are not decreasing despite implementation of and adherence to the aforementioned measures, additional interventions, such as use of active surveillance cultures to identify colonized patients and to place them in contact precautions, may be warranted. When a patient or health care professional is found to be a carrier of *S aureus*, attempts to eradicate carriage with topical nasal mupirocin therapy may be useful. Both low-level (MIC, 8–256 µg/mL) and high-level (MIC, >512 µg/mL) resistance to mupirocin have been identified in *S aureus*, with high-level resistance associated with failure of decolonization therapy. Other topical preparations for intranasal application to be considered if mupirocin fails are ointments containing bacitracin and polymyxin B or a povidone-iodine cream. These preparations have not been studied in children. Minimizing prolonged use of vancomycin will decrease emergence of VISA. Recommendations for investigation and control of VISA and VRSA have been published by the CDC (Table 3.65, p 722). Ongoing review and restriction of vancomycin use is critical in attempts to control the emergence of VISA and VRSA (see Antimicrobial Resistance and Antimicrobial Stewardship: Appropriate and Judicious Use of Antimicrobial Agents, p 874). To date, the use of catheters impregnated with various antimicrobial agents or metals to prevent health care-associated infections has not been evaluated adequately in children.

Nurseries. Outbreaks of *S aureus* infections in newborn nurseries require unique measures of control. Hand hygiene should be emphasized to all personnel and visitors. Application of triple dye or iodophor ointment for umbilical cord care has been used in the past to delay or prevent *S aureus* colonization, although more recent studies suggest limited utility of triple dye, and iodophor ointment no longer is available. The utility of 4% chlorhexidine for cleansing of the umbilical stump has been reported to reduce the risk of omphalitis in resource-limited countries. Other measures recommended during outbreaks include reinforcement of hand hygiene, alleviating overcrowding and understaffing, colonization surveillance cultures of newborn infants at admission and periodically thereafter, use of contact precautions for colonized or infected infants, and cohorting of colonized or infected infants and their caregivers. For hand hygiene, soaps containing chlorhexidine or alcohol-based hand rubs are preferred during an outbreak. Colonized health care professionals epidemiologically

---

[1]Hageman JC, Patel JB, Carey RC, Tenover FC, McDonald LC. *Investigation and Control of Vancomycin-Intermediate and -Resistant Staphylococcus aureus (VISA/VRSA): A Guide for Health Departments and Infection Control Personnel.* Atlanta, GA: Centers for Disease Control and Prevention; 2006. Available at: **www.cdc.gov/hai/pdfs/visa_vrsa/ visa_vrsa_guide.pdf**

[2]Siegel JD, Rhinehart E, Jackson M, Chianello L, and the Healthcare Infection Control Practices Advisory Committee. *2007 Guideline for Isolation Precautions: Preventing Transmission of Infectious Agents in Healthcare Settings. Recommendations of the Healthcare Infection Control Practices Advisory Committee.* Atlanta, GA: Centers for Disease Control and Prevention; 2007. Available at: **www.cdc.gov/hicpac/2007IP/2007isolationPrecautions.html**

implicated in transmission should receive decolonization therapy, but eradication of colonization may not occur.

Group A Streptococcal Infections

CLINICAL MANIFESTATIONS: The most common group A streptococcal (GAS) infection is acute pharyngotonsillitis (pharyngitis), which is heralded by sore throat with tonsillar inflammation and often tender cervical lymphadenopathy. Pharyngitis may be accompanied by palatal petechiae or a strawberry tongue. Purulent complications of pharyngitis usually occur in patients not treated with antimicrobial agents and include otitis media, sinusitis, peritonsillar or retropharyngeal abscesses, and suppurative cervical adenitis. Nonsuppurative complications include acute rheumatic fever (ARF) and acute glomerulonephritis. The goal of antimicrobial therapy for GAS pharyngitis is to reduce acute morbidity, complications, and transmission to close contacts.

Scarlet fever occurs most often in association with pharyngitis and, rarely, with pyoderma or an infected wound. Scarlet fever usually is a mild disease in the modern era and has a characteristic confluent erythematous sandpaper-like rash that is caused by one or more of several erythrogenic exotoxins produced by group A streptococci. Other than occurrence of rash, the epidemiologic features, symptoms, signs, sequelae, and treatment of scarlet fever are the same as those of streptococcal pharyngitis.

Acute streptococcal pharyngitis is uncommon in children younger than 3 years. Instead, they may present with rhinitis and then develop a protracted illness with moderate fever, irritability, and anorexia (streptococcal fever or streptococcosis). The second most common site of GAS infection is skin. Streptococcal skin infections (eg, pyoderma or impetigo) can be followed by acute glomerulonephritis, which occasionally occurs in epidemics. ARF is not a sequela of GAS skin infection.

Other manifestations of GAS infections include erysipelas, cellulitis (including perianal), vaginitis, bacteremia, pneumonia, endocarditis, pericarditis, septic arthritis, necrotizing fasciitis, purpura fulminans, osteomyelitis, myositis, puerperal sepsis, surgical wound infection, mastoiditis, and neonatal omphalitis. Invasive GAS infections often are associated with bacteremia with or without a local focus of infection and can present as streptococcal toxic shock syndrome (STSS) and/or necrotizing fasciitis. Necrotizing fasciitis can follow minor or unrecognized trauma, often involves an extremity, and presents as pain out of proportion to examination findings. An association between GAS infection and sudden onset of obsessive-compulsive behaviors, prepubertal anorexia nervosa, or tic disorders—pediatric autoimmune neuropsychiatric disorders associated with streptococcal infections (PANDAS), also known as pediatric acute-onset neuropsychiatric syndrome (PANS)—has been proposed, but carefully performed prospective studies have not shown that there is a specific relationship between these disorders and GAS infections.

STSS is caused by toxin-producing GAS strains and typically manifests as an acute illness characterized by fever, generalized erythroderma, rapid-onset hypotension, and signs of multiorgan involvement, including rapidly progressive renal failure (see Table 3.68). Evidence of local soft tissue infection (eg, cellulitis, myositis, or necrotizing fasciitis) associated with severe, rapidly increasing pain is common, but STSS can occur without an identifiable focus of infection or with foci such as pneumonia with or without empyema, osteomyelitis, pyarthrosis, or endocarditis.

Table 3.68. Streptococcal Toxic Shock Syndrome: Clinical Case Definition[a]

I. Isolation of group A streptococcus *(Streptococcus pyogenes)*
   A. From a normally sterile site (eg, blood, cerebrospinal fluid, peritoneal fluid, or tissue biopsy specimen)
   B. From a nonsterile site (eg, throat, sputum, vagina, open surgical wound, or superficial skin lesion)
II. Clinical signs of severity
   A. Hypotension: systolic pressure 90 mm Hg or less in adults or lower than the fifth percentile for age in children

   AND

   B. Two or more of the following signs:
   - Renal impairment: creatinine concentration 177 µmol/L (2 mg/dL) or greater for adults or at least 2 times the upper limit of normal for age[b]
   - Coagulopathy: platelet count 100 000/mm^3 or less or disseminated intravascular coagulation
   - Hepatic involvement: elevated alanine transaminase, aspartate transaminase, or total bilirubin concentrations at least 2 times the upper limit of normal for age
   - Adult respiratory distress syndrome
   - A generalized erythematous macular rash that may desquamate
   - Soft tissue necrosis, including necrotizing fasciitis or myositis, or gangrene

Adapted from The Working Group on Severe Streptococcal Infections. Defining the group A streptococcal toxic shock syndrome: rationale and consensus definition. *JAMA*. 1993;269(3):390–339.

[a] An illness fulfilling criteria IA and IIA and IIB can be defined as a *definite* case. An illness fulfilling criteria IB and IIA and IIB can be defined as a *probable* case if no other cause for the illness is identified.

[b] In patients with preexisting renal or hepatic disease, concentrations ≥twofold elevation over patient's baseline.

ETIOLOGY: More than 120 distinct serotypes or genotypes of group A beta-hemolytic streptococci *(Streptococcus pyogenes)* have been identified based on M-protein serotype or M-protein gene sequence *(emm* types). Because of a variety of factors, including M nontypability and *emm* sequence variation within given M types, *emm* typing generally is more discriminating than M-protein serotyping. Epidemiologic studies suggest an association between certain serotypes (eg, types 1, 3, 5, 6, 18, 19, and 24) and rheumatic fever, but a specific rheumatogenic factor has not been identified. Several serotypes (eg, types 49, 55, 57, and 59) more commonly are associated with pyoderma and acute glomerulonephritis. Other serotypes (eg, types 1, 6, and 12) are associated with pharyngitis and acute glomerulonephritis. Most cases of STSS are caused by strains producing at least 1 of several different pyrogenic exotoxins, most commonly streptococcal pyrogenic exotoxin A (SPE A). These toxins act as superantigens that stimulate production of tumor necrosis factor and other inflammatory mediators that cause capillary leak and other physiologic changes, leading to hypotension and organ damage.

EPIDEMIOLOGY: Pharyngitis usually results from contact with the respiratory tract secretions of a person who has GAS pharyngitis. Fomites and household pets, such as dogs, are not vectors of GAS infection. Pharyngitis and impetigo (and their nonsuppurative complications) can be associated with crowding, which often is present in socioeconomically disadvantaged populations. The close contact that occurs in schools, child care centers, contact sports (eg, wrestling), boarding schools, and military installations facilitates transmission. Foodborne outbreaks of pharyngitis occur rarely and are a consequence of human contamination of food in conjunction with improper food preparation or refrigeration procedures.

Streptococcal pharyngitis occurs at all ages but is most common among school-aged children and adolescents, peaking at 7 to 8 years of age. GAS pharyngitis and pyoderma are substantially less common in adults than in children.

Geographically, GAS pharyngitis and pyoderma are ubiquitous. Pyoderma is more common in tropical climates and warm seasons, presumably because of antecedent insect bites and other minor skin trauma. Streptococcal pharyngitis is more common during late autumn, winter, and spring in temperate climates, in part because of close person-to-person contact in schools. Communicability of patients with streptococcal pharyngitis is highest during acute infection and, when untreated, gradually diminishes over a period of weeks. Patients are not considered to be contagious beginning 24 hours after initiation of appropriate antimicrobial therapy.

Throat culture surveys of healthy asymptomatic children during school outbreaks of pharyngitis have yielded group A streptococci prevalence rates as high as 25%. These surveys identified children who were pharyngeal carriers. Carriage of group A streptococci can persist for many months, but risk of transmission from carriers to others is low.

The incidence of ARF in the United States decreased sharply during the 20th century, and rates of this nonsuppurative sequela are low. Focal outbreaks of ARF in school-aged children occurred in several areas in the 1990s, and small clusters continue to be reported periodically. The highest rates of ARF are in Utah, Hawaii, New York, and Pennsylvania, most likely related to circulation of rheumatogenic strains. Their occurrence reemphasizes the importance of diagnosing GAS pharyngitis and treating with a recommended antimicrobial regimen.

In streptococcal impetigo, the organism usually is acquired by direct contact from another person. GAS colonization of healthy skin usually precedes development of impetigo, but group A streptococci do not penetrate intact skin. Impetiginous lesions occur at the site of breaks in skin (eg, insect bites, burns, traumatic wounds, varicella lesions). After development of impetiginous lesions, the upper respiratory tract often becomes colonized with group A streptococci. Infection of surgical wounds and postpartum (puerperal) sepsis usually result from transmission through direct contact. Health care workers who are anal or vaginal carriers and people with skin infection can transmit GAS organisms to surgical and obstetrical patients, resulting in health care-associated outbreaks. Infections in neonates result from intrapartum or contact transmission; in the latter situation, infection can begin as omphalitis, cellulitis, or necrotizing fasciitis.

In the United States, the incidence of invasive GAS infections is highest in infants and the elderly. Fatal cases in children are not common. Before use of varicella vaccine, varicella was the most commonly identified predisposing factor for invasive GAS infection. Other factors increasing risk include exposure to other children and household crowding. The portal of entry is unknown in most invasive GAS infections but is presumed to be skin or mucous membranes. Such infections rarely follow symptomatic GAS pharyngitis. An association between use of nonsteroidal anti-inflammatory drugs and invasive GAS infections in children with varicella has been described, but a causal relationship has not been established.

The incidence of STSS is highest among young children and the elderly, although STSS can occur at any age. Of all cases of invasive streptococcal infections in children, fewer than 5% are associated with STSS. Among children, STSS has been reported with focal lesions (eg, varicella, cellulitis, trauma, osteomyelitis), pneumonia, and bacteremia without a defined focus. Mortality rates are substantially lower for children than for adults with STSS.

The **incubation period** for streptococcal pharyngitis is 2 to 5 days. For impetigo, a 7- to 10-day period between acquisition of group A streptococci on healthy skin and development of lesions has been demonstrated, because GAS organisms do not penetrate intact skin. The **incubation period** for STSS is not known but has been as short as 14 hours in cases associated with subcutaneous inoculation of organisms (eg, childbirth, penetrating trauma).

DIAGNOSTIC TESTS[1]: Children with pharyngitis and obvious viral symptoms (eg, rhinorrhea, cough, hoarseness) should not be tested or treated for GAS infection. Laboratory confirmation is required for cases in children without viral symptoms, because many will not have GAS pharyngitis. A specimen should be obtained by vigorous swabbing of a pair of swabs on both tonsils and the posterior pharynx for culture and/or rapid antigen testing. It is recommended that a throat swab with a negative rapid antigen test result from children be submitted to the laboratory for isolation of group A streptococci; the second swab can be used for this purpose. Culture on sheep blood agar can confirm GAS infection, with latex agglutination differentiating group A streptococci from other beta-hemolytic streptococci. False-negative culture results occur in fewer than 10% of symptomatic patients when an adequate throat swab specimen is obtained and cultured by trained personnel. Recovery of group A streptococci from the pharynx does not distinguish patients with true streptococcal infection (defined by a serologic response to extracellular antigens [eg, streptolysin O]) from streptococcal carriers who have an intercurrent viral pharyngitis. The number of colonies of group A streptococci on an agar culture plate also does not reliably differentiate true infection from carriage. Cultures that are negative for group A streptococci after 18 to 24 hours should be incubated for a second day to optimize recovery of organisms.

Several rapid diagnostic tests for GAS pharyngitis are available. Most are based on nitrous acid extraction of GAS carbohydrate antigen from organisms obtained by throat swab. Specificities of these tests generally are high, but the reported sensitivities vary considerably (ie, false-negative results occur). As with throat swab cultures, sensitivity of these tests is highly dependent on the quality of the throat swab specimen, the experience of the person performing the test, and the rigor of the culture method used for comparison. The US Food and Drug Administration (FDA) has cleared a variety of rapid tests for use in home settings. Parents should be informed that their use is discouraged, and clinicians should be aware that such testing may have an even lower negative predictive value than testing performed in a clinical setting. Because of the high specificity of rapid tests, a positive test result does not require throat culture confirmation. Rapid diagnostic tests using techniques such as polymerase chain reaction (PCR) and chemiluminescent DNA probes have been developed. The FDA recently approved an isothermal nucleic acid amplification test for detection of group A streptococci from throat swab specimens. These tests may be as sensitive as standard throat cultures on sheep blood agar. The diagnosis of ARF is based on the Jones criteria (Table 3.69).

[1]Shulman ST, Bisno AL, Clegg HW, et al. Clinical practice guideline for the diagnosis and management of group a streptococcal pharyngitis: 2012 update by the Infectious Diseases Society of America. *Clin Infect Dis.* 2012;55(10):e86–e102

Table 3.69. Jones Criteria for Diagnosis of Acute Rheumatic Fever[a]

Major Criteria	Minor Criteria	Supporting Evidence
Carditis	Clinical findings:	Positive throat culture or rapid
Polyarthritis	Fever, arthralgia[b]	test for GAS antigen
Chorea	Laboratory findings:	OR
Erythema marginatum	Elevated acute phase	Elevated or rising streptococcal
Subcutaneous nodules	reactants; prolonged PR	antibody test
	interval	

GAS indicates group A streptococcal.
[a]Diagnosis requires 2 major criteria or 1 major and 2 minor criteria with supporting evidence of antecedent group A streptococcal infection.
[b]Arthralgia is not a minor criterion in a patient with arthritis as a major criterion.

Indications for GAS Testing. Factors to be considered in the decision to obtain a throat swab specimen for testing children with pharyngitis are the patient's age, signs and symptoms, season, and family and community epidemiology, including contact with a person with GAS infection or presence in the family of a person with a history of ARF or of post-streptococcal glomerulonephritis. GAS pharyngitis and, therefore, ARF are uncommon in children younger than 3 years, but outbreaks of GAS pharyngitis have been reported in young children in child care settings. The risk of ARF is so remote in young children in industrialized countries that diagnostic studies for GAS pharyngitis generally are not indicated for children younger than 3 years. Children with manifestations highly suggestive of viral infection, such as coryza, conjunctivitis, hoarseness, cough, anterior stomatitis, discrete ulcerative oral lesions, or diarrhea, are unlikely to have GAS pharyngitis and generally should not be tested. In contrast, children with acute onset of sore throat and clinical signs and symptoms such as pharyngeal exudate, pain on swallowing, fever, and enlarged tender anterior cervical lymph nodes or exposure to a person with GAS pharyngitis are more likely to have GAS infection and should have a rapid antigen test, and a throat culture if rapid test result is negative, performed and treatment initiated if a test result is positive.

Testing Contacts for GAS Infection. Indications for testing contacts for GAS infection vary according to circumstances. Testing asymptomatic household contacts for GAS infection is not recommended except when the contacts are at increased risk of developing sequelae of GAS infection, ARF, or acute glomerulonephritis; if test results are positive, contacts should be treated.

In schools, child care centers, or other environments in which a large number of people are in close contact, the prevalence of GAS pharyngeal carriage in healthy children can be as high as 25% in the absence of an outbreak of streptococcal disease. Therefore, classroom or more widespread culture sampling generally are not indicated.

Follow-up Throat Cultures. Post-treatment throat swab cultures are indicated only for patients who are at particularly high risk of ARF or have active symptoms compatible with GAS pharyngitis. Repeated courses of antimicrobial therapy are not indicated for asymptomatic patients with cultures positive for group A streptococci; the exceptions are people who have had or whose family members have had ARF or other uncommon epidemiologic circumstances, such as a community outbreak of ARF or acute poststreptococcal glomerulonephritis.

Patients who have repeated episodes of pharyngitis at short intervals and in whom GAS infection is documented by culture or antigen detection test present a special problem. Most often, these people are chronic GAS carriers who are experiencing frequent viral illnesses and for whom repeated testing and use of antimicrobial agents are unnecessary. In assessing such patients, inadequate adherence to oral treatment also should be considered. Although relatively uncommon, macrolide and azalide resistance among GAS strains occurs, resulting in erythromycin, clarithromycin, or azithromycin treatment failures. Testing asymptomatic household contacts usually is not helpful. However, if multiple household members have pharyngitis or other GAS infections, simultaneous cultures of all household members and treatment of all people with positive cultures or rapid antigen test results may be of value.

Testing for Group A Streptococci in Nonpharyngitis Infections. Cultures of impetiginous lesions often yield both streptococci and staphylococci, and determination of the primary pathogen generally is not possible. Culture is performed when it is necessary to determine susceptibility of the *Staphylococcus aureus* organisms. In suspected invasive GAS infections, cultures of blood and of focal sites of possible infection are indicated. In necrotizing fasciitis, imaging studies may delay, rather than facilitate, establishing the diagnosis. Clinical suspicion of necrotizing fasciitis should prompt surgical evaluation with intervention, including débridement of deep tissues with Gram stain and culture of surgical specimens.

STSS is diagnosed on the basis of clinical findings and isolation of group A streptococci (see Table 3.68, p 733). Blood culture results are positive for *S pyogenes* in approximately 50% of patients with STSS. Culture results from a focal site of infection also usually are positive and can remain so for several days after appropriate antimicrobial agents have been initiated. *S pyogenes* uniformly is susceptible to beta-lactam antimicrobial agents (penicillins and cephalosporins), and susceptibility testing is needed only for non–beta-lactam agents, such as erythromycin or clindamycin, to which *S pyogenes* can be resistant. A significant increase in antibody titers to streptolysin O, deoxyribonuclease B, or other streptococcal extracellular enzymes 4 to 6 weeks after infection can help to confirm the diagnosis if culture results are negative.

TREATMENT[1]:

Pharyngitis.

- Penicillin V is the drug of choice for treatment of GAS pharyngitis. A clinical GAS isolate resistant to penicillin or cephalosporin never has been documented. Prompt administration of penicillin shortens the clinical course, decreases risk of suppurative sequelae and transmission, and prevents acute rheumatic fever even when given up to 9 days after illness onset. For all patients with ARF, a complete course of penicillin or another appropriate antimicrobial agent for GAS pharyngitis should be given to eradicate group A streptococci from the throat, even if group A streptococci are not recovered in the initial throat culture.
- Orally administered amoxicillin as a single daily dose (50 mg/kg; maximum, 1000–1200 mg) for 10 days is as effective as orally administered penicillin V or amoxicillin given multiple times per day for 10 days and comes as a more palatable suspension. This regimen has been endorsed by the American Heart Association in its guidelines

---

[1]Shulman ST, Bisno AL, Clegg HW, et al. Clinical practice guideline for the diagnosis and management of group a streptococcal pharyngitis: 2012 update by the Infectious Diseases Society of America. *Clin Infect Dis.* 2012;55(10):e86–e102

for the treatment of GAS pharyngitis and the prevention of ARF.[1] Compliance is important for once daily dosing regimens.

- The dose of orally administered penicillin V is 400 000 U (250 mg), 2 to 3 times per day, for 10 days for children weighing less than 27 kg (60 lb), and 800 000 U (500 mg), 2 times per day, or 400 000 U (250 mg), 4 times daily, for adolescents and adults. To prevent ARF, oral penicillin should be given for the full 10 days, regardless of the promptness of clinical recovery. Treatment failures may occur more often with oral penicillin than with intramuscular penicillin G benzathine because of inadequate adherence to oral therapy. In addition, short-course treatment (less than 10 days) for GAS pharyngitis, particularly with penicillin V, is associated with inferior bacteriologic eradication rates.

- Intramuscular penicillin G benzathine is appropriate therapy. It ensures adequate blood concentrations and avoids the problem of adherence, but administration is painful. For children who weigh less than 27 kg, penicillin G benzathine is given in a single dose of 600 000 U (375 mg); for heavier children and adults, the dose is 1.2 million U (750 mg). Discomfort is less if the preparation of penicillin G benzathine is brought to room temperature before intramuscular injection. Mixtures containing shorter-acting penicillins (eg, penicillin G procaine) in addition to penicillin G benzathine have not been demonstrated to be more effective than penicillin G benzathine alone but are less painful when administered. Although supporting data are limited, the combination of 900 000 U (562.5 mg) of penicillin G benzathine and 300 000 U (187.5 mg) of penicillin G procaine is satisfactory therapy for most children; however, the efficacy of this combination for heavier patients, such as adolescents and adults, has not been demonstrated.

- For patients who have a history of nonanaphylactic allergy to penicillin, a 10-day course of a narrow-spectrum (first-generation) oral cephalosporin (ie, cephalexin) is indicated. Patients with immediate (anaphylactic) or type I hypersensitivity to penicillin should be treated with oral clindamycin (30 mg/kg per day in 3 divided doses; maximum, 900 mg/day for 10 days) rather than a cephalosporin.

- An oral macrolide or azalide (eg, erythromycin, clarithromycin, or azithromycin) also is acceptable for patients who are allergic to penicillins. Therapy for 10 days is indicated **except** for azithromycin (12 mg/kg/day [maximum, 500 mg]), which is indicated for 5 days. Erythromycin is associated with substantially higher rates of gastrointestinal tract adverse effects compared with clarithromycin or azithromycin. GAS strains resistant to macrolides or azalides have been highly prevalent in some areas of the world and have resulted in treatment failures. In recent years, macrolide resistance rates in most areas of the United States have been 5% to 10%, but resistance rates up to 20% have been reported, and continued monitoring is necessary. Susceptibility testing for macrolide resistance may be helpful in deciding on antibiotic selection for specific penicillin-allergic patients.

Tetracyclines, sulfonamides (including trimethoprim-sulfamethoxazole), and fluoroquinolones should not be used for treating GAS pharyngitis.

Children who have a recurrence of GAS pharyngitis shortly after completing a full course of a recommended oral antimicrobial agent can be retreated with the same

---

[1]Gerber MA, Baltimore RS, Eaton CB, et al. Prevention of rheumatic fever and diagnosis and treatment of acute streptococcal pharyngitis. A scientific statement from the American Heart Association, Rheumatic Fever, Endocarditis, and Kawasaki Disease Committee, Council on Cardiovascular Disease in the Young, and the Quality of Care and Outcomes Research Interdisciplinary Working Group and endorsed by the American Academy of Pediatrics. *Circulation.* 2009;119(11):1541–1551

antimicrobial agent, an alternative oral drug, or an intramuscular dose of penicillin G benzathine, especially if inadequate adherence to oral therapy is suspected. Alternative drugs include a narrow-spectrum cephalosporin (ie, cephalexin), amoxicillin-clavulanate, clindamycin, a macrolide, or azalide. Expert opinions differ about the most appropriate therapy in this circumstance.

Management of a patient who has repeated and frequent episodes of acute pharyngitis associated with positive laboratory tests for group A streptococci is problematic. To determine whether the patient is a long-term streptococcal pharyngeal carrier who is experiencing repeated episodes of intercurrent viral pharyngitis (which is the situation in most cases), the following should be determined: (1) whether the clinical findings are more suggestive of group A streptococci or a virus as the cause; (2) whether epidemiologic factors in the community support group A streptococci or a virus as the cause; (3) the nature of the clinical response to the antimicrobial therapy (in true GAS pharyngitis, response to therapy usually is 24 hours or less); and (4) whether laboratory test results are positive for GAS infection between episodes of acute pharyngitis (suggesting that the patient is a carrier). Measurement of a serial serologic response to GAS extracellular antigens (eg, antistreptolysin O) should be discouraged. Typing (M or *emm* typing) of GAS isolates generally is available only in research laboratories, but if performed, repeated isolation of the same type suggests carriage, and isolation of differing types indicates repeated infections.

Pharyngeal Carriers. Antimicrobial therapy is not indicated for most GAS pharyngeal carriers. The few specific situations in which eradication of carriage may be indicated include the following: (1) a local outbreak of ARF or poststreptococcal glomerulonephritis; (2) an outbreak of GAS pharyngitis in a closed or semiclosed community; (3) a family history of ARF; or (4) multiple ("ping-pong") episodes of documented symptomatic GAS pharyngitis occurring within a family for many weeks despite appropriate therapy.

GAS carriage can be difficult to eradicate with conventional antimicrobial therapy. A number of antimicrobial agents, including clindamycin, cephalosporins, amoxicillin-clavulanate, azithromycin, or a combination that includes either penicillin V or penicillin G benzathine with rifampin for the last 4 days of treatment have been demonstrated to be more effective than penicillin alone in eliminating chronic streptococcal carriage. Of these drugs, oral clindamycin, given as 30 mg/kg per day in 3 doses (maximum, 900 mg/day) for 10 days has been reported to be most effective. Documented eradication of the carrier state is helpful in the evaluation of subsequent episodes of acute pharyngitis; however, carriage can recur after reacquisition of GAS infection, as some individuals appear to be "carrier prone."

Nonbullous Impetigo. Local mupirocin or retapamulin ointment may be useful for limiting person-to-person spread of nonbullous impetigo and for eradicating localized disease. With multiple lesions or with nonbullous impetigo in multiple family members, child care groups, or athletic teams, impetigo should be treated with oral antimicrobials active against both group A streptococci and *S aureus*.

Toxic Shock Syndrome. As outlined in Tables 3.70 and 3.71 (p 740), most aspects of management are the same for toxic shock syndrome caused by group A streptococci or by *S aureus*. Paramount are immediate aggressive fluid replacement management of respiratory and cardiac failure, if present, and aggressive surgical débridement of any deep-seated infection. Because *S pyogenes* and *S aureus* toxic shock syndrome are difficult to distinguish clinically, initial antimicrobial therapy should include an antistaphylococcal agent and a protein synthesis-inhibiting antimicrobial agent, such as clindamycin. The

Table 3.70. Management of Streptococcal Toxic Shock Syndrome Without Necrotizing Fasciitis

- Fluid management to maintain adequate venous return and cardiac filling pressures to prevent end-organ damage
- Anticipatory management of multisystem organ failure
- Parenteral antimicrobial therapy at maximum doses with the capacity to:
  - ◆ Kill organism with bactericidal cell wall inhibitor (eg, beta-lactamase–resistant antimicrobial agent)
  - ◆ Decrease enzyme, toxin, or cytokine production with protein synthesis inhibitor (eg, clindamycin)
- IGIV may be considered for infection refractory to several hours of aggressive therapy or in the presence of an undrainable focus or persistent oliguria with pulmonary edema

IGIV indicates Immune Globulin Intravenous.

Table 3.71. Management of Streptococcal Toxic Shock Syndrome With Necrotizing Fasciitis

- Principles outlined in Table 3.70
- Immediate surgical evaluation
  - ◆ Exploration or incisional biopsy for diagnosis and culture
  - ◆ Resection of all necrotic tissue
- Repeated resection of tissue may be needed if infection persists or progresses

addition of clindamycin to penicillin is recommended for serious GAS infections, because the antimicrobial activity of clindamycin is not affected by inoculum size (does not have the Eagle effect that can be observed with the beta-lactam antibiotics), has a long postantimicrobial effect, and acts on bacteria by inhibiting protein synthesis. Inhibition of protein synthesis results in suppression of synthesis of the *S pyogenes* antiphagocytic M-protein and bacterial toxins. Clindamycin should not be used **alone** as initial antimicrobial therapy in life-threatening situations, because in the United States, 1% to 2% of GAS strains are resistant to clindamycin. Higher resistance rates have been reported for strains associated with invasive infection and may be as high as 10%.

Once GAS infection has been confirmed, antimicrobial therapy should be tailored to penicillin and clindamycin. Intravenous therapy should be continued until the patient is afebrile and stable hemodynamically and blood is sterile as evidenced by negative culture results. The total duration of therapy is based on duration established for the primary site of infection.

Aggressive drainage and irrigation of accessible sites of infection should be performed as soon as possible. If necrotizing fasciitis is suspected, immediate surgical exploration or biopsy is crucial to identify and débride deep soft tissue infection.

The use of Immune Globulin Intravenous (IGIV) can be considered as adjunctive therapy of STSS or necrotizing fasciitis if the patient is severely ill. An IGIV regimen of

1 g/kg on day 1, followed by 0.5 g/kg on days 2 and 3, has been used, but the optimal regimen is unknown.

Other Infections. Parenteral antimicrobial therapy is required for severe infections, such as endocarditis, pneumonia, empyema, abscess, septicemia, meningitis, arthritis, osteomyelitis, erysipelas, necrotizing fasciitis, and neonatal omphalitis. Treatment often is prolonged (2–6 weeks).

Prevention of Sequelae. ARF and acute glomerulonephritis are serious nonsuppurative sequelae of GAS infections. During epidemics of GAS infections on military bases in the 1950s, rheumatic fever developed in 3% of untreated patients with acute GAS pharyngitis. The current incidence after endemic infections is not known but is believed to be substantially less than 1%. The risk of ARF can be eliminated almost completely by adequate treatment of the antecedent GAS infection; however, rare cases have occurred even after apparently appropriate therapy. The effectiveness of antimicrobial therapy for preventing acute poststreptococcal glomerulonephritis after pyoderma or pharyngitis has not been established. Suppurative sequelae, such as peritonsillar abscesses and cervical adenitis, usually are prevented by treatment of the primary infection.

ISOLATION OF THE HOSPITALIZED PATIENT: In addition to standard precautions, droplet precautions are recommended for children with GAS pharyngitis or pneumonia until 24 hours after initiation of appropriate antimicrobial therapy. For burns with secondary GAS infection and extensive or draining cutaneous infections that cannot be covered or contained adequately by dressings, contact precautions should be used for at least 24 hours after initiation of appropriate therapy.

CONTROL MEASURES: The most important means of controlling GAS disease and its sequelae is prompt identification and treatment of infections.

School and Child Care. Children with GAS pharyngitis or skin infections should not return to school or child care until at least 24 hours after beginning appropriate antimicrobial therapy. Close contact with other children during this time should be avoided.

Care of Exposed People. Symptomatic contacts of a child with documented GAS infection who have recent or current clinical evidence of a GAS infection should undergo appropriate laboratory tests and should be treated if test results are positive. Rates of GAS carriage are higher among sibling contacts of children with GAS pharyngitis than among parent contacts in nonepidemic settings; carriage rates as high as 50% for sibling contacts and 20% for parent contacts have been reported during epidemics. Asymptomatic acquisition of group A streptococci may pose some risk of nonsuppurative complications; studies indicate that as many as one third of patients with ARF had no history of recent streptococcal infection and another third had minor respiratory tract symptoms that were not brought to medical attention. However, routine laboratory evaluation of asymptomatic household contacts usually is not indicated except during outbreaks or when contacts are at increased risk of developing sequelae of infection (see Indications for GAS Testing, p 736). In rare circumstances, such as a large family with documented, repeated, intrafamilial transmission resulting in frequent episodes of GAS pharyngitis during a prolonged period, physicians may elect to treat all family members identified by laboratory tests as harboring GAS organisms.

Household contacts of patients with severe invasive GAS disease, including STSS, are at some increased risk of developing severe invasive GAS disease compared with the general population. However, the risk is not sufficiently high to warrant routine testing for GAS colonization, and a clearly effective regimen has not been identified to justify routine chemoprophylaxis of all household contacts. However, because of increased risk of sporadic, invasive GAS disease among certain populations (eg, people with human immunodeficiency virus [HIV] infection) and because of increased risk of death in people 65 years and older who develop invasive GAS disease, physicians may choose to offer targeted chemoprophylaxis to household contacts who are 65 years and older or who are members of other high-risk populations (eg, people with HIV infection, varicella, or diabetes mellitus). Because of the rarity of secondary cases and the low risk of invasive GAS infections in children, chemoprophylaxis is not recommended in schools or child care facilities.

Secondary Prophylaxis for Rheumatic Fever. Patients who have a well-documented history of ARF (including cases manifested solely as Sydenham chorea) and patients who have documented rheumatic heart disease should be given continuous antimicrobial prophylaxis to prevent recurrent attacks (secondary prophylaxis), because asymptomatic and symptomatic GAS infections can result in a recurrence of ARF. Continuous prophylaxis should be initiated as soon as the diagnosis of ARF or rheumatic heart disease is made.

Duration. Secondary prophylaxis should be long-term, perhaps for life, for patients with rheumatic heart disease (even after prosthetic valve replacement), because these patients remain at risk of recurrence of ARF. The risk of recurrence decreases as the interval from the most recent episode increases, and patients without rheumatic heart disease are at a lower risk of recurrence than are patients with residual cardiac involvement. These considerations, as well as the estimate of exposure to GAS infection, influence the duration of secondary prophylaxis in adults but should not alter the practice of secondary prophylaxis for children and adolescents. Secondary prophylaxis for all patients who have had ARF should be continued for at least 5 years or until the person is 21 years of age, whichever is longer (see Table 3.72). Prophylaxis also should be continued if the risk of contact with people with

Table 3.72. Duration of Prophylaxis for People Who Have Had Acute Rheumatic Fever (ARF): Recommendations of the American Heart Association[a]

Category	Duration
Rheumatic fever without carditis	5 y since last episode of ARF or until 21 y of age, whichever is longer
Rheumatic fever with carditis but without residual heart disease (no valvular disease[b])	10 y since last episode of ARF or until age 21 y, whichever is longer
Rheumatic fever with carditis and residual heart disease (persistent valvular disease[b])	10 y since last episode of ARF or until 40 y of age, whichever is longer; consider lifelong prophylaxis for people with severe valvular disease or likelihood of ongoing exposure to group A streptococcal infection

[a]Modified from Gerber M, Baltimore R, Eaton C, et al. Prevention of rheumatic fever and diagnosis and treatment of acute streptococcal pharyngitis. A scientific statement from the American Heart Association, Rheumatic Fever, Endocarditis, and Kawasaki Disease Committee, Council on Cardiovascular Disease in the Young, and the Quality of Care and Outcomes Research Interdisciplinary Working Group. *Circulation.* 2009;119(11):1541–1551.

[b]Clinical or echocardiographic evidence.

GAS infection is high, such as for parents with school-aged children and for people in professions that bring them into contact with children, such as teachers.

The drug regimens in Table 3.73 are effective for secondary prophylaxis. The intramuscular regimen has been shown to be the most reliable, because the success of oral prophylaxis depends primarily on patient adherence; however, inconvenience and pain of injection may cause some patients to discontinue intramuscular prophylaxis. In non-US populations in which the risk of ARF is particularly high, administration of penicillin G benzathine every 3 weeks is justified and recommended, because drug concentrations in serum can decrease below a protective level before the fourth week after administration of a dose. In the United States, administration every 4 weeks seems adequate, except for people who have developed recurrent ARF despite adherence to an every-4-week regimen. Oral sulfadiazine is as effective as oral penicillin for secondary prophylaxis but may not be available readily in the United States. By extrapolating from data demonstrating effectiveness of sulfadiazine, sulfisoxazole has been deemed an appropriate alternative drug; it is available in combination with erythromycin as the generic version of Pediazole.

Allergic reactions to oral penicillin are less common and usually less severe than reactions to parenteral penicillin and occur more often in adults than in children. Severe allergic reactions rarely occur in patients receiving penicillin G benzathine prophylaxis, but the incidence may be higher in patients older than 12 years with severe rheumatic heart disease. Most severe reactions seem to be vasovagal responses rather than anaphylaxis. A serum sickness-like reaction characterized by fever and

Table 3.73. Chemoprophylaxis for Recurrences of Acute Rheumatic Fever[a]

Drug	Dose	Route
Penicillin G benzathine	1.2 million U, every 4 wk[b]; 600 000 U, every 4 wk for patients weighing less than 27.3 kg (60 lb)	Intramuscular
OR		
Penicillin V	250 mg, twice a day	Oral
OR		
Sulfadiazine or sulfisoxazole	0.5 g, once a day for patients weighing 27 kg (60 lb) or less	Oral
	1.0 g, once a day for patients weighing greater than 27 kg (60 lb)	
For people who are allergic to penicillin and sulfonamide drugs		
Macrolide or azalide	Variable (see text)	Oral

[a]Gerber M, Baltimore R, Eaton C, et al. Prevention of rheumatic fever and diagnosis and treatment of acute streptococcal pharyngitis. A scientific statement from the American Heart Association, Rheumatic Fever, Endocarditis, and Kawasaki Disease Committee, Council on Cardiovascular Disease in the Young, and the Quality of Care and Outcomes Research Interdisciplinary Working Group. *Circulation.* 2009;119(11):1541–1551.

[b]In particularly high-risk situations (usually non-US sites), administration every 3 weeks is recommended.

joint pains can occur in people receiving prophylaxis and can be mistaken for recurrence of ARF.

Reactions to continuous sulfadiazine or sulfisoxazole prophylaxis are rare and usually minor; evaluation of blood cell counts may be advisable after 2 weeks of prophylaxis, because leukopenia has been reported in people receiving these drugs. Prophylaxis with a sulfonamide during late pregnancy is contraindicated because of interference with fetal bilirubin metabolism. Febrile mucocutaneous syndromes (erythema multiforme, Stevens-Johnson syndrome, or toxic epidermal necrolysis) have been associated with penicillin and with sulfonamides. When an adverse event occurs with any of these prophylactic regimens, the drug should be stopped immediately and an alternative drug should be selected. For the rare patient who is allergic to both penicillins and sulfonamides, erythromycin is recommended. Other macrolides, such as azithromycin or clarithromycin, also should be acceptable; they have less risk of gastrointestinal tract intolerance but increased cost.

Poststreptococcal Reactive Arthritis. After an episode of acute GAS pharyngitis, reactive arthritis may develop in the absence of sufficient clinical manifestations and laboratory findings to fulfill the Jones criteria for diagnosis of ARF. This syndrome has been termed poststreptococcal reactive arthritis (PSRA). The precise relationship of PSRA to ARF is unclear. In contrast with the arthritis of ARF, PSRA does not respond dramatically to nonsteroidal anti-inflammatory agents. Because a very small proportion of patients with PSRA have been reported to develop valvular heart disease later, these patients should be observed carefully for 1 to 2 years for carditis. Some experts recommend secondary prophylaxis for these patients during the observation period. If carditis occurs, the patient should be considered to have had ARF, and secondary prophylaxis should be initiated (see Secondary Prophylaxis for Rheumatic Fever, p 742).

Bacterial Endocarditis Prophylaxis.[1] The American Heart Association (AHA) has published updated recommendations regarding use of antimicrobial agents to prevent infective endocarditis (see Prevention of Bacterial Endocarditis, p 970). The AHA no longer recommends prophylaxis for patients with rheumatic heart disease without a prosthetic valve. However, use of oral antiseptic solutions and maintenance of optimal oral health through daily oral hygiene and regular dental visits remain important components of an overall health care program. For individuals with a prosthetic valve, infective endocarditis prophylaxis still is recommended, and current AHA recommendations should be followed. If penicillin has been used for secondary prevention of rheumatic fever, an agent other than penicillin should be used for infective endocarditis prophylaxis, because penicillin-resistant alpha-hemolytic streptococci are likely to be present in the oral cavity of such patients.

---

[1]Wilson W, Taubert KA, Gewitz M, et al. Prevention of infective endocarditis. Recommendations by the American Heart Association. A guideline from the American Heart Association Rheumatic Fever, Endocarditis, and Kawasaki Disease Committee, Council on Cardiovascular Disease in the Young, and the Council on Clinical Cardiology, Council on Cardiovascular Surgery and Anesthesia, and the Quality of Care and Outcomes Research Interdisciplinary Working Group. *Circulation.* 2007;116(15):1736–1754

Group B Streptococcal Infections

CLINICAL MANIFESTATIONS: Group B streptococci are a major cause of perinatal infections, including bacteremia, endometritis, and chorioamnionitis; urinary tract infections in pregnant women; and systemic and focal infections in neonates and young infants. Invasive disease in infants is categorized on the basis of chronologic age at onset. Early-onset disease usually occurs within the first 24 hours of life (range, 0–6 days) and is characterized by signs of systemic infection, respiratory distress, apnea, shock, pneumonia, and less often, meningitis (5%–10% of cases). Late-onset disease, which typically occurs at 3 to 4 weeks of age (range, 7–89 days), commonly manifests as occult bacteremia or meningitis (approx 30% of cases); other focal infections, such as osteomyelitis, septic arthritis, necrotizing fasciitis, pneumonia, adenitis, and cellulitis, occur less commonly. Approximately 50% of survivors of early- or late-onset meningitis have long-term neurologic sequelae (encephalomalacia, cortical blindness, cerebral palsy, visual impairment, hearing deficits, or learning disabilities). Late, late-onset disease occurs beyond 89 days of age, usually in very preterm infants requiring prolonged hospitalization. Group B streptococci also cause systemic infections in nonpregnant adults with predisposing medical conditions, such as diabetes mellitus, chronic liver or renal disease, malignancy, or other immunocompromising conditions and in adults 65 years and older.

ETIOLOGY: Group B streptococci *(Streptococcus agalactiae)* are gram-positive, aerobic diplococci that typically produce a narrow zone of beta hemolysis on 5% sheep blood agar. These organisms are divided into 10 types on the basis of capsular polysaccharides (Ia, Ib, II, and III through IX). Types Ia, Ib, II, III, and V account for approximately 95% of cases in infants in the United States. Type III is the predominant cause of early-onset meningitis and the majority of late-onset infections in infants. Capsular polysaccharides and pilus-like structures are important virulence factors and are potential vaccine candidates.

EPIDEMIOLOGY: Group B streptococci are common inhabitants of the human gastrointestinal and genitourinary tracts. Less commonly, they colonize the pharynx. The colonization rate in pregnant women ranges from 15% to 35%. Colonization during pregnancy can be constant or intermittent. Before recommendations were made for prevention of early-onset group B streptococcal (GBS) disease through maternal intrapartum antimicrobial prophylaxis (see Control Measures, p 747), the incidence was 1 to 4 cases per 1000 live births; early-onset disease accounted for approximately 75% of cases in infants and occurred in approximately 1 to 2 infants per 100 colonized women. Following widespread implementation of maternal intrapartum antimicrobial prophylaxis, the incidence of early-onset disease has decreased by approximately 80% to an estimated 0.24 cases per 1000 live births in 2012. The use of intrapartum chemoprophylaxis has had no measurable impact on late-onset GBS disease. In recent years, the incidence of late-onset disease has nearly equaled that of early-onset disease. The case-fatality ratio in term infants ranges from 1% to 3% but is higher in preterm neonates (estimated to be 20% for early-onset disease and 5% for late-onset disease). Approximately 70% of early-onset and 50% of late-onset cases still afflict term neonates.

Transmission from mother to infant occurs shortly before or during delivery. After delivery, person-to-person transmission can occur. Although uncommon, GBS infection can be acquired in the nursery from health care professionals (probably via breaks in hand hygiene) or visitors and more commonly in the community (colonized family members or caregivers). The risk of early-onset disease is increased in preterm infants (less than 37 weeks' gestation), infants born after the amniotic membranes have been ruptured 18 hours or more, and infants born to women with high genital GBS inoculum, intrapartum fever (temperature 38°C [100.4°F] or greater), chorioamnionitis, GBS bacteriuria during the current pregnancy, or a previous infant with invasive GBS disease. A low or an undetectable maternal concentration of type-specific serum antibody to capsular polysaccharide of the infecting strain also is a predisposing factor for neonatal infection. Other risk factors are intrauterine fetal monitoring and maternal age younger than 20 years. Black race is an independent risk factor for both early-onset and late-onset disease. Although the incidence of early-onset disease has declined in all racial groups since the 1990s, rates consistently have been higher among black infants (0.38 cases per 1000 live births in 2012) compared with white infants (0.19 cases per 1000 live births), with the highest incidence observed among preterm black infants. The reason for this racial/ethnic disparity is not known. The period of communicability is unknown but can extend throughout the duration of colonization or disease. Infants can remain colonized for several months after birth and after treatment for systemic infection. Recurrent GBS disease affects an estimated 1% to 3% of appropriately treated infants.

The **incubation period** of early-onset disease is fewer than 7 days. In late-onset and late, late-onset disease, the **incubation period** from GBS acquisition to disease is unknown.

DIAGNOSTIC TESTS: Gram-positive cocci in pairs or short chains by Gram stain of body fluids that typically are sterile (eg, cerebrospinal fluid [CSF], pleural fluid, or joint fluid) provide presumptive evidence of infection. Growth of the organism from cultures of blood, CSF, or if present, a suppurative focus is necessary to establish the diagnosis.

TREATMENT:
- Ampicillin plus an aminoglycoside is the initial treatment of choice for a newborn infant with presumptive early-onset GBS infection. For empirical therapy of late-onset meningitis, ampicillin and an aminoglycoside or cefotaxime are recommended.
- Penicillin G alone is the drug of choice when group B streptococcus has been identified as the cause of the infection and when clinical and microbiologic responses have been documented. Ampicillin is an acceptable alternative therapy.
- For infants with meningitis attributable to group B streptococcus, the recommended dosage of penicillin G for infants 7 days or younger is 250 000 to 450 000 U/kg per day, intravenously, in 3 divided doses; for infants older than 7 days, 450 000 to 500 000 U/kg per day, intravenously, in 4 divided doses is recommended. For ampicillin, the recommended dosage for infants with meningitis 7 days or younger is 200 to 300 mg/kg per day, intravenously, in 3 divided doses; the recommended dosage for infants older than 7 days is 300 mg/kg per day, intravenously, in 4 divided doses.

- For meningitis, some experts believe that a second lumbar puncture approximately 24 to 48 hours after initiation of therapy assists in management and prognosis. If CSF sterility is not achieved, a complicated course (eg, cerebral infarcts) can be expected; also, an increasing protein concentration suggests an intracranial complication (eg, infarction, ventricular obstruction). Additional lumbar punctures are indicated if response to therapy is in doubt, neurologic abnormalities persist, or focal neurologic deficits occur. Failed hearing screen, abnormal neurologic examination, and certain cranial imaging abnormalities at discharge predict an adverse long-term outcome. Consultation with a specialist in pediatric infectious diseases often is useful.
- For infants with bacteremia without a defined focus, treatment should be continued for 10 days. For infants with uncomplicated meningitis, 14 days of treatment is satisfactory, but longer periods of treatment may be necessary for infants with prolonged or complicated courses. Septic arthritis or osteomyelitis requires treatment for 3 to 4 weeks; endocarditis or ventriculitis requires treatment for at least 4 weeks.
- Because of the reported increased risk of infection, the birth mates of a multiple birth index case with early- or late-onset disease should be observed carefully and evaluated and treated empirically for suspected systemic infection if signs of illness occur.

ISOLATION OF THE HOSPITALIZED PATIENT: Standard precautions are recommended, except during a nursery outbreak of disease attributable to group B streptococci (see Control Measures, Nursery Outbreak, p 750).

CONTROL MEASURES:

Chemoprophylaxis. Recommendations from the Centers for Disease Control and Prevention (CDC)[1] and American Academy of Pediatrics[2] have been incorporated into a smart phone app (**www.cdc.gov/groupbstrep/guidelines/prevention-app.html**) and include the following:

- All pregnant women should be screened at 35 to 37 weeks' gestation for vaginal and rectal GBS colonization. For women who present with preterm labor, GBS screening should be performed and parenteral GBS prophylaxis should be initiated. If delivery occurs within 5 weeks and the prior screening result was negative, then no further testing is needed. For those who present >5 weeks after initial preterm labor, then rescreening and management according to the algorithm in the references below is recommended.
- For women who had a previous infant with invasive GBS disease, intrapartum chemoprophylaxis should **always** be given.
- Women with group B streptococci isolated from urine during the current pregnancy should receive intrapartum chemoprophylaxis, because these women usually have a high inoculum of group B streptococci at vaginal sites and are at increased risk of

---

[1]Centers for Disease Control and Prevention. Prevention of perinatal group B streptococcal disease. Revised guidelines from CDC, 2010. *MMWR Recomm Rep.* 2010;59(RR–10):1–36

[2]American Academy of Pediatrics, Committee on Infectious Diseases. Recommendations for the prevention of perinatal group B streptococcal (GBS) disease. *Pediatrics.* 2011;128(3):611–616

delivering an infant with early-onset GBS disease; culture screening at 35 to 37 weeks' gestation is not necessary.

- Intrapartum chemoprophylaxis should be given to **all** pregnant women identified as carriers of group B streptococci. Colonization during a previous pregnancy is *not a*n indication for intrapartum chemoprophylaxis.

- If GBS status is not known at onset of labor or rupture of membranes, intrapartum chemoprophylaxis should be administered to **all** women with gestation less than 37 weeks, duration of membrane rupture 18 hours or longer, or intrapartum temperature of 38.0°C (100.4°F) or greater.

- Oral antimicrobial agents should *not* be used to treat women who are found to have GBS colonization during culture screening. If there is GBS bacteriuria, treatment is warranted according to obstetric standards of care. Such treatment is *not* effective in eliminating carriage of group B streptococci or preventing neonatal disease.

- Intrapartum antimicrobial prophylaxis is *not* recommended for cesarean deliveries performed before labor onset in women with intact amniotic membranes. Women expected to undergo cesarean deliveries should undergo routine culture screening, because onset of labor or rupture of membranes can occur before the planned cesarean delivery, and in this circumstance, intrapartum antimicrobial prophylaxis is recommended if the culture screen is positive.

- Intravenous penicillin G (5 million U initially, then 2.5 to 3.0 million U, every 4 hours, until delivery) is the preferred agent for intrapartum chemoprophylaxis because of its efficacy and narrow spectrum of antimicrobial activity. An alternative drug is intravenous ampicillin (2 g initially, then 1 g every 4 hours until delivery).

- Penicillin-allergic women without a history of anaphylaxis, angioedema, respiratory distress, or urticaria following administration of a penicillin or a cephalosporin should receive intravenous cefazolin (2 g initially, then 1 g every 8 hours). Cefazolin is recommended because of its ability to achieve high amniotic fluid concentrations and effectively prevent early-onset GBS disease.

- Penicillin-allergic women at high risk of anaphylaxis should receive intravenous clindamycin (900 mg every 8 hours) *if* their GBS isolate is documented to be susceptible to clindamycin. Approximately 30% of GBS isolates in the United States were clindamycin resistant in 2010, and the proportion may vary by country. If clindamycin susceptibility testing has not been performed, intravenous vancomycin (1 g every 12 hours) should be administered. The efficacy of clindamycin or vancomycin in preventing early-onset GBS disease is not established.

- Routine use of antimicrobial agents as chemoprophylaxis for neonates born to mothers who have received adequate intrapartum chemoprophylaxis is *not* recommended. Antimicrobial therapy is appropriate only for infants with clinically suspected systemic infection.

- An algorithm for management of newborn infants is provided in Fig 3.11. The recommendations are intended to help clinicians promptly detect and treat cases of early-onset GBS infections.

FIG 3.11. MANAGEMENT OF NEONATES FOR PREVENTION OF EARLY-ONSET GROUP B STREPTOCOCCAL (GBS) DISEASE

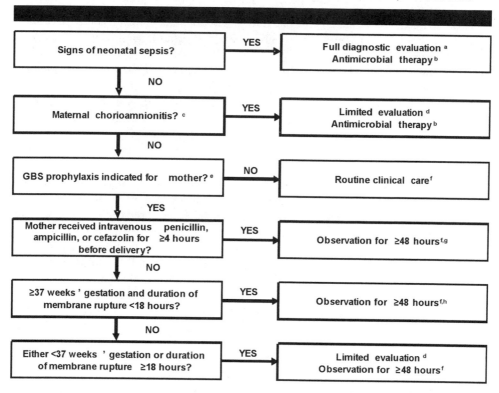

[a] Full diagnostic evaluation includes complete blood cell (CBC) count with differential, platelets, blood culture, chest radiograph (if respiratory abnormalities are present), and lumbar puncture (if patient stable enough to tolerate procedure and sepsis is suspected).

[b] Antimicrobial therapy should be directed toward the most common causes of neonatal sepsis, including GBS and other organisms (including gram-negative pathogens), and should take into account local antimicrobial resistance patterns.

[c] Consultation with obstetric providers is important to determine the level of clinical suspicion for chorioamnionitis. Chorioamnionitis is diagnosed clinically, and some of the signs are nonspecific.

[d] Limited evaluation includes blood culture (at birth) and CBC count with differential and platelets (at birth and/or at 6–12 hours of life).

[e] GBS prophylaxis indicated if one or more of the following: (1) mother GBS positive at 35 to 37 weeks' gestation; (2) GBS status unknown with one or more intrapartum risk factors, including <37 weeks' gestation, rupture of membranes ≥18 hours or temperature ≥100.4°F (38.0°C), or intrapartum nucleic acid amplification test results positive for GBS; (3) GBS bacteriuria during current pregnancy; (4) history of a previous infant with GBS disease.

[f] If signs of sepsis develop, a full diagnostic evaluation should be performed and antimicrobial therapy should be initiated.

[g] If ≥37 weeks' gestation, observation may occur at home after 24 hours if other discharge criteria have been met, if there is a knowledgeable observer and ready access to medical care.

[h] Some experts recommend a CBC with differential and platelets at 6 to 12 hours of age.

- Newborn infants with signs of sepsis should receive a full diagnostic evaluation and initiation of empiric antimicrobial therapy.
- Well-appearing newborn infants whose mothers had suspected chorioamnionitis should undergo a limited evaluation (includes a blood culture and complete blood cell count with differential and platelet counts) and receive empiric antimicrobial therapy pending culture results.
- Well-appearing infants whose mothers had no chorioamnionitis and no indication for GBS prophylaxis should receive routine clinical care.
- Well-appearing infants of any gestational age whose mother received adequate intrapartum GBS prophylaxis (≥4 hours of penicillin, ampicillin, or cefazolin before delivery) should be observed for ≥48 hours; diagnostic testing is *not* recommended. All other maternal antimicrobial agents or durations before delivery are considered inadequate for purposes of neonatal management.
- Well-appearing infants ≥37 weeks' gestation born to mothers who had an indication for GBS prophylaxis but received no or inadequate prophylaxis and in whom duration of membrane rupture before delivery was <18 hours should be observed for ≥48 hours, and *no* diagnostic testing is recommended. Some experts would perform a complete blood count with differential and platelet count at 6 to 12 hours of age in these neonates.
- If the infant was born to a mother who had an indication for GBS prophylaxis but received no or inadequate prophylaxis and is well appearing and either the infant is <37 weeks' gestation or the duration of membrane rupture before delivery was ≥18 hours, then the infant should undergo a limited evaluation and observation for ≥48 hours. Some experts would perform a complete blood count with differential and platelet count at 6 to 12 hours of age.

Neonatal Infection Control. Routine cultures to determine whether infants are colonized with group B streptococci are *not* recommended.

Nursery Outbreak. Cohorting of ill and colonized infants and use of contact precautions during an outbreak are recommended. Other methods of control (eg, treatment of asymptomatic carriers with penicillin) are ineffective. Routine hand hygiene by health care professionals caring for infants colonized or infected with GBS is the best way to prevent spread to other infants.

Non-Group A or B Streptococcal and Enterococcal Infections

CLINICAL MANIFESTATIONS: Streptococci other than Lancefield groups A or B can be associated with invasive disease in infants, children, adolescents, and adults. The principal clinical syndromes of groups C and G streptococci are septicemia, upper and lower respiratory tract infections, skin and soft tissue infections, septic arthritis, meningitis with a parameningeal focus, brain abscess, and endocarditis with various clinical manifestations. Group F streptococcus is an infrequent cause of invasive infection. Viridans streptococci are the most common cause of bacterial endocarditis in children, especially children with congenital or valvular heart disease, and these organisms have become a common cause of bacteremia in neutropenic patients with cancer and in the first 2 weeks after bone marrow transplantation. Among the viridans streptococci, organisms from the *Streptococcus anginosus* group often cause localized infections, such as brain or dental abscesses or abscesses in other sites, including lymph nodes, liver, and lung. Enterococci are associated with bacteremia in neonates and bacteremia, device-associated infections, intra-abdominal abscesses, and urinary tract infections in older children and adults.

ETIOLOGY: Changes in taxonomy and nomenclature of the *Streptococcus* genus have evolved with advances in molecular technology. Among gram-positive organisms that are catalase negative and display chains by Gram stain, the genera associated most often with human disease are *Streptococcus* and *Enterococcus*. The genus *Streptococcus* has been subdivided into 7 species groups on the basis of 16S rRNA gene sequencing. Members of the genus that are beta-hemolytic on blood agar plates include *Streptococcus pyogenes* (see Group A Streptococcal Infections, p 732), *Streptococcus agalactiae* (see Group B Streptococcal Infections, p 745) and groups C and G streptococci, all in the *Streptococcus pyogenes* species group. *Streptococcus dysgalactiae* subspecies *equisimilis* is the group C subspecies most often associated with human infections. Streptococci that are non-beta–hemolytic (alpha-hemolytic or nonhemolytic) on blood agar plates include: (1) *Streptococcus pneumoniae*, a member of the *Streptococcus mitis* group (see Pneumococcal Infections, p 626); (2) the *Streptococcus bovis* group; and (3) viridans streptococci clinically relevant in humans, which include 5 *Streptococcus* species groups (the *anginosus* group, the *mitis* group, the *sanguinis* group, the *salivarius* group, and the *mutans* group). The *anginosus* group (also known as the *Streptococcus milleri* group) includes *Streptococcus anginosus*, *Streptococcus constellatus*, and *Streptococcus intermedius*. This group can have variable hemolysis, and approximately one third possess group A, C, F, or G antigens. Nutritionally variant streptococci, once thought to be viridans streptococci, now are classified in the genera *Abiotrophia* and *Granulicatella*.

The genus *Enterococcus* (previously included with Lancefield group D streptococci) contains at least 18 species, with *Enterococcus faecalis* and *Enterococcus faecium* accounting for most human enterococcal infections. Outbreaks and health care-associated spread in association with *Enterococcus gallinarum* also have occurred occasionally. Nonenterococcal group D streptococci include *S bovis* and *Streptococcus equinus*, both members of the *bovis* group.

EPIDEMIOLOGY: The habitats that non-group A and B streptococci and enterococci occupy in humans include the skin (groups C and G), oropharynx (groups C and G and the *mutans* group), gastrointestinal tract (groups C and G, the *bovis* group, and *Enterococcus* species), and vagina (groups C, D, and G and *Enterococcus* species). Typical human habitats of different species of viridans streptococci are the oropharynx, epithelial surfaces of the oral cavity, teeth, skin, and gastrointestinal and genitourinary tracts. Intrapartum transmission is responsible for most cases of early-onset neonatal infection caused by non-group A and B streptococci and enterococci. Environmental contamination or transmission via hands of health care professionals can lead to colonization of patients. Groups C and G streptococci have been known to cause foodborne outbreaks of pharyngitis.

The **incubation period** and the period of communicability are unknown.

DIAGNOSTIC TESTS: Diagnosis is established by culture of usually sterile body fluids with appropriate biochemical testing and serologic analysis for definitive identification. Antimicrobial susceptibility testing of isolates from usually sterile sites should be performed to guide treatment of infections caused by viridans streptococci or enterococci. The proportion of vancomycin-resistant enterococci among hospitalized patients can be as high as 30%.

TREATMENT: Penicillin G is the drug of choice for groups C and G streptococci. Other agents with good activity include ampicillin, cefotaxime, vancomycin, and linezolid. The combination of gentamicin with a beta-lactam antimicrobial agent (eg, penicillin or ampicillin) or vancomycin may enhance bactericidal activity needed for treatment of life-threatening infections (eg, endocarditis or meningitis).

Many viridans streptococci remain highly susceptible to penicillin (minimal inhibitory concentration [MIC], ≤0.12 µg/mL). Strains with an MIC >0.12 µg/mL and ≤0.5 µg/mL are considered relatively resistant by criteria in the American Heart Association guidelines for determining treatment of streptococcal endocarditis.[1] Strains with a penicillin MIC >0.5 µg/mL are considered resistant. Nonpenicillin antimicrobial agents with good activity against viridans streptococci include cephalosporins (especially ceftriaxone), vancomycin, linezolid, daptomycin, and tigecycline, although pediatric experience with daptomycin and tigecycline is limited. *Abiotrophia* and *Granulicatella* organisms can exhibit relative or high-level resistance to penicillin. The combination of high-dose penicillin or vancomycin and an aminoglycoside can enhance bactericidal activity.

Enterococci exhibit uniform resistance to cephalosporins, and isolates resistant to vancomycin, especially *E faecium*, are increasing in prevalence. In general, children with a central line-associated bloodstream infection caused by enterococci should have the device removed promptly.

Systemic enterococcal infections, such as endocarditis or meningitis, should be treated with ampicillin (if the isolate is susceptible) or vancomycin in combination with an aminoglycoside. Gentamicin is the aminoglycoside recommended for achieving synergy. Gentamicin should be discontinued if in vitro susceptibility testing demonstrates high-level resistance, in which case synergy cannot be achieved. The role of combination therapy for treating central line-associated bloodstream infections is uncertain. Linezolid or daptomycin are options for treatment of infections caused by vancomycin-resistant *E faecium*. Linezolid is approved for use in children, including neonates. Isolates of vancomycin-resistant enterococci (VRE) that also are resistant to linezolid have been described. Resistance to linezolid among VRE isolates also can develop during prolonged treatment. Although most vancomycin-resistant isolates of *E faecalis* and *E faecium* are daptomycin susceptible, daptomycin is approved for use only in adults and experience in children is limited. Data suggest that clearance rates of daptomycin are more rapid in young children compared with adolescents and adults. Daptomycin should not be used

---

[1]Wilson W, Taubert KA, Gewitz M, et al. Prevention of infective endocarditis. Recommendations by the American Heart Association. A guideline from the American Heart Association Rheumatic Fever, Endocarditis, and Kawasaki Disease Committee, Council on Cardiovascular Disease in the Young, and the Council on Clinical Cardiology, Council on Cardiovascular Surgery and Anesthesia, and the Quality of Care and Outcomes Research Interdisciplinary Working Group. *Circulation.* 2007;116(15):1736–1754

to treat pneumonia, as tissue levels are poor and daptomycin is inactivated by surfactants. Quinupristin-dalfopristin is approved for use in adults for treatment of infections attributable to vancomycin-resistant *E faecium* but is not active against *E faecalis*. Microbiologic and clinical cure has been reported in children infected with vancomycin-resistant *E faecium* who were treated with quinupristin-dalfopristin. Tigecycline is approved for use in adults with infections caused by vancomycin-susceptible *E faecalis*. Tigecycline is bacteriostatic against both vancomycin-resistant *E faecalis* and vancomycin-resistant *E faecium*, but experience in children is limited.

Endocarditis. Guidelines for antimicrobial therapy in adults have been formulated by the American Heart Association and should be consulted for regimens that are appropriate for children and adolescents.[1]

ISOLATION OF THE HOSPITALIZED PATIENT: Standard precautions are recommended. For patients with infection or colonization attributable to VRE, contact as well as standard precautions are indicated. Patients harboring vancomycin resistant strains of *Enterococcus gallinarum*, *Enterococcus casseliflavus*, or *Enterococcus flavescens* may be managed using only standard precautions. Common practice is to maintain precautions until the patient no longer harbors the organism or is discharged from the health care facility. Some experts recommend discontinuation of contact precautions if 3 consecutive negative cultures are confirmed from body fluid or tissue specimens from multiple sites (may include stool or rectal swab, perineal area, axilla or umbilicus, wound, and indwelling urinary catheter or colostomy sites, if present). Generally, such cultures should be obtained after cessation of antimicrobial therapy, and each culture is at least 1 week apart from the prior.

CONTROL MEASURES: Patients with a prosthetic valve or prosthetic material used for cardiac valve repair, previous infective endocarditis, or congenital heart disease associated with the highest risk of adverse outcome from endocarditis should receive antimicrobial prophylaxis to prevent endocarditis at the time of dental and other selected surgical procedures (see Prevention of Bacterial Endocarditis, p 970). For these patients, early instruction in proper diet; oral health, including use of dental sealants and adequate fluoride intake; and prevention or cessation of smoking will aid in prevention of dental carries and potentially will lower their risk of recurrent endocarditis.[2]

Use of vancomycin and treatment with broad-spectrum antimicrobial agents are risk factors for colonization and infection with VRE. Hospitals should develop institution-specific guidelines for the proper use of vancomycin.[3]

[1]Wilson W, Taubert KA, Gewitz M, et al. Prevention of infective endocarditis. Recommendations by the American Heart Association. A guideline from the American Heart Association Rheumatic Fever, Endocarditis, and Kawasaki Disease Committee, Council on Cardiovascular Disease in the Young, and the Council on Clinical Cardiology, Council on Cardiovascular Surgery and Anesthesia, and the Quality of Care and Outcomes Research Interdisciplinary Working Group. *Circulation.* 2007;116(15):1736–1754

[2]Hageman JC, Patel JB, Carey RC, Tenover FC, McDonald LC. *Investigation and Control of Vancomycin-Intermediate and -Resistant Staphylococcus aureus (VISA/VRSA): A Guide for Health Departments and Infection Control Personnel.* Atlanta, GA: Centers for Disease Control and Prevention; 2006

[3]Centers for Disease Control and Prevention. Surveillance for dental caries, dental sealants, tooth retention, edentulism, and enamel fluorosis—United States, 1988–1994 and 1999–2002. *MMWR Surveill Summ.* 2005;54(SS-3):1–43

Strongyloidiasis
(Strongyloides stercoralis)

CLINICAL MANIFESTATIONS: Most infections with *Strongyloides stercoralis* are asymptomatic. When symptoms occur, they are most often related to larval skin invasion, tissue migration, and/or the presence of adult worms in the intestine. Infective (filariform) larvae are acquired from skin contact with contaminated soil, producing transient pruritic papules at the site of penetration. Larvae migrate to the lungs and can cause a transient pneumonitis or Löffler-like syndrome. After ascending the tracheobronchial tree, larvae are swallowed and mature into adults within the gastrointestinal tract. Symptoms of intestinal infection include nonspecific abdominal pain, malabsorption, vomiting, and diarrhea. Larval migration from defecated stool can result in migratory pruritic skin lesions in the perianal area, buttocks, and upper thighs, which may present as serpiginous, erythematous tracks called "larva currens." Immunocompromised people, most often those receiving glucocorticoids for underlying malignancy or autoimmune disease, people receiving biologic response modifiers, and people infected with human T-lymphotropic virus 1 (HTLV-1), are at risk of *Strongyloides* hyperinfection syndrome and disseminated disease, in which larvae migrate via the systemic circulation to distant organs, including the brain, liver, kidney, heart, and skin. This condition, which frequently is fatal, is characterized by fever, abdominal pain, diffuse pulmonary infiltrates, and septicemia or meningitis caused by enteric gram-negative bacilli.

ETIOLOGY: *S stercoralis* is a nematode (roundworm).

EPIDEMIOLOGY: Strongyloidiasis is endemic in the tropics and subtropics, including the southeastern United States, wherever suitable moist soil and improper disposal of human waste coexist. Humans are the principal hosts, but dogs, cats, and other animals can serve as reservoirs. Transmission involves penetration of skin by filariform larvae from contact with contaminated soil. Infections rarely can be acquired from intimate skin contact or from inadvertent coprophagy, such as from ingestion of contaminated food or within institutional settings. Adult females release eggs in the small intestine, where they hatch as first-stage (rhabditiform) larvae that are excreted in feces. A small percentage of larvae molt to the infective (filariform) stage during intestinal transit, at which point they can penetrate the bowel mucosa or perianal skin, thus maintaining the life cycle within a single person (autoinfection). Because of this capacity for autoinfection, people can remain infected for decades after leaving an area with endemic infection.

The **incubation period** in humans is unknown.

DIAGNOSTIC TESTS: Strongyloidiasis can be difficult to diagnose in immunocompetent people, because excretion of larvae in feces is highly variable and often of low intensity. At least 3 consecutive stool specimens should be examined microscopically for characteristic larvae (not eggs), but stool concentration techniques may be required to establish the diagnosis. The use of agar plate culture methods may have greater sensitivity than fecal microscopy, and examination of duodenal contents obtained using the string test (Entero-Test) or a direct aspirate through a flexible endoscope also may demonstrate larvae. Eosinophilia (blood eosinophil count greater than $500/\mu L$) is common in chronic infection but may be absent in hyperinfection syndrome. Serodiagnosis is sensitive and should be considered in all people with unexplained eosinophilia (see also Medical Evaluation for Infectious Diseases of Internationally Adopted, Refugee, and Immigrant Children, p 194), especially if immunomodulatory therapy is being considered.

In disseminated strongyloidiasis, filariform larvae may be isolated from sputum or bronchoalveolar lavage fluid as well as spinal fluid. Gram-negative bacillary meningitis is a common associated finding in disseminated disease and carries a high mortality rate.

TREATMENT: Ivermectin is the treatment of choice for both chronic (asymptomatic) strongyloidiasis and hyperinfection with disseminated disease. Ivermectin is approved by the US Food and Drug Administration for the treatment of intestinal strongyloidiasis. An alternative agent is albendazole, although it is associated with lower cure rates (see Drugs for Parasitic Infections, p 927). Prolonged or repeated treatment may be necessary in people with hyperinfection and disseminated strongyloidiasis, and relapse can occur.

ISOLATION OF THE HOSPITALIZED PATIENT: Standard precautions are recommended.

CONTROL MEASURES: Sanitary disposal of human waste is effective at interrupting transmission of *S stercoralis*. Serodiagnosis should be considered in all people with unexplained eosinophilia, especially if immunomodulatory therapy is being considered. If possible, patients should be treated for strongyloidiasis prior to initiation of immunomodulatory therapy.

Syphilis

CLINICAL MANIFESTATIONS:

Congenital Syphilis. Intrauterine infection with *Treponema pallidum* can result in stillbirth, hydrops fetalis, or preterm birth or may be asymptomatic at birth. Infected infants can have hepatosplenomegaly, snuffles (copious nasal secretions), lymphadenopathy, mucocutaneous lesions, pneumonia, osteochondritis and pseudoparalysis, edema, rash, hemolytic anemia, or thrombocytopenia at birth or within the first 4 to 8 weeks of age. Skin lesions or moist nasal secretions of congenital syphilis are highly infectious. However, organisms rarely are found in lesions more than 24 hours after treatment has begun. Untreated infants, regardless of whether they have manifestations in early infancy, may develop late manifestations, which usually appear after 2 years of age and involve the central nervous system (CNS), bones and joints, teeth, eyes, and skin. Some consequences of intrauterine infection may not become apparent until many years after birth, such as interstitial keratitis (5–20 years of age), eighth cranial nerve deafness (10–40 years of age), Hutchinson teeth (peg-shaped, notched central incisors), anterior bowing of the shins, frontal bossing, mulberry molars, saddle nose, rhagades (perioral fissures), and Clutton joints (symmetric, painless swelling of the knees). The first 3 manifestations are referred to as the Hutchinson triad. Late manifestations can be prevented by treatment of early infection.

Acquired Syphilis. Infection with *T pallidum* in childhood or adulthood can be divided into 3 stages. The **primary stage** (or "**primary syphilis**") appears as one or more painless indurated ulcers (chancres) of the skin or mucous membranes at the site of inoculation. Lesions most commonly appear on the genitalia but may appear elsewhere, depending on the sexual contact responsible for transmission (eg, oral). These lesions appear, on average, 3 weeks after exposure (10–90 days) and heal spontaneously in a few weeks. Chancres sometimes are not recognized clinically, and sometimes are still present during the secondary stage of syphilis. The **secondary stage** (or "**secondary syphilis**"), beginning 1 to 2 months later, is characterized by rash, mucocutaneous lesions, and lymphadenopathy. The polymorphic maculopapular rash is generalized and typically includes the palms and soles. In moist areas around the vulva or anus, hypertrophic papular lesions (condyloma lata) can occur and can be confused with condyloma acuminata secondary to human papillomavirus (HPV) infection. Generalized lymphadenopathy, fever, malaise, spleno-megaly, sore throat, headache, alopecia, and arthralgia can be present. Secondary syphilis can be mistaken for other conditions, because its signs and symptoms are nonspecific. This stage also resolves spontaneously without treatment in approximately 3 to 12 weeks, leaving the infected person completely asymptomatic. A variable latent period follows but sometimes is interrupted during the first few years by recurrences of symptoms of secondary syphilis. **Latent syphilis** is defined as the period after infection when patients are seroreactive but demonstrate no clinical manifestations of disease. Latent syphilis acquired within the preceding year is referred to as **early latent syphilis;** all other cases of latent syphilis are **late latent syphilis** (greater than 1 year's duration). Patients who have latent syphilis of unknown duration should be managed clinically as if they have late latent syphilis. The **tertiary stage** of infection occurs 15 to 30 years after the initial infection and can include gumma formation (soft, noncancerous growths that can destroy tissue), cardiovascular involvement (including aortitis), or neurosyphilis. Neurosyphilis is defined as infection of the central nervous system (CNS) with *T pallidum*. Manifestations of neurosyphilis can include syphilitic meningitis, uveitis, and (typically years after infec-tion) dementia and posterior spinal cord degeneration (tabes dorsalis). Neurosyphilis can occur at any stage of infection, especially in people infected with human immunodefi-ciency virus (HIV) and neonates with congenital syphilis.

ETIOLOGY: *T pallidum* is a thin, motile spirochete that is extremely fastidious, surviving only briefly outside the host. The organism has not been cultivated successfully on artifi-cial media.

EPIDEMIOLOGY: Syphilis, which is rare in much of the industrialized world, persists in the United States and in resource-limited countries. The incidence of acquired and congenital syphilis increased dramatically in the United States during the late 1980s and early 1990s but decreased subsequently, and in 2000, the incidence was the lowest since reporting began in 1941. Since 2001, however, the rate of primary and secondary syphilis has increased, primarily among men who have sex with men. Among women, the rate of primary and secondary syphilis increased during 2005–2008, with a concomitant increase in cases of congenital syphilis; rates of primary and secondary syphilis among women and congenital syphilis have since decreased. The highest rates of primary and secondary syphilis and congenital syphilis are in the Southern United States. Late or limited prenatal care and failure of health care providers to follow maternal syphilis screening recommen-dations have been shown to contribute to the incidence of congenital syphilis. In adults, infection with HIV is common among individuals with syphilis, particularly among men who have sex with men. Primary and secondary rates of syphilis are highest in black, non-Hispanic people and in males compared with females.

Congenital syphilis is contracted from an infected mother via transplacental trans-mission of *T pallidum* at any time during pregnancy or possibly at birth from contact with maternal lesions. Among women with untreated early syphilis, as many as 40% of pregnancies result in spontaneous abortion, stillbirth, or perinatal death. Infection can be transmitted to the fetus at any stage of maternal disease. The rate of transmission is 60% to 100% during primary and secondary syphilis and slowly decreases with later stages of maternal infection (approximately 40% with early latent infection and 8% with late latent infection). In 2008, approximately 520 900 adverse outcomes were estimated to be caused by maternal syphilis worldwide, including approximately 212 300 stillbirths (gestational age >28 weeks) or early fetal deaths (gestational age 22 to 28 weeks), 91 800 neonatal deaths, 65 300 infants born preterm or with low birth weight, and 151 500 infected new-born infants.[1]

Acquired syphilis almost always is contracted through direct sexual contact with ulcerative lesions of the skin or mucous membranes of infected people. Open, moist lesions of the primary or secondary stages are highly infectious. Relapses of secondary syphilis with infectious mucocutaneous lesions have been observed 4 years after primary infection.

Sexual abuse must be suspected in any young child with acquired syphilis. In most cases, identification of acquired syphilis in children must be reported to state child protective services agencies. Physical examination for signs of sexual abuse and forensic interviews may be conducted under the auspices of a pediatrician with expertise in child abuse or at a local child advocacy center.

The **incubation period** for acquired primary syphilis typically is 3 weeks but ranges from 10 to 90 days.

DIAGNOSTIC TESTS: Definitive diagnosis is made when spirochetes are identified by microscopic darkfield examination of lesion exudate, nasal discharge, or tissue, such as placenta, umbilical cord, or autopsy specimens. *T pallidum* can be detected by polymerase chain reaction (PCR) assay, but clinical diagnostic PCR assays cleared by the US Food and Drug Administration (FDA) are not yet available. Direct fluorescent antibody (DFA) tests no longer are available in the United States. Specimens should be scraped from moist mucocutaneous lesions or aspirated from a regional lymph node. Specimens from mouth lesions can contain nonpathogenic treponemes that can be difficult to distinguish from *T pallidum* by darkfield microscopy. Although such testing can provide a definitive diagnosis, serologic testing is also necessary.

Presumptive diagnosis is possible using nontreponemal and treponemal serologic tests. Use of only 1 type of test is insufficient for diagnosis, because false-positive nontreponemal test results occur with various medical conditions, and treponemal test results remain positive long after syphilis has been treated adequately (making the diagnosis of reinfection difficult) and can be falsely positive with other spirochetal diseases.

Standard nontreponemal tests for syphilis include the Venereal Disease Research Laboratory (VDRL) slide test and the rapid plasma reagin (RPR) test. These tests measure antibody directed against lipoidal antigen from *T pallidum,* antibody interaction with host tissues, or both. These tests are inexpensive and performed rapidly and provide semi-quantitative results. Quantitative results help define disease activity and monitor response to therapy. Nontreponemal test results (eg, VDRL or RPR) may be falsely negative (ie, nonreactive) in early primary syphilis, latent acquired syphilis of long duration, and late congenital syphilis. Occasionally, a nontreponemal test performed on serum samples containing high concentrations of antibody against *T pallidum* will be weakly reactive or falsely negative, a reaction termed the *prozone* phenomenon. Diluting serum results in a positive test. RPR titers generally are higher than VDRL titers; therefore, when nontreponemal tests are used to monitor treatment response, the same specific test (eg, VDRL or RPR) must be used throughout the follow-up period, preferably performed by the same laboratory, to ensure comparability of results.

[1]Newman L, Kamb M, Hawkes S, et al. Global estimates of syphilis in pregnancy and associated adverse outcomes: analysis of multinational antenatal surveillance data. *PLoS Med.* 2013;10(2):e1001396

A reactive nontreponemal test result from a patient with typical lesions indicates a presumptive diagnosis of syphilis and the need for treatment. However, any reactive nontreponemal test result must be confirmed by one of the specific treponemal tests to exclude a false-positive test result. False-positive results can be caused by certain viral infections (eg, Epstein-Barr virus infection, hepatitis, varicella, measles), lymphoma, tuberculosis, malaria, endocarditis, connective tissue disease, pregnancy, abuse of injection drugs, laboratory or technical error, or Wharton jelly contamination when umbilical cord blood specimens are used. Treatment should not be delayed while awaiting the results of the treponemal test if the patient is symptomatic or at high risk of infection. A sustained fourfold decrease in titer, equivalent to a change of 2 dilutions (eg, from 1:32 to 1:8), of the nontreponemal test result after treatment usually demonstrates adequate therapy, whereas a sustained fourfold increase in titer (eg, from 1:8 to 1:32) after treatment suggests reinfection or relapse. The nontreponemal test titer usually decreases fourfold within 6 to 12 months after therapy for primary or secondary syphilis and usually becomes nonreactive within 1 year after successful therapy if the infection (primary or secondary syphilis) was treated early. The patient usually becomes seronegative within 2 years even if the initial titer was high or the infection was congenital. Some people will continue to have low stable nontreponemal antibody titers despite effective therapy. This serofast state is more common in patients treated for latent or tertiary syphilis.

Treponemal tests in use include the *T pallidum* particle agglutination (TP-PA) test, *T pallidum* enzyme immunoassay (TP-EIA), *T pallidum* chemiluminescent assay (TP-CIA), and fluorescent treponemal antibody absorption (FTA-ABS) test. People who have reactive treponemal test results usually remain reactive for life, even after successful therapy. However, 15% to 25% of patients treated during the primary stage revert to being serologically nonreactive after 2 to 3 years. Treponemal immunoglobulin (Ig) M immunoblotting tests have been developed but are not yet FDA cleared for clinical diagnostic use. Treponemal test antibody titers correlate poorly with disease activity and should not be used to assess response to therapy.

Treponemal tests also are not 100% specific for syphilis; positive reactions occur variably in patients with other spirochetal diseases, such as yaws, pinta, leptospirosis, rat-bite fever, relapsing fever, and Lyme disease. Nontreponemal tests can be used to differentiate Lyme disease from syphilis, because the VDRL test is nonreactive in Lyme disease.

The Centers for Disease Control and Prevention (CDC) recommends syphilis serologic screening with a nontreponemal test, such as the RPR or VDRL test, to identify people with possible untreated infection; this screening is followed by confirmation using one of several available treponemal tests. Some clinical laboratories and blood banks have begun to screen samples using treponemal enzyme immunoassay (EIA) tests rather than beginning with a nontreponemal test; the reasons for this change in sequence of the screening relate to cost and manpower issues. However, this "reverse sequence screening" approach is associated with high rates of false-positive results, and in 2011, the CDC reaffirmed its longstanding recommendation that nontreponemal tests be used to screen for syphilis and that treponemal testing be used to confirm syphilis as the cause of nontreponemal reactivity.[1] The traditional algorithm performs well in identifying people

---

[1] Centers for Disease Control. Discordant results from reverse sequence syphilis screening–five laboratories, United States, 2006–2010. *MMWR Morb Mortal Wkly Rep.* 2011;60(5):133–137

with active infection who require further evaluation and treatment while minimizing false-positive results in low-prevalence populations.

In summary, nontreponemal antibody tests (VDRL and RPR) are used for screening, and treponemal tests (TP-PA, TP-EIA, TP-CIA, and FTA-ABS) are used to establish a presumptive diagnosis. Quantitative nontreponemal antibody tests are useful in assessing the adequacy of therapy and in detecting reinfection. All patients who have syphilis should be tested for HIV infection and other sexually transmitted infections (STIs).

Cerebrospinal Fluid Tests. Cerebrospinal fluid (CSF) abnormalities in patients with neurosyphilis include increased protein concentration, increased white blood cell (WBC) count, and/or a reactive CSF-VDRL test result. The CSF-VDRL is highly specific but is insensitive. Therefore, the CSF VDRL test results should be interpreted cautiously, because a negative result on a VDRL test of CSF does not exclude a diagnosis of neurosyphilis. Alternatively, a reactive CSF-VDRL test in the CSF of neonates can be the result of nontreponemal IgG antibodies that cross the blood-brain barrier. The CSF leukocyte count usually is elevated in neurosyphilis (>5 WBCs/mm^3). CSF test results obtained during the neonatal period can be difficult to interpret; normal values differ by gestational age and are higher in preterm infants. Values as high as 18 WBCs/mm^3 and/or protein up to 130 mg/dL might occur among normal term neonates; some specialists, however, recommend that lower values (ie, 5 WBCs/mm^3 and protein of 40 mg/dL) be considered the upper limits of normal when assessing a term infant for congenital syphilis. Although the FTA-ABS test of CSF is less specific than the CSF-VDRL test, some experts recommend using the FTA-ABS test, believing it to be more sensitive than the CSF-VDRL test. A positive CSF FTA-ABS result can support the diagnosis of neurosyphilis but by itself cannot establish the diagnosis. Fewer data exist for the TP-PA test for CSF, and none exist for the RPR test; these tests should not be used for CSF evaluation.

Testing During Pregnancy. Prevention of congenital syphilis depends on the identification and adequate treatment of pregnant women with syphilis. All women should be screened serologically for syphilis early in pregnancy with a nontreponemal test (RPR or VDRL) and preferably again at delivery.[1] In areas of high prevalence of syphilis and in patients considered at high risk of syphilis, a nontreponemal serum test at the beginning of the third trimester (28 weeks of gestation) and at delivery is indicated. For women treated for syphilis during pregnancy, follow-up nontreponemal serologic testing is necessary to assess the efficacy of therapy. Low-titer false-positive nontreponemal antibody test results occasionally occur in pregnancy. A positive nontreponemal antibody test result should be confirmed with a treponemal antibody test (eg, TP-PA, TP-EIA, TP-CIA, or FTA-ABS). In most cases, if the treponemal antibody test result is negative, the nontreponemal test result is falsely positive, and no further evaluation is necessary. However, in patients with early syphilis, the nontreponemal test result may be positive before the treponemal test result. Therefore, retesting in 2 to 4 weeks and again later if clinically indicated should be considered for pregnant women with a positive nontreponemal test and a negative treponemal test who are at high risk of syphilis. As noted previously, some laboratories are screening pregnant women using an EIA treponemal test, but this reverse-sequence screening approach is not recommended. Pregnant women with reactive treponemal EIA

[1]Wolff T, Shelton E, Sessions C, Miller T. Screening for syphilis infection in pregnant women: evidence for the US Preventive Services Task Force reaffirmation recommendation statement. *Ann Intern Med.* 2009;150(10):710–716

screening tests should have confirmatory testing with a nontreponemal test. Subsequent evaluation and possible treatment of the infant should follow the mother's RPR or VDRL result and her management, as outlined in Fig 3.12. Any woman who delivers a stillborn infant after 20 weeks' gestation should be tested for syphilis.

Evaluation of Infants for Congenital Infection During the Newborn Period and First Months of Life. No newborn infant should be discharged from the hospital without determination of the mother's serologic status for syphilis at least once during pregnancy and also at delivery in communities and populations in which the risk of congenital syphilis is high. All infants born to seropositive mothers require a careful examination and a nontreponemal syphilis test obtained from the infant. The test performed on the infant should be the same as that performed on the mother to enable comparison of titer results. A negative maternal RPR or VDRL test result at delivery does not rule out the possibility of the infant having congenital syphilis, although such a situation is rare. The diagnostic and therapeutic approach to infants being evaluated for congenital syphilis is summarized in Fig 3.12 (p 762) and depends on: (1) identification of maternal syphilis; (2) adequacy of maternal therapy; (3) maternal serologic response to therapy; (4) comparison of maternal and infant serologic titers; and (5) the findings on the infant's physical examination. On the basis of maternal history and initial findings, work-up may include laboratory tests (liver function tests, complete blood cell [CBC] and platelet counts, a CSF-VDRL, and CSF cell count and protein concentration), long-bone and chest radiography, and an ophthalmologic examination. Infants with an abnormal physical examination consistent with congenital syphilis, infants born to mothers with no or inadequate therapy, and infants whose mothers received therapy <4 weeks before delivery will need CSF evaluation to establish the diagnosis of neurosyphilis and aid in planning follow-up evaluations. Additional recommendations for infant evaluation are found in Fig 3.12 (p 762). Other causes of elevated CNS values should be considered when an infant is being evaluated for congenital syphilis.

Infants born to mothers who are coinfected with syphilis and HIV do not require different evaluation, therapy, or follow-up for syphilis than is recommended for all infants.[1]

Evaluation and Treatment of Older Infants and Children. Children who are identified as having reactive serologic tests for syphilis should have maternal serologic test results and records reviewed to assess whether they have congenital or acquired syphilis. The recommended evaluation includes: (1) CSF analysis for CSF-VDRL testing, cell count, and protein concentration; (2) CBC, differential, and platelet count; and (3) other tests as indicated clinically (eg, long-bone or chest radiography, liver function tests, abdominal ultrasonography, ophthalmologic examination, auditory brain stem response testing, and neuroimaging studies).

Cerebrospinal Fluid Testing. CSF should be examined in all patients with neurologic or ophthalmic signs or symptoms, evidence of active tertiary syphilis (eg, aortitis and gumma), treatment failure, or HIV infection with late latent syphilis.

---

[1] Guidelines for prevention and treatment of opportunistic infections in HIV-exposed and HIV-infected children. Recommendations from the National Institutes of Health, Centers for Disease Control and Prevention, the HIV Medicine Association of the Infectious Diseases Society of America, the Pediatric Infectious Diseases Society, and the American Academy of Pediatrics. *Pediatr Infect Dis J.* 2013;32(Suppl 2):i–KK4. Available at: **http://aidsinfo.nih.gov/guidelines/html/5/pediatric-oi-prevention-and-treatment-guidelines/0**

TREATMENT[1]: Parenteral penicillin G remains the preferred drug for treatment of syphilis at any stage. Recommendations for penicillin G use and duration of therapy vary, depending on the stage of disease and clinical manifestations. Parenteral penicillin G is the only documented effective therapy for patients who have neurosyphilis, congenital syphilis, or syphilis during pregnancy and is recommended for HIV-infected patients. Such patients always should be treated with penicillin, even if desensitization for penicillin allergy is necessary.

Penicillin Allergy. Skin testing for penicillin hypersensitivity with the major and minor determinants is reliable in identifying people at high risk of reacting to penicillin, although only the major determinant (benzylpenicilloyl poly-L-lysine [Pre-Pen]) and penicillin G skin tests have been available commercially. Skin testing without the minor determinant misses 3% to 10% of allergic patients who are at risk of serious or fatal reactions. Thus, a cautious approach to penicillin therapy is advised when a patient cannot be tested with all of the penicillin skin test reagents. If the major determinant is not available for skin testing, all patients with IgE-mediated reactions to penicillin should be desensitized in a hospital setting. In patients with non-IgE–mediated reactions, outpatient oral desensitization or monitored test doses may be considered. An oral or intravenous desensitization protocol for patients with a positive skin test result is available and should be performed in a hospital setting. Oral desensitization is regarded as safer and easier to perform. Desensitization usually can be completed in approximately 4 hours, after which the first dose of penicillin can be given.

Congenital Syphilis: Infants in the First Month of Age. The diagnostic and therapeutic approach to neonates delivered to mothers with syphilis is outlined in Fig 3.12 (p 762). For proven or probable congenital syphilis (on the basis of the neonate's physical examination and radiographic and laboratory test results), the preferred treatment is aqueous crystalline penicillin G, administered intravenously for 10 days. The dosage should be based on chronologic age rather than gestational age and is 50 000 U/kg, intravenously, every 12 hours (1 week of age or younger) or every 8 hours (older than 1 week). Alternatively, procaine penicillin G, 50 000 U/kg, intramuscularly, can be administered as a single daily dose for 10 days; no treatment failures have occurred with this formulation despite its low CSF concentrations. When the neonate is at risk of congenital syphilis because of inadequate maternal treatment or response to treatment (or reinfection) during pregnancy but the neonate's physical examination, radiographic imaging, and laboratory analyses are normal (including infant RPR/VDRL titer either the same as or less than fourfold the maternal RPR/VDRL), some experts would treat with a single dose of penicillin G benzathine (50 000 U/kg intramuscularly), but most still would prefer 10 days of treatment. If more than 1 day of therapy is missed, the entire course should be restarted. Data supporting use of other antimicrobial agents (eg, ampicillin) for treatment of congenital syphilis are not available. When possible, a full 10-day course of penicillin is preferred, even if ampicillin initially was provided for possible sepsis. Use of agents other than penicillin requires close serologic follow-up to assess adequacy of therapy.

Infants who have a normal physical examination and a serum quantitative nontreponemal serologic titer less than fourfold higher than the maternal titer (eg, 1:16 is fourfold higher than 1:4) are at minimal risk of syphilis if (1) they are born to mothers who completed appropriate penicillin treatment for syphilis during pregnancy and more than

[1]Centers for Disease Control and Prevention. Sexually transmitted diseases treatment guidelines—United States, 2014. *MMWR Recomm Rep.* 2015; in press

FIG 3.12. ALGORITHM FOR EVALUATION AND TREATMENT OF INFANTS BORN TO MOTHERS WITH REACTIVE SEROLOGIC TESTS FOR SYPHILIS.

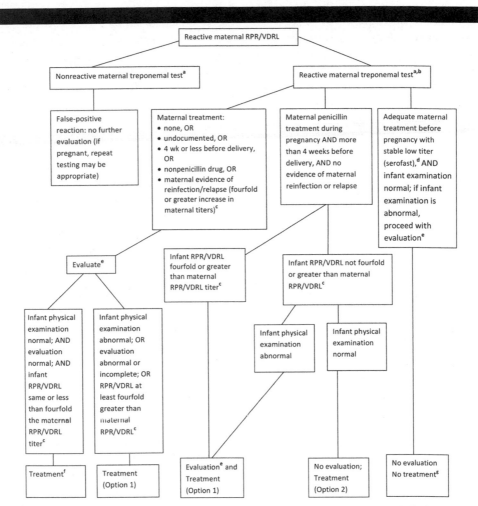

RPR indicates rapid plasma reagin; VDRL, Venereal Disease Research Laboratory; TP-PA, *Treponema pallidum* particle agglutination; FTA-ABS, fluorescent treponemal antibody absorption; TP-EIA, *T pallidum* enzyme immunoassay; MHA-TP, Microhemagglutination test for antibodies to *T pallidum*.

[a] TP-PA, FTA-ABS, TP-EIA, or MHA-TP.

[b] Test for human immunodeficiency virus (HIV) antibody. Infants of HIV-infected mothers do not require different evaluation or treatment for syphilis.

[c] A fourfold change in titer is the same as a change of 2 dilutions. For example, a titer of 1:64 is fourfold greater than a titer of 1:16, and a titer of 1:4 is fourfold lower than a titer of 1:16. When comparing titers, the same type of nontreponemal test should be used (eg, if the initial test was an RPR, the follow-up test should also be an RPR).

[d] Women who maintain a VDRL titer 1:2 or less or an RPR 1:4 or less beyond 1 year after successful treatment are considered serofast.

[e] Complete blood cell (CBC) and platelet count; cerebrospinal fluid (CSF) examination for cell count, protein, and quantitative VDRL; other tests as clinically indicated (eg, chest radiographs, long-bone radiographs, eye examination, liver function tests, neuroimaging, and auditory brainstem response).

[f] Treatment (Option 1 or Option 2, below), with most experts recommending Treatment Option 1. If a single dose of benzathine penicillin G is used, then the infant must be fully evaluated, full evaluation must be normal, and follow-up must be certain. If any part of the infant's evaluation is abnormal or not performed, or if the CSF analysis is rendered uninterpretable, then a 10-day course of penicillin is required.

[g] Some experts would consider a single intramuscular injection of benzathine penicillin (Treatment Option 2), particularly if follow-up is not certain.

Treatment Options:

(1) Aqueous penicillin G, 50 000 U/kg, intravenously, every 12 hours (1 week of age or younger) or every 8 hours (older than 1 week); or procaine penicillin G, 50 000 U/kg, intramuscularly, as a single daily dose for 10 days. If 24 or more hours of therapy is missed, the entire course must be restarted.

(2) Benzathine penicillin G, 50 000 U/kg, intramuscularly, single dose.

4 weeks before delivery; and (2) the mother had no evidence of reinfection or relapse. Although a full evaluation may be unnecessary, these infants should be treated with a single intramuscular injection of penicillin G benzathine, because fetal treatment failure can occur despite adequate maternal treatment during pregnancy. Alternatively, these infants may be examined carefully, preferably monthly, until their nontreponemal serologic test results are negative.

Infants who have a normal physical examination and a serum quantitative nontreponemal serologic titer either the same as or lower than the maternal titer and (1) whose mother's treatment was adequate before pregnancy; and (2) whose mother's nontreponemal serologic titer remained low and stable before and during pregnancy and at delivery (VDRL less than 1:2; RPR less than 1:4) require no evaluation. Some experts, however, would treat with penicillin G benzathine as a single intramuscular injection if follow-up is uncertain.

Congenital Syphilis: Older Infants and Children. Because establishing the diagnosis of neurosyphilis is difficult, infants older than 1 month who possibly have congenital syphilis or who have neurologic involvement should be treated with intravenous aqueous crystalline penicillin for 10 days (see Table 3.74, p 764). This regimen also should be used to treat children older than 2 years who have late and previously untreated congenital syphilis. Some experts suggest giving such patients a single dose of penicillin G benzathine, 50 000 U/kg, intramuscularly, after the 10-day course of intravenous aqueous crystalline penicillin. If the patient has no clinical manifestations of disease, the CSF examination is normal, and the result of the CSF-VDRL test is negative, some experts would treat with 3 weekly doses of penicillin G benzathine (50 000 U/kg, intramuscularly).

Syphilis in Pregnancy. Regardless of stage of pregnancy, women should be treated with penicillin according to the dosage schedules appropriate for the stage of syphilis as recommended for nonpregnant patients (see Table 3.74, p 764). For penicillin-allergic patients, no proven alternative therapy has been established. A pregnant woman with a history of penicillin allergy should be treated with penicillin after desensitization. Desensitization should be performed in consultation with a specialist and only in facilities in which emergency assistance is available (see Penicillin Allergy, p 761).

Erythromycin, azithromycin, or any other nonpenicillin treatment of syphilis during pregnancy cannot be considered reliable to cure infection in the fetus. Tetracycline is not recommended for pregnant women because of potential adverse effects on the fetus.

Early Acquired Syphilis (Primary, Secondary, Early Latent Syphilis). A single intramuscular dose of penicillin G benzathine is the preferred treatment for children and adults (see Table 3.74, p 764). All children should have a CSF examination before treatment to exclude a diagnosis of neurosyphilis. Evaluation of CSF in adolescents and adults is necessary only if clinical signs or symptoms of neurologic or ophthalmic involvement are present. Neurosyphilis should be considered in the differential diagnosis of neurologic disease in HIV-infected people.

For nonpregnant patients who are allergic to penicillin, doxycycline or tetracycline should be given for 14 days. Children younger than 8 years should not be given tetracycline or doxycycline unless the benefits of therapy are greater than the risks of dental staining. Tetracycline-based antimicrobial agents, including doxycycline, may cause permanent tooth discoloration for children younger than 8 years if used for repeated treatment courses. However, doxycycline binds less readily to calcium compared with older tetracyclines, and in some studies, doxycycline was not associated with visible teeth staining in younger children

Table 3.74. Recommended Treatment for Syphilis in People Older Than 1 Month

Status	Children	Adults
Congenital syphilis	Aqueous crystalline penicillin G, 200 000–300 000 U/kg/day, IV, administered as 50 000 U/kg, every 4–6 h for 10 days[a]	
Primary, secondary, and early latent syphilis[b]	Penicillin G benzathine,[c] 50 000 U/kg, IM, up to the adult dose of 2.4 million U in a single dose	Penicillin G benzathine, 2.4 million U, IM, in a single dose **OR** *If allergic to penicillin and not pregnant,* Doxycycline, 100 mg, orally, twice a day for 14 days **OR** Tetracycline, 500 mg, orally, 4 times/day for 14 days
Late latent syphilis[d]	Penicillin G benzathine, 50 000 U/kg, IM, up to the adult dose of 2.4 million U, administered as 3 single doses at 1-wk intervals (total 150 000 U/kg, up to the adult dose of 7.2 million U)	Penicillin G benzathine, 7.2 million U total, administered as 3 doses of 2.4 million U, IM, each at 1-wk intervals **OR** *If allergic to penicillin and not pregnant,* Doxycycline, 100 mg, orally, twice a day for 4 wk **OR** Tetracycline, 500 mg, orally, 4 times/day for 4 wk
Tertiary	…	Penicillin G benzathine 7.2 million U total, administered as 3 doses of 2.4 million U, IM, at 1-wk intervals *If allergic to penicillin and not pregnant, consult an infectious diseases expert*
Neurosyphilis[e]	Aqueous crystalline penicillin G, 200 000–300 000 U/kg/day, IV, every 4–6 h for 10–14 days, in doses not to exceed the adult dose	Aqueous crystalline penicillin G, 18–24 million U per day, administered as 3–4 million U, IV, every 4 h for 10–14 days[f] **OR** Penicillin G procaine,[c] 2.4 million U, IM, once daily **PLUS** probenecid, 500 mg, orally, 4 times/day, both for 10–14 days[f]

IV indicates intravenously; IM, intramuscularly.

[a] If the patient has no clinical manifestations of disease, the cerebrospinal fluid (CSF) examination is normal, and the CSF Venereal Disease Research Laboratory (VDRL) test result is negative, some experts would treat with up to 3 weekly doses of penicillin G benzathine, 50 000 U/kg, IM. Some experts also suggest giving these patients a single dose of penicillin G benzathine, 50 000 U/kg, IM, after the 10-day course of intravenous aqueous penicillin.

[b] Early latent syphilis is defined as being acquired within the preceding year.

[c] Penicillin G benzathine and penicillin G procaine are approved for intramuscular administration only.

[d] Late latent syphilis is defined as syphilis beyond 1 year's duration.

[e] Patients who are allergic to penicillin should be desensitized.

[f] Some experts administer penicillin G benzathine, 2.4 million U, IM, once per week for up to 3 weeks after completion of these neurosyphilis treatment regimens.

(see Tetracyclines, p 873). Clinical studies (along with biologic and pharmacologic considerations) suggest that ceftriaxone at 1 g once daily, either intramuscularly or intravenously, for 10 to 14 days (for adolescents and adults) is effective for early-acquired syphilis, but the optimal dose and duration of therapy have not been defined. Single-dose therapy with ceftriaxone is not effective. Preliminary data suggest that azithromycin might be effective as a single oral dose of 2 g. However, several cases of azithromycin treatment failures have been reported, and resistance to azithromycin has been documented in several geographic areas.

Close follow-up of people receiving any alternative therapy is essential. When follow-up cannot be ensured, especially for children younger than 8 years, consideration must be given to hospitalization and desensitization followed by administration of penicillin G (see Penicillin Allergy, p 761).

Syphilis of More Than 1 Year's Duration (Late Latent Syphilis and Late Syphilis). Penicillin G benzathine should be given intramuscularly, weekly, for 3 successive weeks (see Table 3.74, p 764). In patients who are allergic to penicillin, doxycycline or tetracycline for 4 weeks should be given only with close serologic and clinical follow-up. Limited clinical studies suggest that ceftriaxone might be effective, but the optimal dose and duration have not been defined. Patients who have syphilis and who demonstrate any of the following criteria should have a prompt CSF examination:
1. Neurologic or ophthalmic signs or symptoms
2. Evidence of active tertiary syphilis (eg, aortitis, gumma, iritis, uveitis)
3. Serologic treatment failure

If dictated by circumstances and patient or parent preferences, a CSF examination may be performed for patients who do not meet these criteria. Some experts recommend performing a CSF examination on all patients who have latent syphilis and a nontreponemal serologic test result of 1:32 or greater or if the patient is HIV infected and has a serum CD4+ T-lymphocyte count of 350 or less. The risk of asymptomatic neurosyphilis in these circumstances is increased approximately threefold. If a CSF examination is performed and the results indicate abnormalities consistent with neurosyphilis, the patient should be treated for neurosyphilis (see Neurosyphilis). Children younger than 8 years should not be given tetracycline or doxycycline unless the benefits of therapy are greater than the risks of dental staining. Tetracycline-based antimicrobial agents, including doxycycline, may cause permanent tooth discoloration for children younger than 8 years if used for repeated treatment courses. However, doxycycline binds less readily to calcium compared with older tetracyclines, and in some studies, doxycycline was not associated with visible teeth staining in younger children (see Tetracyclines, p 873).

Neurosyphilis. The recommended regimen for adults is aqueous crystalline penicillin G, intravenously, for 10 to 14 days (see Table 3.74, p 764). If adherence to therapy can be ensured, patients may be treated with an alternative regimen of daily intramuscular penicillin G procaine plus oral probenecid for 10 to 14 days. Some experts recommend following both of these regimens with penicillin G benzathine, 2.4 million U, intramuscularly, weekly, for 1 to 3 doses. For children, intravenous aqueous crystalline penicillin G for 10 to 14 days is recommended, and some experts recommend additional therapy with intramuscular penicillin G benzathine, 50 000 U/kg per dose (not to exceed 2.4 million U), for up to 3 single weekly doses.

If the patient has a history of allergy to penicillin, consideration should be given to desensitization, and the patient should be managed in consultation with an allergy specialist (see Penicillin Allergy, p 761).

Other Considerations.

- Mothers of infants with congenital syphilis should be tested for other STIs, including *Neisseria gonorrhoeae, Chlamydia trachomatis,* HIV, and hepatitis B. If injection drug use is suspected, the mother also may be at risk of hepatitis C virus infection.
- All recent sexual contacts of people with acquired syphilis should be evaluated for other STIs as well as syphilis (see Control Measures, p 767). Partners who were exposed within 90 days preceding the diagnosis of primary, secondary, or early latent syphilis in the index patient should be treated presumptively for syphilis, even if they are seronegative.
- All patients with syphilis should be tested for other STIs, including *N gonorrhoeae, C trachomatis,* HIV, and hepatitis B. Patients who have primary syphilis should be retested for HIV after 3 months if the first HIV test result is negative.
- For HIV-infected patients with syphilis, careful follow-up is essential. Patients infected with HIV who have early syphilis may be at increased risk of neurologic complications and higher rates of treatment failure with currently recommended regimens.[1]
- Children with acquired primary, secondary, or latent syphilis should be evaluated for possible sexual assault or abuse.

Follow-up and Management.

Congenital Syphilis. All infants who have reactive serologic tests for syphilis or were born to mothers who were seroreactive at delivery should receive careful follow-up evaluations during regularly scheduled well-child care visits at 2, 4, 6, and 12 months of age. Serologic nontreponemal tests should be performed every 2 to 3 months until the nontreponemal test becomes nonreactive or the titer has decreased at least fourfold (ie, 1:16 to 1:4). Nontreponemal antibody titers should decrease by 3 months of age and should be nonreactive by 6 months of age if the infant was infected and adequately treated or was not infected and initially seropositive because of transplacentally acquired maternal antibody. The serologic response after therapy may be slower for infants treated after the neonatal period. Patients with increasing titers or with persistent stable titers 6 to 12 months after initial treatment should be reevaluated, including a CSF examination, and treated with a 10-day course of parenteral penicillin G, even if they were treated previously.

Treponemal tests should not be used to evaluate treatment response, because results for an infected child can remain positive despite effective therapy. Passively transferred maternal treponemal antibodies can persist in an infant until 15 months of age. A reactive treponemal test after 18 months of age is diagnostic of congenital syphilis. If the nontreponemal test is nonreactive at this time, no further evaluation or treatment is necessary. If the nontreponemal test is reactive at 18 months of age, the infant should be evaluated (or reevaluated) fully and treated for congenital syphilis.

Treated infants with congenital neurosyphilis and initially positive results of CSF-VDRL tests or abnormal CSF cell counts and/or protein concentrations should undergo repeated clinical evaluation and CSF examination at 6-month intervals until their CSF examination is normal. A reactive CSF-VDRL test or abnormal CSF indices that cannot

---

[1] Guidelines for prevention and treatment of opportunistic infections in HIV-exposed and HIV-infected children. Recommendations from the National Institutes of Health, Centers for Disease Control and Prevention, the HIV Medicine Association of the Infectious Diseases Society of America, the Pediatric Infectious Diseases Society, and the American Academy of Pediatrics. *Pediatr Infect Dis J.* 2013;32(Suppl 2):i–KK4. Available at: **http://aidsinfo.nih.gov/guidelines/html/5/ pediatric-oi-prevention-and-treatment-guidelines/0**

be attributed to another ongoing illness at the 6-month interval are indications for retreatment. Neuroimaging studies, such as magnetic resonance imaging, should be considered in these children.

Acquired Syphilis. Treated pregnant women with syphilis should have quantitative nontreponemal serologic tests repeated at 28 to 32 weeks of gestation, at delivery, and according to recommendations for the stage of disease. Serologic titers may be repeated monthly in women at high risk of reinfection or in geographic areas where the prevalence of syphilis is high. The clinical and antibody response should be appropriate for stage of disease, but most women will deliver before their serologic response to treatment can be assessed definitively. Inadequate maternal treatment is likely if clinical signs of infection are present at delivery or if maternal antibody titer is fourfold higher than the pretreatment titer. Fetal treatment is considered inadequate if delivery occurs within 28 days of maternal therapy.

Indications for Retreatment.

Primary/Secondary Syphilis.

- If clinical signs or symptoms persist or recur or if a fourfold increase in titer of a nontreponemal test occurs, evaluate CSF and HIV status and repeat therapy.
- If the nontreponemal titer fails to decrease fourfold within 6 months after therapy, evaluate for HIV; repeat therapy unless follow-up for continued clinical and serologic assessment can be ensured. Some experts recommend CSF evaluation.

Latent Syphilis. In the following situations, CSF examination should be performed and retreatment should be provided:

- Titers increase at least fourfold (ie, 1:4 to 1:16);
- An initially high titer (greater than 1:32) fails to decrease at least fourfold (ie, 1:32 to 1:8) within 12 to 24 months; or
- Signs or symptoms attributable to syphilis develop.

In all these instances, retreatment should be performed with 3 weekly injections of penicillin G benzathine, 2.4 million U, intramuscularly, unless CSF examination indicates that neurosyphilis is present, at which time treatment for neurosyphilis should be initiated. Retreated patients should be treated with the schedules recommended for patients with syphilis for more than 1 year. In general, only 1 retreatment course is indicated. The possibility of reinfection or concurrent HIV infection should always be considered when retreating patients with early syphilis, and repeat HIV testing should be performed in such cases.

Patients with neurosyphilis associated with acquired syphilis must have periodic serologic testing, clinical evaluation at 6-month intervals, and repeat CSF examinations. If the CSF white blood cell count has not decreased after 6 months or if the CSF white blood cell count or protein are not normal after 2 years, retreatment should be considered. CSF abnormalities may persist for extended periods of time in HIV-infected people with neurosyphilis. Close follow-up is warranted.

ISOLATION OF THE HOSPITALIZED PATIENT: Standard precautions are recommended for all patients, including infants with suspected or proven congenital syphilis. Because moist open lesions, secretions, and possibly blood are contagious in all patients with syphilis, gloves should be worn when caring for patients with congenital, primary, and secondary syphilis with skin and mucous membrane lesions until 24 hours of treatment has been completed.

CONTROL MEASURES:

- All women should be screened for syphilis early in pregnancy. For communities and populations in which the prevalence of syphilis is high or for patients at high risk, serologic testing also should be performed at 28 to 32 weeks of gestation and at delivery. No newborn infant should leave the hospital without the maternal serologic status having been determined at least once during the pregnancy.

- Education of patients and populations about STIs, treatment of sexual contacts, reporting of each case to local public health authorities for contact investigation and appropriate follow-up, and serologic screening of high-risk populations are indicated.
- All recent sexual contacts of a person with acquired syphilis should be identified, examined, serologically tested, and treated appropriately. Sexual contacts of people with primary, secondary, or early latent syphilis who were exposed within the preceding 90 days may be infected even if seronegative and should be treated for early-acquired syphilis. People exposed more than 90 days previously should be treated presumptively if serologic test results are not available immediately and follow-up is uncertain. For identification of at-risk sexual partners, the periods before treatment are as follows: (1) 3 months plus duration of symptoms for primary syphilis; (2) 6 months plus duration of symptoms for secondary syphilis; and (3) 1 year for early latent syphilis. Recommendations for partner service programs provided to partners of people with syphilis are available.[1]
- All people, including hospital personnel, who have had close unprotected contact with a patient with early congenital syphilis before identification of the disease or during the first 24 hours of therapy should be examined clinically for the presence of lesions 2 to 3 weeks after contact. Serologic testing should be performed and repeated 3 months after contact or sooner if symptoms occur. If the degree of exposure is considered substantial, immediate treatment should be considered.

Tapeworm Diseases
(Taeniasis and Cysticercosis)

CLINICAL MANIFESTATIONS:
Taeniasis. Infection with adult tapeworms often is asymptomatic; however, mild gastrointestinal tract symptoms, such as nausea, diarrhea, and pain, can occur. Tapeworm segments can be seen migrating from the anus or in feces.

Cysticercosis. In contrast, cysticercosis caused by larval pork tapeworm infection can have serious consequences. Manifestations depend on the location and number of pork tapeworm larval cysts (cysticerci) and the host response. Cysticerci may be found anywhere in the body. The most common and serious manifestations are caused by cysticerci in the central nervous system. Larval cysts of *Taenia solium* in the brain (neurocysticercosis) can cause seizures, behavioral disturbances, obstructive hydrocephalus, and other neurologic signs and symptoms. Neurocysticercosis is the leading infectious cause of epilepsy in the developing world. The host reaction to degenerating cysticerci can produce signs and symptoms of meningitis. Cysts in the spinal column can cause gait disturbance, pain, or transverse myelitis. Subcutaneous cysticerci produce palpable nodules, and ocular involvement can cause visual impairment.

ETIOLOGY: Taeniasis is caused by intestinal infection by the adult tapeworm, *Taenia saginata* (beef tapeworm) or *T solium* (pork tapeworm). *Taenia asiatica* causes taeniasis in Asia. Human cysticercosis is caused only by the larvae of *T solium (Cysticercus cellulosae).*

---

[1]Centers for Disease Control and Prevention. Recommendations for partner service programs for HIV infection, syphilis, gonorrhea, and chlamydial infection. *MMWR Recomm Rep.* 2008;57(RR-9):1–83

EPIDEMIOLOGY: These tapeworm diseases have worldwide distribution. Prevalence is high in areas with poor sanitation and human fecal contamination in areas where cattle graze or swine are fed. Most cases of *T solium* infection in the United States are imported from Latin America or Asia, although the disease is prevalent in sub-Saharan Africa as well. High rates of *T saginata* infection occur in Mexico, parts of South America, East Africa, and central Europe. *T asiatica* is common in China, Taiwan, and Southeast Asia. Taeniasis is acquired by eating undercooked beef *(T saginata)* or pork *(T solium)*. *T asiatica* is acquired by eating viscera of infected pigs that contain encysted larvae. Infection often is asymptomatic.

Cysticercosis in humans is acquired by ingesting eggs of the pork tapeworm *(T solium)*, through direct fecal-oral contact with a person harboring the adult tapeworm, or through ingestion of fecally contaminated food. Autoinfection is possible. Eggs are found only in human feces, because humans are the obligate definitive host. Eggs liberate oncospheres in the intestine that migrate through the blood and lymphatics to tissues throughout the body, including the central nervous system, where the oncospheres develop into cysticerci. Although most cases of cysticercosis in the United States have been imported, cysticercosis can be acquired in the United States from tapeworm carriers who emigrated from an area with endemic infection and still have *T solium* intestinal-stage infection. *T saginata* and *T asiatica* do not cause cysticercosis.

The **incubation period** for taeniasis (the time from ingestion of the larvae until segments are passed in the feces) is 2 to 3 months. For cysticercosis, the time between infection and onset of symptoms may be several years.

DIAGNOSIS: Diagnosis of taeniasis (adult tapeworm infection) is based on demonstration of the proglottids or ova in feces or the perianal region. However, these techniques are insensitive. Species identification of the parasite is based on the different structures of gravid proglottids and scolex. Diagnosis of neurocysticercosis typically requires both imaging of the central nervous system and serologic testing. Computed tomography (CT) scanning or magnetic resonance imaging (MRI) of the brain or spinal cord are used to demonstrate lesions compatible with cysticerci. Antibody assays that detect specific antibodies to larval *T solium* in serum and cerebrospinal fluid (CSF) are useful to confirm the diagnosis but can have limited sensitivity if few cysticerci are present. In the United States, antibody tests are available through the Centers for Disease Control and Prevention and a few commercial laboratories. In general, antibody tests are more sensitive with serum specimens than with CSF specimens. Serum antibody assay results often are negative in children with solitary parenchymal lesions but usually are positive in patients with multiple lesions.

TREATMENT:

Taeniasis. Praziquantel is highly effective for eradicating infection with the adult tapeworm, and niclosamide is an alternative (see Drugs for Parasitic Infections, p 927). Praziquantel is not approved for this indication, but dosing is provided for children older than 4 years for other indications. Niclosamide is not approved for treatment of *T solium* infection but is approved for treatment of *T saginata* infection. However, niclosamide is not available commercially in the United States.

Cysticercosis. Neurocysticercosis treatment should be individualized on the basis of the number, location, and viability of cysticerci as assessed by neuroimaging studies (MRI or CT scan) and the clinical manifestations. Management generally is aimed at symptoms and should include anticonvulsants for patients with seizures and insertion of shunts for patients with hydrocephalus. Two antiparasitic drugs—albendazole and praziquantel—are available (see Drugs for Parasitic Infections, p 927). Praziquantel is not approved for this indication, but dosing is provided for children older than 4 years for some other indications. Although both drugs are cysticercidal and hasten radiologic resolution of cysts, most symptoms result from the host inflammatory response and may be exacerbated by treatment. In some clinical trials, patients treated with albendazole had better radiologic and clinical responses than patients treated with low doses of praziquantel. Several studies have indicated that patients with single inflamed cysts within brain parenchyma do well without antiparasitic therapy, although treating enhancing cysts as opposed to granulomas may be beneficial. Most experts recommend therapy with albendazole or praziquantel for patients with nonenhancing or multiple cysticerci. Albendazole is preferred over praziquantel, because it has fewer drug-drug interactions with anticonvulsants. Coadministration of corticosteroids during antiparasitic therapy may decrease adverse effects if more extensive viable central nervous system cysticerci are suspected, and a prolonged course may be required for some forms of the disease (eg, basal or subarachnoid). Corticosteroids can affect the tissue concentrations of albendazole. Arachnoiditis, vasculitis, or diffuse cerebral edema (cysticercal encephalitis) is treated with corticosteroid therapy until the cerebral edema is controlled.

The medical and surgical management of cysticercosis can be highly complex and often needs to be conducted in consultation with a neurologist or neurosurgeon. Seizures may recur for months or years. Anticonvulsant therapy is recommended until there is neuroradiologic evidence of resolution and seizures have not occurred for 1 to 2 years. Calcification of cysts may require prolonged or indefinite use of anticonvulsants. Intraventricular cysticerci and hydrocephalus usually require surgical therapy. Intraventricular cysticerci often can be removed by endoscopic surgery, which is the treatment of choice. If cysticerci cannot be removed easily, hydrocephalus should be corrected with placement of intraventricular shunts. Adjunctive chemotherapy with antiparasitic agents and corticosteroids may decrease the rate of subsequent shunt failure. Ocular cysticercosis is treated by surgical excision of the cysticerci. Ocular and spinal cysticerci generally are not treated with anthelmintic drugs, which can exacerbate inflammation. An ophthalmic examination should be performed before treatment to rule out intraocular cysticerci.

ISOLATION OF THE HOSPITALIZED PATIENT: Standard precautions are recommended.

CONTROL MEASURES: Eating raw or undercooked beef or pork should be avoided. Whole cuts of meat should be cooked to at least 145°F (63°C) then allowed to rest for 3 minutes before consuming, and ground meat and wild game meat should be cooked to at least 160°F (71°C). People known to harbor the adult tapeworm of *T solium* should be treated immediately. Careful attention to hand hygiene and appropriate disposal of fecal material is important.

Examination of stool specimens obtained from food handlers who recently have emigrated from countries with endemic infection for detection of eggs and proglottids is advisable. To prevent fecal-oral transmission of *T solium* eggs, people traveling to developing countries with high endemic rates of cysticercosis should avoid eating uncooked vegetables and fruits that cannot be peeled.

Other Tapeworm Infections
(Including Hydatid Disease)

Most tapeworm infections are asymptomatic, but nausea, abdominal pain, and diarrhea have been observed in people who are heavily infected.

ETIOLOGIES, DIAGNOSIS, AND TREATMENT

Hymenolepis nana. This tapeworm, also called the dwarf tapeworm because it is the smallest of the adult human tapeworms, can complete its entire life cycle within humans. New infection may be acquired by ingestion of eggs passed in feces of infected people or of infected arthropods (fleas). More problematic is autoinfection, which perpetuates infection in the host, because eggs can hatch within the intestine and reinitiate the life cycle, leading to development of new worms and a large worm burden. Diagnosis is made by recognition of the characteristic eggs passed in stool. Praziquantel is the treatment of choice, with nitazoxanide as an alternative drug (see Drugs for Parasitic Infections, p 927). If infection persists after treatment, retreatment with praziquantel is indicated. Praziquantel and nitazoxanide are not approved for this indication, but dosing recommendations are available for children 4 years and older (praziquantel) and 1 year and older (nitazoxanide) for other indications.

Dipylidium caninum. This tapeworm is the most common and widespread adult tapeworm of dogs and cats. *Dipylidium caninum* infects children when they inadvertently swallow a dog or cat flea, which serves as the intermediate host. Diagnosis is made by finding the characteristic eggs or motile proglottids in stool. Proglottids resemble rice kernels. Therapy with praziquantel is effective. Niclosamide is an alternative therapeutic option but is not available in the United States (see Drugs for Parasitic Infections, p 927). Praziquantel and niclosamide are not approved for this indication, but dosing recommendations are available for children 4 years and older (praziquantel) and 2 years and older (niclosamide) for other indications.

Diphyllobothrium latum *(and related species).* Fish are one of the intermediate hosts of the *Diphyllobothrium latum* tapeworm, also called fish tapeworm. Consumption of infected, raw freshwater fish (including trout and pike) leads to infection. Three to 5 weeks are needed for the adult tapeworm to mature and begin to lay eggs. The worm sometimes causes mechanical obstruction of the bowel or diarrhea, abdominal pain, or rarely, megaloblastic anemia secondary to vitamin B_{12} deficiency. Infection with other related species of fish tapeworm are associated with consumption of anadromous or saltwater fish, such as salmon. Diagnosis is made by recognition of the characteristic proglottids or eggs passed in stool. Therapy with praziquantel is effective; niclosamide is an alternative but is not available in the United States (see Drugs for Parasitic Infections, p 927). Praziquantel is not approved for this indication, but dosing recommendations are available for children 4 years and older for other indications.

Echinococcus granulosus *and* Echinococcus multilocularis. The larval forms of these tapeworms cause cystic echinococcosis, also known as hydatid disease, and alveolar echinococcosis, respectively. The distribution of *Echinococcus granulosus* is related to sheep or cattle herding. Areas of high prevalence include parts of Central and South America, East Africa, Eastern Europe, the Middle East, the Mediterranean region, China, and Central

Asia. The parasite also is endemic in Australia and New Zealand. In the United States, small foci of endemic transmission have been reported in Arizona, California, New Mexico, and Utah, and a strain of the parasite is adapted to wolves, moose, and caribou in Alaska and Canada. Dogs, coyotes, wolves, dingoes, and jackals can become infected by swallowing protoscolices of the parasite within hydatid cysts in the organs of sheep or other intermediate hosts. Dogs pass embryonated eggs in their stools, and sheep become infected by swallowing the eggs. If humans swallow *Echinococcus* eggs, they can become inadvertent intermediate hosts, and cysts can develop in various organs, such as the liver, lungs, kidneys, and spleen. Cysts caused by larvae of *E granulosus* usually grow slowly (1 cm in diameter per year) and eventually can contain several liters of fluid. If a cyst ruptures, anaphylaxis and multiple secondary cysts from seeding of protoscolices can result. Clinical diagnosis often is difficult. A history of contact with dogs in an area with endemic infection is helpful. Cystic lesions can be demonstrated by radiography, ultrasonography, or computed tomography of various organs. Serologic testing, available at the Centers for Disease Control and Prevention, is helpful, but false-negative results occur; conversely, tests at commercial labs may provide false-positive results. Treatment depends on ultrasonographic staging and may include watchful waiting, antiparasitic therapy, PAIR (**p**uncture **a**spiration, **i**njection of protoscolicidal agents, and **r**easpiration), surgical excision, or no treatment. In uncomplicated cases, treatment of choice is PAIR. Contraindications to PAIR include communication of the cyst with the biliary tract (eg, bile staining after initial aspiration), superficial cysts, and heavily septated cysts. Surgical therapy is indicated for complicated cases and requires meticulous care to prevent spillage, including preparations such as soaking of surgical drapes in hypertonic saline. In general, the cyst should be removed intact, because leakage of contents is associated with a higher rate of complications. Patients are at risk of anaphylactic reactions to cyst contents. Treatment with albendazole generally should be initiated days to weeks before surgery or PAIR and continued for several weeks to months afterward (see Drugs for Parasitic Infections, p 927).

Echinococcus multilocularis, a species for which the life cycle involves foxes, dogs, and rodents, causes alveolar echinococcosis, which is characterized by invasive growth of the larvae in the liver with occasional metastatic spread. Alveolar echinococcosis is limited to the northern hemisphere and usually is diagnosed in people 50 years of age or older. The disease has been reported frequently from Western China. The preferred treatment is surgical removal of the entire larval mass. In nonresectable cases, continuous treatment with albendazole has been associated with clinical improvement (see Drugs for Parasitic Infections, p 927).

ISOLATION OF THE HOSPITALIZED PATIENT: Standard precautions are recommended.

CONTROL MEASURES: Preventive measures for *H nana* include educating the public about personal hygiene and sanitary disposal of feces.

Infection with *D caninum* is prevented by keeping dogs and cats free of fleas and worms.

Thorough cooking to an internal temperature of 63°C [145°F], freezing (−35°C [−31°F]) until solid, or irradiation of freshwater fish ensures protection against *D latum*.

Control measures for prevention of *E granulosus* and *E multilocularis* include educating the public about hand hygiene and avoiding exposure to dog and wild canid feces. Prevention and control of infection in dogs decreases the risk.

Tetanus
(Lockjaw)

CLINICAL MANIFESTATIONS: Tetanus is caused by neurotoxin produced by the anaerobic bacterium *Clostridium tetani* in a contaminated wound and can manifest in 4 overlapping clinical forms: generalized, local, neonatal, and cephalic.

Generalized tetanus (lockjaw) is a neurologic disease manifesting as trismus and severe muscular spasms, including risus sardonicus. Onset is gradual, occurring over 1 to 7 days, and symptoms progress to severe painful generalized muscle spasms, which often are aggravated by any external stimulus. Autonomic dysfunction, manifesting as diaphoresis, tachycardia, labile blood pressure, arrhythmias, often is present. Severe spasms persist for 1 week or more and subside over several weeks in people who recover. Neonatal tetanus is a form of generalized tetanus occurring in newborn infants lacking protective passive immunity because their mothers are not immune.

Local tetanus manifests as local muscle spasms in areas contiguous to a wound. Cephalic tetanus is a dysfunction of cranial nerves associated with infected wounds on the head and neck. Local and cephalic tetanus can precede generalized tetanus.

ETIOLOGY: *C tetani* is a spore-forming, obligate anaerobic, gram-positive bacillus. This organism is a wound contaminant that causes neither tissue destruction nor an inflammatory response. The vegetative form of *C tetani* produces a potent plasmid-encoded exotoxin (tetanospasmin), which binds to gangliosides at the myoneural junction of skeletal muscle and on neuronal membranes in the spinal cord, blocking inhibitory impulses to motor neurons. The action of tetanus toxin on the brain and sympathetic nervous system is less well documented. *C tetani* also produces tetanolysin, a toxin with hemolytic and cytolytic properties; however, its effect on clinical presentation of tetanus has not been elucidated.

EPIDEMIOLOGY: Tetanus occurs worldwide and is more common in warmer climates and during warmer months, in part because of higher frequency of contaminated wounds associated with those locations and seasons. The organism, a normal inhabitant of soil and animal and human intestines, is ubiquitous in the environment, especially where contamination by excreta is common. Organisms multiply in wounds, recognized or unrecognized, and elaborate toxins in the presence of anaerobic conditions. Contaminated wounds, especially wounds with devitalized tissue and deep-puncture trauma, are at greatest risk. Neonatal tetanus is common in many developing countries where pregnant women are not immunized appropriately against tetanus and nonsterile umbilical cord-care practices are followed. More than 250 000 deaths from neonatal tetanus were estimated to have occurred worldwide each year between 2000 and 2003. Widespread active immunization against tetanus has modified the epidemiology of disease in the United States, where 40 or fewer cases have been reported annually since 1999. Tetanus is not transmissible from person to person.

The **incubation period** ranges from 3 to 21 days, with most cases occurring within 8 days. Shorter incubation periods have been associated with more heavily contaminated wounds, more severe disease, and a worse prognosis. In neonatal tetanus, symptoms usually appear from 4 to 14 days after birth, averaging 7 days.

DIAGNOSTIC TESTS: The diagnosis of tetanus is made clinically by excluding other causes of tetanic spasms, such as hypocalcemic tetany, phenothiazine reaction, strychnine poisoning, and conversion disorder. Attempts to culture *C tetani* are associated with poor yield, and a negative culture does not rule out disease. A protective serum antitoxin concentration should not be used to exclude the diagnosis of tetanus.

TREATMENT: Human Tetanus Immune Globulin (TIG), 3000 to 6000 U, given in a single dose, is recommended for treatment; however, the optimal therapeutic dose has not been established. Some experts recommend 500 U, which appears to be as effective as higher doses and causes less discomfort. Available preparations must be given intramuscularly. Infiltration of part of the dose locally around the wound is recommended, although the efficacy of this approach has not been proven. Results of studies on the benefit from intrathecal administration of TIG are conflicting. The TIG preparation in use in the United States is not licensed or formulated for intrathecal or intravenous use.

- In countries where TIG is not available, equine tetanus antitoxin may be available. Equine antitoxin, 1500 to 3000 U, is administered after appropriate testing for sensitivity and desensitization if necessary. This product no longer is available in the United States.
- Immune Globulin Intravenous (IGIV) contains antibodies to tetanus and can be considered for treatment in a dose of 200 to 400 mg/kg if TIG is not available. The US Food and Drug Administration has not licensed IGIV for this use, and antitetanus antibody concentrations are not assessed routinely in IGIV.
- All wounds should be cleaned and débrided properly, especially if extensive "necrosis is present. In neonatal tetanus, wide excision of the umbilical stump is not indicated.
- Supportive care and pharmacotherapy to control tetanic spasms are of major importance.
- Oral (or intravenous) metronidazole (30 mg/kg per day, given at 6-hour intervals; maximum, 4 g/day) is effective in decreasing the number of vegetative forms of *C tetani* and is the antimicrobial agent of choice. Parenteral penicillin G (100 000 U/kg per day, given at 4- to 6-hour intervals; maximum 12 million U/day) is an alternative treatment. Therapy for 7 to 10 days recommended.
- Active immunization against tetanus always should be undertaken during convalescence from tetanus. Because of the extreme potency of tiny amounts of toxin, tetanus disease may not result in immunity.

ISOLATION OF THE HOSPITALIZED PATIENT: Standard precautions are recommended.

CONTROL MEASURES:

Care of Exposed People (see Table 3.75). Following a dose of tetanus toxoid, anti-tetanus antibody begins to be detectable at 4 to 7 days and reaches maximum concentrations by 2 to 4 weeks (although protective concentrations can be achieved by 1 to 2 weeks in previously immunized people, depending on which order dose is being given and how long it has been since the previous dose). The maximum response following a dose varies by individual and the order of dose (eg, first, second, third, etc) being administered. Protective anti-tetanus antibody is not reliably achieved following a first dose of tetanus toxoid and occurs too late to reliably prevent tetanus disease. Following intramuscular administration, the circulating half-life of TIG is approximately 28 days. After completion of the primary immunization with tetanus toxoid, antitoxin persists at protective concentrations in most people for at least 10 years and for a longer time after a booster immunization.

- The use of tetanus toxoid with or without TIG in management of wounds depends on the nature of the wound and the history of immunization with tetanus toxoid, as described in Table 3.75.

- In the unusual circumstance that an infant is born outside the hospital and the umbilical cord likely is contaminated (eg, cut with nonsterile equipment), maternal history of tetanus immunization should be confirmed. If the mother's tetanus immunization status is unknown and she is unlikely to have been immunized, TIG should be administered to the neonate unless tetanus serostatus can be confirmed quickly. Infant diphtheria and tetanus toxoids and acellular pertussis vaccine (DTaP) should be given on the standard schedule.

- For infants younger than 6 months who have not received a full 3-dose primary series of tetanus toxoid-containing vaccine, decisions on the need for TIG with wound care should be based on the mother's tetanus toxoid immunization history at the time of delivery, applying the guidelines in Table 3.75.

Table 3.75. Guide to Tetanus Prophylaxis in Routine Wound Management

History of Adsorbed Tetanus Toxoid (Doses)	Clean, Minor Wounds		All Other Wounds[a]	
	DTaP, Tdap, or Td[b]	TIG[c]	DTaP, Tdap, or Td[b]	TIG[c]
Fewer than 3 or unknown	Yes	No	Yes	Yes
3 or more	No if <10 y since last tetanus-containing vaccine dose	No	No[d] if <5 y since last tetanus-containing vaccine dose	No
	Yes if ≥10 y since last tetanus-containing vaccine dose	No	Yes if ≥5 y since last tetanus-containing vaccine dose	No

Tdap indicates booster tetanus toxoid, reduced diphtheria toxoid, and acellular pertussis vaccine; DTaP, diphtheria and tetanus toxoids and acellular pertussis vaccine; Td, adult-type diphtheria and tetanus toxoids vaccine; TIG, Tetanus Immune Globulin (human).

[a] Such as, but not limited to, wounds contaminated with dirt, feces, soil, and saliva (eg, following animal bites); puncture wounds; avulsions; and wounds resulting from missiles, crushing, burns, and frostbite.

[b] DTaP is used for children younger than 7 years. Tdap is preferred over Td for underimmunized children 7 years and older who have not received Tdap previously.

[c] Immune Globulin Intravenous should be used when TIG is not available.

[d] More frequent boosters are not needed and can accentuate adverse effects.

- Although any open wound is a potential source of tetanus, wounds contaminated with dirt, feces, soil, or saliva (eg, animal bites) are at increased risk. Punctures and wounds containing devitalized tissue, including necrotic or gangrenous wounds, frostbite, crush and avulsion injuries, and burns particularly are conducive to *C tetani* infection.
- If tetanus immunization is incomplete at the time of wound treatment, a dose of vaccine should be given, and the immunization series should be completed according to the age-appropriate primary immunization schedule. TIG should be administered for tetanus-prone wounds in patients infected with HIV or other severe immunodeficiency, regardless of the history of tetanus immunizations.
- DTaP is the recommended and preferred vaccine for children 6 weeks through 6 years of age and for catch-up immunization for children 4 months through 6 years of age (see **http://aapredbook.aappublications.org/site/resources/izschedules. xhtml**). When a booster injection is indicated for wound prophylaxis in a child younger than 7 years, DTaP should be used unless pertussis vaccine is contraindicated (see Pertussis, p 608), in which case immunization with diphtheria and tetanus toxoids (DT) vaccine is recommended.
- When tetanus toxoid is required for wound prophylaxis in a child 7 through 10 years of age, use of adult-type diphtheria and tetanus toxoids (Td) vaccine instead of tetanus toxoid alone is advisable so that diphtheria immunity also is maintained. If the child is previously underimmunized for pertussis, tetanus toxoid, reduced diphtheria toxoid, and acellular pertussis vaccine (Tdap) should be administered.
- Adolescents 10 through 18 years of age who require a tetanus toxoid-containing vaccine as part of wound management should receive a single dose of Tdap instead of Td if they have not received Tdap previously (see Pertussis, p 608). People 19 years and older who require a tetanus toxoid-containing vaccine as part of wound management should receive Tdap instead of Td if they previously have not received Tdap.
- When TIG is required for wound prophylaxis, it is administered intramuscularly in a dose of 250 U (regardless of age or weight). IGIV is recommended if TIG is unavailable. If tetanus toxoid and TIG or IGIV are administered concurrently, separate syringes and sites should be used. Administration of TIG or IGIV does not preclude initiation of active immunization with adsorbed tetanus toxoid. Efforts should be made to initiate immunization and arrange for its completion. Administration of tetanus toxoid simultaneously with or at an interval after receipt of IG does not impair development of protective antibody substantially.
- Regardless of immunization status, wounds should be cleaned and débrided properly if dirt or necrotic tissue is present. Wounds should receive prompt surgical treatment to remove all devitalized tissue and foreign material as an essential part of tetanus prophylaxis. It is not necessary or appropriate to débride puncture wounds extensively.

Immunization. Active immunization with tetanus toxoid is recommended for all people. For all appropriate indications, tetanus immunization is administered with diphtheria toxoid-containing vaccines or with diphtheria toxoid- and acellular pertussis-containing vaccines. Vaccine is administered intramuscularly and may be given concurrently with other vaccines (see Simultaneous Administration of Multiple Vaccines, p 35). Conjugate vaccines containing tetanus toxoid (eg, *Haemophilus influenzae* type b and a meningococcal conjugate vaccine) are not substitutes for tetanus toxoid immunization. Recommendations for use of tetanus toxoid-containing vaccines (**http://aapredbook.aappublications.org/site/ resources/izschedules.xhtml**) are as follows:

- Immunization for children from 6 weeks of age to the seventh birthday should consist of 5 doses of tetanus and diphtheria toxoid-containing vaccine. All doses are given as DTaP (or DTaP-containing vaccines). The initial 3 doses are administered at 2-month intervals beginning at approximately 2 months of age. A fourth dose is recommended 6 to 12 months after the third dose, usually at 15 through 18 months of age (see Pertussis, p 608). The final dose of DTaP is recommended before school entry (kindergarten or elementary school) at 4 through 6 years of age, unless the fourth dose was given after the fourth birthday in which case the preschool (fifth) dose is omitted. DTaP can be given concurrently with other vaccines (see Simultaneous Administration of Multiple Vaccines, p 35).
- For children younger than 7 years who have received fewer than the recommended number of doses of pertussis vaccine but who have received the recommended number of DT doses for their age (ie, children in whom immunization was started with DT and who then were given DTaP [or diphtheria and tetanus toxoid and whole-cell pertussis vaccine, DTwP, outside the United States]), dose(s) of DTaP should be given to complete the recommended pertussis immunization schedule (see Pertussis, p 608). However, the total number of doses of diphtheria and tetanus toxoids (as DT, DTaP, or DTwP) should not exceed 6 before the seventh birthday.
- Immunization against tetanus and diphtheria for children younger than 7 years in whom pertussis immunization is contraindicated (see Pertussis, p 608) should be accomplished with DT instead of DTaP, as follows:
  - For children younger than 1 year, 3 doses of DT are administered at 2-month intervals; a fourth dose should be administered 6 to 12 months after the third dose, and the fifth dose should be administered before school entry at 4 through 6 years of age.
  - For children 1 through 6 years of age who have not received previous doses of DT, DTaP, or DTwP, 2 doses of DT approximately 2 months apart should be administered, followed by a third dose 6 to 12 months later to complete the initial series. DT can be given concurrently with other vaccines. An additional dose is recommended before school entry at 4 through 6 years of age unless the preceding dose was given after the fourth birthday.
  - For children 1 through 6 years of age who have received 1 or 2 doses of DTaP, DTwP, or DT during the first year of life and for whom further pertussis immunization is contraindicated, additional doses of DT should be administered until a total of 5 doses of diphtheria and tetanus toxoids are received by the time of school entry. The fourth dose is administered 6 to 12 months after the third dose. The preschool (fifth) dose is omitted if the fourth dose was given after the fourth birthday.

Other recommendations for tetanus immunization, including recommendations for older children, are as follows:

- For catch-up immunization for children 7 through 10 years of age, Tdap vaccine should be substituted for a single dose of Td in the catch-up series (see **http://aapredbook.aappublications.org/site/resources/izschedules.xhtml**).[1]
- Adolescents 11 years and older should receive a single dose of Tdap instead of Td for booster immunization against tetanus, diphtheria, and pertussis. The preferred age for Tdap immunizations is 11 through 12 years of age.

[1]American Academy of Pediatrics, Committee on Infectious Diseases. Additional recommendations for use of tetanus toxoid, reduced-content diphtheria toxoid, and acellular pertussis vaccine (Tdap). *Pediatrics.* 2011;128(4):809–812

- Adolescents 11 years and older who received Td but not Tdap should receive a single dose of Tdap to provide protection against pertussis. Tdap can be administered regardless of time since receipt of last tetanus- or diphtheria-containing vaccine.
- If more than 5 years have elapsed since the last dose, a booster dose of a tetanus-containing vaccine should be considered for people at risk of occupational exposure in locations where tetanus boosters may not be available readily. Tdap is preferred over Td if the person has not received Tdap previously.
- Prevention of neonatal tetanus can be accomplished by prenatal immunization of the previously unimmunized women and those for whom 10 years have passed since their previous tetanus-containing vaccine.
- Pregnant women who have not completed their primary series should receive 3 vaccinations containing tetanus and reduced diphtheria toxoids, if time permits. The recommended schedule is 0, 4 weeks, and 6 through 12 months. If there is insufficient time, 2 doses of Td should be administered at least 4 weeks apart, and the second dose should be given at least 2 weeks before delivery. Tdap should replace 1 of the Td doses, preferably between 27 and 36 weeks of gestation (see Pertussis, p 608).
- Active immunization against tetanus always should be undertaken during convalescence from tetanus, because this exotoxin-mediated disease usually does not confer immunity.

Adverse Events, Precautions, and Contraindications. Severe anaphylactic reactions, Guillain-Barré syndrome (GBS), and brachial neuritis attributable to tetanus toxoid have been reported but are rare. No increased risk of GBS has been observed with use of DTaP in children, and therefore, no special precautions are recommended when immunizing children with a history of GBS.

An immediate anaphylactic reaction to tetanus and diphtheria toxoid-containing vaccines (ie, DTaP, Tdap, DT, or Td, or conjugate vaccine containing diphtheria or tetanus toxoid) is a contraindication to further doses unless the patient can be desensitized to these toxoids (see Pertussis, p 608).

People who experienced Arthus-type hypersensitivity reactions or temperature greater than 39.4°C (103°F) after a previous dose of a tetanus toxoid-containing preparation usually have very high serum tetanus antibody concentrations and should not receive even emergency doses of tetanus toxoid-containing preparation more frequently than every 10 years, even if they have a wound that is neither clean nor minor.

Other Control Measures. Sterilization of hospital supplies will prevent the rare instances of tetanus that may occur in a hospital from contaminated sutures, instruments, or plaster casts.

For prevention of neonatal tetanus, preventive measures (in addition to maternal immunization) include community immunization programs for adolescent girls and women of childbearing age and appropriate training of midwives in recommendations for immunization and sterile technique.

Tinea Capitis
(Ringworm of the Scalp)

CLINICAL MANIFESTATIONS: Dermatophytic fungal infections of the scalp have 3 major forms: "black dot," "gray patch," and favus:

- "Black dot" tinea capitis is the most common manifestation in the United States. It begins as an erythematous scaling patch over the scalp that slowly enlarges and often is recognized only when hair loss becomes noticeable. The name comes from the areas of alopecia in which the hair is broken off flush with the scalp, giving the appearance of black dots. Inflammation, which may be accompanied by tender lymphadenopathy, can be prominent and can be confused for pyoderma or discoid lupus erythematosus. Scarring with permanent alopecia can occur in the absence of treatment.

- "Gray patch" tinea capitis also begins as a well-demarcated erythematous, scaling patch over the scalp and spreads centrifugally. Lesions can be singular or multiple and are accompanied by hair breakage a few millimeters above the scalp.
- Favus (tinea favosa) primarily manifests as a perifollicular erythema of the scalp that can progress to yellow crusting known as scutula, which can coalesce into confluent, adherent masses overlying severe hair loss.
- Both "black dot and "gray patch" tinea capitis can evolve into kerion, a boggy erythematous nodule lacking hair, which can become suppurative and drain. Kerion can be mistaken for a primary bacterial abscess or cellulitis but, in fact, represents an extreme inflammatory response to the fungus. However, secondary bacterial infection also can occur. As with other forms of tinea, a dermatophytic or id reaction can develop and can involve a papular, vesicular, or "eczema-like" eruption that often is pruritic and may be extensive, involving the face, trunk, and/or extremities. When this reaction develops following initiation of therapy, it sometimes is mistaken for a drug eruption.

The differential diagnosis for tinea capitis includes atopic dermatitis, seborrheic dermatitis, psoriasis, bacterial folliculitis or abscess, trichotillomania, alopecia areata, head lice, and scarring alopecia, such as discoid lupus.

ETIOLOGY: Tinea capitis develops when dermatophyte fungal elements invade the scalp hair follicle and shaft. The specific pathogen varies by geographic region and mode of transmission. The prime causes of the disease are fungi of the genus *Trichophyton*, including *Trichophyton tonsurans* (commonly associated with "black dot" tinea capitis) and *Trichophyton schoenleinii* (commonly associated with favus). An endemic form of "gray patch" tinea capitis is caused by *Microsporum canis*.

EPIDEMIOLOGY: "Black dot" tinea capitis predominantly is a disease of young African American school-aged children but has been reported in all racial and ethnic groups as well as in infants and postmenopausal female caregivers. "Gray patch" tinea capitis is rare in North America, as is tinea favus, which remains more common in areas such as Iran, China, and Nigeria. Pathogenic dermatophytes can be transmitted to affected people by other humans, animals (especially pet cats or dogs), or the environment. The organism remains viable for prolonged periods on fomites (eg, brushes, combs, hats), and the rate of asymptomatic carriage and infected individuals among family members of index cases is high. The role of asymptomatic carriers is unclear, but they may to serve as a reservoir of infection within families, schools, and communities.

The **incubation period** is unknown but is thought to be 1 to 3 weeks. Symptoms are caused by hypersensitivity reaction of the host. Dermatophyte infections have been reported in infants as young as 1 week of age.

DIAGNOSTIC TESTS: The presence of alopecia, scale, and neck lymphadenopathy makes the diagnosis of tinea capitis almost certain, and most clinicians will choose to treat empirically prior to laboratory confirmation. Dermoscopic evaluation of areas of alopecia with a lighted magnifier may show comma- or corkscrew-shaped hairs. Hairs and scale obtained by gentle scraping of a moistened area of the scalp with a blunt scalpel, toothbrush, brush, or tweezers are used for potassium hydroxide wet mount examination. The dermatophyte test medium also is a reliable, simple, and inexpensive method of diagnosing tinea capitis. Skin scrapings from lesions are inoculated directly onto culture medium and incubated at room temperature. After 1 to 2 weeks, a phenol red indicator in the agar will turn from yellow to red in the area surrounding a dermatophyte colony. When necessary, the diagnosis also can be confirmed by culture on Sabouraud dextrose agar, although this often requires an incubation for 3 to 4 weeks.

Scalp scales and hairs may be scraped or plucked from the scalp for immediate evaluation utilizing potassium hydroxide prep mounts. Arthroconidia can be visualized within the hair shaft in endothrix infections, such as *T tonsurans*, while ectothrix infections, such as *M canis*, exhibit conidia on the outside of the hair shaft. In both forms, septate hyphae may be visualized in scrapings from the scalp surface. Woods lamp evaluation is only useful if a *Microsporum* infection is present, in which case affected areas will fluoresce yellow-green. Polymerase chain reaction and periodic acid-Schiff stain evaluation of specimens are possible but are not generally used.

TREATMENT: Optimal treatment of tinea capitis is controversial, and current treatment options are summarized in Table 3.76. Experts generally use higher doses of griseofulvin than have been approved by the US Food and Drug Administration or that were used in clinical trials. Griseofulvin is approved by the FDA for children 2 years or older, is available in either liquid or tablet form, can be dosed on a daily basis, and should be taken with fatty foods. Although high-dose griseofulvin is considered standard of care for *M canis* infections, many experts believe that terbinafine is a better choice for *T tonsurans* infections because of the shorter duration of therapy required for cure. Shorter (usually

Table 3.76. Recommended Therapy for Tinea Capitis

Drug	Dosage	Duration
Griseofulvin microsize (liquid 125 mg/5 mL)	20–25 mg/kg/day	≥6 wk; continue until clinically clear
Griseofulvin ultramicrosize (tablets of varying size)	10–15 mg/kg/day	≥6 wk; continue until clinically clear
Terbinafine tablets (250 mg)	4–6 mg/kg/day 10–20 kg: 62.5 mg 20–40 kg: 125 mg >40 kg: 250 mg	*T tonsurans:* 2–6 wk *M canis:* 8–12 wk
Terbinafine granules (125 mg and 187.5 mg)	<25 kg: 125 mg 25–35 kg: 187.5 mg >35 kg: 250 mg	FDA approved for children ≥4 y 6-wk duration for all species
Fluconazole	6 mg/kg/day	3–6 wk FDA approved for children >2 y

4 weeks) courses of terbinafine are either equal to or superior to longer-term griseofulvin therapy for *T tonsurans* infection. Terbinafine granules are approved by the FDA for the treatment of tinea capitis in children 4 years and older for 6 weeks. The capsules can be opened and mixed in nonacidic food, such as pudding or peanut butter, when required. Terbinafine dosing is weight-based (Table 3.76). Off-label use in younger children and alternate therapy using terbinafine tablets, which can be split and mixed with foods, are therapeutic options. The granule dosing is higher than that traditionally recommended for the tablets, reflecting the finding that terbinafine clearance of drug is higher in children. The FDA recommends baseline liver function testing before instituting therapy. Some practitioners perform follow-up testing 4 to 6 weeks later. Fluconazole is the only oral antifungal that is approved by the FDA for children younger than 2 years, and azole agents also have been used for tinea capitis. Laboratory evaluation is not required for healthy children who receive 8 weeks or less of therapy.

Topical treatment may be useful as an adjunct to systemic therapy in order to decrease carriage of viable conidia. Selenium sulfide, ketoconazole, or ciclopirox shampoos (although not FDA approved for this use and ineffective by themselves) can be applied 2 to 3 times per week and left in place for 5 to 10 minutes; duration of therapy should continue for at least 2 weeks; some experts recommend continuing topical treatments until clinical and mycologic cure occurs.

Kerion is managed by systemic treatment as outlined previously; combined antifungal and corticosteroid therapy (either oral or intralesional) has not been shown to be superior to antifungal therapy alone. Unless secondary bacterial infection has occurred, treatment with antibiotics generally is unnecessary.

ISOLATION OF THE HOSPITALIZED PATIENT: Standard precautions apply.

CONTROL MEASURES: Infected children should receive systemic therapy and generally also should receive adjunct topical management. They should not be excluded from school once therapy has been instituted. Family members and close contacts should be questioned regarding symptoms, and anyone with symptoms should be evaluated. Some experts recommend topical antifungal shampoo therapy for asymptomatic family members, but evidence is lacking regarding the efficacy of this intervention. Sharing of fomites such as hats and combs/brushes should be avoided in households with an affected person. If pets are suspected as a source of infection, treatment of the affected animal should be implemented.

Tinea Corporis
(Ringworm of the Body)

CLINICAL MANIFESTATIONS: Superficial tinea infections of the nonhairy (glabrous) skin, termed tinea corporis, involve the face, trunk, or limbs. The lesion often is ring-shaped or circular (hence, the lay term "ringworm"), slightly erythematous, and well demarcated with a scaly, vesicular, or pustular border and central clearing. Small confluent plaques or papules as well as multiple lesions can occur, particularly in wrestlers (tinea gladiatorum). Lesions can be mistaken for psoriasis, pityriasis rosea, nummular eczema, erythema annulare centrifugum, or atopic, seborrheic, or contact dermatitis. A frequent source of confusion is an alteration in the appearance of lesions as a result of application of a topical corticosteroid preparation, termed tinea incognito. Such patients also may develop Majocchi granuloma, a follicular fungal infection associated with a granulomatous dermal reaction. In patients with diminished T-lymphocyte function (eg, human immunodeficiency virus infection), skin lesions may appear as grouped papules or pustules unaccompanied by scaling or erythema.

A pruritic, fine, papular or vesicular eruption (dermatophytic or id reaction) involving the trunk, hands, or face, caused by a hypersensitivity response to infecting fungus, may accompany skin lesions. Tinea corporis can occur in association with tinea capitis, and examination of the scalp should be performed.

ETIOLOGY: The prime causes of the disease are fungi of the genus *Trichophyton,* especially *Trichophyton tonsurans, Trichophyton rubrum,* and *Trichophyton mentagrophytes*; the genus *Microsporum,* especially *Microsporum canis*; and *Epidermophyton floccosum. Microsporum gypseum* also occasionally can cause infection.

EPIDEMIOLOGY: These causative fungi occur worldwide and are transmissible by direct contact with infected humans, animals, soil or fomites. Fungi in lesions are communicable.

The **incubation period** is thought to be 1 to 3 weeks but can be shorter, as documented infections have occurred at 6 days of life in infants with unaffected mothers. Symptoms are caused by hypersensitivity reaction of the host.

DIAGNOSTIC TESTS: Fungi responsible for tinea corporis can be detected by microscopic examination of a potassium hydroxide wet mount of skin scrapings. Use of dermatophyte test medium also is a reliable, simple, and inexpensive method of diagnosing tinea corporis. Skin scrapings from lesions are inoculated directly onto culture medium and incubated at room temperature. After 1 to 2 weeks, a phenol red indicator in the agar will turn from yellow to red in the area surrounding a dermatophyte colony. When necessary, the diagnosis also can be confirmed by culture on Sabouraud dextrose agar, although this often requires an incubation for 3 to 4 weeks. Histopathologic diagnosis using periodic acid-Schiff staining and polymerase chain reaction diagnostic tools are available but are expensive and generally unnecessary.

TREATMENT: Topical application of a miconazole, clotrimazole, terbinafine (12 years of age and older), tolnaftate, or ciclopirox (10 years of age and older) preparation twice a day or of a ketoconazole, econazole, naftifine, oxiconazole, sertaconazole, butenafine (12 years of age and older), or sulconazole preparation once a day is recommended (see Topical Drugs for Superficial Fungal Infections, p 913). Topical econazole, ketoconazole, naftifine, and sulconazole are not approved by the US Food and Drug Administration (FDA) for use as antifungal agents in children. Although clinical resolution may be evident within 2 weeks of therapy, continuing therapy for another 2 to 4 weeks generally is recommended. If significant clinical improvement is not observed after 4 to 6 weeks of treatment, an alternate diagnosis should be considered. Topical preparations of antifungal medication mixed with high-potency corticosteroids should not be used, because these often are less effective and can lead to a more deep-seated follicular infection (Majocchi granuloma); in addition, local and systemic adverse events from the corticosteroids can occur.

If lesions are extensive or unresponsive to topical therapy, griseofulvin may be administered orally for 6 weeks (see Tinea Capitis, p 778). Oral itraconazole, fluconazole, and terbinafine are alternative effective options for more severe cases; these agents are not approved by the FDA for this purpose in children and have a much different benefit-to-risk profile. If Majocchi granulomas are present, oral antifungal therapy is recommended, because topical therapy is unlikely to penetrate deeply enough to eradicate infection.

ISOLATION OF THE HOSPITALIZED PATIENT: Standard precautions are recommended.

CONTROL MEASURES: Direct contact with known or suspected sources of infection should be avoided. Periodic inspections of contacts for early lesions and prompt therapy are recommended. Athletic mats and equipment should be cleaned frequently, and actively infected athletes in sports with person-to-person contact must be excluded from competitions. Athletes with tinea corporis cannot participate in matches for 72 hours after commencement of topical therapy unless the affected area can be covered. Infected pets also should receive antifungal treatment.

Tinea Cruris
(Jock Itch)

CLINICAL MANIFESTATIONS: Tinea cruris is a common superficial fungal disorder of the groin and upper thighs. Concomitant tinea pedis has been reported in patients with tinea cruris as well as previous episodes of tinea cruris. The eruption usually is bilaterally symmetric and sharply marginated, often with polycyclic borders. Involved skin is erythematous and scaly and varies from red to brown; occasionally, the eruption is accompanied by central clearing and can have a vesiculopapular border. In chronic infections, the margin may be subtle, and lichenification may be present. Tinea cruris skin lesions may be extremely pruritic. The appearance of tinea cruris may be altered in patients who have erroneously been treated with topical corticosteroids (tinea incognito), including diminished erythema, absence of typical scaling border, and development of folliculitis (Majocchi granuloma). These lesions should be differentiated from candidiasis, intertrigo, seborrheic dermatitis, psoriasis, atopic dermatitis, irritant or allergic contact dermatitis (generally caused by therapeutic agents applied to the area), and erythrasma. The latter is a superficial bacterial infection of the skin caused by *Corynebacterium minutissimum*.

ETIOLOGY: The fungi *Epidermophyton floccosum*, *Trichophyton rubrum*, and *Trichophyton mentagrophytes* are the most common causes. *Trichophyton tonsurans*, *Trichophyton verrucosum*, and *Trichophyton interdigitale* also have been identified.

EPIDEMIOLOGY: Tinea cruris occurs predominantly in adolescent and adult males, mainly via indirect contact from desquamated epithelium or hair. Moisture, close-fitting garments, friction, and obesity are predisposing factors. Direct or indirect person-to-person transmission may occur. This infection commonly occurs in association with tinea pedis, and all infected patients should be evaluated for this possibility, with careful evaluation of the interdigital web spaces. Onychomycosis also is a possible association, particularly in adolescents and adults.

The **incubation period** is unknown but is thought to be approximately 1 to 3 weeks. Symptoms are caused by hypersensitivity reaction of the host.

DIAGNOSTIC TESTS: Fungi responsible for tinea cruris may be detected by microscopic examination of a potassium hydroxide wet mount of scales. Use of dermatophyte test medium also is a reliable, simple, and inexpensive method of diagnosing tinea cruris. Skin scrapings from lesions are inoculated directly onto culture medium and incubated at room temperature. After 1 to 2 weeks, a phenol red indicator in the agar will turn from yellow to red in the area surrounding a dermatophyte colony. When necessary, the diagnosis also can be confirmed by culture on Sabouraud dextrose agar, although this often requires an incubation for 3 to 4 weeks. Polymerase chain reaction assay is a more expensive diagnostic tool that generally is not required. A characteristic coral-red fluorescence under Wood light can identify the presence of erythrasma (an eruption of reddish brown patches attributable to the presence of *Corynebacterium minutissimum*) and, thus, exclude tinea cruris.

TREATMENT: Twice-daily topical application for 4 to 6 weeks of a clotrimazole, miconazole, terbinafine (12 years and older), tolnaftate, or ciclopirox (10 years and older) preparation rubbed or sprayed onto the affected areas and surrounding skin is effective. Once-daily therapy with topical econazole, ketoconazole, naftifine, oxiconazole, butenafine (12 years and older), or sulconazole preparation also is effective (see Topical Drugs for Superficial Fungal Infections, p 913). Topical econazole, ketoconazole, and sulconazole are not approved by the US Food and Drug Administration for use as antifungal agents in children. Tinea pedis, if present, should be treated concurrently (see Tinea Pedis and Tinea Unguium, p 784). Treatment of concurrent onychomycosis (tinea unguium) also may reduce the risk of recurrence.

Topical preparations of antifungal medication mixed with high-potency corticosteroids should be avoided because of the potential for prolonged infections and local and systemic adverse corticosteroid-induced events. Loose-fitting, washed cotton underclothes to decrease chafing, avoidance of hot baths, and use of an absorbent powder can be helpful adjuvants to therapy. Griseofulvin, given orally for 6 weeks, may be effective in unresponsive cases (see Tinea Capitis, p 778). Oral itraconazole, fluconazole, and terbinafine are more effective therapies in adults but may have a less advantageous benefit-to-risk profile. If Majocchi granulomas are present, oral antifungal therapy is recommended as topical therapy is unlikely to penetrate deeply enough to eradicate infection. Because many conditions mimic tinea cruris, a differential diagnosis should be considered if primary treatments fail, and a fungal culture should be performed if the diagnosis is in question.

ISOLATION OF THE HOSPITALIZED PATIENT: Standard precautions are recommended.

CONTROL MEASURES: Infections should be treated promptly. Potentially involved areas should be kept dry to prevent recurrences, and loose undergarments should be worn. Patients should be advised to dry the groin area before drying their feet to avoid inoculating dermatophytes of tinea pedis into the groin area.

Tinea Pedis and Tinea Unguium
(Athlete's Foot, Ringworm of the Feet)

CLINICAL MANIFESTATIONS: Tinea pedis manifests as a fine scaly or vesiculopustular eruption that commonly is pruritic. Lesions can involve all areas of the foot but usually are patchy in distribution, with a predisposition to fissures and scaling between toes, particularly in the third and fourth interdigital spaces or distributed around the sides of the feet. Toenails may be infected and can be thickened with subungual debris and yellow or white discoloration (tinea unguium). Toenails may be the source for recurrent tinea pedis. Tinea pedis must be differentiated from dyshidrotic eczema, atopic dermatitis, contact dermatitis, juvenile plantar dermatosis, palmoplantar keratoderma, and erythrasma (an eruption of reddish brown patches caused by *Corynebacterium minutissimum*). Tinea pedis commonly occurs in association with tinea cruris and onychomycosis (tinea unguium). Dermatophyte infections commonly affect otherwise healthy people, but immunocompromised people have increased susceptibility.

Tinea pedis and many other fungal infections can be accompanied by a hypersensitivity reaction to the fungi (the dermatophytid or id reaction), with resulting papular or papulovesicular eruptions on the palms and the sides of fingers and, occasionally, by an erythematous vesicular eruption on the extremities, trunk, and face.

ETIOLOGY: The fungi *Trichophyton rubrum, Trichophyton mentagrophytes,* and *Epidermophyton floccosum* are the most common causes of tinea pedis.

EPIDEMIOLOGY: Tinea pedis is a common infection worldwide in adolescents and adults but is less common in young children. Fungi are acquired by contact with skin scales containing fungi or with fungi in damp areas, such as swimming pools, locker rooms, and showers. Tinea pedis can spread throughout a household among family members and is communicable for as long as infection is present.

The **incubation period** is unknown but is thought to be approximately 1 to 3 weeks. Symptoms are caused, in part, by hypersensitivity reaction of the host.

DIAGNOSTIC TESTS: Tinea pedis usually is diagnosed by clinical manifestations and may be confirmed by microscopic examination of a potassium hydroxide wet mount of cutaneous scrapings. Use of dermatophyte test medium is a reliable, simple, and inexpensive method of diagnosing tinea pedis and tinea unguium. Skin scrapings from lesions are inoculated directly onto the culture medium and incubated at room temperature. After 1 to 2 weeks, a phenol red indicator in the agar will turn from yellow to red in the area surrounding a dermatophyte colony. When necessary, the diagnosis also can be confirmed by culture on Sabouraud dextrose agar, although this often requires an incubation of 3 to 4 weeks. Infection of the nail can be verified by direct microscopic examination with potassium hydroxide, fungal culture of desquamated subungual material, or fungal stain of a nail clipping fixed in formalin. Periodic acid-Schiff stain has the highest sensitivity for detecting fungus but does not identify the associated species, and cannot necessarily differentiate other mold infections from dermatophyte infections.

TREATMENT: Topical application of terbinafine, twice daily; ciclopirox; or an azole agent (clotrimazole, miconazole, econazole, oxiconazole, sertaconazole, ketoconazole), once or twice daily, usually is adequate for milder cases of tinea pedis. Acute vesicular lesions may be treated with intermittent use of open wet compresses (eg, with Burrow solution, 1:80). Dermatophyte infections in other locations, if present, should be treated concurrently (see Tinea Cruris, p 783).

Tinea pedis that is severe, chronic, or refractory to topical treatment may be treated with oral therapy. Oral itraconazole or terbinafine is the most effective, with griseofulvin next and fluconazole least effective. None are approved by the US Food and Drug Administration (FDA) for treatment of tinea pedis. Id (hypersensitivity response) reactions are treated by wet compresses, topical corticosteroids, occasionally systemic corticosteroids, and eradication of the primary source of infection.

Recurrence is prevented by proper foot hygiene, which includes keeping the feet dry and cool, gentle cleaning, drying between the toes, use of absorbent antifungal foot powder, frequent airing of affected areas, and avoidance of occlusive footwear and nylon socks or other fabrics that interfere with dissipation of moisture.

In people with onychomycosis (tinea unguium), topical therapy should be used only when the infection is confined to the distal ends of the nail; however, even topical therapy for 48 weeks typically has a cure rate less than 20%. Topical ciclopirox (8% [approved by the FDA for people 12 years and older]) may be applied to affected toenail(s) once daily in combination with a comprehensive nail management program. Studies in adults have demonstrated the best cure rates after therapy with oral itraconazole or terbinafine; however, safety and effectiveness in children has not been established. Terbinafine is approved by the FDA as 250 mg, daily, for 12 weeks in adults for toenail infection and 250 mg, daily, for 6 weeks for fingernail infection.

Guidelines for dosing of terbinafine for children are based on studies for tinea capitis and are weight based: children weighing 10 to 20 kg, 62.5 mg/day, orally; children weighing 20 to 40 kg, 125 mg/day, orally; and children weighing >40 kg, 250 mg/day, orally (Table 3.76, p 780). The duration of therapy is the same as in adults. Pediatric dosing of itraconazole is less well established. Recurrences are common. Removal of the nail plate followed by use of oral therapy during the period of regrowth can help to affect a cure in resistant cases.

ISOLATION OF THE HOSPITALIZED PATIENT: Standard precautions are recommended.

CONTROL MEASURES: Treatment of patients with active infections should decrease transmission. Public areas conducive to transmission (eg, swimming pools) should not be used by people with active infection. Chemical foot baths are of no value and can facilitate spread of infection. Because recurrence after treatment is common, proper foot hygiene is important (as described in Treatment). People should be advised to dry the groin area before drying their feet to avoid inoculating tinea pedis dermatophytes into the groin area.

Toxocariasis
(Visceral Toxocariasis [previously Visceral Larva Migrans]; Ocular Toxocariasis [previously Ocular Larva Migrans])

CLINICAL MANIFESTATIONS: The severity of symptoms depends on the number of larvae ingested and the degree of the inflammatory response. Most people who are infected are asymptomatic. Characteristic manifestations of visceral toxocariasis include fever, leukocytosis, eosinophilia, hypergammaglobulinemia, wheezing, abdominal pain, and hepatomegaly. Other manifestations include malaise, anemia, cough, and in rare instances, pneumonia, myocarditis, and encephalitis. Atypical manifestations include hemorrhagic rash and seizures. When ocular invasion (resulting in endophthalmitis or retinal granulomas) occurs, other evidence of infection usually is lacking, suggesting that the visceral and ocular manifestations are distinct syndromes.

ETIOLOGY: Toxocariasis is caused by *Toxocara* species, which are common roundworms of dogs and cats (especially puppies or kittens), specifically *Toxocara canis* and *Toxocara cati* in the United States; most cases are caused by *T canis*. Other nematodes of animals also can cause this syndrome, although rarely.

EPIDEMIOLOGY: On the basis of a nationally representative survey, 14% of the US population has serologic evidence of *Toxocara* infection. Visceral toxocariasis typically occurs in children 2 to 7 years of age, often with a history of pica, but can occur in older children and adults. Ocular toxocariasis usually occurs in older children and adolescents. Humans are infected by ingestion of soil containing infective eggs of the parasite. Eggs may be found wherever dogs and cats defecate, often in sandboxes and playgrounds. Eggs become infective after 2 to 4 weeks in the environment and may persist long term in the soil. Direct contact with dogs is of secondary importance, because eggs are not infective immediately when shed in the feces. Infection risk is highest in hot, humid regions where eggs persist in soil.

The **incubation period** cannot be accurately determined.

DIAGNOSTIC TESTS: Hypereosinophilia and hypergammaglobulinemia associated with increased titers of isohemagglutinin to the A and B blood group antigens are presumptive evidence of infection. An enzyme immunoassay for *Toxocara* antibodies in serum, available at the Centers for Disease Control and Prevention and some commercial laboratories, can provide confirmatory evidence of toxocariasis but does not distinguish between past and current, active infection. This assay is specific and sensitive for diagnosis of visceral toxocariasis but is less sensitive for diagnosis of ocular toxocariasis. Microscopic identification of larvae in a liver biopsy specimen is diagnostic, but this finding is rare. A liver biopsy negative for larvae, therefore, does not exclude the diagnosis.

TREATMENT: Albendazole is the recommended drug for treatment of toxocariasis (see Drugs for Parasitic Infections, p 927). The drug has been approved by the US Food and Drug Administration, but not for this indication. Alternate drugs include mebendazole and ivermectin, although mebendazole no longer is available in the United States. In severe cases with myocarditis or involvement of the central nervous system, corticosteroid therapy should be considered. Correcting the underlying causes of pica helps prevent reinfection.

Antiparasitic treatment of ocular toxocariasis may not be effective. Inflammation may be decreased by topical or systemic corticosteroids, and secondary damage may be decreased with ophthalmologic surgery.

ISOLATION OF THE HOSPITALIZED PATIENT: Standard precautions are recommended.

CONTROL MEASURES: Proper disposal of cat and dog feces is essential. Regular veterinary care and treatment of dogs and cats, and especially puppies and kittens, with anthelmintics prevents excretion of eggs by worms acquired from the environment, transplacentally, or through the mother's milk. Covering sandboxes when not in use is helpful. No specific management of exposed people is recommended.

Toxoplasma gondii Infections
(Toxoplasmosis)

The term *Toxoplasma gondii* infection is reserved for the asymptomatic presence of the parasite in the setting of an acute or chronic infection. In contrast, the term toxoplasmosis is used when the parasite causes symptoms and/or signs during the primary or acute infection (eg, congenital infection, infectious mononucleosis presentation) or reactivation of *T gondii* in an immunosuppressed patient or ocular reactivation in those with congenital or postnatally acquired infection.

CLINICAL MANIFESTATIONS:

Congenital Infection. Although infants with congenital infection can be born without clinical manifestations at birth, visual or hearing impairment, learning disabilities, or mental retardation will become apparent in a large proportion of these children several months to years later. The incidence of chorioretinitis later in life is affected by whether a person's mother was screened and treated during gestation at the time of acute maternal infection.

Major clinical signs of congenital toxoplasmosis include chorioretinitis, cerebral calcifications, and hydrocephalus; they can be present alone or in combination. The concomitant presence of these 3 major signs ("classic triad") is rare but is highly suggestive of congenital toxoplasmosis; it historically was seen primarily in babies whose mothers were not treated for toxoplasmosis during gestation. More than 70% of congenitally infected children develop chorioretinitis later in life if born to mothers who were not treated during gestation, and up to 30% do so if born to mothers who received treatment. Additional signs of congenital toxoplasmosis at birth include microcephaly, seizures, hearing loss, strabismus, a maculopapular rash, generalized lymphadenopathy, hepatomegaly, splenomegaly, jaundice, pneumonitis, diarrhea, hypothermia, anemia, petechiae, and thrombocytopenia. As a consequence of intrauterine infection, meningoencephalitis with cerebrospinal fluid (CSF) abnormalities can develop. Some severely affected fetuses/infants die in utero or within a few days of birth. Cerebral calcifications can be demonstrated by plain radiograph, ultrasonography, or computed tomography (CT) imaging of the head. CT is the radiologic technique of choice, because it is the most sensitive for calcifications and can reveal brain abnormalities when plain radiographic and/or ultrasonographic studies are normal.

Postnatally Acquired Primary Infection. *T gondii* infection acquired after birth is asymptomatic in most immunocompetent patients. When symptoms develop, they may be nonspecific and can include malaise, fever, headache, sore throat, arthralgia, and myalgia. Lymphadenopathy, frequently cervical, is the most common sign. Patients occasionally have a mononucleosis-like illness associated with a macular rash and hepatosplenomegaly. The clinical course usually is benign and self-limited. In a subset of immunocompetent individuals and in immunocompromised patients, primary infection presents with persistent fever, myocarditis, myositis, hepatitis, pericarditis, pneumonia, encephalitis with and without brain abscesses, and skin lesions. These syndromes and a more aggressive clinical course, including life-threatening pneumonia, have been documented in patients who acquired primary toxoplasmosis in certain tropical countries in South America, such as French Guiana, Brazil, and Colombia. Toxoplasmosis should be included in the differential diagnosis of ill travelers who return home with these unexplained syndromes.

Ocular toxoplasmosis also occurs in the setting of postnatally acquired infection. In Brazil and Canada, up to 17% of patients diagnosed with postnatally acquired toxoplasmosis have toxoplasmic chorioretinitis. Acute ocular involvement manifests as blurred vision, eye pain, decreased visual acuity, floaters, scotoma, photophobia, or epiphora. The most common late finding is chorioretinitis, which can result in vision loss. Ocular disease can become reactivated years after the initial infection in healthy and immunocompromised people.

Reactivation of Chronic Infection in Immunocompromised Patients. In chronically infected immunodeficient patients, including people with human immunodeficiency virus (HIV) infection, reactivation of *T gondii* can result in life-threatening encephalitis, pneumonitis, toxoplasmic chorioretinitis (a posterior uveitis), fever of unknown origin, or disseminated toxoplasmosis. In patients with acquired immunodeficiency syndrome (AIDS), toxoplasmic encephalitis (TE) is the most common cause of encephalitis and typically presents with acute to subacute neurologic or psychiatric symptoms and multiple ring-enhancing brain lesions. In these patients, a clear improvement in their symptoms and signs within

7 to 10 days of beginning empiric antitoxoplasma drugs is considered diagnostic of TE. However, immunocompromised patients without AIDS (eg, transplant or cancer patients, patients taking immunosuppressive drugs) who are chronically infected with *T gondii* and who present with multiple ring-enhancing brain lesions should undergo an immediate brain biopsy to confirm the diagnosis rather than receiving empiric treatment only. In this latter group of patients, the differential diagnosis should be widened to other pathogens, such as molds and *Nocardia* species. TE also can present as a single brain lesion by magnetic resonance imaging (MRI) or as a diffuse and rapidly progressive process in the setting of apparently negative brain MRI studies. MRI is superior to CT for the diagnosis of TE and can detect lesions not revealed by CT. However, MRI is less likely than CT to detect calcifications in the brain of a toxoplasma-infected newborn infant.

Seropositive hematopoietic stem cell and solid organ transplant patients are at risk of their latent *T gondii* infection being reactivated. In these patients, toxoplasmosis may manifest as pneumonia, unexplained fever or seizures, myocarditis, hepatosplenomegaly, lymphadenopathy, or skin lesions in addition to brain abscesses and diffuse encephalitis. *T gondii*-seropositive solid organ donors (D+) can transmit the parasite via the allograft to seronegative recipients (R–). Thirty percent of D+/R– heart transplant recipients develop toxoplasmosis in the absence of anti-*T gondii* prophylaxis.

ETIOLOGY: *T gondii* is a protozoan and obligate intracellular parasite. *T gondii* organisms exist in nature in 3 primary clonal lineages (types I, II, and III) and several infectious forms (tachyzoite, tissue cysts containing bradyzoites, and oocysts containing sporozoites). The tachyzoite and the host immune response are responsible for symptoms observed during the acute infection or during the reactivation of a latent infection in immunocompromised patients. The tissue cyst is responsible for latent infection and usually is present in brain, skeletal muscle, cardiac tissue, brain, and eyes of humans and other vertebrate animals. It is the tissue cyst form that is transmitted through ingestion of undercooked or raw meat. The oocyst is present in the small intestine of cats and other members of the feline family; it is responsible for transmission through ingestion of soil, water, or food contaminated with cat feces that contain the organism.

EPIDEMIOLOGY: *T gondii* is worldwide in distribution and infects most species of warm-blooded animals. The seroprevalence of *T gondii* infection (a reflection of the chronic infection and measured by the presence of *T gondii*-specific IgG antibodies) varies by geographic locale and the socioeconomic strata of the population. The age-adjusted seroprevalence of infection in the United States has been estimated at 11% among women 15 to 44 years old. Members of the feline family are definitive hosts. Cats generally acquire the infection by ingestion of infected animals (eg, mice), uncooked household meats, soil organic matter, and water or food contaminated with their own oocysts. The parasite replicates sexually in the feline small intestine. Cats may begin to excrete millions of oocysts in their stools 3 to 30 days after primary infection and may shed oocysts for 7 to 14 days. After excretion, oocysts require a maturation phase (sporulation) of 1 to 5 days in temperate climates before they are infective by the oral route. Sporulated oocysts survive for long periods under most ordinary environmental conditions, for example, surviving in moist soil for months and even years. Intermediate hosts (including sheep, pigs, and cattle) can have tissue cysts in the brain, myocardium, skeletal muscle, and other organs. These cysts remain viable for the lifetime of the host. Humans usually become infected by consumption of raw or undercooked meat that contains cysts or by accidental ingestion of sporulated oocysts from soil or in contaminated food or water. A large outbreak linked epidemiologically to contamination of a municipal water supply also has been reported. A recent epidemiologic study revealed the following risk factors associated with acute infection in the United States: eating raw ground beef; eating rare lamb; eating locally produced cured, dried, or smoked meat; working with meat; drinking unpasteurized goat milk; and owning 3 or more kittens. In this study, eating raw oysters, clams, or mussels also was identified as a novel risk factor. Drinking untreated water also was found to have a trend toward increased risk for acute infection in the United States. Although the risk factors for acute infection have been reported in studies from Europe, South America, and the United States, up to 50% of acutely infected people do not recall identifiable risk factors or symptoms. Thus, *T gondii* infection and toxoplasmosis may occur even in patients without a suggestive epidemiologic history or illness. Only appropriate laboratory testing can establish or rule out the diagnosis of *T gondii* infection or toxoplasmosis. There is no evidence of human-to-human transmission except through vertical transmission, blood products or organ transplantation.

Transmission of *T gondii* has been documented in the setting of solid organ (eg, heart, kidney, liver) or hematopoietic stem cell transplantation from a seropositive donor with latent infection to a seronegative recipient. Infection rarely has occurred as a result of a laboratory accident or from blood or blood product transfusion. In most cases, congenital transmission occurs as a result of primary maternal infection during gestation. In utero infection rarely occurs as a result of reactivated parasitemia during pregnancy in chronically infected immunocompromised women. The incidence of congenital toxoplasmosis in the United States has been estimated to be 1 in 1000 to 1 in 10 000 live births

The **incubation period** of acquired infection, on the basis of a well-studied outbreak, is estimated to be approximately 7 days, with a range of 4 to 21 days.

DIAGNOSTIC TESTS: Serologic tests are the primary means of diagnosing primary and latent infection. Polymerase chain reaction (PCR) testing of body fluids and staining of a biopsy specimen with *T gondii*-specific immunoperoxidase are valuable for confirming the diagnosis of toxoplasmosis. Isolation of the parasite occasionally is attempted for the purpose of genotyping the infecting strain. Correlation of genotype with clinical manifestations may be attempted, but results must be interpreted carefully in the context of each clinical scenario. Laboratories with special expertise in *Toxoplasma* serologic assays and their interpretation, such as the Palo Alto Medical Foundation Toxoplasma Serology Laboratory (PAMF-TSL; Palo Alto, CA; **www.pamf.org/serology/**; telephone: (650) 853-4828; e-mail toxolab@pamf.org), are useful to clinicians and nonreference laboratories.

Immunoglobulin (Ig) G-specific antibodies achieve a peak concentration 1 to 2 months after infection and remain positive indefinitely. The vast majority of patients will have low-positive IgG antibody titers 6 months after the acute infection. To determine the approximate time of infection in IgG-positive adults, specific IgM antibody determinations should be performed. The lack of *T gondii*-specific IgM antibodies in a person with low-positive titers of IgG antibodies (eg, a Dye test at PAMF-TSL ≤512) indicates infection of at least 6 months' duration. Detectable *T gondii*-specific IgM antibodies can indicate recent infection, chronic infection or a false-positive reaction. Sera with positive *T gondii*-specific IgM test results may be sent to PAMF-TSL for confirmatory testing and to establish whether the patient has an acute or a chronic infection. Enzyme immunoassays (EIAs) are the most sensitive tests for IgM, and indirect fluorescent antibody tests are the least sensitive tests for detecting IgM. IgM-specific antibodies can be detected 2 weeks after infection (IgG-specific antibodies usually are negative during this period), achieve peak concentrations in 1 month, decrease thereafter, and usually become undetectable within 6 to 9 months. However, in some people, a positive IgM test result may persist for years without apparent clinical significance. In adults, a positive IgM test should be followed by confirmatory testing at a laboratory with special expertise in *Toxoplasma* serology when determining the timing of infection is important clinically (eg, in a pregnant woman).

Laboratory tests that have been found to be helpful in determining timing of infection in patients with positive IgM test results include an IgG avidity test, the AC/HS or differential agglutination test, and IgA- and IgE-specific antibody tests. The presence of high-avidity IgG antibodies indicates that infection occurred at least 12 to 16 weeks prior. However, the presence of low-avidity antibodies is not a reliable indication of more recent infection, and treatment may affect the maturation of IgG avidity and prolong the presence of low-avidity antibodies. A nonacute pattern in the AC/HS test usually is indicative of an infection that was acquired at least 12 months before the serum was obtained. Tests to detect IgA and IgE antibodies, which decrease to undetectable concentrations sooner than IgM antibodies do, also are useful for diagnosis of congenital infections and infections in pregnant women, for whom more precise information about the duration of infection is needed. *T gondii*-specific IgA and IgE antibody tests are available in *Toxoplasma* reference laboratories but generally not in other laboratories. Diagnosis of *Toxoplasma* infection during pregnancy should be made on the basis of results of serologic assays performed in a reference laboratory.

PCR assay and *T gondii*-specific immunoperoxidase staining can be attempted with virtually any body fluid or tissue, depending on the clinical scenario. Specimens on which PCR assay can be performed include amniotic fluid, CSF, whole blood, bronchoalveolar lavage fluid, vitreous fluid, aqueous humor, peritoneal fluid, ascitic fluid, pleural fluid, bone marrow, and urine. Essentially any tissue can be stained with *T gondii*-specific immunoperoxidase; the presence of extracellular antigens and a surrounding inflammatory response also are diagnostic of toxoplasmosis. A positive PCR test result in tissue must be interpreted with caution, because it does not distinguish reactivation from inactive chronic latent infection.

Special Situations.

Prenatal. A definitive diagnosis of congenital toxoplasmosis can be made prenatally by detecting parasite DNA in amniotic fluid by PCR assay. Isolation of the parasite by mouse or tissue culture inoculation also can be attempted from amniotic fluid. Serial fetal ultrasonographic examinations can be performed in cases of suspected congenital infection to detect any increase in size of the lateral ventricles of the central nervous system or other signs of fetal infection, such as brain, hepatic, or splenic calcifications. Some states routinely screen all newborn infants for the presence of antibody to *T gondii*.

Postnatal. Congenital toxoplasmosis should be considered in infants born to: (1) women suspected of having or who have been diagnosed with primary *T gondii* infection during gestation; (2) women infected shortly before conception (eg, within 3 months of conception); (3) immunocompromised women (HIV-infected or otherwise) with serologic evidence of past infection with *T gondii;* or (4) any infant with clinical signs or laboratory abnormalities suggestive of congenital infection.

Toxoplasma-specific IgG, IgM (by the immunosorbent agglutination assay [ISAGA] method), and IgA tests should be performed for all newborn infants suspected of having congenital toxoplasmosis in a laboratory with expertise in *Toxoplasma* serologic assays. Infected newborn infants can have any combination of positive or negative IgM and IgA antibodies. Although placental leak occasionally can lead to false-positive IgM or IgA reactions in the newborn infant, repeat testing after approximately 10 days of life can help confirm the diagnosis, because the half-life of these immunoglobulins is short and the titers in an infant who is not infected should decrease rapidly. The sensitivity of *T gondii*-specific IgM as determined by an ISAGA is 87% in newborn infants born to mothers not treated during gestation; sensitivity for IgA antibodies is 77%; and when both are taken into consideration, the sensitivity increases to 93%. The indirect fluorescent assay or EIA for IgM should not be relied on to diagnose congenital infection.

If the mother was not tested during pregnancy, a maternal serum sample also should be tested for IgG and IgM, and the AC/HS test should be performed as soon as it is feasible. Maternal test results can help in the interpretation of newborn test results. In newborn infants with clinical signs, peripheral blood, CSF, and urine specimens should be assayed for *T gondii* by PCR assay in a reference laboratory. Evaluation of the infant should include ophthalmologic, auditory, and neurologic examinations; lumbar puncture; and CT of the head. An attempt may be made to isolate *T gondii* by mouse inoculation from placenta, umbilical cord blood, CSF, urine, or peripheral blood specimens. Examination of the placenta by histologic tools and PCR assay can be helpful, but a positive result does not necessarily indicate that the newborn is infected.

Congenital infection is confirmed serologically by persistently positive IgG titers beyond the first 12 months of life. Conversely, in an uninfected infant, a continuous decrease in IgG titer before 12 months without detection of IgM or IgA antibodies will occur. Transplacentally transmitted IgG antibody usually becomes undetectable by 6 to 12 months of age. Congenital toxoplasmosis can be confirmed before 12 months of age in infants with the following laboratory test results: (1) a persistently positive or increasing IgG antibody concentration compared with the mother; (2) a positive *Toxoplasma*-specific IgM (after 5 days of life) or IgA assay (after 10 days of life); (3) a positive PCR test result in CSF, peripheral blood, or urine; or (4) a positive IgG antibody test accompanied by clinical signs in a newborn infant born to a mother who was infected during gestation.

Immunocompromised Patients. Immunocompromised patients (eg, patients with AIDS, solid organ transplant recipients, patients with cancer, or people taking immunosuppressive drugs) who are infected latently with *T gondii* have variable titers of IgG antibody to *T gondii* but rarely have IgM antibody. Immunocompromised patients should be tested for *T gondii*-specific IgG before commencing immunosuppressive therapy or as soon as their status of immunosuppression is diagnosed to determine whether they are chronically infected with *T gondii* and at risk of reactivation of latent infection. Active disease in immunosuppressed patients may or may not result in seroconversion and a fourfold increase in IgG antibody titers; consequently, serologic diagnosis in these patients often is difficult. Previously seropositive patients may have changes in their IgG titers in any direction (increase, decrease, or no change) without any clinical relevance. In these patients, PCR testing, histologic examination, and attempts to isolate the parasite become the laboratory methods of choice to diagnose toxoplasmosis.

In HIV-infected patients who are seropositive for *T gondii* IgG, reactivation of their latent infection usually is manifested by TE. TE can be diagnosed presumptively on the basis of characteristic clinical and radiographic findings. MRI usually reveals the presence of multiple brain-occupying and ring-enhancing lesions. If there is no clinical response within 10 days to an empiric trial of anti-*T gondii* therapy, demonstration of *T gondii* organisms, antigen, or DNA in specimens such as blood, CSF, or bronchoalveolar fluid may be necessary to confirm the diagnosis. TE also can present as diffuse encephalitis without space-occupying lesions on brain MRI. Prompt recognition of this syndrome and confirmation of the diagnosis by PCR testing in CSF is crucial, because these patients usually exhibit a rapidly progressive and fatal clinical course.

Diagnosis of TE in immunocompromised patients other than HIV-infected people requires confirmation by brain biopsy or PCR testing of CSF. In this group of patients, other organisms, such as invasive mold infections and nocardiosis, should be considered before beginning an empiric trial of anti-*T gondii* therapy.

Infants born to women who are infected simultaneously with HIV and *T gondii* should be evaluated for congenital toxoplasmosis because of an increased likelihood of maternal reactivation and congenital transmission in this setting. Expert advice is available at the PAMF-TSL (**www.pamf.org/serology/**; telephone [650] 853-4828; e-mail toxolab@pamf.org) and the National Collaborative Chicago-Based Congenital Toxoplasmosis Study [NCCCTS]; Chicago, IL; **www.uchospitals.edu/specialties/infectious-diseases/toxoplasmosis/;** telephone [773] 834-4131; e-mail rmcleod@midway.uchicago.edu).

Ocular Toxoplasmosis. Toxoplasmic chorioretinitis usually is diagnosed on the basis of characteristic retinal lesions in conjunction with a positive serum *T gondii*-specific IgG test result. All patients with eye disease should have an IgM test performed; if a positive IgM test result is confirmed at a reference laboratory and eye lesions are consistent with toxoplasmic chorioretinitis, ocular disease is the result of an acute *T gondii* infection rather than reactivation of a chronic infection. Patients who have atypical retinal lesions or who fail to respond to anti-*T gondii* therapy should undergo examination of vitreous fluid or aqueous humor by PCR, and antibody testing (by using the Goldmann-Witmer coefficient, which compares the levels of intraocular antibody production to that of serum, as measured by enzyme-linked immunosorbent assay [ELISA] or radioimmunoassay) should be considered.

TREATMENT[1]: Most cases of acquired infection in an immunocompetent host do not require specific antimicrobial therapy unless infection occurs during pregnancy or symptoms are severe or persistent. When indicated (eg, chorioretinitis or significant organ damage), the combination of pyrimethamine and sulfadiazine,[2] with supplemental leucovorin (folinic acid) to minimize pyrimethamine-associated hematologic toxicity, is the regimen most widely accepted for children and adults with acute symptomatic disease (see Drugs for Parasitic Infections, p 927). Trimethoprim-sulfamethoxazole (TMP-SMX) has been reported to be equivalent to pyrimethamine/sulfadiazine in the treatment of patients with toxoplasmic chorioretinitis. In addition, pyrimethamine can be used in combination with clindamycin, atovaquone, or azithromycin if the patient does not tolerate sulfonamide compounds. Corticosteroids appear to be useful in management of ocular complications, central nervous system disease (CSF protein >1000 mg/dL), and focal lesions with substantial mass effects in certain patients.

---

[1]American Academy of Pediatrics, Committee on Infectious Diseases. Technical report: the prevention and treatment of congenital toxoplasmosis. *Pediatrics.* 2015; in press

[2]Available from Sandoz Inc, Princeton, NJ (800-526-0225).

HIV-infected adolescents and children 6 years or older who have completed initial therapy (at least 6 weeks and clinical response) for TE should receive suppressive therapy (secondary prophylaxis; see Table 3.77) to prevent recurrence until their CD4+ T-lymphocyte count recovers above 200 cells/μL and their HIV viral load is nondetectable for at least 6 months. HIV-infected children 1 through 5 years of age also should receive suppressive therapy after completion of initial therapy; discontinuation may be considered after they have been on stable antiretroviral therapy (ART) for longer than 6 months, are asymptomatic, and have demonstrated an increase in CD4+ T-lymphocyte percentage above 15% for more than 3 consecutive months. Prophylaxis should be reinstituted whenever these parameters are not met. Regimens for primary treatment also are effective for suppressive therapy.

Table 3.77. Prophylaxis to Prevent First Episode and Recurrence of Toxoplasmosis in Children

Prevention of	Indication	First Choice	Alternatives
First episode of toxoplasmosis[a]	Severe immuno-suppression and presence of immunoglobulin G antibody to *Toxoplasma*	Trimethoprim-sulfamethoxazole, 150–750 mg/m^2/day in 2 divided doses, orally, every day	Dapsone (children 1 mo of age or older), 2 mg/kg or 15 mg/m^2 (max 25 mg), orally, every day; **PLUS** pyrimethamine, 1 mg/kg, orally every day (max 25 mg); **PLUS** leucovorin, 5 mg, orally, every 3 days Atovaquone, children 1 through 3 mo or older than 24 mo of age; 30 mg/kg, orally, every day; children 4–24 mo of age: 45 mg/kg, orally, every day
Recurrence of toxoplasmosis[b]	Prior to toxoplasmic encephalitis or toxoplasmosis	Sulfadiazine, 85–120 mg/kg/day (max 2–4 g) in 2–4 divided doses, orally, every day, **PLUS** pyrimethamine, 1 mg/kg or 15 mg/m^2 (maximum, 25 mg), orally, every day; **PLUS** leucovorin, 5 mg, orally, every 3 days	Clindamycin, 20–30 mg/kg/day in 3–4 divided doses, orally, every day, **PLUS** pyrimethamine 1 mg/kg, orally, every day (max 25 mg); **PLUS** leucovorin, 5 mg, orally, every 3 days Atovaquone, children 1 through 3 mo or older than 24 mo of age; 30 mg/kg, orally, every day; children 4–24 mo of age: 45 mg/kg, orally, every day

[a]Protection against toxoplasmosis is provided by the preferred antipneumocystis regimen (TMP-SMX) and possibly by atovaquone but not by pentamidine. Atovaquone may be used with or without pyrimethamine. Pyrimethamine alone provides little, if any, protection (for information about severe immunosuppression, see Table 3.57, p 641).

[b]Only pyrimethamine plus sulfadiazine confers protection against *Pneumocystis jirovecii* pneumonia as well as toxoplasmosis. Although the clindamycin plus pyrimethamine regimen is recommended in adults, this regimen has not been tested in children and has been found to have high rates of relapses in adults. However, these drugs are safe and are used for other infections.

Primary prophylaxis to prevent the first episode of toxoplasmosis generally is recommended for HIV-infected adolescents and children 6 years or older who are *T gondii*-seropositive and have CD4+ T-lymphocyte counts less than 100/μL (see Table 3.77, p 794). HIV-infected children 1 through 5 years of age should initiate primary prophylaxis when CD4+ T-lymphocyte percentage falls below 15%. Alternative regimens and recommendations for discontinuation of prophylaxis after the CD4+ T-lymphocyte count recovers in association with antiretroviral therapy are available.[1] TMP-SMX, when administered for *Pneumocystis jirovecii* pneumonia (PCP) prophylaxis, also provides prophylaxis against toxoplasmosis. Dapsone plus pyrimethamine or atovaquone also may provide protection. Children older than 12 months who qualify for PCP prophylaxis and who are receiving an agent other than TMP-SMX or atovaquone should have serologic testing for *Toxoplasma* antibodies, because alternative drugs for PCP prophylaxis such as pentamidine are not effective against *T gondii*. Severely immunosuppressed children who are not receiving TMP-SMX or atovaquone and who are found to be seropositive for *Toxoplasma* infection should receive prophylaxis for both PCP and toxoplasmosis (ie, dapsone plus pyrimethamine).

Primary prophylaxis with TMP-SMX or atovaquone also is recommended for previously seropositive patients who undergo allogeneic hematopoietic stem cell or bone marrow transplantation. In addition, D+/R− heart transplant recipients also must receive primary prophylaxis with TMP-SMX, atovaquone, or pyrimethamine. For immunocompromised patients without HIV infection, suppressive therapy should be continued lifelong or until the patient no longer is significantly immunosuppressed.

For symptomatic and asymptomatic congenital infections, pyrimethamine combined with sulfadiazine (supplemented with folinic acid) is recommended as initial therapy. Duration of therapy is prolonged and often is 1 year. However, the optimal dosage and duration are not established definitively and should be determined in consultation with an infectious diseases specialist. Some experts alternate pyrimethamine/sulfadiazine/folinic acid monthly with spiramycin during months 7 through 12 of treatment in infants with mild disease. Children with moderate or severe congenital toxoplasmosis should receive pyrimethamine/sulfadiazine for the full 12 months.

Treatment: of primary *T gondii* infection in pregnant women, including women with HIV infection, is recommended. Appropriate specialists should be consulted for management. Spiramycin treatment of primary infection during gestation is used in an attempt to prevent transmission of *T gondii* from the mother to the fetus but does not treat the fetus if in utero infection already has occurred because spiramycin does not cross the placenta. Maternal therapy may decrease the severity of sequelae in the fetus once congenital toxoplasmosis has occurred. Spiramycin is available only as an investigational drug in the United States but may be obtained from the manufacturer, at no cost, following the advice of PAMF-TSL and with authorization from the US Food and Drug Administration.[2] If

---

[1] Guidelines for prevention and treatment of opportunistic infections in HIV-exposed and HIV-infected children. Recommendations from the National Institutes of Health, Centers for Disease Control and Prevention, the HIV Medicine Association of the Infectious Diseases Society of America, the Pediatric Infectious Diseases Society, and the American Academy of Pediatrics. *Pediatr Infect Dis J.* 2013;32(Suppl 2):i–KK4. Available at: **http://aidsinfo.nih.gov/guidelines/html/5/ pediatric-oi-prevention-and-treatment-guidelines/0**

[2] US Food and Drug Administration, Division of Antiinfective Products. Telephone: (301) 796-1400; fax: (301) 796-9881.

fetal infection is confirmed at or after 18 weeks of gestation or if the mother acquires infection during the third trimester, consideration should be given to starting therapy with pyrimethamine and sulfadiazine.

ISOLATION OF THE HOSPITALIZED PATIENT: Standard precautions are recommended.

CONTROL MEASURES: Consideration should be given to testing of household or close family members of individuals diagnosed with acute *Toxoplasma* infection in settings where individuals at high risk (eg, pregnant women, immunocompromised patients) can be identified.

Pregnant women and immunocompromised patients whose serostatus for *T gondii* is negative or unknown should avoid activities that potentially expose them to cat feces (such as changing litter boxes, gardening, landscaping, or visiting the zoo if lions or tigers are present), or they should wear gloves and wash their hands if such activities are unavoidable. Daily changing of cat litter will decrease the chance of infection, because oocysts are not infective during the first 1 to 2 days after passage. Domestic cats can be protected from infection by feeding them commercially prepared cat food and preventing them from eating undercooked meat and hunting wild rodents and birds.

Oral ingestion of viable *T gondii* can be avoided by: (1) avoiding consumption of raw or undercooked meat and cooking meat—particularly pork, lamb, and venison—to an internal temperature of 65.5°C to 76.6°C (150°F–170°F [no longer pink]) before consumption (smoked meat and meat cured in brine are not considered safe); (2) freezing meat to −12°C (10°F) for 48 hours; (3) washing fruits and vegetables; (4) washing hands and cleaning kitchen surfaces after handling fruits, vegetables, and raw meat; (5) washing hands after gardening or other contact with soil; (6) preventing contamination of food with raw or undercooked meat or soil; (7) avoiding ingestion of raw shellfish such as oysters, clams, and mussels; (8) avoiding ingestion of raw goat milk; and (9) avoiding ingestion of untreated water, particularly in resource-limited countries. All HIV-infected people and pregnant women should be counseled about the various sources of toxoplasmic infection. There currently is no vaccine available for prevention of *T gondii* infection or toxoplasmosis. Additional resources for health care personnel may be found at **www. cdc.gov/parasites/toxocariasis/health_professionals/index.html.**

Trichinellosis
(*Trichinella spiralis* and Other Species)

CLINICAL MANIFESTATIONS: The clinical spectrum of infection ranges from inapparent to fulminant and fatal illness, but most infections are asymptomatic. The severity of disease is proportional to the infective dose. During the first week after ingesting infected meat, a person may experience abdominal discomfort, nausea, vomiting, and/or diarrhea as excysted larvae infect the intestine. Two to 8 weeks later, as progeny larvae migrate into tissues, fever, myalgia, periorbital edema, urticarial rash, and conjunctival and subungual hemorrhages may develop. In severe infections, myocarditis, neurologic involvement, and pneumonitis can occur in 1 or 2 months. Larvae may remain viable in tissues for years; calcification of some larvae in skeletal muscle usually occurs within 6 to 24 months and may be detected on radiographs.

ETIOLOGY: Infection is caused by nematodes (roundworms) of the genus *Trichinella*. At least 5 species capable of infecting only warm-blooded animals have been identified. Worldwide, *Trichinella spiralis* is the most common cause of human infection.

EPIDEMIOLOGY: Infection is enzootic worldwide in carnivores and omnivores, especially scavengers. Infection occurs as a result of ingestion of raw or insufficiently cooked meat containing encysted larvae of *Trichinella* species. Commercial and home-raised pork remain a source of human infections, but meats other than pork, such as venison, horse meat, and particularly meats from wild carnivorous or omnivorous game (especially bear, boar, seal, and walrus) are now the most common sources of infection. The disease is not transmitted from person to person.

The **incubation period** usually is less than 1 month.

DIAGNOSTIC TESTS: Eosinophilia up to 70%, in conjunction with compatible symptoms and dietary history, suggests the diagnosis. Increases in concentrations of muscle enzymes, such as creatinine phosphokinase and lactic dehydrogenase, occur. Identification of larvae in suspect meat can be the most rapid source of diagnostic information. Encapsulated larvae in a skeletal muscle biopsy specimen (particularly deltoid and gastrocnemius) can be visualized microscopically beginning 2 weeks after infection by examining hematoxylin-eosin stained slides or sediment from digested muscle tissue. Serologic tests are available through commercial and state laboratories and the Centers for Disease Control and Prevention. Serum antibody titers generally take 3 or more weeks to become positive and may remain positive for years. Testing paired acute and convalescent serum specimens usually is diagnostic.

TREATMENT: Albendazole and mebendazole have comparable efficacy for treatment of trichinellosis (see Drugs for Parasitic Infections, p 927). However, albendazole and mebendazole are less effective for *Trichinella* larvae already in the muscles, and neither drug is approved by the US Food and Drug Administration for trichinellosis. Mebendazole no longer is available in the United States. Coadministration of corticosteroids with mebendazole or albendazole often is recommended when systemic symptoms are severe. Corticosteroids can be lifesaving when the central nervous system or heart is involved.

ISOLATION OF THE HOSPITALIZED PATIENT: Standard precautions are recommended.

CONTROL MEASURES: Transmission to pigs can be prevented by not feeding pigs garbage, by preventing cannibalism among animals, and by effective rat control. The public should be educated about the necessity of cooking pork and meat of wild animals thoroughly (>160°F [71°C] internal temperature). Specific recommendations:

* For whole cuts of meat (excluding poultry and wild game): cook to at least 145°F (63°C) as measured with a food thermometer placed in the thickest part of the meat, then allow the meat to rest for 3 minutes before carving or consuming.
* For ground meat (including wild game, excluding poultry): cook to at least 160°F (71°C); ground meats do not require a rest time.
* For all wild game (whole cuts and ground): cook to at least 160°F (71°C).

Freezing pork less than 6 inches thick at 5°F (−15°C) for 20 days kills *T spiralis*. However, *Trichinella* organisms in wild animals, such as bears and raccoons, are resistant to freezing. People known to have ingested undercooked contaminated meat recently should be treated with albendazole (or mebendazole, but this no longer is available in the United States).

Trichomonas vaginalis Infections
(Trichomoniasis)

CLINICAL MANIFESTATIONS: *Trichomonas vaginalis* infection is asymptomatic in 70% to 85% of infected people. Clinical manifestations in symptomatic pubertal or postpubertal females may include a diffuse vaginal discharge, odor, and vulvovaginal pruritus and irritation. Dysuria and, less often, lower abdominal pain can occur. Vaginal discharge may be any color, but classically is yellow-green, frothy, and malodorous. The vulva and vaginal mucosa can be erythematous and edematous. The cervix can be inflamed and sometimes is covered with numerous punctate cervical hemorrhages and swollen papillae, referred to as "strawberry" cervix. This finding occurs in less than 5% of infected females but is highly suggestive of trichomoniasis. Clinical manifestations in symptomatic men include urethritis and, rarely, epididymitis or prostatitis. Reinfection is common, and resistance to treatment is rare but increasing. Rectal infections are uncommon, and oral infections have not been described.

T vaginalis infections in pregnant women have been associated with premature rupture of the membranes and preterm delivery. Perinatal infection may occur in up to 5% of children of infected mothers. *T vaginalis* in female newborn infants may cause vaginal discharge during the first weeks of life but usually is self-limited, resolving as maternal hormones are metabolized. Respiratory infections in newborn infants may occur as well.

ETIOLOGY: *T vaginalis* is a flagellated protozoan approximately the size of a leukocyte. It requires adherence to host cells for survival. The genome of *T vaginalis* has been sequenced.

EPIDEMIOLOGY: Although formal surveillance programs are not in place, several studies suggest that *T vaginalis* infection is the most common curable sexually transmitted infection (STI) in the United States and globally. Prevalence in a nationally representative sample of sexually experienced 14- to 19-year-old females in the United States was 3.6%. It commonly coexists with other conditions, particularly with *Neisseria gonorrhoeae* and *Chlamydia trachomatis* infections and bacterial vaginosis. Transmission results almost exclusively from sexual contact, and the presence of *T vaginalis* in a child or preadolescent beyond the perinatal period is considered highly suspicious for sexual abuse. *T vaginalis* infection can increase both the acquisition and transmission of human immunodeficiency virus (HIV).

The **incubation period** averages 1 week but ranges from 5 to 28 days.

DIAGNOSTIC TESTS: Diagnosis in a symptomatic female typically is established by careful and immediate examination of a wet-mount preparation of vaginal discharge. The jerky motility of the protozoan and the movement of the flagella are distinctive. Microscopy has 50% to 65% sensitivity for *T vaginalis* diagnosis in females and is less sensitive in males; test sensitivity declines if the evaluation is delayed.[1] The presence of symptoms and the identification of the organism are related directly to the number of organisms present. The nucleic acid amplification test (NAAT) is the most sensitive means

---

[1] Centers for Disease Control and Prevention. Sexually transmitted diseases treatment guidelines, 2014. *MMWR Recomm Rep.* 2015; in press

of diagnosing *T vaginalis* infection and is encouraged for detection in females and males. The APTIMA *Trichomonas vaginalis* assay (Hologic Gen-Probe, San Diego, CA) is a commercially available, US Food and Drug Administration (FDA)-cleared product available for testing vaginal specimens, endocervical specimens, female urine, and liquid cytology specimens. The BD Probe Tec TV Q^x Amplified DNA Assay (Becton Dickinson, Franklin Lakes, NJ) is FDA-cleared for detection of *T vaginalis* infection from endocervical, vaginal, or female urine specimens. The NAAT for *T vaginalis* also has demonstrated superior sensitivity for trichomoniasis diagnosis in men but it is not licensed for male specimens. Laboratories that have met Clinical Laboratory Improvement Amendments (CLIA) requirements and validated their *T vaginalis* NAAT performance on male specimens may offer this test. Culture of *T vaginalis* in Diamond media or other trichomoniasis-specific culture systems (eg, InPouch, BioMed Diagnostics, White City, OR) is a sensitive and specific method of diagnosis in females but has lower sensitivity in males.

Two point-of-care tests are available for testing female vaginal swab specimens in settings where no microscope is available and rapid results are desirable. The OSOM Trichomonas Rapid Test (OSOM, Sekisui Diagnostics, LLC, Exton, PA) is a CLIA-waived, antigen-detection, point-of-care test that uses immunochromatographic capillary flow dipstick technology. Results are available within 10 minutes. The Affirm VPIII (Becton, Dickinson and Company, Franklin Lakes, NJ) is a nucleic acid probe test for *T vaginalis*, *Gardnerella vaginalis*, and *Candida albicans*. Although the Affirm VPIII is considered a point-of-care diagnostic tool, test results are available in 45 minutes. Vaginal specimens can also be sent to a clinical laboratory for Affirm VPIII testing. Both of these vaginitis tests are reported to be more sensitive than microscopy (63% when compared with culture) and to have a specificity of 99%. False-positive results may occur in populations with a low prevalence of disease.

TREATMENT[1]: Treatment of adults with metronidazole (2 g, orally, in a single dose) results in cure rates of approximately 90% to 95%. Treatment with tinidazole (2 g, orally, in a single dose) appears to be similar or even superior to metronidazole. Both drugs are approved for this indication in adults and adolescents, and metronidazole is approved in children. Topical vaginal preparations should not be used, because they do not achieve therapeutic concentrations in the urethra or perivaginal glands. Sexual partners should be treated, even if asymptomatic, because reinfection is a major factor in treatment failures. *T vaginalis* strains with decreased susceptibility to metronidazole have been reported; most of these infections respond to tinidazole or higher doses of metronidazole. If treatment failure occurs with a single 2-g dose of metronidazole and reinfection is excluded, metronidazole, 500 mg, orally, twice daily for 7 days, should be used. If treatment failure occurs following this regimen, a course of either metronidazole or tinidazole, 2 g daily, for 7 days, may be used. If several 1-week regimens have failed in a person who is unlikely to have nonadherence or reinfection, testing of the organism for metronidazole and tinidazole susceptibility is recommended. The CDC (**www.cdc.gov/std**) has accumulated experience with testing and treatment of nitroimidazole-resistant *T vaginalis* and can offer susceptibility testing and management assistance.

Treatment of symptomatic pregnant females should be considered regardless of week of gestation. Metronidazole (2 g, in a single dose) may be used at any stage of pregnancy.

---

[1]Centers for Disease Control and Prevention. Sexually transmitted diseases treatment guidelines, 2014. *MMWR Recomm Rep.* 2015; in press

Although metronidazole treatment produces parasitologic cure, several trials have shown no significant difference in perinatal morbidity following metronidazole treatment. One trial suggested the possibility of increased preterm delivery in women with *T vaginalis* infection who received metronidazole treatment, but study limitations prevented definitive conclusions regarding the risks of treatment. Other studies have shown no positive or negative association between metronidazole use during pregnancy and adverse outcomes of pregnancy. Metronidazole is a pregnancy category B drug (animal studies have revealed no evidence of harm to the fetus, but no adequate and well-controlled studies in pregnant women have been conducted). Tinidazole is a pregnancy category C drug (animal studies have demonstrated an adverse effect, but no adequate and well-controlled studies in pregnant women have been conducted). In lactating women to whom metronidazole is administered, withholding breastfeeding during treatment and for 12 to 24 hours after the last dose will reduce the exposure of metronidazole to the infant. While using tinidazole, interruption of breastfeeding is recommended during treatment and for 3 days after the last dose.

People infected with *T vaginalis* should be evaluated for other STIs, including syphilis, gonorrhea, chlamydia, HIV, and hepatitis B. For newborn infants, infection with *T vaginalis* acquired maternally is self-limited, and treatment generally is not recommended.

ISOLATION OF THE HOSPITALIZED PATIENT: Standard precautions are recommended.

CONTROL MEASURES: Measures to prevent STIs, particularly the consistent and correct use of condoms, are indicated. Patients should be instructed to avoid sexual activity until they and their sexual partners are treated and asymptomatic. In states where it is allowed, patient-delivered partner treatment should be offered (**www.cdc.gov/std/ept/**).

Routine Screening Tests[1]: Although routine *T vaginalis* screening of asymptomatic adolescents is not recommended, screening may be considered for adolescent and young adult females at high risk of infection. Risk factors that may put females at higher risk of *T vaginalis* infection include new or multiple partners, or a history of STIs.

Management of Sexual Partners. All people with a known exposure to *T vaginalis* infection should be treated routinely, regardless of a diagnostic test result. Expedited partner therapy might have a role in partner management for trichomoniasis and may be used in states where this approach is permissible.

Trichuriasis
(Whipworm Infection)

CLINICAL MANIFESTATIONS: Disease caused by the whipworm *Trichuris trichiura* generally is proportional to the intensity of the infection. Although most infected children are asymptomatic, those with heavy infestations can develop a colitis that mimics inflammatory bowel disease and can lead to anemia, physical growth restriction, and clubbing. *T trichiura* dysentery syndrome is more intense and characterized by abdominal pain, tenesmus, and bloody diarrhea with mucus; it can be associated with rectal prolapse.

ETIOLOGY: *T trichiura*, the human whipworm, is the causative agent. Adult worms are 30 to 50 mm long with a large, thread-like anterior end that embeds in the mucosa of the large intestine.

---

[1]American Academy of Pediatrics, Committee on Adolescence, and Society for Adolescent Health and Medicine. Screening for nonviral sexually transmitted infections in adolescents and young adults. *Pediatrics.* 2014;134(1):e302–e311

EPIDEMIOLOGY: The parasite is the second most common soil-transmitted helminth in the world, occurring mainly in tropical regions with poor sanitation. It is coendemic with *Ascaris* and hookworm species. Humans are the natural reservoir. Eggs require a minimum of 10 days of incubation in the soil before they are infectious. The disease is not communicable from person to person.

The **incubation period** is approximately 12 weeks.

DIAGNOSTIC TESTS: Eggs may be found on direct examination of stool, although diagnosis of light to moderate infections may require concentration techniques.

TREATMENT: Albendazole, ivermectin, or mebendazole administered for 3 days provide only moderate rates of cure. Albendazole is considered the treatment of choice in the United States because mebendazole no longer is available in this country. Either albendazole or mebendazole are treatments of choice where mebendazole is available (see Drugs for Parasitic Infections, p 927). In 1-year-old children, the World Health Organization recommends reducing the albendazole dose to half of that given to older children and adults for single-dose and 3-day treatment. Albendazole and ivermectin are not approved by the US Food and Drug Administration for treatment of trichuriasis. Reexamination of stool specimens 2 weeks after therapy to determine whether the worms have been eliminated is helpful for assessing the effectiveness of therapy. A recent study suggests that combination therapy with mebendazole and ivermectin is associated with a higher cure rate than any currently available monotherapy.

ISOLATION OF THE HOSPITALIZED PATIENT: Only standard precautions are recommended, because there is no direct person-to-person transmission.

CONTROL MEASURES: Proper disposal of fecal material is the most effective means of control for whipworm and other soil transmitted helminths. Mass drug administration of benzimidazoles to high-risk groups is recommended by the World Health Organization for the community-based control of trichuriasis and other soil-transmitted helminth infections, although evidence of sustained benefit or reductions in prevalence of infections is limited.

African Trypanosomiasis
(African Sleeping Sickness)

CLINICAL MANIFESTATIONS: The clinical course of human African trypanosomiasis has 2 stages: the first is the hemolymphatic stage in which the parasite multiplies in subcutaneous tissues, lymph, and blood; once the parasite crosses the blood-brain barrier and infects the central nervous system (CNS), the disease enters the second stage, known as the neurologic stage. The rapidity of disease progression and clinical manifestations vary with the infecting subspecies. With *Trypanosoma brucei gambiense* infection (West African sleeping sickness), initial symptoms may be mild and include fever, muscle aches, and malaise. Pruritus, rash, weight loss, and generalized lymphadenopathy can occur. Posterior cervical lymphadenopathy, known as Winterbottom sign, may be present. CNS involvement typically develops after 1 to 2 years with development of behavioral changes, cachexia, headache, hallucinations, delusions, and daytime somnolence followed by nighttime insomnia. In contrast, *Trypanosoma brucei rhodesiense* infection (East African sleeping sickness) is an acute, generalized illness that develops days to weeks after parasite inoculation, with manifestations including high fever, lymphadenopathy, rash, muscle and joint aches, thrombocytopenia, hepatitis, anemia, myocarditis, and rarely, laboratory evidence of disseminated intravascular coagulopathy.

A chancre may develop at the site of the tsetse fly bite. Clinical meningoencephalitis can develop as early as 3 weeks after onset of the untreated systemic illness. Both forms of African trypanosomiasis have high fatality rates; without treatment, infected patients usually die within weeks to months after clinical onset of disease caused by *T brucei rhodesiense* and within a few years from disease caused by *T brucei gambiense.*

ETIOLOGY: Human African trypanosomiasis (sleeping sickness) occurs in sub-Saharan Africa. It is caused by the protozoan parasite *Trypanosoma brucei*, transmitted by blood-feeding tsetse flies. The west and central African (Gambian) form progresses more slowly and is caused by *T brucei gambiense.* The east and southern African (Rhodesian) form is more acute and is caused by *T brucei rhodesiense.* Both are extracellular protozoan hemoflagellates that live in blood and tissue of the human host.

EPIDEMIOLOGY: Approximately 7000 human cases are reported annually worldwide, although only a few cases, which are acquired in Africa, are reported every year in the United States. Transmission is confined to an area in Africa between the latitudes of 15° north and 20° south, corresponding precisely with the distribution of the tsetse fly vector (*Glossina* species). In West and Central Africa, humans are the main reservoir of *T brucei gambiense*, although the parasite sometimes can be found in domestic animals, such as dogs and pigs. In East Africa, wild animals, such as antelope, bush buck, and hartebeest, constitute the major reservoirs for sporadic infections with *T brucei rhodesiense*, although cattle serve as reservoir hosts in local outbreaks. In addition to the bite of the tsetse fly, *T brucei* can also be transmitted congenitally and through blood transfusions or organ transplantation, although these modes are uncommon.

The **incubation period** for *T brucei rhodesiense* infection ranges from 3 to 21 days, and for most cases is 5 to 14 days; for *T brucei gambiense* infection, the incubation period usually is longer but is not well defined.

DIAGNOSTIC TESTS: Diagnosis is made by identification of trypanosomes in specimens of blood, cerebrospinal fluid (CSF), or fluid aspirated from a chancre or lymph node or by inoculation of susceptible laboratory animals (mice) with heparinized blood. Examination of CSF is critical to management and should be performed using the double-centrifugation technique. Concentration and Giemsa staining of the buffy coat layer of peripheral blood also can be helpful and is easier for *T brucei rhodesiense*, because the density of organisms in circulating blood is higher than for *T brucei gambiense*. *T brucei gambiense* is more likely to be found in lymph node aspirates. Identification of trypanosomes or a white blood cell count of 6 or higher in the CSF is the most widely used criteria for CNS involvement; elevated protein and an increase in immunoglobulin M may also suggest second stage disease. Serologic testing is available outside the United States for *T brucei gambiense*; there is no serologic screening test for *T brucei rhodesiense.*

TREATMENT: The choice of drug used for treatment will be dependent on the type and stage of African trypanosomiasis. When no evidence of CNS involvement is present, the drug of choice for the acute hemolymphatic stage of infection is pentamidine for *T brucei gambiense* infection and suramin for *T brucei rhodesiense* infection. For treatment of infection with CNS involvement, the drug of choice is eflornithine for *T brucei gambiense* infection and melarsoprol for *T brucei rhodesiense* infection. Suramin, eflornithine, and melarsoprol can be obtained from the Centers for Disease Control and Prevention (404-718-4745). In certain cases, nifurtimox is added to eflornithine or melarsoprol. For specific dosing recommendations, see Drugs for Parasitic Infections (p 929). Because of the risk of relapse, patients who have had CNS involvement should undergo repeated CSF examinations every 6 months for 2 years.

ISOLATION OF THE HOSPITALIZED PATIENT: Standard precautions are recommended.

CONTROL MEASURES: Travelers to areas with endemic infection should avoid known foci of sleeping sickness and tsetse fly infestation and minimize fly bites by wearing long-sleeved shirts and pants of medium-weight material in neutral colors. Infected patients should not breastfeed or donate blood.

American Trypanosomiasis
(Chagas Disease)

CLINICAL MANIFESTATIONS: The acute phase of *Trypanosoma cruzi* infection lasts 2 to 3 months, followed by the chronic phase that, in the absence of successful antiparasitic treatment, is lifelong. The acute phase, when parasites circulate in the blood, commonly is asymptomatic or characterized by mild, nonspecific symptoms. Young children are more likely to exhibit symptoms than are adults. In some patients, a red, indurated nodule known as a *chagoma* develops at the site of the original inoculation, usually on the face or arms. Unilateral edema of the eyelids, known as the Romaña sign, may occur if the portal of entry was the conjunctiva; it usually is not present. The edematous skin may be violaceous and associated with conjunctivitis and enlargement of the ipsilateral preauricular lymph node. Fever, malaise, generalized lymphadenopathy, and hepatosplenomegaly may develop. In rare instances, acute myocarditis and/or meningoencephalitis can occur. The symptoms of acute Chagas disease resolve without treatment within 3 months, and patients pass into the chronic phase of the infection, during which few or no parasites are found in the blood. Most people with chronic *T cruzi* infection have no signs or symptoms and are said to have the indeterminate form of chronic Chagas disease. In 20% to 30% of cases, serious progressive sequelae affecting the heart and/or gastrointestinal tract develop years to decades after the initial infection (called determinate forms of chronic Chagas disease). Chagas cardiomyopathy is characterized by conduction system abnormalities, especially right bundle branch block, and ventricular arrhythmias and may progress to dilated cardiomyopathy and congestive heart failure. Patients with Chagas cardiomyopathy may die suddenly from ventricular arrhythmias, complete heart block, or emboli phenomena; death also may occur from intractable congestive heart failure. Although cardiac manifestations are more common, some patients with chronic Chagas disease may develop digestive disease with dilatation of the colon and/or esophagus with swallowing difficulties accompanied by severe weight loss. Congenital Chagas disease occurs in 1% to 10% of infants born to infected mothers and may be characterized by low birth weight, hepatosplenomegaly, myocarditis, and/or meningoencephalitis with seizures and tremors, but most infants with congenital *T cruzi* infection have no signs or symptoms of disease. Reactivation of chronic *T cruzi* infection with parasites found in the circulating blood, which may be life threatening, may occur in immunocompromised people, including people infected with human immunodeficiency virus and those who are immunosuppressed after transplantation.

ETIOLOGY: *T cruzi*, a protozoan hemoflagellate, is the cause.

EPIDEMIOLOGY: Parasites are transmitted in feces of infected triatomine insects (sometimes called "kissing bugs"; local Spanish/Portuguese names include *vinchuca, chinche picuda, or barbeiro*). The bugs defecate during or after taking blood. The bitten person is inoculated through inadvertent rubbing of insect feces containing the parasite into the site of the bite or mucous membranes of the eye or the mouth. The parasite also can be transmitted congenitally, during solid organ transplantation, through blood transfusion, and by ingestion of food or drink contaminated by the vector's excreta. Accidental laboratory infections can result from handling parasite cultures or blood from infected people or laboratory animals, usually through needlestick injuries. Vectorborne transmission of the disease is limited to the Western hemisphere, predominantly Mexico and Central and South America. The southern United States has established enzootic cycles of *T cruzi* involving several triatomine vector species and mammalian hosts, such as raccoons, opossums, rodents, and domestic dogs. Nevertheless, most *T cruzi*-infected individuals in the United States are immigrants from areas of Latin America with endemic infection. There are an estimated 300 000 individuals with *T cruzi* infection in the United States. Assuming a 1% to 5% risk of congenital transmission, based on estimates of maternal infection, approximately 63 to 315 infants are born with Chagas disease in the United States every year. Several transfusion- and transplantation-associated cases have been documented in the United States.

The disease is an important cause of morbidity and death in Latin America, where an estimated 8 million people are infected, of whom approximately 30% to 40% either have or will develop cardiomyopathy and/or gastrointestinal tract disorders.

The **incubation period** for the acute phase of disease is 1 to 2 weeks or longer. Chronic manifestations do not appear for years to decades.

DIAGNOSTIC TESTS: During the acute phase of disease, the parasite is demonstrable in blood specimens by Giemsa staining after a concentration technique or in direct wet-mount or buffy coat preparations. Molecular techniques and hemoculture in special media (available at the Centers for Disease Control and Prevention [CDC]) also have high sensitivity in the acute phase. The chronic phase of *T cruzi* infection is characterized by low-level parasitemia; the sensitivity of culture and polymerase chain reaction (PCR) assay generally is less than 50%. Diagnosis in the chronic phase relies on serologic tests to demonstrate immunoglobulin (Ig) G antibodies against *T cruzi*. Serologic tests include indirect immunofluorescent and enzyme immunosorbent assays; however, no single serologic test is sufficiently sensitive or specific for confirmed diagnosis of chronic *T cruzi* infection. The Pan American Health Organization and the World Health Organization recommend that samples be tested using 2 assays of different formats before diagnostic decisions are made.

The diagnosis of congenital Chagas disease can be made during the first 3 months of life by identification of motile trypomastigotes by direct microscopy of fresh anticoagulated blood specimens. PCR testing has higher sensitivity than microscopy. All infants born to seropositive mothers should be screened using conventional serologic testing after 9 months of age, when IgG measurements reflect infant response rather than maternal antibody. Diagnostic testing and consultation are available from the CDC Division of Parasitic Diseases and Malaria (phone: 404-718-4745; e-mail: parasites@cdc.gov;mailto: CDC Emergency Operator [after business hours and on weekends]: 770-488-7100).

TREATMENT: Antitrypanosomal treatment is recommended for all cases of acute and congenital Chagas disease, reactivated infection attributable to immunosuppression, and chronic *T cruzi*-infection in children younger than 18 years. Treatment of chronic *T cruzi* infection in adults without advanced cardiomyopathy also generally is recommended. The only drugs with proven efficacy are benznidazole and nifurtimox (see Drugs for Parasitic Infections, p 927). Neither drug is approved by the US Food and Drug Administration (FDA) for use in the United States, but both drugs can be obtained from the CDC

(Division of Parasitic Diseases and Malaria, 404-718-4745) for treatment of patients under compassionate use protocols.

ISOLATION OF THE HOSPITALIZED PATIENT: Standard precautions should be followed.

CONTROL MEASURES: Risk to travelers is low. Travelers to areas with endemic infection should avoid contact with triatomine bugs (also called "reduviid") by avoiding habitation in buildings vulnerable to infestation, particularly those constructed of mud, palm thatch, or adobe brick. The use of insecticide-impregnated bed nets also may be beneficial. Camping or sleeping outdoors in areas with endemic transmission is not recommended. Travelers to regions with endemic infection also should avoid ingestion of unpasteurized juices, such as sugar cane or açai palm fruit juice, which have been linked to oral transmission of Chagas disease. Diagnostic testing should be performed on members of households with an infected patient if they have had exposure to the vector similar to that of the patient. All children of women with *T cruzi* infection should be tested for Chagas disease.

Education about the mode of spread and methods of prevention is warranted in areas with endemic infection. Homes should be examined for the presence of the vectors, and if found, measures to eliminate the vector should be taken.

Since late 2006, the FDA has cleared 2 screening tests to detect antibodies to *T cruzi* in donated blood (Ortho *T cruzi* ELISA Test System and the Abbott Prism Chagas assay). The American Red Cross and Blood Systems Inc voluntarily began screening all blood donations in January 2007. Recommendations to all blood collection agencies for the appropriate use of serologic tests to reduce the risk of transfusion-transmitted *T cruzi* infection were issued by the FDA in December 2010 (**www.fda. gov/BiologicsBloodVaccines/GuidanceComplianceRegulatoryInformation/ Guidances/Blood/ucm235855.htm**). The Ortho *T cruzi* ELISA Test System also is cleared by the FDA for use to screen organ donors when specimens are obtained while the donor's heart is still beating, and in testing blood specimens to screen cadaveric (non-heart-beating) donors.

Tuberculosis

CLINICAL MANIFESTATIONS: Tuberculosis disease is caused by infection with organisms of the *Mycobacterium tuberculosis* complex. Most infections caused by *M tuberculosis* complex in children and adolescents are asymptomatic. When tuberculosis disease occurs, clinical manifestations most often appear 1 to 6 months after infection (up to 18 months for osteoarticular disease) and include fever, weight loss or poor weight gain, growth delay, cough, night sweats, and chills. Chest radiographic findings after infection rarely are specific for tuberculosis and range from normal to diverse abnormalities, such as lymphadenopathy of the hilar, subcarinal, paratracheal, or mediastinal nodes; atelectasis or infiltrate of a segment or lobe; pleural effusion that can conceal small interstitial lesions; interstitial cavities; or miliary-pattern infiltrates. In selected instances, computed tomography or magnetic resonance imaging of the chest can resolve indistinct radiographic findings, but these methods are not necessary for routine diagnosis. Although cavitation is common in reactivation "adult" tuberculosis, cavitation is uncommon in childhood tuberculosis. Necrosis and cavitation can result from a progressive primary focus in very young or immunocompromised patients and in the setting of lymphobronchial disease. Extrapulmonary manifestations include meningitis and granulomatous inflammation of the lymph nodes, bones, joints, skin, and middle ear and mastoid. Gastrointestinal tuberculosis can mimic inflammatory bowel disease. Renal tuberculosis and progression to disease from latent *M tuberculosis* infection ("adult-type pulmonary tuberculosis") are unusual in younger children but can occur in adolescents. In addition, chronic abdominal pain with peritonitis and intermittent partial intestinal obstruction can be present in disease caused by *M bovis*. Congenital tuberculosis can mimic neonatal sepsis, or the infant may come to medical attention in the first 90 days of life with bronchopneumonia and hepatosplenomegaly. Clinical findings in patients with drug-resistant tuberculosis disease are indistinguishable from manifestations in patients with drug-susceptible disease.

ETIOLOGY: The causative agent is *M tuberculosis* complex, a group of closely related acid-fast bacilli, which routinely includes the human pathogens *M tuberculosis, Mycobacterium bovis,* and *Mycobacterium africanum. M africanum* is rare in the United States, so clinical laboratories do not distinguish it routinely, and treatment recommendations are the same as for *M tuberculosis. M bovis* can be distinguished from *M tuberculosis* in reference laboratories, and although the spectrum of illness caused by *M bovis* is similar to that of *M tuberculosis,* the epidemiology, treatment, and prevention are different, as detailed later in the chapter.

Definitions:

- **Positive tuberculin skin test (TST).** A positive TST result (see Table 3.78) indicates possible infection with *M tuberculosis* complex. Tuberculin reactivity appears

Table 3.78. Definitions of Positive Tuberculin Skin Test (TST) Results in Infants, Children, and Adolescents[a]

Induration 5 mm or greater

Children in close contact with known or suspected contagious people with tuberculosis disease
Children suspected to have tuberculosis disease:
- Findings on chest radiograph consistent with active or previous tuberculosis disease
- Clinical evidence of tuberculosis disease[b]

Children receiving immunosuppressive therapy[c] or with immunosuppressive conditions, including human immunodeficiency (HIV) infection

Induration 10 mm or greater

Children at increased risk of disseminated tuberculosis disease:
- Children younger than 4 years
- Children with other medical conditions, including Hodgkin disease, lymphoma, diabetes mellitus, chronic renal failure, or malnutrition (see Table 3.79, p 812)

Children with likelihood of increased exposure to tuberculosis disease:
- Children born in high-prevalence regions of the world
- Children who travel to high-prevalence regions of the world
- Children frequently exposed to adults who are HIV infected, homeless, users of illicit drugs, residents of nursing homes, incarcerated, or institutionalized

Induration 15 mm or greater

Children age 4 years or older without any risk factors

---

[a]These definitions apply regardless of previous bacille Calmette-Guérin (BCG) immunization (see also Testing for *M tuberculosis* Infection, p 810); erythema alone at TST site does not indicate a positive test result. Tests should be read at 48 to 72 hours after placement.

[b]Evidence by physical examination or laboratory assessment that would include tuberculosis in the working differential diagnosis (eg, meningitis).

[c]Including immunosuppressive doses of corticosteroids (see Corticosteroids, p 824) or tumor necrosis factor-alpha antagonists or blockers (see Biologic Response Modifiers Used to Decrease Inflammation, p 83).

2 to 10 weeks after initial infection; the median interval is 3 to 4 weeks (see The Tuberculin Skin Test, p 810). Bacille Calmette-Guérin (BCG) immunization can produce a positive TST result (see Diagnostic Tests, Testing for *M tuberculosis* Infection).

- **Positive interferon-gamma release assay (IGRA).** A positive IGRA result indicates probable infection with *M tuberculosis* complex. IGRAs measure ex vivo interferon-gamma production from T lymphocytes in response to stimulation with antigens specific to *M tuberculosis* complex, which includes *M tuberculosis* and *Mycobacterium bovis*. However, the IGRA antigens used are not found in BCG or most pathogenic nontuberculous mycobacteria (eg, are not found in *M avium* complex but are found in *Mycobacterium kansasii*, *Mycobacterium szulgai*, and *Mycobacterium marinum*).

- **Exposed person** refers to a person who has had recent (eg, within 3 months) contact with another person with suspected or confirmed contagious tuberculosis disease (ie, pulmonary, laryngeal, tracheal, or endobronchial disease) and who has a negative TST or IGRA result, normal physical examination findings, and chest radiographic findings that are normal or not compatible with tuberculosis. Some exposed people are or become infected (and subsequently develop a positive TST or IGRA result), while others do not become infected after exposure; the 2 groups cannot be distinguished initially.

- **Source case** is defined as the person who has transmitted infection with *M tuberculosis* complex to another person who subsequently develops either latent *M tuberculosis* infection (LTBI) or tuberculosis disease.

- **Latent tuberculosis infection (LTBI)** is defined as *M tuberculosis* complex infection in a person who has a positive TST or IGRA result, no physical findings of disease, and chest radiograph findings that are normal or reveal evidence of healed infection (eg, calcification in the lung, hilar lymph nodes, or both).

- **Tuberculosis disease** is defined as illness in a person with infection in whom symptoms, signs, or radiographic manifestations caused by *M tuberculosis* complex are apparent; disease can be pulmonary, extrapulmonary, or both.

- **Contagious tuberculosis** refers to tuberculosis disease typical of the lungs or airway in a person where there is the potential to transmit *M tuberculosis* to other people.

- **Directly observed therapy (DOT)** is defined as an intervention by which medications are administered directly to the patient by a health care professional or trained third party (not a relative or friend) who observes and documents that the patient ingests each dose of medication.

- **Multiply drug-resistant (MDR) tuberculosis** is defined as infection or disease caused by a strain of *M tuberculosis* complex that is resistant to at least isoniazid and rifampin, the 2 first-line drugs with greatest efficacy.

- **Extensively drug-resistant (XDR) tuberculosis** is a subset of MDR tuberculosis. It is defined as infection or disease caused by a strain of *M tuberculosis* complex that is resistant to isoniazid and rifampin, at least a fluoroquinolone, and at least 1 of the following parenteral drugs: amikacin, kanamycin, or capreomycin.

- **Bacille Calmette-Guérin (BCG)** is a live-attenuated vaccine strain of *M bovis*. BCG vaccine rarely is administered to children in the United States but is one of the most widely used vaccines in the world. An isolate of BCG can be distinguished from wild-type *M bovis* only in a reference laboratory.

EPIDEMIOLOGY: Case rates of tuberculosis in all ages are higher in urban, low-income areas and in nonwhite racial and ethnic groups; more than 80% of reported cases in the

United States occur in Hispanic and nonwhite people. In recent years, 60% of all US cases have been in people born outside the United States. Almost 75% of all childhood TB is associated with some form of foreign contact of the child, parent, or a household member. Specific groups with greater LTBI and disease rates include immigrants, international adoptees, refugees from or travelers to high-prevalence regions (eg, Asia, Africa, Latin America, and countries of the former Soviet Union), homeless people, people who use alcohol excessively or illicit drugs, and residents of correctional facilities and other congregate settings. Several published studies document increased risk of infection in children with exposure to secondhand smoke.

Infants and postpubertal adolescents are at increased risk of progression of LTBI to tuberculosis disease. Other predictive factors for development of disease include recent infection (within the past 2 years); immunodeficiency, especially from HIV infection; use of immunosuppressive drugs, such as prolonged or high-dose corticosteroid therapy or chemotherapy; intravenous drug use; and certain diseases or medical conditions, including Hodgkin disease, lymphoma, diabetes mellitus, chronic renal failure, and malnutrition. There have been reports of tuberculosis disease in adolescents and adults being treated for arthritis, inflammatory bowel disease, and other conditions with tumor necrosis factor-alpha (TNF-alpha) antagonists or blockers, such as infliximab and etanercept (see Biologic Response Modifiers Used to Decrease Inflammation, p 83). A positive TST or IGRA result should be accepted as indicative of infection in individuals receiving/about to receive these medications.[1]

A diagnosis of LTBI or tuberculosis disease in a young child is a public health sentinel event often representing recent transmission. Transmission of *M tuberculosis* complex is airborne, with inhalation of droplet nuclei usually produced by an adult or adolescent with contagious pulmonary, endobronchial, or laryngeal tuberculosis disease. *M bovis* is transmitted most often by unpasteurized dairy products,[2] but airborne human-to-human transmission can occur. The duration of contagiousness of an adult receiving effective treatment depends on drug susceptibilities of the organism, adherence to an appropriate drug regimen by the patient, the number of organisms in sputum, and frequency of cough. Although contagiousness usually lasts only a few days to weeks after initiation of effective drug therapy, it can last longer, especially when the adult patient has pulmonary cavities, does not adhere to medical therapy, or is infected with a drug-resistant strain. If the sputum smear is negative for acid-fast bacilli (AFB) on 3 separate specimens at least 8 hours apart and the patient has improved clinically with resolution of cough, the treated person can be considered at low risk of transmitting *M tuberculosis*. Children younger than 10 years with small pulmonary lesions (paucibacillary disease) and nonproductive cough rarely are contagious. Unusual cases of adult-form pulmonary disease in young children, particularly with lung cavities and positive sputum-smear microscopy for AFB, and cases of congenital tuberculosis can be highly contagious.

The **incubation period** from infection to development of a positive TST or IGRA result is 2 to 10 weeks. The risk of developing tuberculosis disease is highest during the

---

[1]Starke JR; American Academy of Pediatrics, Committee on Infectious Diseases. Clinical report: Interferon-γ release assays for diagnosis of tuberculosis infection and disease in children. *Pediatrics.* 2014;134(6):e1763–e1773

[2]American Academy of Pediatrics, Committee on Infectious Diseases and Committee on Nutrition. Consumption of raw or unpasteurized milk and milk products by pregnant women and children. *Pediatrics.* 2014;133(1):175–179

6 months after infection and remains high for 2 years; however, many years can elapse between initial *M tuberculosis* infection and subsequent disease.

DIAGNOSTIC TESTS:

Assessing for* M tuberculosis *Disease. Patients testing positive for *M tuberculosis* infection (below) should have a chest radiograph and physical examination completed to assess for tuberculosis disease. Most experts recommend that children younger than 12 months who are suspected of having pulmonary or extrapulmonary tuberculosis disease (eg, have a positive TST <u>and</u> symptoms, physical examination signs, or chest radiograph abnormalities consistent with tuberculosis disease), with or without neurologic symptoms, should have a lumbar puncture to evaluate for tuberculous meningitis. Some experts also recommend performing a lumbar puncture in children 12 through 23 months of age with tuberculosis disease, with or without neurologic symptoms. Children 24 months of age and older with tuberculosis disease require a lumbar puncture only if they have neurologic signs or symptoms.

Laboratory isolation of *M tuberculosis* complex by culture from specimens of sputum, gastric aspirates, bronchial washings, pleural fluid, cerebrospinal fluid (CSF), urine, or other body fluids or a tissue biopsy specimen establishes the diagnosis. Children older than 5 years and adolescents frequently can produce sputum spontaneously or by induction with aerosolized hypertonic saline. Studies have demonstrated successful collections of induced sputum from infants with pulmonary tuberculosis, but this requires special expertise. The best specimen for diagnosis of pulmonary tuberculosis in any child or adolescent in whom cough is absent or nonproductive and sputum cannot be induced is an early-morning gastric aspirate. Gastric aspirate specimens should be obtained with a nasogastric tube on awakening the child and before ambulation or feeding, and the acid pH of the gastric secretions should be neutralized as soon as possible.[1] Aspirates collected on 3 separate mornings should be submitted for testing by staining and culture. Fluorescent staining methods for specimen smears are more sensitive than AFB smears and are preferred. The overall diagnostic yield of microscopy of gastric aspirates and induced sputum is low in children with clinically suspected pulmonary tuberculosis, and false-positive smear results caused by the presence of nontuberculous mycobacteria can occur. Histologic examination for and demonstration of AFB and granulomas in biopsy specimens from lymph node, pleura, mesentery, liver, bone marrow, or other tissues can be useful, but *M tuberculosis* complex organisms cannot be distinguished reliably from other mycobacteria in stained specimens. Regardless of results of the AFB smears, each specimen should be cultured.

Because *M tuberculosis* complex organisms are slow growing, detection of these organisms may take as long as 10 weeks using solid media; use of liquid media allows detection within 1 to 6 weeks and usually within 3 weeks. Even with optimal culture techniques, *M tuberculosis* complex organisms are isolated from fewer than 50% of children and 75% of infants with pulmonary tuberculosis diagnosed by other clinical criteria. Current methods for species identification of isolates from culture include molecular probes, genetic sequencing, mass spectroscopy, and biochemical tests. *M bovis* usually is suspected because of pyrazinamide resistance, which is characteristic of almost all *M bovis* isolates,

---

[1] **www.nationaltbcenter.ucsf.edu/catalogue/epub/index.cfm?tableName=GAP**

but further biochemical or molecular testing is required to distinguish *M bovis* from *M tuberculosis*.

Several nucleic acid amplification tests (NAATs) for rapid diagnosis of tuberculosis are available and can be either tests that are cleared by the US Food and Drug Administration (FDA) or laboratory-developed tests that are not FDA reviewed and have been validated for use in that laboratory only. NAATs have varying sensitivity and specificity for sputum, gastric aspirate, cerebrospinal fluid (CSF), and tissue specimens, with false-negative and false-positive results reported. Further research is needed before NAATs can be recommended routinely for the diagnosis of tuberculosis in children when specimens other than sputum are submitted to the laboratory. For a child with clinically suspected tuberculosis disease, finding the culture-positive source case supports the child's presumptive diagnosis and provides the likely drug susceptibility of the child's organism. Culture material should be collected from children with evidence of tuberculosis disease, especially when (1) an isolate from a source case is not available; (2) the presumed source case has drug-resistant tuberculosis; (3) the child is immunocompromised or ill enough to require hospital admission; or (4) the child has extrapulmonary disease. Traditional methods of determining drug susceptibility require bacterial isolation. Several new molecular methods of rapidly determining drug resistance directly from clinical samples now are available and being used in reference laboratories and soon are expected to be used in hospital laboratories. GeneXpert MTB-RIF is a cartridge-based automated NAAT that can detect the presence in patient specimens of genetic material both for *M tuberculosis* and rifampin resistance within 2 hours. It is widely available in countries with a high prevalence of tuberculosis but in the United States is limited mostly to reference laboratories.

Testing for M tuberculosis *Infection*

The Tuberculin Skin Test. The TST is an indirect method for detecting *M tuberculosis* infection. It is one of 2 methods for diagnosing LTBI in asymptomatic people, the other method being IGRA (p 811). Both methods rely on specific cellular sensitization after infection. Conditions that decrease lymphocyte numbers or functionality can reduce the sensitivity of these tests. The routine (ie, Mantoux) technique of administering the skin test consists of 5 tuberculin units of purified protein derivative (PPD; 0.1 mL) injected intradermally using a 27-gauge needle and a 1.0-mL syringe into the volar aspect of the forearm. Creation of a palpable wheal 6 to 10 mm in diameter is crucial to accurate testing.

Administration of TSTs and interpretation of results should be performed by trained and experienced health care personnel, because administration and interpretation by unskilled people and family members are unreliable. The recommended time for assessing the TST result is 48 to 72 hours after administration. The diameter of induration in millimeters is measured transversely to the long axis of the forearm. Positive TST results, as defined in Table 3.78, can persist for several weeks.

Lack of reaction to a TST does not exclude LTBI or tuberculosis disease. Approximately 10% to 40% of immunocompetent children with culture-documented tuberculosis disease do not react initially to a TST. Host factors, such as young age, poor nutrition, immunosuppression, viral infections (especially measles, varicella, and influenza), recent *M tuberculosis* infection, and disseminated tuberculosis disease can decrease

TST reactivity. Many children and adults coinfected with HIV and *M tuberculosis* complex do not react to a TST. Control skin tests to assess cutaneous anergy are not recommended routinely, because the diagnostic significance of sensitivity and anergy to the control antigens is unknown, and selective anergy to tuberculin is a feature of tuberculosis disease, which renders reactivity to anergy tests meaningless.

Classification of TST results is based on epidemiologic and clinical factors. Interpretation of the size of induration (mm) as a positive result varies with the person's risk of LTBI and likelihood of progression to tuberculosis disease. Current guidelines from the Centers for Disease Control and Prevention (CDC), the American Thoracic Society, and the American Academy of Pediatrics (AAP) that recommend interpretation of TST findings on the basis of an individual's risk stratification are summarized in Table 3.78 (p 806). Prompt clinical and radiographic evaluation of all children and adolescents with a positive TST result is recommended.

Generally, interpretation of TST results in BCG recipients who are known contacts of a person with tuberculosis disease or who are at high risk of tuberculosis disease is the same as for people who have not received BCG vaccine. After BCG immunization, distinguishing between a positive TST result caused by pathogenic *M tuberculosis* complex infection and that caused by BCG is difficult. Reactivity of the TST after receipt of BCG vaccine does not occur in some patients. The size of the TST reaction (ie, mm of induration) attributable to BCG immunization depends on many factors, including age at BCG immunization, quality and strain of BCG vaccine used, number of doses of BCG vaccine received, nutritional and immunologic status of the vaccine recipient, frequency of TST administration, and time lapse between immunization and TST. Evidence that increases the probability that a positive TST result is attributable to LTBI includes known contact with a person with contagious tuberculosis, a family history of tuberculosis disease, a long interval (more than 5 years) since neonatal BCG immunization, and a TST reaction 15 mm or greater.

Blood-Based Testing with Interferon-Gamma Release Assays (IGRAs).[1,2] QuantiFERON-TB Gold In-Tube and T-SPOT.*TB* are IGRAs and are the preferred tests for tuberculosis infection in asymptomatic children 5 years and older who have been vaccinated with BCG. These FDA-approved blood tests measure ex vivo interferon-gamma production from T lymphocytes in response to stimulation with antigens specific to *M tuberculosis* complex, which includes *M tuberculosis* and *M bovis*. However, the IGRA antigens used are not found in BCG. As with TSTs, IGRAs cannot distinguish between latent infection and disease, and a negative result from these tests cannot exclude the possibility of tuberculosis disease in a patient with suggestive findings. The sensitivity of IGRA tests is similar to that of TSTs for detecting infection in adults and older children who have untreated culture-confirmed tuberculosis. In many clinical settings, the specificity of IGRAs is higher than that for the TST, because the antigens used are not found in BCG or most pathogenic nontuberculous mycobacteria (eg, are not found in *M avium* complex but are found in *M kansasii,*

---

[1]Centers for Disease Control and Prevention. Updated guidelines for using interferon gamma release assays to detect *Mycobacterium tuberculosis* infection—United States. *MMWR Recomm Rep.* 2010;59(RR-5):1–26

[2]Starke JR; American Academy of Pediatrics, Committee on Infectious Diseases. Clinical report: Interferon-γ release assays for diagnosis of tuberculosis infection and disease in children. *Pediatrics.* 2014;134(6):e1763–e1773

M szulgai, and *M marinum*). IGRAs are recommended by the CDC for all indications in which TST would be used, and some experts prefer IGRAs for use in adults. The published experience testing children with IGRAs demonstrates that IGRAs consistently perform well in children 5 years and older, and some data support their use for children as young as 3 years. The negative predictive value of IGRAs is not clear, but in general, if the IGRA result is negative and the TST result is positive in an asymptomatic child, the diagnosis of LTBI is unlikely. A negative result for a TST or an IGRA should be considered as especially unreliable in infants younger than 3 months.

At this time, neither an IGRA nor the TST can be considered "the gold standard" for diagnosis of LTBI. Current recommendations for use of IGRAs in children for LTBI are shown in Tables 3.79 and Fig 3.13:

- Children with a positive result from an IGRA should be considered infected with *M tuberculosis* complex. A negative IGRA result cannot be interpreted universally as absence of infection.
- Indeterminate IGRA results have several possible causes that could be related to the patient, the assay itself, or its performance. Indeterminate results do not exclude *M tuberculosis* infection and may necessitate repeat testing, possibly with a different test. Indeterminate IGRA results should not be used to make clinical decisions.

Table 3.79. Tuberculin Skin Test (TST) and IGRA Recommendations for Infants, Children, and Adolescents[a]

Children for whom immediate TST or IGRA is indicated[b]:
- Contacts of people with confirmed or suspected contagious tuberculosis (contact investigation)
- Children with radiographic or clinical findings suggesting tuberculosis disease
- Children immigrating from countries with endemic infection (eg, Asia, Middle East, Africa, Latin America, countries of the former Soviet Union), including international adoptees
- Children with travel histories to countries with endemic infection and substantial contact with indigenous people from such countries[c]

Children who should have annual TST or IGRA:
- Children infected with HIV infection (TST only)

Children at increased risk of progression of LTBI to tuberculosis disease: Children with other medical conditions, including diabetes mellitus, chronic renal failure, malnutrition, congenital or acquired immunodeficiencies, and children receiving tumor necrosis factor (TNF) antagonists deserve special consideration. Without recent exposure, these people are not at increased risk of acquiring *M tuberculosis* infection. Underlying immune deficiencies associated with these conditions theoretically would enhance the possibility for progression to severe disease. Initial histories of potential exposure to tuberculosis should be included for all of these patients. If these histories or local epidemiologic factors suggest a possibility of exposure, immediate and periodic TST or IGRA should be considered. **A TST or IGRA should be performed before initiation of immunosuppressive therapy, including prolonged systemic corticosteroid administration, organ transplantation, use of TNF-alpha antagonists or blockers, or other immunosuppressive therapy in any child requiring these treatments.**

IGRA indicates interferon-gamma release assay; HIV, human immunodeficiency virus; LTBI, latent *M tuberculosis* infection.
[a]Bacille Calmette-Guérin immunization is not a contraindication to a TST.
[b]Beginning as early as 3 months of age for TST, 3 years of age for IGRAs for LTBI and disease.
[c]If the child is well and has no history of exposure, the TST or IGRA should be delayed for up to 10 weeks after return.

Fig 3.13. Guidance on Strategy for Use of TST and IGRA by Age and BCG-Immunization Status

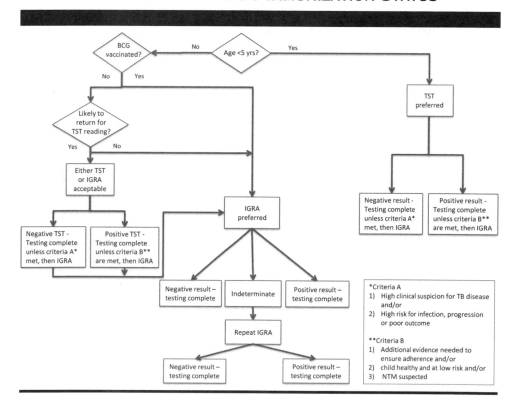

Use of Tests for M tuberculosis *Infection.* A TST or IGRA should be performed in children who are at increased risk of infection with *M tuberculosis* (see Table 3.79, p 812). Universal testing with TST or IGRA, including programs based at schools, child care centers, and camps that include populations at low risk, is discouraged, because it results in either a low yield of positive results or a large proportion of false-positive results, leading to an inefficient use of health care resources. However, using a questionnaire to determine risk factors for LTBI can be effective in health care settings. Simple questionnaires can identify children with risk factors for LTBI (see Table 3.80, p 814) who then should have a TST or IGRA performed. Risk assessment for tuberculosis should be performed at first health care encounter with a child and every 6 months thereafter for the first year of life (eg, 2 weeks and 6 and 12 months of age). After 1 year of age, risk assessment for tuberculosis should be performed at the time of routine care, annually if possible. The most reliable strategies for identifying LTBI and preventing tuberculosis disease in children are based on thorough and expedient contact investigations rather than nonselective skin testing of large populations. Contact investigations are public-health interventions that should be coordinated through the local public health department. Specific recommendations for TST and IGRA use are provided in Table 3.79 and Fig 3.13. Only children deemed to have increased risk of contact with people with contagious tuberculosis or

Table 3.80. Validated Questions for Determining Risk of LTBI in Children in the United States

- Has a family member or contact had tuberculosis disease?
- Has a family member had a positive tuberculin skin test result?
- Was your child born in a high-risk country (countries other than the United States, Canada, Australia, New Zealand, or Western and North European countries)?
- Has your child traveled (had contact with resident populations) to a high-risk country for more than 1 week?

LTBI indicates latent *M tuberculosis* infection.

children with suspected tuberculosis disease should be considered for a TST or IGRA. Household investigation of children for tuberculosis is indicated whenever a TST or IGRA result of a household member converts from a negative to positive test (indicating recent infection).

HIV Infection. Children with HIV infection are considered at high risk of tuberculosis, and an annual TST beginning at 3 through 12 months of age is recommended, or if older, when HIV infection is diagnosed. Children who have tuberculosis disease should be tested for HIV infection. The clinical manifestations and radiographic appearance of tuberculosis disease in children with HIV infection tend to be similar to those in immunocompetent children, but manifestations in these children can be more severe and unusual and can include extrapulmonary involvement of multiple organs. In HIV-infected patients, a TST induration of ≥5 mm is considered a positive result (see Table 3.78, p 806); however, a negative TST result attributable to HIV-related immunosuppression also can occur. An IGRA test also can be used, but a negative result does not exclude tuberculosis. Specimens for culture should be obtained from all HIV-infected children with suspected tuberculosis.

Organ Transplant Patients. The risk of tuberculosis in organ transplant patients is several-fold greater than in the general population. A careful history of previous exposure to tuberculosis should be taken from all transplant candidates, including details about previous TST results and exposure to individuals with active TB. All transplant candidates should undergo evaluation by TST or IGRA for LTBI. A positive result of either test should be taken as evidence of *M tuberculosis* infection.

Patients Receiving Immunosuppressive Therapies Including Tumor Necrosis Factor Antagonists or Blockers. Patients should be screened for risk factors for *M tuberculosis* complex infection and have a TST and/or IGRA performed before the initiation therapy with of systemic corticosteroids, antimetabolite agents, and tumor necrosis factor antagonists or blockers (eg, infliximab and etanercept; see Biologic Response Modifiers Used to Decrease Inflammation, p 83). A positive result of either test should be taken as evidence of *M tuberculosis* infection.

Other Considerations. Testing for tuberculosis at any age is not required before administration of live-virus vaccines. Measles vaccine temporarily can suppress tuberculin reactivity for at least 4 to 6 weeks. If indicated, a TST can be applied at the same visit during which these vaccines are administered (ie, before substantial replication of the vaccine virus). The effects of vaccination on IGRA characteristics have not been determined; the same precautions as for TST should be followed. The effect of live-virus varicella, yellow fever, and live-attenuated influenza vaccines on TST reactivity and IGRA results is not known. In the absence of data, the same spacing recommendation should be applied to these vaccines as described for measles-mumps-rubella (MMR) vaccine. There is no evidence that inactivated vaccines, polysaccharide vaccines, or recombinant or subunit vaccines or toxoids interfere with clinical interpretation of TST or IGRAs.

Chest radiographic findings of a granuloma, calcification, or adenopathy can be caused by infection with *M tuberculosis* complex but not by BCG immunization. BCG can cause suppurative lymphadenitis in the regional lymph node drainage of the inoculation site of a healthy child and can cause disseminated disease in children with severe forms of immunodeficiency.

Sensitivity to PPD tuberculin antigen persists for years in most instances, even after effective treatment. The durability of positive IGRA results has not been determined. Studies seeking to show reversion of TST or IGRA results after treatment of LTBI or tuberculosis disease have had inconclusive findings. Currently, repeat testing with either TST or IGRA has no known clinical utility for assessing the effectiveness of treatment or for diagnosing new infection in patients who previously were infected with *M tuberculosis* and who are reexposed.

TREATMENT:

Specific Drugs. Antituberculosis drugs kill or inhibit multiplication of *M tuberculosis* complex organisms, thereby arresting progression of infection and preventing most complications. Chemotherapy does not cause rapid disappearance of already caseous or granulomatous lesions (eg, mediastinal lymphadenitis). Dosage recommendations and the more commonly reported adverse reactions of major antituberculosis drugs are summarized in Tables 3.81 (p 816) and 3.82 (p 817). For treatment of tuberculosis disease, these drugs always must be used in recommended combination and dosage to minimize emergence of drug-resistant strains. Use of nonstandard regimens for any reason (eg, drug allergy or drug resistance) should be undertaken only in consultation with an expert in treating tuberculosis.

Isoniazid (INH) is bactericidal, rapidly absorbed, and well tolerated and penetrates into body fluids, including CSF. Isoniazid is metabolized in the liver and excreted primarily through the kidneys. Hepatotoxic effects are rare in children but can be life threatening. Caution should be used in storing and administering isoniazid, because accidental or deliberate overdose is dangerous. In children and adolescents given recommended doses, peripheral neuritis or seizures caused by inhibition of pyridoxine metabolism are rare, and most do not need pyridoxine supplements. Pyridoxine supplementation is recommended for exclusively breastfed infants and for children and adolescents on meat- and milk-deficient diets; children with nutritional deficiencies, including all symptomatic HIV-infected children; and pregnant adolescents and women. For infants and young children, isoniazid tablets can be pulverized.

Rifampin (RIF) is a bactericidal agent in the rifamycin class of drugs that is absorbed rapidly and penetrates into body fluids, including CSF. Other drugs in the rifamycin class approved for treating tuberculosis are rifabutin and rifapentine. Rifampin is metabolized by the liver and can alter the pharmacokinetics and serum concentrations of many other drugs. Rare adverse effects include hepatotoxicity, influenza-like symptoms, pruritus, and thrombocytopenia. Rifampin is excreted in bile and urine and can cause orange urine, sweat, and tears, with discoloration of soft contact lenses. Rifampin can make oral contraceptives ineffective, so nonhormonal birth-control methods should be

Table 3.81. Recommended Usual Treatment Regimens for Drug-Susceptible Tuberculosis in Infants, Children, and Adolescents

Infection or Disease Category	Regimen	Remarks
Latent *M tuberculosis* infection (positive TST or IGRA result, no disease)[a]		
• Isoniazid susceptible	9 mo of isoniazid, once a day	If daily therapy is not possible, DOT twice a week can be used for 9 mo.
• Isoniazid resistant	4 mo of rifampin, once a day	If daily therapy is not possible, DOT twice a week can be used for 4 mo.
• Isoniazid-rifampin resistant	Consult a tuberculosis specialist	
Pulmonary and extrapulmonary (except meningitis)[b]	2 mo of isoniazid, rifampin, pyrazinamide, and ethambutol daily or twice weekly, followed by 4 mo of isoniazid and rifampin[c] by DOT[d] for drug-susceptible *Mycobacterium tuberculosis*	Some experts recommend a 3-drug initial regimen (isoniazid, rifampin, and pyrazinamide) if the risk of drug resistance is low. DOT is highly desirable.
	9 to 12 mo of isoniazid and rifampin for drug-susceptible *Mycobacterium bovis*	If hilar adenopathy only and the risk of drug resistance is low, a 6-mo course of isoniazid and rifampin is sufficient.
		Drugs can be given 2 or 3 times/wk under DOT.
Meningitis	2 mo of isoniazid, rifampin, pyrazinamide, and an aminoglycoside or ethionamide, once a day, followed by 7–10 mo of isoniazid and rifampin, once a day or twice a week (9–12 mo total) for drug-susceptible *M tuberculosis*	For patients who may have acquired tuberculosis in geographic areas where resistance to streptomycin is common, kanamycin, amikacin, or capreomycin can be used instead of streptomycin.
	At least 12 mo of therapy without pyrazinamide for drug-susceptible *M bovis*	

TST indicates tuberculin skin test; IGRA, interferon-gamma release assay; DOT, directly observed therapy.

[a] See text for additional acceptable or alternative regimens.

[b] Duration of therapy may be longer for human immunodeficiency virus (HIV)-infected people, and additional drugs and dosing intervals may be indicated (see Tuberculosis Disease and HIV Infection, p 824).

[c] Medications should be administered daily for the first 2 weeks to 2 months of treatment and then can be administered 2 to 3 times per week by DOT. (Twice-weekly therapy is not recommended for HIV-infected people.)

[d] If initial chest radiograph shows pulmonary cavities and sputum culture after 2 months of therapy remains positive, the continuation phase is extended to 7 months, for a total treatment duration 9 months.

Table 3.82. Commonly Used Drugs for Treatment of Tuberculosis in Infants, Children, and Adolescents

Drugs	Dosage Forms	Daily Dosage, (Range), mg/kg	Twice a Week Dosage, mg/kg per Dose	Maximum Dose	Adverse Reactions
Ethambutol	Tablets 100 mg 400 mg	20 (15–25)	50	2.5 g	Optic neuritis (usually reversible), decreased red-green color discrimination, gastrointestinal tract disturbances, hypersensitivity
Isoniazid[a]	Scored tablets 100 mg 300 mg	10 (10–15)[b]	20–30	Daily, 300 mg Twice a week, 900 mg	Mild hepatic enzyme elevation, hepatitis,[b] peripheral neuritis, hypersensitivity
Pyrazinamide[a]	Scored tablets 500 mg	35 (30–40)	50	2 g	Hepatotoxic effects, hyperuricemia, arthralgia, gastrointestinal tract upset
Rifampin[a]	Capsules 150 mg 300 mg Syrup formulated capsules	15 (10–20)	15 (10–20)	600 mg	Orange discoloration of secretions or urine, staining of contact lenses; vomiting, hepatitis, influenza-like reaction, thrombocytopenia, pruritus; oral contraceptives may be ineffective

[a]Rifamate is a capsule containing 150 mg of isoniazid and 300 mg of rifampin. Two capsules provide the usual adult (greater than 50 kg) daily doses of each drug. Rifater, in the United States, is a capsule containing 50 mg of isoniazid, 120 mg of rifampin, and 300 mg of pyrazinamide. Isoniazid and rifampin also are available for parenteral administration.

[b]When isoniazid in a dosage exceeding 10 mg/kg/day is used in combination with rifampin, the incidence of hepatotoxic effects may be increased.

adopted when rifampin is administered to sexually active female adolescents and adults. For infants and young children, the contents of the capsules can be suspended in cherry-flavored syrup or sprinkled on semisoft foods (eg, pudding). *M tuberculosis* complex isolates that are resistant to rifampin are almost always resistant to isoniazid. Rifabutin is a suitable alternative to rifampin in HIV-infected children receiving antiretroviral therapy that restricts the use of rifampin because of drug interactions; however, experience in children is limited. Major toxicities of rifabutin include leukopenia, gastrointestinal tract upset, polyarthralgia, rash, increased transaminase concentrations, and skin and secretion discoloration (pseudojaundice). Anterior uveitis has been reported among children receiving rifabutin as prophylaxis or as part of a combination regimen for treatment, usually when administered at high doses. Rifabutin also increases hepatic metabolism of many drugs but is a less potent inducer of cytochrome P450 enzymes than rifampin and has fewer problematic drug interactions than rifampin. However, adjustments in doses of rifabutin and coadministered antiretroviral drugs may be necessary for certain combinations. Rifapentine is a long-acting rifamycin that permits weekly dosing in selected adults and adolescents, but its evaluation in younger pediatric patients has been limited.

Pyrazinamide (PZA) attains therapeutic CSF concentrations, is detectable in macrophages, is administered orally, and is metabolized by the liver. Administration of pyrazinamide for the first 2 months with isoniazid and rifampin allows for 6-month regimens in immunocompetent patients with drug-susceptible tuberculosis. Almost all isolates of *M bovis* are resistant to pyrazinamide, precluding 6-month therapy for this pathogen. In daily doses of 40 mg/kg per day or less, pyrazinamide seldom has hepatotoxic effects and is well tolerated by children. Some adolescents and many adults develop arthralgia and hyperuricemia because of inhibition of uric acid excretion. Pyrazinamide must be used with caution in people with underlying liver disease; when administered with rifampin, pyrazinamide is associated with somewhat higher rates of hepatotoxicity.

Ethambutol (EMB) is well absorbed after oral administration, diffuses well into tissues, and is excreted in urine. However, concentrations in CSF are low. At 20 mg/kg per day, ethambutol is bacteriostatic, and its primary therapeutic role is to prevent emergence of drug resistance. Ethambutol can cause reversible or irreversible optic neuritis, but reports in children with normal renal function are rare. Children who are receiving ethambutol should be monitored monthly for visual acuity and red-green color discrimination if they are old enough to cooperate. Use of ethambutol in young children whose visual acuity cannot be monitored requires consideration of risks and benefits, but it can be used routinely to treat tuberculosis disease in infants and children unless otherwise contraindicated.

The less commonly used (eg, "second-line") antituberculosis drugs, their doses, and adverse effects are listed in Table 3.83 (p 819). These drugs have limited usefulness because of decreased effectiveness and greater toxicity and should be used only in consultation with a specialist familiar with childhood tuberculosis. **Ethionamide** is an orally administered antituberculosis drug that is well tolerated by children, achieves therapeutic CSF concentrations, and may be useful for treatment of people with meningitis or drug-resistant tuberculosis. **Fluoroquinolones** have antituberculosis activity and can be used in special circumstances including drug-resistant organisms but are not FDA approved for this indication. Because some fluoroquinolones are approved by the FDA for use only in

Table 3.83. Drugs for Treatment of Drug-Resistant Tuberculosis in Infants, Children, and Adolescents[a]

Drugs	Dosage, Forms	Daily Dosage	Maximum Dose	Adverse Reactions
Amikacin[b]	Vials, 500 mg and 1 g	15–30 mg/kg (intravenous or intramuscular administration)	1 g	Auditory and vestibular toxic effects, nephrotoxic effects
Capreomycin[b]	Vials, 1 g	15–30 mg/kg (intramuscular administration)	1 g	Auditory and vestibular toxicity and nephrotoxic effects
Cycloserine	Capsules, 250 mg	10–20 mg/kg, given in 2 divided doses	1 g	Psychosis, personality changes, seizures, rash
Ethionamide	Tablets, 250 mg	15–20 mg/kg, given in 2–3 divided doses	1 g	Gastrointestinal tract disturbances, hepatotoxic effects, hypersensitivity reactions, hypothyroid
Kanamycin	Vials 75 mg/2 mL 500 mg/2 mL 1 g/3 mL	15–30 mg/kg (intramuscular or intravenous administration)	1 g	Auditory and vestibular toxic effects, nephrotoxic effects
Levofloxacin[c]	Tablets 250 mg 500 mg 750 mg Oral solution 25 mg/mL Vials 5 mg/mL 25 mg/mL	Adults: 750–1000 mg (once daily) Children: 15–20 mg/kg	1 g	Theoretical effect on growing cartilage, tendonitis, gastrointestinal tract disturbances, cardiac disturbances, peripheral neuropathy, rash, headache, restlessness, confusion

continued

Table 3.83. Drugs for Treatment of Drug-Resistant Tuberculosis in Infants, Children, and Adolescents,[a] continued

Drugs	Dosage, Forms	Daily Dosage, mg/kg	Maximum Dose	Adverse Reactions
Para-aminosalicylic acid (PAS)	Packets, 3 g	200–300 mg/kg (2–4 times a day)	10 g	Gastrointestinal tract disturbances, hypersensitivity, hepatotoxic effects
Streptomycin[b]	Vials 1 g 4 g	20–40 mg/kg (intramuscular administration)	1 g	Auditory and vestibular toxic effects, nephrotoxic effects (which must be preemptively monitored) and rash

[a] These drugs should be used in consultation with a specialist in tuberculosis.
[b] Dose adjustment in renal insufficiency.
[c] Levofloxacin is not approved for use in children younger than 18 years; its use in younger children necessitates assessment of the potential risks and benefits (see Antimicrobial Agents and Related Therapy, p 871).

people 18 years and older, their use in younger patients necessitates careful assessment of the potential risks and benefits (see Antimicrobial Agents and Related Therapy, p 871).

Occasionally, a patient cannot tolerate oral medications. Isoniazid, rifampin, **streptomycin** and related drugs, and fluoroquinolones can be administered parenterally.

Treatment Regimens for LTBI

Isoniazid Therapy for LTBI. A 9-month course of isoniazid is the preferred regimen in the United States for treatment of LTBI in most children. Isoniazid given to adults who have LTBI (ie, no clinical or radiographic abnormalities suggesting tuberculosis disease) provides substantial protection (54%–88%) against development of tuberculosis disease for at least 20 years. Among children, efficacy approaches 100% if adherence to therapy is high. Unfortunately, many studies have shown the adherence rate to be 50% to 75% over 9 months when families give isoniazid on their own. All infants and children who have LTBI but no evidence of tuberculosis disease and who never have received antituberculosis therapy should be considered for isoniazid unless resistance to isoniazid is suspected (ie, known exposure to a person with isoniazid-resistant tuberculosis), or a specific contraindication exists. Isoniazid, in this circumstance, is therapeutic and prevents development of disease. A physical examination and chest radiograph should be performed prior to when isoniazid therapy is initiated to exclude tuberculosis disease.

Duration of Isoniazid Therapy for LTBI. For infants, children, and adolescents, including those with HIV infection or other immunocompromising conditions, the recommended duration of isoniazid therapy in the United States is 9 months. The World Health Organization recommends a 6-month course of isoniazid, but modeling studies have shown that the efficacy of 6 months of treatment is approximately 30% less than that of a 9-month course. Isoniazid usually is given daily in a single dose. Physicians who treat LTBI should educate patients and their families about the adverse effects of isoniazid, provide written information about adverse drug effects, and prescribe it in monthly allocations with clinic visits scheduled for periodic face-to-face monitoring. Successful completion of therapy is based on total number of doses taken. When adherence with daily therapy with isoniazid cannot be ensured, twice-a-week DOT can be considered. The twice-weekly regimen should not be prescribed unless each dose is documented by DOT. Routine determination of serum transaminase concentrations during the 9 months of therapy for LTBI is not indicated except for children and adolescents who: (1) have concurrent or recent liver or biliary disease; (2) are pregnant or in the first 12 weeks postpartum; (3) are having clinical evidence of hepatotoxic effects; or (4) concurrently are taking other hepatotoxic drugs (eg, anticonvulsant or HIV agents). If therapy is completed successfully, there is no need to perform additional tests or chest radiographs unless a new exposure to tuberculosis is documented or the child develops a clinical illness consistent with tuberculosis.

Isoniazid-Rifapentine Therapy for LTBI.[1] In 2011, on the basis of a large clinical trial, the CDC recommended a 12-week, once-weekly dose of isoniazid and rifapentine, **given under DOT by a health department**, as an alternative regimen for treating LTBI in people 12 years or older. This regimen was shown to be at least as effective with fewer adverse reactions than 9 months of isoniazid given by self-supervision. Children between 2 and 11 years of age were enrolled in the trial, and the regimen was shown to be safe and well tolerated.

---

[1]Centers for Disease Control and Prevention. Recommendations for use of an isoniazid-rifapentine regimen with direct observation to treat latent *Mycobacterium tuberculosis* infection. *MMWR Morb Mortal Wkly Rep.* 2011;60(48):1650–1653

However, efficacy of this regimen in this age group could not be determined because of the study design. This regimen should not be used routinely for children younger than 12 years but can be considered when the likelihood of completing another regimen is low. This regimen should not be used in children younger than 2 years.

Additional Regimens for Treatment of LTBI. Additional possible regimens for treatment of LTBI are: (1) 3 months of daily isoniazid and rifampin, with the isoniazid dosage the same as when used alone and the rifampin dosage of 10 to 15 mg/kg/day (maximum 600 mg); or (2) 2 months of daily rifampin and pyrazinamide when given as part of RIPE (rifampin, isoniazid, pyrazinamide, and ethambutol) therapy for suspected tuberculosis disease (which subsequently is determined to be *M tuberculosis* infection only). The rifampin dose is 10 to 20 mg/kg day, maximum 600 mg; and the pyrazinamide dose is 30 to 40 mg/kg/day, maximum 2 g.

Therapy for Contacts of Patients With Isoniazid-Resistant M tuberculosis *and When Isoniazid Cannot Be Given.* The incidence of isoniazid resistance among *M tuberculosis* complex isolates from US patients is approximately 9%. Risk factors for drug resistance are listed in Table 3.84. Most experts recommend that isoniazid be used to treat LTBI in children unless the child has had contact with a person known to have isoniazid-resistant tuberculosis or the infection was acquired in a locale known to have a high prevalence of isoniazid resistance (**wwwnc.cdc.gov/travel/yellowbook/2014/chapter-3-infectious-diseases-related-to-travel/tuberculosis**). If the source case is found to have isoniazid-resistant, rifampin-susceptible organisms, isoniazid should be discontinued and rifampin should be given daily for a total course of 4 months. Some experts would choose to treat children younger than 12 years with rifampin daily for 6 months. Rifampin also can be used when isoniazid cannot be given because of patient intolerance or when isoniazid is unavailable. Optimal therapy for children with LTBI caused by organisms with resistance to isoniazid and rifampin (ie, multidrug resistant [MDR]) is not known. In these circumstances, fluoroquinolones alone and multidrug regimens have been used, but the safety and the efficacy of these empiric regimens have not been assessed in clinical trials. Drugs to consider include pyrazinamide, a fluoroquinolone, and ethambutol, depending on susceptibility of the isolate. Consultation with a tuberculosis specialist is indicated.

Treatment of Tuberculosis Disease. The goal of treatment is to achieve killing of replicating organisms in the tuberculous lesion in the shortest possible time. Achievement of this goal minimizes the possibility of development of resistant organisms. The major problem limiting successful treatment is poor adherence to prescribed treatment regimens. The use of

Table 3.84. People at Increased Risk of Drug-Resistant Tuberculosis Infection or Disease

- People with a history of treatment for tuberculosis disease (or whose source case for the contact received such treatment)
- Contacts of a patient with drug-resistant contagious tuberculosis disease
- People from countries with high prevalence of drug-resistant tuberculosis
- Infected people whose source case has positive smears for acid-fast bacilli or cultures after 2 months of appropriate antituberculosis therapy and patients who do not respond to a standard treatment regimen
- Residence in geographic area with a high percentage of drug-resistant isolates

DOT decreases the rates of relapse, treatment failures, and drug resistance; therefore, DOT is recommended strongly for treatment of all children and adolescents with tuberculosis disease in the United States.

For tuberculosis disease, a 6-month, 4-drug regimen consisting of rifampin, isoniazid, pyrazinamide, and ethambutol (RIPE) for the first 2 months and isoniazid and rifampin for the remaining 4 months is recommended for treatment of pulmonary disease, pulmonary disease with hilar adenopathy, and hilar adenopathy disease in infants, children, and adolescents when an MDR case is not suspected as the source of infection or when drug-susceptibility results are available from the patient or the likely source case. Some experts would administer 3 drugs (isoniazid, rifampin, and pyrazinamide) as the initial regimen if a source case has been identified with known pansusceptible *M tuberculosis* or if the presumed source case has no risk factors for drug-resistant *M tuberculosis*. For children with hilar adenopathy in whom drug resistance is not a consideration, a 6-month regimen of only isoniazid and rifampin is considered adequate by some experts. If the chest radiograph shows one or more pulmonary cavities and sputum culture result remains positive after 2 months of therapy, the duration of therapy should be extended to 9 months.

In the 6-month regimen with 4-drug therapy, rifampin, isoniazid, pyrazinamide, and ethambutol (RIPE) are given once a day for at least the first 2 weeks by DOT daily (at least 5 days per week). An alternative to daily dosing between 2 weeks and 2 months of treatment is to give these drugs twice or 3 times a week by DOT (except in HIV-infected people, in whom twice-weekly dosing is not recommended). After the initial 2-month period, a DOT regimen of isoniazid and rifampin given 2 or 3 times a week is acceptable (see Table 3.81, p 816, for doses). Several alternative regimens with differing durations of daily therapy and total therapy have been used successfully in adults and children. These alternative regimens should be prescribed and managed by a specialist in tuberculosis.

Therapy for Drug-Resistant Tuberculosis Disease. Drug resistance is more common in the following groups: (1) people previously treated for tuberculosis disease; (2) people born in areas with a high prevalence of drug resistance, such as Russia and the nations of the former Soviet Union, Asia, Africa, and Latin America (**wwwnc.cdc.gov/travel/yellowbook/2014/chapter-3-infectious-diseases-related-to-travel/tuberculosis**); and (3) contacts, especially children, with tuberculosis disease whose source case is a person from one of these groups (see also Table 3.84, p 822). When **resistance to drugs other than isoniazid** is likely (see Table 3.84, p 822), initial therapy should be adjusted by adding at least 2 drugs to match the presumed drug susceptibility pattern until drug susceptibility results are available. If an isolate from the pediatric case under treatment is not available, drug susceptibilities can be inferred by the drug susceptibility pattern of isolates from the adult source case. Data for guiding drug selection may not be available for foreign-born children or in circumstances of international travel or adoption. If this information is not available, a 4- or 5-drug initial regimen is recommended with close monitoring for clinical response.

Most cases of pulmonary tuberculosis in children that are caused by an isoniazid-resistant but rifampin- and pyrazinamide-susceptible strain of *M tuberculosis* complex can be treated with a 6-month regimen of rifampin, pyrazinamide, and ethambutol. For cases of MDR tuberculosis disease, the treatment regimen needed for cure should include at least 4 or 5 antituberculosis drugs to which the organism is susceptible. Bedaquiline recently was approved by the FDA as treatment for adults with MDR tuberculosis for whom an effective 4-drug regimen could not be instituted without the use of bedaquiline; unfortunately, there currently are no safety, tolerability, efficacy or pharmacokinetic data for children for this drug.[1] Therapy for MDR tuberculosis is administered for 12 to 24 months from the time of culture conversion to negativity. An injectable drug such as kanamycin or capreomycin should be used for the first 4 to 6 months of treatment, as tolerated. Regimens in which drugs are administered 2 or 3 times per week are not recommended for drug-resistant disease; daily DOT is critical to prevent emergence of additional resistance. An expert in drug-resistant tuberculosis should be consulted for all drug-resistant cases.

Extrapulmonary Tuberculosis Disease. In general, extrapulmonary tuberculosis—with the exception of meningitis—can be treated with the same regimens as used for pulmonary tuberculosis. For suspected drug-susceptible tuberculous meningitis, daily treatment with isoniazid, rifampin, pyrazinamide, and ethionamide, if possible, or an aminoglycoside should be initiated. When susceptibility to all drugs is established, the ethionamide or aminoglycoside can be discontinued. Pyrazinamide is given for a total of 2 months, and isoniazid and rifampin are given for a total of 9 to 12 months. Isoniazid and rifampin can be given daily or 2 or 3 times per week after the first 2 months of treatment if the child has responded well.

Other Treatment Considerations

Corticosteroids. The evidence supporting adjuvant treatment with corticosteroids for children with tuberculosis disease is incomplete. Corticosteroids are definitely indicated for children with tuberculous meningitis, because corticosteroids decrease rates of mortality and long-term neurologic impairment. Corticosteroids can be considered for children with pleural and pericardial effusions (to hasten reabsorption of fluid), severe miliary disease (to mitigate alveolocapillary block), endobronchial disease (to relieve obstruction and atelectasis), and abdominal tuberculosis (to decrease the risk of strictures). Corticosteroids should be given only when accompanied by appropriate antituberculosis therapy. Most experts consider 2 mg/kg per day of prednisone (maximum, 60 mg/day) or its equivalent for 4 to 6 weeks followed by tapering.

Tuberculosis Disease and HIV Infection.[2] Most HIV-infected adults with drug-susceptible tuberculosis respond well to standard treatment regimens when appropriate therapy is initiated early. However, optimal therapy for tuberculosis in children with HIV infection has not been established. Treating tuberculosis in an HIV-infected child is complicated by antiretroviral drug interactions with the rifamycins and overlapping toxicities. Therapy always should include at least 4 drugs initially, should be administered daily via DOT, and should be continued for at least 6 months. Isoniazid, rifampin, and pyrazinamide, usually with ethambutol or an aminoglycoside, should be given for at least the first 2 months. Ethambutol can be discontinued once drug-resistant tuberculosis disease is excluded. Rifampin may be contraindicated in people who are receiving antiretroviral therapy. Rifabutin can be substituted for rifampin in some circumstances. Consultation with a specialist who has experience in managing HIV-infected patients with tuberculosis is advised.

Evaluation and Monitoring of Therapy in Children and Adolescents. Careful monthly monitoring of clinical and bacteriologic responses to therapy is important. With DOT, clinical evaluation is an integral component of each visit for drug administration. For patients with

---

[1]Centers for Disease Control and Prevention. Provisional CDC guidelines for the use and safety monitoring of bedaquiline fumarate (Sirturo) for the treatment of multidrug-resistant tuberculosis. *MMWR Recomm Rep.* 2013;62(RR-9):1–11

[2]Guidelines for the prevention and treatment of opportunistic infections in HIV infected adults and adolescents: Recommendations from CDC, NIH, IDSA. December 2014. Available at: **http://aidsinfo.nih. gov/e-news**

pulmonary tuberculosis, chest radiographs should be obtained after 2 months of therapy to evaluate response. Even with successful 6-month regimens, hilar adenopathy can persist for 2 to 3 years; normal radiographic findings are not necessary to discontinue therapy. Follow-up chest radiography beyond termination of successful therapy usually is not necessary unless clinical deterioration occurs.

If therapy has been interrupted, the date of completion should be extended. Although guidelines cannot be provided for every situation, factors to consider when establishing the date of completion include the following: (1) length of interruption of therapy; (2) time during therapy (early or late) when interruption occurred; and (3) the patient's clinical, radiographic, and bacteriologic status before, during, and after interruption of therapy. The total doses administered by DOT should be calculated to guide the duration of therapy. Consultation with a specialist in tuberculosis is advised.

Untoward effects of isoniazid therapy, including severe hepatitis in otherwise healthy infants, children, and adolescents, are rare. Routine determination of serum transaminase concentrations is not recommended. However, for children with severe tuberculosis disease, especially children with meningitis or disseminated disease, transaminase concentrations should be monitored approximately monthly during the first several months of treatment. Other indications for testing include the following: (1) having concurrent or recent liver or biliary disease; (2) being pregnant or in the first 12 weeks postpartum; (3) having clinical evidence of hepatotoxic effects; or (4) concurrently using other hepatotoxic drugs (eg, anticonvulsant or HIV agents). In most other circumstances, monthly clinical evaluations to observe for signs or symptoms of hepatitis and other adverse effects of drug therapy without routine monitoring of transaminase concentrations is appropriate follow-up. In all cases, regular physician-patient contact to assess drug adherence, efficacy, and adverse effects is an important aspect of management. Patients should be provided with written instructions and advised to call a physician immediately if symptoms of adverse events, in particular hepatotoxicity (ie, nausea, vomiting, abdominal pain, jaundice), develop.

Immunizations. Patients who are receiving treatment for tuberculosis can be given measles and other age-appropriate attenuated live-virus vaccines unless they are receiving high-dose systemic corticosteroids, are severely ill, or have other specific contraindications to immunization.

Tuberculosis During Pregnancy and Breastfeeding. Tuberculosis treatment during pregnancy is complex. If tuberculosis disease is diagnosed during pregnancy, a regimen of isoniazid, rifampin, and ethambutol is recommended. Pyrazinamide commonly is used in a 3- or 4-drug regimen, but safety during pregnancy has not been established. At least 6 months of therapy is indicated for drug-susceptible tuberculosis disease if pyrazinamide is used; at least 9 months of therapy is indicated if pyrazinamide is not used. Prompt initiation of therapy is mandatory to protect mother and fetus.

Asymptomatic pregnant women with a positive TST or IGRA result, normal chest radiographic findings, and recent contact with a contagious person should be considered for isoniazid therapy. The recommended duration of therapy is 9 months. Therapy in these circumstances should begin after the first trimester. Pyridoxine supplementation is indicated for all pregnant and breastfeeding women receiving isoniazid.

Isoniazid, ethambutol, and rifampin are relatively safe for the fetus. The benefit of ethambutol and rifampin for therapy of tuberculosis disease in the mother outweighs the risk to the infant. Because streptomycin can cause ototoxic effects in the fetus, it should not be used unless administration is essential for effective treatment. The effects of other second-line drugs on the fetus are unknown, and ethionamide has been demonstrated to be teratogenic, so its use during pregnancy is contraindicated.

Although isoniazid is secreted in human milk, no adverse effects of isoniazid on nursing infants have been demonstrated (see Human Milk, p 125). Breastfed infants do not require pyridoxine supplementation unless they are receiving isoniazid. The isoniazid dosage of a breastfed baby whose mother is taking isoniazid does not require adjustment for the small amount of drug in the milk.

Congenital Tuberculosis. Women who have only pulmonary tuberculosis are not likely to infect the fetus but can infect their infant after delivery. Congenital tuberculosis is rare, but in utero infections can occur after maternal bacillemia and have been reported following in vitro fertilization of women from endemic countries in whom infertility likely was related to subclinical maternal genitourinary tract tuberculosis.

If a newborn infant is suspected of having congenital tuberculosis, a TST and IGRA test, chest radiography, lumbar puncture, and appropriate cultures and radiography should be performed promptly. The TST result usually is negative in newborn infants with congenital or perinatally acquired infection. Hence, regardless of the TST or IGRA results, treatment of the infant should be initiated promptly with isoniazid, rifampin, pyrazinamide, and an aminoglycoside (eg, amikacin). The placenta should be examined histologically for granulomata and AFB, and a specimen should be cultured for *M tuberculosis* complex. The mother should be evaluated for presence of pulmonary or extrapulmonary disease, including genitourinary tuberculosis. If the physical examination and chest radiographic findings support the diagnosis of tuberculosis disease, the newborn infant should be treated with regimens recommended for tuberculosis disease. If meningitis is confirmed, corticosteroids should be added (see Corticosteroids, p 824). Drug susceptibility testing of the organism recovered from the mother or household contact, infant, or both should be performed.

Management of the Newborn Infant Whose Mother (or Other Household Contact) Has LTBI or Tuberculosis Disease. Management of the newborn infant is based on categorization of the maternal (or household contact) infection. Although protection of the infant from exposure and infection is of paramount importance, contact between infant and mother should be allowed when possible. Differing circumstances and resulting recommendations are as follows:

- **Mother (or household contact) has a positive TST or IGRA result and normal chest radiographic findings.** If the mother (or household contact) is asymptomatic, no separation is required. The mother usually is a candidate for treatment of LTBI after the initial postpartum period. The newborn infant needs no special evaluation or therapy. Because of the young infant's exquisite susceptibility, and because the mother's positive TST or IGRA result could be a marker of an unrecognized case of contagious tuberculosis within the household, other household members should have a TST or IGRA and further evaluation; this should not delay the infant's discharge from the hospital. These mothers can breastfeed their infants.

- **Mother (or household contact) has clinical signs and symptoms or abnormal findings on chest radiograph consistent with tuberculosis disease.** Cases of suspected or proven tuberculosis disease in mothers (or household contacts) should be reported immediately to the local health department, and investigation of all household members should start as soon as possible. If the mother has tuberculosis disease, the infant should be evaluated for congenital tuberculosis (see Congenital Tuberculosis), and the mother should be tested for HIV infection. The mother (or household contact) and the infant should be separated until the mother (or household contact) has been evaluated and, if tuberculosis disease is suspected, until the mother (or household contact) and infant are receiving appropriate antituberculosis therapy, the mother wears a mask, and the mother understands and is willing to adhere to infection-control measures. Once the infant is receiving isoniazid, separation is not necessary unless the mother (or household contact) has possible MDR tuberculosis disease or has poor adherence to treatment and DOT is not possible. If the mother is suspected of having MDR tuberculosis disease, an expert in tuberculosis disease treatment should be consulted. Women with drug-susceptible tuberculosis disease who have been treated appropriately for 2 or more weeks and who are not considered contagious can breastfeed.

If congenital tuberculosis is excluded, isoniazid is given until the infant is 3 or 4 months of age when a TST should be performed. If the TST result is positive, the infant should be reassessed for tuberculosis disease. If tuberculosis disease is excluded in an infant with a positive TST result, isoniazid alone should be continued for a total of 9 months. The infant should be evaluated monthly during treatment for signs of illness or poor growth. If the TST result is negative at 3 to 4 months of age and the mother (or household contact) has good adherence and response to treatment and no longer is contagious, isoniazid should be discontinued.

- **Mother (or household contact) has a positive TST or IGRA and abnormal findings on chest radiography but no evidence of tuberculosis disease.** If the chest radiograph of the mother (or household contact) appears abnormal but is not suggestive of tuberculosis disease and the history, physical examination, and sputum smear indicate no evidence of tuberculosis disease, the infant can be assumed to be at low risk of *M tuberculosis* infection and need not be separated from the mother (or household contact). The mother and her infant should receive follow-up care and the mother should be treated for LTBI. Other household members should have a TST or IGRA and further evaluation.

ISOLATION OF THE HOSPITALIZED PATIENT: Most children with tuberculosis disease, especially children younger than 10 years, are not contagious. Exceptions are the following: (1) children with pulmonary cavities; (2) children with positive sputum AFB smears; (3) children with laryngeal involvement; (4) children with extensive pulmonary infection; or (5) neonates or infants with congenital tuberculosis undergoing procedures that involve the oropharyngeal airway (eg, endotracheal intubation). In these instances, airborne infection isolation precautions for tuberculosis are indicated until effective therapy has been initiated, sputum smears are negative, and coughing has abated. Additional criteria apply to MDR tuberculosis. Children with no cough and negative sputum AFB smears can be hospitalized in an open ward. Infection-control measures for hospital personnel and visitors exposed to contagious patients should include the use of personally "fit tested" and "sealed" particulate respirators for all patient contacts (see Infection Control and Prevention for Hospitalized Children, p 161). The contagious patient should be placed in an airborne infection isolation room in the hospital.

The major concern in infection control relates to adult household members and contacts that can be the source of infection. Visitation should be limited to people who have been evaluated medically. Household members and contacts should be managed with tuberculosis precautions when visiting until they are demonstrated not to have contagious tuberculosis. Nonadherent household contacts should be excluded from hospital visitation until evaluation is complete and tuberculosis disease is excluded or treatment has rendered source cases noncontagious.

Tuberculosis Caused by M bovis. Infections with *M bovis* account for approximately 1% to 2% of tuberculosis cases in the United States. Children who come from countries where *M bovis* is prevalent in cattle or whose parents come from those countries are more likely to be infected. Most infections in humans are transmitted from cattle by unpasteurized milk and its products, such as fresh cheese,[1] although human-to-human transmission by the airborne route has been documented. In children, *M bovis* more commonly causes cervical lymphadenitis, intestinal tuberculosis disease and peritonitis, and meningitis. In adults, latent *M bovis* infection can progress to advanced pulmonary disease, with a risk of transmission to others.

The TST result typically is positive in a person infected with *M bovis*; IGRAs have not been studied systematically for diagnosing *M bovis* infection in particular, but theoretically they should have acceptable test characteristics. The definitive diagnosis of *M bovis* infection requires a culture isolate. The commonly used methods for identifying a microbial isolate as *M tuberculosis* complex do not distinguish *M bovis* from *M tuberculosis, M africanum,* and BCG; *M bovis* is suspected in clinical laboratories by its typical resistance to pyrazinamide. This approach can be unreliable, and species confirmation at a reference laboratory should be requested when *M bovis* is suspected. Molecular genotyping through the state health department may assist in identifying *M bovis*. Resistance to first-line drugs in addition to pyrazinamide has been reported. BCG rarely is isolated from pediatric clinical specimens in the United States; however, it should be suspected from the characteristic lesions or localized BCG suppuration or draining lymphadenitis in children who have received BCG vaccine. Only a reference laboratory can distinguish an isolate of BCG from an isolate of *M bovis.*

Therapy for M bovis Disease. Controlled clinical trials for treatment of *M bovis* disease have not been conducted, and treatment recommendations for *M bovis* disease in adults and children are based on results from treatment trials for *M tuberculosis* disease. Although most strains of *M bovis* are pyrazinamide-resistant and resistance to other first-line drugs has been reported, MDR strains are rare. Initial therapy disease caused by *M bovis* should include 3 or 4 drugs, excluding pyrazinamide, that would be used to treat disease attributable to *M tuberculosis*. For isoniazid- and rifampin-susceptible strains, a total treatment course of at least 9 to 12 months is recommended.

Parents should be counseled about the many infectious diseases transmitted by unpasteurized milk and its products,[1] and parents who might import traditional dairy products from countries where *M bovis* infection is prevalent in cattle should be advised against giving those products to their children. When people are exposed to an adult who has pulmonary disease caused by *M bovis* infection, they should be evaluated by the same methods as for *M tuberculosis.*

CONTROL MEASURES[2,3]: Reporting of suspected and confirmed cases of tuberculosis disease is mandated by law in all states. LTBI is reportable in some states. Control of

[1]American Academy of Pediatrics, Committee on Infectious Diseases and Committee on Nutrition. Consumption of raw or unpasteurized milk and milk products by pregnant women and children. *Pediatrics.* 2014;133(1):175–179

[2]American Thoracic Society, Centers for Disease Control and Prevention, and Infectious Diseases Society of America. Controlling tuberculosis in the United States. Recommendations from the American Thoracic Society, CDC, and the Infectious Diseases Society of America. *MMWR Recomm Rep.* 2005;54(RR-12):1–81

[3]Starke JR; American Academy of Pediatrics, Committee on Infectious Diseases. Clinical report: interferon-γ release assays for diagnosis of tuberculosis infection and disease in children. *Pediatrics.* 2014;134(6): e1763–e1773

tuberculosis disease in the United States requires collaboration between health care providers and health department personnel, obtaining a thorough history of exposure(s) to people with contagious tuberculosis, timely and effective contact investigations, proper interpretation of TST or IGRA results, and appropriate antituberculosis therapy, including DOT services. A plan to control and prevent extensively drug-resistant tuberculosis has been published.[1] Eliminating ingestion of unpasteurized dairy products will prevent most *M bovis* infection.[2]

Management of Contacts, Including Epidemiologic Investigation.[3,4] Children with a positive TST or IGRA result or tuberculosis disease ideally should be the starting point for epidemiologic investigation by the local health department, if adequate resources are available. Close contacts of a TST- or IGRA-positive child, if the test was performed because the child has 1 or more risk factors, should have a TST or IGRA, and people with a positive TST or IGRA result or with symptoms consistent with tuberculosis disease should be investigated further. Because children with tuberculosis usually are not contagious unless they have an adult-type multibacillary form of pulmonary or laryngeal disease, their contacts are not likely to be infected unless they also have been in contact with an adult source case. After the presumptive adult source of the child's tuberculosis is identified, other contacts of that adult should be evaluated.

Therapy for Contacts. Children and adolescents recently exposed to a contagious case of tuberculosis disease should have a TST or IGRA test performed and an evaluation for tuberculosis disease (chest radiography and physical examination) undertaken. For exposed contacts with impaired immunity (eg, HIV infection) and all contacts younger than 4 years, treatment for presumptive LTBI should be initiated, even if the initial TST or IGRA result is negative, once tuberculosis disease is excluded (see Treatment Regimens for LTBI, p 821). Infected people can have a negative TST or IGRA result because a cellular immune response has not yet developed or because of cutaneous anergy. People with a negative TST or IGRA result should be retested 8 to 10 weeks after the last exposure to a source of infection. If the TST or IGRA result still is negative in an immunocompetent person, isoniazid can be discontinued. If the contact is immunocompromised and LTBI cannot be excluded, after an evaluation for TB disease, treatment should be continued to the completion of the regimen. If a TST or IGRA result of a contact becomes positive, the regimen for LTBI should be completed after an evaluation for TB disease.

Child Care and Schools. Children with tuberculosis disease can attend school or child care if they are receiving therapy (see Children in Out-of-Home Child Care, p 132). They can return to regular activities as soon as effective therapy has been instituted, adherence to therapy has been documented, and clinical symptoms have diminished. Children with LTBI can participate in all activities whether they are receiving treatment or not.

---

[1]Centers for Disease Control and Prevention. Plan to combat extensively drug-resistant tuberculosis: recommendations of the Federal Tuberculosis Task Force. *MMWR Recomm Rep.* 2009;58(RR-3):1–43

[2]American Academy of Pediatrics, Committee on Infectious Diseases and Committee on Nutrition. Consumption of raw or unpasteurized milk and milk products by pregnant women and children. *Pediatrics.* 2014;133(1):175–179

[3]National Tuberculosis Controllers Association and Centers for Disease Control and Prevention. Guidelines for the investigation of contacts of persons with infectious tuberculosis. Recommendations from the National Tuberculosis Controllers Association and CDC. *MMWR Recomm Rep.* 2005;54(RR-15):1–47

[4]Starke JR; American Academy of Pediatrics, Committee on Infectious Diseases. Clinical report: interferon-γ release assays for diagnosis of tuberculosis infection and disease in children. *Pediatrics.* 2014;134(6):e1763–e1773

BCG Vaccines. BCG vaccine is a live vaccine originally prepared from attenuated strains of *M bovis.* Use of BCG vaccine[1] is recommended by the Expanded Programme on Immunization of the World Health Organization for administration at birth (see Table 1.6, p 15) and is used in more than 100 countries to reduce the incidence of disseminated and other life-threatening manifestations of tuberculosis in infants and young children. Although BCG immunization appears to decrease the risk of serious complications of tuberculosis disease in children, the various BCG vaccines used throughout the world differ in composition and efficacy.

Two meta-analyses of published clinical trials and case-control studies concerning the efficacy of BCG vaccines concluded that BCG vaccine has relatively high protective efficacy (approximately 80%) against meningeal and miliary tuberculosis in children. The protective efficacy against pulmonary tuberculosis differed significantly among the studies, precluding a specific conclusion. Protection afforded by BCG vaccine in one meta-analysis was estimated to be 50%. One BCG vaccine manufactured by Organon Teknika Corp and distributed by Merck/Schering-Plough is licensed in the United States for the prevention of tuberculosis. Comparative evaluations of this and other BCG vaccines have not been performed.

Indications. In the United States, administration of BCG vaccine should be considered only in limited and select circumstances, such as unavoidable risk of exposure to tuberculosis and failure or unfeasibility of other control methods. Recommendations for use of BCG vaccine for control of tuberculosis among children and health care personnel have been published by the Advisory Committee on Immunization Practices of the CDC and the Advisory Council for the Elimination of Tuberculosis.[2] For infants and children, BCG immunization should be considered only for people with a negative TST result who are not infected with HIV in the following circumstances:

- The child is exposed continually to a person or people with contagious pulmonary tuberculosis resistant to isoniazid and rifampin, and the child cannot be removed from this exposure.
- The child is exposed continually to a person or people with untreated or ineffectively treated contagious pulmonary tuberculosis and the child cannot be removed from such exposure or given antituberculosis therapy.

Careful assessment of the potential risks and benefits of BCG vaccine and consultation with personnel in local tuberculosis control programs are recommended strongly before use of BCG vaccine.

Healthy infants from birth to 2 months of age may be given BCG vaccine without a TST unless congenital infection is suspected; thereafter, BCG vaccine should be given only to children with a negative TST result.

Adverse Reactions. Uncommonly (1%–2% of immunizations), BCG vaccine can result in local adverse reactions, such as subcutaneous abscess and regional lymphadenopathy, which generally are not serious. One rare complication, osteitis affecting the epiphysis of long bones, can occur as long as several years after BCG immunization. Disseminated fatal infection occurs rarely (approximately 2 per 1 million people), primarily in people who are immunocompromised, such as children with poorly controlled HIV infection.

---

[1] **www.bcgatlas.org**

[2] Centers for Disease Control and Prevention. The role of BCG vaccine in the prevention and control of tuberculosis in the United States: a joint statement by the Advisory Committee for the Elimination of Tuberculosis and the Advisory Committee on Immunization Practices. *MMWR Recomm Rep.* 1996;45(RR-4):1–18

Antituberculosis therapy is recommended to treat osteitis and disseminated disease caused by BCG vaccine. Pyrazinamide is not believed to be effective against BCG and should not be included in treatment regimens.

Most localized complications of BCG vaccination self-resolve. Internationally, some experts advise observation without treatment, while others manage these infections with at least isoniazid and rifampin. In the United States, if treatment is undertaken, the regimen should consist of 2 or 3 drugs to which the isolate is susceptible. Most experts do not recommend treatment of draining skin lesions or chronic suppurative lymph-adenitis caused by BCG vaccine, because spontaneous resolution occurs in most cases. Large-needle aspiration of suppurative lymph nodes can hasten resolution. People with complications caused by BCG vaccine should be referred for management, if possible, to a tuberculosis expert and also should have consideration of evaluation for an immune deficiency.

Contraindications. People with burns, skin infections, and primary or secondary immu-nodeficiencies, including HIV infection, should not receive BCG vaccine. Because an increasing number of cases of localized and disseminated BCG have been described in infants and children with HIV infection, the World Health Organization no longer rec-ommends BCG in healthy, HIV-infected children. Use of BCG vaccine is contraindicated for people receiving immunosuppressive medications including high-dose corticosteroids (see Corticosteroids, p 824). Although no untoward effects of BCG vaccine on the fetus have been observed, immunization of women during pregnancy is not recommended.

Diseases Caused by Nontuberculous Mycobacteria
(Environmental Mycobacteria, Mycobacteria Other Than *Mycobacterium tuberculosis*)

CLINICAL MANIFESTATIONS: Several syndromes are caused by nontuberculous mycobac-teria (NTM). In children, the most common of these syndromes is cervical lymphadenitis. Cutaneous infection may follow soil- or water-contaminated traumatic wounds, surgeries, or cosmetic procedures (eg, tattoos, pedicures, body piercings).[1,2] Less common syndromes include soft tissue infection, osteomyelitis, otitis media, central catheter-associated blood-stream infections, and pulmonary infections, especially in adolescents with cystic fibrosis. NTM, especially *Mycobacterium avium* complex (MAC [including *M avium* and *Mycobacterium avium-intracellulare*]) and *Mycobacterium abscessus,* can be recovered from sputum in 10% to 20% of adolescents and young adults with cystic fibrosis and can be associated with fever and declining clinical status. Disseminated infections almost always are associated with impaired cell-mediated immunity, as found in children with congenital immune defects (eg, interleukin-12 deficiency, NF-kappa-B essential modulator [NEMO] mutation and related disorders, and interferon-gamma receptor defects), hematopoietic stem cell transplants, or advanced human immunodeficiency virus (HIV) infection. Disseminated MAC is rare in HIV-infected children during the first year of life. The frequency of dis-seminated MAC increases with increasing age and declining CD4+ T-lymphocyte counts,

---

[1]Wentworth AB, Drage LA, Wengenack NL, Wilson JW, Lohse CM. Increased incidence of cutaneous nontu-berculous mycobacterial infection, 1980 to 2009: a population-based study. *Mayo Clin Proc.* 2013;88(1):38–45

[2]Notes from the field: rapidly growing nontuberculous Mycobacterium wound infections among medical tour-ists undergoing cosmetic surgeries in the Dominican Republic—multiple states, March 2013–February 2014. *MMWR Morb Mortal Wkly Rep.* 2014;63(9):201–202

Table 3.85. Diseases Caused by Nontuberculous *Mycobacterium* Species

Clinical Disease	Common Species	Less Common Species in the United States
Cutaneous infection	*M chelonae, M fortuitum, M abscessus, M marinum*	*M ulcerans*[a]
Lymphadenitis	MAC; *M haemophilum; M lentiflavum*	*M kansasii, M fortuitum, M malmoense*[b]
Otologic infection	*M abscessus*	*M fortuitum*
Pulmonary infection	MAC, *M kansasii, M abscessus*	*M xenopi, M malmoense,*[b] *M szulgai, M fortuitum, M simiae*
Catheter-associated infection	*M chelonae, M fortuitum*	*M abscessus*
Skeletal infection	MAC, *M kansasii, M fortuitum*	*M chelonae, M marinum, M abscessus, M ulcerans*[a]
Disseminated	MAC	*M kansasii, M genavense, M haemophilum, M chelonae*

MAC indicates *Mycobacterium avium* complex.

[a]Not endemic in the United States.

[b]Found primarily in Northern Europe.

typically less than 50 cells/μL, in children older than 6 years.[1] Manifestations of disseminated NTM infections depend on the species and route of infection but include fever, night sweats, weight loss, abdominal pain, fatigue, diarrhea, and anemia. These signs and symptoms also are found in advanced immunosuppressed HIV-infected children without disseminated MAC. For HIV-infected children who have disseminated MAC, respiratory symptoms and isolated pulmonary disease are uncommon. In HIV-infected patients developing immune restoration with initiation of antiretroviral therapy (ART), local MAC symptoms can worsen temporarily. This immune reconstitution syndrome usually occurs 2 to 4 weeks after initiation of ART. Symptoms can include worsening fever, swollen lymph nodes, local pain, and laboratory abnormalities.

ETIOLOGY: Of the more than 130 species of NTM that have been identified, only a few account for most human infections. The species most commonly infecting children in the United States are MAC, *Mycobacterium fortuitum, M abscessus,* and *Mycobacterium marinum* (see Table 3.85). Several new species, which can be detected by nucleic acid amplification testing but cannot be grown by routine culture methods, have been identified in lymph nodes of children with cervical adenitis. NTM disease in patients with HIV infection usually is

---

[1]Guidelines for prevention and treatment of opportunistic infections in HIV-exposed and HIV-infected children. Recommendations from the National Institutes of Health, Centers for Disease Control and Prevention, the HIV Medicine Association of the Infectious Diseases Society of America, the Pediatric Infectious Diseases Society, and the American Academy of Pediatrics. *Pediatr Infect Dis J.* 2013;32(Suppl 2):i–KK4. Available at: **http://aidsinfo.nih.gov/guidelines/html/5/pediatric-oi-prevention-and-treatment-guidelines/0**

caused by MAC. *M fortuitum, Mycobacterium chelonae, M smegmatis,* and *M abscessus* commonly are referred to as "rapidly growing" mycobacteria (RGM), because sufficient growth and identification can be achieved in the laboratory within 3 to 7 days, whereas MAC, *M marinum, M szulgai* usually require several weeks before sufficient growth occurs for identification (SGM). Rapidly growing mycobacteria have been implicated in wound, soft tissue, bone, pulmonary, central venous catheter, and middle-ear infections. Other mycobacterial species that usually are not pathogenic have caused infections in immunocompromised hosts or have been associated with the presence of a foreign body.

EPIDEMIOLOGY: Many NTM species are ubiquitous in nature and are found in soil, food, water, and animals. Tap water is the major reservoir for *Mycobacterium kansasii, Mycobacterium lentiflavum, Mycobacterium xenopi, Mycobacterium simiae,* and health care-associated infections attributable to the rapidly growing mycobacteria *M abscessus* and *M fortuitum.* Outbreaks have been associated with contaminated water used for pedicures and inks used for tattooing. For *M marinum,* water in a fish tank or aquarium or an injury in a salt-water environment are the major sources of infection. The environmental reservoir for *M abscessus* and MAC causing pulmonary infection is unknown. Although many people are exposed to NTM, it is unknown why some exposures result in acute or chronic infection. Usual portals of entry for NTM infection are believed to be abrasions in the skin (eg, cutaneous lesions caused by *M marinum*), penetrating trauma (needles and organic material most often associated with *M abscessus* and *M fortuitum*), surgical sites (especially for central vascular catheters), oropharyngeal mucosa (the presumed portal of entry for cervical lymphadenitis), gastrointestinal or respiratory tract for disseminated MAC, and respiratory tract (including tympanostomy tubes for otitis media). Pulmonary disease and rare cases of mediastinal adenitis and endobronchial disease do occur. NTM can be an important pathogen in patients with cystic fibrosis and is an emerging pathogen in individuals receiving biologic response modifiers, such as anti-tumor necrosis factor-alpha (see Biologic Response Modifiers Used to Decrease Inflammation, p 83). Most infections remain localized at the portal of entry or in regional lymph nodes. Dissemination to distal sites primarily occurs in immunocompromised hosts. No definitive evidence of person-to-person transmission of NTM exists. Outbreaks of otitis media caused by *M abscessus* have been associated with polyethylene ear tubes and use of contaminated equipment or water. A waterborne route of transmission has been implicated for MAC infection in some immunodeficient hosts. Buruli ulcer disease is a skin and bone infection caused by *Mycobacterium ulcerans,* an emerging disease causing significant morbidity and disability in tropical areas such as Africa, Asia, South America, Australia, and the western Pacific.

The **incubation periods** are variable.

DIAGNOSTIC TESTS: Routine screening of respiratory or gastrointestinal tract specimens for MAC microorganisms is not recommended. Definitive diagnosis of NTM disease requires isolation of the organism. Consultation with the laboratory should occur to ensure that culture specimens are handled correctly. For example, isolation of *Mycobacterium haemophilum* requires that the culture be maintained at 30°C and that heme-containing medium is added for isolation. Because these organisms commonly are found in the environment, contamination of cultures or transient colonization can occur. Caution must be exercised in interpretation of cultures obtained from nonsterile sites, such as gastric washing specimens, endoscopy material, a single expectorated sputum sample, or urine specimens, and also when the species cultured usually is non-pathogenic (eg, *Mycobacterium terrae* complex or *Mycobacterium gordonae*). An acid-fast bacilli smear-positive sample and repeated isolation on culture media of a single species from any site are more likely to indicate disease than culture contamination or transient colonization. Diagnostic criteria for NTM lung disease in adults include 2 or more separate sputum samples that grow NTM or 1 bronchial alveolar lavage specimen that grows NTM.[1] These criteria have not been validated in children and apply best to MAC, *M kansasii,* and *M abscessus.* NTM isolates from draining sinus tracts or wounds almost always are significant clinically. Recovery of NTM from sites that usually are sterile, such as cerebrospinal fluid, pleural fluid, bone marrow, blood, lymph node aspirates, middle ear or mastoid aspirates, or surgically excised tissue, is the most reliable diagnostic test. With radiometric or nonradiometric broth techniques, blood cultures are highly sensitive in recovery of disseminated MAC and other bloodborne NTM species. Disseminated MAC disease should prompt a search for underlying immunodeficiency.

Patients with NTM infection, such as *M marinum* or MAC cervical lymphadenitis, can have a positive tuberculin skin test (TST) result, because the purified protein derivative preparation, derived from *M tuberculosis,* shares a number of antigens with NTM species. These TST reactions usually measure less than 10 mm of induration but can measure more than 15 mm (see Tuberculosis, p 804). The interferon-gamma release assays use 2 or 3 antigens to detect infection with *M tuberculosis.* Although these antigens are not found on *M avium-intracellulare* and most other NTM species, cross reactions can occur with infection caused by *M kansasii, M marinum,* and *Mycobacterium szulgai* (see Tuberculosis, p 804).

TREATMENT: Many NTM are relatively resistant in vitro to antituberculosis drugs. In vitro resistance to these agents, however, does not necessarily correlate with clinical response, especially with MAC infections. Only limited controlled trials of drug treatment have been performed in patients with NTM infections. The approach to therapy should be directed by the following: (1) the species causing the infection; (2) the results of drug-susceptibility testing; (3) the site(s) of infection; (4) the patient's immune status; and (5) the need to treat a patient presumptively for tuberculosis while awaiting culture reports that subsequently reveal NTM.

For NTM lymphadenitis in otherwise healthy children, especially when the disease is caused by MAC, complete surgical excision is curative. Antimicrobial therapy has been shown in a randomized, controlled trial to provide no additional benefit. Therapy with clarithromycin or azithromycin combined with ethambutol or rifampin or rifabutin may be beneficial for children in whom surgical excision is incomplete or for children with recurrent disease (see Table 3.86, p 835).

Isolates of rapidly growing mycobacteria (*M fortuitum, M abscessus,* and *M chelonae*) should be tested in vitro against drugs to which they commonly are susceptible and that have been used with some therapeutic success (eg, amikacin, imipenem, sulfamethoxazole or trimethoprim-sulfamethoxazole, cefoxitin, ciprofloxacin, clarithromycin, linezolid, and doxycycline). Clarithromycin and at least 1 other agent is the treatment of choice for cutaneous (disseminated) infections attributable to *M chelonae* or *M abscessus.* Indwelling foreign bodies should be removed, and surgical débridement for serious localized disease is optimal. The choice of drugs, dosages, and duration should be reviewed with a consultant experienced in the management of NTM infections.

---

[1]American Thoracic Society and Infectious Disease Society of America. An official ATS/IDSA statement: diagnosis, treatment, and prevention of nontuberculous mycobacterial diseases. *Am J Respir Crit Care Med.* 2007;175(4):367–416

Table 3.86. Treatment of Nontuberculous Mycobacteria Infections in Children

Organism	Disease	Initial Treatment
Slowly Growing Species		
Mycobacterium avium complex (MAC); *Mycobacterium haemophilum*; *Mycobacterium lentiflavum*	Lymphadenitis	Complete excision of lymph nodes; if excision incomplete or disease recurs, clarithromycin or azithromycin plus ethambutol and/or rifampin (or rifabutin).
	Pulmonary infection	Clarithromycin or azithromycin plus ethambutol with rifampin or rifabutin (pulmonary resection in some patients who fail to respond to drug therapy). For severe disease, an initial course of amikacin or streptomycin often is included. Clinical data in adults support that 3-times-weekly therapy is as effective as daily therapy, with less toxicity for adult patients with mild to moderate disease. For patients with advanced or cavitary disease, drugs should be given daily.
	Disseminated	See text.
Mycobacterium kansasii	Pulmonary infection	Rifampin plus ethambutol with isoniazid daily. If rifampin-resistance is detected, a 3-drug regimen based on drug susceptibility testing should be used.
	Osteomyelitis	Surgical débridement and prolonged antimicrobial therapy using rifampin plus ethambutol with isoniazid.
Mycobacterium marinum	Cutaneous infection	None, if minor; rifampin, trimethoprim-sulfamethoxazole, clarithromycin, or doxycycline[a] for moderate disease; extensive lesions may require surgical débridement. Susceptibility testing not routinely required.
Mycobacterium ulcerans	Cutaneous and bone infections	Daily intramuscular streptomycin and oral rifampin for 8 weeks; excision to remove necrotic tissue, if present; disability prevention

continued

Table 3.86. Treatment of Nontuberculous Mycobacteria Infections in Children, continued

Organism	Disease	Initial Treatment
Rapidly Growing Species		
Mycobacterium fortuitum group	Cutaneous infection	Initial therapy for serious disease is amikacin plus meropenem, IV, followed by clarithromycin, doxycycline[a] or trimethoprim-sulfamethoxazole, or ciprofloxacin, orally, on the basis of in vitro susceptibility testing; may require surgical excision. Up to 50% of isolates are resistant to cefoxitin.
	Catheter infection	Catheter removal and amikacin plus meropenem, IV; clarithromycin, trimethoprim-sulfamethoxazole, or ciprofloxacin, orally, on the basis of in vitro susceptibility testing.
Mycobacterium abscessus	Otitis media; cutaneous infection	There is no reliable antimicrobial regimen because of variability in drug susceptibility. Clarithromycin plus initial course of amikacin plus cefoxitin or meropenem; may require surgical débridement on the basis of in vitro susceptibility testing (50% are amikacin resistant).
	Pulmonary infection (in cystic fibrosis)	Serious disease, clarithromycin, amikacin, and cefoxitin or meropenem on the basis of susceptibility testing; may require surgical resection.
Mycobacterium chelonae	Catheter infection	Catheter removal and tobramycin (initially) plus clarithromycin.
	Disseminated cutaneous infection	Tobramycin and meropenem or linezolid (initially) plus clarithromycin.

IV indicates intravenously.

[a] Tetracycline-based antimicrobial agents, including doxycycline, may cause permanent tooth discoloration for children younger than 8 years if used for repeated treatment courses. However, doxycycline binds less readily to calcium compared with older tetracyclines, and in some studies, doxycycline was not associated with visible teeth staining in younger children (see Tetracyclines, p 873). Only 50% of isolates of *M marinum* are susceptible to doxycycline.

For patients with cystic fibrosis and isolation of MAC species, treatment is suggested only for those with clinical symptoms not attributable to other causes, worsening lung function, and chest radiographic progression. The decision to embark on therapy should take into consideration susceptibility testing results and should involve consultation with an expert in cystic fibrosis care. *M abscessus* is difficult to treat, and the role of therapy in clinical benefit is unknown.

In patients with acquired immunodeficiency syndrome (AIDS) and in other immunocompromised people with disseminated MAC infection, multidrug therapy is recommended. Clinical isolates of MAC usually are resistant to many of the approved antituberculosis drugs, including isoniazid, but are susceptible to clarithromycin and azithromycin and often are susceptible to combinations of ethambutol, rifabutin or rifampin, and amikacin or streptomycin. Susceptibility testing to these other agents has not been standardized and, thus, is not recommended routinely. The optimal regimen is yet to be determined. Treatment of disseminated MAC infection should be undertaken in consultation with an expert. In addition, the following treatment guidelines should be considered:

- Susceptibility testing to drugs other than the macrolides is not predictive of in vivo response and should not be used to guide therapy.
- Unless there is clinical or laboratory evidence of macrolide resistance, treatment regimens should contain clarithromycin or azithromycin, combined with ethambutol. This 2-drug regimen is the foundation for any MAC treatment.
- Many clinicians have added a third agent (rifampin or rifabutin), especially for pulmonary disease, and in some situations, a fourth agent (amikacin or streptomycin).
- Drug-drug interactions can occur between medications used to treat disseminated MAC and HIV infections. Protease inhibitors (PIs) can increase and efavirenz can decrease clarithromycin concentrations. Available data are not adequate to make recommendations for clarithromycin dose adjustments in these circumstances. Azithromycin is not metabolized by the cytochrome P450 (CYP 450) system, and drug-drug interactions with PIs and efavirenz is not a concern. Rifampin and rifabutin increase CYP 450 activity and lead to more rapid clearance of PIs and efavirenz and increase toxicity. Rifampin and rifabutin should be avoided in HIV-infected children receiving PIs or efavirenz.[1,2]
- The optimal time to initiate ART in a child in whom HIV and disseminated MAC are newly diagnosed is not established. Many experts would provide treatment of disseminated MAC for 2 weeks before initiating ART in an attempt to minimize occurrence of the immune reconstitution syndrome and minimize confusion relating to the cause of drug-associated toxicity.
- Clofazimine is ineffective for treatment of MAC infection and should not be used.

---

[1]Centers for Disease Control and Prevention. Guidelines for the prevention and treatment of opportunistic infections among HIV-exposed and HIV-infected children: recommendations from the CDC, the National Institutes of Health, the HIV Medicine Association of the Infectious Diseases Society of America, the Pediatric Infectious Diseases Society, and the American Academy of Pediatrics. *MMWR Recomm Rep.* 2009;58(RR-11):1–166

[2]Guidelines for prevention and treatment of opportunistic infections in HIV-exposed and HIV-infected children. Recommendations from the National Institutes of Health, Centers for Disease Control and Prevention, the HIV Medicine Association of the Infectious Diseases Society of America, the Pediatric Infectious Diseases Society, and the American Academy of Pediatrics. *Pediatr Infect Dis J.* 2013;32(Suppl 2):i–KK4. Available at: **http://aidsinfo.nih.gov/guidelines/html/5/pediatric-oi-prevention-and-treatment-guidelines/0**

- Patients receiving therapy should be monitored. Considerations are as follows:
  - Most patients who respond ultimately show substantial clinical improvement in the first 4 to 6 weeks of therapy. Elimination of the organisms from blood cultures can take longer, often up to 12 weeks.
  - Patients receiving clarithromycin plus rifabutin or high-dose rifabutin (with another drug) should be observed for the rifabutin-related development of leukopenia, uveitis, polyarthralgia, and pseudojaundice.

The duration of therapy for NTM infections will depend on host status, site(s) of involvement, and severity. Most experts recommend a minimum of 3 to 6 months or longer. **Chemoprophylaxis.** The most effective way to prevent disseminated MAC in HIV-infected children is to preserve their immune function through use of combination ART. HIV-infected children with advanced immunosuppression should be offered prophylaxis against disseminated MAC with azithromycin or clarithromycin.[1,2] Age-related advanced immunosuppression is defined according to the following CD4+ T-lymphocyte thresholds:

- 6 years or older: <50 cells/μL;
- 2 through 5 years of age: <75 cells/μL;
- 1 to 2 years of age: <500 cells/μL; and
- Younger than 1 year: <750 cells/μL.

Rifabutin is a less effective alternative agent that should not be used until tuberculosis disease has been excluded. Disseminated MAC should be excluded by a negative blood culture result before prophylaxis is initiated. Combination therapy for prophylaxis should be avoided in children, if possible, because it has not been shown to be cost effective and increases rates of adverse events. Children with a history of disseminated MAC and continued immunosuppression should receive lifelong prophylaxis to prevent recurrence.

Oral suspensions of clarithromycin and azithromycin are available in the United States. Appropriate doses are: clarithromycin, 7.5 mg/kg (maximum, 500 mg), orally, twice daily; azithromycin, 20 mg/kg (maximum, 1200 mg), orally, weekly; or azithromycin, 5 mg/kg (maximum, 250 mg), orally, daily. No pediatric formulation of rifabutin is available, but a dosage of 5 mg/kg per day (maximum, 300 mg) seems appropriate. Rifabutin should be used only for children 6 years or older. Prophylaxis can be discontinued in some HIV-infected children after immune reconstitution.[2]

ISOLATION OF THE HOSPITALIZED PATIENT: Standard precautions are recommended.

---

[1]Centers for Disease Control and Prevention. Guidelines for the prevention and treatment of opportunistic infections among HIV-exposed and HIV-infected children: recommendations from the CDC, the National Institutes of Health, the HIV Medicine Association of the Infectious Diseases Society of America, the Pediatric Infectious Diseases Society, and the American Academy of Pediatrics. *MMWR Recomm Rep.* 2009;58(RR-11):1–166

[2]Guidelines for prevention and treatment of opportunistic infections in HIV-exposed and HIV-infected children. Recommendations from the National Institutes of Health, Centers for Disease Control and Prevention, the HIV Medicine Association of the Infectious Diseases Society of America, the Pediatric Infectious Diseases Society, and the American Academy of Pediatrics. *Pediatr Infect Dis J.* 2013;32(Suppl 2):i–KK4. Available at: **http://aidsinfo.nih.gov/guidelines/html/5/pediatric-oi-prevention-and-treatment-guidelines/0**

CONTROL MEASURES: Control measures include chemoprophylaxis for high-risk patients with HIV infection (see Treatment, p 834)[1]; avoidance of tap water contamination of central venous catheters surgical wounds, skin, or endoscopic equipment; and use of sterile equipment for middle-ear instrumentation, including otoscopic equipment, for prevention of *M abscessus* otitis media. Because MAC and *M abscessus* are common in environmental sources, current information does not support specific recommendations about avoidance of exposure for HIV-infected people (MAC) or adolescents with cystic fibrosis (MAC or *M abscessus*).

Tularemia

CLINICAL MANIFESTATIONS: Most patients with tularemia have abrupt onset of fever, chills, myalgia, and headache. Illness usually conforms to one of several tularemic syndromes. Most common is the ulceroglandular syndrome, characterized by a maculopapular lesion at the entry site with subsequent ulceration and slow healing, associated with painful, acutely inflamed regional lymph nodes that can drain spontaneously. The glandular syndrome (regional lymphadenopathy with no ulcer) also is common. Less common disease syndromes are: respiratory (flu-like symptoms often without chest radiograph abnormalities), oculoglandular (severe conjunctivitis and preauricular lymphadenopathy), oropharyngeal (severe exudative stomatitis, pharyngitis, or tonsillitis and cervical lymphadenopathy), vesicular skin lesions that can be mistaken for herpes simplex virus or varicella zoster virus cutaneous infections, typhoidal (systemic infection, high fever, hepatomegaly, splenomegaly, and possibly septicemia), and intestinal (intestinal pain, vomiting, and diarrhea). Respiratory tularemia, characterized by fever, dry cough, chest pain, and hilar adenopathy, normally is associated with farming or lawn maintenance activities that create aerosols and dust. This would also be the anticipated syndrome after intentional aerosol release of organisms.

ETIOLOGY: *Francisella tularensis* is a small, weakly-staining, gram-negative pleomorphic coccobacillus. Two subspecies cause human infection in North America, *F tularensis* subspecies *tularensis* (type A), and *F tularensis* subspecies *holarctica* (type B). Type A can be further subdivided into 4 distinct genotypes (A1a, A1b, A2a, A2b), with A1b appearing to produce more serious disease in humans. Type A generally is considered more virulent, although either can be lethal, especially if inhaled.

EPIDEMIOLOGY: *F tularensis* can infect more than 100 animal species; vertebrates considered most important in enzootic cycles are rabbits, hares, and rodents, especially muskrats, voles, beavers, and prairie dogs. Domestic cats are another source of infection. In the United States, human infection usually is associated with direct contact with one of these species, or with the bite of arthropod vectors such as ticks and deer flies. Infection has been reported in commercially traded hamsters and in a child bitten by a pet hamster. Infection also can be acquired following ingestion of contaminated water or inadequately

[1]Guidelines for prevention and treatment of opportunistic infections in HIV-exposed and HIV-infected children. Recommendations from the National Institutes of Health, Centers for Disease Control and Prevention, the HIV Medicine Association of the Infectious Diseases Society of America, the Pediatric Infectious Diseases Society, and the American Academy of Pediatrics. *Pediatr Infect Dis J.* 2013;32(Suppl 2):i–KK4. Available at: **http://aidsinfo.nih.gov/guidelines/html/5/pediatric-oi-prevention-and-treatment-guidelines/0**

cooked meat, inhalation of contaminated aerosols generated during lawn mowing, brush cutting, or certain farming activities, such as baling contaminated hay. At-risk people have occupational or recreational exposure to infected animals or their habitats, such as rabbit hunters and trappers, people exposed to certain ticks or biting insects, and laboratory technicians working with *F tularensis*, which is highly infectious and may be aerosolized when grown in culture. In the United States, most cases occur during May through September. Approximately two thirds of cases occur in males, and one quarter of cases occur in children 1 to 14 years of age. Tularemia has been reported in all US states except Hawaii. Six states accounted for 59% of reported cases: Missouri (19%), Arkansas (13%), Oklahoma (9%), Massachusetts (7%), South Dakota (5%), and Kansas (5%). Among the 10 states with the highest incidence of tularemia, all but Massachusetts were located in the central or western United States. Tularemia has been a nationally notifiable disease since 2000. During 2001–2010, 1208 cases were reported (median: 126.5 cases per year; range: 90–154).[1] Organisms can be present in blood during the first 2 weeks of disease, and in cutaneous lesions for as long as 1 month if untreated. Person-to-person transmission has not been reported.

The **incubation period** usually is 3 to 5 days, with a range of 1 to 21 days.

DIAGNOSTIC TESTS: Diagnosis is established most often by serologic testing. Most clinical laboratories are not equipped to perform the generally accepted diagnostic tests for tularemia, and suspect samples may need to be processed by a designated reference laboratory. Patients do not develop antibodies until the second week of illness. A single serum antibody titer of 1:128 or greater determined by microagglutination (MA) or of 1:160 or greater determined by tube agglutination (TA) is consistent with recent or past infection and constitutes a presumptive diagnosis. Confirmation by serologic testing requires a fourfold or greater titer change between serum samples obtained at least 2 weeks apart, with 1 of the specimens having a minimum titer of 1:128 or greater by MA or 1:160 or greater by TA. Nonspecific cross-reactions can occur with specimens containing heterophile antibodies or antibodies to *Brucella* species, *Legionella* species, or other gram-negative bacteria. However, cross-reactions rarely result in MA or TA titers that are diagnostic. Some clinical laboratories presumptively can identify *F tularensis* in ulcer exudate or aspirate material by polymerase chain reaction (PCR) assay or direct fluorescent antibody assay. Immunohistochemical staining is specific for detection of *F tularensis* in fixed tissues; however, this method is not available in most clinical laboratories. Isolation of *F tularensis* from specimens of blood, skin, ulcers, lymph node drainage, gastric washings, or respiratory tract secretions is best achieved by inoculation of cysteine-enriched media such as that used for clinical isolation of *Legionella*. Suspect growth on culture can be identified presumptively by PCR or direct fluorescent antibody assays. Because of its propensity for causing laboratory-acquired infections, laboratory personnel should be alerted when *F tularensis* infection is suspected.

TREATMENT: Gentamicin (5 mg/kg/day, divided twice or 3 times/day, intravenously or intramuscularly) is the drug of choice for the treatment of tularemia in children because of the limited availability of streptomycin (30–40 mg/kg/day, divided twice/day, intramuscularly) and the fewer adverse effects of gentamicin. Duration of therapy usually is 7 to 10 days. A 5- to 7-day course may be sufficient in mild disease, but a longer

---

[1]Centers for Disease Control and Prevention. Tularemia—United States, 2001–2010. *MMWR Morb Mortal Wkly Rep.* 2013;62(47):963–966

course is required for more severe illness (eg, meningitis). Ciprofloxacin is an alternative for mild disease but is not approved by the US Food and Drug Administration for this indication, and data supporting its use in patients younger than 18 years are limited. Doxycycline is another alternative agent but is associated with a higher rate of relapses when compared with other therapies, and longer courses (14 days) of therapy should be used. Tetracycline-based antimicrobial agents, including doxycycline, may cause permanent tooth discoloration for children younger than 8 years if used for repeated treatment courses. However, doxycycline binds less readily to calcium compared with older tetracyclines, and in some studies, doxycycline was not associated with visible teeth staining in younger children (see Tetracyclines, p 873). Suppuration of lymph nodes can occur despite antimicrobial therapy. *F tularensis* is resistant to beta-lactam drugs and carbapenems.

ISOLATION OF THE HOSPITALIZED PATIENT: Standard precautions are recommended.

CONTROL MEASURES:
- People should protect themselves against arthropod bites by wearing protective clothing, by frequent inspection for and removal of ticks from the skin and scalp, and by using insect repellents (see Prevention of Tickborne Infections, p 210).
- Gloves should be worn by those handling the carcasses of wild rabbits and other potentially infected animals. Children should not handle sick or dead animals, including pets.
- Game meats should be cooked thoroughly.
- Primary clinical specimens may be handled in the laboratory using Biological Safety Level 2 (BSL2) precautions. Work with suspected cultures requires BSL3 precautions. Note that *F tularensis* is a tier 1 select agent and must be handled as such after it has been identified.
- Standard precautions should be used for handling clinical materials.
- A 14-day course of doxycycline or ciprofloxacin is recommended for children and adults after exposure to an intentional release of tularemia and for laboratory workers with inadvertent exposure to *F tularensis*.
- A live-attenuated vaccine derived from *F tularensis* subspecies *holarctica* (type B) strain to protect at-risk personnel, including people routinely working with *F tularensis* in the laboratory, is available via the Special Immunization Program administered by the US Department of Defense.

Endemic Typhus
(Murine Typhus)

CLINICAL MANIFESTATIONS: Endemic typhus resembles epidemic (louseborne) typhus but usually has a less abrupt onset with less severe systemic symptoms. In young children, the disease can be mild. Fever, present in almost all patients, can be accompanied by a persistent, usually severe, headache and myalgia. Nausea and vomiting also develop in approximately half of patients. A rash typically appears on day 4 to 7 of illness, is macular or maculopapular, lasts 4 to 8 days, and tends to remain discrete, with sparse lesions and no hemorrhage. Rash is present in approximately 50% of patients. Illness seldom lasts longer than 2 weeks; visceral involvement is uncommon. Laboratory findings include thrombocytopenia, elevated liver transaminases, and hyponatremia. Fatal outcome is rare except in untreated severe disease.

ETIOLOGY: Endemic typhus is caused by *Rickettsia typhi* and *Rickettsia felis*.

EPIDEMIOLOGY: Rats, in which infection is unapparent, are the natural reservoirs for *Rickettsia typhi*. The primary vector for transmission among rats and to humans is the rat flea, *Xenopsylla cheopis*, although other fleas and mites have been implicated. Cat fleas and opossums have been implicated as the source of some cases of endemic typhus caused by *Rickettsia felis*. Infected flea feces are rubbed into broken skin or mucous membranes or are inhaled. The disease is worldwide in distribution and tends to occur most commonly in adults, in males, and during the months of April to October in the United States; in children, males and females are affected equally. Exposure to rats and their fleas is the major risk factor for infection, although a history of such exposure often is absent. Endemic typhus is rare in the United States, with most cases occurring in southern California, southern Texas, the southeastern Gulf Coast, and Hawaii.

The **incubation period** is 6 to 14 days.

DIAGNOSTIC TESTS: Antibody titers determined with *R typhi* antigen by an indirect fluorescent antibody (IFA) assay, enzyme immunoassay, or latex agglutination test peak around 4 weeks after infection, but results of these test often are negative early in the course of illness. A fourfold immunoglobulin (Ig) G titer change between acute and convalescent serum specimens taken 2 to 3 weeks apart is diagnostic. Although more prone to false-positive results, immunoassays demonstrating increases in specific IgM antibody can aid in distinguishing clinical illness from previous exposure if interpreted with a concurrent IgG test; use of IgM assays alone is not recommended. Serologic tests may not differentiate murine typhus from epidemic (louseborne) typhus, *Rickettsia felis* infection, or from infection with spotted fever rickettsiosis, such as *R rickettsii*, without antibody cross-absorption for IFA or western blotting analyses, which are not available routinely. Isolation of the organism in cell culture potentially is hazardous and is best performed by specialized laboratories, such as the Centers for Disease Control and Prevention (CDC). Routine hospital blood cultures are not suitable for culture of *R typhi*. Molecular diagnostic assays on infected whole blood and skin biopsies can distinguish endemic and epidemic typhus and other rickettsioses and are performed at the CDC. Immunohistochemical procedures on formalin-fixed skin biopsy tissues can be performed at the CDC.

TREATMENT: Doxycycline is the treatment of choice for endemic typhus, regardless of patient age. The recommended dosage of doxycycline is 4 mg/kg per day, divided every 12 hours, intravenously or orally (maximum 100 mg/dose [see Tetracyclines, p 873]). Doxycycline has not been demonstrated to cause cosmetic staining of developing permanent teeth when used in the dose and duration recommended to treat rickettsial diseases. Treatment should be continued for at least 3 days after defervescence and evidence of clinical improvement is documented, and the total treatment course is usually for 7 to 14 days. Fluoroquinolones or chloramphenicol are alternative medications but may not be as effective; fluoroquinolones are not approved for this use in children younger than 18 years (see Fluoroquinolones, p 872).

ISOLATION OF THE HOSPITALIZED PATIENT: Standard precautions are recommended.

CONTROL MEASURES: Fleas should be controlled by appropriate insecticides before use of rodenticides, because fleas will seek alternative hosts, including humans. Suspected animal populations should be controlled by species-appropriate means. No prophylaxis is recommended for exposed people. The disease should be reported to local or state public health departments.

Epidemic Typhus
(Louseborne or Sylvatic Typhus)

CLINICAL MANIFESTATIONS: Clinically, epidemic typhus should be considered when people in crowded conditions develop abrupt onset of high fever, chills, and myalgia accompanied by severe headache and malaise. Although epidemic typhus patients often develop a rash by day 4 to 7 after the start of illness, rash may not always be present and should not be relied on for diagnosis. When present, the rash usually begins on the trunk, spreads to the limbs, and generally spares the face, palms, and soles. The rash typically is macular to maculopapular, but in advanced stages can become petechial or hemorrhagic. There is no eschar, as often is present in many other rickettsial diseases. Abdominal complaints (stomach pain, nausea) and changes in mental status are common, and delirium or coma may occur. Myocardial and renal failure can occur when the disease is severe. The fatality rate in untreated people is as high as 30%. Mortality is less common in children, and the rate increases with advancing age. Untreated patients who recover typically have an illness lasting 2 weeks. Brill-Zinsser disease is a relapse of epidemic typhus that can occur years after the initial episode. Factors that reactivate the rickettsiae are unknown, but relapse often is more mild and of shorter duration.

ETIOLOGY: Epidemic typhus is caused by *Rickettsia prowazekii*.

EPIDEMIOLOGY: Humans are the primary reservoir of the organism, which is transmitted from person to person by the human body louse, *Pediculus humanus corporis*. Infected louse feces are rubbed into broken skin or mucous membranes or are inhaled. All ages are affected. Poverty, crowding, and poor sanitary conditions contribute to the spread of body lice and, hence, the disease. Cases of epidemic typhus are rare in the United States but have occurred throughout the world, including the colder, mountainous areas of Asia, Africa, some parts of Europe, and Central and South America, particularly in refugee camps and jails of resource-limited countries. Epidemic typhus is most common during winter, when conditions favor person-to-person transmission of the vector, the body louse. Rickettsiae are present in the blood and tissues of patients during the early febrile phase but are not found in secretions. Direct person-to-person spread of the disease does not occur in the absence of the louse vector.

In the United States, sporadic human cases associated with close contact with infected flying squirrels (*Glaucomys volans*), their nests, or their ectoparasites occasionally are reported in the eastern United States. Cases have been reported in people who reside or work in flying squirrel-infested dwellings, even when direct contact is not reported. Flying squirrel-associated disease, called sylvatic typhus, typically presents with a similar illness to that observed with body louse-transmitted infection. Illness can be severe, although fatalities are uncommonly reported with sylvatic typhus; the later development of Brill Zinsser disease has been confirmed in at least 1 case of untreated sylvatic typhus. *Amblyomma* ticks in the Americas and in Ethiopia have been shown to carry *R prowazekii*, but their vector potential is unknown.

The **incubation period** is 1 to 2 weeks.

DIAGNOSTIC TESTS: Epidemic typhus may be diagnosed by the detection of *R prowazekii* DNA in acute blood and serum specimens by polymerase chain reaction (PCR) assay. The specimen should preferably be taken within the first week of symptoms and before (or within 24 hours of) doxycycline administration, and a negative result does not rule out

R prowazekii infection. Diagnosis may also be attained by the detection of rickettsial DNA in biopsy or autopsy specimens by PCR assay or immunohistochemical (IHC) visualization of rickettsiae in tissues. The gold standard for serologic diagnosis of epidemic typhus is a fourfold increase in immunoglobulin (Ig) G antibody titer by the indirect fluorescent antibody (IFA) test. A negative acute serologic test does not rule out a diagnosis of epidemic typhus. Both IgG and IgM antibodies begin to increase around day 7 to 10 after onset of symptoms; therefore, an elevated acute titer may represent past exposure rather than acute infection. Low-level elevated antibody titers can be an incidental finding in a significant proportion of the general population in some regions. IgM antibodies may remain elevated for months and are not highly specific for acute epidemic typhus. A confirmed case, therefore, is one that shows a fourfold or greater increase in antigen-specific IgG between acute and convalescent sera obtained 2 to 6 weeks apart. Cross-reactivity may be observed to antibodies to *R typhi* (the agent of endemic typhus), *R rickettsii* (the agent of Rocky Mountain spotted fever), and other spotted fever group rickettsiae. Testing of acute and convalescent sera by enzyme immunoassays or dot blot immunoassay tests can also be used for assessing presence of antibody but are less useful for quantifying changes in titer. *R prowazekii* may also be isolated from acute blood specimens by animal passage or through tissue culture, but this can be hazardous, and culture is restricted to specialized procedures (not routine blood culture) at reference laboratories with at minimum Biosafety Level 3 containment facilities. Cell culture cultivation of the organism must be confirmed by molecular methods.

TREATMENT: Doxycycline is the drug of choice to treat epidemic typhus, regardless of patient age. The recommended dosage of doxycycline is 4 mg/kg per day, divided every 12 hours, intravenously or orally (maximum 100 mg/dose [see Tetracyclines, p 873]). Doxycycline is available in both oral and intravenous formulations (see Tetracyclines, p 873). Doxycycline has not been demonstrated to cause cosmetic staining of developing permanent teeth when used in the dose and duration recommended to treat rickettsial diseases. Treatment should be continued for at least 3 days after defervescence and evidence of clinical improvement is documented, and the total treatment course is usually for 5 to 10 days. Other broad-spectrum antibiotics, including ciprofloxacin, are not recommended and may be more likely to result in fatal outcome. Chloramphenicol may be used in cases of absolute contraindication of doxycycline (life-threatening allergy) but also carries significant risks (ie, aplastic anemia). To halt the spread of disease to other people, louse-infested patients should be treated with cream or gel pediculicides containing pyrethrins or permethrin; malathion is prescribed most often when pyrethroids fail. In epidemic situations in which antimicrobial agents may be limited (eg, refugee camps), a single dose of doxycycline may provide effective treatment (100 mg for children; 200 mg for adults) and facilitate outbreak control when combined with delousing efforts.

ISOLATION OF THE HOSPITALIZED PATIENT: Standard precautions are recommended. Precautions should be taken to delouse hospitalized patients with louse infestations.

CONTROL MEASURES: Thorough delousing in epidemic situations, particularly among exposed contacts of cases, is recommended. Several applications of pediculicides may be needed, because lice eggs are resistant to most insecticides. Washing clothes in hot water kills lice and eggs. During epidemics, insecticides dusted onto clothes of louse-infested populations are effective. Prevention and control of flying squirrel-associated typhus requires application of insecticides and precautions to prevent contact with these animals and their ectoparasites and to exclude them from human dwellings. No prophylaxis is recommended for people exposed to flying squirrels. In situations involving outbreaks of epidemic typhus in prisons and refugee settings, active surveillance for fever is important to assess efficacy of control measures and to ensure rapid and effective treatment. Cases should be reported to local, state/regional, or national public health departments.

Ureaplasma urealyticum and *Ureaplasma parvum* Infections

CLINICAL MANIFESTATIONS: The role of *Ureaplasma* species in human disease is controversial. There has been an inconsistent association with *Ureaplasma urealyticum* infections and nongonococcal urethritis (NGU). Although 15% to 40% of cases of NGU are caused by *Chlamydia trachomatis* and an additional 15% to 25% by *Mycoplasma genitalium*, *U urealyticum*, but not *Ureaplasma parvum*, has been implicated as an etiologic agent in some cases in the United States. Without treatment, the disease usually resolves within 1 to 6 months, although asymptomatic infection may persist. There also has been an inconsistent relationship of infection by *Ureaplasma* species with prostatitis and epididymitis in men and salpingitis and endometritis in women. *Ureaplasma* organisms commonly are detected in placentas with histologic chorioamnionitis. Some reports also describe an association between *Ureaplasma* infection with recurrent pregnancy loss and preterm birth.

U urealyticum and *U parvum* have been isolated from the lower respiratory tract and from lung biopsy specimens of preterm infants; their contribution to intrauterine pneumonia and chronic lung disease of prematurity remains controversial. Although these organisms have been recovered from respiratory tract secretions of infants 3 months of age or younger with pneumonia, their role in development of lower respiratory tract disease in otherwise healthy young infants is controversial. *Ureaplasma* species have been isolated from the bloodstream of newborn infants with bacteremia and from cerebrospinal fluid of infants with meningitis, intraventricular hemorrhage, and hydrocephalus. The contribution of *U urealyticum* to the outcome of infants with infections of the central nervous system is unclear given the confounding effects of preterm birth and intraventricular hemorrhage. Numerous cases of *U urealyticum* or *U parvum* arthritis, osteomyelitis, pneumonia, pericarditis, meningitis, and progressive sinopulmonary disease, mainly in immunocompromised patients, have been reported.

ETIOLOGY: *Ureaplasma* organisms are small pleomorphic bacteria that lack a cell wall. The genus contains 2 species capable of causing human infection, *U urealyticum* and *U parvum*. At least 14 serotypes have been described, 4 for *U parvum* and 10 for *U urealyticum*.

EPIDEMIOLOGY: The principal reservoir of human *Ureaplasma* species is the genital tract of sexually active adults. Colonization occurs in approximately half of sexually active women; the incidence in sexually active men is lower. Colonization is uncommon in prepubertal children and adolescents who are not sexually active, but a positive genital tract culture is not clearly definitive of sexual abuse. Transmission during delivery is likely from an asymptomatic colonized mother to her newborn infant, and infection also may occur in utero. *Ureaplasma* species may colonize the throat, eyes, umbilicus, and perineum of newborn infants and may persist for several months after birth. *U parvum* generally is more common than *U urealyticum* as a colonizer in pregnant women and their offspring.

Because *Ureaplasma* species commonly are isolated from the female lower genital tract and neonatal respiratory tract in the absence of disease, a positive culture does not establish its causative role in acute infection. However, recovery of these organisms from an upper genital tract or lower respiratory tract specimen is much more indicative of true infection.

The **incubation period** after sexual transmission is 10 to 20 days.

DIAGNOSTIC TESTS: Specimens for culture require specific *Ureaplasma* transport media with refrigeration at 4°C (39°F). Dacron or calcium alginate swabs should be used; cotton swabs should be avoided. Several rapid, sensitive real-time polymerase chain reaction assays for detection of *U urealyticum* and *U parvum* have been developed. Many of these assays have greater sensitivity than culture, but they are not widely available outside of reference laboratories. *Ureaplasma* species can be cultured in urea-containing broth and agar in 1 to 2 days. Serologic testing is of limited value and is not available commercially for diagnostic purposes

TREATMENT: A positive *Ureaplasma* culture does not indicate need for therapy if the patient is asymptomatic. *Ureaplasma* species generally are susceptible to chloramphenicol, macrolides, tetracyclines, and quinolones, but because they lack a cell wall, they are not susceptible to penicillins or cephalosporins. They also are not affected by trimethoprim-sulfamethoxazole. For symptomatic older children, adolescents, and adults, doxycycline can be used for treatment. Persistent urethritis after doxycycline treatment can be attributable to doxycycline-resistant *U urealyticum* or *M genitalium*. Recurrences are common, and tetracycline resistance may occur in up to 50% of *Ureaplasma* isolates in some patient populations. Azithromycin is the preferred antimicrobial agent for children younger than 8 years, people who are allergic to tetracyclines, and people with infections caused by tetracycline-resistant strains. A recent randomized placebo-controlled trial in adult men with NGU using single-dose azithromycin (1 g, orally) versus doxycycline (100 mg, twice daily for 7 days) showed no difference in clinical or microbiologic cure rates.[1] Antimicrobial treatment with erythromycin has failed to prevent preterm delivery and in preterm infants to prevent pulmonary disease both in small randomized trials and in reports of cohort studies in pregnant women. Although in vitro efficacy against *Ureaplasma* species is observed with clarithromycin, azithromycin, and fluoroquinolones, lack of evidence of benefit precludes recommendations on treatment for preterm infants. Definitive evidence of efficacy of antimicrobial agents in the treatment of central nervous system infections caused by *Ureaplasma* species in infants and children also is lacking. There are reports of preterm infants with *Ureaplasma* species identified in cerebrospinal fluid who have or have not received antimicrobial therapy and who have had documentation of sterilization of cerebrospinal fluid.

ISOLATION OF THE HOSPITALIZED PATIENT: Standard precautions are recommended.

CONTROL MEASURES: Partners of patients with NGU attributable to *U urealyticum* should be offered treatment.

Varicella-Zoster Virus Infections

CLINICAL MANIFESTATIONS: Primary infection results in varicella (chickenpox), manifesting in unvaccinated people as a generalized, pruritic, vesicular rash typically consisting of 250 to 500 lesions in varying stages of development (papules, vesicles) and resolution (crusting), low-grade fever, and other systemic symptoms. Complications include bacterial

---

[1]Manhart LE, Gillespie CW, Lowens MS, et al. Standard treatment options for nongonococcal urethritis have similar but declining cure rates: a randomized controlled trial. *Clin Infect Dis.* 2013;56(7):934–942

superinfection of skin lesions with or without bacterial sepsis, pneumonia, central nervous system involvement (acute cerebellar ataxia, encephalitis, stroke/vasculopathy), thrombocytopenia, and other rare complications, such as glomerulonephritis, arthritis, and hepatitis. Primary viral pneumonia is not common among immunocompetent children but is the most common complication in adults. Varicella tends to be more severe in infants, adolescents, and adults than in children. Before the introduction of routine immunization against varicella, an average of 100 to 125 people died of chickenpox in the United States each year. Breakthrough varicella cases can occur in immunized children, as described later in Active Immunization (p 855), and usually are mild and clinically modified. Reye syndrome may follow cases of varicella, although this outcome has become rare since the recommendation not to use salicylate-containing compounds (eg, aspirin, bismuth-subsalicylate) for children during varicella illness. In immunocompromised children, progressive, severe varicella may occur with continuing eruption of lesions and high fever, persisting into the second week of illness, and visceral dissemination (ie, encephalitis, hepatitis, and pneumonia) can develop. Hemorrhagic varicella is more common among immunocompromised patients than among immunocompetent hosts. In children with human immunodeficiency virus (HIV) infection, recurrent varicella or disseminated herpes zoster can develop. Severe and even fatal varicella has been reported in otherwise healthy children receiving courses of high-dose corticosteroids (greater than 2 mg/kg/day of prednisone or equivalent) for treatment of asthma and other illnesses. The risk especially is high when corticosteroids are given during the incubation period for varicella.

Varicella-zoster virus (VZV) establishes latency in sensory (dorsal root, cranial nerve, and autonomic including enteric) ganglia during infection. Latency in sensory ganglia can occur as a result of primary infection with wild type VZV in an unvaccinated individual, infection with wild type VZV in a previously vaccinated individual, or after vaccination with vaccine-strain VZV. Reactivation results in herpes zoster ("shingles"), characterized by grouped vesicular skin lesions in the distribution of 1 to 3 sensory dermatomes, frequently accompanied by pain and/or itching localized to the area. *Postherpetic neuralgia*, pain that persists after resolution of the zoster rash, may last for weeks to months. Childhood zoster tends to be milder than disease in adults and rarely is associated with postherpetic neuralgia. Zoster occasionally can become disseminated in immunocompromised patients, with lesions appearing outside the primary dermatomes and resulting in visceral complications. VZV reactivation less frequently may occur in the absence of skin rash (zoster sine herpete); these patients may present with aseptic meningitis or encephalitis as well as with gastrointestinal tract involvement. Visceral zoster can arise from reactivation of latent VZV in the enteric (gastrointestinal) nervous system. Some, but not all, of these patients may eventually develop a zosteriform skin rash.

The attenuated VZV in the varicella vaccine may establish latent infection and reactivate as herpes zoster. However, prelicensure data from immunocompromised children indicate that the risk of developing zoster is lower among vaccine recipients than among children who have experienced natural varicella. Postlicensure studies also have documented a lower risk of herpes zoster among healthy children who received varicella vaccines compared with unvaccinated children.

Fetal infection after maternal varicella during the first or early second trimester of pregnancy occasionally results in fetal death or varicella embryopathy, characterized by limb hypoplasia, cutaneous scarring, eye abnormalities, and damage to the central nervous system (congenital varicella syndrome). The incidence of the congenital varicella syndrome among infants born to mothers who experience gestational varicella is approximately 1% to 2% when infection occurs between 8 and 20 weeks of gestation. Rarely, cases of congenital varicella syndrome have been reported in infants of women infected after 20 weeks of pregnancy, the latest occurring at 28 weeks gestation. Children infected with VZV in utero may develop zoster early in life without having had extrauterine varicella. Varicella infection has a higher case-fatality rate in infants when the mother develops varicella from 5 days before to 2 days after delivery, because there is little opportunity for development and transfer of antibody from mother to infant and the infant's cellular immune system is immature. When varicella develops in a mother more than 5 days before delivery and gestational age is 28 weeks or more, the severity of disease in the newborn infant is modified by transplacental transfer of VZV-specific maternal immunoglobulin (Ig) G antibody.

ETIOLOGY: VZV (also known as human herpesvirus 3) is a member of the *Herpesviridae* family, the subfamily *Alphaherpesviridae*, and the genus *Varicellovirus*.

EPIDEMIOLOGY: Humans are the only source of infection for this highly contagious virus. Humans are infected when the virus comes in contact with the mucosa of the upper respiratory tract or the conjunctiva of a susceptible person. Person-to-person transmission occurs by the airborne route from direct contact with patients with vesicular VZV lesions (varicella and herpes zoster); vesicles contain infectious virus that can be aerosolized. Skin lesions appear to be the major source of transmissible VZV; transmission from infected respiratory tract secretions is possible but probably less common than from skin vesicles. There is no evidence of VZV spread from fomites; the virus is extremely labile and is unable to survive for long in the environment. In utero infection occurs as a result of transplacental passage of virus during viremic maternal varicella infection. VZV infection in a household member usually results in infection of almost all susceptible people in that household. Children who acquire their infection at home (secondary family cases) often have more skin lesions than the index case. Health care-associated transmission is well-documented in pediatric units, but transmission is rare in newborn nurseries.

In temperate climates in the prevaccine era, varicella was a childhood disease with a marked seasonal distribution, with peak incidence during late winter and early spring and among children younger than 10 years. High rates of vaccine coverage in the United States have effectively eliminated discernible seasonality of varicella. In tropical climates, the epidemiology of varicella is different; acquisition of disease occurs at later ages, resulting in a higher proportion of adults being susceptible to varicella compared with adults in temperate climates. Following implementation of universal immunization in the United States in 1995, varicella declined in all age groups, providing evidence of herd protection. In areas with active surveillance and with high vaccine coverage, the rate of varicella disease decreased by approximately 90% between 1995 and 2005. Since recommendation of a routine second dose of vaccine in 2006, the incidence of varicella has declined further in children. The age of peak varicella incidence is shifting from children younger than 10 years to children 10 through 14 years of age, although the incidence in this and all age groups is lower than in the prevaccine era. Immunity to varicella generally is lifelong. Cellular immunity is more important than humoral immunity for limiting the extent of primary infection with VZV and for preventing reactivation of virus with herpes zoster. Symptomatic reinfection is uncommon in immunocompetent people, in whom asymptomatic reinfection is more frequent. Asymptomatic primary infection is unusual.

Since 2007, coverage with 1 or more doses of varicella vaccine among 19- through 35-month-old children in the United States has been >90%. As of 2013, more than 78% of 13- to 17-year-old adolescents have received 2 doses of varicella vaccine. As the majority of children are vaccinated against varicella and the incidence of wild-type varicella decreases, a greater proportion of varicella cases are occurring in immunized people as breakthrough disease. This should not be confused as an increasing rate of breakthrough disease or as evidence of increasing vaccine failure.

Immunocompromised people with primary (varicella) or recurrent (herpes zoster) infection are at increased risk of severe disease. Severe varicella and disseminated zoster are more likely to develop in children with congenital T-lymphocyte defects or acquired immunodeficiency syndrome than in people with B-lymphocyte abnormalities. Other groups of pediatric patients who may experience more severe or complicated disease include infants, adolescents, patients with chronic cutaneous or pulmonary disorders, and patients receiving systemic corticosteroids, other immunosuppressive therapy, or long-term salicylate therapy.

Patients are contagious from 1 to 2 days before onset of the rash until all lesions have crusted.

The **incubation period** usually is 14 to 16 days, with a range of 10 to 21 days after exposure to rash. The incubation period may be prolonged for as long as 28 days after receipt of Varicella-Zoster Immune Globulin (VariZIG [Cangene Corp, Winnipeg, Canada]) or Immune Globulin Intravenous (IGIV) and can be shortened in immunocompromised patients. Varicella can develop between 2 and 16 days after birth in infants born to mothers with active varicella around the time of delivery; the usual interval from onset of rash in a mother to onset in her neonate is 9 to 15 days.

DIAGNOSTIC TESTS: Diagnostic tests for VZV are summarized in Table 3.87, p 850. Vesicular fluid or a scab can be used to identify VZV using a polymerase chain reaction (PCR) test, which currently is the diagnostic method of choice. This testing may be used to distinguish between wild-type and vaccine-strain VZV (genotyping). During the acute phase of illness, VZV also can be identified by PCR assay of saliva or buccal swabs, from both unimmunized and immunized patients, although VZV is more likely to be detected in vesicular fluid or scabs. VZV can be demonstrated by direct fluorescent antibody (DFA) assay, using scrapings of a vesicle base during the first 3 to 4 days of the eruption or by viral isolation in cell culture from vesicular fluid. Viral culture and DFA assay both are less sensitive than PCR assay, and neither test has the capacity to distinguish vaccine-strain from wild-type viruses. Genotyping is available free of charge through the specialized reference laboratory at the Centers for Disease Control and Prevention (CDC [404-639-0066]) and also through a safety research program sponsored by Merck & Co (1-800-672-6372). A significant increase in serum varicella IgG antibody between acute and convalescent samples by any standard serologic assay can confirm a diagnosis retrospectively. These antibody tests are reliable for diagnosing natural infection in healthy hosts but may not be reliable in immunocompromised people (see Care of Exposed People, p 851). However, diagnosis of VZV infection by serologic testing seldom is necessary. Commercially available enzyme immunoassay (EIA) tests usually are not sufficiently sensitive to demonstrate reliably a vaccine-induced antibody response, and therefore, routine postvaccination serologic testing is not recommended. IgM tests are not reliable for routine confirmation or ruling out of acute infection. All VZV IgM assays are prone to false-positive results, but in the presence of a rash, positive results can indicate current or recent VZV infection or reactivation.

Table 3.87. Diagnostic Tests for Varicella-Zoster Virus (VZV) Infection

Test	Specimen	Comments
PCR	Vesicular swabs or scrapings, scabs from crusted lesions, biopsy tissue, CSF	Very sensitive method. Specific for VZV. Methods have been designed that distinguish vaccine strain from wild-type (see text).
DFA	Vesicle scraping, swab of lesion base (must include cells)	Specific for VZV. More rapid and more sensitive than culture, less sensitive than PCR.
Viral culture	Vesicular fluid, CSF, biopsy tissue	Distinguishes VZV from HSV. Cost, limited availability, requires up to a week for result. Least sensitive method.
Tzanck smear	Vesicle scraping, swab of lesion base (must include cells)	Observe multinucleated giant cells with inclusions. Not specific for VZV. Less sensitive and accurate than DFA.
Serology (IgG)	Acute and convalescent serum specimens for IgG	Specific for VZV. Commercial assays generally have low sensitivity to reliably detect vaccine-induced immunity. gpELISA and FAMA are the only IgG methods that can readily detect vaccine seroconversion, but these tests are not commercially available.
Capture IgM	Acute serum specimens for IgM	Specific for VZV. IgM inconsistently detected. Not reliable method for routine confirmation but positive result indicates current/recent VZV activity. Requires special equipment.

PCR indicates polymerase chain reaction; CSF, cerebrospinal fluid; VZV, varicella-zoster virus; DFA, direct fluorescent antibody; HSV, herpes simplex virus; IgG, immunoglobulin G; gpELISA, glycoprotein enzyme-linked immunoassay; FAMA, fluorescent antibody to membrane antigen (assay); IgM, immunoglobulin M.

TREATMENT: The decision to use antiviral therapy and the route and duration of therapy should be determined by specific host factors, extent of infection, and initial response to therapy. Antiviral drugs have a limited window of opportunity to affect the outcome of VZV infection. In immunocompetent hosts, most virus replication has stopped by 72 hours after onset of rash; the duration of replication may be extended in immunocompromised hosts. Oral acyclovir or valacyclovir are not recommended for routine use in otherwise healthy children with varicella. Administration within 24 hours of onset of rash in healthy children results in only a modest decrease in symptoms. Oral acyclovir or valacyclovir should be considered for otherwise healthy people at increased risk of moderate to severe varicella, such as unvaccinated people older than 12 years, people with chronic cutaneous or pulmonary disorders, people receiving long-term salicylate therapy, and people receiving short, intermittent, or aerosolized courses of corticosteroids. Some experts also recommend use of oral acyclovir or valacyclovir for secondary household cases in which the disease usually is more severe than in the primary case. For recommendations on dosage and duration of therapy, see Non-HIV Antiviral Drugs (p 919).

Acyclovir is a category B drug based on US Food and Drug Administration (FDA) Drug Risk Classification in pregnancy. Some experts recommend oral acyclovir or valacyclovir for pregnant women with varicella, especially during the second and third trimesters. Intravenous acyclovir is recommended for the pregnant patient with serious complications of varicella.

Intravenous acyclovir therapy is recommended for immunocompromised patients, including patients being treated with high-dose corticosteroid therapy for more than 14 days. Therapy initiated early in the course of the illness, especially within 24 hours of rash onset, maximizes benefit. Oral acyclovir should not be used to treat immunocompromised children with varicella because of poor oral bioavailability. In 2008, valacyclovir (20 mg/kg per dose, with a maximum dose of 1000 mg, administered 3 times daily for 5 days) was licensed for treatment of varicella in children 2 through 17 years of age. Some experts have used valacyclovir, with its improved bioavailability compared with oral acyclovir, in selected immunocompromised patients perceived to be at low to moderate risk of developing severe varicella, such as HIV-infected patients with relatively normal concentrations of CD4+ T-lymphocytes and children with leukemia in whom careful follow-up is ensured. Famciclovir is available for treatment of VZV infections in adults, but its efficacy and safety have not been established for children. Although VariZIG or, if not available, IGIV given shortly after exposure can prevent or modify the course of disease, Immune Globulin preparations are not effective treatment once disease is established (see Care of Exposed People).

Infections caused by acyclovir-resistant VZV strains, which generally are rare and limited to immunocompromised hosts, should be treated with parenteral foscarnet.

Children with varicella should not receive salicylates or salicylate-containing products, because administration of salicylates to such children increases the risk of Reye syndrome. Salicylate therapy should be stopped in an unimmunized child who is exposed to varicella.

ISOLATION OF THE HOSPITALIZED PATIENT: In addition to standard precautions, airborne and contact precautions are recommended for patients with varicella until all lesions are crusted, typically at least 5 days after onset of rash but a week or longer in immunocompromised patients. For immunized patients with breakthrough varicella with only maculopapular lesions, isolation is recommended until no new lesions appear within a 24-hour period, even if lesions have not resolved completely. For exposed patients without evidence of immunity (see Evidence of Immunity to Varicella, p 857), airborne and contact precautions from 8 until 21 days after exposure to the index patient also are indicated; these precautions should be maintained until 28 days after exposure for those who received VariZIG or IGIV.

Airborne and contact precautions are recommended for neonates born to mothers with varicella and, if still hospitalized, should be continued until 21 days of life, or until 28 days of age if VariZIG or IGIV was administered. Infants with varicella embryopathy do not require isolation if they do not have active skin lesions.

Immunocompromised patients who have zoster (localized or disseminated) and immunocompetent patients with disseminated zoster require airborne and contact precautions for the duration of illness. For immunocompetent patients with localized zoster, standard precautions and complete covering of the lesions are indicated until all lesions are crusted.

CONTROL MEASURES:

Child Care and School. Children with uncomplicated varicella who have been excluded from school or child care may return when the rash has crusted or, in immunized people without crusts, until no new lesions appear within a 24-hour period.

Exclusion of children with zoster whose lesions cannot be covered is based on similar criteria. Children who are excluded may return after the lesions have crusted. Lesions that are covered pose little risk to susceptible people, although transmission has been reported.

CARE OF EXPOSED PEOPLE: Potential interventions for people without evidence of immunity exposed to a person with varicella include either varicella vaccine, administered ideally within 3 days but up to 5 days after exposure (followed by a second dose of vaccine at the age-appropriate interval after the first dose) or, when indicated, VariZIG. VariZIG, a purified immune globulin preparation made from human plasma containing high levels of anti-VZV antibodies (IgG) was approved by the US Food and Drug Administration (FDA) in December 2012 and is the only varicella-zoster immune globulin preparation currently available in the United States. VariZIG should be administered as soon as possible following VZV exposure, ideally within 96 hours for greatest effectiveness; limited data suggest benefit when given up to 10 days after exposure. If VariZIG is not available, IGIV can be used (see Unavailability of Varicella-Zoster Immune Globulin, p 855). Prophylactic administration of oral acyclovir beginning 7 days after exposure also may prevent or attenuate varicella in healthy children. There is little information on whether prophylactic oral acyclovir is protective for immunocompromised people.

Hospital Exposure. If an inadvertent exposure occurs in the hospital to an infected person by a patient, health care professional, or visitor, the following control measures are recommended:

- Health care professionals, patients, and visitors who have been exposed (see Fig 3.14) and who lack evidence of immunity to varicella should be identified.
- Varicella immunization is recommended for people without evidence of immunity, provided there are no contraindications to vaccine use.
- VariZIG should be administered to appropriate candidates (see Fig 3.14). If VariZIG is not available, IGIV should be considered as an alternative (see Unavailability of Varicella-Zoster Immune Globulin, p 855).
- All exposed patients without evidence of immunity should be discharged as soon as possible.
- All exposed patients without evidence of immunity who cannot be discharged should be placed in isolation from day 8 to day 21 after exposure to the index patient. For people who received VariZIG or IGIV, isolation should continue until day 28.
- Health care professionals who have received 2 doses of vaccine and who are exposed to VZV should be monitored daily during days 8 through 21 after exposure through the employee health program or by an infection-control nurse to determine clinical status. They should be placed on sick leave immediately if symptoms such as fever, headache, other constitutional symptoms, or any atypical skin lesions occur.
- Health care professionals who have received only 1 dose of vaccine and who are exposed to VZV should receive the second dose with a single-antigen varicella vaccine within 3 to 5 days of exposure, provided 4 weeks have elapsed after the first dose. After immunization, management is similar to that of 2-dose vaccine recipients. For more information, see the recommendations of the CDC.[1]
- Immunized health care professionals who develop breakthrough infection should be considered infectious until vesicular lesions have crusted or, if they had maculopapular lesions, until no new lesions appear within a 24-hour period.

Postexposure Immunization. Varicella vaccine should be administered to healthy people without evidence of immunity who are 12 months or older, including adults, as soon as possible, preferably within 3 days and possibly up to 5 days after varicella or herpes zoster exposure, if there are no contraindications to vaccine use. This approach may prevent or modify disease. Patients should be counseled that not all close exposures result in

---

[1]Centers for Disease Control and Prevention. Immunization of health-care personnel: recommendations of the Advisory Committee on Immunization Practices (ACIP). *MMWR Recomm Rep.* 2011;60(RR-7):1–45

FIG 3.14. MANAGEMENT OF EXPOSURES TO VARICELLA-ZOSTER VIRUS

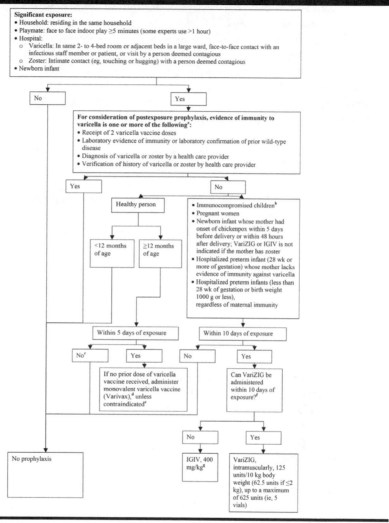

Significant exposure:
- Household: residing in the same household
- Playmate: face to face indoor play ≥5 minutes (some experts use >1 hour)
- Hospital:
  - Varicella: In same 2- to 4-bed room or adjacent beds in a large ward, face-to-face contact with an infectious staff member or patient, or visit by a person deemed contagious
  - Zoster: Intimate contact (eg, touching or hugging) with a person deemed contagious
- Newborn infant

No / Yes

For consideration of postexposure prophylaxis, evidence of immunity to varicella is one or more of the following[a]:
- Receipt of 2 varicella vaccine doses
- Laboratory evidence of immunity or laboratory confirmation of prior wild-type disease
- Diagnosis of varicella or zoster by a health care provider
- Verification of history of varicella or zoster by health care provider

Yes / No

Healthy person

- Immunocompromised children[b]
- Pregnant women
- Newborn infant whose mother had onset of chickenpox within 5 days before delivery or within 48 hours after delivery; VariZIG or IGIV is not indicated if the mother has zoster
- Hospitalized preterm infant (28 wk or more of gestation) whose mother lacks evidence of immunity against varicella
- Hospitalized preterm infants (less than 28 wk of gestation or birth weight 1000 g or less), regardless of maternal immunity

<12 months of age / ≥12 months of age

Within 5 days of exposure / Within 10 days of exposure

No[c] / Yes / No / Yes

If no prior dose of varicella vaccine received, administer monovalent varicella vaccine (Varivax),[d] unless contraindicated[e]

Can VariZIG be administered within 10 days of exposure?[f]

No / Yes

No prophylaxis

IGIV, 400 mg/kg[g]

VariZIG, intramuscularly, 125 units/10 kg body weight (62.5 units if ≤2 kg), up to a maximum of 625 units (ie, 5 vials)

[a] People who receive hematopoietic stem cell transplants should be considered nonimmune regardless of previous history of varicella disease or varicella vaccination in themselves or in their donors.

[b] Immunocompromised children include those with congenital or acquired T-lymphocyte immunodeficiency, including leukemia, lymphoma, and other malignant neoplasms affecting the bone marrow or lymphatic system; children receiving immunosuppressive therapy, including ≥2 mg/kg/day of systemic prednisone (or its equivalent) for ≥14 days; all children with human immunodeficiency virus (HIV) infection regardless of CD4+ T-lymphocyte percentage; and all hematopoietic stem cell transplant patients regardless of pretransplant immunity status.

[c] No postexposure prophylaxis, but age-appropriate vaccination still recommended for protection against subsequent exposures. If the exposure occurred during an outbreak, 2-dose vaccination is recommended for preschool-aged children younger than 4 years for outbreak control.

[d] If 1 prior dose of varicella vaccine has been received, a second dose should be administered at ≥4 years of age. If the exposure occurred during an outbreak, a second dose is recommended for preschool-aged children younger than 4 years for outbreak control.

[e] Contraindications include patients who are allergic to a vaccine component, or who are immunocompromised (see above footnote), or pregnant. Caution should be used in patients receiving salicylates. Vaccine may not be as effective if patient has recently received Immune Globulin Intravenous, whole blood, or plasma transfusions, and for this reason, it is recommended that varicella vaccine be withheld for 3 to 11 months, depending on the dose, after administration of these products.

[f] Varicella Zoster Immune Globulin (VariZIG) was approved by the US Food and Drug Administration in December 2012. The product is manufactured by Cangene Corporation (Winnipeg, Canada) and distributed in the United States by FFF Enterprises (Temecula, California; 800-843-7477; **www.fffenterprises.com**) and ASD Healthcare (Frisco, TX) (telephone, 800-746-6273; online at **www.asdhealthcare.com**).

[g] If VariZIG and IGIV are not available, some experts recommend prophylaxis with oral acyclovir (20 mg/kg per dose administered 4 times per day, with a maximum daily dose of 3200 mg) or oral valacyclovir (if >3 months of age; 20 mg/kg per dose administered 3 times per day, with a maximum daily dose of 3000 mg) beginning 7 to 10 days after exposure and continuing for 7 days.

infection, so vaccination even 3 days after exposure is still warranted. A second vaccine dose should be given at the age-appropriate interval after the first dose. Physicians should advise parents and their children that the vaccine may not protect against disease in all cases, because some children may have been exposed at the same time as the index case. However, if exposure to varicella does not cause infection, postexposure immunization with varicella vaccine will result in protection against subsequent exposure. There is no evidence that administration of varicella vaccine during the presymptomatic or prodromal stage of illness increases the risk of vaccine-associated adverse events or more severe natural disease.

Passive Immunoprophylaxis. The decision to administer VariZIG depends on 3 factors: (1) the likelihood that the exposed person has no evidence of immunity to varicella; (2) the probability that a given exposure to varicella or zoster will result in infection; and (3) the likelihood that complications of varicella will develop if the person is infected. Currently, VariZIG is the only licensed varicella-zoster immune globulin product in the United States.

Data are unavailable regarding the sensitivity and specificity of serologic tests in immunocompromised patients. Detection of VZV IgG after one dose of varicella vaccine might not correspond to adequate protection in immunocompromised people, and false-positive results can occur. Therefore, regardless of serologic test results, careful questioning of children's parents about potential past exposure to disease or clinical description of disease can be helpful in determining immunity. Administration of VariZIG or IGIV as soon as possible within 10 days to immunocompromised children who are exposed with no history of varicella or vaccination and/or unknown or negative serologic test results is recommended. The degree and type of immunosuppression should be considered in making this decision. VariZIG is given intramuscularly at the recommended dose of 62.5 units (0.5 vial) for children weighing ≤2.0 kg; 125 units (1 vial) for children weighing 2.1 to 10 kg; 250 units (2 vials) for children weighing 10.1 to 20 kg; 375 units (3 vials) for children weighing 20.1 to 30 kg; 500 units (4 vials) for children weighing 30.1 to 40 kg; and 625 units (5 vials) for all people weighing >40 kg. IGIV is given intravenously at the dose of 400 mg/kg.

Patients receiving monthly high-dose IGIV (400 mg/kg or greater) at regular intervals are likely to be protected if the last dose of IGIV was given 3 weeks or less before exposure.

Where to Obtain VariZIG. In July 2013, the CDC published updated recommendations for use of VariZIG.[1] At the time of the report, VariZIG could be ordered only from the exclusive US distributor, FFF Enterprises (Temecula, CA; telephone 800-843-7477; **www.fffenterprises.com**). A second distributor for VariZIG now is available in the United States. VariZIG will continue to be available from FFF Enterprises, but it is now also available through ASD Healthcare (Frisco, TX; telephone 800-746-6273; **www. asdhealthcare.com**).

Recommended Use of Varicella-Zoster Immune Globulin. Fig 3.14 indicates people without evidence of immunity who should receive VariZIG if exposed, including immunocompromised people, pregnant women, and certain newborn infants. Because of challenges in assessing immunity against varicella in immunocompromised patients, postexposure VariZIG for selected VZV-seropositive people, such as hematopoietic stem cell

[1]Centers for Disease Control and Prevention. Updated recommendations for use of VariZIG—United States, 2013. *MMWR Morb Mortal Wkly Rep.* 2013;62(28):574–576

transplantation recipients, has been recommended by some experts. Clinicians may consider use of postexposure prophylaxis among profoundly immunocompromised patients on an individual basis.

For healthy term infants exposed postnatally to varicella, including infants whose mother's rash developed more than 48 hours after delivery, VariZIG is not indicated. However, some experts advise use of VariZIG for exposed newborn infants within the first 2 weeks of life whose mothers do not have evidence of immunity to VZV.

Subsequent Exposures and Follow-up of Varicella-Zoster Immune Globulin Recipients. Any patient to whom VariZIG is administered to prevent varicella subsequently should receive age-appropriate varicella vaccine, provided that receipt of live vaccines is not contraindicated. Varicella immunization should be delayed until 5 months after VariZIG administration. Varicella vaccine is not needed if the patient develops varicella after administration of VariZIG.

Unavailability of Varicella-Zoster Immune Globulin. If VariZIG is not available, IGIV can be used (Fig 3.14). The recommendation for use of IGIV is based on "best judgment of experts" and is supported by reports comparing VZV IgG antibody titers measured in both IGIV and VariZIG preparations and patients given IGIV and VariZIG. Although licensed IGIV preparations contain antivaricella antibodies, the titer of any specific lot of IGIV is uncertain, because IGIV is not tested routinely for antivaricella antibodies. No clinical data demonstrating effectiveness of IGIV for postexposure prophylaxis of varicella are available. The recommended IGIV dose for postexposure prophylaxis of varicella is 400 mg/kg, administered once intravenously.

Chemoprophylaxis. If VariZIG or IGIV are not available, some experts recommend prophylaxis with acyclovir (20 mg/kg per dose, administered 4 times per day, with a maximum daily dose of 3200 mg) or valacyclovir (20 mg/kg per dose, administered 3 times per day, with a maximum daily dose of 3000 mg) beginning 7 to 10 days after exposure and continuing for 7 days for immunocompromised patients without evidence of immunity who have been exposed to varicella or herpes zoster (Fig 3.14). A 7-day course of acyclovir or valacyclovir also may be given to adults without evidence of immunity if vaccine is contraindicated. Limited data on acyclovir as postexposure prophylaxis are available for healthy children, and no studies have been performed for adults or immunocompromised people. However, these clinical experiences support use of acyclovir or valacyclovir as postexposure prophylaxis, and clinicians may choose this option if active or passive immunization is not possible.

Active Immunization.[1]

Vaccine. Varicella vaccine is a live-attenuated preparation of the serially propagated and attenuated wild Oka strain. The product contains gelatin and trace amounts of neomycin. The monovalent vaccine was developed in the early 1970s by Professor Michiaki Takahashi and was licensed in March 1995 by the FDA for use in healthy people 12 months or older who have not had varicella illness. Quadrivalent measles-mumps-rubella-varicella (MMRV) vaccine was licensed in September 2005 by the FDA for use in healthy children 12 months through 12 years of age.

Dose and Administration. The recommended dose of vaccine is 0.5 mL, administered subcutaneously.

---

[1]Centers for Disease Control and Prevention. Prevention of varicella: recommendations of the Advisory Committee on Immunization Practices (ACIP). *MMWR Recomm Rep.* 2007;56(RR-4):1–40

Immunogenicity. Approximately 76% to 85% of immunized healthy children older than 12 months develop a humoral immune response to VZV at levels considered associated with protection (using ≥5 glycoprotein enzyme-linked immunosorbent assay [gpELISA] units/mL or fluorescent antibody to membrane antigen [FAMA] ≥1:4) after a single dose of varicella vaccine. Seroprotection rates are significantly higher (approaching 100% for ≥5 gpELISA units/mL) after 2 doses. Cell-mediated immune response also is higher after 2 doses.

Effectiveness. The efficacy of 1 dose of varicella vaccine in open-label studies ranged from 70% to 90% against infection and 95% against severe disease. In general, postlicensure effectiveness studies have reported a similar range for prevention against infection (median 85%), with a few studies yielding lower or higher values. The vaccine is highly effective (97% or greater) in preventing severe varicella in postlicensure evaluations. Recipients of 2 doses of varicella vaccine are 3.3-fold less likely to have breakthrough varicella as compared with recipients of 1 dose during the first 10 years after immunization. A study evaluating postlicensure effectiveness of the current 2-dose varicella vaccine schedule demonstrated 98% effectiveness for 2 doses, compared with 86% for 1 dose.

Simultaneous Administration With Other Vaccines or Antiviral Agents. Varicella-containing vaccines may be administered simultaneously with other childhood immunizations recommended for children 12 through 15 months of age and 4 through 6 years of age (see **http://aapredbook.aappublications.org/site/resources/izschedules. xhtml**). If not administered at the same visit or as MMRV vaccine, the interval between administration of a varicella-containing vaccine and measles-mumps-rubella (MMR) vaccine should be at least 28 days. The minimal interval between MMRV vaccine doses is 3 months. Because of susceptibility of vaccine virus to acyclovir, valacyclovir, or famciclovir, these antiviral agents usually should be avoided from 1 day before to 21 days after receipt of a varicella-containing vaccine.

Adverse Events. Varicella vaccine is safe; reactions generally are mild and occur with an overall frequency of approximately 5% to 35%. Approximately 20% to 25% of immunized people will experience minor injection site reactions (eg, pain, redness, swelling). In approximately 1% to 3% of immunized children, a localized rash develops, and in an additional 3% to 5%, a generalized varicella-like rash develops. These rashes typically consist of 2 to 5 lesions and may be maculopapular rather than vesicular; lesions usually appear 5 to 26 days after immunization. However, not all observed postimmunization rashes can be attributable to vaccine. After MMRV or monovalent varicella vaccine plus MMR, a measles-like rash was reported in 2% to 3% of recipients. After 1 dose among children 12 to 23 months of age, fever was reported in 22% of recipients of MMRV and 15% of recipients of monovalent varicella vaccine and MMR given at separate injections. Both fever and measles-like rash usually occurred within 5 to 12 days of immunization, were of short duration, and resolved without long-term sequelae. In a 2-dose regimen of monovalent vaccine separated by 3 months, injection site complaints were slightly higher after the second dose.

A slightly increased risk of febrile seizures is associated with the higher likelihood of fever following the first dose of MMRV compared with MMR and monovalent varicella. After dose 1 of MMRV vaccine, 1 additional febrile seizure is expected to occur per approximately 2300 to 2600 young children immunized, compared with MMR and monovalent varicella. After the second vaccine dose administered in older children (4 to 6 years of age), there were no differences in incidence of fever, rash, or febrile seizures among recipients of MMRV vaccine compared with recipients of simultaneous MMR and varicella vaccines.[1]

Breakthrough Disease. Breakthrough disease is defined as a case of infection with wild-type VZV occurring more than 42 days after immunization. Varicella in vaccine recipients usually is milder than that occurring in unimmunized children, with rash frequently atypical, predominantly maculopapular with a median of fewer than 50 lesions; lower rate of fever; and faster recovery. In contrast, the median number of lesions in unimmunized children with varicella is more than 250. Breakthrough varicella may be so mild that it is not recognizable easily as varicella, because skin lesions may resemble insect bites. Vaccine recipients with mild breakthrough disease are approximately one third as contagious as unimmunized children. Nonetheless, transmission from mild breakthrough disease has been documented. Approximately 25% to 30% of breakthrough cases are not mild, with clinical features more similar to those in unvaccinated people that can include rash, complications, and hospitalization.

Herpes Zoster After Immunization. Vaccine-strain VZV has been associated with development of herpes zoster in immunocompetent and immunocompromised people. However, data from postlicensure surveillance indicate that the age-specific risk of herpes zoster is lower among immunocompetent children immunized with varicella vaccine than among children who have had natural varicella infection. Wild-type VZV has been identified in skin lesion specimens in people with herpes zoster after immunization, indicating that herpes zoster in immunized people also may result from natural VZV infection that occurred before or after immunization.

Transmission of Vaccine-Strain VZV. Vaccine-strain VZV transmission to contacts is rare (documented in only 9 immunized people, resulting in 11 secondary cases), and the documented risk of transmission exists only if the immunized person develops a rash. Postexposure prophylaxis with VariZIG, IGIV, acyclovir, or valacyclovir in high-risk people exposed to immunized people with lesions has not been studied. However, some experts believe that immunocompromised people in whom skin lesions develop, possibly related to vaccine virus, should receive acyclovir or valacyclovir treatment. Attempts to confirm the presence of VZV by laboratory means, particularly by PCR assay, should be made in these patients.

Evidence of Immunity to Varicella. Evidence of immunity to varicella includes any of the following:
1. Documentation of age-appropriate immunization.
   - Preschool-aged children (ie, ≥12 months of age): 1 dose
   - School-aged children, adolescents, and adults: 2 doses
2. Laboratory evidence of immunity or laboratory confirmation of disease.
3. Varicella diagnosed by a physician or verification of history of varicella disease.
4. History of herpes zoster diagnosed by a physician.

Recommendations for Immunization.

Children 12 Months Through 12 Years of Age. Both monovalent varicella vaccine and MMRV have been licensed for use for healthy children 12 months through 12 years of age.[1] Children in this age group should receive two 0.5-mL doses of monovalent varicella vaccine or MMRV administered subcutaneously, separated by at least 3 months. The recommendation for at least a 3-month interval between doses is based on the design of the studies evaluating

---

[1]Centers for Disease Control and Prevention. Use of combination measles, mumps, rubella, and varicella vaccine: recommendations of the Advisory Committee on Immunization Practices (ACIP). *MMWR Recomm Rep.* 2010;59(RR-3):1–12

2 doses in this age group; if the second dose inadvertently is administered between 28 days and 3 months after the first dose, the second dose does not need to be repeated.

All healthy children routinely should receive the first dose of varicella-containing vaccine at 12 through 15 months of age. The second dose of vaccine is recommended routinely when children are 4 through 6 years of age (ie, before a child enters kindergarten or first grade) but can be administered at an earlier age. Because of the minimal potential for increased febrile seizures after the first dose of MMRV vaccine in children 12 through 15 months of age, the American Academy of Pediatrics recommends a choice of either MMR plus monovalent varicella vaccine or MMRV for toddlers receiving their first immunization of this kind. Parents should be counseled about the rare possibility of their child developing a febrile seizure 1 to 2 weeks after immunization with MMRV for the first immunizing dose. For the second dose at 4 through 6 years of age, MMRV generally is preferred over MMR plus monovalent varicella to minimize the number of injections. Varicella vaccine should be administered to all children in this age range unless there is evidence of immunity to varicella or a contraindication to administration of the vaccine. A catch-up second dose of varicella vaccine should be offered to all children 7 years and older who have received only 1 dose. A routine health maintenance visit at 11 through 12 years of age is recommended for all adolescents to evaluate immunization status and administer necessary vaccines, including the varicella vaccine.

People 13 Years or Older. Healthy individuals 13 years or older without evidence of immunity should receive two 0.5-mL doses of monovalent varicella vaccine, separated by at least 28 days. The recommendation for at least a 28-day interval between doses is based on the design of the studies evaluating 2 doses in this age group. For people who previously received only 1 dose of varicella vaccine, a second dose is necessary. Only monovalent varicella vaccine is licensed for use in this age group.

Contraindications and Precautions.

Intercurrent Illness. As with other vaccines, varicella vaccine should not be administered to people who have moderate or severe illnesses, with or without fever (see Vaccine Contraindications and Precautions, p 52).

Immunization of Immunocompromised Patients.

General recommendations.[1] Varicella vaccine should not be administered routinely to children who have congenital or acquired T-lymphocyte immunodeficiency, including people with leukemia, lymphoma, and other malignant neoplasms affecting the bone marrow or lymphatic systems, as well as children receiving long-term immunosuppressive therapy. An exception includes certain children infected with HIV, as discussed below. Children with impaired humoral immunity alone may be immunized. Immunodeficiency should be excluded before immunization in children with a family history of hereditary immunodeficiency.

In people with possible altered immunity, only monovalent varicella vaccine should be used for immunization against varicella. The Oka vaccine strain remains susceptible to acyclovir, and if a high-risk patient develops vaccine-related varicella, then acyclovir or valacyclovir should be used as treatment.

Acute lymphocytic leukemia. Although recommendations for vaccination of children with acute lymphocytic leukemia in remission have become increasingly conservative, current clinical recommendations from pediatric oncologists are to avoid VZV

[1]Rubin LG, Levin MJ, Ljungman P, et al. 2013 IDSA clinical practice guideline for vaccination of the immunocompromised host. *Clin Infect Dis.* 2014;58(3):e44–e100

immunization. Most deaths from varicella, although rare, occur within the first year of diagnosis and, thus, would not be prevented by immunization. Ensuing delay of chemotherapy for 2 weeks also is a practical constraint. Immunization of children with leukemia without evidence of immunity and in remission should be undertaken only with expert guidance and with availability of antiviral therapy, should complications occur.

Live-virus vaccines usually are withheld for an interval of at least 3 months after cancer chemotherapy has been discontinued. However, the interval until immune reconstruction varies with the intensity and type of immunosuppressive therapy, radiation therapy, underlying disease, and other factors. Therefore, it often is not possible to make a definitive recommendation for an interval after cessation of immunosuppressive therapy when live-virus vaccines can be administered safely and effectively.

Recommendations for vaccination of recipients of hematopoietic stem cell or bone marrow transplant include optional administration of varicella vaccine 24 months after transplantation. However, nonimmune family members, close contacts, and health care workers associated with the patient should be immunized.

HIV infection.[1] Screening for HIV infection is not indicated before routine VZV immunization. Monovalent varicella vaccine should be considered for HIV-infected children without evidence of immunity and with a CD4+ T-lymphocyte percentage of 15% or greater, especially if they are receiving antiretroviral therapy. Eligible children should receive 2 doses of monovalent varicella vaccine with a 3-month interval between doses and return for evaluation if they experience a postimmunization varicella-like rash. Varicella vaccine has been shown to protect these children not only against varicella but also against developing herpes zoster, possibly by preventing infection with wild-type VZV.

Children receiving corticosteroids. Varicella vaccine should not be administered to people who are receiving high doses of systemic corticosteroids (2 mg/kg per day or more of prednisone or its equivalent or 20 mg/day of prednisone or its equivalent) for 14 days or more. The recommended interval between discontinuation of corticosteroid therapy and immunization with varicella vaccine is at least 1 month. Varicella vaccine may be administered to individuals receiving inhaled, nasal, and topical steroids.

Children with nephrotic syndrome. The results of one small study indicate that 2 doses of the varicella vaccine in 29 children between 12 months and 18 years of age generally were well tolerated and immunogenic, including children receiving low-dose, alternate-day prednisone.

Households with potential contact with immunocompromised people. Household contacts of immunocompromised people should be immunized if they have no evidence of immunity to decrease the likelihood that wild-type VZV will be introduced into the household. No precautions are needed following immunization of healthy people who do not develop a rash. Immunized people in whom a rash develops should avoid direct contact with immunocompromised hosts without evidence of immunity for the duration of the rash.

---

[1]Guidelines for prevention and treatment of opportunistic infections in HIV-exposed and HIV-infected children. Recommendations from the National Institutes of Health, Centers for Disease Control and Prevention, the HIV Medicine Association of the Infectious Diseases Society of America, the Pediatric Infectious Diseases Society, and the American Academy of Pediatrics. *Pediatr Infect Dis J.* 2013;32(Suppl 2):i–KK4. Available at: **http://aidsinfo.nih.gov/guidelines/html/5/pediatric-oi-prevention-and-treatment-guidelines/0**

Pregnancy and Lactation. Varicella vaccine should not be administered to pregnant women, because the possible effects on fetal development are unknown, although no cases of congenital varicella syndrome or patterns of malformation have been identified after inadvertent immunization of pregnant women. When postpubertal females are immunized, pregnancy should be avoided for at least 1 month after immunization. A pregnant mother or other household member is not a contraindication for immunization of a child in the household. Reporting of instances of inadvertent immunization with a varicella-zoster–containing vaccine during pregnancy by telephone is encouraged (1-877-888-4231 [see Immunization in Pregnancy, p 70–74]).

A study of nursing mothers and their infants showed no evidence of excretion of vaccine strain in human milk or of transmission to infants who are breastfeeding. Varicella vaccine should be administered to nursing mothers who lack evidence of immunity.

Immune Globulin. Whether Immune Globulin (IG) can interfere with varicella vaccine-induced immunity is unknown, although IG can interfere with immunity induction by measles vaccine. Pending additional data, varicella vaccine should be withheld for the same intervals after receipt of any form of IG or other blood product as measles vaccine (see Measles, p 535; and Table 1.10, p 39). Conversely, IG should be withheld for at least 2 weeks after receipt of varicella vaccine. Transplacental antibodies to VZV do not interfere with the immunogenicity of varicella vaccine administered at 12 months or older.

Salicylates. No cases of Reye syndrome have been reported in children who receive the varicella vaccine while receiving salicylates. However, because of the association with Reye syndrome, natural varicella infection, and salicylates, the vaccine manufacturer recommends that salicylates be avoided for 6 weeks after administration of varicella vaccine. Physicians need to weigh the theoretical risks associated with varicella vaccine against the known risks of wild-type virus in children receiving long-term salicylate therapy.

Allergy to Vaccine Components. Varicella vaccine should not be administered to people who have had an anaphylactic-type reaction to any component of the vaccine, including gelatin and neomycin. Most people with allergy to neomycin have resulting contact dermatitis, a reaction that is not a contraindication to immunization. Monovalent varicella vaccine does not contain preservatives or egg protein, and although the measles and mumps vaccines included in MMRV vaccine are produced in chick embryo culture, the amounts of egg cross-reacting proteins are not significant. Therefore, children with egg allergy routinely may be given MMRV without previous skin testing.

VIBRIO INFECTIONS

Cholera
(Vibrio cholerae)

CLINICAL MANIFESTATIONS: Cholera is characterized by voluminous watery diarrhea and rapid onset of life-threatening dehydration. Hypovolemic shock may occur within hours of the onset of diarrhea. Stools have a characteristic rice-water appearance, are white-tinged and contains small flecks of mucus, and contain high concentrations of sodium, potassium, chloride, and bicarbonate. Vomiting is a common feature of cholera. Fever and abdominal cramps usually are absent. In addition to dehydration and hypovolemia, common complications of cholera include hypokalemia, metabolic acidosis, and hypoglycemia, particularly in children. Although severe cholera is a distinctive illness characterized by profuse diarrhea and rapid dehydration, most people infected with toxigenic *Vibrio cholerae* O1 have either no symptoms or mild to moderate diarrhea lasting 3 to 7 days.

ETIOLOGY: *V cholerae* is a curved or comma-shaped motile gram-negative rod. There are more than 200 *V cholerae* serogroups, some of which carry the cholera toxin (CT) gene. Although those serogroups with the CT gene and others without the CT gene can cause acute watery diarrhea, only toxin-producing serogroups O1 and O139 cause epidemic cholera, with O1 causing the vast majority of cases of cholera. *V cholerae* O1 is classified into 2 biotypes, classical and El Tor, and 2 major serotypes, Ogawa and Inaba. Since 1992, toxigenic *V cholerae* serogroup O139 has been recognized as a cause of epidemic cholera in Asia. Aside from the substitution of the O139 for the O1 antigen, the organism is almost identical to *V cholerae* O1 El Tor. All other serogroups of *V cholerae* are collectively known as *V cholerae* non-O1/non-O139. Toxin-producing strains of *V cholerae* non-O1/non-O139 can cause sporadic cases of severe dehydrating diarrheal illness but have not caused large outbreaks of epidemic cholera. Non–toxin-producing strains of *V cholerae* non-O1/non-O139 are associated with sporadic cases of gastroenteritis, sepsis, and rare cases of wound infection (discussed in Other Vibrio Infections, p 863).

EPIDEMIOLOGY: Since the early 1800s, there have been 7 cholera pandemics. The current pandemic began in 1961 and is caused by *V cholerae* O1 El Tor. Molecular epidemiology shows that this pandemic has occurred in 3 successive waves, with each one spreading from South Asia to other regions in Asia, Africa, and the Western Pacific Islands (Oceania). In 1991, epidemic cholera caused by toxigenic *V cholerae* O1 El Tor appeared in Peru and spread to most countries in South, Central, and North America, causing more than 1 million cases of cholera before subsiding. In 2010, *V cholerae* O1 El Tor was introduced into Haiti, initiating a massive epidemic of cholera. In the United States, sporadic cases resulting from travel to or ingestion of contaminated food transported from regions with endemic cholera are reported, including several cases imported from Hispaniola since 2010.

Humans are the only documented natural host, but free-living *V cholerae* organisms can persist in the aquatic environment. Infection primarily is acquired by ingestion of large numbers of organisms from contaminated water or food (particularly raw or undercooked shellfish, raw or partially dried fish, or moist grains or vegetables held at ambient temperature). People with low gastric acidity and with blood group O are at increased risk of severe cholera infection.

The **incubation period** usually is 1 to 3 days, with a range of a few hours to 5 days.

DIAGNOSTIC TESTS: *V cholerae* can be cultured from fecal specimens (preferred) or vomitus plated on thiosulfate citrate bile salts sucrose agar. Because most laboratories in the United States do not culture routinely for *V cholerae* or other *Vibrio* organisms, clinicians should request appropriate cultures for clinically suspected cases. Isolates of *V cholerae* should be sent to a state health department laboratory for confirmation and then forwarded to the Centers for Disease Control and Prevention (CDC) for confirmation, serogrouping, and detection of the cholera toxin gene **(www.cdc.gov/laboratory/specimen-submission/detail.html?CDCTestCode=CDC-10119).** Tests to detect serum antibodies to *V cholerae*, such as the vibriocidal assay and an anticholera toxin enzyme-linked immunoassay, are available at the CDC subject to preapproval. Both assays require submission of acute and convalescent serum specimens and, thus, provide

Table 3.88. Antibiotics for Suspected Cholera

Antibiotic	Pediatric Dose[a]	Adult Dose	Comment(s)
Doxycycline	4-6 mg/kg, single dose	300 mg, single dose	Use should be in epidemics caused by susceptible isolates. Not recommended for pregnant women and children younger than 8 y.
Ciprofloxacin	15 mg/kg, twice daily for 3 days (single dose 20 mg/kg has been used[b])	500 mg, twice daily for 3 days	Decreased susceptibility to fluoroquinolones is associated with treatment failure. Ciprofloxacin is not recommended in children and pregnant women.
Azithromycin	20 mg/kg, single dose	1 g, single dose	
Erythromycin	12.5 mg/kg, 4 times/day for 3 days	250 mg, 4 times/day for 3 days	
Tetracycline	12.5 mg/kg, 4 times/day for 3 days	500 mg, 4 times/day for 3 days	

[a]Not to exceed adult dose.
[b]Saha D, Khan WA, Karim MM, Chowdhury HR, Salam MA, Bennish ML, Single-dose ciprofloxacin versus 12-dose erythromycin for childhood cholera: a randomised controlled trial. *Lancet.* 2005;366(9491):1085–1093

a retrospective diagnosis. A fourfold increase in vibriocidal or anticholera toxin antibody titers between acute and convalescent sera suggests the diagnosis of cholera. Several commercial tests for rapid antigen detection of *V cholerae* O1 and O139 in stool specimens have been developed. These *V cholerae* O1 and O139 rapid diagnostic tests (RDTs) have sensitivities ranging from approximately 80% to 97% and specificities of approximately 70% to 90% compared with culture on thiosulfate citrate bile salts sucrose agar. RDTs are not a substitute for stool culture but potentially provide a rapid presumptive indication of a suspect cholera outbreak in regions where stool culture is not immediately available.

TREATMENT: Appropriate rehydration therapy is the cornerstone of management of cholera and reduces the mortality of severe cholera to less than 0.5%. Rehydration therapy should be based on World Health Organization standards, with the goal of replacing the estimated fluid deficit within 3 to 4 hours of initial presentation. In patients with severe dehydration, isotonic intravenous fluids should be used, and lactated Ringer solution is the preferred widely commercially available option.[1] For patients without severe dehydration, oral rehydration therapy using the World Health Organization's reduced-osmolality oral rehydration solution (ORS) has been the standard, but data suggest that rice-based ORS or amylase-resistant starch ORS is more effective.

Prompt initiation of antimicrobial therapy decreases the duration and volume of diarrhea and decreases the shedding of viable bacteria. Antimicrobial therapy should be considered for people who are moderately to severely ill. The choice of antimicrobial therapy

[1]World Health Organization. *The Treatment of Diarrhoea, a Manual for Physicians and Other Senior Health Workers.* 4th Rev. WHO/FCH/CAH/05.1. Geneva, Switzerland: World Health Organization; 2005

should be made on the basis of the age of the patient as well as prevailing patterns of antimicrobial resistance (Table 3.88). In cases in which prevailing patterns of resistance are unknown, antimicrobial susceptibility testing should be performed and monitored.

ISOLATION OF THE HOSPITALIZED PATIENT: In addition to standard precautions, contact precautions are indicated for diapered or incontinent children for the duration of illness.

CONTROL MEASURES:

Hygiene. Disinfection of drinking water through chlorination or boiling prevents water-borne transmission of *V cholerae*. Thoroughly cooking crabs, oysters, and other shellfish from the Gulf Coast before eating is recommended to decrease the likelihood of transmission. Foods such as fish, rice, or grain gruels should be refrigerated promptly after meals and thoroughly reheated before eating. Appropriate hand hygiene after defecating and before preparing or eating food is important for preventing transmission.

Treatment of Contacts. Although administration of appropriate antibiotics within 24 hours of identification of the index case may prevent additional cases of cholera among household contacts, chemoprophylaxis of contacts is not currently recommended by the World Health Organization, except in special circumstances in which the probability of fecal exposure is high and medication can be delivered rapidly.

Vaccine. No cholera vaccines are available in the United States. Two inactivated oral vaccines are available in other countries. Dukoral (Crucell, The Netherlands), licensed in 1992, is a monovalent vaccine based on heat-killed whole cells of serogroup O1 plus recombinant cholera toxin B subunit. The second vaccine, licensed in 2009 as mORC-Vax in Ha Noi, Vietnam (VaBiotech), and Shanchol in Hyderabad, India (Shanthol Biotechnics), is a bivalent (O1 and O139) vaccine. Cholera immunization is not required for travelers entering the United States from cholera-affected areas, and the World Health Organization no longer recommends immunization for travel to or from areas with cholera infection. No country requires cholera vaccine for entry.

Public Health Reporting. Confirmed cases of cholera must be reported to health authorities in any country in which they occur and were contracted. Local and state health departments should be notified immediately of presumed or known cases of cholera.

Other *Vibrio* Infections

CLINICAL MANIFESTATIONS: Illnesses attributable to nontoxigenic species of the *Vibrionaceae* family are considered vibriosis. This includes infections attributable to: (1) toxigenic *V cholerae* O75 and O141; (2) nontoxigenic *V cholerae* O1; (3) members of the *Vibrionaceae* family that are not in the genus *Vibrio* (eg, *Grimontia hollisae*); and (4) other *Vibrio* species. Associated clinical syndromes include gastroenteritis, wound infection, and septicemia. Gastroenteritis is the most common syndrome and is characterized by acute onset of watery stools and crampy abdominal pain. Approximately half of those afflicted will have low-grade fever, headache, and chills; approximately 30% will have vomiting. Spontaneous recovery follows in 2 to 5 days. Primary septicemia is uncommon but can develop in immunocompromised people with preceding gastroenteritis or wound infection. Wound infections can be severe in people with liver disease or people who are immunocompromised. Septicemia and hemorrhagic bullous or necrotic skin lesions can be seen in people with infections caused by *Vibrio vulnificus*, with associated high morbidity and mortality rates.

ETIOLOGY: *Vibrio* organisms are facultatively anaerobic, motile, gram-negative bacilli that are tolerant of salt. The most commonly reported nontoxigenic *Vibrio* species associated with diarrhea are *Vibrio parahaemolyticus* and *Vibrio cholerae* non-O1/non-O139. *V vulnificus* typically causes primary septicemia and severe wound infections; the other species can also cause these syndromes. *Vibrio alginolyticus* typically causes wound infections.

EPIDEMIOLOGY: *Vibrio* species are natural inhabitants of marine and estuarine environments. In temperate climates, most noncholera *Vibrio* infections occur during summer and autumn months, when *Vibrio* populations in seawater are highest. Gastroenteritis usually follows ingestion of raw or undercooked seafood, especially oysters, clams, crabs, and shrimp. Wound infections can result from exposure of a preexisting wound to contaminated seawater or from punctures resulting from handling of contaminated shellfish. Exposure to contaminated water during natural disasters, such as hurricanes, has resulted in wound infections. Person-to-person transmission of infection has not been reported. People with liver disease, low gastric acidity, and immunodeficiency have increased susceptibility to infection with *Vibrio* species. Infections associated with noncholera *Vibrio* organisms became nationally notifiable in January 2007.

The **incubation period** for gastroenteritis is typically 24 hours, with a range of 5 to 92 hours.

DIAGNOSTIC TESTS: *Vibrio* organisms can be isolated from stool of patients with gastroenteritis, from blood specimens, and from wound exudates. Extraintestinal specimens may be cultured according to standard clinical practice, because *Vibrio* species grow well on most nonselective plating media with sodium chloride, such as blood or chocolate agar. Fecal specimens should be cultured on thiosulfate citrate bile salts sucrose agar, which inhibits background fecal flora. Because identification of the organism requires special techniques, laboratory personnel should be notified when infection with *Vibrio* species is suspected.

TREATMENT: Most episodes of diarrhea are mild and self-limited and do not require treatment other than oral rehydration. Antimicrobial therapy can benefit people with severe diarrhea, wound infection, or septicemia. Septicemia with or without hemorrhagic bullae should be treated with a third-generation cephalosporin plus doxycycline (see Tetracyclines, p 873). In younger children, a combination of trimethoprim-sulfamethoxazole and an aminoglycoside is an alternative regimen. Wound infections require surgical débridement of necrotic tissue, if present.

ISOLATION OF THE HOSPITALIZED PATIENT: In addition to standard precautions, contact precautions are recommended for diapered or incontinent children.

CONTROL MEASURES: Seafood should be fully cooked and, if not ingested immediately, should be refrigerated. Cross-contamination of cooked seafood by contact with surfaces and containers contaminated by raw seafood should be avoided. Uncooked mollusks and crustaceans should be handled with care, and gloves can be worn during preparation. Abrasions suffered by ocean bathers should be rinsed with clean fresh water. All children, immunocompromised people, and people with chronic liver disease should avoid eating raw oysters or clams, and all individuals should be advised of risks associated with seawater exposure if a wound is present or likely to occur. Vibriosis is a nationally notifiable disease, and cases should be reported to local or state health departments.

West Nile Virus

CLINICAL MANIFESTATIONS: An estimated 70% to 80% of people infected with West Nile virus (WNV) are asymptomatic. Most symptomatic people experience an acute systemic febrile illness that often includes headache, myalgia, or arthralgia; gastrointestinal tract symptoms and a transient maculopapular rash also are reported commonly. Less than 1% of infected people develop neuroinvasive disease, which typically manifests as meningitis, encephalitis, or acute flaccid paralysis. WNV meningitis is indistinguishable clinically from aseptic meningitis caused by most other viruses. Patients with WNV encephalitis usually present with seizures, mental status changes, focal neurologic deficits, or movement disorders. WNV acute flaccid paralysis often is clinically and pathologically identical to poliovirus-associated poliomyelitis, with damage of anterior horn cells, and may progress to respiratory paralysis requiring mechanical ventilation. WNV-associated Guillain-Barré syndrome also has been reported and can be distinguished from WNV acute flaccid paralysis by clinical manifestations and electrophysiologic testing. Cardiac dysrhythmias, myocarditis, rhabdomyolysis, optic neuritis, uveitis, chorioretinitis, orchitis, pancreatitis, and hepatitis have been described rarely after WNV infection.

Routine clinical laboratory results are generally nonspecific in WNV infections. In patients with neuroinvasive disease, cerebrospinal fluid (CSF) examination generally shows lymphocytic pleocytosis, but neutrophils may predominate early in the illness. Brain magnetic resonance imaging frequently is normal, but signal abnormalities may be seen in the basal ganglia, thalamus, and brainstem with WNV encephalitis and in the spinal cord with WNV acute flaccid paralysis.

Most patients with WNV nonneuroinvasive disease or meningitis recover completely, but fatigue, malaise, and weakness can linger for weeks or months. Patients who recover from WNV encephalitis or acute flaccid paralysis often have residual neurologic deficits. Among patients with neuroinvasive disease, the overall case-fatality rate is approximately 10% but is significantly higher in WNV encephalitis and myelitis than in WNV meningitis.

Most women known to have been infected with WNV during pregnancy have delivered infants without evidence of infection or clinical abnormalities. In the single known instance of confirmed congenital WNV infection, the mother developed WNV encephalitis during week 27 of gestation, and the infant was born with cystic destruction of cerebral tissue and chorioretinitis. If WNV disease is diagnosed during pregnancy, a detailed examination of the fetus and of the newborn infant should be performed.[1]

ETIOLOGY: WNV is an RNA virus of the *Flaviviridae* family (genus *Flavivirus*) that is related antigenically to St. Louis encephalitis and Japanese encephalitis viruses.

EPIDEMIOLOGY: WNV is an arthropodborne virus (arbovirus) that is transmitted in an enzootic cycle between mosquitoes and amplifying vertebrate hosts, primarily birds. WNV is transmitted to humans primarily through bites of infected *Culex* mosquitoes. Humans usually do not develop a level or duration of viremia sufficient to infect mosquitoes. Therefore,

---

[1]Centers for Disease Control and Prevention. Interim guidelines for the evaluation of infants born to mothers infected with West Nile virus during pregnancy. *MMWR Morb Mortal Wkly Rep.* 2004;53(7):154–157. Available at: **www.cdc.gov/mmwr/preview/mmwrhtml/mm5307a4.htm**

humans are dead-end hosts. However, person-to-person WNV transmission can occur through blood transfusion and solid organ transplantation. Intrauterine and probable breastfeeding transmission have been described rarely. Transmission through percutaneous and mucosal exposure has occurred in laboratory workers and occupational settings.

WNV transmission has been documented on every continent except Antarctica. Since the 1990s, the largest outbreaks of WNV neuroinvasive disease have occurred in the Middle East, Europe, and North America. WNV first was detected in the Western Hemisphere in New York City in 1999 and subsequently spread across the continental United States and Canada. From 1999 through 2012, 16 196 cases of WNV neuroinvasive disease were reported in the United States, including 605 (4%) cases among children younger than 18 years. The national incidence of WNV neuroinvasive disease peaked in 2002 (1.02 per 100 000) and 2003 (0.98). During 2004–2011, annual incidence was relatively low (median: 0.31; range: 0.13–0.50). In 2012, the national incidence of WNV neuroinvasive disease increased to 0.92 per 100 000. WNV remains the leading cause of neuroinvasive arboviral disease in the United States; in 2013, 2469 cases of WNV neuroinvasive disease were reported, more than 20 times the number of neuroinvasive disease cases reported than for all other domestic arboviruses combined (eg, Eastern equine encephalitis, La Crosse, Powassan, and St. Louis encephalitis viruses). A map of the distribution of WNV neuroinvasive disease across the United States can be found on the Centers for Disease Control and Prevention Web site (**www.cdc.gov/westnile/statsMaps**).

In temperate and subtropical regions, most human WNV infections occur in summer or early autumn. Although all age groups and both genders are susceptible to WNV infection, the incidence of severe disease (eg, encephalitis and death) is highest among adults older than 60 years. Chronic renal failure, history of cancer, history of alcohol abuse, diabetes, and hypertension have been associated with developing severe WNV disease (eg, hospitalization) or acquiring encephalitis.

The **incubation period** usually is 2 to 6 days but ranges from 2 to 14 days and can be up to 21 days in immunocompromised people.

DIAGNOSTIC TESTS: Detection of anti-WNV immunoglobulin (Ig) M antibodies in serum or CSF is the most common way to diagnose WNV infection. The presence of anti-WNV IgM usually is good evidence of recent WNV infection but may indicate infection with another closely related flavivirus. Because anti-WNV IgM can persist in the serum of some patients for longer than 1 year, a positive test result occasionally may reflect past infection. Detection of WNV IgM in CSF is generally indicative of recent neuroinvasive infection. WNV IgM antibodies are detectable in most WNV-infected patients within 7 days of symptom onset. For patients in whom serum collected within 10 days of illness lacks detectable IgM, testing should be repeated on a convalescent-phase sample. IgG antibody generally is detectable shortly after IgM and can persist for years. Plaque-reduction neutralization tests can be performed to measure virus-specific neutralizing antibodies and to discriminate between cross-reacting antibodies from closely related flaviviruses. A fourfold or greater increase in virus-specific neutralizing antibodies between acute- and convalescent-phase serum specimens collected 2 to 3 weeks apart may be used to confirm recent WNV infection.

Viral culture and WNV nucleic acid amplification tests (including reverse transcriptase-polymerase chain reaction) can be performed on acute-phase serum, CSF, or tissue specimens. However, by the time most immunocompetent patients present with clinical symptoms, WNV RNA usually is no longer detectable, thus polymerase chain reaction assay is not recommended for diagnosis in immunocompetent hosts. The sensitivity of these tests is likely higher in immunocompromised patients. Immunohistochemical staining can detect WNV antigens in fixed tissue, but negative results are not definitive.

WNV disease should be considered in the differential diagnosis of febrile or acute neurologic illnesses associated with recent exposure to mosquitoes, blood transfusion, or solid organ transplantation and of illnesses in neonates whose mothers were infected with WNV during pregnancy or while breastfeeding. In addition to other more common causes of aseptic meningitis and encephalitis (eg, herpes simplex virus and enteroviruses), other arboviruses should also be considered in the differential diagnosis (see Arboviruses, p 240).

TREATMENT: Management of WNV disease is supportive. Although various therapies have been evaluated or used for WNV disease, none has shown specific benefit thus far. Information regarding previous clinical trials is available online **(http://clinicaltrials. gov/ct2/results?term=west+nile).**

ISOLATION OF THE HOSPITALIZED PATIENT: Standard precautions are recommended.

CONTROL MEASURES: Candidate WNV vaccines are being evaluated, but none are licensed for use in humans. In the absence of a vaccine, prevention of WNV disease depends on community-level mosquito control programs to reduce vector densities, on personal protective measures to decrease exposure to infected mosquitoes, and on screening of blood and organ donors. Personal protective measures include use of mosquito repellents, wearing long-sleeved shirts and long pants, and limiting outdoor exposure from dusk to dawn (see Prevention of Mosquitoborne Infections, p 213). Using air conditioning, installing window and door screens, and reducing peridomestic mosquito breeding sites can further decrease the risk of WNV exposure. Blood donations in the United States are screened for WNV infection using tests with different sensitivities depending on the seasons, but physicians should remain vigilant for the possible transmission of WNV through blood transfusion or organ transplantation. Any suspected WNV infections temporally associated with blood transfusion or organ transplantation should be reported promptly to the appropriate state health department.

Pregnant women should take aforementioned precautions to avoid mosquito bites. Products containing N,N-diethyl-meta-toluamide (DEET) can be used in pregnancy without adverse effects. Pregnant women who develop meningitis, encephalitis, flaccid paralysis, or unexplained fever in areas of ongoing WNV transmission should be tested for WNV infection. Confirmed WNV infections should be reported to the local or state health department, and women should be followed to determine the outcomes of their pregnancies. Although WNV probably has been transmitted through human milk, such transmission appears rare and no adverse effects on infants have been described. Because the benefits of breastfeeding outweigh the risk of WNV disease in breastfeeding infants, mothers should be encouraged to breastfeed even in areas on ongoing WNV transmission.

Yersinia enterocolitica and *Yersinia pseudotuberculosis* Infections
(Enteritis and Other Illnesses)

CLINICAL MANIFESTATIONS: *Yersinia enterocolitica* causes several age-specific syndromes and a variety of other less commonly reported clinical illnesses. Infection with *Y entero-colitica* typically manifests as fever and diarrhea in young children; stool often contains leukocytes, blood, and mucus. Relapsing disease and, rarely, necrotizing enterocolitis also have been described. In older children and adults, a pseudoappendicitis syndrome (fever, abdominal pain, tenderness in the right lower quadrant of the abdomen, and leukocyto-sis) predominates. Bacteremia with *Y enterocolitica* most often occurs in children younger than 1 year and in older children with predisposing conditions, such as excessive iron storage (eg, desferrioxamine use, sickle cell disease, and beta-thalassemia) and immu-nosuppressive states. Focal manifestations of *Y enterocolitica* are uncommon and include pharyngitis, meningitis, osteomyelitis, pyomyositis, conjunctivitis, pneumonia, empyema, endocarditis, acute peritonitis, abscesses of the liver and spleen, and primary cutaneous infection. Postinfectious sequelae with *Y enterocolitica* infection include erythema nodosum, reactive arthritis, and proliferative glomerulonephritis. These sequelae occur most often in older children and adults, particularly people with HLA-B27 antigen.

Major manifestations of *Yersinia pseudotuberculosis* infection include fever, scarlatiniform rash, and abdominal symptoms. Acute pseudoappendiceal abdominal pain is common, resulting from ileocecal mesenteric adenitis or terminal ileitis. Other findings include diar-rhea, erythema nodosum, septicemia, and sterile pleural and joint effusions. Clinical fea-tures can mimic those of Kawasaki disease; in Hiroshima, Japan, nearly 10% of children with a diagnosis of Kawasaki disease have serologic or culture evidence of *Y pseudotubercu-losis* infection.

ETIOLOGY: The genus *Yersinia* consists of 11 species of gram-negative bacilli. *Y enterocolitica*, *Y pseudotuberculosis*, and *Yersinia pestis* are the 3 most recognized human pathogens; however, other *Yersinia* species have also been isolated from clinical specimens. *Y enterocolitica* biosero-types most often associated with human illness are 1B/O:8, 2/O:5,27, 2/O:9, 3/O:3, and 4/O:3, with bioserotype 4/O:3 now predominating as the most common type in the United States. Differences in virulence gene distribution exist among the bioserotypes of *Y enteroco-litica* and also different degrees of pathogenicity. Virulence can be attributed to adhesion/invasion genes, enterotoxins, iron-scavenging genomic islands, and secretion systems. Highly pathogenic *Yersinia* are known to carry a 70 kb pYV virulence plasmid, which encodes a type III secretion system that is activated at human body temperatures and promotes entry into lymph tissues and subsequent evasion of host defense mechanisms.

EPIDEMIOLOGY: *Yersinia* infections are uncommonly reported in the United States, and infection is not nationally notifiable. *Y enterocolitica* and *Y pseudotuberculosis* are isolated most often during the cool months of temperate climates. According to the Foodborne Disease Active Surveillance Network, which conducts active surveillance for infections caused by 9 pathogens, including *Yersinia* species, during 2012, 3.3 laboratory-confirmed infections per 1 million people were reported to surveillance sites. During FoodNet surveillance from 1996-2009, 47% of infections were in children younger than 5 years; 28% were hospi-talized, and 1% died. Most isolates were recovered from stool. In contrast, the average annual incidence of *Y pseudotuberculosis* was 0.04 cases per 1 million people; the median age was 47 years, 72% were hospitalized, and 11% died. Two-thirds of *Y pseudotuberculosis* isolates were recovered from blood.

The principal reservoir of *Y enterocolitica* is swine; feral *Y pseudotuberculosis* has been isolated from ungulates (deer, elk, goats, sheep, cattle), rodents (rats, squirrels, beaver), rabbits, and many bird species. Infection with *Y enterocolitica* is believed to be transmitted by ingestion of contaminated food (raw or incompletely cooked pork products, tofu, and unpasteurized or inadequately pasteurized milk[1]), by contaminated surface or well water, by direct or indirect contact with animals, and rarely by transfusion with contaminated packed red blood cells and by person-to-person transmission. Cross-contamination has been documented to lead to infection in infants if their caregivers handle raw pork intestines (ie, chitterlings) and do not cleanse their hands adequately before handling the infant or the infant's toys, bottles, or pacifiers. Recent outbreaks of *Y pseudotuberculosis* infection in Finland have been associated with eating fresh produce, presumably contaminated by wild animals carrying the organism.

The **incubation period** typically is 4 to 6 days, with a range of 1 to 14 days. Organisms are typically excreted for 2 to 3 weeks and up to 2 to 3 months in untreated cases. Prolonged asymptomatic carriage is possible.

DIAGNOSTIC TESTS: *Y enterocolitica* and *Y pseudotuberculosis* can be recovered from stool, throat swab specimens, mesenteric lymph nodes, peritoneal fluid, and blood. *Y enterocolitica* also has been isolated from synovial fluid, bile, urine, cerebrospinal fluid, sputum, pleural fluid, and wounds. Stool cultures generally yield bacteria during the first 2 weeks of illness, regardless of the nature of gastrointestinal tract manifestations. *Yersinia* organisms are not sought routinely in stool specimens by most laboratories in the United States. Consequently, laboratory personnel should be notified when *Yersinia* infection is suspected so that stool can be cultured on suitable media (eg, CIN agar); however, strains of *Y enterocolitica* 3/O:3 and *Y pseudotuberculosis* may be inhibited on CIN agar and MacConkey is preferred. Biotyping and serotyping for further identification of pathogenic strains are available through public health reference laboratories. Infection also can be confirmed by demonstrating increases in serum antibody titer after infection, but these tests generally are available only in reference or research laboratories. Cross-reactions of these antibodies with *Brucella, Vibrio, Salmonella, Rickettsia* organisms, and *Escherichia coli* can lead to false-positive *Y enterocolitica* and *Y pseudotuberculosis* titers. In patients with thyroid disease, persistently increased *Y enterocolitica* antibody titers can result from antigenic similarity of the organism with antigens of the thyroid epithelial cell membrane. Characteristic ultrasonographic features demonstrating edema of the wall of the terminal ileum and cecum help to distinguish pseudoappendicitis from appendicitis and can help avoid exploratory surgery.

TREATMENT: Neonates, immunocompromised hosts, and all patients with septicemia or extraintestinal disease require treatment for *Yersinia* infection. Parenteral therapy with a third-generation cephalosporin is appropriate, and evaluation of cerebrospinal fluid should be performed for infected neonates. Otherwise healthy nonneonates with enterocolitis can be treated symptomatically. Other than decreasing the duration of fecal excretion of *Y enterocolitica* and *Y pseudotuberculosis*, a clinical benefit of antimicrobial therapy for immunocompetent patients with enterocolitis, pseudoappendicitis syndrome, or mesenteric adenitis

---

[1]American Academy of Pediatrics, Committee on Infectious Diseases and Committee on Nutrition. Consumption of raw or unpasteurized milk and milk products by pregnant women and children. *Pediatrics.* 2014;133(1):175–179

has not been established. In addition to third-generation cephalosporins, *Y enterocolitica* and *Y pseudotuberculosis* usually are susceptible to trimethoprim-sulfamethoxazole, aminoglycosides, fluoroquinolones (for patients 18 years and older [see Fluoroquinolones, p 872), chloramphenicol, tetracycline, or doxycycline. Tetracycline-based antimicrobial agents, including doxycycline, may cause permanent tooth discoloration for children younger than 8 years if used for repeated treatment courses. However, doxycycline binds less readily to calcium compared with older tetracyclines, and in some studies, doxycycline was not associated with visible teeth staining in younger children (see Tetracyclines, p 873). *Y enterocolitica* isolates usually are resistant to first-generation cephalosporins and most penicillins.

ISOLATION OF THE HOSPITALIZED PATIENT: In addition to standard precautions, contact precautions are indicated for diapered or incontinent children for the duration of diarrheal illness.

CONTROL MEASURES: Ingestion of uncooked or undercooked meat, unpasteurized milk, or contaminated water should be avoided. People who handle raw meat products should minimize contact with young children and their possessions while handling raw products. Meticulous hand hygiene should be practiced before and after handling and preparation of uncooked products.

Antimicrobial Agents and Related Therapy

······························
INTRODUCTION

The product label (package insert) approved by the US Food and Drug Administration (FDA) for a given antimicrobial drug provides information on indications (the clinical infections that require antimicrobial treatment, such as "complicated urinary tract infection") based on clinical trial data reviewed by the FDA. Virtually all current antimicrobial product labels are available at **http://dailymed.nlm.nih.gov/dailymed/about.cfm.** The FDA also maintains a general Web site (**www.accessdata.fda.gov/scripts/cder/ob/default.cfm**) of approved drug products with therapeutic equivalence evaluations that can be searched by active ingredient or proprietary names.

An FDA-approved indication means that statistically adequate and well-controlled studies were conducted, reviewed, and approved by the FDA. However, accepted medical practice (ie, when to use which antimicrobial agent for a specific infection or "indication") often includes use of drugs that are not reflected in approved indications found in the drug label. These additional uses of antimicrobial agents are usually based on studies that may or may not have been supported by the drug's manufacturer (the sponsor). These studies are not always presented formally to the FDA by the clinical investigators or the sponsor for review because of the substantial cost of conducting the clinical trials, collecting and analyzing the data, and presenting the data to the FDA for approval for that specific indication. Lack of FDA approval for an indication, therefore, does not necessarily mean lack of effectiveness, but signifies either that FDA-required studies have not been performed or that they have not been submitted to the FDA for approval for that specific indication. Therefore, unapproved use does not imply improper use, provided that reasonable supporting medical evidence exists and that use of the drug is deemed to be in the best interest of the patient. Conversely, many vaccines or drugs are not recommended for use by the American Academy of Pediatrics (AAP) or Centers for Disease Control and Prevention (CDC), despite licensed indications noted in the package label. The decision to prescribe a drug is the responsibility of the physician, who must weigh risks and benefits of using the drug for the specific situation.

Despite FDA approval of certain agents and their recommended use for specific clinical situations by professional societies like the AAP, manufacturing of drugs is the responsibility of the pharmaceutical industry, which is regulated by the FDA. On occasion, drug shortages can occur. The pharmaceutical company may share information about the shortage with the FDA (**www.fda.gov/cder/drug/shortages/default.htm**). Alternative, nonstandard therapy may be required when drug shortages occur.

Some antimicrobial agents with proven therapeutic benefit in adults are not approved by the FDA for use in pediatric patients or, more rarely, are considered contraindicated in children because of possible toxicity. Drugs such as fluoroquinolones (in people younger than 18 years), tetracyclines (in children younger than 8 years), and other agents approved for use in adults may be used in special circumstances after careful assessment of risks and benefits.

The following information delineates general principles for use of fluoroquinolones, tetracy-clines, and other agents that are approved for adults with serious bacterial infections.

Fluoroquinolones

Fluoroquinolones (eg, ciprofloxacin, levofloxacin, gemifloxacin, moxifloxacin) should not be routinely used as first line agents in children younger than 18 years except where specific indi-cations exist or in specific conditions for which there are no alternative agents (including oral agents) and the drug is known to be effective for the specific situation. Current information on the safety of fluoroquinolones for children was reviewed and published by the AAP.[1]

Although generally well tolerated, transient arthralgia has been reported in patients treated with fluoroquinolones. This adverse event also has been noted in some chil-dren treated with control antibiotics in these studies, making it difficult to assess the fluoroquinolone-attributable contribution to this adverse effect. For some fluoroquinolones, cartilage damage in animal models occurs at doses that approximate therapeutic doses in humans. The mechanism of damage remains speculative. In some pediatric studies, an increased incidence of reversible adverse events involving joints or surrounding tissues has been observed. To date, however, no child treated with fluoroquinolone agents has developed physician-documented, drug-attributable long-term sequelae related to bone or joint toxicity.

There is an increased risk of *Clostridium difficile* disease in patients treated with fluoroquinolone-class antibiotics. Certain fluoroquinolones (ciprofloxacin, moxifloxacin) have been shown to potentially prolong the QT interval and should be avoided in patients with long QT syndrome, those with hypokalemia or hypomagnesemia, those with organic heart disease including congestive heart failure, those receiving an antiarrhythmic agent from class Ia (particularly quinidine), and those who are receiving a concurrent drug that prolongs the QTc interval independently.

Two black box warnings have been issued by the FDA related to fluoroquinolones. Fluoroquinolones are associated with an increased risk of tendon rupture, particularly in people older than 60 years, especially in those with underlying diabetes; in those who have received renal, heart, or lung transplants; and with concurrent use of corticosteroids. Neurologic complications associated with fluoroquinolone use include peripheral neu-ropathy, dizziness, and headaches.

Circumstances in which use of systemic fluoroquinolones may be justified in children include the following: (1) parenteral therapy is not practical and no other safe and effec-tive oral agent is available; and (2) infection is caused by a multidrug-resistant pathogen, such as certain *Pseudomonas* or *Mycobacterium* strains, for which there is no other effective intravenous or oral agent available. The only indications for which a fluoroquinolone is approved by the FDA for use in patients younger than 18 years are complicated urinary tract infection or pyelonephritis (ciprofloxacin) and postexposure prophylaxis for inhala-tion anthrax (ciprofloxacin, levofloxacin). Accordingly, potential uses of fluoroquinolones for pediatric patients include the following:

- Urinary tract infections caused by *Pseudomonas aeruginosa* or other multidrug-resistant, gram-negative bacteria;
- Multidrug-resistant pneumococcal infections (eg, caused by serotype 19A);
- Chronic suppurative otitis media or malignant otitis externa caused by *P aeruginosa*;

---

[1]American Academy of Pediatrics, Committee on Infectious Diseases. The use of systemic and topical fluoro-quinolones. *Pediatrics* 2011;128(4):e1034–e1045

- Chronic or acute osteomyelitis or osteochondritis caused by *P aeruginosa*, or other multi-drug-resistant, gram-negative bacterial infection caused by isolates known to be susceptible to fluoroquinolones but resistant to standard, nonfluoroquinolone agents;
- Gram-negative bacterial infections in immunocompromised hosts in which oral therapy is desired or antibacterial resistance to alternative agents is present;
- Gastrointestinal tract infection caused by suspected or documented multidrug-resistant *Shigella* species, *Salmonella* species, *Vibrio cholerae*, *Campylobacter jejuni*, or *Campylobacter coli*.
- Serious infections attributable to fluoroquinolone-susceptible pathogen(s) in children with severe allergy to alternative agents.
- Topical fluoroquinolone-containing agents are preferred as safer alternatives to aminoglycoside-containing agents for treatment of otorrhea associated with tympanic membrane perforation, and tympanostomy tube otorrhea.

Inappropriate use of fluoroquinolones in children and adults is likely to be associated with increasing resistance to these agents.

Tetracyclines

Use of tetracyclines in pediatric patients has been limited because these drugs can cause permanent dental discoloration in children younger than 8 years. Studies have documented that tetracyclines and their colored degradation products are incorporated in enamel. The period of odontogenesis to completion of formation of enamel in permanent teeth appears to be the critical time for effects of these drugs and virtually ends by 8 years of age, at which time the drug can be given without concern for dental staining. The degree of staining appears to depend on dosage, duration of therapy, and which drug in the tetracycline class is used. Doxycycline binds less readily to calcium compared with older tetracyclines, and in some studies, doxycycline was not associated with visible teeth staining in younger children. In addition to dental discoloration, tetracyclines can cause tooth enamel hypoplasia and reversible delay in rate of bone growth. These tetracycline-related adverse effects have resulted in recommendations for the use of alternative, equally effective antimicrobial agents in most circumstances in young children.

Even with these constraints, in some cases the benefits of therapy with a tetracycline can exceed the risks, particularly if alternative drugs provide less effective therapy for serious infections or if pathogens are only susceptible to tetracyclines. In these cases, use of tetracyclines for a single therapeutic course in young children is justified. Examples include life-threatening infections caused by pathogens in the *Rickettsia/Ehrlichia/Anaplasma* group, including Rocky Mountain spotted fever (see p 682) and ehrlichiosis (see p 329) and also cholera (see p 860) and anthrax (see p 234). Doxycycline usually is the tetracycline-class agent of choice in children with these infections, because it is less likely to cause staining of developing permanent teeth compared with tetracycline.

Other Agents

Other antimicrobial agents in a variety of classes have been studied and approved by the FDA for use in adults for certain indications but still are under investigation for pharmacokinetics, safety, and efficacy in children. These agents include but are not limited to ceftaroline, daptomycin, doripenem, and tigecycline. These drugs should be used in children only when no other safe and effective agents that are FDA approved for use in children are available and when benefits are expected to exceed risks for that patient. For these agents with relatively undefined safety and efficacy in pediatrics, consultation with an expert in pediatric infectious diseases should be considered.

··

ANTIMICROBIAL RESISTANCE AND ANTIMICROBIAL STEWARDSHIP: APPROPRIATE AND JUDICIOUS USE OF ANTIMICROBIAL AGENTS[1]

Antimicrobial Resistance

The Centers for Disease Control and Prevention (CDC), World Health Organization (WHO), and other international agencies have identified antimicrobial resistance as one of the world's most pressing public health threats. It is estimated that more than 2 million people in the United States are infected with antimicrobial-resistant bacteria, and at least 23 000 people die each year because of these infections. Highly resistant gram-negative pathogens *(Pseudomonas aeruginosa, Acinetobacter* species, extended-spectrum beta-lactamase–producing *Escherichia coli*, carbapenemase-producing *Klebsiella pneumoniae*, and *Burkholderia cepacia)* and gram-positive pathogens (methicillin-resistant *Staphylococcus aureus*, and *Enterococcus* resistant to ampicillin and vancomycin) increasingly are associated with invasive infections. *Clostridium difficile* infection, the most common cause of diarrhea acquired in a health care facility and an infection that usually results from antimicrobial exposure, causes approximately 250 000 hospitalizations and at least 14 000 deaths annually. Although *C difficile* infection often is considered to affect predominately adults, recent evidence suggests an increase in infection rates and mortality in children.

The presence of resistant pathogens complicates patient management, increases morbidity and mortality, and increases medical expenses for patients and the health care system. Studies have estimated that antimicrobial resistance in the United States adds as much as $20 billion in excess costs to the health care system each year, and costs to society as a result of lost productivity are as high as $35 billion.

Factors Contributing to Resistance

The use of antimicrobial agents is the single most important factor leading to the development of resistance. Antimicrobial agents are among the most commonly prescribed drugs used in human medicine. However, up to 50% of all prescribed antimicrobial agents are unnecessary or are prescribed inappropriately.

The number of antibiotic-resistant bacteria and the diversity of molecular mechanisms of resistance have increased sharply in recent years, but the development of newer, effective antimicrobial agents has not kept pace. The loss of effective antimicrobial agents will hamper clinicians' efforts to treat potentially life-threatening infections.

At the same time, many advances in medical treatment involve immunosuppression; subsequently, patients' ability to control infections depends even more so on the receipt of effective antimicrobial agents. When first-line and second-line treatment options are limited by

[1]Dellit TH, Owens RC, McGowan JE Jr, et al. Infectious Diseases Society of America and the Society for Healthcare Epidemiology of America guidelines for developing an institutional program to enhance antimicrobial stewardship. *Clin Infect Dis.* 2007;44(2):159–177

resistance or are unavailable, health care providers are forced to use antimicrobial agents that may be more toxic to the patient and frequently also are more expensive and less effective.

In addition to overuse in humans, the overuse of antimicrobial agents in animal agriculture contributes substantially to the problem of antimicrobial resistance. The vast majority of antimicrobial use in animals is not intermittent or to treat infections; rather, animals are fed antibiotics regularly to speed growth and to compensate for unsanitary and crowded conditions. The CDC has determined that antimicrobial use in animals is linked to resistance in humans. The US Food and Drug Administration recently described a pathway toward reducing inappropriate antimicrobial use in animals, and many major medical and public health organizations, including the American Academy of Pediatrics (AAP), have called for stronger action.

Antimicrobial Resistance Threats

The CDC released a landmark report, "Antibiotic Resistance Threats in the United States, 2013" (**www.cdc.gov/drugresistance/threat-report-2013/**), which describes the burden and threats posed by antimicrobial resistance and outlines immediate actions that must be taken to address the problem. The CDC report ranked the antimicrobial-resistant bacteria (and fungi) that have the most impact on human health in categories of urgent, serious, and concerning threats (Table 4.1). The threats were

Table 4.1. Antibiotic-Resistant Bacteria Posing Health Threats

Urgent Threats	Serious Threats	Concerning Threats
Carbapenem-resistant *Enterobacteriaceae*	Methicillin-resistant *Staphylococcus aureus*	Vancomycin-resistant *S aureus*
Antibiotic-resistant gonorrhea	Drug-resistant tuberculosis	Erythromycin-resistant group A streptococci
Clostridium difficile	Drug-resistant *Streptococcus pneumoniae*	Clindamycin-resistant group B streptococci
	Extended-spectrum beta-lactamase-producing *Enterobacteriaceae*	
	Multidrug-resistant *Acinetobacter* species	
	Drug-resistant *Campylobacter* species	
	Fluconazole-resistant *Candida* species (fungus)	
	Vancomycin-resistant *Enterococcus* species	
	Multidrug-resistant *Pseudomonas aeruginosa*	
	Drug-resistant nontyphoidal *Salmonella* species	
	Drug-resistant *Salmonella Typhi*	
	Drug-resistant *Shigella* species	

Adapted from Zaoutis T. CDC highlights threats posed by antibiotic resistance, calls for action. *AAP News.* 2013;34(11):11. See the CDC Web site for further details (**www.cdc.gov/drugresistance/threat-report-2013/**)

assessed according to 7 factors associated with resistant infections: health impact, economic impact, prevalence of the infection, 10-year projection of prevalence, ease of transmission, availability of effective antimicrobial agents, and barriers to prevention.

Actions to Prevent or Slow Antimicrobial Resistance

Antimicrobial resistance can be addressed only through concerted and collaborative efforts. To combat the threat posed by antibiotic resistance, the CDC has identified 4 core actions that must be taken:

1. **Prevent infections and prevent the spread of resistance.** Antimicrobial-resistant infections can be prevented by immunization, infection prevention in health care settings, safe food preparation and handling, and handwashing.

2. **Track antibiotic resistant infections.** The CDC gathers data on antimicrobial-resistant infections to help inform strategies and interventions for prevention.

3. **Improve antimicrobial use and promote antimicrobial stewardship.** The most important action is to modify the way antimicrobial agents are used in humans and animals. Inappropriate use of antimicrobial agents is common in hospitalized patients and often is a result of errors in dosing or duration of therapy. Unnecessary exposure to antimicrobial agents results in adverse drug reactions, complications including *C difficile* infections, and subsequent treatment challenges related to the development of antimicrobial resistance. Every hospital should have a formal antimicrobial stewardship program built on validated core elements.

4. **Develop drugs and improved diagnostic tests.** Antibiotic resistance develops as a part of a natural process in which bacteria evolve. Therefore, discovery of new antimicrobial agents is needed to keep pace with the emergence of resistance. Unfortunately, the number of antimicrobial agents in late-phase clinical development is low; in particular, few agents are being developed with a new mechanism of action to treat resistant gram-negative infections. Additionally, new diagnostic tests are needed to track the development of resistance.

Antimicrobial Stewardship

The primary goal of antimicrobial stewardship is to optimize antimicrobial use, with the aim of decreasing inappropriate use that leads to unwarranted toxicity and to selection and spread of resistant organisms. Core members of an inpatient antimicrobial stewardship program include infectious diseases specialists, clinical pharmacists, clinical microbiologists, hospital epidemiologists, infection prevention professionals, and information systems specialists.[1,2] The core strategies of antimicrobial stewardship that can be implemented in the inpatient setting are postprescription audit and feedback and/or preprescription authorization. Additional strategies include education, development of clinical practice guidelines, facilitation of conversion from intravenous to oral agents, dose optimization, and implementation of electronic decision support. Pediatricians should support infectious diseases experts and hospital administrators to ensure effective stewardship

[1]Dellit TH, Owens RC, McGowan JE Jr, et al. Infectious Diseases Society of America and the Society for Healthcare Epidemiology of America guidelines for developing an institutional program to enhance antimicrobial stewardship. *Clin Infect Dis.* 2007;44(2):159–177

[2]Newland JG, Banerjee R, Gerber JS, Hersh AL, Steinke L, Weissman SJ. Antimicrobial stewardship in pediatric care: strategies and future directions. *Pharmacotherapy.* 2012;32(8):735–743

programs that protect patients and preserve the therapeutic effectiveness of antimicrobial agents. Core elements that should be ensured in every program include institutional leadership support, with an identified physician director and clinical pharmacist with dedicated time to accomplish the programmatic goals. The program should provide tracking of antimicrobial usage and resistance patterns with defined interventions to improve use, followed by direct reporting to and education of staff. Efforts in the hospitalized patients should particularly target and eliminate inappropriate use of vancomycin and/or broad-spectrum agents (eg, meropenem).

Many different strategies have been used for improving antimicrobial use in the outpatient setting. Common approaches include patient education, provider education, provider audit and feedback, and clinical decision support. Interventions that incorporate active clinician education or a combination of approaches tend to be most effective.

Role of the Pediatrician

At the practice level, pediatricians can integrate key recommendations that focus on antibiotic prescribing for common infections in children. These include the following:

1. Confirm urinary tract infection by documenting that the patient is symptomatic and has a properly obtained a urinalysis and quantitative culture with each episode, with a positive result based on the strain of bacteria isolated and the colony count. Once the infection is established, susceptibility data should be used to prescribe the narrowest spectrum appropriate antimicrobial agent.
2. Before treating a patient for bacterial pneumonia, ensure that there is not an alternate diagnosis or explanation for radiologic findings. The vast majority of respiratory syncytial virus infections in infants are not complicated by bacterial infection, but migratory atelectasis is common. For infants with uncomplicated bronchiolitis, antimicrobial agents are not indicated.[1]
3. Limit the use of vancomycin for treatment of methicillin-resistant *Staphylococcus aureus* (MRSA) infections or other methicillin-resistant pathogens to those cases when there is no suitable alternative. Pediatricians should standardize their own processes and ensure that appropriate cultures and other diagnostic tests are obtained before antimicrobial agents are administered. They also should know how to access their local antibiograms and be aware of antimicrobial resistance patterns. Antimicrobial agents should be initiated promptly for suspected or proven infection, and indication, dose, timing, and anticipated duration should be documented.
4. Reassess response to therapy within 48 hours, taking into account new clinical and laboratory data. Focus definitive therapy to use the most appropriate narrow-spectrum agent, and discontinue therapy when a treatable infection is excluded. Pediatricians also can collaborate with their antibiotic stewardship team and use formal infectious diseases consultation for cases in which the patient has comorbidities or a severe illness or if the diagnosis is uncertain.

Additional information for health care professionals and parents on judicious use of antimicrobial agents (The Get Smart Campaign) and antimicrobial resistance is available on the CDC Web site (**www.cdc.gov/getsmart/** and **www.cdc.gov/drugresistance**).

---

[1] Ralston SL, Lieberthal AS, Meissner HC, et al. Clinical practice guideline: the diagnosis, management, and prevention of bronchiolitis. *Pediatrics*. 2014;134(5):e1474–e1502

Principles of Appropriate Use of Antimicrobial Therapy for Upper Respiratory Tract Infections[1]

More than half of all outpatient prescriptions for antimicrobial agents for children are given for 5 conditions: otitis media, sinusitis, cough illness/bronchitis, pharyngitis, and nonspecific upper respiratory tract infection (the common cold). Antimicrobial agents often are prescribed, even though many of these illnesses are caused by viruses, which are unresponsive to antibiotic therapy. Children treated with an antimicrobial agent for respiratory tract infections are at increased risk of becoming colonized with resistant respiratory tract flora, including *Streptococcus pneumoniae* and *Haemophilus influenzae*. Children who subsequently develop respiratory tract infections are more likely to experience failure of antimicrobial therapy and are likely to spread resistant bacteria to close contacts, both children and adults. The following principles, with supporting evidence, were published by the AAP and CDC to identify clinical conditions for which antimicrobial therapy could be curtailed without compromising patient care (**www.cdc.gov/getsmart/**).

OTITIS MEDIA

- Antimicrobial agents are indicated for treatment of children with the definitive diagnosis acute otitis media (AOM)—that is, the presence of middle ear effusion and moderate-to-severe bulging of the tympanic membrane—or new onset of otorrhea not attributable to otitis externa. Clinicians may diagnose acute otitis media in children who have mild bulging of the tympanic membrane and recent onset of ear pain or intense erythema of the tympanic membrane.[2] Observation without use of an antimicrobial agent in a child with uncomplicated AOM is an option for selected children on the basis of diagnostic certainty, age, illness severity, and assurance of follow-up.[2]
- When antimicrobial agents are used for AOM, a narrow-spectrum antimicrobial agent (eg, amoxicillin, 80–90 mg/kg per day) in 2 divided doses for 5 to 7 days should be used for episodes in most children 2 years or older.[2] Microbiologic and clinical failure with high-dose amoxicillin has been associated with highly penicillin-resistant pneumococci (uncommon currently with widespread use of the 13-valent pneumococcal conjugate vaccine [PCV13]) and with beta-lactamase–producing *Haemophilus* species and *Moraxella* species (an increasing problem as the proportion of cases of AOM caused by pneumococci decreases). Additional β-lactamase coverage for AOM is indicated if the child has received amoxicillin in the last 30 days or has concurrent purulent conjunctivitis or a history of recurrent AOM unresponsive to amoxicillin.[2]
- Younger children and children with underlying medical conditions, craniofacial abnormalities, chronic or recurrent otitis media, or perforation of the tympanic membrane represent a more complicated and diverse population. Initial therapy with a 10-day course of an antimicrobial agent is likely to be more effective than shorter courses for many of these children.

---

[1]Hersh AL, Jackson MA, Hicks LA; American Academy of Pediatrics, Committee on Infectious Diseases. Clinical report: principles of judicious antibiotic prescribing for upper respiratory tract infections in pediatrics. *Pediatrics.* 2013;132(6):1146–1154

[2]Lieberthal AS, Carroll AE, Chonmaitree T, et al. Clinical practice guideline: the diagnosis and management of acute otitis media. *Pediatrics.* 2013;131(3):e964–e999

- Persistent middle ear effusion (MEE) is common and can be detected by pneumatic otoscopy (with or without verification by tympanometry) after resolution of acute symptoms. Two weeks after successful antibiotic treatment of AOM, 60% to 70% of children have MEE, decreasing to 40% at 1 month and 10% to 25% at 3 months after successful antibiotic treatment. The presence of MEE without clinical symptoms is defined as otitis media with effusion (OME). OME must be differentiated clinically from AOM and requires infrequent additional monitoring but not antibiotic therapy.[1] Assurance that OME resolves is particularly important for parents of children with cognitive or developmental delays that may be affected adversely by transient hearing loss associated with MEE.

ACUTE SINUSITIS

- Clinical practice guidelines from the AAP[2] and the Infectious Diseases Society of America[3] delineate evidence-based criteria for the diagnosis and treatment of acute bacterial sinusitis. Clinical diagnosis of acute bacterial sinusitis requires the presence of one of the following criteria: (1) persistent nasal discharge (of any quality) or daytime cough (which may be worse at night) without evidence of clinical improvement for ≥10 days; (2) body temperature of ≥39°C (102°F) or higher and purulent nasal discharge or facial pain present concurrently for at least 3 consecutive days in a child who seems ill; or (3) a worsening course (worsening or new onset of nasal discharge, daytime cough, or fever after initial improvement.[2]
- Findings on sinus radiographs correlate poorly with disease and should not be used. Computed tomography of sinuses may be indicated when complications are suspected.
- Antimicrobial therapy is indicated for children with severe onset or a worsening course. For children with nonsevere, persistent illness, either observation for an additional 3 days or antimicrobial therapy is indicated.[2]
- Initial antimicrobial treatment of acute sinusitis with amoxicillin (80–90 mg/kg per day in 2 divided doses) is preferred for most children. Amoxicillin-clavulanate (14:1 formulation) may be indicated when antimicrobial resistance is likely (eg, treatment with amoxicillin within 30 days). Treatment duration should be at least 7 days after resolution of symptoms.
- Guidelines from the Infectious Diseases Society of America address the inability of existing clinical criteria to differentiate accurately bacterial from viral acute rhinosinusitis, gaps in knowledge, and quality of evidence regarding empiric recommendations, changing prevalence and antimicrobial susceptibility profiles of bacterial-associated isolates, and the impact of pneumococcal conjugate vaccines on pneumococcal organisms associated with sinusitis.[3]

---

[1]Lieberthal AS, Carroll AE, Chonmaitree T, et al. Clinical practice guideline: the diagnosis and management of acute otitis media. *Pediatrics.* 2013;131(3):e964–e999

[2]Wald ER, Applegate KE, Bordley C, et al; American Academy of Pediatrics. Clinical practice guidelines for the diagnosis and management of acute bacterial sinusitis in children aged 1 to 18 years. *Pediatrics.* 2013;132(1):e262–e280

[3]Chow AW, Benninger MS, Brook I, et al; Infectious Disease Society of America. IDSA clinical practice guideline for acute bacterial rhinosinusitis in children and adults. *Clin Infect Dis.* 2012;54(8):e72–e112

COUGH ILLNESS/BRONCHITIS

- Nonspecific cough illness/bronchitis in children does not warrant antimicrobial treatment.
- Prolonged cough (10–14 days or more) may be caused by *Bordetella pertussis, Bordetella parapertussis, Mycoplasma pneumoniae,* or *Chlamydophila pneumoniae.* When infection caused by one of these organisms is suspected clinically or is confirmed, appropriate antimicrobial therapy is indicated (see Pertussis, p 608, *Mycoplasma pneumoniae* Infections, p 568, and Chlamydial Infections, p 284).

PHARYNGITIS

(See Group A Streptococcal Infections, p 732.)
- Diagnosis of group A streptococcal pharyngitis should be made on the basis of results of appropriate laboratory tests in conjunction with clinical and epidemiologic findings.
- Group A streptococcal testing should only be performed in patients with signs and symptoms of pharyngitis without evidence of rhinorrhea and cough.
- Most cases of pharyngitis are viral in origin. Antimicrobial therapy should not be given to a child with pharyngitis in the absence of positive group A streptococcal testing. Rarely, other bacteria may cause pharyngitis (eg, *Corynebacterium diphtheriae, Francisella tularensis,* groups G and C hemolytic streptococci, *Neisseria gonorrhoeae, Arcanobacterium haemolyticum*), and treatment should be provided according to recommendations in disease-specific chapters in section 3.
- Penicillin remains the drug of choice for treating group A streptococcal pharyngitis. Amoxicillin and other oral antimicrobial agents may be better tolerated and have improved efficacy of microbiologic eradication of group A streptococci from the pharynx, but this potential advantage must be considered against the disadvantage of increased antimicrobial pressure from use of more broad-spectrum antimicrobial agents.

THE COMMON COLD

- Antimicrobial agents should not be given for the common cold.
- Mucopurulent rhinitis (thick, opaque, or discolored nasal discharge that begins a few days into a viral upper respiratory tract infection) commonly accompanies the common cold and is not an indication for antimicrobial treatment unless it persists without signs of improvement for ≥10 days, suggesting possible acute bacterial sinusitis.

DRUG INTERACTIONS

Use of multiple drugs for treatment of seriously ill patients increases the probability of drug-drug interactions. Drug-drug interactions can be considered as producing either changes in drug concentrations (pharmacokinetics) or changes in the drug effect/toxicity profile (pharmacodynamics). Pharmacokinetic interactions result from alterations in the absorption, distribution, metabolism, or excretion of a drug, resulting in a change in concentration in the body. Pharmacodynamic drug-drug interactions may produce synergistic, additive, or antagonistic drug effects or toxicities. Many of the serious adverse interactions between drugs are attributable to inhibition (some macrolides, quinolones, and azole agents) or induction (rifabutin, rifampin) of hepatic intestinal cytochrome P450 (CYP) isoenzymes, especially CYP3A, which is thought to be involved in metabolism of more than 50% of prescribed drugs. Drug interactions related to inhibition of transporter proteins increasingly are being recognized. P-glycoprotein probably is the best understood of these transport proteins. Examples of transporter-based effects include interactions of penicillin with probenecid and of digoxin with quinidine.

Complete drug interaction software programs are used by most hospital and health care system pharmacies. The scope and cost of these programs usually is beyond the needs of most physicians. A more detailed description of drug interactions can be found on the Food and Drug Administration Web site (**www.fda. gov/Drugs/DevelopmentApprovalProcess/DevelopmentResources/ DrugInteractionsLabeling/ucm080499.htm**). Labels for individual drugs often include information about clinically significant drug interactions. Individual drug labels can be found online through the DailyMed (**http://dailymed.nlm.nih.gov/ dailymed/about.cfm**) or Drugs@FDA (**www.accessdata.fda.gov/scripts/ cder/drugsatfda/**) Web sites.

TABLES OF ANTIBACTERIAL DRUG DOSAGES

Recommended dosages for antibacterial agents commonly used for neonates (see Table 4.2, p 882) and for infants and children (see Table 4.3, p 884) are provided separately because of differences in drug disposition and elimination in neonates and resulting differences in pharmacokinetics and tissue site drug exposure. The table for neonates is divided by postnatal age and weight to reflect maturational changes that occur with time from conception (best described by postconceptional age or postmenstrual age) and those that are accelerated after birth (best described by chronologic age).

Recommended dosages are not absolute and are intended only as a guide. Clinical judgment about the disease, alterations in renal or hepatic function, coadministration of other drugs, and other factors affecting pharmacokinetics, patient response, and laboratory results may dictate modifications of these recommendations in an individual patient. In some cases, monitoring of serum drug concentrations is recommended to avoid toxicity and to ensure therapeutic efficacy.

With an increasing prevalence of multidrug resistance for both gram-negative and gram-positive pathogens, antimicrobial drugs that previously were reserved for severe infections now should be used to treat less severe infections if a safer alternative drug with a more narrow spectrum is not available. For antimicrobial agents not yet approved by the US Food and Drug Administration (FDA) but under study, the infections and dosages used for investigational treatments may be found at **http://ClinicalTrials.gov**.

Product label information or a pediatric pharmacist should be consulted for details, such as the appropriate diluent for reconstitution of injectable preparations, measures to be taken to avoid incompatibilities, drug interactions, and other precautions. FDA-approved drug labels can be found online at DailyMed (**http://dailymed.nlm.nih. gov/dailymed/about.cfm**) or Drugs@FDA (**www.accessdata.fda.gov/scripts/ cder/drugsatfda/**).

Table 4.2 Antibacterial Drugs for Neonates (≤28 Postnatal Days of Age)[a]

Drug	Route	Body Weight ≤2 kg		Body Weight >2 kg	
		≤7 days of age	8–28 days of age[b]	≤7 days of age	8–28 days of age
Aminoglycosides[c,d]					
Amikacin	IV, IM	15 mg every 48 h	15 mg every 24h	15 mg every 24 h	17.5 mg every 24 h
Gentamicin	IV, IM	5 mg every 48 h	5 mg every 36 h	4 mg every 24 h	4–5 mg every 24 h
Tobramycin	IV, IM	5 mg every 48 h	5 mg every 36 h	4 mg every 24 h	4–5 mg every 24 h
Carbapenems					
Imipenem/cilastatin[e]	IV	20 mg every 12 h	25 mg every 12 h	25 mg every 12 h	25 mg every 8 h
Meropenem[f]	IV	20 mg every 12 h (≤14 days of age)	20 mg every 8 h (>14 days of age)	20 mg every 8 h (>14 days of age)	30 mg every 8 h (≤14 days of age)
Cephalosporins[f]					
Cefepime[g]	IV, IM	30 mg every 12 h	30 mg every 12 h	30 mg every 12 h	30 mg every 12 h
Cefotaxime	IV, IM	50 mg every 12 h	50 mg every 8–12 h	50 mg every 12 h	50 mg every 8 h
Cefazolin	IV, IM	25 mg every 12 h	25 mg every 12 h	25 mg every 12 h	25 mg every 8 h
Ceftazidime	IV, IM	50 mg every 12 h	50 mg every 8–12 h	50 mg every 12 h	50 mg every 8 h
Cefoxitin	IV, IM	35 mg every 12 h	35 mg every 8 h	35 mg every 8 h	30 mg every 6 h
Ceftriaxone[h]	IV, IM	50 mg every 24 h	50 mg every 24 h	50 mg every 24 h	50 mg every 24 h
Cefuroxime	IV, IM	50 mg every 12 h	50 mg every 8–12 h	50 mg every 12 h	50 mg every 8 h
Penicillins					
Ampicillin[f]	IV, IM	50 mg every 12 h[h,i,j]	50 mg every 8 h[i]	50 mg every 8 h[h,i,j]	50 mg every 6 h[i]
Nafcillin, oxacillin[f]	IV, IM	25 mg every 12 h	25 mg every 8 h	25 mg every 8 h	25 mg every 6 h
Penicillin G crystalline[f]	IV, IM	25 000–50 000 U every 12 h	25 000–50 000 U every 8 h	25 000–50 000 U every 8 h	25 000–50 000 U every 8 h
Penicillin G procaine	IM only	50 000 U every 24 h	50 000 U every 24 h	50 000 U every 24 h	50 000 U every 24 h
Piperacillin-tazobactam	IV	100 mg piperacillin component every 12 h	100 mg piperacillin component every 8 h	100 mg piperacillin component every 12 h	100 mg piperacillin component every 8 h
Ticarcillin-clavulanate	IV	75 mg every 12 h	75 mg every 8 h	75 mg every 12 h	75 mg every 8 h

Table 4.2 Antibacterial Drugs for Neonates (≤28 Postnatal Days of Age),ᵃ continued

Drug	Route	Dose per kg and Frequency of Administration			
		Body Weight ≤2 kg		Body Weight >2 kg	
		≤7 days of age	8–28 days of ageᵇ	≤7 days of age	8–28 days of age
Other agents					
Azithromycin	PO	10–20 mg every 24 h	10–20 mg every 24	10–20 mg every 24 h	10–20 mg every 24 h
	IV	10 mg every 24 h	10 mg every 24 h	10 mg every 24 h	10 mg every 24 h
Aztreonamᵍ	IV, IM	30 mg every 12 h	30 mg every 8–12 h	30 mg every 8 h	30 mg every 6 h
Clindamycin	IV, IM, PO	5 mg every 12 h	5 mg every 8 h	5 mg every 8 h	5 mg every 6 h
Erythromycin	IV, PO	10 mg every 12 h	10 mg every 8 h	10 mg every 12 h	10 mg every 8 h
Linezolid	IV	10 mg every 12 h	10 mg every 8 h	10 mg every 8 h	10 mg every 8 h
Metronidazoleᵏ [15 mg/kg loading dose all categories (for body weight ≤2 kg or >2 kg, and for ≤7 days of age or 8–28 days of age)]	IV	7.5 mg every 12 h	7.5 mg every 12 h	7.5 mg every 8 h	7.5 mg every 6 h
Vancomycin	IV	See commentˡ			

IV indicates intravenous; IM, intramuscular; PO, oral.

We gratefully acknowledge the review and comments on this Table by John Van den Anker, MD, PhD.

ᵃ Adapted from American Academy of Pediatrics. 2015 Nelson's Pediatric Antimicrobial Therapy. Bradley JS, Nelson JD, Cantey JB, Kimberlin DW, Leake JAD, Palumbo PE, Sauberan J, Steinbach WJ, eds. 21st ed. Elk Grove Village, IL: American Academy of Pediatrics; 2015

ᵇ May use the longer dosing interval in extremely low birth weight (less than 1000 g) neonates until 2 weeks of life.

ᶜ Dosages for aminoglycosides may differ from those recommended by the manufacturer and approved by the US Food and Drug Administration.

ᵈ Optimal, individualized dosage should be based on determination of serum concentrations.

ᵉ Accumulation of cilastatin may occur in neonates with multiple doses.

ᶠ Higher doses than those listed may be required for meningitis.

ᵍ 50 mg/kg/dose may be required for Pseudomonas infections.

ʰ Neonates should not receive ceftriaxone intravenously if they also are receiving, or are expected to receive, intravenous calcium in any form, including parenteral nutrition. See Bradley JS, Wassel RT, Lee L, Nambiar S. Intravenous ceftriaxone and calcium in the neonate: assessing the risk for cardiopulmonary adverse events. Pediatrics. 2009;123(4):e609–e613.

ⁱ Some experts recommend 75 mg/kg/dose every 6 h for group B streptococcal meningitis for all weight groups.

ʲ 100 mg/kg/dose every 12 hours also is acceptable for treatment of presumed early-onset group B streptococcal septicemia without meningitis.

ᵏ Metronidazole kinetics are best described by postmenstrual (postconceptional) age, which is equivalent to gestational age plus chronologic age. For postmenstrual age <34 weeks, 7.5 mg/kg every 12 h; for 34–40 weeks, 7.5 mg/kg every 8 h; for >40 weeks, 7.5 mg/kg every 6 h. All categories should receive a 15-mg/kg loading dose.

ˡ Dosing algorithm for vancomycin is based on serum creatinine concentration (which will take approximately 5 days after birth to reasonably reflect neonatal renal function); if <0.7 mg/dL, then 15 mg/kg every 12 h; if 0.7–0.9 mg/dL, then 20 mg/kg every 24 h; if 1–1.2 mg/dL, then 15 mg/kg every 24 h; if 1.3–1.6 mg/dL, then 10 mg/kg every 24 h; if >1.6 mg/dL, then 10 mg/kg every 48 h.

Table 4.3. Antibacterial Drugs for Pediatric Patients Beyond the Newborn Period[a]

Drug Generic (Trade Name)	Generic Available	Route	Dosage per kg per Day		Comments
			Mild to Moderate Infections	Severe Infections	
Aminoglycosides[b]					Individualize dose and frequency based on analysis of serum concentrations.[b]
Amikacin	Y	IV, IM	Inappropriate	15–22.5 mg in 2–3 doses, or 15–20 mg in 1 dose	Aminoglycosides may be given once daily, or in divided doses. Measured serum concentrations should guide ongoing therapy. Higher doses are appropriate for patients with cystic fibrosis.
Gentamicin	Y	IV, IM	Inappropriate	6–7.5 mg in 3 doses, or 5–7.5 mg in 1 dose	Aminoglycosides may be given once daily, or in divided doses. Measured serum concentrations should guide ongoing therapy.
Neomycin	Y	PO	100 mg in 4 doses	100 mg in 4 doses	For some enteric infections.
Tobramycin	Y	IV, IM	Inappropriate	6–7.5 mg in 3–4 doses, or 5–7.5 mg in 1 dose	Aminoglycosides may be given once daily, or in divided doses. Measured serum concentrations should guide ongoing therapy. Higher doses are appropriate for patients with cystic fibrosis.
Carbapenems[c]					
Doripenem (Doribax)	N	IV	Inappropriate	60 mg in 3 doses (daily adult dose, 1500 mg in 3 doses)	Not yet FDA approved for children, but under study. Not studied in meningitis.
Cephalosporins[c]					The generation of each agent is listed as a rough guide to antimicrobial spectrum.
Imipenem/cilastatin (Primaxin)	Y	IV	Inappropriate	60–100 mg in 4 doses (daily adult dose, 1–4 g)	Caution in use for treatment of CNS infections because of increased risk of seizures. Higher doses for more severe infections or *Pseudomonas aeruginosa* infections.

Table 4.3. Antibacterial Drugs for Pediatric Patients Beyond the Newborn Period,[a] continued

Drug Generic (Trade Name)	Generic Available	Route	Dosage per kg per Day		Comments
			Mild to Moderate Infections	Severe Infections	
Meropenem (Merrem)	Y	IV	Inappropriate	30–60 mg in 3 doses (daily adult dose, 1.5–6 g)	Higher dose (120 mg in 3 doses) used for treatment of meningitis.
Ertapenem (Invanz)	N	IV/IM	Inappropriate	30 mg in 2 doses (adult dose, 1 g, once daily)	Poor activity against *Pseudomonas* and *Acinetobacter* species.
Cefaclor (Ceclor)	Y	PO	20–40 mg in 2 or 3 doses (daily adult dose, 750 mg–1.5 g)	Inappropriate	Second-generation.
Cefadroxil (Duricef)	Y	PO	30 mg in 2 doses (daily adult dose, 1–2 g)	Inappropriate	First-generation.
Cefazolin	Y	IV, IM	25–50 mg in 3 doses (daily adult dose, 3 g)	100–150 mg in 3 doses (daily adult dose, 4–6 g)	First-generation. Limited data on dosages above 100 mg/kg/day.
Cefdinir (Omnicef)	Y	PO	14 mg in 1 or 2 doses (max, 600 mg/day)	Inappropriate	Extended-spectrum third generation. Inadequate activity against penicillin-resistant pneumococci.
Cefditoren (Spectracef)	Y	PO	≥12 y: 400–800 mg total daily dose (not per kg) in 2 doses	Inappropriate	Extended-spectrum third general. Contraindicated in patients with carnitine deficiency.
Cefepime (Maxipime)	Y	IV, IM	100 mg in 2 doses (daily adult dose, 2–4 g)	100–150 mg in 2–3 doses (daily adult dose, 4–6 g)	Extended-spectrum fourth generation. Higher dose (150 mg in 3 doses) used for *Pseudomonas* infections, or for febrile neutropenia.
Cefixime (Suprax)	N	PO	8 mg in 1 or 2 doses (daily adult dose, 400 mg)	Inappropriate	Extended-spectrum third generation. Inadequate activity against penicillin-resistant pneumococci.

Table 4.3. Antibacterial Drugs for Pediatric Patients Beyond the Newborn Period,[a] continued

Drug Generic (Trade Name)	Generic Available	Route	Dosage per kg per Day		Comments
			Mild to Moderate Infections	Severe Infections	
Cefotaxime (Claforan)	Y	IV, IM	50–180 mg in 3 or 4 doses (daily adult dose, 3–6 g)	200–225 mg in 4 or 6 doses (daily adult dose, 8–12 g)	Extended-spectrum third generation. Up to 300 mg in 4 or 6 doses for meningitis.
Cefotetan	Y	IV, IM	60 mg in 2 doses (daily adult dose, 2–4 g)	100 mg in 2 doses (daily adult dose, 4–6 g)	Second-generation. A cephamycin, with enhanced anaerobic activity. Not FDA approved for use in children.
Cefoxitin (Mefoxin)	Y	IV, IM	80 mg in 3–4 doses (daily adult dose, 3–4 g)	160 mg in 4 doses (daily adult dose, 6–12 g)	Second-generation. A cephamycin, with enhanced anaerobic activity. Active against *Bacteroides fragilis*.
Cefpodoxime (Vantin)	Y	PO	10 mg in 2 doses (daily adult dose, 200–400 mg, 800 mg for SSTIs)	Inappropriate	Extended-spectrum third generation.
Cefprozil (Cefzil)	Y	PO	15–30 mg in 2 doses (daily adult dose, 0.5–1 g)	Inappropriate	Second-generation.
Ceftaroline (Teflaro)	N	IV	Inappropriate	Adults, 1200 mg per day in 2–3 doses	Extended-spectrum fifth generation with activity against CA MRSA. Not yet FDA approved for children, but under study.
Ceftazidime (Fortaz)	Y	IV, IM	90–150 mg in 3 doses (daily adult dose, 3 g)	200 mg in 3 doses for patients without cystic fibrosis 300 mg in 3 doses for patients with cystic fibrosis (for both populations, daily adult dose, 6 g)	Extended-spectrum third generation. Anti-*Pseudomonas* activity.

Table 4.3. Antibacterial Drugs for Pediatric Patients Beyond the Newborn Period,ª continued

Drug Generic (Trade Name)	Generic Available	Route	Dosage per kg per Day		Comments
			Mild to Moderate Infections	Severe Infections	
Ceftibuten (Cedax)	Y	PO	9 mg once daily (daily adult dose, 400 mg)	Inappropriate	Extended-spectrum third generation. Inadequate activity against penicillin-resistant pneumococci.
Ceftriaxone (Rocephin)	Y	IV, IM	50–75 mg once daily (daily adult dose, 1 g)	100 mg in 1 or 2 doses (daily adult dose, 2–4 g)	Extended-spectrum third generation. Larger dosage (up to that used for meningitis) appropriate for penicillin-resistant pneumococcal pneumonia. 50 mg/kg, IM, for 1–3 days for AOM (up to 1 g).
Cefuroxime (Zinacef)	Y	IV, IM	75–100 mg in 3 doses (daily adult dose, 2.25–4.5 g)	100–200 mg in 3–4 doses (daily adult dose, 3–6 g)	Second-generation. Less active than parenteral extended-spectrum cephalosporins against penicillin-resistant pneumococcus.
Cefuroxime (Ceftin)	Y	PO	20–30 mg in 2 doses (daily adult dose, 0.5–1 g)	Inappropriate	Second-generation. Limited activity against penicillin-resistant pneumococcus.
Cephalexin (Keflex)	Y	PO	25–50 mg in 2 or 4 doses (daily adult dose, 1–2 g)	75–100 mg in 3–4 doses (daily adult dose, 2–4 g)	First-generation. The 100 mg/kg/day dosage has been studied for osteoarticular infections.
Chloramphenicol (oral formulation not available in the US)	Y	IV only	Inappropriate	50–100 mg in 4 doses (daily adult dose, 2–4 g)	Individualize dose and frequency based on analysis of serum concentrations. Usually reserved for serious infections because of rare risk of aplastic anemia.

Table 4.3. Antibacterial Drugs for Pediatric Patients Beyond the Newborn Period,[a] continued

Drug Generic (Trade Name)	Generic Available	Route	Dosage per kg per Day		Comments
			Mild to Moderate Infections	Severe Infections	
Clindamycin (Cleocin)	Y	IM, IV	20–30 mg in 3 doses (daily adult dose, 0.9–1.8 g)	40 mg in 3–4 doses (daily adult dose, 1.8–2.7 g)	Active against anaerobes, especially *Bacteroides* species. Active against many multidrug-resistant pneumococci and CA-MRSA.
		PO	10–25 mg in 3 doses (daily adult dose, 600 mg–1.8 g)	30–40 mg in 3–4 doses (daily adult dose, 1.2–1.8 g)	The 30–40 mg dosage recommended for AOM and CA-MRSA.
Daptomycin (Cubicin)	N	IV	Inappropriate	6–10 mg, once daily (daily adult dose, 4–6 mg/kg of total body weight)	Not yet FDA-approved for children, but under study
Fluoroquinolones[d]					
Ciprofloxacin (Cipro)	Y Tablet only	PO	20 mg in 2 doses (daily adult dose, 0.5–1 g)	30–40 mg in 2 doses (daily adult dose, 1–1.5 g)	20 mg one time for *Neisseria meningitidis* prophylaxis (adult dose 500 mg). Also see Fluoroquinolones, p 872.
	Y	IV	Inappropriate	20–30 mg in 2 or 3 doses (daily adult dose, 0.8–1.2 g)	
Levofloxacin (Levaquin)	Y	IV, PO	Inappropriate	16–20 mg in 2 doses (daily adult dose, 500–750 mg)	Also see Fluoroquinolones, p 872.

Table 4.3. Antibacterial Drugs for Pediatric Patients Beyond the Newborn Period,[a] continued

Drug Generic (Trade Name)	Generic Available	Route	Dosage per kg per Day		Comments
			Mild to Moderate Infections	Severe Infections	
Macrolides					
Azithromycin (Zithromax, Zmax)	Y	PO	5–12 mg once daily (adult single or total course dose, 1.5–2 g); 60-mg single dose of extended-release formulation, Zmax (adult dose 2 g)	Inappropriate	All doses once daily: AOM: 10 mg/kg/day for 3 days; or 30 mg/kg for 1 day; or 10 mg/kg/day for 1 day, then 5 mg/kg/day for 4 days. Pharyngitis: 12 mg/kg/day for 5 days (maximum 1.5 g total course). Sinusitis: 10 mg/kg/day for 3 days or 10 mg/kg/day for 1 day, then 5 mg/kg/day for 4 days. Community associated pneumonia: 10 mg/kg × 1 day; then 5 mg/kg/day for 4 days or 60 mg/kg for 1 day of Zmax extended-release suspension for infants and children >6 months of age. Shigellosis: 12 mg/kg × 1 day, 6 mg/kg/day for 4 days.
	Y	IV	Inappropriate	10 mg/kg, once daily	Administer over at least 60 minutes to potentially prevent local reactions.
Clarithromycin (Biaxin)	Y	PO	15 mg in 2 doses (daily adult dose, 0.5–1 g)	Inappropriate	Similar activity to erythromycin; more activity against *Mycobacterium avium* and *Helicobacter pylori*.

Table 4.3. Antibacterial Drugs for Pediatric Patients Beyond the Newborn Period,[a] continued

Drug Generic (Trade Name)	Generic Available	Route	Dosage per kg per Day		Comments
			Mild to Moderate Infections	Severe Infections	
Erythromycin (numerous)	Y	PO	40–50 mg in 3–4 doses (daily adult dose, 1–2 g)	Inappropriate	Available in base, stearate, and ethylsuccinate preparations.
	N	IV	Inappropriate	20 mg in 4 doses (daily adult dose, 2–4 g)	Administer over at least 60 minutes to potentially prevent cardiac arrhythmias. Minimal systemic absorption;
Fidaxomicin (Dificid)	N	PO	Adults: 400 mg total daily dose (not per kg) in 2 doses	Inappropriate	Used for treatment of *Clostridium difficile*-associated diarrhea. Not yet FDA approved for children, but under study.
Metronidazole (Flagyl)	Y	PO	30–50 mg in 3 doses (daily adult dose, 0.75–2.25 g)	Same	30 mg in 4 doses for *C difficile* infection
	Y	IV	22.5–40 mg in 3 doses (daily adult dose, 1.5 g)	Same	
Monobactam					
Aztreonam (Azactam)	Y	IV, IM	90 mg in 3 doses (daily adult dose, 3 g)	90–120 mg in 3 or 4 doses (maximum daily adult dose, 8 g)	…
Nitrofurantoin (Furadantin, Macrodantin)	Y	PO	5–7 mg in 4 doses (daily adult dose, 200–400 mg)	Inappropriate	For treatment of cystitis; not appropriate for pyelonephritis. UTI prophylaxis: 1–2 mg once daily.

Table 4.3. Antibacterial Drugs for Pediatric Patients Beyond the Newborn Period,[a] continued

Drug Generic (Trade Name)	Generic Available	Route	Dosage per kg per Day		Comments
			Mild to Moderate Infections	Severe Infections	
Oxazolidinones					
Linezolid (Zyvox)	N	PO, IV	For children <12 y of age: 30 mg in 3 doses For adolescents ≥12 y and adults: 1200 mg per day in 2 doses	Same	Myelosuppression increases with duration of therapy over 10 days.
PENICILLINS[c]					
Broad-spectrum penicillins					
Amoxicillin (Amoxil)	Y	PO	25–50 mg in 3 doses (daily adult dose, 750 mg–1.5 g)	High dosage for oral step-down therapy of invasive, non-AOM infections: 80–100 mg in 3 doses, or for highly susceptible pathogens, 90 mg in 2 doses	90 mg/kg in 2 doses recommended for initial therapy of AOM.
Amoxicillin-clavulanic acid (Augmentin)	Y	PO	14:1 Formulation: 90 mg amoxicillin component in 2 doses (<40 kg) for recurrent AOM, treatment failures 7:1 Formulation: 25–45 mg amoxicillin component in 2 doses (daily adult dose, 1750 mg) 4:1 Formulation: 20–40 mg amoxicillin component in 3 doses (daily adult dose, 1500 mg)	Inappropriate	

Table 4.3. Antibacterial Drugs for Pediatric Patients Beyond the Newborn Period,[a] continued

Drug Generic (Trade Name)	Generic Available	Route	Dosage per kg per Day		Comments
			Mild to Moderate Infections	Severe Infections	
Ampicillin	Y	IV, IM	100–150 mg in 4 doses (daily adult dose, 2–4 g)	200–400 mg in 4 doses (daily adult dose, 6–12 g)	Highest doses in treatment of CNS infections
	Y	PO	50–100 mg in 4 doses (daily adult dose, 2–4 g)	Inappropriate	
Ampicillin-sulbactam (Unasyn)	Y	IV	100–200 mg of ampicillin component in 4 doses (daily adult dose, 4 g)	200 mg ampicillin component in 4 doses (daily adult dose, 8 g)	
Piperacillin-tazobactam (Zosyn)	Y	IV	Inappropriate	For children ≥9 months of age: 300 mg piperacillin component in 3 doses (daily adult dose, 9–16 g)	Lower dose (240 mg piperacillin component in 3 doses) recommended for patients 2–9 mo of age.
Ticarcillin-clavulanate (Timentin)	N	IV	Inappropriate	200–300 mg ticarcillin component in 4–6 doses (daily adult dose, 12–18 g)	
Penicillin[c]					
Penicillin G, crystalline potassium or sodium	Y	IV, IM	100 000–150 000 units in 4 doses (daily adult dose, 4–8 million units)	200 000–300 000 units in 4–6 doses (daily adult dose, 12–24 million units)	Use highest doses in treatment of CNS infections.
Penicillin G procaine	Y	IM	50 000 units in 1–2 doses (daily adult dose, 300 000–1.2 million units)	Inappropriate	Not safe for IV administration.
Penicillin G benzathine (Bicillin LA)	N	IM	<27 kg (60 lb) 300 000–600 000 units (not dosed per kg) one time ≥27 kg (60 lb) 900 000 units (not dosed per kg) one time	Inappropriate	Not safe for IV administration. Very low but prolonged serum concentrations. 50 000 U/kg for newborns and infants. Major use is treatment of rheumatic fever prophylaxis and treponemal infections.

Table 4.3. Antibacterial Drugs for Pediatric Patients Beyond the Newborn Period,[a] continued

Drug Generic (Trade Name)	Generic Available	Route	Dosage per kg per Day		Comments
			Mild to Moderate Infections	Severe Infections	
Penicillin G benzathine/procaine (Bicillin CR)[e]	N	IM	<14 kg (30 lb) 600 000 units (not dosed per kg) one time 14–27 kg (30–60 lb) 900 000–1 200 000 units (not dosed per kg) one time ≥27 kg (60 lb) 2 400 000 units (not dosed per kg) one time		Not safe for IV administration. Major use is treatment of group A streptococcal infections.
Penicillin V	Y	PO	25–75 mg in 3 or 4 doses (daily adult dose, 1–2 g)	Inappropriate	
Penicillinase-resistant penicillins[e]					
					Methicillin (oxacillin)-resistant staphylococci usually are resistant to all semisynthetic antistaphylococcal penicillins and cephalosporins except ceftaroline.
Oxacillin	Y	IV, IM	100–150 mg in 4 doses (daily adult dose, 4 g)	150–200 mg in 4–6 doses (daily adult dose, 6–12 g)	
Nafcillin	Y	IV, IM	100–150 mg in 4 doses (daily adult dose, 4 g)	150–200 mg in 4–6 doses (daily adult dose, 6–12 g)	
Dicloxacillin (suspension no longer available in the US)	Y	PO	12–25 mg in 4 doses (daily adult dose, 0.5–1 g)	100 mg in 4 divided doses (for step-down therapy of osteoarticular infections)	
Rifamycins					
Rifampin (Rifadin)	Y	IV, PO	10–20 mg in 1–2 doses (daily adult dose, 600 mg)	20 mg in 2 doses (daily adult dose, 600 mg)	Should not be used routinely as monotherapy because of rapid emergence of resistance. See p 815–816 for *M tuberculosis* dosing.

Table 4.3. Antibacterial Drugs for Pediatric Patients Beyond the Newborn Period,[a] continued

Drug Generic (Trade Name)	Generic Available	Route	Dosage per kg per Day		Comments
			Mild to Moderate Infections	Severe Infections	
Rifaximin (Xifaxan)	N	PO	≥12 y of age: 600 mg/day (not per kg) in 3 doses	Inappropriate	Treatment of travelers' diarrhea caused by noninvasive *Escherichia coli*; should not be used for bloody diarrhea with risk of bacteremia.
Streptogramin					
Quinupristin/ dalfopristin (Synercid)	N	IV	Inappropriate	For children ≥12 y of age: 15 mg in 2 doses (daily adult dose, same)	Moderate activity against *Staphylococcus aureus*. Limited experience in children.
Sulfonamides					
Sulfadiazine	Y	PO	120–150 mg in 4–6 doses (daily adult dose, 4–6 g)	120–150 mg in 4–6 doses (daily adult dose, 4–6 g)	
Trimethoprim (TMP)-sulfamethoxazole (SMX) in 1:5 ratio (Bactrim, Septra)	Y	PO, IV	6–12 mg of TMP component in 2 doses (daily adult dose, 320 mg TMP)	same	2 mg of TMP component once daily for UTI prophylaxis. See p 641 for *Pneumocystis jirovecii* dosing.
Tetracyclines					
Tetracycline (Sumycin)	Y	PO	25–50 mg in 4 doses (daily adult dose, 1–2 g)	25–50 mg in 4 doses (daily adult dose, 1–2 g)	Responsible for staining of developing teeth; routine use only in children 8 y or older. Exceptions for circumstances in which the benefits of therapy exceed the risks and alternative drugs are less effective or more toxic found on p 873.

Table 4.3. Antibacterial Drugs for Pediatric Patients Beyond the Newborn Period,[a] continued

Drug Generic (Trade Name)	Generic Available	Route	Dosage per kg per Day		Comments
			Mild to Moderate Infections	Severe Infections	
Doxycycline (Vibramycin)	Y	PO, IV	2–4 mg in 1–2 doses (daily adult dose, 50–200 mg)	4 mg/kg per day, divided every 12 hours, intravenously or orally (maximum 100 mg/dose)	Adverse effects similar to those of other tetracycline products except that risk of dental staining in children younger than 8 y with doxycycline is unlikely at the dose and duration recommended to treat serious infections.
Minocycline (Dynacin, Minocin)	Y	PO, IV	4 mg in 2 doses (daily adult dose, 200 mg)	4 mg in 2 doses (daily adult dose, 200 mg)	Responsible for staining of developing teeth; routine use only in children 8 y or older.
Vancomycin (Vancocin)	Y	IV	40–45 mg in 3–4 doses (daily adult dose, 1–2 g)	45–60 mg in 3–4 doses (daily adult dose, 2–4 g)	Measured serum concentrations should guide ongoing therapy.
		PO		40 mg in 4 doses (daily adult dose, 2 g)	For *C difficile* infection.

IV, indicates intravenous; IM, intramuscular; PO, oral; FDA, US Food and Drug Administration; CNS, central nervous system; SSTI, skin and soft tissue infection; CA MRSA; community-associated methicillin-resistant *Staphylococcus aureus*; AOM, acute otitis media; UTI, urinary tract infection.

[a] Adapted from American Academy of Pediatrics. *2015 Nelson's Pediatric Antimicrobial Therapy.* Bradley JS, Nelson JD, Cantey JB, Kimberlin DW, Leake JAD, Palumbo PE, Sauberan J, Steinbach WJ, eds. 21st ed. Elk Grove Village, IL: American Academy of Pediatrics; 2015

[b] Once-daily aminoglycoside dosing may provide equal efficacy with reduced toxicity and may be used as an alternative to multiple daily dosing. See Contopoulos-Iannidis DG, Giotis ND, Baliatsa DV, Iannidis JP. Extended-interval aminoglycoside administration for children: a meta-analysis. *Pediatrics.* 2004;114(1):e111–e118, and Best EJ, Gazarian M, Cohn R, Wilkinson M, Palasanthiran P. Once-daily gentamicin in infants and children: a prospective cohort study evaluating safety and the role of therapeutic drug monitoring in minimizing toxicity. *Pediatr Infect Dis J.* 2011;30(10):827–832.

[c] Children with a history of an IgE-mediated, immediate hypersensitivity reaction to penicillins (urticaria, angioedema, bronchospasm, anaphylaxis) who require treatment with an alternate b-lactam should be considered for skin testing (if available) to confirm the allergy, and/or undergo supervised graded clinical challenge or desensitization with the alternate b-lactam agent under the supervision of an expert in drug allergy and desensitization.

[d] Ciprofloxacin is FDA approved for use in patients younger than 18 years for complicated UTI and postexposure inhalation anthrax but also has been studied in other infections. Levofloxacin is FDA approved for postexposure inhalation anthrax and plague, but has been studied in children and adolescents for treatment of AOM, community acquired pneumonia (see Fluoroquinolones, p 872).

[e] Available in 2-mL prefilled syringes. Each 1 mL contains 300 000 units benzathine plus 300 000 units procaine (600 000 total units per mL).

SEXUALLY TRANSMITTED INFECTIONS

Table 4.4. Guidelines for Treatment of Sexually Transmitted Infections in Children and Adolescents According to Syndrome

Preferred regimens are listed. For further information concerning other acceptable regimens and diseases not included, see recommendations in disease-specific chapters in Section 3. In addition, revised recommendations on treatment of sexually transmitted infections have been issued by the Centers for Disease Control and Prevention in 2015[a]; updates are posted at **www.cdc.gov/std/treatment.**

Syndrome	Organisms/Diagnoses	Treatment of Adolescent[a]	Treatment of Infant/Child
Urethritis and cervicitis Urethritis: Inflammation of urethra with erythema and/or mucoid, mucopurulent, or purulent discharge Cervicitis: Inflammation of cervix with erythema, friability and/or mucopurulent or purulent cervical discharge. Cervicitis occurs rarely in prepubertal girls (see Prepubertal vaginitis, below)	*Neisseria gonorrhoeae, Chlamydia trachomatis* Other causes of urethritis and cervicitis include *Mycoplasma genitalium,* possibly *Ureaplasma urealyticum,* and sometimes *Trichomonas vaginalis* and herpes simplex virus (HSV)	Ceftriaxone, 250 mg, IM, in a single dose[b] **PLUS EITHER** Azithromycin, 1 g, orally, in a single dose **OR** Doxycycline, 100 mg, orally, twice a day for 7 days	*Children <45 kg and <8 y of age:* Ceftriaxone, 125 mg, IM, in a single dose[b] **PLUS** Erythromycin base or ethylsuccinate, 50 mg/kg per day, orally, in 4 divided doses (maximum 2 g/day) for 14 days *Children ≥45 kg but <8 y of age:* Ceftriaxone, 250 mg, IM, in a single dose[b] **PLUS** Azithromycin, 1 g, orally, in a single dose *Children ≥45 kg and ≥8 y of age:* Ceftriaxone, 250 mg, IM, in a single dose[b] **PLUS EITHER** Azithromycin, 1 g, orally, in a single dose **OR** Doxycycline, 100 mg, orally, twice a day for 7 days

Table 4.4. Guidelines for Treatment of Sexually Transmitted Infections in Children and Adolescents According to Syndrome, continued

Syndrome	Organisms/Diagnoses	Treatment of Adolescent	Treatment of Infant/Child
Prepubertal vaginitis (STI related):	*N gonorrhoeae*[a]	…	***Children <45 kg:*** Ceftriaxone, 125 mg, in a single dose ***Children ≥45 kg but <8 y of age:*** Ceftriaxone, 250 mg, IM, in a single dose[b] **PLUS** Azithromycin, 1 g, orally, in a single dose ***Children ≥45 kg and ≥8 y of age:*** Ceftriaxone, 250 mg, IM, in a single dose[b] **PLUS EITHER** Azithromycin, 1 g, orally, in a single dose **OR** Doxycycline, 100 mg, orally, twice a day for 7 days
	C trachomatis[a]	…	***Children <45 kg:*** Erythromycin base or ethylsuccinate, 50 mg/kg per day, orally, in 4 divided doses (maximum 2 g/day) for 14 days ***Children ≥45 kg but <8 y of age:*** Azithromycin, 1 g, orally, in a single dose ***Children ≥45 kg and ≥8 y of age:*** Azithromycin, 1 g, orally, in a single dose **OR** Doxycycline, 100 mg, orally, twice a day for 7 days

Table 4.4. Guidelines for Treatment of Sexually Transmitted Infections in Children and Adolescents According to Syndrome, continued

Syndrome	Organisms/ Diagnoses	Treatment of Adolescent	Treatment of Infant/Child
	T vaginalis	…	**Children <45 kg:** Metronidazole, 45 mg/kg per day, orally, in 3 divided doses (maximum 2 g/day) for 7 days
	Bacterial vaginosis	…	**Children <45 kg:** Metronidazole, 45 mg/kg per day, orally, in 3 divided doses (maximum 2 g/day) for 7 days
	HSV—1st clinical episode		**Children <45 kg:** Acyclovir, 80 mg/kg per day, orally, in 4 divided doses (maximum 3.2 g/day) for 7–10 days **OR** Valacyclovir, 40 mg/kg per day, orally, in 2 divided doses for 7–10 days **Children ≥45 kg:** Acyclovir 400 mg, orally, 3 times/day for 7–10 days **OR** Acyclovir 200 mg, orally, 5 times/day for 7–10 days **OR** Famciclovir 250 mg, orally, 3 times/day for 7–10 days **OR** Valacyclovir 1 g, orally, twice daily for 7–10 days

Table 4.4. Guidelines for Treatment of Sexually Transmitted Infections in Children and Adolescents According to Syndrome, continued

Syndrome	Organisms/Diagnoses	Treatment of Adolescent	Treatment of Infant/Child
Adolescent vulvovaginitis	*T vaginalis*	Metronidazole, 2 g, orally, in a single dose **OR** Tinidazole, 2 g, orally, in a single dose	…
	Bacterial vaginosis	Metronidazole, 500 mg, orally, twice daily for 7 days **OR** Metronidazole gel 0.75%, 1 full applicator (5 g), intravaginally, once a day for 5 days **OR** Clindamycin cream 2%, 1 full applicator (5 g), intravaginally at bedtime, for 7 days	…
	Candida species	See Table 4.5, Recommended Regimens for Vulvovaginal Candidiasis (p 904)	…
	HSV—1st clinical episode	Acyclovir 400 mg, orally, 3 times/day for 7–10 days **OR** Acyclovir 200 mg, orally, 5 times/day for 7–10 days **OR** Famcyclovir 250 mg, orally, 3 times/day for 7–10 days **OR** Valacyclovir 1 g, orally twice daily for 7–10 days	…

Table 4.4. Guidelines for Treatment of Sexually Transmitted Infections in Children and Adolescents According to Syndrome, continued

Syndrome	Organisms/Diagnoses	Treatment of Adolescent	Treatment of Infant/Child
Pelvic inflammatory disease (PID)	*N gonorrhoeae, C trachomatis,* anaerobes, coliform bacteria, and *Streptococcus* species	See Pelvic Inflammatory Disease (Table 3.48, p 607)	PID occurs rarely, if at all, in prepubertal girls
Syphilis	*Treponema pallidum*	Penicillin G benzathine, 50 000 U/kg, IM up to the adult dose of 2.4 million U in a single dose. See Syphilis, p 755, for treatment of late latent syphilis, tertiary syphilis or neurosyphilis.	Aqueous crystalline penicillin G 200 000-300 000 U/kg/day IV, administered as 50 000 U/kg/dose, every 4–6 hours for 10 days.
Genital ulcer disease	*T pallidum*	Penicillin G benzathine, 50,000 U/kg, IM up to the adult dose of 2.4 million U in a single dose. See Syphilis, p 755, for treatment of late latent syphilis, tertiary syphilis or neurosyphilis.	Aqueous crystalline penicillin G 200 000-300 000 U/kg/day IV, administered as 50 000 U/kg/dose, every 4–6 hours for 10 days.
	HSV—1st clinical episode	Acyclovir, 400 mg, orally, 3 times/day for 7–10 days **OR** Acyclovir, 200 mg, orally, 5 times/day for 7–10 days **OR** Famciclovir, 250 mg, orally, 3 times/day for 7–10 days **OR** Valacyclovir, 1 g, orally, twice daily for 7–10 days	***Children <45 kg:*** See prepubertal vaginitis, above

Table 4.4. Guidelines for Treatment of Sexually Transmitted Infections in Children and Adolescents According to Syndrome, continued

Syndrome	Organisms/Diagnoses	Treatment of Adolescent	Treatment of Infant/Child
	Haemophilus ducreyi (chancroid)	Azithromycin, 1 g, orally, in a single dose **OR** Ceftriaxone, 250 mg, IM, in a single dose **OR** Ciprofloxacin, 500 mg, orally, twice daily for 3 days[c] **OR** Erythromycin base, 500 mg, orally, 3 times/day for 7 days	***Children <45 kg:*** Ceftriaxone, 50 mg/kg, IM, in a single dose (maximum 250 mg) **OR** ***Children <45 kg:*** Azithromycin, 20 mg/kg, orally, in a single dose (maximum 1 g)
	Klebsiella granulomatis (granuloma inguinale [Donovanosis])[a,d]	Doxycycline, 100 mg, orally, twice a day for at least 3 wk and until all lesions have healed completely (preferred) **OR** Azithromycin, 1 g, orally, once/wk for at least 3 wk and until all lesions have healed completely **OR** Ciprofloxacin, 750 mg, orally, twice a day for at least 3 wk and until all lesions have healed completely **OR** Erythromycin base, 500 mg, orally, 4 times/day for at least 3 wk and until all lesions have healed completely **OR** Trimethoprim-sulfamethoxazole, 1 double-strength (160 g/800 mg) tablet, orally, twice a day for at least 3 wk and until all lesions have healed completely	

Table 4.4. Guidelines for Treatment of Sexually Transmitted Infections in Children and Adolescents According to Syndrome, continued

Syndrome	Organisms/ Diagnoses	Treatment of Adolescent	Treatment of Infant/Child
Epididymitis	C trachomatis, N gonorrhoeae	Ceftriaxone, 250 mg, IM, in a single dose **PLUS EITHER** Doxycycline, 100 mg, orally, twice daily for 10 days **OR** Tetracycline, 500 mg, orally, 4 times/day for 10 days **OR** Azithromycin, 1 g, orally, each wk for 2 wk	…
	Enteric organisms (for patients allergic to cephalosporins and/or tetracycline)	Levofloxacin, 500 mg, orally, once daily for 10 days **OR** Ofloxacin, 300 mg, orally, twice a day for 10 days	
Gonococcal infections of the pharynx	N gonorrhoeae	Ceftriaxone, 250 mg, IM, in a single dose **PLUS** Azithromycin, 1 g, orally, in a single dose	Ceftriaxone, 125 mg, IM, in a single dose

Table 4.4. Guidelines for Treatment of Sexually Transmitted Infections in Children and Adolescents According to Syndrome, continued

Syndrome	Organisms/ Diagnoses	Treatment of Adolescent	Treatment of Infant/Child
Anogenital warts	Human papillomavirus	*Patient-applied:* Podofilox 0.5% solution or gel[c] **OR** Imiquimod 3.75% or 5% cream **OR** Sinecatechins 15% ointment *Provider-administered:* Cryotherapy **OR** Trichloroacetic acid or bichloroacetic acid 80%–90% **OR** Surgical removal	***Children <45 kg:*** Same as for adolescents

IM indicates intramuscularly; STI, sexually transmitted infection.

[a] For additional information and recommendations, see Centers for Disease Control and Prevention. Sexually transmitted diseases treatment guidelines, 2014. *MMWR Morb Mortal Wkly Rep.* 2015; in press (see **www.cdc.gov/std/treatment**).

[b] If ceftriaxone is not feasible, may substitute cefixime 400 mg orally in a single dose plus azithromycin 1 gram orally in a single dose (cefixime 8 mg/kg for a child <45 kg). Providers treating patients with a severe cephalosporin allergy should consult an infectious disease specialist. Dual treatment is recommended for adolescent patients with gonococcal infections. In these patients, the use of azithromycin as the second antimicrobial in adolescents is preferred because of the high prevalence of tetracycline resistance among gonococcal isolates in the United States. However, when azithromycin is not available or when the patient is allergic to azithromycin, doxycycline 100 mg orally twice a day for 7 days can be used as an alternative second antimicrobial in adolescents.

[c] Not tested for safety in children and contraindicated in pregnancy.

[d] For infections that do not respond to therapy within several days, consider the addition of intravenous gentamicin.

Table 4.5. Recommended Regimens for Vulvovaginal Candidiasis

Intravaginal Agents[a]

Butoconazole, 2% cream, 5 g, intravaginally, for 3 days[b]

OR

Butoconazole, 2% cream (sustained release), 5 g, single-dose intravaginal application for 1 day

OR

Clotrimazole, 1% cream, 5 g, intravaginally, for 7–14 days[b]

OR

Clotrimazole 2% cream, 5 g, intravaginally, for 3 days[b]

OR

Miconazole, 2% cream, 5 g, intravaginally, for 7 days[b]

OR

Miconazole, 4% cream, 5 g, intravaginally, for 3 days[a,b]

OR

Miconazole, 100-mg vaginal suppository, 1 suppository for 7 days[b]

OR

Miconazole, 200-mg vaginal suppository, 1 suppository for 3 days[b]

OR

Miconazole, 1200-mg vaginal suppository, 1 suppository for 1 day[b]

OR

Nystatin, 100 000-unit vaginal tablet, 1 tablet for 14 days

OR

Tioconazole, 6.5% ointment, 5 g, intravaginally, in a single application[b]

OR

Terconazole, 0.4% cream, 5 g, intravaginally, for 7 days

OR

Terconazole, 0.8% cream, 5 g, intravaginally, for 3 days

OR

Terconazole, 80-mg vaginal suppository, 1 suppository for 3 days

Oral agent:

Fluconazole, 150-mg oral tablet, 1 tablet in single dose

---

[a] These creams and suppositories are oil-based and might weaken latex condoms and diaphragms. Refer to condom or diaphragm product labeling for additional information.
[b] Over-the-counter preparations.

Antifungal Drugs for Systemic Fungal Infections

Polyenes

Amphotericin B is a fungicidal agent that is effective against a broad array of fungal species. Amphotericin B, especially the "conventional" deoxycholate formulation, can cause adverse reactions, particularly renal toxicity, so its use is limited in certain patients. Lipid-associated formulations of amphotericin B, especially liposomal amphotericin B, limit renal toxicity but also can cause adverse effects and does not achieve optimal concentrations in some sites of infection (eg, kidney).

Amphotericin B deoxycholate is the preferred formulation for treatment of neonates with systemic candidiasis because of better penetration into the central nervous system, urinary tract, and eye, which often are involved in *Candida* species infections; lipid-associated formulations do not penetrate as well into these body sites. Amphotericin B deoxycholate is given intravenously in a single daily dose of 1 mg/kg or up to 1.5 mg/kg when administered on alternate days (maximum, 1.5 mg/kg/day). Amphotericin B is administered in 5% dextrose in water at a concentration of 0.1 mg/mL and delivered through a central or peripheral venous catheter. Infusion times of 1 to 2 hours have been shown to be well tolerated in adults and older children and theoretically increase the blood-to-tissue gradient, thereby improving drug delivery. After completing 1 week of daily therapy, adequate serum concentrations of the drug usually can be maintained by administering 1.5 mg/kg on alternate days due to the long half-life. The total dose and duration of therapy depends on the type and extent of the specific fungal infection.

Amphotericin B deoxycholate is eliminated by a renal mechanism for approximately 2 weeks after therapy is discontinued. No adjustment in dose is required for neonates or for children with impaired renal function, because serum concentrations are not increased significantly in these patients. If renal toxicity occurs, alternate-day dosing is preferred to a decrease in daily dose. Neither hemodialysis nor peritoneal dialysis significantly decreases serum concentrations of the drug.

Infusion-related reactions to amphotericin B deoxycholate include fever, chills, and sometimes nausea, vomiting, headache, generalized malaise, hypotension, and arrhythmias; these reactions are rare in neonates. Onset usually is within 1 to 3 hours after starting the infusion; duration typically is less than an hour. Hypotension and arrhythmias are idiosyncratic reactions that are unlikely to occur if not observed after the initial dose but also can occur in association with rapid infusion. Multiple regimens have been used to prevent infusion-related reactions, but few have been studied in controlled clinical trials. Pretreatment with acetaminophen, alone or combined with diphenhydramine, may alleviate febrile reactions; these reactions appear to be less common in children than in adults. Hydrocortisone (25–50 mg in adults and older children) also can be added to the infusion to decrease febrile and other systemic reactions. Tolerance to febrile reactions develops with time, allowing tapering and eventual discontinuation of the hydrocortisone and often diphenhydramine and antipyretic agents. Meperidine and ibuprofen have been effective in preventing or treating fever and chills in some patients who are refractory to the conventional premedication regimen.

Toxicity from amphotericin B deoxycholate can include nephrotoxicity, hepatotoxicity, anemia, or neurotoxicity. Nephrotoxicity is caused by decreased renal blood flow and can be prevented or ameliorated by hydration, saline solution loading (0.9% saline solution over 30 minutes) before infusion of amphotericin B, and avoidance of diuretic drugs. Hypokalemia is common and can be exacerbated by sodium loading. Renal tubular acidosis can occur but usually is mild. Permanent nephrotoxicity is related to cumulative dose. Nephrotoxicity is increased by concomitant administration of amphotericin B and aminoglycosides, cyclosporine, tacrolimus, cisplatin, nitrogen mustard compounds, and acetazolamide. Anemia is secondary to inhibition of erythropoietin production. Neurotoxicity occurs rarely and can manifest as confusion, delirium, obtundation, psychotic behavior, seizures, blurred vision, or hearing loss.

Lipid-associated and liposomal formulations of amphotericin B have a role in children who are intolerant of or refractory to amphotericin B deoxycholate or who have renal insufficiency or are at risk of significant renal toxicity from concomitant medications. In adults, none of the lipid-associated formulations have been demonstrated to be more effective than has conventional amphotericin B deoxycholate. Amphotericin B lipid formulations approved by the US Food and Drug Administration (FDA) for treatment of invasive fungal infections in children and adults who are refractory to or intolerant of amphotericin B deoxycholate therapy are amphotericin B lipid complex (ABLC, Abelcet) and liposomal amphotericin B (L-AmB, AmBisome). Acute infusion-related reactions occur with both formulations but are less frequent with AmBisome. Nephrotoxicity is less common with lipid-associated products than with amphotericin B deoxycholate. Liver toxicity, which generally is not associated with amphotericin B deoxycholate, has been reported with the lipid formulations.

Pyrimidines

Among pyrimidine antifungal agents, only flucytosine (5-fluorocytosine) is approved by the FDA for use in children. Flucytosine has a limited spectrum of activity against fungi and has potential for toxicity, and when flucytosine is used as a single agent resistance often emerges rapidly. Flucytosine can be used in combination with amphotericin B for cryptococcal meningitis. It is important to monitor serum concentrations of flucytosine to avoid bone marrow toxicity. Flucytosine is only available in oral formulation in the United States.

Azoles

Five oral azoles are available in the United States: ketoconazole, fluconazole, itraconazole, voriconazole, and posaconazole. All have relatively broad activity against common fungi but differ in their in vitro activity (see Table 4.6, p 907), bioavailability, adverse effects, and potential for drug interactions. Fewer data are available regarding the safety and efficacy of azoles in pediatric than in adult patients, and trials comparing these agents to amphotericin B have been limited. Azoles are easy to administer and have little toxicity, but their use can be limited by the frequency of their interactions with co-administered drugs. These drug interactions can result in decreased serum concentrations of the azole (ie, poor therapeutic activity) or unexpected toxicity from the co-administered drug (caused by increased serum concentrations of the co-administered drug). When considering use of azoles, the patient's concurrent medications should be reviewed to avoid

Table 4.6. Relative in Vitro Activity of Drugs for Invasive and Other Serious Fungal Infections Antifungal Spectrum of Activity

Fungal Species	Amphotericin B Formulations	Fluconazole	Itraconazole	Voriconazole	Posaconazole	Flucytosine	Caspofungin, Micafungin, or Anidulafungin
Candida albicans	+	++	+	+	+	+	++
Candida tropicalis	+	++	+	+	+	+	++
Candida parapsilosis	++	++	+	+	+	+	+/–
Candida glabrata	+	–	–	+/–	+/–	+	++
Candida krusei	+	–	+	+	+	–	++
Candida lusitaniae	–	++	+	+	+	+	+
Candida guilliermondii	+	+	+	+	+	+	+/–
Cryptococcus species	++	+	+	+	+	++	–
Aspergillus fumigatus	+	–	+	++	+	–	+
Aspergillus terreus	–	–	+	++	+	–	+
Aspergillus calidoustus	++	–	+	–	–	–	++
Fusarium species	+	–	+	++	+	–	–
Mucor species	++	–	+/–	–	+	–	–
Rhizopus species	++	–	–	–	+	–	–
Scedosporium apiospermum	–	–	+	++	+	–	–
Scedosporium prolificans	–	–	+/–	+/–	+/–	–	–
Histoplasma capsulatum	++	+	++	+	+	–	–
Coccidioides immitis	++	+	++	+	+	–	–
Blastomyces dermatitidis	++	+	++	+	+	–	–
Paracoccidioides species	+	+	++	+	+	–	–
Sporothrix species	+	+	++	+	+	–	–
Penicillium species	+/–	–	++	+	+	–	–
Trichosporon species	–	+	+	++	+	–	–

NOTE: ++ = more active, scenario dependent; + = usually active; +/– = variably active; – = usually not active.

potential adverse clinical outcomes. Another potential limitation of azoles is emergence of resistant fungi, especially *Candida* species resistant to fluconazole. *Candida krusei* intrinsically are resistant to fluconazole and strains of *Candida glabrata* increasingly are resistant to both fluconazole and voriconazole. Itraconazole is approved by the FDA for treatment of blastomycosis, histoplasmosis (nonmeningeal), and aspergillosis in patients who are intolerant to amphotericin B, and for empiric therapy of febrile neutropenic patients with suspected fungal infection. Itraconazole does not cross the blood-brain barrier and should not be used for infections of the central nervous system. Voriconazole has been approved by the FDA for primary treatment of invasive *Aspergillus* species, for candidemia in non-neutropenic patients, for esophageal candidiasis, and for refractory infection with *Fusarium* species and some *Scedosporium* species, such as *Scedosporium apiospermum*. Therapeutic monitoring of voriconazole with measurement of serum trough concentrations is important in patients with serious infections. Posaconazole is approved for use in adults for prophylaxis of invasive aspergillosis and candidiasis and treatment of oropharyngeal candidiasis. The drug is available only by the oral route and strategies to enhance absorption are necessary (eg, administration with high fat meal, avoidance of proton pump inhibitors). Ketoconazole seldom is used because other azoles have fewer adverse effects and generally are preferred.

Echinocandins

Caspofungin, micafungin, and anidulafungin are the only echinocandins approved by the FDA. Caspofungin is approved for treatment of pediatric patients 3 months and older with esophageal candidiasis, empiric therapy for presumed fungal infections in febrile neutropenic patients, invasive candidiasis, and aspergillosis in adults who are refractory to or intolerant of other antifungal drugs. Clinical trials have demonstrated safety and efficacy in pediatric patients down to 3 months of age; noncomparative anecdotal experience in neonatal infections also is reported. Micafungin is approved by the FDA for intravenous treatment of pediatric patients four months and older with candidemia, acute disseminated candidiasis, Candida peritonitis and abscesses, esophageal candidiasis and prophylaxis of invasive *Candida* infections in patients undergoing hematopoietic stem cell transplantation. Although micafungin in not FDA-approved for the aspergillosis, data are available to support its use in the treatment of refractory disease. Anidulafungin is approved by the FDA for use in children but is FDA approved for the intravenous treatment of candidemia, *Candida* infections, and esophageal candidiasis in adults. Table 4.6 (p 907) provides data on the relative in vitro susceptibilities of specific fungal species with amphotericin B, azoles, echinocandins, and flucytosine.

RECOMMENDED DOSES OF PARENTERAL AND ORAL ANTIFUNGAL DRUGS

Table 4.7. Recommended Doses of Parenteral and Oral Antifungal Drugs

Drug	Route	Dose (per day)	Adverse Reactions[a,b]
Amphotericin B deoxycholate (see Antifungal Drugs for Systemic Fungal Infections, p 905, for detailed information)	IV	1.0–1.5 mg/kg per day; infuse as a single dose over 2 h	Fever, chills, gastrointestinal tract symptoms, headache, hypotension, renal dysfunction, hypokalemia, anemia, cardiac arrhythmias, neurotoxicity, anaphylaxis
	IT	0.025 mg, increase to 0.5 mg, twice/wk	Headache, gastrointestinal tract symptoms, arachnoiditis/radiculitis
Amphotericin B lipid complex (Abelcet)[c,d]	IV	5 mg/kg per day, infused over 2 h	Fever, chills, other reactions associated with amphotericin B deoxycholate, but less nephrotoxicity; hepatotoxicity has been reported with lipid complex
Anidulafungin[c,d]	IV	Adults: 100–200 mg loading dose, then 50–100 mg once daily (higher dose for candidemia) Children: load with 1.5 to 3 mg/kg once, then 0.75–1.5 mg/kg per day	Fever, headache, nausea, vomiting, diarrhea, leukopenia, hepatic enzyme elevations, and phlebitis
Liposomal amphotericin B (AmBisome)[c,d]	IV	3–5 mg/kg, infused over 1–2 h	Fever, chills, other reactions associated with amphotericin B, but less nephrotoxicity; hepatotoxicity has been reported
Caspofungin[c,d]	IV	Adults: 70 mg loading dose, then 50 mg once daily Children: 70 mg/m² loading dose, then 50 mg/m² once daily	Fever, rash, pruritus, phlebitis, headache, gastrointestinal tract symptoms, anemia; concomitant use with cyclosporine is not recommended unless potential benefits outweigh potential risks
Clotrimazole	PO	10-mg tablet, 5 times per day (dissolved slowly in mouth	Gastrointestinal tract symptoms, hepatotoxicity

Table 4.7. Recommended Doses of Parenteral and Oral Antifungal Drugs, continued

Drug	Route	Dose (per day)	Adverse Reactions[a,b]
Fluconazole[b,d]	IV	Children: 3–6 mg/kg per day, single dose (up to 12 mg/kg per day for serious infections)	Rash, gastrointestinal tract symptoms, hepatotoxicity, Stevens-Johnson syndrome, anaphylaxis
	PO	Children: 6 mg/kg once, then 3 mg/kg per day for oropharyngeal or esophageal candidiasis; 6–12 mg/kg per day for invasive fungal infections; 6 mg/kg per day for suppressive therapy in HIV-infected children with cryptococcal meningitis Adults: 200 mg once, followed by 100 mg/day for oropharyngeal or esophageal candidiasis; 400–800 mg/day for other invasive fungal infections; 400 mg/day for suppressive therapy in HIV-infected patients with cryptococcal meningitis	
Flucytosine	PO	50–150 mg/kg per day in 4 doses at 6-h intervals (adjust dose if renal dysfunction); follow trough levels closely	Bone marrow suppression, renal dysfunction, gastrointestinal tract symptoms, rash, neuropathy, hepatotoxicity, confusion, hallucinations
Griseofulvin	PO	Ultramicrosize: 5–15 mg/kg, single dose; maximum dose, 750 mg Microsize: 10–20 mg/kg per day divided in 2 doses; maximum dose, 1000 mg	Rash, paresthesias, leukopenia, gastrointestinal tract symptoms, proteinuria, hepatotoxicity, mental confusion, headache

Table 4.7. Recommended Doses of Parenteral and Oral Antifungal Drugs, continued

Drug	Route	Dose (per day)	Adverse Reactions[a,b]
Itraconazole[b,d]	IV, PO	Children: 5–10 mg/kg per day divided into 2 doses; confirm therapeutic trough level after 2 wk of therapy to ensure adequate drug exposure (≥1 µg/mL but <10 µg/mL) Adults: 200–400 mg/day once or twice a day; 200 mg, once a day, for suppressive therapy in HIV-infected patients with histoplasmosis	Gastrointestinal tract symptoms, rash, edema, headache, hypokalemia, hepatotoxicity, thrombocytopenia, leukopenia; cardiac toxicity is possible in patients also taking terfenadine or astemizole
Ketoconazole[b,d]	PO	Children[e]: 3.3–6.6 mg/kg per day, single dose Adults: 200 mg, twice a day for 4 doses, then 200 mg, once a day	Hepatotoxicity, gastrointestinal tract symptoms, rash, anaphylaxis, thrombocytopenia, hemolytic anemia, gynecomastia, adrenal insufficiency; cardiac toxicity is possible in patients also taking terfenadine or astemizole
Micafungin[e,d]	IV	Adults: 50–150 mg once daily Children: 2–10 mg/kg per day once daily (higher dose needed for patients <8 y of age), maximum 200 mg per day	Fever, headache, nausea, vomiting, diarrhea, leukopenia, hepatic enzyme elevations, and phlebitis
Nystatin	PO	Infants: 200 000 U, 4 times a day, after meals Children and adults: 400 000–600 000 U, 3 times a day, after meals	Gastrointestinal tract symptoms, rash
Posaconazole[e,d]	PO	Adults: 400 mg, 2 times a day with fatty meals (or liquid nutritional supplement) for treatment; 200 mg, 3 times a day for prophylaxis Children: not known	Gastrointestinal tract symptoms, rash, edema, headache, anemia, neutropenia, thrombocytopenia, fatigue, arthralgia, myalgia, fever

Table 4.7. Recommended Doses of Parenteral and Oral Antifungal Drugs, continued

Drug	Route	Dose (per day)	Adverse Reactions[a,b]
Terbinafine[c]	PO	Adults: 250 mg, once a day Children: <20 kg: 67.5 mg/day; 20–40 kg: 125 mg/day; >40 kg: 250 mg/day	Gastrointestinal tract symptoms, rash, taste abnormalities, cholestatic hepatitis
Voriconazole[d]	IV	Children 2–12 y: 9 mg/kg, IV, every 12 h for 1 day, then 8 mg/kg, IV, every 12 h (maximum dose, 350 mg, every 12 h); follow trough levels closely (>2 µg/mL) Adults and children ≥12 y: 6 mg/kg, every 12 h for 1 day (loading dose), then 4 mg/kg, every 12 h; follow trough levels closely (>1 µg/mL)	Visual disturbance, hallucinations, photosensitive rash, increased liver function tests, encephalopathy; recent reports of aggressive cutaneous malignancy associated with prolonged voriconazole use
	PO	Children 2–12 y: 9 mg/kg, every 12 h; follow trough levels closely (much lower bioavailability in children than adults) Adults: <40 kg: 200 mg, every 12 h for 1 day, then 100 mg, every 12 h; >40 kg: 400 mg, every 12 h for 1 day, then 200-300 mg, every 12 h	

IV indicates intravenous; IT, intrathecal; PO, oral; HIV, human immunodeficiency virus.

[a] See package insert or listing in current edition of the *Physicians' Desk Reference* or www.pdr.net (for registered users only).

[b] Interactions with other drugs are common. Consult www.fda.gov/Drugs/DevelopmentApprovalProcess/DevelopmentResources/DrugInteractionsLabeling/default.htm?utm_campaign=Google2&utm_source=fdaSearch&utm_medium=website&utm_term=drug%20interactions&utm_content=1 and the *Physicians' Desk Reference* (a drug interaction reference or database) or a pharmacist before prescribing these medications.

[c] Experience with drug in children is limited; 3 mg/kg doses generally used.

[d] Limited or no information about use in newborn infants is available. Voriconazole has now been identified as an independent risk factor for development of cutaneous malignancies in lung transplant patients.

[e] For children 2 years and younger, the daily dose has not been established.

TOPICAL DRUGS FOR SUPERFICIAL FUNGAL INFECTIONS

Table 4.8. Topical Drugs for Superficial Fungal Infections

Drug	Strength	Formulation	Trade Name Examples	Application(s) per Day	Adverse Reactions/Notes
Amorolfine (OTC)	5%	NL	Loceryl; Curanail	1–2 weekly (mild onychomycosis)	Well tolerated; minor local, not FDA approved.
Basic fuchsin, phenol, resorcinol, and acetone (Rx)		S	Castellani Paint Modified	1	Excellent for intertriginous areas. Stains everything. Also available as a colorless solution with alcohol and without basic fuchsin. This is an alternative if the patient cannot tolerate other topical antifungals. Not FDA approved. Must be compounded.
Butenafine HCl (Rx and OTC)	1%	C	Mentax; Lotrimin Ultra	1, typically for 2 wk	Safety and efficacy in patients younger than 12 y of age have not been established. Do not occlude. Sensitivity to allylamines. Not to be used on scalp or nails.
Ciclopirox olamine (Rx)	0.77%	C, L, S, P, G, NL	Loprox; Penlac nail lacquer; Ciclodan	2	Irritant dermatitis, hair discoloration; shake lotion vigorously before application; safety and efficacy in children younger than 10 y of age have not been established. Precautions: diabetes mellitus; immune compromise; seizures. Do not occlude.
Clioquinol (Rx and OTC)		C, O (F available in Canada)	Vioform	2–4/day for 4 wk	Can stain skin, hair, nails, and clothing yellow in color. Irritant dermatitis.
Clotrimazole (Rx and OTC)	1%	C, L, S, P, Com, SpP, SpL; check with pharmacist	Topical solution (more than 10 preparations); Lotrimin, Mycelex, Desenex	1 (Rx) 2 (OTC)	Irritant dermatitis. Avoid topical steroid combinations.[a]

Table 4.8. Topical Drugs for Superficial Fungal Infections, continued

Drug	Strength	Formulation	Trade Name Examples	Application(s) per Day	Adverse Reactions/Notes
Clotrimazole and betamethasone dipropionate (Rx)	1%/0.05%	C, L	Lotrisone[b]	2[a]	Irritant dermatitis: Not generally intended for patients younger than 17 y or for diaper dermatitis. In two studies in pediatric subjects, 39.5% of tinea pedis patients and 47.1% of tinea cruris patients demonstrated adrenal suppression as determined by co-syntropin testing. If used in the groin area, patients should use medication for 2 wk only and use sparingly. Do not occlude. Contraindication: varicella.
Econazole nitrate (Rx)	1%	C, L, P, S, F	Spectazole, Pevaryl-Ecreme	1 (dermatophyte) 2 (candidiasis)	Irritant dermatitis; safety and efficacy in children have not been established.
Iodoquinol and 2% hydrocortisone acetate (Rx)	1%	G	Alcortin A	3–4	Burning/itching sensation. Local allergic reaction. Can stain skin and clothes. Can interfere with results of thyroid function tests. Not to be used under occlusion in the diaper area. Not intended for use on infants. Not FDA approved.
Iodoquinol and 1% aloe polysaccharides (Rx)	1.25%	G	Aloquin	3–4	Can interfere with thyroid function tests. False-positive ferric chloride test (used for PKU) if present in the diaper or urine. Discoloration of skin, hair, and fabric, which can be removed with normal cleansing. Not intended for use on infants, under occlusions or in the diaper area. Safety and efficacy in pediatric patients younger than 12 y not established. Not FDA approved.

Table 4.8. Topical Drugs for Superficial Fungal Infections, continued

Drug	Strength	Formulation	Trade Name Examples	Application(s) per Day	Adverse Reactions/Notes
Ketoconazole (Rx and OTC)	1, 2%	C, Sh, G, F	Nizoral, Nizoral AD, Sebizol, Xolegel, Extina, Ketodan	1 (tinea dermatophyte) 2 (candidiasis)	Potential sulfite reaction with anaphylactic or asthmatic reaction; shampoo can cause dry or oily hair and increase hair loss; irritant dermatitis. May interfere with permanent waving or changes in hair texture. Intended for patients over 12 y; safety and efficacy not established for younger than 12 y. Foam must not be applied directly to hands, but on a cool surface and applied using fingertips.
Miconazole (Rx and OTC)	2%	O, C, P, S, SpP, SpL; check with pharmacist[e]	More than 10 preparations; Monistat-Derm, Zeasorb AF, Micatin, Daktarin tincture	2 (seborrhea), apply 2–3 times/day for several months 2 (C, L) 2 (P, L) 1 (tinea versicolor)	Irritant and allergic contact dermatitis. Generally not recommended for children younger than 2 y.
Miconazole nitrate and 15% Zinc oxide (Rx)	0.25%	O	Vusion	Every diaper change for 1 wk	Skin irritation. Can be used in children 4 wk and older. Do not routinely use for more than 7 days.
Naftifine HCl (Rx)	1%, 2% gel	C, G	Naftin	1 (C) 2 (Gel)	Burning/stinging, irritant dermatitis, safety and efficacy in children have not been established. Do not occlude.

Table 4.8. Topical Drugs for Superficial Fungal Infections, continued

Drug	Strength	Formulation	Trade Name Examples	Application(s) per Day	Adverse Reactions/Notes
Nystatin (Rx and OTC	100 000 U/mL or 100 000 U/g	C, P, O, Com	Nystatin, Nystop powder, Pedi-Dri powder, My-costatin, Nyamyc	2 (C) 2–3 (P)	Nontoxic except with topical steroid combinations.[d]
Nystatin and triamcinolone acetonide (Rx)		C, O	Mytrex cream, Mytrex ointment, Mycolog-II	2	Pediatric patients may demonstrate greater susceptibility to topical corticosteroid-induced hypothalamic-pituitary-adrenal (HPA) axis suppression and Cushing syndrome than mature patients because of a larger ratio of skin surface area to body weight. Contraindications: varicella or vaccinia. Do not occlude. Use lowest effective dose.
Oxiconazole (Rx)	1%	C, L	Oxistat	1–2 (tinea dermatophyte)	Pruritus, burning, irritant dermatitis. Do not occlude.
Sertaconazole (Rx)	2%	C	Ertaczo	2	Dry skin, skin tenderness, contact dermatitis, local hypersensitivity; safety and efficacy in children younger than 12 y have not been established.
Sulconazole (Rx)	1%	C, S	Exelderm	1–2 (tinea vesicular) 2 (tinea pedis)	Irritant dermatitis; safety and efficacy in children have not been established.
Terbinafine (Rx and OTC)	1%	C, G, S, Sp	Lamisil, Lamisil AT	1–2	Irritant dermatitis; avoid use of occlusive clothing or dressings. Do not apply spray to face. Safety and efficacy in children younger than 12 y have not been established.

Table 4.8. Topical Drugs for Superficial Fungal Infections, continued

Drug	Strength	Formulation	Trade Name Examples	Application(s) per Day	Adverse Reactions/Notes
Tolnaftate (OTC)	1%	C, P, S, G, SpP, SpL; check with pharmacist[e]	>10 preparations; Tinactin, Fungi-cure	1–2	Irritant and allergic contact dermatitis. Not recommended if younger than 2 y of age.
Undecylenic acid and derivatives (OTC)	8%–25%	C, O, S, F, SpP, P, soap	See pharmacist for formulations and applications[e]	2 (tincture); spray 1–2 sec	Irritant dermatitis. Generally not recommended for children younger than 2 y.
Undecylenic acid and chloroxy-lenol	25% 3%	S	Gordochom solution	2 for 4 wk	Local hypersensitivity. Generally not recommended for children younger than 2 y.
Other Remedies					
Benzoic acid and salicylic acid (OTC)	12%	O	Whitfields Ointment, Bensal HP	2	Warm, burning sensation. Avoid eyes, mouth and, nose. Keep out of the reach of children. Safety and efficacy in children not established. Not FDA approved.
Gentian violet (OTC)	2%	S	…	2	Staining. Keep out of the reach of children. Safety and efficacy in children not established OTC monograph not final.

Table 4.8. Topical Drugs for Superficial Fungal Infections, continued

Drug	Strength	Formulation	Trade Name Examples	Application(s) per Day	Adverse Reactions/Notes
Selenium sulfide (Rx and OTC)	2.5%	Sh, L	Selsun 2.5%	Use twice weekly for 2 wk 1, for 7 days (L)	Irritant dermatitis and ulceration. For tinea capitis, to decrease spore formation and to decrease the potential spread of the dermatophyte. Hair loss; discoloration of hair; oiliness or dryness of scalp. Safety and efficacy in children not established. May damage jewelry. Not to be used when inflammation or exudation is present.
	1%	Sh, L	Head & Shoulders, Selsun Blue	Use twice weekly for at least 2 wk	For tinea capitis, to decrease spore formation and to decrease the potential spread of the dermatophyte.
Sodium thiosulfate		L	Versiclear Lotion	2	Safety and effectiveness in children younger than 12 y has not been established.

OTC indicates over the counter; NL, nail lacquer; FDA, US Food and Drug Administration; Rx, prescription; S, solution; C, cream; L, lotion; P, powder; G, gel; O, ointment; F, foam; Com, combinations; SpP, spray powder; SpL, spray lotion; PKU, phenylketonuria; Sh, shampoo; Sp, spray.

a Topical steroids must be used with caution in young children and in areas of thin skin (eg, diaper area). In these circumstances, high systemic exposure may occur, resulting in endogenous synthesis suppression with the potential for serious adverse effects. Potential adverse effects include irritant dermatitis, folliculitis, hypertrichosis, acneform eruptions, hypopigmentation, perioral dermatitis, allergic contact dermatitis, maceration, secondary infection, skin atrophy, striae, and miliaria.

b Lotrisone cream no longer is available; lotion is available. Also available are Lotrim and Fungizid spray.

c Pharmacists are the best resource to verify formulations that are available and new (they use *Facts and Comparisons* reference products).

d Any topical preparation has the potential to irritate the skin and cause itching, burning stinging, erythema, edema, vesicles, and blister formation.
For more information on individual drugs, see *Physician's Desk Reference* or **www.pdr.net** (for registered users only).

Non-HIV Antiviral Drugs

Table 4.9. Non-HIV Antiviral Drugs[a]

Generic (Trade Name)	Indication	Route	Age	Usually Recommended Dosage
Acyclovir[b,c,d,e] (Zovirax)	Neonatal herpes simplex virus (HSV) infection	IV	Birth to 3 mo	Treatment dosing: 60 mg/kg per day, in 3 divided doses for 14–21 days
		PO	2 wk to 8 mo	Suppressive dosing following completion of treatment dosing: 300 mg/m² , 3 times per day for 6 months
	HSV encephalitis	IV	≥3 mo to 12 y	30–45 mg/kg per day, in 3 divided doses for 14–21 days; FDA-approved dose for this indication and age range is 60 mg/kg per day, in 3 divided doses, but nephrotoxicity may be increased at this higher dose[f]
		IV	≥12 y	30 mg/kg per day, in 3 divided doses for 14–21 days
	Varicella in immunocompetent host[g]	Oral	≥2 y	≤40 kg: 80 mg/kg per day, in 4 divided doses for 5 days; maximum daily dose, 3200 mg/day >40 kg: 3200 mg, in 4 divided doses for 5 days
	Varicella in immunocompetent host requiring hospitalization	IV	≥2 y	30 mg/kg per day for 7–10 days or 1500 mg/m² per day in 3 doses for 7–10 days
	Varicella in immunocompromised host	IV	<1 y	30 mg/kg per day, in 3 divided doses for 7–10 days
		IV	≥1 y	1500 mg/m² per day, in 3 doses for 7–10 days; some experts recommend the 30 mg/kg per day dose
	Zoster in immunocompetent host	IV (if requiring hospitalization)	All ages	Same as for varicella in immunocompromised host
		Oral	≥12 y	4000 mg/day, in 5 divided doses for 5–7 days
	Zoster in immunocompromised host	IV	<12 y	30 mg/kg per day, in 3 divided doses, for 7–10 days
		IV	≥12 y	30 mg/kg per day, in 3 divided doses, for 7–10 days

Table 4.9. Non-HIV Antiviral Drugs,[a] continued

Generic (Trade Name)	Indication	Route	Age	Usually Recommended Dosage
	HSV infection in immunocompromised host (localized, progressive, or disseminated)	IV	All ages	30 mg/kg per day, in 3 divided doses for 7–14 days
		Oral	≥2 y	1000 mg/day, in 3–5 divided doses for 7–14 days
	Prophylaxis of HSV in immunocompromised hosts who are HSV seropositive	Oral	≥2 y	600–1000 mg/day, in 3–5 divided doses during period of risk
		IV	All ages	15 mg/kg, in 3 divided doses during period of risk
	Genital HSV infection: first episode	Oral	≥12 y	1000–1200 mg/day, in 3–5 divided doses for 7–10 days. Oral pediatric dose: 40–80 mg/kg per day, divided in 3–4 doses for 5–10 days (maximum 1.0 g/day)
	Genital HSV infection: recurrence	IV	≥12 y	15 mg/kg per day, in 3 divided doses for 5–7 days
		Oral	≥12 y	1000 mg in 5 divided doses for 5 days, or 1600 mg in 2 divided doses for 5 days, or 2400 mg in 3 divided doses for 2 days
	Chronic suppressive therapy for recurrent genital and cutaneous (ocular) HSV episodes	Oral	≥12 y	800 mg/day, in 2 divided doses for as long as 12 continuous mo
Adefovir (Hepsera)	Chronic hepatitis B	Oral	≥12 y	10 mg, once daily, in patients with adequate renal function; optimal duration of therapy unknown
Amantadine (Symmetrel)[n]	Influenza A: treatment and prophylaxis (see Influenza, p 476)[n]	Oral	1–9 y	Treatment or prophylaxis: 5 mg/kg per day, maximum 150 mg/day, in 2 divided doses
		Oral	≥10 y	Treatment or prophylaxis: <40 kg: 5 mg/kg per day, in 2 divided doses; ≥40 kg: 200 mg/day, in 2 divided doses
		Oral	Dose by weight, not age	Alternative prophylactic dose for children >20 kg and adults: 100 mg/day

Table 4.9. Non-HIV Antiviral Drugs,ᵃ continued

Generic (Trade Name)	Indication	Route	Age	Usually Recommended Dosage
Boceprevir (Victrelis)	Chronic hepatitis C	Oral	Adult dose (≥18 years)[i]	800 mg, 3 times per day for 24–44 wk in combination with pegylated interferon alfa and ribavirin for 28–48 wk of total treatment, depending on prior HCV treatment status and HCV viral load during therapy; Initiate therapy with pegylated interferon and ribavirin for 4 wk prior to initiating boceprevir
Cidofovir (Vistide)	Cytomegalovirus (CMV) retinitis	IV	Adult dose[i]	Induction: 5 mg/kg, once weekly, × 2 doses with probenecid and hydration; Maintenance: 5 mg/kg, once every 2 wk, with probenecid and hydration
Entecavir (Baraclude)	Chronic hepatitis B	Oral	≥16 y[i]	0.5 mg, once daily, in patients who have not received prior nucleoside therapy; 1 mg once daily in patients who are previously treated (not first choice in this setting); optimum duration of therapy unknown
Famciclovir (Famvir)	Genital HSV infection, episodic recurrent episodes	Oral	Adult dose[i]	Immunocompetent: 2000 mg/day, in 2 divided doses for 1 day; HIV-infected patients: 1000 mg, in 2 divided doses for 7 days
	Daily suppressive therapy	Oral	Adult dose[i]	Immunocompetent: 500 mg/day, in 2 divided doses for 1 y; then reassess for recurrence of HSV infection
	Recurrent herpes labialis	Oral	Adult dose[i]	Immunocompetent: 1500 mg as a single dose; HIV-infected patients: 1000 mg/day, in 2 divided doses for 7 days
	Herpes zoster	Oral	Adult dose[i]	1500 mg/day, in 3 divided doses for 7 days

Table 4.9. Non-HIV Antiviral Drugs,[a] continued

Generic (Trade Name)	Indication	Route	Age	Usually Recommended Dosage
Foscarnet[b] (Foscavir)	CMV retinitis in patients with acquired immunodeficiency syndrome	IV	Adult dose[i]	180 mg/kg per day, in 2–3 divided doses for 14–21 days, then 90–120 mg/kg once a day as maintenance dose
	HSV infection resistant to acyclovir in immunocompromised host	IV	Adult dose[i]	80–120 mg/kg per day, in 2–3 divided doses until infection resolves
	VZV infection resistant to acyclovir	IV	Adult dose[i]	120 mg/kg per day, divided every 8 h, up to 3 wk
Ganciclovir[b] (Cytovene)	Symptomatic congenital CMV disease	IV	Birth to 2 mo	12 mg/kg per day, divided every 12 h; duration of treatment is 6 months, but most or all of the treatment should be accomplished with oral valganciclovir (see below)
	Acquired CMV retinitis in immunocompromised host[j]	IV	Adult dose[i]	Treatment: 10 mg/kg per day, in 2 divided doses for 14–21 days; Long-term suppression; 5 mg/kg per day for 7 days/wk or 6 mg/kg per day for 5 days/wk
	Prophylaxis of CMV in high-risk host	IV	Adult dose[i]	10 mg/kg per day, in 2 divided doses for 1–2 wk, then 5 mg/kg per day, in 1 dose for 100 days or 6 mg/kg per day for 5 days/wk
Interferon alfa-2b (Intron A)	Chronic hepatitis B	SC	1–18 y / >18 y	6 million IU/m², 3 times/wk for 16–24 wk / 5 million IU/day; or 10 million IU, 3 times/wk, for 16 wk
	Chronic hepatitis C	SC; IM	>18 y[i]	3 million IU, 3 times/wk, for 24–48 wk, depending on HCV genotype Note: pegylated interferon preferred over interferon alfa-2b
Lamivudine (Epivir-HBV)	Treatment of chronic hepatitis B	Oral	≥2 y	3 mg/kg once day (maximum 100 mg/day) (children coinfected with HIV and hepatitis B should use the approved dose for HIV)

Table 4.9. Non-HIV Antiviral Drugs,[a] continued

Generic (Trade Name)	Indication	Route	Age	Usually Recommended Dosage
Oseltamivir[k] (Tamiflu)	Influenza A and B: treatment (see Influenza, p 476)	Oral	Birth to <9 mo[l]	3 mg/kg, twice daily for 5 days[l]
		Oral	9–12 mo	3.5 mg/kg, twice daily for 5 days
		Oral	1–12 y	≤15 kg: 30 mg, twice daily; 15.1–23 kg: 45 mg, twice daily; 23.1–40 kg: 60 mg, twice daily; >40 kg: 75 mg, twice daily for 5 days
		Oral	≥13 y	75 mg, twice daily for 5 days
	Influenza A and B: prophylaxis	Oral	1–12 y	Same as treatment for patients 1–12 y of age, except dose given once daily for 10 days (following known exposure) or for up to 6 wk (preexposure during community outbreak)
		Oral	≥13 y	75 mg once daily for 10 days (following known exposure) or for up to 6 wk (preexposure during community outbreak)
Peglated interferon alfa-2a (Pegasys)	Chronic hepatitis B	SC	>18 y[i]	180 μg, once weekly for 48 wk
	Chronic hepatitis C	SC	≥23 kg	180 μg/1.73 m², once weekly for 24–48 wk, depending on HCV genotype, given concomitantly with oral ribavirin[m]
	Chronic hepatitis C	SC	>18 y[i]	180 μg, once weekly for 24–48 wk, depending on HCV genotype
Peglated interferon-alfa-2b (PegIntron)	Chronic hepatitis C	SC	>18 y	1.5 μg/kg, once weekly for 24–48 wk, depending on HCV genotype
			>3 to 17 y	60 μg/m², once weekly for 24–48 wk, depending on HCV genotype

Table 4.9. Non-HIV Antiviral Drugs,[a] continued

Generic (Trade Name)	Indication	Route	Age	Usually Recommended Dosage
Ribavirin (Rebetol or Copegus)	Treatment of hepatitis C in combination with an alfa interferon	Oral/capsule	≥3 y (Note: capsule doses recommended for use with pegylated interferon alfa-2a and alfa-2b are different)	Fixed dose by weight is suggested for 24–48 wk, depending on HCV genotype 23–33 kg: 200 mg AM and PM >34–46 kg: 200 mg AM and 400 mg PM >47–59 kg: 400 mg AM and PM >60–74 kg: 400 mg AM and 600 mg PM >75 kg: 600 mg AM and PM
		Oral/solution (Rebetol)	≥3 y	15 mg/kg per day, in 2 divided doses for 24–48 wk, depending on HCV genotype
Rimantadine (Flumadine)[h]	Influenza A: treatment[i]	Oral	≥13 y	200 mg/day, in 2 divided doses
	Influenza A: prophylaxis (see Influenza, p 476)[h]	Oral	≥1 y	1–9 y of age: 5 mg/kg per day, maximum 150 mg/day, once daily ≥10 y of age, <40 kg: 5 mg/kg per day, in 2 divided doses; ≥40 kg: 200 mg/day in 2 divided doses
Simeprevir	Chronic hepatitis C	Oral	Adult dose[i]	150 mg, taken once daily with food, as a component of combination therapy with both pegylated interferon alfa and ribavirin
Sofosbuvir	Chronic hepatitis C	Oral	Adult dose[i]	400 mg, taken once daily with or without food, as a component of combination therapy with ribavirin or with ribavirin plus pegylated interferon
Telaprevir	Chronic hepatitis C	Oral	Adult dose[i]	750 mg, 3 times per day for 12 wk in combination with pegylated interferon alfa and ribavirin for 24–48 wk of total treatment, depending on prior HCV treatment status and HCV viral load during therapy

Table 4.9. Non-HIV Antiviral Drugs,[a] continued

Generic (Trade Name)	Indication	Route	Age	Usually Recommended Dosage
Telbivudine (Tyzeka)	Chronic hepatitis B	Oral	Adult dose[i]	600 mg, once daily
Tenofovir (Viread)	Chronic hepatitis B	Oral	>12 y dose	300 mg, once daily
Valacyclovir (Valtrex)	Varicella	Oral	2 to <18 y	20 mg/kg, 3 times daily for 5 days, not to exceed 1 g per dose 3 times daily
	Genital HSV infection, first episode	Oral	Adult dose[i]	2 g/day, in 2 divided doses for 10 days
	Episodic recurrent genital HSV infection	Oral	Adult dose[i]	1 g/day, in 2 divided doses for 3 days
	Daily suppressive therapy for recurrent genital HSV infection	Oral	Adult dose[i]	1000 mg, once daily for 1 year, then reassess for recurrences
	Recurrent herpes labialis	Oral	>12 y	4 g/day, in 2 divided doses for 1 day
	Herpes zoster	Oral	Adult dose[i]	3 g/day, in 3 divided doses for 7 days
Valganciclovir (Valcyte)	Symptomatic congenital CMV disease	Oral	Birth to 2 mo	32 mg/kg per day; in 2 divided doses for 6 mo
	Acquired CMV retinitis in immunocompromised host	Oral	Adult dose[i]	Treatment: 900 mg, twice daily for 3 wk Long-term suppression: 900 mg, once daily
	Prevention of CMV disease in kidney or heart transplant patients	Oral	4 mo–16 y	Dose once a day within 10 days of transplantation until 100 days post-transplantation according to dosage algorithm based on body surface area and creatinine clearance Dose (mg) = 7 × body surface area × creatinine clearance (see drug package insert)

Table 4.9. Non-HIV Antiviral Drugs,[a] continued

Generic (Trade Name)	Indication	Route	Age	Usually Recommended Dosage
Zanamivir (Relenza)	Influenza A and B: treatment (see Influenza, p 476)	Inhalation	≥7 y (treatment)	10 mg, twice daily for 5 days
	Influenza A and B: prophylaxis	Inhalation	≥5 y (prophylaxis)	10 mg, once daily for as long as 28 days (community outbreaks) or 10 days (household setting)

IV indicates intravenous; FDA, US Food and Drug Administration; VZV, varicella-zoster virus; SC, subcutaneous; IM, intramuscular; HCV, hepatitis C virus; HIV, human immunodeficiency virus.

[a] Drugs for human immunodeficiency virus infection are not included. See **http://aidsinfo.nih.gov** for current information on HIV drugs and treatment recommendations.

[b] Dose should be decreased in patients with impaired renal function.

[c] Oral dosage of acyclovir in children should not exceed 80 mg/kg per day (3200 mg/day).

[d] Acyclovir doses listed in this table are based on clinical trials and clinical experience and may not be identical to doses approved by the FDA.

[e] In times of shortage of intravenous acyclovir, the American Academy of Pediatrics Committee on Infectious Diseases recommends that existing supplies of intravenous acyclovir be conserved to improve availability for neonatal HSV infections, herpes simplex encephalitis, or HSV and varicella-zoster virus infections in immunocompromised patients, including more ill pregnant women with visceral dissemination of either virus. If acyclovir is not available, intravenous ganciclovir should be substituted. Alternative regimens to the use of intravenous acyclovir and other options for priority and nonpriority conditions are outlined in an exclusive *Red Book* Online Intravenous Acyclovir Shortage Table (**http://redbook.solutions.aap.org/selfserve/ssPage.aspx?SelfServeContentId=acyclovir-shortage**).

[f] Monitor for nephrotoxicity and neurologic irritation. Consider involving an infectious diseases or pharmacology specialist if weight-based dosing exceeds 800 mg per dose or if being administered with other nephrotoxic medications.

[g] Selective indications; see Varicella-Zoster Infections (p 846).

[h] Since 2005–2006, almost all influenza A (H3N2) strains and 2009 pandemic H1N1 strains tested have been resistant to adamantanes, and adamantane use therefore has not been recommended. See Influenza (p 476) for specific recommendations.

[i] There are not sufficient clinical data to identify the appropriate dose for use in children.

[j] Some experts use ganciclovir in immunocompromised hosts with CMV gastrointestinal tract disease and CMV pneumonitis (with or without CMV Immune Globulin Intravenous).

[k] See Influenza (p 476) and **www.cdc.gov/flu/professionals/antivirals/index.htm** for specific recommendations, which may vary on the basis of most recent influenza virus susceptibility patterns.

[l] Preterm, <38 weeks' postmenstrual age, 1.0 mg/kg/dose, orally, twice daily; preterm, 38 through 40 weeks' postmenstrual age, 1.5 mg/kg/dose, orally, twice daily; preterm >40 weeks' postmenstrual age through 8 months' chronologic age, 3.0 mg/kg/dose, orally, twice daily.

[m] See approved product label for PEGASYS (pegylated interferon alfa-2a).

For more information on individual drugs, see *Physician's Desk Reference* or **www.pdr.net** (for registered users only).

DRUGS FOR PARASITIC INFECTIONS

Table 4.10. Drugs for Parasitic Infections

Disease	Drug	Adult Dosage	Pediatric Dosage	CDC Web Site, including listings of adverse events
African trypanosomiasis (African sleeping sickness)				
Trypanosoma brucei rhodesiense, hemo-lymphatic stage	Suramin[1]	1 g, IV, on days 1, 3, 5, 14, and 21[2]	20 mg/kg (max 1 g), IV, on days 1, 3, 5, 14, and 21[3]	**www.cdc.gov/parasites/ sleepingsickness/health_profession-als/index.html**
T brucei rhodesiense, CNS involvement	Melarsoprol[4]	2–3.6 mg/kg/day (max 200 mg), IV, × 3 days[5] After 7 days, 3.6 mg/kg/day × 3 days Give a 3rd series of 3.6 mg/kg/day after 7 days	2–3.6 mg/kg/day (max 200 mg), IV, × 3 days[5] After 7 days, 3.6 mg/kg/day × 3 days Give a 3rd series of 3.6 mg/kg/day after 7 days	
T brucei gambiense, he-molymphatic stage	Pentamidine[6]	4 mg/kg/day, IV or IM, × 7–10 days	4 mg/kg/day, IV or IM, × 7–10 days	
T brucei gambiense, CNS involvement	Eflornithine[7]	400 mg/kg/day, IV, in 4 doses × 14 days	400 mg/kg/day, IV, in 4 doses × 14 days	
American trypano-somiasis (Chagas disease; *Trypanosoma cruzi* infection)	Benznidazole[8]	<12 y 5–7.5 mg/kg per day, orally, in 2 divided doses for 60 days 12 y or older 5–7 mg/kg per day, orally, in 2 divided doses for 60 days	5–7.5 mg/kg per day, orally, in 2 divided doses for 60 days	**www.cdc.gov/parasites/chagas/health_professionals/index.html**

CDC indicates Centers for Disease Control and Prevention; IV, intravenous; CNS, central nervous system; IM, intramuscular; FDA, US Food and Drug Administration.

[1]Pentamidine is also effective against *T b rhodesiense* in the hemolymphatic stage, but suramin may have somewhat higher efficacy. Suramin is not approved by the FDA but is available through the CDC Drug Service.

[2]A suramin test dose of 100 mg should be given prior to the first dose and the patient should be monitored for hemodynamic stability.

[3]A suramin test dose of 2 mg/kg (max 100 mg) should be given prior to the first dose and the patient should be monitored for hemodynamic stability.

[4]Corticosteroids have been used to prevent melarsoprol encephalopathy. Melarsoprol is not approved by the FDA but is available through the CDC Drug Service.

[5]The dose of melarsoprol is progressively increased during the first series.

Table 4.10. Drugs for Parasitic Infections, continued

Disease	Drug	Adult Dosage	Pediatric Dosage	CDC Web Site, including listings of adverse events
	OR			
	Nifurtimox[8]	1–10 y	15–20 mg/kg per day, orally, in 3 or 4 divided doses for 90 days	
		11–16 y	12.5–15 mg/kg per day, orally, in 3 or 4 divided doses for 90 days	
		17 y or older	8–10 mg/kg per day, orally, in 3 or 4 divided doses for 90–120 days	
Ascariasis (*Ascaris lumbricoides*; intestinal roundworm)	Albendazole[9]	400 mg, orally, once		
	OR			
	Mebendazole[10]	100 mg, orally, twice daily for 3 days, or 500 mg, orally, once		**www.cdc.gov/parasites/ascariasis/ health_professionals/index.html**
	OR			
	Ivermectin[11]	150–200 µg/kg, orally, once		
Babesiosis[12]	Atovaquone	750 mg orally twice a day	40 mg/kg/day, orally, in 2 doses (max 750 mg/ dose)	

[6]Suramin is also effective against *T b gambiense* in the hemolymphatic stage but should be used only in patients in whom onchocerciasis has been excluded. Suramin is not approved by the FDA but is available through the CDC Drug Service.

[7]Eflornithine (400 mg/kg/day, IV, in 2 doses × 7 days) given in combination with oral nifurtimox (15 mg/kg/day, in 3 divided doses × 10 days) is also highly effective against *T b gambiense* with CNS involvement; eflornithine is not approved by the FDA but is available through the CDC Drug Service. Nifurtimox is not FDA-approved, nor is this use covered by CDC's Investigational New Drug (IND) protocol for nifurtimox, which solely covers treatment of Chagas disease; permission for other uses would need to be obtained.

[8]The 2 drugs used to treat infection with *Trypanosoma cruzi* are benznidazole and nifurtimox. In the United States, these drugs are not FDA approved and are available only from CDC under investigational protocols. For both drugs, adverse effects are fairly common and tend to be more frequent and more severe with increasing age. Questions regarding treatment should be directed to Parasitic Diseases Public Inquiries (404-718-4745; e-mail **chagas@cdc.gov**).

Table 4.10. Drugs for Parasitic Infections, continued

Disease	Drug	Adult Dosage	Pediatric Dosage	CDC Web Site, including listings of adverse events
	PLUS			
	Azithromycin	On the first day, give a total dose in the range of 500–1000 mg, orally; on subsequent days, give a total daily dose in the range of 250–1000 mg	10 mg/kg (max 500 mg/dose), orally, on day 1, then 5 mg/kg/day (max 250 mg/dose), orally, on subsequent days	**www.cdc.gov/parasites/babesiosis/health_professionals/index.html**
	OR			
	Clindamycin	600 mg, orally, 3 times a day, **or** 300–600 mg, IV, 4 times a day	20–40 mg/kg/day (max 600 mg/dose), orally, in 3 doses	
	PLUS			
	Quinine	650 mg, orally, 3 times a day	30 mg/kg/day, orally, in 3 doses (max 650 mg/dose)	

[9] The safety of albendazole in children younger than 6 years is not certain. Studies of the use of albendazole in children as young as 1 year suggest that its use is safe.

[10] The safety of mebendazole in children has not been established. There are limited data in children 2 years and younger.

[11] Safety of ivermectin for treating children who weigh less than 15 kg has not been established.

[12] Usually treat for at least 7 to 10 days. The combination of clindamycin plus quinine is the standard of care for babesiosis patients who are severely ill.

[13] In cases in which suspicion of exposure is high, immediate treatment with albendazole (25–50 mg/kg per day by mouth for 10–20 days) may be appropriate. Treatment is successful when administered soon after exposure to abort the migration of larvae. Treatment should be initiated as soon as possible after ingestion of infectious material, ideally within 3 days. For clinical baylisascariasis, treatment with albendazole with concurrent corticosteroids to help reduce the inflammatory reaction is indicated to attempt to control the disease.

[14] The clinical significance of *Blastocystis* species is controversial.

[15] Praziquantel is not approved for treatment of children younger than 4 years, but this drug has been used successfully to treat cases of *D caninum* infection in children as young as 6 months.

[16] Niclosamide is unavailable in the United States.

[17] Treatment of cystic echinococcosis depends on the World Health Organization classification of the cysts. Albendazole is not appropriate for all forms of the infection.

[18] Triclabendazole is not approved by the FDA but is available through the CDC Drug Service. It requires an individual IND from the FDA for administration.

Table 4.10. Drugs for Parasitic Infections, continued

Disease	Drug	Adult Dosage	Pediatric Dosage	CDC Web Site, including listings of adverse events
Balantidiasis (*Balantidium coli*)	Tetracycline	500 mg, orally, 4 times daily for 10 days	Age ≥8 y, 40 mg/kg/day (max 2 g), orally, in 4 doses for 10 days	**www.cdc.gov/parasites/balantidium/ health_professionals/index.html**
	OR			
	Metronidazole	500–750 mg, orally, 3 times daily for 5 days	35–50 mg/kg/day, orally, in 3 doses for 5 days	
	OR			
	Iodoquinol	650 mg, orally, 3 times daily for 20 days	30–40 mg/kg/day (max 2 g), orally, in 3 doses for 20 days	
	OR			
	Nitazoxanide	500 mg, orally, twice daily for 3 days	Age 4–11 y: 200 mg, orally, twice daily for 3 days Age 1–3 y: 100 mg, orally, twice daily for 3 days	
Baylisascariasis (raccoon roundworm infection)	Albendazole[9]	25–50 mg/kg per day, orally, for 10–20 days[13]		**www.cdc.gov/parasites/baylisascaris/ health_professionals/index.html**

[19]Sodium stibogluconate is not approved by the FDA but is available through the CDC Drug Service. Only selected treatments and regimens are provided. Expert consultation about these and other potential treatment options for leishmaniasis is encouraged. For some cases of cutaneous leishmaniasis, no therapy may be needed or local (vs systemic) therapy may suffice or other systemic treatments may be considered. Miltefosine (IMPAVIDO) was approved in March 2014 by the FDA for treatment of visceral leishmaniasis attributable to *L donovani*, mucosal leishmaniasis attributable to *L braziliensis*, and cutaneous leishmaniasis attributable to *L braziliensis*, *L guyanensis*, and *L panamensis* (ie, some new world cutaneous leishmaniasis species, but no old world cutaneous leishmaniasis species) for patients who are at least 12 years of age and at least 30 kg of weight.

[20]Pediculicides should not be used for infestations of the eyelashes. Such infestations are treated with petrolatum ointment applied 2 to 4 times/day for 8 to 10 days. For pubic lice, treat with 1% permethrin, pyrethrins with piperonyl butoxide, or ivermectin.

[21]Permethrin and pyrethrin are pediculicidal; retreatment in 7 to 10 days is needed to eradicate the infestation. Some lice are resistant to pyrethrins and permethrin. Pyrethrins with piperonyl butoxide are recommended for use in children >2 years old; permethrin for children >2 months old.

[22]Ivermectin is not ovicidal, but lice that hatch from treated eggs die within 48 hours after hatching. Recommended for use in children >6 months old.

[23]Spinosad is not ovicidal, but causes neuronal excitation in insects leading to paralysis and death. The formulation also includes benzyl alcohol, which is pediculicidal. Two applications 7 days apart are needed. Recommended for children >4 years old.

Table 4.10. Drugs for Parasitic Infections, continued

Disease	Drug	Adult Dosage	Pediatric Dosage	CDC Web Site, including listings of adverse events
Blastocystis hominis infection[14]	Metronidazole	750 mg, orally, 3 times daily for 10 days	35–50 mg/kg/day, orally, in 3 doses for 10 days	www.cdc.gov/parasites/blastocystis/health_professionals/index.html
	OR			
	Trimethoprim (TMP)/sulfamethoxazole (SMX)	160 mg TMP, 800 mg SMX twice daily for 7 days	Age >2 mo: 8 mg TMP/kg and 40 mg/kg SMX per day in 2 divided doses for 7 days	
	OR			
	Nitazoxanide	500 mg, orally, twice daily for 3 days	Age 4–11 y: 200 mg, orally, twice daily for 3 days Age 1–3 y: 100 mg, orally, twice daily for 3 days	
Capillariasis	Mebendazole[10]	200 mg, orally, twice a day for 20 days		www.cdc.gov/parasites/capillaria/health_professionals/index.html
	OR			
	Albendazole[9]	400 mg, orally, once a day for 10 days		
Chilomastix mesnili infection	No treatment is necessary; this protozoan is harmless			www.cdc.gov/parasites/nonpathprotozoa/health_professionals/index.html
Clonorchiasis	Praziquantel	75 mg/kg/day, orally, 3 doses per day for 2 days		www.cdc.gov/parasites/clonorchis/health_professionals/index.html
	OR			
	Albendazole[9]	10 mg/kg/day for 7 days		

[24] Benzyl alcohol prevents lice from closing their respiratory spiracles and the lotion vehicle then obstructs their airway causing them to asphyxiate. It is not ovicidal. Two applications at least 7 days apart are needed. Recommended for use in children >6 months old. Resistance, which is a problem with other drugs, is unlikely to develop.

[25] Malathion is both ovicidal and pediculicidal; 2 applications at least 7 days apart are generally necessary to kill all lice and nits. Recommended for children >6 years old.

[26] Ivermectin is pediculicidal, but not ovicidal; more than 1 dose is generally necessary to eradicate the infestation. The number of doses and interval between doses has not been established; animal studies have shown adverse effects on the fetus. In one study of treatment of head lice, 2 doses of ivermectin (400 µg/kg) 7 days apart were more effective than treatment with topical malathion. In one study of treatment of body lice, a regimen of 3 doses of ivermectin (12 mg each) administered at 7-day intervals was effective.

Table 4.10. Drugs for Parasitic Infections, continued

Disease	Drug	Adult Dosage	Pediatric Dosage	CDC Web Site, including listings of adverse events
Cutaneous larva migrans (zoonotic hookworm)	Albendazole[9]	400 mg/day, orally, once a day for 3 to 7 days	Age >2 y: 400 mg/day, orally, for 3 days	**www.cdc.gov/parasites/zoonotichookworm/health_professionals/index.html**
	OR			
	Ivermectin	200 µg/kg orally, as a single dose	Weight >15 kg: 200 µg/kg, orally, as a single dose	
Cyclosporiasis	TMP/SMX	160 mg TMP/800 mg SMX, orally, 2 times/day × 7–10 days	8–10 mg TMP/kg/day, orally, divided 2 times/day for 7–10 days	**www.cdc.gov/parasites/cyclosporiasis/health_professionals/index.html**
Cystoisosporiasis (*Cystoisospora* infection; formerly isosporiasis)	TMP/SMX	160 mg TMP/800 mg SMX, orally, 2 times/day × 7–10 days	8–10 mg TMP/kg/day, orally, divided 2 times/day for 7–10 days	**www.cdc.gov/parasites/cystoisospora/health_professionals/index.html**
	OR			
	Ciprofloxacin (second-line alternate)	500 mg, orally, 2 times/day × 7 days	—	
Dientamoeba fragilis infection	Iodoquinol	650 mg, orally, 3 times/day for 20 days	30–40 mg/kg/day (max 2 g), orally, divided 3 times/day × 20 days	**www.cdc.gov/parasites/dientamoeba/health_professionals/index.html**
	OR			
	Paromomycin	25–35 mg/kg/day, orally, divided 3 times/day for 7 days		
	OR			
	Metronidazole	500–750 mg, orally, 3 times/day for 10 days	35–50 mg/kg/day, orally, divided 3 times/day × 10 days	

Table 4.10. Drugs for Parasitic Infections, continued

Disease	Drug	Adult Dosage	Pediatric Dosage	CDC Web Site, including listings of adverse events
Diphyllobothrium infection	Praziquantel[15]	5–10 mg/kg, orally, in a single dose		www.cdc.gov/parasites/ diphyllobothrium/ health_professionals/index.html
	OR			
	Niclosamide[16]	2 g, orally, once	50 mg/kg (max 2 g), orally, once	
Dipylidium caninum infection (dog or cat flea tapeworm)	Praziquantel[15]	5–10 mg/kg, orally, in a single dose		www.cdc.gov/parasites/dipylidium/ health_professionals/index.html
	OR			
	Niclosamide[16]	2 g, orally, once	50 mg/kg (max 2 g), orally, once	
Echinococcosis[17]	Albendazole[9]	400 mg, orally, twice a day for 1–6 mo	10–15 mg/kg/day (max 800 mg), orally, in 2 doses for 1–6 mo	www.cdc.gov/parasites/ echinococcosis/health_professionals/ index.html
Endolimax nana infection	No treatment is necessary; this protozoan is harmless			www.cdc.gov/parasites/nonpathprotozoa/ health_professionals/index.html
Entamoeba coli infection	No treatment is necessary; this protozoan is harmless			www.cdc.gov/parasites/nonpathprotozoa/ health_professionals/index.html
Entamoeba dispar infection	No treatment is necessary; this protozoan is harmless			www.cdc.gov/parasites/nonpathprotozoa/ health_professionals/index.html

[27] Diethylcarbamazine (DEC) is not approved by the FDA, but is available from the CDC Drug Service through an IND after confirmed positive lab results. DEC is contraindicated in patients who may also have onchocerciasis. Prior to DEC treatment for lymphatic filariasis, onchocerciasis should be excluded in all patients with a consistent exposure history because of the possibility of severe exacerbations of skin and eye involvement (Mazzotti reaction). People coinfected with loiasis and *O volvulus* should not be treated with DEC until the onchocerciasis is treated; their onchocerciasis should not be treated with ivermectin if it is unsafe to treat their loiasis.

[28] If a person develops malaria despite taking chemoprophylaxis, that particular medicine should not be used as a part of their treatment regimen. Use one of the other options instead.

[29] There are 4 options (A, B, C, or D) available for treatment of uncomplicated malaria caused by chloroquine-resistant *P falciparum*. Options A, B, and C are equally recommended. Because of a higher rate of severe neuropsychiatric reactions seen at treatment doses, option D (mefloquine) is not recommended unless the other options cannot be used. For option C, because there are more data on the efficacy of quinine in combination with doxycycline or tetracycline, these treatment combinations are generally preferred to quinine in combination with clindamycin.

[30] Atovaquone-proguanil or artemether-lumefantrine should be taken with food or whole milk. If patient vomits within 30 minutes of taking a dose, the dose should be repeated.

[31] The US-manufactured quinine sulfate capsule is in a 324-mg dosage; therefore, 2 capsules should be sufficient for adult dosing. Pediatric dosing may be difficult because of unavailability of noncapsule forms of quinine.

Table 4.10. Drugs for Parasitic Infections, continued

Disease	Drug	Adult Dosage	Pediatric Dosage	CDC Web Site, including listings of adverse events
Entamoeba hartmanni infection	No treatment is necessary; this protozoan is harmless			**www.cdc.gov/parasites/nonpathprotozoa/ health_professionals/index.html**
Entamoeba polecki	No treatment is necessary; this protozoan is harmless			**www.cdc.gov/parasites/nonpathprotozoa/ health_professionals/index.html**
Enterobiasis (pinworm)	Mebendazole[10]		100 mg, orally, once; repeat in 2 wk	
	OR			
	Pyrantel pamoate		11 mg/kg base, orally, once (max 1 g); repeat in 2 wk	**www.cdc.gov/parasites/pinworm/ health_professionals/index.html**
	OR			
	Albendazole[9]		For children 20 kg or greater: 400 mg PO once; repeat in 2 wk	
			For children <20 kg: 200 mg PO once; repeat in 2 wk	
Fascioliasis (*Fasciola hepatica*; sheep liver fluke)	Triclabendazole[18]	10 mg/kg, orally, once or twice		
	OR			
	Nitazoxanide	500 mg, orally, 2 times/ day × 7 days	Age 1–3 y: 100 mg, orally, 2 times/day × 7 days Age 4–11 y: 200 mg, orally, 2 times/day × 7 days Age ≥12 y: 500 mg, orally, 2 times/day × 7 days	**www.cdc.gov/parasites/fasciola/ health_professionals/index.html**
Fasciolopsiasis	Praziquantel[15]	75 mg/kg/day, orally, in 3 divided doses for 1 day		**www.cdc.gov/parasites/fasciolopsis/ health_professionals/index.html**
Gnathostomiasis (cutaneous)	Albendazole[9]	400 mg, orally, 2 times/day × 21 days		**www.cdc.gov/parasites/gnathostoma/ health_professionals/index.html**

Table 4.10. Drugs for Parasitic Infections, continued

Disease	Drug	Adult Dosage	Pediatric Dosage	CDC Web Site, including listings of adverse events
	OR			
	Ivermectin		200 μg, orally, once daily × 2 days	
Heterophyiasis	Praziquantel[15]		75 mg/kg/day, divided 3 times/day × 1 day, orally	www.cdc.gov/dpdx/heterophyiasis/tx.html
Hymenolepiasis (*Hymenolepis nana;* dwarf tapeworm)	Praziquantel[15]		25 mg/kg in a single-dose therapy, orally	www.cdc.gov/parasites/hymenolepis/health_professionals/index.html
	OR			
	Niclosamide[16]	2 g in a single dose for 7 days, orally	Weight 11–34 kg: 1 g in a single dose on day 1, then 500 mg per day, orally, for 6 days Weight >34 kg: 1.5 g in a single dose on day 1, then 1 g per day, orally, for 6 days	
	OR			
	Nitazoxanide	500 mg, orally, 2 times/day × 3 days	Age 1–3 y: 100 mg, orally, 2 times/day × 3 days Age 4–11 y: 200 mg, orally, 2 times/day × 3 days Age ≥12 y: 500 mg, orally, 2 times/day × 3 days	

[32] For infections acquired in Southeast Asia, quinine treatment should continue for 7 days. For infections acquired elsewhere, quinine treatment should continue for 3 days.

[33] Doxycycline and tetracycline are not indicated for use in children younger than 8 years. For children younger than 8 years with chloroquine-resistant *P falciparum*, atovaquone-proguanil and artemether-lumefantrine are recommended treatment options; mefloquine can be considered if no other options are available. For children younger than 8 years with chloroquine-resistant *P vivax*, mefloquine is the recommended treatment. If it is not available or is not being tolerated and if the treatment benefits outweigh the risks, atovaquone-proguanil or artemether-lumefantrine should be used instead.

[34] Treatment with mefloquine is not recommended in people who have acquired infections from Southeast Asia because of drug resistance.

Table 4.10. Drugs for Parasitic Infections, continued

Disease	Drug	Adult Dosage	Pediatric Dosage	CDC Web Site, including listings of adverse events
Hookworm (Human; *Ancylostoma duodenale, Necator americanus*)	Albendazole[9]	400 mg, orally, once		**www.cdc.gov/parasites/hookworm/health_professionals/index.html**
	OR			
	Mebendazole[10]	100 mg, orally, twice a day for 3 days, or 500 mg, orally, once		
	OR			
	Pyrantel pamoate	11 mg/kg (up to a maximum of 1 g), orally, daily for 3 days		
Iodamoeba buetschlii Infection	No treatment is necessary; this protozoan is harmless			**www.cdc.gov/parasites/nonpathprotozoa/health_professionals/index.html**
Leishmaniasis[19]				
Visceral (Kala-azar)	Liposomal amphotericin B	3 mg/kg/day, IV, on days 1–5, 14, and 21		**www.cdc.gov/parasites/leishmaniasis/health_professionals/index.html**
	OR			
	Sodium stibogluconate	20 mg pentavalent antimony (Sb)/kg/day, IV or IM, × 28 days		
	OR			
	Miltefosine	30 through 44 kg; 50 mg, twice daily, for 28 consecutive days		
		≥ 45 kg; 50 mg, 3 times daily, for 28 consecutive days		
	OR			
	Amphotericin B deoxycholate	1 mg/kg, IV, daily × 15–20 days or every second day for up to 8 wk (total usually 15–20 mg/kg)		
Cutaneous	Sodium stibogluconate	20 mg Sb/kg/day, IV or IM, × 20 days		

Table 4.10. Drugs for Parasitic Infections, continued

Disease	Drug	Adult Dosage	Pediatric Dosage	CDC Web Site, including listings of adverse events
	OR			
	Miltefosine	30 through 44 kg: 50 mg, twice daily, for 28 consecutive days; ≥ 45 kg: 50 mg, 3 times daily, for 28 consecutive days		
Mucosal	Sodium stibogluconate	20 mg Sb/kg/day, IV or IM, × 28 days		
	OR			
	Amphotericin B	0.5–1 mg/kg, IV, daily × 15–20 days or every second day for up to 8 wk		
	OR			
	Miltefosine	30 through 44 kg: 50 mg, twice daily, for 28 consecutive days; ≥45 kg: 50 mg, 3 times daily, for 28 consecutive days		

35 When treating chloroquine-sensitive infections, chloroquine and hydroxychloroquine are recommended options. However, regimens used to treat chloroquine-resistant infections may also be used if available, more convenient, or preferred.

36 Primaquine is used to eradicate any hypnozoites that may remain dormant in the liver and, thus, prevent relapses in *P vivax* and *P ovale* infections. Because primaquine can cause hemolytic anemia in glucose-6-phosphate dehydrogenase (G6PD)–deficient people, G6PD screening must occur prior to starting treatment with primaquine. For people with borderline G6PD deficiency or as an alternate to the above regimen, primaquine, 45 mg, orally, once per week for 8 weeks may be given; consultation with an expert in infectious disease and/or tropical medicine is advised if this alternative regimen is considered in G6PD-deficient people. Primaquine must not be used during pregnancy.

37 There are 3 options (A, B, or C) available for treatment of uncomplicated malaria caused by chloroquine-resistant *P vivax*. High treatment failure rates attributable to chloroquine-resistant *P vivax* have been well documented in Papua New Guinea and Indonesia. Rare case reports of chloroquine-resistant *P vivax* have also been documented in Burma (Myanmar), India, and Central and South America. People acquiring *P vivax* infections outside of Papua New Guinea or Indonesia should be started on chloroquine. If the patient does not respond, the treatment should be changed to a chloroquine-resistant *P vivax* regimen and the CDC should be notified (Malaria Hotline number listed previously). For treatment of chloroquine-resistant *P vivax* infections, options A, B, and C are equally recommended.

38 For pregnant women diagnosed with uncomplicated malaria caused by chloroquine-resistant *P falciparum* or chloroquine-resistant *P vivax* infection, treatment with doxycycline or tetracycline is generally not indicated. However, doxycycline or tetracycline may be used in combination with quinine (as recommended for nonpregnant adults) if other treatment options are not available or are not being tolerated, and the benefit is judged to outweigh the risks.

39 Atovaquone-proguanil and artemether-lumefantrine are generally not recommended for use in pregnant women, particularly in the first trimester, because of lack of sufficient safety data. For pregnant women diagnosed with uncomplicated malaria caused by chloroquine-resistant *P falciparum* infection, atovaquone-proguanil or artemether-lumefantrine may be used if other treatment options are not available or are not being tolerated, and if the potential benefit is judged to outweigh the potential risks.

Table 4.10. Drugs for Parasitic Infections, continued

Disease	Drug	Adult Dosage	Pediatric Dosage	CDC Web Site, including listings of adverse events
Lice infestation (*Pediculus humanus*, *P. capitis*, *Phthirus pubis*)[20]	Pyrethrins with piperonyl butoxide[21]	Topically, twice, at least 7 days apart	Topically, twice at least 7 days apart	**www.cdc.gov/parasites/lice/body/ health_professionals/index.html**
	OR			
	0.5% Ivermectin lotion[22]	Topically, once	Topically, once	
	OR			
	0.9% Spinosad suspension[23]	Topically, twice, at least 7 days apart	Topically, twice, at least 7 days apart	**www.cdc.gov/parasites/gnathostoma/ health_professionals/index.html**
	OR			
	1% Permethrin[21]	Topically, twice, at least 7 days apart	Topically, twice, at least 7 days apart	**www.cdc.gov/parasites/lice/pubic/ health_professionals/index.html**
	OR			
	5% Benzyl alcohol lotion[24]	Topically, twice, at least 7 days apart	Topically, twice, at least 7 days apart	
	OR			
	0.5% Malathion[25]	Topically, twice, at least 7 days apart	Topically, twice, at least 7 days apart	
	OR			
	Ivermectin[26]	200 or 400 µg /kg, orally	≥15 kg: 200 or 400 µg / kg, orally	

[40] For *P. vivax* and *P. ovale* infections, primaquine phosphate for radical treatment of hypnozoites should not be given during pregnancy. Pregnant patients with *P. vivax* and *P. ovale* infections should be maintained on chloroquine prophylaxis for the duration of their pregnancy. The chemoprophylactic dose of chloroquine phosphate is 300 mg base (=500 mg salt), orally, once per week. After delivery, pregnant patients who do not have G6PD deficiency should be treated with primaquine.

Table 4.10. Drugs for Parasitic Infections, continued

Disease	Drug	Adult Dosage	Pediatric Dosage	CDC Web Site, including listings of adverse events
Loiasis (*Loa loa*)		*Indication:*		www.cdc.gov/parasites/loiasis/health_professionals/index.html
		Symptomatic loiasis with microfilariae of L loa/mL <8000		
	Diethylcarbamazine (DEC)[27]	8–10 mg/kg, orally, in 3 divided doses daily for 21 days		
		Indication:		
		Symptomatic loiasis, with microfilariae of L loa/mL <8000 and failed 2 rounds DEC		
		OR		
		Symptomatic loiasis, with microfilariae of L loa/mL ≥8000 to reduce level to <8000 prior to treatment with DEC		
	Albendazole[9]	200 mg, orally, twice daily for 21 days		
Lymphatic filariasis (elephantiasis; *Wuchereria bancrofti, Brugia malayi, Brugia timori*)	Diethylcarbamazine (DEC)[27]	Treatment of lymphatic filariasis: Adults and children >18 mo: 6 mg/kg/day, orally, divided in 3 doses for 12 consecutive days OR 6 mg/kg/day as a single oral dose Treatment of tropical pulmonary eosinophilia (TPE): Adults and children >18 mo: 6 mg/kg/day, orally, divided in 3 doses for 14–21 days		www.cdc.gov/parasites/lymphaticfilariasis/health_professionals/index.html

[41] People with a positive blood smear OR history of recent possible exposure and no other recognized pathologic abnormality who have 1 or more of the following clinical criteria (impaired consciousness/coma, severe normocytic anemia, renal failure, pulmonary edema, acute respiratory distress syndrome, circulatory shock, disseminated intravascular coagulation, spontaneous bleeding, acidosis, hemoglobinuria, jaundice, repeated generalized convulsions, and/or parasitemia of >5%) are considered to have manifestations of more severe disease. Severe malaria is most often caused by *P falciparum*.

[42] Patients with a diagnosis of severe malaria should be treated aggressively with parenteral antimalarial therapy. Treatment with IV quinidine should be initiated as soon as possible after the diagnosis has been made. Patients with severe malaria should be given an intravenous loading dose of quinidine unless they have received more than 40 mg/kg of quinine in the preceding 48 hours or if they have received mefloquine within the preceding 12 hours. Consultation with a cardiologist and a physician with experience treating malaria is advised when treating malaria patients with quinidine. During administration of quinidine, blood pressure monitoring (for hypotension) and cardiac monitoring (for widening of the QRS complex and/or lengthening of the QTc interval) should be monitored continuously and blood glucose (for hypoglycemia) should be monitored periodically. Cardiac complications, if severe, may warrant temporary discontinuation of the drug or slowing of the intravenous infusion.

Table 4.10. Drugs for Parasitic Infections, continued

Disease	Drug	Adult Dosage	Pediatric Dosage	CDC Web Site, including listings of adverse events www.cdc.gov/malaria/resources/pdf/treatmenttable.pdf
Malaria (*Plasmodium* species)	Region infection acquired			CDC Malaria Hotline: (770) 488-7788 or (855) 856-4713 toll-free Monday–Friday 9 am to 5 pm EST; (770) 488-7100 after hours, weekends, and holidays
Uncomplicated malaria *P falciparum* or species not identified	Chloroquine-resistant or unknown resistance[28,29] (All malarious regions except those specified as chloroquine-sensitive listed below.)			
If "species not identified" subsequently diagnoses as *P vivax* or *P ovale*, see below re: treatment with primaquine	Atovaquone-proguanil[30]	1000 mg atovaquone/400 mg proguanil, orally, once daily × 3 days	Weight 5–8 kg: 2 pediatric tablets, orally, once daily × 3 days Weight 9–10 kg: 3 pediatric tablets, orally, once daily × 3 day Weight 11–20 kg: 1 adult tab, orally, once daily × 3 d Weight 21–30 kg: 2 adult tablets, orally, once daily × 3d 31–40 kg: 3 adult tablets, orally, once daily × 3d >40 kg: 4 adult tablets, orally, once daily × 3d	

[43] Pregnant women diagnosed with severe malaria should be treated aggressively with parenteral antimalarial therapy.

[44] Albendazole is currently the treatment of choice for neurocysticercosis. Longer courses may be needed for subarachnoid disease. Steroids are almost always required when albendazole or praziquantel is used. Not all forms of neurocysticercosis should be treated with anthelmintics. Some forms require only symptom control.

[45] People coinfected with *O volvulus* and loiasis should not be treated with diethylcarbamazine (DEC) until the onchocerciasis is treated; their onchocerciasis should not be treated with ivermectin if it is unsafe to treat their loiasis. Patients should only be treated with doxycycline if they no longer live in areas with endemic infection unless there is a contraindication for ivermectin.

[46] Doxycycline is not standard therapy; but several studies support its use and safety. Treatment with ivermectin should be given 1 week prior to treatment with doxycycline to provide symptom relief to the patient. If the patient cannot tolerate the dosage of 200 mg, orally, daily of doxycycline, 100 mg, orally, daily is sufficient to sterilize female *Onchocerca organisms*.

Table 4.10. Drugs for Parasitic Infections, continued

Disease	Drug	Adult Dosage	Pediatric Dosage	CDC Web Site, including listings of adverse events
	OR			
	Artemether-lumefantrine[30] 1 tablet = 20 mg artemether and 120 mg lumefantrine	A 3-day treatment schedule with a total of 6 oral doses is recommended for both adult and pediatric patients based on weight. The patient should receive the initial dose, followed by the second dose 8 h later, then 1 dose, orally, 2 times/day; for the following 2 days. Weight 5–<15 kg: 1 tablet per dose Weight 15–<25 kg: 2 tablets per dose Weight 25–<35 kg: 3 tablets per dose Weight ≥35 kg: 4 tablets per dose		
	OR			
	Quinine sulfate[31,32] plus one of the following: Doxycycline,[33] Tetracycline,[33] or Clindamycin	Quinine sulfate: 542 mg base (=650 mg salt),[4] orally, 3 times/day × 3 or 7 days[5] Doxycycline: 100 mg, orally, 2 times/day × 7 days Tetracycline: 250 mg, orally, 4 times/day × 7 days Clindamycin: 20 mg base/kg/day, orally, divided 3 times/day × 7 days	Quinine sulfate: 8.3 mg base/kg (=10 mg salt/kg), orally, 3 times/day × 3 or 7 days Doxycycline: 2.2 mg/kg, orally, every 12 h × 7 days Tetracycline: 25 mg/kg/day, orally, divided 4 times/day × 7 days Clindamycin: 20 mg base/kg/day, orally, divided 3 times/day × 7 days	

[47] For treatment and chronic suppression of toxoplasmosis in human immunodeficiency virus (HIV) infected children, see Guidelines for the Prevention and Treatment of Opportunistic Infections Among HIV-Exposed and HIV-Infected Children, 2013 at **http://aidsinfo.nih.gov/contentfiles/lvguidelines/oi_guidelines_pediatrics.pdf.**

[48] Plus leucovorin, 10–25 mg, with each dose of pyrimethamine.

Table 4.10. Drugs for Parasitic Infections, continued

Disease	Drug	Adult Dosage	Pediatric Dosage	CDC Web Site, including listings of adverse events
	OR	Mefloquine[34] 684 mg base (=750 mg salt), orally, as initial dose, followed by 456 mg base (=500 mg salt), orally, given 6–12 h after initial dose Total dose = 1250 mg salt	13.7 mg base/kg (=15 mg salt/kg), orally, as initial dose, followed by 9.1 mg base/kg (=10 mg salt/kg), orally, given 6–12 h after initial dose Total dose = 25 mg salt/kg	
Uncomplicated malaria *P falciparum* or species not identified	Chloroquine-sensitive (Central America west of Panama Canal; Haiti; the Dominican Republic; and most of the Middle East)			
	Chloroquine phosphate[35]	600 mg base (=1000 mg salt), orally, immediately, followed by 300 mg base (=500 mg salt), orally, at 6, 24, and 48 h Total dose: 1500 mg base (=2500 mg salt)	10 mg base/kg, orally, immediately, followed by 5 mg base/kg, orally, at 6, 24, and 48 h Total dose: 25 mg base/kg	
	OR			
	Hydroxychloroquine	620 mg base (=800 mg salt), orally, immediately, followed by 310 mg base (=400 mg salt), orally, at 6, 24, and 48 h Total dose: 1550 mg base (=2000 mg salt)	10 mg base/kg, orally, immediately, followed by 5 mg base/kg, orally, at 6, 24, and 48 h Total dose: 25 mg base/kg	

Table 4.10. Drugs for Parasitic Infections, continued

Disease	Drug	Adult Dosage	Pediatric Dosage	CDC Web Site, including listings of adverse events
All regions	Chloroquine phosphate[35]	600 mg base (=1000 mg salt), orally, immediately; followed by 300 mg base (=500 mg salt), orally, at 6, 24, and 48 h Total dose: 1500 mg base (=2500 mg salt)	10 mg base/kg, orally, immediately; followed by 5 mg base/kg, orally, at 6, 24, and 48 hours Total dose: 25 mg base/kg	
Uncomplicated malaria *P malariae or P knowlesi*	OR Hydroxychloroquine	620 mg base (=800 mg salt), orally, immediately; followed by 310 mg base (=400 mg salt), orally, at 6, 24, and 48 h Total dose: 1550 mg base (=2000 mg salt)	10 mg base/kg, orally, immediately; followed by 5 mg base/kg, orally, at 6, 24, and 48 h Total dose: 25 mg base/kg	

[49] Women who develop toxoplasmosis during the first trimester of pregnancy should be treated with spiramycin (3–4 g/day). After the first trimester, if there is no documented transmission to the fetus, spiramycin can be continued until term. Spiramycin is not currently available in the United States but can be obtained at no cost from Aventis through an IND from the FDA (301-796-1600, -1400, –0563, or -3763) following confirmation of the diagnosis by a recognized laboratory (ie, Palo Alto Medical Foundation, Toxoplasmosis Laboratory 650-853-4828). If transmission has occurred in utero, therapy with pyrimethamine and sulfadiazine should be started. Pyrimethamine is a potential teratogen and should be used only after the first trimester (Montoya JG, Remington JS. Management of Toxoplasma gondii infection during pregnancy. *Clin Infect Dis.* 2008;47[4]:554). Congenitally infected newborns should be treated with pyrimethamine every 2 or 3 days and a sulfonamide daily for approximately 1 year (Remington JS, McLeod R, Wilson CB, Desmonts G. Toxoplasmosis. Remington JS, Klein J, Wilson C, Nizet V, Maldonado Y, eds. *Infectious Disease of the Fetus and Newborn Infant.* 7th ed. Philadelphia, PA: Saunders; 2011:918-1041).

Table 4.10. Drugs for Parasitic Infections, continued

Disease	Drug	Adult Dosage	Pediatric Dosage	CDC Web Site, including listings of adverse events
	All regions			
	Note: for suspected chloroquine-resistant *P vivax*, see row below			
	Chloroquine phosphate[35]	600 mg base (=1000 mg salt), orally, immediately, followed by 300 mg base (=500 mg salt), orally, at 6, 24, and 48 h Total dose: 1500 mg base (=2500 mg salt)	10 mg base/kg, orally, immediately, followed by 5 mg base/kg, orally, at 6, 24, and 48 h Total dose: 25 mg base/kg	
	PLUS			
Uncomplicated malaria *P vivax* or *P ovale*	Primaquine phosphate[36]	30 mg base, orally, once daily × 14 days	0.5 mg base/kg, orally, once daily × 14 days	
	OR			
	Hydroxychloro-quine	620 mg base (=800 mg salt), orally, immediately, followed by 310 mg base (=400 mg salt), orally, at 6, 24, and 48 h Total dose: 1550 mg base (=2000 mg salt)	10 mg base/kg, orally, immediately, followed by 5 mg base/kg, orally, at 6, 24, and 48 h Total dose: 25 mg base/kg	
	PLUS			
	Primaquine phosphate[36]	30 mg base, orally, once daily × 14 days	0.5 mg base/kg, orally, once daily × 14 days	

Table 4.10. Drugs for Parasitic Infections, continued

Disease	Drug	Adult Dosage	Pediatric Dosage	CDC Web Site, including listings of adverse events
Uncomplicated malaria *P vivax*	Chloroquine-resistant[37] (Papua New Guinea and Indonesia)			
	Quinine sulfate plus either Doxycycline or Tetracycline plus Primaquine phosphate[36]	Quinine sulfate: 542 mg base (=650 mg salt),[4] orally, 3 times/day × 3 or 7 days[32] Doxycycline: 100 mg, orally, 2 times/day × 7 days Tetracycline: 250 mg, orally, 4 times/day × 7 days Primaquine phosphate: 30 mg base, orally, once daily × 14 days	Quinine sulfate: 8.3 mg base/kg (=10 mg salt/kg), orally, 3 times/day × 3 or 7 days[32] Doxycycline: 2.2 mg/kg, orally, every 12 h × 7 days Tetracycline: 25 mg/kg/day, orally, divided 4 times/day × 7 days Primaquine Phosphate: 0.5 mg base/kg, orally, once daily × 14 days	
	OR			

Table 4.10. Drugs for Parasitic Infections, continued

Disease	Drug	Adult Dosage	Pediatric Dosage	CDC Web Site, including listings of adverse events
	Atovaquone-proguanil plus Primaquine phosphate[36]	Atovaquone-proguanil: 1000 mg atovaquone/ 400 mg proguanil, orally, once daily × 3 days	Atovaquone-proguanil: 5–8 kg: 2 pediatric tablets, orally, once daily × 3 days 9–10 kg: 3 pediatric tablets, orally, once daily x 3 days 11–20 kg: 1adult tablet, orally, once daily × 3 days 21–30 kg: 2 adult tablets, orally, once daily x 3days 31–40 kg: 3 adult tablets, orally, once daily × 3days >40 kg: 4 adult tablets, orally, once daily × 3 days	
		Primaquine phosphate: 30 mg base, orally, once daily × 14 days	Primaquine phosphate: 0.5 mg base/kg, orally, once daily × 14 days	

OR

Table 4.10. Drugs for Parasitic Infections, continued

Disease	Drug	Adult Dosage	Pediatric Dosage	CDC Web Site, including listings of adverse events
	Mefloquine plus Primaquine phosphate[36]	Mefloquine: 684 mg base (=750 mg salt), orally, as initial dose, followed by 456 mg base (=500 mg salt), orally, given 6–12 h after initial dose Total dose =1250 mg salt Primaquine phosphate: 30 mg base, orally, once daily × 14 days	Mefloquine: 13.7 mg base/kg (=15 mg salt/kg), orally, as initial dose, followed by 9.1 mg base/kg (=10 mg salt/kg), orally, given 6–12 h after initial dose Total dose =25 mg salt/kg Primaquine phosphate: 0.5 mg base/kg, orally, once daily × 14 days	
Uncomplicated malaria: alternatives for pregnant women[38,39,40]	Chloroquine-sensitive (see uncomplicated malaria sections above for chloroquine-sensitive species by region)			
	Chloroquine phosphate[35]	600 mg base (=1000 mg salt), orally, immediately; followed by 300 mg base (=500 mg salt), orally, at 6, 24, and 48 h Total dose: 1500 mg base (=2500 mg salt)	Not applicable	

Table 4.10. Drugs for Parasitic Infections, continued

Disease	Drug	Adult Dosage	Pediatric Dosage	CDC Web Site, including listings of adverse events
	OR			
	Hydroxychloro-quine	620 mg base (=800 mg salt), orally, immediately, followed by 310 mg base (=400 mg salt), orally, at 6, 24, and 48 h Total dose: 1550 mg base (=2000 mg salt)	Not applicable	
Chloroquine-resistant (see sections above for regions with chloroquine resistant *P. falciparum and P. vivax*)				
	Quinine sulfate plus Clindamycin	Quinine sulfate: 542 mg base (=650 mg salt),[4] orally, 3 times/day × 3 or 7 days[5] Clindamycin: 20 mg base/kg/day, orally, divided 3 times/day × 7 days	Not applicable	
	OR			
	Mefloquine	684 mg base (=750 mg salt), orally, as initial dose, followed by 456 mg base (=500 mg salt), orally, given 6–12 h after initial dose Total dose =1250 mg salt	Not applicable	

Table 4.10. Drugs for Parasitic Infections, continued

Disease	Drug	Adult Dosage	Pediatric Dosage	CDC Web Site, including listings of adverse events
Severe malaria[41,42,43]	All regions			
	Quinidine gluconate[31] plus one of the following: Doxycycline, Tetracycline, or Clindamycin	Quinidine gluconate: 6.25 mg base/kg (=10 mg salt/kg) loading dose, IV over 1–2 h, then 0.0125 mg base/kg/min (=0.02 mg salt/kg/min) continuous infusion for at least 24 h. An alternative regimen is 15 mg base/kg (=24 mg salt/kg) loading dose, IV infused over 4 h, followed by 7.5 mg base/kg (=12 mg salt/kg) infused over 4 h every 8 h, starting 8 h after the loading dose (see package insert). Once parasite density <1% and patient can take oral medication, complete treatment with oral quinine, dose as above. Quinidine/quinine course = 7 days in Southeast Asia; = 3 days in Africa or South America.	Quinidine gluconate: Same mg/kg dosing and recommendations as for adults. Doxycycline: 2.2 mg/kg, orally, every 12 h × 7 days. If patient not able to take oral medication, may give IV. For children <45 kg, give 2.2 mg/kg, IV, every 12 h and then switch to oral doxycycline (dose as above) as soon as patient can take oral medication. For children >45 kg, use same dosing as for adults. For IV use, avoid rapid administration. Treatment course = 7 days. Tetracycline: 25 mg/kg/day, orally, divided 4 times/day × 7 days	

Table 4.10. Drugs for Parasitic Infections, continued

Disease	Drug	Adult Dosage	Pediatric Dosage	CDC Web Site, including listings of adverse events
		Doxycycline: 100 mg, orally, 2 times/day × 7 days If patient not able to take oral medication, give 100 mg, IV, every 12 h and then switch to oral doxycycline (as above) as soon as patient can take oral medication. For IV use, avoid rapid administration. Treatment course = 7 days.	Clindamycin: 20 mg base/kg/day, orally, divided 3 times/day × 7 days. If patient not able to take oral medication, give 10 mg base/kg loading dose, IV, followed by 5 mg base/kg, IV, every 8 h. Switch to oral clindamycin (oral dose as above) as soon as patient can take oral medication. For IV use, avoid rapid administration. Treatment course = 7 days.	
		Tetracycline: 250 mg, orally, 4 times/day × 7 days	*Investigational new drug (contact CDC for information):*	

Table 4.10. Drugs for Parasitic Infections, continued

Disease	Drug	Adult Dosage	Pediatric Dosage	CDC Web Site, including listings of adverse events
		Clindamycin: 20 mg base/ kg/day, orally, divided 3 times/day × 7 days. If patient not able to take oral medication, give 10 mg base/kg loading dose, IV, followed by 5 mg base/kg, IV, every 8 h. Switch to oral clindamycin (oral dose as above) as soon as patient can take oral medication. For IV use, avoid rapid administration. Treatment course = 7 days. *Investigational new drug (contact CDC for information):* Artesunate followed by one of the following: atovaquone-proguanil, doxycycline (clindamycin in pregnant women), or mefloquine	Artesunate followed by one of the following: atovaquone-proguanil, clindamycin, or mefloquine	

Table 4.10. Drugs for Parasitic Infections, continued

Disease	Drug	Adult Dosage	Pediatric Dosage	CDC Web Site, including listings of adverse events
Neurocysticercosis[44]	Albendazole[9]	400 mg, orally, 2 times/day × 15 days; can be repeated as necessary	15 mg/kg/day (max 800 mg), orally, in divided 2 times/day × 15 days; can be repeated as necessary	www.cdc.gov/parasites/cysticercosis/health_professionals/index.html
	OR			
	Praziquantel[15]	100 mg/kg/day, orally, in 3 divided doses × 1 day, then 50 mg/kg/day in 3 divided doses × 29 days		
Onchocerciasis (*Onchocerca volvulus*; River Blindness)[45]	Ivermectin	150 µg/kg, orally, in 1 dose every 6 mo until asymptomatic		www.cdc.gov/parasites/onchocerciasis/health_professionals/index.html
	OR			
	Doxycycline[46]	200 mg, orally, daily for 6 wk		
Opisthorchis Infection (Southeast Asian liver fluke)	Praziquantel[15]	75 mg/kg/day, orally, divided 3 times/day for 2 days		www.cdc.gov/parasites/opisthorchis/health_professionals/index.html
	OR			
	Albendazole[9]	10 mg/kg/day, orally, for 7 days		
Paragonimiasis	Praziquantel[15]	75 mg/kg/day, orally, divided 3 times/day for 2 days		www.cdc.gov/parasites/paragonimus/health_professionals/index.html
	OR			
	Triclabendazole[18]	10 mg/kg, orally, once or twice		

Table 4.10. Drugs for Parasitic Infections, continued

Disease	Drug	Adult Dosage	Pediatric Dosage	CDC Web Site, including listings of adverse events
Scabies (Mite Infestation)	Permethrin cream 5%	Topically, twice, at least 7 days apart		www.cdc.gov/parasites/scabies/health_professionals/meds.html
	OR			
	Crotamiton lotion 10% and Crotamiton cream 10%	Topically, overnight, on days 1, 2, 3, and 8		
	OR			
	Ivermectin	200 µg/kg, orally, twice, at least 7 days apart		
Schistosomiasis (Bilharzia)	*Schistosoma mansoni, S haematobium, S intercalatum*			www.cdc.gov/parasites/schistosomiasis/health_professionals/index.html
	Praziquantel[15] *S japonicum, S mekongi*	40 mg/kg/day, orally, divided 2 times/day for 1 day		
	Praziquantel[15]	60 mg/kg/day, orally, divided 3 times/day for 1 day		
Strongyloidiasis	Ivermectin	200 µg/kg, orally, daily for 1–2 days; for patients unable to take ivermectin orally, a parenteral formulation is available commercially for veterinary use and may be used under a single patient investigational new drug application on request to FDA		www.cdc.gov/parasites/strongyloides/health_professionals/index.html
	OR			
	Albendazole[9]	400 mg, orally, divided 2 times/day for 7 days		

Table 4.10. Drugs for Parasitic Infections, continued

Disease	Drug	Adult Dosage	Pediatric Dosage	CDC Web Site, including listings of adverse events
Taeniasis [*Taenia saginata* (beef tapeworm), *Taenia solium* (pork tapeworm), and *Taenia asiatica* (Asian tapeworm)]	Praziquantel[15]	5–10 mg/kg, orally, once		www.cdc.gov/parasites/taeniasis/health_professionals/index.html
	OR			
	Niclosamide[16]	2 g, orally, once	50 mg/kg, orally, once	
Toxocariasis (Ocular Larva Migrans, Visceral Larva Migrans)	Albendazole[9]	400 mg, orally, 2 times/day × 5 days		www.cdc.gov/parasites/toxocariasis/health_professionals/index.html
	OR			
	Mebendazole[10]	100–200 mg, orally, 2 times/day × 5 days		
Toxoplasmosis CNS disease (*Toxoplasma gondii*)[47]	Pyrimethamine[48]	200 mg, orally, once, then 50–75 mg/day, orally × 3–6 wk	2 mg/kg/day, orally, × 2 days, then 1 mg/kg/day (max 25 mg/day) × 3–6 wk	www.cdc.gov/parasites/toxoplasmosis/health_professionals/index.html
	PLUS			
	Sulfadiazine	1.5 g, orally, 4 times/day × 3–6 wk	100–200 mg/kg/day, orally, divided every 6 h × 3–6 wk	
	OR			
	Pyrimethamine[48]	200 mg, orally, once, then 50–75 mg/day, orally, × 3–6 wk	2 mg/kg/day, orally, × 2 days, then 1 mg/kg/day (max 25 mg/day) × 3–6 wk	
	PLUS			

Table 4.10. Drugs for Parasitic Infections, continued

Disease	Drug	Adult Dosage	Pediatric Dosage	CDC Web Site, including listings of adverse events
	Clindamycin	1.8–2.4 g/day, IV or orally, divided 3 or 4 times/day × 3–6 wk	5–7.5 mg/kg/dose (max 600 mg/dose), orally, divided 3 or 4 times/day × 3–6 wk	
	OR			
	Pyrimeth-amine[48]	200 mg, orally, once, then 50–75 mg/day, orally, × 3–6 wk	2 mg/kg/day, orally, × 2 days, then 1 mg/kg/day (max 25 mg/day) × 3–6 wk	
	PLUS			
	Atovaquone	1500 mg, orally, 2 times/day	See footnote 47	
	OR			
	Trimethoprim/Sulfamethox-azole	15–20 mg/kg TMP and 75–100 mg/kg SMX per day divided 3 or 4 times/day × 3–6 wk	15–20 mg/kg TMP and 75–100 mg/kg SMX per day divided 3 or 4 times/day × 3–6 wk	

Table 4.10. Drugs for Parasitic Infections, continued

Disease	Drug	Adult Dosage	Pediatric Dosage	CDC Web Site, including listings of adverse events
Toxoplasmosis in pregnancy and neonates (*Toxoplasma gondii*)	See footnote 49.			www.cdc.gov/parasites/toxoplasmosis/health_professionals/index.html
Trichinellosis (trichinosis; *Trichinella species*)	Albendazole[9]	400 mg, orally, twice a day for 8 to 14 days		www.cdc.gov/parasites/trichinellosis/health_professionals/index.html
	OR			
	Mebendazole[10]	200–400 mg, orally, 3 times a day for 3 days, then 400–500 mg, orally, 3 times a day for 10 days		
Trichuriasis (whipworm infection; *Trichuris trichiura*)	Albendazole[9]	400 mg, orally, for 3 days		www.cdc.gov/parasites/whipworm/health_professionals/index.html
	OR			
	Mebendazole[10]	100 mg, orally, twice a day for 3 days		
	OR			
	Ivermectin	200 µg/kg/day, orally, for 3 days		

MedWatch–The FDA Safety Information and Adverse Event-Reporting Program

MedWatch, the Food and Drug Administration (FDA) Safety Information and Adverse Event Reporting Program, serves as a gateway for clinically important safety information and reporting serious problems with human medical products, including FDA-regulated drugs, biologics (including human cells, tissues, and cellular and tissue-based products), medical devices (including in vitro diagnostics), special nutritional products, and cosmetics. Serious adverse events include those that are reported as fatal, disabling, life threatening, requiring hospital admission, prolonging a hospital stay, resulting in a congenital anomaly, or requiring medical intervention to prevent such an outcome. Reports are used by the FDA as a data source to identify and evaluate new safety concerns with drugs and devices after they are approved and more widely used in clinical practice. Many prelicensure clinical trials are not large enough to reveal rare adverse events. Based on information from postmarketing safety surveillance, the FDA may take regulatory actions, such as revising and strengthening warnings, precautions, contraindications, and adverse reaction descriptions in the package insert; issuing "Dear Health Care Professional" letters; and posting safety notifications on the agency's Web site.

Health care professionals and consumers are encouraged to report product quality problems and adverse events. The MedWatch voluntary form is a 1-page, postage-paid form (see Fig 4.1, p 958). Adverse events can be reported online at **www.fda.gov/ MedWatch/report.htm.** The MedWatch form can also be sent by fax (800-FDA-0178) or mail. A toll-free number (800-FDA-1088) is available to report by phone or request blank forms with instructions.

Vaccine-related adverse events should be reported to the Vaccine Adverse Event Reporting System **(http://vaers.hhs.gov/)** (see p 46).

FIG 4.1 MEDWATCH REPORTING FORM

Reset Form

U.S. Department of Health and Human Services

MEDWATCH

The FDA Safety Information and
Adverse Event Reporting Program

For VOLUNTARY reporting of
adverse events, product problems and
product use errors

Page 1 of 3

Form Approved: OMB No. 0910-0291, Expires: 6/30/2015
See PRA statement on reverse.

FDA USE ONLY

Triage unit
sequence #

A. PATIENT INFORMATION

1. Patient Identifier | 2. Age at Time of Event or Date of Birth: | 3. Sex | 4. Weight

☐ Female lb

☐ Male or kg

In confidence

B. ADVERSE EVENT, PRODUCT PROBLEM OR ERROR

Check all that apply:

1. ☐ Adverse Event ☐ Product Problem (e.g., defects/malfunctions)

☐ Product Use Error ☐ Problem with Different Manufacturer of Same Medicine

2. Outcomes Attributed to Adverse Event
(Check all that apply)

☐ Death: _____ (mm/dd/yyyy)

☐ Life-threatening

☐ Hospitalization - initial or prolonged

☐ Required Intervention to Prevent Permanent Impairment/Damage (Devices)

☐ Disability or Permanent Damage

☐ Congenital Anomaly/Birth Defect

☐ Other Serious (Important Medical Events)

3. Date of Event (mm/dd/yyyy) | 4. Date of this Report (mm/dd/yyyy)

5. Describe Event, Problem or Product Use Error

(Continue on page 3)

6. Relevant Tests/Laboratory Data, Including Dates

(Continue on page 3)

7. Other Relevant History, Including Preexisting Medical Conditions (e.g., allergies, race, pregnancy, smoking and alcohol use, liver/kidney problems, etc.)

(Continue on page 3)

C. PRODUCT AVAILABILITY

Product Available for Evaluation? (Do not send product to FDA)

☐ Yes ☐ No ☐ Returned to Manufacturer on: _____ (mm/dd/yyyy)

D. SUSPECT PRODUCT(S)

1. Name, Strength, Manufacturer (from product label)

#1 Name:
Strength:
Manufacturer:

#2 Name:
Strength:
Manufacturer:

FORM FDA 3500 (2/13) Submission of a report does not constitute an admission that medical personnel or the product caused or contributed to the event.

---

2. Dose or Amount | Frequency | Route

#1

#2

3. Dates of Use (If unknown, give duration) from/to (or best estimate)

#1

#2

4. Diagnosis or Reason for Use (Indication)

#1

#2

5. Event Abated After Use Stopped or Dose Reduced?

#1 ☐ Yes ☐ No ☐ Doesn't Apply

#2 ☐ Yes ☐ No ☐ Doesn't Apply

8. Event Reappeared After Reintroduction?

#1 ☐ Yes ☐ No ☐ Doesn't Apply

#2 ☐ Yes ☐ No ☐ Doesn't Apply

6. Lot #
#1
#2

7. Expiration Date
#1
#2

9. NDC # or Unique ID

E. SUSPECT MEDICAL DEVICE

1. Brand Name

2. Common Device Name | 2b. Procode

3. Manufacturer Name, City and State

4. Model # | Lot # | 5. Operator of Device
   ☐ Health Professional

Catalog # | Expiration Date (mm/dd/yyyy) | ☐ Lay User/Patient

Serial # | Unique Identifier (UDI) # | ☐ Other:

6. If Implanted, Give Date (mm/dd/yyyy) | 7. If Explanted, Give Date (mm/dd/yyyy)

8. Is this a Single-use Device that was Reprocessed and Reused on a Patient?
☐ Yes ☐ No

9. If Yes to Item No. 8, Enter Name and Address of Reprocessor

F. OTHER (CONCOMITANT) MEDICAL PRODUCTS

Product names and therapy dates (exclude treatment of event)

(Continue on page 3)

G. REPORTER (See confidentiality section on back)

1. Name and Address

Name:
Address:

City: State: ZIP:

Phone # | E-mail

2. Health Professional? | 3. Occupation | 4. Also Reported to:
☐ Yes ☐ No | | ☐ Manufacturer

5. If you do NOT want your identity disclosed to the manufacturer, place an "X" in this box: ☐ | ☐ User Facility
 ☐ Distributor/Importer

PLEASE TYPE OR USE BLACK INK

Available for download at **www.fda.gov/downloads/AboutFDA/ReportsManualsForms/Forms/UCM163919.pdf.**

Antimicrobial Prophylaxis

ANTIMICROBIAL PROPHYLAXIS

Antimicrobial prophylaxis is defined as the use of antimicrobial drugs in the absence of suspected or documented infection to prevent development of infection or disease and is a common practice in pediatrics. The efficacy of such prophylactic antimicrobial agents has been documented for some conditions but not for many more for which it is used. "Antibiotic solutions" for irrigation or instillation should not be considered prophylaxis and generally are unproven as efficacious for prevention of infection.

Effective chemoprophylaxis should be directed at pathogens common in the infection-prone body sites (Table 5.1). When using prophylactic antimicrobial therapy, the risk of emergence of antimicrobial-resistant organisms and the possibility of an adverse event from the drug must be weighed against potential benefits. Ideally, prophylactic agents should have a narrow spectrum of activity and should be used for as brief a period as possible.

Table 5.1. Antimicrobial Chemoprophylaxis[a]

Anatomic Site-Related Infections	Exposed Host; Time-Limited Exposure	Vulnerable Host (Pathogen); Ongoing Exposure
Otitis media	*Bordetella pertussis* exposure	Immunosuppressed patients because
Urinary tract	*Neisseria meningitidis* exposure	of treatment of conditions, eg, on-
infection	Traveler's diarrhea (*Escherichia coli*,	cologic, rheumatologic (*Pneumocystis*
Endocarditis	*Shigella* species, *Salmonella* species,	*jirovecii*, fungi)
	Campylobacter species)	Organ transplant patients (CMV,
	Perinatal group B *Streptococcus* (mother/	*P jirovecii*, fungi)
	infant) exposure	HIV-infected children (*P jirovecii*; poly-
	Bite wound (human, animal, reptile)	saccharide-encapsulated bacteria)
	Infants born to HIV-infected moth-	Preterm neonates (*Candida* species)
	ers, to decrease the risk of HIV	Anatomic or functional asplenia
	transmission.	(polysaccharide-encapsulated bacteria)
	Influenza virus, following close family	Chronic granulomatous disease
	exposure in those unimmunized	(*Staphylococcus aureus* and certain
	Susceptible contacts of index cases of	other catalase-positive bacteria and
	invasive *Haemophilus influenzae* type	fungi)
	b disease	Congenital immune deficiencies
	Exposure to aerosolized spores of	(various pathogens)
	Bacillus anthracis	Rheumatic fever (group A streptococcus)
		Infant with neonatal HSV disease[b]

HIV indicates human immunodeficiency virus; CMV, cytomegalovirus; HSV, herpes simplex virus.

[a] Antimicrobial prophylactic regimens for exposed hosts and vulnerable hosts (pathogens) are described in each pathogen or disease-specific chapter in Section 3. Immune globulin prophylaxis is not discussed in this Section but should be considered for specific bacteria (eg, *Clostridium tetani* or viruses [eg, respiratory syncytial virus]).

[b] 6-month post-treatment suppressive therapy to prevent reactivation within the brain or on the skin.

Infection-Prone Body Sites

Antibiotic prophylaxis in vulnerable body sites is most successful if: (1) the period of risk is defined and brief; (2) the expected pathogens have predictable antimicrobial susceptibility; and (3) the site is accessible to adequate antimicrobial concentrations.

ACUTE OTITIS MEDIA

Acute otitis media recurs less frequently in otitis-prone children treated prophylactically with antimicrobial agents. Studies have demonstrated that amoxicillin, sulfisoxazole, and trimethoprim-sulfamethoxazole are effective. However, antimicrobial prophylaxis may alter the nasopharyngeal flora and foster colonization with resistant organisms, compromising long-term efficacy of the prophylactic drug and treatment options if disease occurs while a person is receiving prophylaxis. Continuous orally administered antimicrobial prophylaxis should be reserved for control of recurrent acute otitis media, only when defined as 3 or more distinct and well-documented episodes during a period of 6 months or 4 or more episodes during a period of 12 months. Although prophylactic administration of an antimicrobial agent limited to a period of time when a person is at high risk of otitis media, such as during acute viral respiratory tract infection, has been suggested, this method has not been evaluated critically.

The use of pneumococcal conjugate vaccines (eg, PCV13) has been effective in reducing acute bacterial otitis media in vaccine recipients. The risks and benefits of other methods of preventing recurrent otitis media in high risk children, such as placement of tympanostomy tubes, has not been systematically compared with antimicrobial prophylaxis.

URINARY TRACT INFECTION[1]

The role of chemoprophylaxis for urinary tract infection (UTI) has come under increasing scrutiny. The effectiveness of prophylactic therapy depends on the rate of emergence of antimicrobial resistance in the gastrointestinal tract flora, which is the usual source of bacteria causing urinary tract infection. Resistance usually will develop to any agent used for prophylaxis. Careful consideration of the anatomic abnormalities of the urinary tract, the consequences of recurrent infection, the risks of infection caused by a resistant pathogen, and the anticipated duration of prophylaxis need to be individually assessed. Data do not support use of antimicrobial prophylaxis to prevent febrile recurrent UTIs in infants without vesicoureteral reflux (VUR),[1] but among children with grade I through IV VUR, chemoprophylaxis decreases recurrent UTIs by 50% following a first or second febrile or symptomatic UTI, albeit with an increase in detection of resistant organisms.[2,3]

---

[1]American Academy of Pediatrics, Subcommittee on Urinary Tract Infections, Steering Committee on Quality Improvement and Management. Urinary tract infection: clinical practice guideline for the diagnosis and management of the initial UTI in febrile infants and children 2 to 24 months. *Pediatrics.* 2011;128(3):595–610

[2]Craig JC, Simpson JM, Williams GJ, et al; Prevention of Recurrent Urinary Tract Infection in Children with Vesicoureteric Reflux and Normal Renal Tracts (PRIVENT) Investigators. Antibiotic prophylaxis and recurrent urinary tract infection in children. *N Engl J Med.* 2009;361(18):1748–1759

[3]The RIVUR Trial Investigators. Antimicrobial prophylaxis for children with vesicoureteral reflux. *N Engl J Med.* 2014;370(25):2367–2376

Exposure to Specific Pathogens

Prophylaxis may be appropriate or indicated if an increased risk of serious infection with a specific pathogen exists and a specific antimicrobial agent has been demonstrated to decrease the risk of infection by that pathogen. It is assumed that the benefit of prophylaxis is greater than the risk of adverse effects of the antimicrobial agent or the risk of subsequent infection by antimicrobial-resistant organisms. For some pathogens that colonize the upper respiratory tract, elimination of the carrier state can be difficult and may require use of a specific antimicrobial agent that achieves microbiologically effective concentrations in nasopharyngeal secretions (eg, rifampin).

Vulnerable Hosts

Attempts to prevent serious infections in specific populations of vulnerable patients with antimicrobial prophylaxis have been successful in some carefully defined populations that are known to be at risk of infection caused by defined pathogens. In some situations, such as prophylaxis of pneumococcal bacteremia in asplenic children, resistance to beta-lactam agents may lead to decreased effectiveness of continuous prophylaxis. In other situations, such as prophylaxis of *Pneumocystis* infection in immune-compromised children with trimethoprim-sulfamethoxazole, resistance has not appeared to develop despite years of continuous prophylaxis.

ANTIMICROBIAL PROPHYLAXIS IN PEDIATRIC SURGICAL PATIENTS

Surgical site infections (SSIs) complicate 2% to 5% of inpatient surgeries, prolong the length of hospitalization, and increase the risk of death. Prevention of SSIs should be a priority for children's hospitals. Active surveillance targeting high-risk, high-volume procedures should be performed and requires education of surgeons and perioperative personnel, technological infrastructure, and use of a multidisciplinary team of trained personnel who are knowledgeable regarding SSI criteria. Institutions should monitor compliance with basic process measures and provide feedback to surgical personnel and leadership.

Prevention of postoperative wound infections through perioperative prophylaxis generally is recommended for procedures with moderate or high infection rates, such as appendectomy for a ruptured appendix, and for procedures in which the consequences of infection are likely to be serious, such as implantation of prosthetic material. Consensus recommendations for prevention of SSIs in adults and children have been developed. Although few data exist specifically for pediatric surgical prophylaxis, the principles of antimicrobial agent selection and exposure at surgical sites in adults should apply to children. Additional consequences of inappropriate prophylactic use of antimicrobial agents include increased costs and adverse events as a result of unnecessary drug use and potential emergence of resistant organisms, posing a risk not only to the recipient but also to other hospitalized patients in whom a health care-associated infection could develop.

Guidelines for Appropriate Use

Guidelines for prevention of SSIs have been published.[1,2] General principles include that agents use for antimicrobial prophylaxis should prevent SSIs and related morbidity and mortality, should reduce the duration and cost of care, should produce no adverse effects, and should minimize adverse consequences on the microbial flora. Recommendations address indications, appropriate drug selection, dosing, preoperative timing and need for intraoperative redosing, and duration of prophylaxis.

Indications for Prophylaxis

Major determinants of postoperative surgical site infection include the number of micro-organisms in the wound during the procedure, the virulence of the microorganisms, the presence of foreign material in the wound, and host risk factors. The classification of surgical procedures is based on an estimation of bacterial contamination and, thus, risk of subsequent infection. The 4 classes are: (1) clean wounds; (2) clean-contaminated wounds; (3) contaminated wounds; and (4) dirty and infected wounds. Additional independent factors include the operation site, the duration of procedure, and the patient's preoperative health status. A patient risk index, which incorporates the American Society of Anesthesiologists' preoperative physical status assessment score, the duration of the operation, and the aforementioned wound classification, has been demonstrated to be a good predictor of postoperative surgical site infection.[3] Others have summarized those at "high risk" of surgical site infection.[2] Although a high-risk pediatric patient is not clearly defined, high-risk factors in adult patients may include obesity, coexistent infections at a remote body site, altered immune response, colonization with pathogenic microorganisms, and diabetes mellitus. Limited data are available on optimal dosing in the obese child.

CLEAN WOUNDS

Clean wounds are uninfected operative wounds in which no inflammation is encountered; the respiratory, alimentary, and genitourinary tracts or oropharyngeal cavity are not entered; and no break in aseptic technique occurred. The operative procedures are elective, and wounds are closed primarily and, if necessary, drained with closed drainage. Operative incisional wounds that follow nonpenetrating (blunt) abdominal trauma should be included in this category, provided that the surgical procedure does not entail entry into the gastrointestinal or genitourinary tracts. The benefits of systemic antimicrobial prophylaxis do not justify the potential risks associated with antimicrobial use in most

---

[1]Antimicrobial prophylaxis for surgery. *Treat Guidel Med Lett.* 2012;10(122):73–78

[2]Bratzler DW, Dellinger EP, Olsen KM, et al; American Society of Health-System Pharmacists; Infectious Disease Society of America; Surgical Infection Society; Society for Healthcare Epidemiology of America. Clinical practice guidelines for antimicrobial prophylaxis in surgery. *Am J Health Syst Pharm.* 2013;70(3):195–283

[3]Gaynes RP, Culver DH, Horan TC, Edwards JR, Richards C, Tolson JS. Surgical site infection (SSI) rates in the United States, 1992-1998: the National Nosocomial Surveillance System basic SSI risk index. *Clin Infect Dis.* 2001;33(suppl2):S69–S77

clean wound procedures, because the risk of infection is low (1%–2%). Some exceptions exist in which prophylaxis is given because the risks or consequences of infection are high. Examples include implantation of intravascular prosthetic material (eg, insertion of a prosthetic heart valve) or a prosthetic joint, open-heart surgery for repair of structural defects, body cavity exploration in neonates, and most neurosurgical operations.

CLEAN-CONTAMINATED WOUNDS

In clean-contaminated wounds, the respiratory, alimentary, or genitourinary tracts are entered under controlled conditions without significant contamination. Operations involving the gastrointestinal tract, the biliary tract, appendix, vagina, or oropharynx and urgent or emergency surgery in an otherwise clean procedure are included in this category, provided that no evidence of infection is encountered and no major break in aseptic technique occurs. Prophylaxis is limited to procedures in which a substantial amount of wound contamination is expected. The overall risk of infection for these surgical sites is 3% to 15%. On the basis of data from adults, procedures for which prophylaxis is indicated for pediatric patients include: (1) all gastrointestinal tract procedures in which there is obstruction, when the patient is receiving H_2 receptor antagonists or proton pump blockers, or when the patient has a permanent foreign body; (2) selected biliary tract operations (eg, when there is obstruction from common bile duct stones); and (3) urinary tract surgery or instrumentation in the presence of bacteriuria or obstructive uropathy.

CONTAMINATED WOUNDS

Contaminated wounds are previously sterile tissue sites that are likely to be heavily contaminated with bacteria and include open, fresh wounds; operative wounds in the setting of major breaks in aseptic technique or gross spillage from the gastrointestinal tract; exposed viscera at birth from congenital anomalies; penetrating trauma of fewer than 4 hours' duration; and incisions in which acute nonpurulent inflammation is encountered. The estimated rate of infection for these surgical sites is 15%. In contaminated wound procedures, antimicrobial prophylaxis is appropriate for some patients with acute nonpurulent inflammation isolated to, and contained within, an inflamed viscus (such as acute, nonperforated appendicitis or cholecystitis). For wounds in which contaminating bacteria have had an opportunity to establish inflammation and ongoing infection, antimicrobial therapy should be considered as treatment rather than prophylaxis.

DIRTY AND INFECTED WOUNDS

Dirty and infected wounds include penetrating trauma of more than 4 hours' duration from time of occurrence, wounds with retained devitalized tissue, and wounds involving existing clinical infection or perforated viscera. This definition suggests that the organisms causing postoperative infection were present in the operative field before surgery. The estimated rate of infection for these surgical sites is 40%. In dirty and infected wound procedures, such as procedures for a perforated abdominal viscus (eg, ruptured appendix), a compound fracture, a laceration attributable to an animal or human bite, or major break in sterile technique, antimicrobial agents are given as treatment rather than prophylaxis.

Surgical Site Infection Criteria

Specific classification criteria for SSIs have been developed by the National Healthcare Safety Network.

SUPERFICIAL INCISIONAL SSI

A superficial incisional SSI is diagnosed if a superficial wound appearance is consistent with infection, occurs within 30 days of operation, and consists of one of the following: (1) purulent drainage from the superficial incision; (2) organism growth from an aseptically obtained culture of fluid or tissue; (3) surgical wound exploration with no culture or positive culture; or (4) surgeon diagnosis of incisional wound infection.

DEEP INCISIONAL SSI

A deep incisional SSI occurs within 30 days after the operative procedure if no implant is left in place or within 1 year if an implant is in place, the infection appears to be related to the operative procedure, and the patient has at least one of the following: (1) purulent drainage from the deep incision but not from the organ/space component of the surgical site; (2) a deep incision that spontaneously dehisces or is deliberately opened by a surgeon and is culture positive or not cultured and the patient has at least 1 of the following signs or symptoms: fever (>38°C) or localized pain or tenderness (a culture-negative finding does not meet this criterion); (3) an abscess or other evidence of infection involving the deep incision that is found on direct examination, during reoperation, or by histopathologic or radiologic examination; or (4) diagnosis of a deep incisional SSI by a surgeon or attending physician.

ORGAN/SPACE SSI

An organ or space SSI is defined by the specific site of infection (eg, endocarditis, mediastinitis, osteomyelitis) and excludes the skin incision, fascia, or muscle layers that have been manipulated during the procedure. Organ/space SSI must occur within 30 days of the operation or within 1 year if an implant is in place, and the patient must have 1 or more of the following: (1) purulent drainage from a drain that is placed through a stab wound into the organ/space; (2) organisms isolated from an aseptically obtained culture of fluid or tissue in the organ/space; (3) an abscess or other evidence of infection involving the organ/space that is found on direct examination, during reoperation, or by histopathologic or radiologic examination; or (4) diagnosis of an organ/space SSI by a surgeon or attending physician.

Timing of Administration of Prophylactic Antimicrobial Agents

Effective chemoprophylaxis occurs only when adequate antimicrobial drug concentrations are present in tissues at sufficient local concentrations at the time of intraoperative bacterial contamination. Administration of an antimicrobial agent within 1 or 2 hours before surgery has been demonstrated to decrease the risk of wound infection. Accordingly, administration of the prophylactic agent is recommended within 60 minutes before surgical incision to ensure adequate tissue concentrations at the start of the procedure. When antimicrobial agents require longer administration times, such as with glycopeptides (eg, vancomycin) or fluoroquinolones, administration should begin within 120 minutes before the surgery begins.

Dosing and Duration of Administration of Antimicrobial Agents

Weight-based dosing for pediatric patients is routine, but preoperative doses should not exceed the usual dose for adults. Many hospitals currently use 2 g of cefazolin as the standard dose for adult patients and 3 g for patients weighing >120 kg.

Adequate antimicrobial concentrations should be maintained throughout the surgical procedure; in most instances, a single dose of an antimicrobial agent is sufficient. Intraoperative dosing is required if the duration of the procedure is greater than 2 times the half-life of the antimicrobial agent or if there is excessive blood loss (eg, >1500 mL in adults). For example, cefazolin may be administered every 3 to 4 hours during a prolonged surgical procedure that involves large-volume blood loss. Postoperative doses after closure generally are not recommended. Duration of prophylaxis should be 24 hours after the procedure for all procedures.

Preoperative Screening and Decolonization

The use of preoperative surveillance to identify carriers of methicillin-susceptible *Staphylococcus aureus* (MSSA) or methicillin-resistant *S aureus* (MRSA) has been explored in the adult population. Use of preoperative nasal mupirocin and chlorhexidine baths for *S aureus* carriers may reduce the risk of deep SSI and is recommended as an adjunct to intravenous prophylaxis in adult cardiac and orthopedic surgery patients.

Recommended Antimicrobial Agents

An antimicrobial agent is chosen on the basis of bacterial pathogens most likely to cause infectious complications during and after the specific procedure, the antimicrobial susceptibility pattern of these pathogens, and the safety and efficacy of the drug. Newer, more broad-spectrum, and more costly antimicrobial agents generally are not recommended unless prophylactic efficacy has been proven to be superior to drugs of established benefit or there is a shift in organisms and/or their antimicrobial resistance patterns causing surgical site infections. Antimicrobial agents administered prophylactically do not have to be active in vitro against every potential organism to be effective, because it is unlikely that all potential organisms are actually contaminating the wound. Doses and routes of administration are determined on the basis of the need to achieve therapeutic blood and tissue concentrations throughout the procedure. Antimicrobial prophylaxis for most surgical procedures (including gastric, biliary, thoracic [noncardiac], vascular, neurosurgical, and orthopedic operations) can be achieved effectively using an agent such as a first-generation cephalosporin (eg, cefazolin) unless the risk for MRSA infection is high, in which case vancomycin may be indicated. For colorectal surgery or appendectomy, effective prophylaxis requires antimicrobial agents that are active against aerobic and anaerobic intestinal flora. Table 5.2 (p 967) provides recommendations for drugs, including preoperative doses, to be used in children undergoing surgical manipulation or invasive procedures. Physicians should be aware of potential interactions and adverse effects associated with prophylactic antimicrobial agents and other medications the patient may be receiving. Routine use of extended-spectrum cephalosporins for surgical prophylaxis generally is not recommended. Hospital systems should be regularly evaluated to ensure that the process for provision, delivery, and maintenance of appropriate antimicrobial prophylaxis is in place. There are no data to support the practice of continuing antibiotic prophylaxis in cardiac surgery patients until all invasive lines, drains, and indwelling catheters have been removed.

Routine use of vancomycin for prophylaxis is not recommended. For children known to be colonized or previously infected by MRSA or for children living in a community with a high rate of MRSA infections, vancomycin prophylaxis may be considered.

Special considerations should be given to patients with congenital heart disease who undergo surgery or patients who undergo certain orthopedic procedures (eg, spinal procedures, implantation of foreign materials). Recommendations are found in Prevention of Bacterial Endocarditis, p 970.

Table 5.2. Recommendations for Preoperative Antimicrobial Prophylaxis[a]

Operation	Likely Pathogens	Recommended Drugs	Preoperative Dose
Neonatal (≤72 h of age)—all major procedures	Group B streptococci, enteric gram-negative bacilli,[b] enterococci, coagulase-negative Staphylococci	Ampicillin **PLUS** Gentamicin	50 mg/kg 2.5 mg/kg
Neonatal (>72 h of age)—all major procedures	Prophylaxis targeted to colonizing organisms, nosocomial organisms, and operative site		
Cardiac (cardiac surgical procedures, prosthetic valve or pacemaker, ventricular assist devices)	*Staphylococcus epidermidis*, *Staphylococcus aureus*, *Corynebacterium* species, enteric gram-negative bacilli[b]	Cefazolin **OR** (if MRSA or MRSE is likely)[a] Vancomycin	30 mg/kg 15 mg/kg
Gastrointestinal			
Esophageal and gastroduodenal	Enteric gram-negative bacilli,[b] gram-positive cocci	Cefazolin (high risk only[c])	30 mg/kg
Biliary tract	Enteric gram-negative bacilli,[b] enterococci,	Cefazolin[d]	30 mg/kg
Colorectal or appendectomy (uncomplicated, nonperforated)	Enteric gram-negative bacilli,[b] enterococci, anaerobes (*Bacteroides* species)[e]	Cefoxitin **OR** Metronidazole **PLUS** Gentamicin **OR** Cefazolin **PLUS** Metronidazole **OR** Clindamycin **PLUS** Gentamicin **OR** Ciprofloxacin	40 mg/kg 15 mg/kg 2.5 mg/kg 30 mg/kg 15 mg/kg 10 mg/kg 2.5 mg/kg (gentamicin); 10 mg/kg (ciprofloxacin)

Table 5.2. Recommendations for Preoperative Antimicrobial Prophylaxis,[a] continued

Operation	Likely Pathogens	Recommended Drugs	Preoperative Dose
Ruptured viscus (treatment, not prophylaxis)	Enteric gram-negative bacilli,[b] enterococci anaerobes (*Bacteroides* species)[e]	Cefoxitin	40 mg/kg
		WITH OR WITHOUT	
		Gentamicin	2 mg/kg
		OR	
		Gentamicin	2.5 mg/kg
		PLUS	
		Metronidazole	10 mg/kg
		PLUS	
		Ampicillin	50 mg/kg
		OR	
		Meropenem	20 mg/kg
		OR	
		Other regimens for complicated appendicitis[f]	
Genitourinary	Enteric gram-negative bacilli,[b] enterococci	Ampicillin	50 mg/kg
		PLUS	
		Gentamicin **OR** Cefazolin	2 mg/kg (gentamicin); 30 mg/kg (cefazolin)
Head and neck surgery (incision through oral or pharyngeal mucosa)	Anaerobes, enteric gram-negative bacilli,[b] *S aureus*	Clindamycin	10 mg/kg
		WITH OR WITHOUT	
		Gentamicin	2.5 mg/kg
		OR	
		Cefazolin	30 mg/kg
		PLUS	
		Metronidazole	15 mg/kg

Table 5.2. Recommendations for Preoperative Antimicrobial Prophylaxis,[a] continued

Operation	Likely Pathogens	Recommended Drugs	Preoperative Dose
Neurosurgery (craniotomy, intrathecal baclofen shunt or ventricular shunt placement)	*S epidermidis, S aureus*	Cefazolin **OR** (if MRSA or MRSE is likely)[a] Vancomycin	30 mg/kg 15 mg/kg
Ophthalmic	*S epidermidis, S aureus,* streptococci, enteric gram-negative bacilli[b] *Pseudomonas* species	Gentamicin, ciprofloxacin, ofloxacin, moxifloxacin, tobramycin **OR** Neomycin-gramicidin-polymyxin B **OR** Cefazolin	Multiple drops topically for 2–24 h before procedure Multiple drops topically for 2–24 h before procedure 100 mg, subconjunctivally 30 mg/kg
Orthopedic (internal fixation of fractures, implantation of materials including prosthetic joint and spinal procedures with and without instrumentation)	*S epidermidis, S aureus*	Cefazolin **OR** (if MRSA or MRSE is likely)[a] Vancomycin	30 mg/kg 15 mg/kg
Thoracic (noncardiac)	*S epidermidis, S aureus,* streptococci, gram-negative enteric bacilli[b]	Cefazolin **OR** (if MRSA or MRSE is likely)[a] Vancomycin	30 mg/kg 15 mg/kg
Traumatic wound (nonbites)	*S aureus,* group A streptococci, *Clostridium* species	Cefazolin	30 mg/kg

[a]MRSA indicates methicillin-resistant *Staphylococcus aureus*; MRSE indicates methicillin-resistant *S epidermidis*.

[b]Selection of antibiotics should take into consideration the institution-specific and patient-specific colonization/infection isolate susceptibility patterns.

[c] Esophageal obstruction, decreased gastric acidity or gastrointestinal motility; see text for additional high risk factors.

[d]Acute cholecystitis, nonfunctioning gallbladder, obstructive jaundice, common duct stones.

[e]High rates of resistance to clindamycin (approx 30%) now reported for *Bacteroides fragilis.* Lowest rates of resistance to carbapenems, ampicillin/sulbactam, and piperacillin/tazobactam. Resistance to cefoxitin reported at 3.5% to 9.4% (Snydman DR, Jacobus NV, McDermott LA, et al. Update on resistance of *Bacteroides fragilis* group and related species with special attention to carbapenems 2006-2009. *Anaerobe.* 2011;17[4]:147–151).

[f]Solomkin JS, Mazuski JE, Bradley JS, et al. Diagnosis and management of complicated intra-abdominal infection in adults and children: guidelines by the Surgical Infection Society and the Infectious Diseases Society of America (erratum in *Clin Infect Dis.* 2010;50[12]:1695; dosage error in article text). *Clin Infect Dis.* 201015;50(2):133–164.

PREVENTION OF BACTERIAL ENDOCARDITIS

The Committee on Rheumatic Fever, Endocarditis, and Kawasaki Disease of the American Heart Association periodically issues detailed recommendations on the rationale, indications, and antimicrobial regimens for prevention of bacterial endocarditis for people at increased risk. The most recent recommendations were published in 2007.[1] The committee noted that data have cast doubt on benefits of antimicrobial prophylaxis at time of dental procedures to prevent endocarditis, because bacteremia associated with most dental procedures represents only a small fraction of bacteremia episodes that occur with events of daily living, such as brushing teeth, chewing, and other oral hygiene measures. The committee has restricted recommendations for endocarditis prophylaxis to a considerably narrower group of people who have cardiac abnormalities and for fewer procedures than in the past. Although previous recommendations stressed endocarditis prophylaxis for people undergoing procedures most likely to produce bacteremia, this revision stresses those cardiac conditions in which an episode of infective endocarditis would have high risk of an adverse outcome. Furthermore, prophylaxis is recommended only for certain dental procedures. Prophylaxis no longer is recommended solely to prevent endocarditis for procedures involving the gastrointestinal and genitourinary tracts. The cardiac conditions and procedures for which endocarditis prophylaxis is recommended are discussed in this section, and specific prophylactic regimens are presented in Table 5.3 (p 971). Antibiotic prophylaxis is reasonable for patients who undergo an invasive procedure of the respiratory tract that involves incision of the respiratory tract mucosa. Physicians should consult the published recommendations for further details **(http://circ.ahajournals.org/cgi/content/full/116/15/1736).**

　　Cardiac conditions associated with the highest risk of adverse outcome from endocarditis for which prophylaxis with dental procedures is reasonable include the following[2]:

- Prosthetic cardiac valve or prosthetic material used for repair of valve.
- Previous infective endocarditis.
- Congenital heart disease (CHD)[2]:
  - ◆ Unrepaired cyanotic CHD, including palliative shunts and conduits.
  - ◆ Completely repaired congenital heart defect with prosthetic material or device, whether placed by surgery or by catheter intervention, during the first 6 months after the procedure.[3]
  - ◆ Repaired CHD with residual defect(s) at the site or adjacent to the site of a prosthetic patch or prosthetic device (which inhibit endothelialization).
- Cardiac transplantation with subsequent cardiac valvulopathy.

---

[1] Wilson W, Taubert KA, Gewitz M, et al. Prevention of Infective Endocarditis. Guidelines from the American Heart Association. A Guideline From the American Heart Association Rheumatic Fever, Endocarditis, and Kawasaki Diseases Committee, Council on Cardiovascular Disease in the Young, and the Council on Clinical Cardiology, Council on Cardiovascular Surgery and Anesthesia, and the Quality of Care and Outcomes Research Interdisciplinary Working Group. *Circulation.* 2007;116(15):1736–1754

[2] Except for the conditions listed, antimicrobial prophylaxis no longer is recommended for any other form of CHD.

[3] Prophylaxis is recommended, because endothelialization of prosthetic material occurs within 6 months after the procedure.

Table 5.3. Regimens for Antimicrobial Prophylaxis for a Dental Procedure

Situation	Agent	Regimen: Single Dose 30 to 60 min Before Procedure	
		Children	Adults
Oral	Amoxicillin	50 mg/kg	2 g
Unable to take oral medication	Ampicillin	50 mg/kg, IM or IV	2 g, IM or IV
	OR		
	Cefazolin or ceftriaxone	30 mg/kg, IM or IV (cefazolin); 50 mg/kg, IM or IV (ceftriaxone)	1 g, IM or IV
Allergic to penicillins or oral ampicillin	Cephalexin[a,b]	50 mg/kg	2 g
	OR		
	Clindamycin	10 mg/kg	900 mg
	OR		
	Azithromycin or clarithromycin	15 mg/kg	500 mg
Allergic to penicillins or ampicillin and unable to take oral medication	Cefazolin or ceftriaxone[b]	30 mg/kg, IM or IV (cefazolin); 50 mg/kg, IM or IV (ceftriaxone)	1 g, IM or IV
	OR		
	Clindamycin	10 mg/kg, IM or IV	900 mg, IM or IV

IM, indicates intramuscular; IV, intravenous.

[a] Or other first- or second-generation oral cephalosporin in equivalent pediatric or adult dosage.

[b] Cephalosporins should not be used in a person with a history of anaphylaxis, angioedema, or urticaria with penicillins or ampicillin.

Dental procedures for which endocarditis prophylaxis is reasonable for patients listed above include the following:

- All dental procedures that involve manipulation of gingival tissue or the periapical region of teeth or perforation of the oral mucosa.
- The following procedures and events do not require prophylaxis: routine anesthetic injections through noninfected tissue, taking dental radiographs, placement of removable prosthodontic or orthodontic appliances, adjustment of orthodontic appliances, placement of orthodontic brackets, shedding of deciduous teeth, and bleeding from trauma to the lips or oral mucosa.

PREVENTION OF NEONATAL OPHTHALMIA

Ophthalmia neonatorum is defined as conjunctivitis occurring within the first 4 weeks of life. Routine prophylaxis is mandated in most jurisdictions in the United States. The causes of ophthalmia neonatorum are presented in Table 5.4 (p 974). Neonates with ophthalmia neonatorum require clinical evaluation with appropriate laboratory testing and prompt initiation of therapy. Pregnant females at high risk of gonorrhea or *C trachomatis* infection, in particular females 24 years or younger and females with new or multiple sexual partners or living in an area in which the prevalence of *N gonorrhoeae* is high, should be targeted for screening. The Centers for Disease Control and Prevention recommends routine testing of all pregnant women during the first trimester and advises retesting of all pregnant females younger than 25 years during the third trimester to prevent perinatal complications. Pregnant females diagnosed with a chlamydial infection during the first trimester not only should receive a test to document chlamydial eradication 3 to 4 weeks after treatment but also should be tested 3 months after treatment as well as in the third trimester (see Chlamydial Infections, p 284, and Gonococcal Infections, p 356). If a pregnant female has not been evaluated for *Chlamydia trachomatis* and/or *Neisseria gonorrhoeae* prior to labor/delivery, these women should be evaluated during labor/delivery or immediately postpartum for *C trachomatis* and *N gonorrhoeae* infections. If either agent is identified, the infant should receive therapy as outlined in the following sections on gonococcal ophthalmia or chlamydial ophthalmia. A prophylactic agent should be instilled into the eyes of all newborn infants to prevent sight-threatening gonococcal ophthalmia, including infants born by cesarean delivery. Although infections usually are transmitted during passage through the birth canal, ascending infection can occur.

Gonococcal Ophthalmia

For prevention of gonococcal ophthalmia in newborn infants, 0.5% erythromycin ophthalmic ointment should be instilled in each eye in a single application. Although 1% silver nitrate solution and 1% tetracycline ophthalmic ointment are equally effective, they are no longer manufactured in the United States. Bacitracin is not effective, and povidone iodine has not been studied adequately. Healthy infants born to females with untreated gonococcal infection should receive 1 dose of ceftriaxone (25–50 mg/kg, intravenously [IV] or intramuscularly [IM], not to exceed 125 mg). Topical antimicrobial therapy alone is inadequate for *N gonorrhoeae*-exposed or infected infants and is not necessary when systemic antimicrobial therapy is administered. Infants who have gonococcal ophthalmia should be hospitalized, evaluated for disseminated infection, and treated (see Gonococcal Infections, p 356). Appropriate chlamydial testing should be performed simultaneously. Frequent eye irrigations with saline solution should be performed until resolution of the discharge. One dose of ceftriaxone is adequate therapy for gonococcal conjunctivitis. Evaluation by a pediatric ophthalmologist should be considered.

Chlamydial Ophthalmia

Recommended topical prophylaxis with erythromycin for all newborn infants for prevention of gonococcal ophthalmia will not prevent neonatal chlamydial conjunctivitis or extraocular infection, and it does not eliminate nasopharyngeal colonization by *C trachomatis*. Neonatal ophthalmia attributable to *C trachomatis* is not as clinically severe as gonococcal conjunctivitis. Chlamydial conjunctivitis in the neonate is characterized by a mucopurulent discharge, eyelid swelling, a propensity to form membranes on the palpebral conjunctiva, and lack of a follicular response and should be in the differential diagnosis for infants younger than 30 days who have conjunctivitis if the mother has a history of treated chlamydia infection. Most sensitive and specific nonculture tests, such as nucleic acid amplification tests (NAATs), are not cleared by the US Food and Drug Administration for detection of chlamydia from conjunctival swab specimens. However, laboratories that have met Clinical Laboratory Improvement Amendment (CLIA) requirements and validated chlamydia NAAT performance on conjunctival swab specimens may offer these tests. Infants with chlamydial conjunctivitis are treated with oral erythromycin base or ethylsuccinate (50 mg/kg/day in 4 divided doses daily) for 14 days or with azithromycin (20 mg/kg as a single daily dose) for 3 days. Because the efficacy of erythromycin therapy is approximately 80% for both of these conditions, a second course may be required, and follow-up of infants is recommended. A diagnosis of *C trachomatis* infection in an infant should prompt treatment of the mother and her sexual partner(s). The need for treatment of infants can be avoided by screening pregnant females to detect and treat *C trachomatis* infection before delivery.

An association between orally administered erythromycin and infantile hypertrophic pyloric stenosis (IHPS) has been reported in infants younger than 6 weeks. The risk of IHPS after treatment with other macrolides (eg, azithromycin and clarithromycin) is unknown, although IHPS has been reported after use of azithromycin. Because confirmation of erythromycin as a contributor to cases of IHPS will require additional investigation and because alternative therapies are not as well studied, the American Academy of Pediatrics continues to recommend use of erythromycin for treatment of diseases caused by *C trachomatis*. Physicians who prescribe erythromycin to newborn infants should inform parents about the signs and potential risks of developing IHPS. Cases of pyloric stenosis after use of oral erythromycin or azithromycin should be reported to MedWatch (see MedWatch, p 957). Topical therapy is unnecessary and does not prevent development of chlamydial pneumonia (see Chlamydial Infections, p 284). Infants born to mothers known to have untreated chlamydial infection are at high risk of infection; however, prophylactic antimicrobial treatment is not indicated, because the efficacy of such treatment is unknown. Infants should be monitored clinically to ensure appropriate treatment if infection develops. If adequate follow-up cannot be ensured, preemptive therapy should be considered.

Nongonococcal, Nonchlamydial Ophthalmia

Neonatal ophthalmia can be caused by many different bacterial pathogens (see Table 5.4). Silver nitrate, povidone-iodine, and erythromycin are effective for preventing nongono-coccal, nonchlamydial conjunctivitis during the first 2 weeks of life.

Administration of Neonatal Ophthalmic Prophylaxis

Before administering local prophylaxis, each eyelid should be wiped gently with sterile cotton. Two drops of a 1% silver nitrate solution or a 1-cm ribbon of antimicrobial oint-ment (0.5% erythromycin or 1% tetracycline) is placed in each lower conjunctival sac. The eyelids then should be massaged gently to spread the ointment. After 1 minute, oint-ment may be wiped away with sterile cotton. None of the prophylactic agents should be flushed from the eyes after instillation, because flushing can decrease efficacy.

Prophylaxis should be given shortly after birth. Efficacy is unlikely to be influenced by delaying prophylaxis for as long as 1 hour to facilitate parent-infant bonding. Longer delays have not been studied for efficacy. Hospitals should establish a process to ensure that infants are given prophylaxis appropriately.

Table 5.4. Major and Minor Etiologies in Ophthalmia Neonatorum

Etiology of Ophthalmia Neonatorum	Proportion of Cases	Incubation Period (Days)	Severity of Conjunctivitis[a]	Associated Problems
Chlamydia trachomatis	2%–40%	5–12	+	Pneumonitis 3 wk–3 mo (see Chlamydial Infec-tions, p 284)
Neisseria gonorrhoeae	Less than 1%	2–5	+++	Disseminated infection (see Gonococcal Infec-tions, p 356)
Other bacterial microbes[b]	30%–50%	5–14	+	Variable
Herpes simplex virus	Less than 1%	6–14	+	Disseminated infection, meningoencephalitis (see Herpes simplex, p 432); keratitis and ulceration also possible
Chemical	Varies with silver nitrate use	1	+	...

[a] + indicates mild; +++, severe.
[b] Includes skin, respiratory, vaginal and gastrointestinal tract pathogens such as *Staphylococcus aureus*; *Streptococcus pneumoniae*; *Hae-mophilus influenzae*, nontypeable; group A and B streptococci; *Corynebacterium* species; *Moraxella catarrhalis*; *Escherichia coli*; *Klebsiella pneumoniae*; *Pseudomonas aeruginosa*.

APPENDIX I

Directory of Resources[a]

Organization	Telephone/Fax Number	Web site
AIDSinfo	1-800-HIV-0440 (1-800-448-0440, US) 1-301-315-2816 (Outside US) TTY: 1-888-480-3739 Fax: 1-301-315-2818	www.aidsinfo.nih.gov
American Academy of Pediatrics (AAP)	1-847-434-4000 or 1-800-433-9016 Fax: 1-847-434-8000 Publications/Customer Service: 1-866-THE-AAP1 (1-866-843-2271)	www.aap.org
American Sexual Health Association	1-919-361-8400 919-361-8425 (facsimile)	www.ashastd.org
Canadian Paediatric Society (CPS)	1-613-526-9397 Fax: 1-613-526-3332	www.cps.ca
Centers for Disease Control and Prevention (CDC)	1-800-232-4636 TTY: 888-232-6348	www.cdc.gov
24-Hour Service	1-404-639-2888	
Advisory Committee on Immunization Practices	1-404-639-8836	www.cdc.gov/vaccines/acip/index.html
Botulism case consultation and antitoxin	1-770-488-7100	
Division of Foodborne, Waterborne, and Environmental Diseases	1-404-639-1603	www.cdc.gov/ncezid/dfwed/
Division of Parasitic Diseases	1-770-488-7775 OR 1-770-488-7760	www.cdc.gov/parasites
Division of Tuberculosis Elimination	1-404-639-8120	www.cdc.gov/tb
Division of Vector-Borne Infectious Diseases	1-970-221-6400	www.cdc.gov/ncidod/dvbid/index.htm
Division of Viral Hepatitis	1-888-4-HEP-CDC (1-888-443-7232)	www.cdc.gov/hepatitis/index.htm

Directory of Resources,[a] continued

Organization	Telephone/Fax Number	Web site
Division of High-Consequence Pathogens and Pathology	1-404-639-3574	www.cdc.gov/ncezid/dhcpp/
Contact Center	1-800-CDC-INFO (1-800-232-4636)	www.cdc.gov/netinfo.htm
Drug Service (weekdays, 8 AM to 4:30 PM ET)	1-404-639-3670	www.cdc.gov/ncezid/dsr/office-director. html#drugservice
Drug Service (weekends, nights, holidays)	1-404-639-2888	www.cdc.gov/ncezid/dsr/office-director. html#drugservice
Immunization, Infectious Diseases, and other Health Information—Voice Information System	1-800-232-SHOT (1-800-232-7468)	
Influenza (seasonal) materials		www.cdc.gov/flu
Malaria Hotline	1-770-488-7788	www.cdc.gov/malaria
National Center for Immunization and Respiratory Diseases	1-404-639-8200 English Hotline: 1-800-232-4636 Spanish Hotline: 1-800-232-0233 Fax: 1-888-CDC-FAXX (1-888-232-3299)	www.cdc.gov/ncird/index.html
National Prevention Information Network	1-800-458-5231	www.cdcnpin.org
Public Inquiries	1-404-639-3534	
Publications	1-800-232-2522 Fax: 1-404-639-8828	www.cdc.gov/publications.htm#pubs
Traveler's Health Hotline and Fax	1-877-FYI-TRIP (877-394-8747) Fax (toll free): 1-888-232-3299	www.cdc.gov/travel
Vaccines and Immunizations Web Site		www.cdc.gov/vaccines
Vaccine safety information		www.cdc.gov/vaccinesafety/index.html

Directory of Resources,[a] continued

Organization	Telephone/Fax Number	Web site
Vaccine Information Statements		www.cdc.gov/vaccines/hcp/vis/index.html
VFC Operations Guide		www.cdc.gov/vaccines/programs/vfc/index.html
Voice/Fax Information Service (including international travel and immunization)	1-404-332-4555 Fax: 1-404-332-4565	www.cdc.gov/travel
Food and Drug Administration (FDA)		
Center for Biologics Evaluation and Research	1-888-463-6332	www.fda.gov
	1-301-827-2000 or 1-800-835-4709	www.fda.gov/cber
Center for Drug Evaluation and Research	1-301-827-4570	www.fda.gov/cder
Division of Special Pathogen and Immunologic Drug Products	1-301-796-1600 Fax: 1-301-827-2475	
Safety Report on products presented to the Pediatric Advisory Committee		www.fda.gov/PedDrugSafety
HIV/AIDS Office of Special Health Issues	1-301-827-4460	www.fda.gov/oashi/aids/hiv.html
New Pediatric Labeling Information Database		www.fda.gov/NewPedLabeling
Pediatric Studies Characteristics Database		www.fda.gov/PedStudies
Vaccines, Blood, and Biologics		www.fda.gov/BiologicsBloodVaccines/default.htm
MedWatch	1-800-FDA-1088 (1-800-332-1088) Fax: 1-800-FDA-0178 (1-800-332-0178)	www.fda.gov/medwatch
Vaccine Adverse Event Reporting System (VAERS)	1-800-822-7967	www.fda.gov/cber/vaers/vaers.htm
Vaccine Package Inserts		www.fda.gov/BiologicsBloodVaccines/Vaccines/ApprovedProducts/ucm093830.htm

Directory of Resources,[a] continued

Organization	Telephone/Fax Number	Web site
Immunization Action Coalition (IAC)	1-651-647-9009 Fax: 1-651-647-9131	www.immunize.org
Infectious Diseases Society of America (IDSA)	1-703-299-0200 Fax: 1-703-299-0204	www.idsociety.org
Institute of Medicine (IOM)	1-202-334-2352	www.iom.edu
Institute for Vaccine Safety		www.vaccinesafety.edu
National Institutes of Health (NIH)	1-301-496-4000	www.nih.gov
National Institute of Allergy and Infectious Diseases (NIAID)	1-301-496-5717 or toll-free: 1-866-284-4107	www.niaid.nih.gov
AIDS Therapies Resource Guide		www.niaid.nih.gov/labsandresources/resources/ atrg/Pages/default.aspx
National Library of Medicine	1-888-346-3656	www.nlm.nih.gov
National Network for Immunization Information (NNii)	1-702-200-0201 Fax: 1-409-772-5208	www.immunizationinfo.org
National Resource Center for Safety and Health in Child Care		www.nrckids.org
National Vaccine Injury Compensation Program (for information on filing claims)	1-800-338-2382	www.hrsa.gov/vaccinecompensation/index.html
National Vaccine Program Office (NVPO)	1-202-690-5566	www.hhs.gov/nvpo/
Parents of Kids with Infectious Diseases (PKIDS)		www.pkids.org
Pediatric Branch, National Cancer Institute	1-301-496-4256 1-877-624-4878	http://pediatrics.cancer.gov/
Pediatric Infectious Diseases Society	1-703-299-6764 Fax: 1-703-299-0473	www.pids.org

Directory of Resources,[a] continued

Organization	Telephone/Fax Number	Web site
Sociedad Latinoamericana de Infectologia Pediátrica (SLIPE)		www.slipe.org
Vaccine Education Center of the Childdren's Hospital of Pennsylvania		www.vaccine.chop.edu
Voices for Vaccines		www.voicesforvaccines.org
Women, Children, and HIV		www.womenchildrenhiv.org/
World Health Organization (WHO)	(+41 22) 791 21 11 Fax: (+41 22) 791 31 11	www.who.int

[a]Internet addresses and telephone/fax numbers are current at the time of publication.

APPENDIX II

Codes for Commonly Administered Pediatric Vaccines/Toxoids and Immune Globulins

Immune Globulin	Separately report the administration with code 96372	Manufacturer	Brand	ICD-9-CM[a] / ICD-10-CM[a]
90375	Rabies immune globulin (RIG), human, for intramuscular and/or subcutaneous use	Novartis	HyperRAB S/D	V04.5[b] / Z20.3[b]
90376	Rabies immune globulin, heat treated (RIG-HT), human, for intramuscular and/or subcutaneous use	Sanofi Pasteur	IMOGAM Rabies-HT	V04.5[b] / Z20.3[b]
90378	Respiratory syncytial virus immune globulin (RSV-IGIM), for intramuscular use, 50 mg, each	MedImmune	Synagis	V04.82[c]

Vaccine	Separately report the administration with codes 90460–90461 or 90471–90474 [Please see table below]	Manufacturer	Brand	ICD-9-CM[a] / ICD-10-CM[a]	Number of Vaccine Components
90630	Influenza virus vaccine, quadrivalent (IIV4), split virus, preservative free, for intradermal use	✓	✓	V04.81/Z23	1
90633	Hepatitis A vaccine (HepA), pediatric/adolescent dosage, 2 doses, for intramuscular use	GlaxoSmithKline Merck	HAVRIX VAQTA	V05.3/Z23	1
90644	Meningococcal conjugate vaccine, serogroups C & Y and *Haemophilus influenzae* type b vaccine, tetanus toxoid conjugate (Hib-MenCY-TT), 4-dose schedule, when administered to children 2-15 months of age, for intramuscular use	GlaxoSmithKline	MenHibrix	V06.8/Z23	2
90647	*Haemophilus influenzae* type b vaccine (Hib), PRP-OMP conjugate, 3 doses, for intramuscular use	Merck	PedvaxHIB	V03.81/Z23	1
90648	*Haemophilus influenzae* type b vaccine (Hib), PRP-T conjugate, 4 doses, for intramuscular use	Sanofi Pasteur GlaxoSmithKline	ActHIB	V03.81/Z23	1

Commonly Administered Pediatric Vaccines/Toxoids and Immune Globulins, continued

Vaccine	Separately report the administration with codes 90460–90461 or 90471–90474 [Please see table below]	Manufacturer	Brand	ICD-9-CM[a]/ ICD-10-CM[a]	Number of Vaccine Components
90649	Human papillomavirus vaccine, types 6, 11, 16, 18 quadrivalent (HPV4), 3-dose schedule, for intramuscular use	Merck	GARDASIL	V04.89/Z23	1
90650	Human papillomavirus vaccine, types 16 and 18, bivalent (HPV2), 3-dose schedule, for intramuscular use	GlaxoSmithKline	CERVARIX	V04.89/Z23	1
90651	Human papillomavirus vaccine types 6, 11, 16, 18, 31, 33, 45, 52, 58, nonavalent (HPV), 3 dose schedule, for intramuscular use	✔	✔	V04.89/Z23	1
90655	Influenza virus vaccine, trivalent (IIV3), split virus, preservative free, for children 6–35 months of age, for intramuscular use	Sanofi Pasteur	Fluzone No Preservative Pediatric	V04.81/Z23	1
90656	Influenza virus vaccine, trivalent (IIV3), split virus, preservative free, when administered to 3 years of age and above, for intramuscular use	Merck Sanofi Pasteur Novartis GlaxoSmithKline	AFLURIA Fluzone No Preservative Fluvirin FLUARIX	V04.81/Z23	1
90657	Influenza virus vaccine, trivalent (IIV3), split virus, 6–35 months dosage, for intramuscular use	Sanofi Pasteur	Fluzone	V04.81/Z23	1
90658	Influenza virus vaccine, trivalent(IIV3), split virus, 3 years and older dosage, for intramuscular use	Merck GlaxoSmithKline Sanofi Pasteur Novartis	AFLURIA FLULAVAL Fluzone Fluvirin	V04.81/Z23 V04.81/Z23	1

Commonly Administered Pediatric Vaccines/Toxoids and Immune Globulins, continued

Vaccine	Separately report the administration with codes 90460–90461 or 90471–90474 [Please see table below]	Manufacturer	Brand	ICD-9-CM[a]/ ICD-10-CM[a]	Number of Vaccine Components
90670	Pneumococcal conjugate vaccine, 13-valent(PCV13), for intramuscular use	Pfizer	PREVNAR 13	V03.82/Z23	1
90672	Influenza virus vaccine, quadrivalent (LAIV), live, intranasal use	MedImmune	FluMist Quadrivalent	V04.81/Z23	1
90675	Rabies vaccine, for intramuscular use	Sanofi Pasteur Novartis	IMOVAX RabAvert	V04.5[b] / Z20.3[b]	1
90680	Rotavirus vaccine, pentavalent (RV5), 3-dose schedule, live, for oral use	Merck	RotaTeq	V04.89/Z23	1
90681	Rotavirus vaccine, human, attenuated (RV1), 2-dose schedule, live, for oral use	GlaxoSmithKline	ROTARIX	V04.89/Z23	1
90685	Influenza virus vaccine, quadrivalent (IIV4), split virus, preservative-free, for children 6–35 months of age, for intramuscular use	Sanofi Pasteur	Fluzone Quadrivalent	V04.89/Z23	1
90686	Influenza virus vaccine, quadrivalent (IIV4), split virus, preservative free, when administered to 3 years of age and above, for intramuscular use	Sanofi Pasteur GlaxoSmithKline	Fluzone Quadrivalent FLUARIX Quadrivalent	V04.89/Z23	1
90687	Influenza virus vaccine, quadrivalent (IIV4), split virus, 6–35 months dosage, for intramuscular use	Sanofi Pasteur	Fluzone Quadrivalent	V04.89/Z23	1
90688	Influenza virus vaccine, quadrivalent (IIV4), split virus, 3 years and older dosage, for intramuscular use	Sanofi Pasteur GlaxoSmithKline	Fluzone Quadrivalent FLULAVAL Quadrivalent	V04.89/Z23	1

Commonly Administered Pediatric Vaccines/Toxoids and Immune Globulins, continued

Vaccine	Separately report the administration with codes 90460–90461 or 90471–90474 [Please see table below]	Manufacturer	Brand	ICD-9-CM[a]/ ICD-10-CM[a]	Number of Vaccine Components
90696	Diphtheria, tetanus toxoids, and acellular pertussis vaccine and inactivated poliovirus vaccine (DTaP-IPV), when administered to children 4 years through 6 years of age, for intramuscular use	GlaxoSmithKline	KINRIX	V06.3/Z23	4
90697	Diphtheria, tetanus toxoids, acellular pertussis vaccine, inactivated poliovirus vaccine, Haemophilus influenza type b PRP-OMP conjugate vaccine, and hepatitis B vaccine (DTaP-IPV-HibHepB), for intramuscular use	✔	✔	V06.8/Z23	6
90698	Diphtheria, tetanus toxoids, acellular pertussis vaccine, Haemophilus influenzae type b, and inactivated poliovirus vaccine (DTaP-IPV/Hib), for intramuscular use	Sanofi Pasteur	Pentacel	V06.8/Z23	5
90700	Diphtheria, tetanus toxoids, and acellular pertussis vaccine (DTaP), when administered to children younger than 7 years, for intramuscular use	Sanofi Pasteur GlaxoSmithKline	DAPTACEL INFANRIX	V06.1/Z23	3
90702	Diphtheria and tetanus toxoids, adsorbed (DT) when administered to children younger than 7 years, for intramuscular use	Sanofi Pasteur	Diphtheria and Tetanus Toxoids Adsorbed	V06.5/Z23	2
90707	Measles, mumps, and rubella virus vaccine (MMR), live, for subcutaneous use	Merck	M-M-R II	V06.4/Z23	3
90710	Measles, mumps, rubella, and varicella vaccine (MMRV), live, for subcutaneous use	Merck	ProQuad	V06.8/Z23	4
90713	Poliovirus vaccine (IPV), inactivated, for subcutaneous or intramuscular use	Sanofi Pasteur	IPOL	V04.0/Z23	1

Commonly Administered Pediatric Vaccines/Toxoids and Immune Globulins, continued

Vaccine	Separately report the administration with codes 90460–90461 or 90471–90474 [Please see table below]	Manufacturer	Brand	ICD-9-CMª/ ICD-10-CMª	Number of Vaccine Components
90714	Tetanus and diphtheria toxoids adsorbed (Td), preservative free, when administered to people 7 years of age or older, for intramuscular use	Sanofi Pasteur	Tenivac	V06.5/Z23	2
90715	Tetanus, diphtheria toxoids and acellular pertussis vaccine (Tdap), when administered to people 7 years of age or older, for intramuscular use	Sanofi Pasteur GlaxoSmithKline	ADACEL BOOSTRIX	V06.1/Z23	3
90716	Varicella virus vaccine (VAR), live, for subcutaneous use	Merck	VARIVAX	V05.4/Z23	1
90723	Diphtheria, tetanus toxoids, acellular pertussis vaccine, hepatitis B, and inactivated poliovirus vaccine (DTaP-Hep B-IPV), for intramuscular use	GlaxoSmithKline	PEDIARIX	V06.8/Z23	5
90732	Pneumococcal polysaccharide vaccine, 23-valent (PPSV23), adult or immunosuppressed patient dosage, when administered to 2 years or older, for subcutaneous or intramuscular use	Merck	PNEUMOVAX 23	V03.82/Z23	1
90733	Meningococcal polysaccharide vaccine, serogroups A, C, Y, W-135, quadrivalent (MenACWY or MPSV4), for subcutaneous use	Sanofi Pasteur	Menomune	V03.89/Z23	1
90734	Meningococcal conjugate vaccine, serogroups A, C, Y and W-135 quadrivalent (MenACWY or MCV4), for intramuscular use	Sanofi Pasteur Novartis	Menactra Menveo	V03.89/Z23	1
90740	Hepatitis B vaccine (HepB), dialysis or immunosuppressed patient dosage, 3 dose, for intramuscular use	Merck	RECOMBIVAX HB	V05.3/Z23	1

Commonly Administered Pediatric Vaccines/Toxoids and Immune Globulins, continued

Vaccine	Separately report the administration with codes 90460–90461 or 90471–90474 [Please see table below]	Manufacturer	Brand	ICD-9-CM[a]/ ICD-10-CM[a]	Number of Vaccine Components
90743	Hepatitis B vaccine (HepB), adolescent, 2 doses, for intramuscular use	Merck	RECOMBIVAX HB	V05.3/Z23	1
90744	Hepatitis B vaccine (HepB), pediatric/adolescent dosage, 3 doses, for intramuscular use	Merck GlaxoSmithKline	RECOMBIVAX HB ENERGIX-B	V05.3/Z23	1
90746	Hepatitis B vaccine (HepB), adult dosage, for intramuscular use	Merck GlaxoSmithKline	RECOMBIVAX HB ENERGIX-B	V05.3/Z23	1
90747	Hepatitis B vaccine (HepB), dialysis or immunosuppressed patient dosage, 4 doses, for intramuscular use	GlaxoSmithKline	ENERGIX-B	V05.3/Z23	1
90749	Unlisted vaccine or toxoid				

Immunization Administration Codes

Immunization Administration Through Age 18 With Counseling

| | | | Please See ICD Manual |

90460   Immunization administration (IA) through 18 years of age via any route of administration, with counseling by physician or other qualified health care professional; first vaccine/toxoid component (Do not report with 90471 or 90473)

+90461   IA, through 18 years of age via any route of administration, with counseling by physician or other qualified health care professional; each additional vaccine/toxoid component (Report with 90460)

^CPT 2013 manual has defined an "**other qualified healthcare profession-al**" as one who is qualified by education and training, licensure/regulation, and facility privileging who performs a professional service within his/her scope of practice and independently reports that service. These professionals are distinct from "clinical staff." A **clinical staff** member is a person who works under the supervision of a physician or other qualified healthcare professional and who is allowed by law, regulation and facility policy to perform or assist in the performance of a specified professional service, but who does not individually report that professional service. Therefore, based on these new restrictions, if clinical staff alone performs vaccine counseling, you must defer to codes **90471-90474.**

Commonly Administered Pediatric Vaccines/Toxoids and Immune Globulins, continued

Immunization Administration Codes

Immunization Administration

90471	IA, one vaccine (Do not report with 90460 or 90473)
+90472	IA, each additional vaccine (Report with 90460: 90471, 90473)
90473	IA by intranasal/oral route; one vaccine (Do not report with 90460 or 90471)
+90474	IA by intranasal/oral route; each additional vaccine (Report with 90460, 90471, 90473)

^a *ICD-9-CM* guidelines indicate that immunizations administered as part of a routine well baby or child check should be reported with code **V20.2**. The codes listed above can be reported in addition to the **V20.2** code if specific payers request them. Immunizations administered in *encounters other than those for a routine well baby or child check* should be reported only with the codes listed above. When reporting vaccines administered report *ICD-10-CM* code **Z23** regardless of which vaccine is given or the reason for the encounter. If, however, an *ICD-10-CM* code is listed next to an immune globulin or vaccine, use the *ICD-10-CM* code. Note at time of publication, *ICD-10-CM* was set to be released on **October 1, 2015.**

^b For rabies reporting, it is important to also include the *ICD-9-CM* codes to describe the injuries (eg, puncture wound to leg) and the E code for the animal bite. When reporting the rabies vaccine after the *ICD-10-CM* implementation date, you will also need to report the nature of the injuries and the circumstances surrounding the injury, including type of animal along with the Z20.3 for contact with and suspected exposure to rabies

^c **For the RSV (Synagis) immune globulin, remember to also list the gestation age of the patient to support the medical necessity.**

* Vaccine pending FDA approval (**www.ama-assn.org/ama/pub/physician-resources/solutions-managing-your-practice/coding-billing-insurance/cpt/about-cpt/category-i-vaccine-codes.page?**).

+ **Denotes an add-on CPT code. Only report these codes with their appropriate primary procedure code.**

CPT Copyright 2014 American Medical Association. All rights reserved.

Developed and maintained by the American Academy of Pediatrics (AAP). For reporting purposes only. For specific vaccine recommendations, please refer to AAP policy within the *Red Book*.

APPENDIX III

National Childhood Vaccine Injury Act Reporting and Compensation Tables[a]

Vaccine	Adverse Event and Interval From Vaccination to Onset of Event	
	For Reporting[b]	For Compensation[c]
I. Tetanus toxoid-containing vaccines in any combination (eg, DTaP, DTaP-IPV, DTaP-IPV/Hib, DTP, DTP-Hib, Tdap, DT, Td, or TT)	A. Anaphylaxis or anaphylactic shock (**7 days**) B. Brachial neuritis (**28 days**) C. Any acute complication or sequela, including death, of above events that occurred within the time period prescribed (**No applicable time interval**) D. Events described in manufacturer's package insert as contraindications to the vaccine (**See package insert**)	A. Anaphylaxis or anaphylactic shock (**4 hours**) B. Brachial neuritis (**2–28 days**) C. Any acute complication or sequela, including death, of above events that occurred within the time period prescribed (**No applicable time interval**)
II. Pertussis antigen-containing vaccines in any combination (eg, DTaP, DTaP-IPV, DTaP-IPV/Hib, DTP, DTP-Hib, P, DTP-Hib)	A. Anaphylaxis or anaphylactic shock (**7 days**) B. Encephalopathy or encephalitis (**7 days**) C. Any acute complication or sequela, including death, of above events that occurred within the time period prescribed (**No applicable time interval**) D. Events described in manufacturer's package insert as contraindications to the vaccine (**See package insert**)	A. Anaphylaxis or anaphylactic shock (**4 hours**) B. Encephalopathy or encephalitis (**72 hours**) C. Any acute complication or sequela, including death, of above events that occurred within the time period prescribed (**No applicable time interval**)
III. Measles, mumps, and rubella virus-containing vaccines in any combination (eg, MMR, MMRV, MR, M, R)	A. Anaphylaxis or anaphylactic shock (**7 days**) B. Encephalopathy or encephalitis (**15 days**) C. Any acute complication or sequela, including death, of above events that occurred within the time period prescribed (**No applicable time interval**) D. Events described in manufacturer's package insert as contraindications to the vaccine (**See package insert**)	A. Anaphylaxis or anaphylactic shock (**4 hours**) B. Encephalopathy or encephalitis (**5–15 days**) C. Any acute complication or sequela, including death, of above events that occurred within the time period prescribed (**No applicable time interval**)

National Childhood Vaccine Injury Act Reporting and Compensation Tables,[a] continued

Vaccine	Adverse Event and Interval From Vaccination to Onset of Event	
	For Reporting[b]	For Compensation[c]
IV. Rubella virus-containing vaccines in any combination (eg, MMR, MMRV, MR, R)	A. Chronic arthritis (42 days) B. Any acute complication or sequela, including death, of above event that occurred within the time period prescribed (No applicable time interval) C. Events described in manufacturer's package insert as contraindications to the vaccine (See package insert)	A. Chronic arthritis (7–42 days) B. Any acute complication or sequela, including death, of above event that occurred within the time period prescribed (No applicable time interval)
V. Measles virus-containing vaccines in any combination (eg, MMR, MMRV, MR, M)	A. Thrombocytopenic purpura (30 days) B. Vaccine-strain measles viral infection in an immunodeficient recipient (6 months) C. Any acute complication or sequela, including death, of above events that occurred within the time period prescribed (No applicable time interval) D. Events described in manufacturer's package insert as contraindications to the vaccine (See package insert)	A. Thrombocytopenic purpura (7–30 days) B. Vaccine-strain measles viral infection in an immunodeficient recipient (6 months) C. Any acute complication or sequela, including death, of above events that occurred within the time period prescribed (No applicable time interval)

National Childhood Vaccine Injury Act Reporting and Compensation Tables,ᵃ continued

Vaccine	Adverse Event and Interval From Vaccination to Onset of Event	
	For Reportingᵇ	**For Compensationᶜ**
VI. Polio live virus-containing vaccines (eg, OPV)	A. Paralytic polio — in a nonimmunodeficient recipient **(30 days)** — in an immunodeficient recipient **(6 months)** — in a vaccine-associated community case **(No applicable time interval)** B. Vaccine-strain polio viral infection — in a nonimmunodeficient recipient **(30 days)** — in an immunodeficient recipient **(6 months)** — in a vaccine-associated community case **(No applicable time interval)** C. Any acute complication or sequela, including death, of above events that occurred within the time period prescribed **(No applicable time interval)** D. Events described in manufacturer's package insert as contraindications to the vaccine **(See package insert)**	A. Paralytic polio — in a nonimmunodeficient recipient **(30 days)** — in an immunodeficient recipient **(6 months)** — in a vaccine-associated community case **(No applicable time interval)** B. Vaccine-strain polio viral infection — in a nonimmunodeficient recipient **(30 days)** — in an immunodeficient recipient **(6 months)** — in a vaccine-associated community case **(No applicable time interval)** C. Any acute complication or sequela, including death, of above events that occurred within the time period prescribed **(No applicable time interval)**
VII. Polio inactivated-virus containing vaccines in any combination (eg, IPV, DTaP-IPV, DTaP-IPV/Hib)	A. Anaphylaxis or anaphylactic shock **(7 days)** B. Any acute complication or sequela, including death, of above event that occurred within the time period prescribed **(No applicable time interval)** C. Events described in manufacturer's package insert as contraindications to the vaccine **(See package insert)**	A. Anaphylaxis or anaphylactic shock **(0–4 hours)** B. Any acute complication or sequela, including death, of above event that occurred within the time period prescribed **(No applicable time interval)**

National Childhood Vaccine Injury Act Reporting and Compensation Tables,[a] continued

Vaccine	Adverse Event and Interval From Vaccination to Onset of Event	
	For Reporting[b]	For Compensation[c]
VIII. Hepatitis B antigen-containing vaccines in any combination (eg, HBV, HAV-HBV)	A. Anaphylaxis or anaphylactic shock (7 days) B. Any acute complication or sequela, including death, of above event that occurred within the time period prescribed (No applicable time interval) C. Events described in manufacturer's package insert as contraindications to the vaccine (See package insert)	A. Anaphylaxis or anaphylactic shock (0–4 hours) B. Any acute complication or sequela, including death, of above event that occurred within the time period prescribed (No applicable time interval)
IX. *Haemophilus influenzae* type b (conjugate vaccines) in any combination (eg, Hib, DTaP-IPV/Hib, Hib-MenCY)	Events described in manufacturer's package insert as contraindications to the vaccine (See package insert)	No condition specified for compensation
X. Varicella vaccine in any combination (eg, VZV, MMRV)	Events described in manufacturer's package insert as contraindications to the vaccine (See package insert)	No condition specified for compensation
XI. Rotavirus vaccine	Events described in manufacturer's package insert as contraindications to the vaccine (See package insert)	No condition specified for compensation
XII. Pneumococcal conjugate vaccines (eg, PCV7, PCV13)	Events described in manufacturer's package insert as contraindications to the vaccine (See package insert)	No condition specified for compensation
XIII. Hepatitis A vaccine in any combination (eg, HAV, HAV-HBV)	Events described in manufacturer's package insert as contraindications to the vaccine (See package insert)	No condition specified for compensation
XIV. Trivalent influenza vaccine (eg, TIV, LAIV)	Events described in manufacturer's package insert as contraindications to the vaccine (See package insert)	No condition specified for compensation

National Childhood Vaccine Injury Act Reporting and Compensation Tables,[a] continued

Vaccine	Adverse Event and Interval From Vaccination to Onset of Event	
	For Reporting[b]	For Compensation[c]
XV. Meningococcal vaccine (eg, MCV4, MPSV4, Hib-MenCY)	Events described in manufacturer's package insert as contraindications to the vaccine **(See package insert)**	No condition specified for compensation
XVI. Human papillomavirus vaccine (eg, HPV4, HPV2)	Events described in manufacturer's package insert as contraindications to the vaccine **(See package insert)**	No condition specified for compensation
XVII. Any new vaccine recommended by the Centers for Disease Control and Prevention for routine administration to children, after publication by Secretary, HHS of a notice of coverage.	Events described in manufacturer's package insert as contraindications to the vaccine **(See package insert)**	No condition specified for compensation

DTaP indicates diphtheria and tetanus toxoids and acellular pertussis vaccine; IPV, inactivated poliovirus vaccine; Hib, *Haemophilus influenzae* type b vaccine; DTP, diphtheria and tetanus toxoids and pertussis; Tdap, tetanus and diphtheria toxoids and pertussis vaccine for adolescent/adult use; DT, diphtheria and tetanus toxoids vaccine; Td, tetanus and diphtheria toxoids vaccine for adolescent/adult use; TT, tetanus toxoid vaccine; MMR, measles-mumps-rubella vaccine; MMRV, measles-mumps-rubella-varicella vaccine; MR, measles-rubella vaccine; M, measles vaccine; R, rubella vaccine; OPV, oral poliovirus vaccine; HBV, hepatitis B virus vaccine; HAV, hepatitis A virus vaccine; VZV, varicella-zoster virus vaccine; PCV, pneumococcal conjugate vaccine; TIV, trivalent inactivated influenza vaccine; LAIV, live-attenuated influenza vaccine; MCV, meningococcal conjugate vaccine; MPSV, meningococcal polysaccharide vaccine; HPV, quadrivalent or bivalent human papillomavirus vaccines; HHS, Health and Human Services.

[a] Effective date March 13, 2014.

[b] Taken from the Reportable Events Table (RET), which lists conditions reportable by law (42 USC § 300aa-25) to the Vaccine Adverse Event Reporting System (VAERS), including conditions found in the manufacturer's package insert. In addition, individuals are encouraged to report **any** clinically significant or unexpected events (even if you are not certain the vaccine caused the event) for **any** vaccine, whether or not it is listed on the RET. Manufacturers also are required by regulation (21 CFR 600.80) to report to the VAERS program all adverse events made known to them for any vaccine. VAERS reporting forms and information can be obtained by calling 1-(800) 822-7967 or from the VAERS Web site (**http://vaers.hhs.gov**).

[c] Taken from the Vaccine Injury Table (VIT) used in adjudication of claims filed with the National Vaccine Injury Compensation Program (VICP) on or after July 22, 2011 (42 CFR 100.3(a)). Claims filed for a condition with onset outside the designated time intervals or a condition not included in the Table may be compensable as a non-Table injury, provided they are filed within the statute of limitations period (42 USC § 300aa-16(a)) and meet other eligibility requirements. Information on filing a claim can be obtained by calling 1-(800) 338-2382 or through the VICP Web site (**www.hrsa.gov/vaccinecompensation**).

······················
APPENDIX IV

Nationally Notifiable Infectious Diseases in the United States

Nationally notifiable infectious diseases are those that public health officials from state and territorial public health departments voluntarily report to the Centers for Disease Control and Prevention (CDC). Notifiable disease data are based on data collected at the state, territorial, and local levels as a result of legislation and regulations in those jurisdictions that require health care providers, medical laboratories, and other entities to submit health-related data on reportable conditions to public health departments. Notifiable disease surveillance helps federal, state, and local public health monitor the occurrence and spread of disease across the nation and to evaluate prevention and control measures, among other purposes. To ensure consistency, national public health surveillance case definitions are established and used for each disease. The Council of State and Territorial Epidemiologists (CSTE), with advice from the CDC, reviews the list of nationally notifiable infectious diseases on an annual basis and may recommend that a disease be added or deleted from the list or that a case definition be revised. The current list is included in Table 1. Provisional data are published weekly and finalized data are published annually in the *Morbidity and Mortality Weekly Report* and the *Summary of Notifiable Diseases, United States*, respectively.

Because the list of reportable diseases and conditions is determined by state or territorial law and varies by jurisdiction, health care providers are strongly encouraged to obtain specific reporting requirements from the appropriate local, state, or territorial public health department, including the timeliness required for case reporting. Case reporting to local, state or territorial public health officials provides them the information needed to investigate these diseases or conditions and to implement prevention and control strategies, among other purposes.

If a reportable disease or condition meets the criteria for a nationally notifiable condition, the state or territorial health department will submit a case notification to the CDC. The timeliness of case notifications sent to CDC from the state or territory CDC varies by condition, and notifications are summarized on the CDC National Notifiable Diseases Surveillance System Web site (**wwwn.cdc.gov/nndss/document/NNC_2015_Notification_Requirements_By_Category.pdf**).
Notifications are categorized as:

1. **Immediate, extremely urgent:** The state/territorial health department must notify the CDC by phone within 4 hours of a case meeting the notification criteria, followed by submission of an electronic case notification to CDC by the next business day (eg, paralytic poliomyelitis; SARS-associated coronavirus; smallpox; anthrax attributable to an intentional release, unrecognized source, or naturally occurring source resulting in serious illness).

2. **Immediate, urgent:** The state/territorial health department must notify the CDC by phone within 24 hours of a case meeting the notification criteria, followed by submission of an electronic case notification in the next regularly scheduled electronic transmission (eg, measles, rubella, diphtheria, yellow fever, novel influenza A virus infection, brucellosis, naturally occurring anthrax).

3. **Standard:** The state/territorial health department must submit electronic case notification within the next reporting cycle (eg, mumps, pertussis, tuberculosis, shigellosis).

Table 1. Infectious Diseases Designated as Notifiable at the National Level—United States, 2015[1]

Anthrax

Arboviral diseases, neuroinvasive and nonneuroinvasive
- California serogroup virus diseases
- Chikungunya virus disease
- Eastern equine encephalitis virus disease
- Powassan virus disease
- St. Louis encephalitis virus disease
- West Nile virus disease
- Western equine encephalitis virus disease

Babesiosis

Botulism
- Foodborne
- Infant
- Wound and other unspecified

Brucellosis

Campylobacteriosis

Chancroid

Chlamydia trachomatis infection

Cholera

Coccidioidomycosis

Congenital syphilis

Cryptosporidiosis

Cyclosporiasis

Dengue virus infections
- Dengue fever
- Dengue hemorrhagic fever
- Dengue shock syndrome
- Dengue-like syndrome
- Severe dengue

Diphtheria

Ehrlichiosis and Anaplasmosis
- *Anaplasma phagocytophilum* infection
- *Ehrlichia chaffeensis* infection
- *Ehrlichia ewingii* infection
- Undetermined human ehrlichiosis/anaplasmosis

Giardiasis

Gonorrhea

Haemophilus influenzae, invasive disease

Hansen disease

Hantavirus pulmonary syndrome

Hemolytic uremic syndrome, postdiarrheal

Hepatitis A, acute

Hepatitis B, acute

Hepatitis B, chronic

Hepatitis B, perinatal infection

Hepatitis C, acute

Hepatitis C, past or present

HIV infection (AIDS has been reclassified as HIV stage III)

Influenza-associated pediatric mortality

Invasive pneumococcal disease

Legionellosis

Leptospirosis

Listeriosis

Lyme disease

Malaria

Measles

Meningococcal disease

Mumps

Novel influenza A virus infections

Pertussis

Plague

Poliomyelitis, paralytic

Poliovirus infection, nonparalytic

Psittacosis

Q fever

Rabies, animal

Rabies, human

Rubella

Rubella, congenital syndrome

Salmonellosis

Severe acute respiratory syndrome-associated coronavirus disease

Shiga toxin-producing *Escherichia coli*

Shigellosis

Smallpox

Spotted fever rickettsiosis

Streptococcal toxic-shock syndrome

Syphilis
- Syphilis, primary
- Syphilis, secondary
- Syphilis, latent (including early latent, late latent, and latent syphilis of unknown duration)
- Neurosyphilis
- Late syphilis with clinical manifestations other than neurosyphilis
- Syphilitic stillbirth

Tetanus

Toxic shock syndrome (other than streptococcal)

Trichinellosis

Tuberculosis

Tularemia

Typhoid fever

Vancomycin-intermediate *Staphylococcus aureus* and vancomycin-resistant *Staphylococcus aureus*

Varicella

Varicella deaths

Vibriosis

Viral hemorrhagic fever
- Crimean-Congo hemorrhagic fever virus
- Ebola virus
- Lassa virus
- Lujo virus
- New World arenavirus:
  - Guanarito virus
  - Junin virus
  - Machupo virus
  - Sabia virus

Yellow fever

[1] wwwn.cdc.gov/nndss/script/ConditionList.aspx?Type=0&Yr=2015

....
Appendix V

Guide to Contraindications and Precautions to Immunizations, 2015

A **contraindication** to vaccination is a condition in a patient that increases the risk of a serious adverse reaction and for whom this increased risk of an adverse reaction outweighs the benefit of the vaccine. A vaccine should **not** be administered when a contraindication is present. The only contraindication applicable to all vaccines is a history of anaphylaxis to a previous dose or to a vaccine component, unless the patient has undergone desensitization. A **precaution** is a condition in a recipient that might increase the risk or seriousness of an adverse reaction or complicate making another diagnosis because of a possible vaccine-related reaction. A precaution also may exist for conditions that might compromise the ability of the vaccine to produce immunity (eg, administering measles vaccine to a person with passive immunity to measles from a blood transfusion).

This information is based on recommendations of the Advisory Committee on Immunization Practices (ACIP) of the Centers for Disease Control and Prevention (CDC) and the Committee on Infectious Diseases of the American Academy of Pediatrics (AAP). Sometimes, these recommendations vary from those in the manufacturers' package inserts. For more detailed information, physicians should consult published recommendations of the ACIP and AAP, manufacturers' package inserts, and **www.cdc.gov/vaccines/recs/vac-admin/contraindications.htm.** These guidelines, originally issued in 1993, have been updated to give recommendations as of 2015 (on the basis of information available as of January 2015).

Guide to Contraindications and Precautions to Immunizations, 2015

Vaccine	Contraindications	Precautions[a]	Not Contraindications (Vaccines May Be Given if Indicated)
General for all vaccines (DTaP, DT, Td, Tdap, IPV, MMR, MMRV, Hib, pneumococcal, meningococcal, hepatitis B, varicella, hepatitis A, influenza, zoster, rotavirus, HPV)	Anaphylactic reaction to a vaccine contraindicates further doses of that vaccine Anaphylactic reaction to a vaccine constituent contraindicates the use of vaccines containing that substance	Moderate or severe illnesses with or without fever Latex allergy[b]	Mild to moderate local reaction (soreness, redness, swelling) after a dose of an injectable antigen. Low-grade or moderate fever after a previous vaccine dose. Mild acute illness with or without low-grade fever. Current antimicrobial therapy. Convalescent phase of illnesses. Preterm birth (same dosage and indications as for healthy, full-term infants); hepatitis B is the exception for healthy, full-term infants; hepatitis B is the exception (see Hepatitis B, p 400). Recent exposure to an infectious disease. History of penicillin or other nonspecific allergies or fact that relatives have such allergies. Pregnancy of mother or household contact. Unimmunized household contact. Immunodeficient household contact. Breastfeeding (nursing infant OR lactating mother). Lack of a physical examination.
DTaP	Severe allergic reaction (eg, anaphylaxis) after a previous dose or to a vaccine component Encephalopathy (eg, coma, decreased level of consciousness, or prolonged seizures) not attributable to another identifiable cause) within 7 days of administration of previous dose of DTaP/DTP	Moderate or severe illnesses with or without fever Progressive neurologic disorder, including infantile spasms, uncontrolled epilepsy, progressive encephalopathy; generally have DTaP immunization deferred temporarily until neurologic status clarified and stabilized; children with a stable neurologic condition (well-controlled seizures, a history of seizure disorder, cerebral palsy) should receive pertussis immunization on schedule.	Family history of seizures[c] Family history of sudden infant death syndrome. Family history of an adverse event after DTaP/DTP administration. Fever <105°F (<40°C), fussiness, or mild drowsiness after a previous dose of DTP/DTaP

Guide to Contraindications and Precautions to Immunizations, 2015, continued

Vaccine	Contraindications	Precautions[a]	Not Contraindications (Vaccines May Be Given if Indicated)
		Temperature of 40.5°C (105°F) or greater within 48 h after immunization with a previous dose of DTaP/DTP Collapse or shock-like state (hypotonic-hyporesponsive episode) within 48 h of receiving a previous dose of DTaP/DTP Seizures within 3 days of receiving a previous dose of DTaP/DTP[c] Persistent inconsolable crying lasting 3 h, within 48 h of receiving a previous dose of DTaP/DTP GBS within 6 wk after a dose[d] History of Arthus-type hypersensitivity reaction after a previous dose of a tetanus- or diphtheria toxoid- containing vaccine (defer for 10 years after last tetanus toxoid-containing vaccine)	
DT, Td	Severe allergic reaction (eg, anaphylaxis) after a previous dose or to a vaccine component	Moderate or severe acute illness with or without fever GBS 6 wk or less after previous dose of tetanus toxoid-containing vaccine History of Arthus-type hypersensitivity reaction after a previous dose of tetanus or diphtheria toxoid-containing vaccine; defer vaccination until at least 10 years have elapsed since the last tetanus toxoid-containing vaccine (see DTaP)	

Guide to Contraindications and Precautions to Immunizations, 2015, continued

Vaccine	Contraindications[a]	Precautions[a]	Not Contraindications (Vaccines May Be Given if Indicated)
IPV	Severe allergic reaction (eg, anaphylaxis) after a previous dose or to a vaccine component, including neomycin, streptomycin, or polymyxin B	Moderate or severe acute illness with or without fever Pregnancy	Previous receipt of one or more doses of oral polio vaccine.
MCV4 and MPSV4	Severe allergic reaction (eg, anaphylaxis) after a previous dose or to a vaccine component, including diphtheria toxoid, or to dry natural rubber latex	Moderate or severe acute illness with or without fever	
MMR[e,f]	Severe allergic reaction (eg, anaphylaxis) after a previous dose or to a vaccine component, including neomycin or gelatin Pregnancy Known severe immunodeficiency (eg, from hematologic and solid tumors, receipt of chemotherapy, long-term immunosuppressive therapy,[k] congenital immunodeficiency, or patients with HIV infection who are severely immunocompromised[l]	Moderate or severe acute illness with or without fever Recent (within 11 mo, depending on product and dose) Immune Globulin administration[g] (see Table 1.10, p 39) Thrombocytopenia or history of thrombocytopenic purpura[g] Tuberculosis or positive PPD test result[h] Personal or family history of seizure if provided as MMRV (consider giving as separate administrations [MMR+V]	Simultaneous tuberculin skin testing or IGRA.[i] Breastfeeding. Pregnancy of mother of recipient. Immunodeficient family member or household contact. Nonanaphylactic reactions to gelatin or neomycin. Allergy to egg Recipient is a female of child-bearing age

Guide to Contraindications and Precautions to Immunizations, 2015, continued

Vaccine	Contraindications	Precautions[a]	Not Contraindications (Vaccines May Be Given if Indicated)
Hib	Severe allergic reaction (eg, anaphylaxis) after a previous dose or to a vaccine component Age <6 wk	... Moderate or severe acute illness with or without fever	...
Hepatitis B	Severe allergic reaction (eg, anaphylaxis) after a previous dose or to a vaccine component	Moderate or severe acute illness with or without fever Preterm birth[j]	Pregnancy. Autoimmune disease (eg, systemic lupus erythematosis or rheumatoid arthritis).
PCV13 and PPSV23	Severe allergic reaction (eg, anaphylaxis) to previous dose or vaccine component, including for PCV7, PCV13, or any vaccine containing diphtheria-toxoid	Moderate or severe acute illness with or without fever	History of invasive pneumococcal disease or pneumonia.
Tdap	Severe allergic reaction (eg, anaphylaxis) to a previous dose or vaccine component History of encephalopathy (eg, coma, prolonged seizures) within 7 days of administration of a pertussis vaccine that is not attributable to another identifiable cause	Moderate or severe acute illness, with or without fever GBS 6 wk or less after previous dose of a tetanus toxoid vaccine Progressive neurologic disorder; uncontrolled epilepsy; or progressive encephalopathy until the condition has stabilized History of Arthus-type hypersensitivity reaction (see DTaP)	Temperature 105°F (40.5°C) or greater within 48 h after DTP/ DTaP immunization not attributable to another cause. Collapse or shock-like state (hypotonic hyporesponsive episode) within 48 h after DTP/DTaP immunization. Persistent crying lasting 3 h or longer; occurring within 48 h after DTP/DTaP immunization. Convulsions with or without fever, occurring within 3 days after DTP/DTaP immunization. History of extensive limb swelling reaction after pediatric DTP/DTaP or Td immunization that was not an Arthus-type hypersensitivity reaction.

Guide to Contraindications and Precautions to Immunizations, 2015, continued

Vaccine	Contraindications	Precautions[a]	Not Contraindications (Vaccines May Be Given if Indicated)
			Stable neurologic disorder, including well-controlled seizures, history of seizure disorder, and cerebral palsy.
			Brachial neuritis.
			Latex allergy other than anaphylactic allergies (eg, a history of contact to latex gloves). The tip and rubber plunger of the Boostrix needleless syringe contain latex. This Boostrix product should not be administered to adolescents with a history of a severe (anaphylactic) allergy to latex but may be administered to people with less severe allergies (eg, contact allergy to latex gloves). The Boostrix single-dose vial and Adacel preparations do not contain latex.
			Pregnancy.
			Breastfeeding.
			Immunosuppression, including people with human immunodeficiency virus infection (Tdap poses no known safety concern for immunosuppressed people; the immunogenicity of Tdap in people with immunosuppression has not been studied and could be suboptimal).
			Intercurrent minor illness.
			Antimicrobial use.

Guide to Contraindications and Precautions to Immunizations, 2015, continued

Vaccine	Contraindications	Precautions[a]	Not Contraindications (Vaccines May Be Given if Indicated)
Varicella[e]	Pregnancy Severe allergic reaction (eg, anaphylaxis) after a previous dose or to a vaccine component (eg, neomycin or gelatin) Known severe immunodeficiency (hematologic and solid tumors, receipt of chemotherapy, long-term immunosuppressive therapy, congenital immunodeficiency, or patients with HIV infection who are severely immunocompromised[l])	Moderate or severe acute illness with or without fever Recent Immune Globulin administration (see Table 1.10, p 39) Family history of immunodeficiency[m] Infection with HIV[l] Personal or family history of seizure if provided as MMRV (consider giving as separate administrations [MMR+V])	Pregnancy of mother of recipient. Immunodeficiency in a household contact. Household contact with HIV.
Hepatitis A	Severe allergic reaction (eg, anaphylaxis) after a previous dose or to a vaccine component (ie, to 2-phenoxyethanol or alum)	Moderate or severe acute illness with or without fever	…
Influenza (inactivated)	Severe allergic reaction (eg, anaphylaxis) to a previous dose or vaccine component including egg protein For RIV, severe allergic reaction (eg, anaphylaxis) after a previous dose of RIV or to a vaccine component. RIV does not contain egg protein	Moderate or severe acute illness with or without fever GBS within 6 wk after a previous influenza immunization People who experience only hives with exposure to eggs may receive RIV (if age 19–49 y) or, with additional safety precautions, may receive IIV[n]	Pregnancy. Nonsevere (eg, contact) allergy to latex, thimerosal, or egg. Current administration of coumadin or theophylline.

Guide to Contraindications and Precautions to Immunizations, 2015, continued

Vaccine	Contraindications	Precautions[a]	Not Contraindications (Vaccines May Be Given if Indicated)
Influenza (live-attenuated)	Severe allergic reaction (eg, anaphylaxis) to a previous dose or vaccine component (including egg protein) Pregnancy Conditions for which the ACIP recommends against use, but which are not contraindications in the vaccine package insert: immune suppression, certain chronic medical conditions such as: asthma, diabetes, heart or kidney disease, or pregnancy Children 2 through 4 y of age with health care professional or medical history documentation of wheezing within the past 12 mo; receiving aspirin;	Moderate or severe acute illness with or without fever GBS within 6 wk after a previous influenza immunization Receipt of specific antivirals (ie, amantadine, rimantadine, zanamavir, or oseltamavir) 48 hours before vaccination. Avoid use of these antiviral drugs for 14 days after vaccination	Health care providers that see patients with chronic diseases or altered immunocompetence (an exception is providers for severely immunocompromised patients requiring care in a protected environment). Breastfeeding. Contacts of people with chronic disease or altered immunocompetence (an exception is contacts of severely immunocompromised patients requiring care in a protected environment).
Rotavirus	Severe allergic reaction (eg, anaphylaxis) after a previous dose or to a vaccine component Severe combined immune deficiency (SCID) History of previous episode of intussusception	Moderate or severe acute illness, with or without fever Altered immunocompetence other than SCID Chronic gastrointestinal disease Spina bifida or bladder exstrophy	Breastfeeding. Immunodeficient family member or household contact. Preterm infants. Pregnant household contacts.

Guide to Contraindications and Precautions to Immunizations, 2015, continued

Vaccine	Contraindications	Precautions[a]	Not Contraindications (Vaccines May Be Given if Indicated)
HPV	Severe allergic reaction (eg, anaphylaxis) after a previous dose or to a vaccine component	Moderate or severe acute illness with or without fever Pregnancy	Administration to people with minor acute illnesses. Immunosuppression. Previous equivocal or abnormal papanicolau test. Known HPV infection. Breastfeeding. History of genital warts.
Zoster	Severe allergic reaction after any component of the vaccine Known severe immunodeficiency (hematologic or solid tumors, receipt of chemotherapy, congenital immunodeficiency, or patients with HIV infection who are severely immunocompromised, and long-term immunosuppressive therapy Pregnancy	Moderate or severe acute illness with or without fever Receipt of specific antivirals (ie, acyclovir, famciclovir, or valacyclovir) 24 hours before vaccination: avoid use of these antiviral drugs for 14 days after vaccination.	Mild acute illness. Therapy with low-dose methotrexate (≤0.4 mg/kg/week), azathioprine (≤3.0 mg/kg/day) or 6-mercaptopurine (≤1.5 mg/kg/day) for treatment of rheumatoid arthritis, psoriasis, polymyositis, sarcoidosis, inflammatory bowel disease, or other conditions. Health-care providers of patients with chronic diseases or altered immunocompetence. Contacts of patients with chronic diseases or altered immunocompetence. Unknown or uncertain history of varicella in a US-born person.

DTaP indicates diphtheria and tetanus toxoids and acellular pertussis; DT, pediatric diphtheria-tetanus toxoid; Td, adult tetanus-diphtheria toxoid; Tdap, tetanus toxoid, reduced diphtheria toxoid, and acellular pertussis; IPV, inactivated poliovirus; MMR, measles-mumps-rubella; MMRV, measles-mumps-rubella-varicella; Hib, *Haemophilus influenzae type* b; HPV, human papillomavirus; DTP, diphtheria and tetanus toxoids and pertussis; GBS, Guillain-Barré syndrome; MCV4, tetravalent (A, C, Y, W-135) meningococcal conjugate vaccine; MPSV4, tetravalent meningococcal polysaccharide vaccine; HIV, human immunodeficiency virus; PPD, purified protein derivative (tuberculin); PCV7, pneumococcal conjugate vaccine; PPSV23, pneumococcal polysaccharide vaccine.

[a] The events or conditions listed as precautions, although not contraindications, should be reviewed carefully. The benefits and risks of administering a specific vaccine to a person under the circumstances should be considered. If the risks are believed to outweigh the benefits, the immunization should be withheld; if the benefits are believed to outweigh the risks (eg, during an outbreak or foreign travel), the immunization should be given. Whether and when to administer DTaP to children with proven or suspected underlying neurologic disorders should be decided on an individual basis.

[b] If a person reports a severe (anaphylactic) allergy to latex, vaccines supplied in vials or syringes that contain natural rubber should not be administered unless the benefits of immunization outweigh the risks of an allergic reaction to the vaccine. For latex allergies other than anaphylactic allergies (eg, a history of contact allergy to latex gloves), vaccines supplied in vials or syringes that contain dry natural rubber or latex can be administered.

Guide to Contraindications and Precautions to Immunizations, 2015, continued

Vaccine	Contraindications	Precautions[a]	Not Contraindications (Vaccines May Be Given if Indicated)

[c] Acetaminophen given before administering DTaP and thereafter every 4 hours for 24 hours should be considered for children with a personal or family (ie, siblings or parents) history of seizures.

[d] The decision to give additional doses of DTaP should be made on the basis of consideration of the benefit of further immunization versus the risk of recurrence of GBS. For example, completion of the primary series in children is justified.

[e] The administration of multiple live-virus vaccines within 28 days (4 weeks) of one another if not given on the same day may result in suboptimal immune response. Data substantiate this risk for MMR and possibly varicella vaccine, which should, therefore, be given on the same day or more than 4 weeks apart.

[f] Egg allergy is not considered a contraindication or precaution.

[g] The decision to immunize should be made on the basis of consideration of the benefits of immunity to measles, mumps, and rubella versus the risk of recurrence or exacerbation of thrombocytopenia after immunization or from natural infections of measles or rubella. In most instances, the benefits of immunization will be much greater than the potential risks and justify giving MMR, particularly in view of the even greater risk of thrombocytopenia after measles or rubella disease. However, if a previous episode of thrombocytopenia occurred in temporal proximity to immunization, not giving a subsequent dose may be prudent.

[h] A theoretical basis exists for concern that measles vaccine might exacerbate tuberculosis. Consequently, before administering MMR to people with untreated active tuberculosis, initiating antituberculosis therapy is advisable.

[i] Measles immunization may suppress tuberculin reactivity temporarily. MMR vaccine may be given after, or on the same day as, tuberculin skin testing. If MMR has been given recently, postpone the tuberculin skin test until 4 to 6 weeks after administration of MMR. The effect of MMR on IGRA test results is unknown.

[j] For infants weighing less than 2 kg at birth and born to hepatitis B surface antigen (HBsAg)-negative mothers, initiation of immunization should be delayed until just before hospital discharge if the infant weighs 2 kg or more, or until approximately 2 months of age, when other routine immunizations are given, to improve response. All infants weighing less than 2 kg born to HBsAg-positive mothers should receive immunoprophylaxis (Hepatitis B Immune Globulin and vaccine) beginning as soon as possible after birth, followed by appropriate postimmunization testing and receipt of 3 doses of hepatitis B vaccine.

[k] Immunosuppressive steroid dose is considered to be 2 or more weeks of daily receipt of 20 mg prednisone or the equivalent. Vaccination should be deferred for at least 1 month after discontinuation of such therapy.

[l] Absence of severe immunosuppression is defined as CD4 percentages of $\geq$15% for $\geq$6 months for people 5 years or younger and CD4+ T-lymphocyte percentages $\geq$15% and CD4+ T-lymphocyte counts $\geq$200 lymphocytes/cubic mm for $\geq$6 months for people older than 5 years. When only CD4+ T-lymphocyte counts or CD4+ T-lymphocyte percentages are available for those older than 5 years, the assessment of severe immunosuppression can be on the basis of the CD4+ T-lymphocyte values (count or percentage) that are available. When CD4+ T-lymphocyte percentages are not available for those 5 years or younger, the assessment of severe immunosuppression can be on the basis of age-specific CD4+ T-lymphocyte counts at the time they were measured (ie, absence of severe immunosuppression is defined as $\geq$6 months above age-specific CD4+ T-lymphocyte count criteria: CD4+ T-lymphocyte count >750 lymphocytes/mm^3 while 12 months or younger, and CD4+ T-lymphocyte counts $\geq$500 while age 1 through 5 years).

[m] Varicella vaccine should not be administered to a person who has a family history of congenital or hereditary immunodeficiency in parents or siblings unless that person's immune competence has been substantiated clinically or verified by a laboratory.

[n] Refer to influenza chapter.

APPENDIX VI

Prevention of Infectious Disease From Contaminated Food Products[1]

Foodborne diseases are associated with significant morbidity and mortality in people of all ages. The Centers for Disease Control and Prevention (CDC) estimates that there are 48 million cases of foodborne illness in the United States each year, resulting in approximately 128 000 hospitalizations and 3000 deaths.[2,3] Young children, the elderly, and immunocompromised people are especially susceptible to illnesses and complications caused by many of the organisms associated with foodborne illness. Norovirus is the most common cause of foodborne illness in the United States.

The Foodborne Disease Active Surveillance Network (FoodNet) of the CDC's Emerging Infections Program conducts active, population-based surveillance in 10 states for all laboratory-confirmed infections with select enteric pathogens transmitted commonly through food. The FoodNet program conducts surveillance for illnesses attributable to *Campylobacter* species, *Listeria monocytogenes*, *Salmonella enterica*, Shiga toxin-producing *Escherichia coli* (STEC) O157:H7, *Shigella* species, *Vibrio* species, and *Yersinia enterocolitica* (since 1996); *Cryptosporidium* species and *Cyclospora* species since 1997; and STEC non-O157 since 2000. FoodNet also conducts surveillance for hemolytic-uremic syndrome (HUS), a complication of STEC infection. Additional information about FoodNet can be found at **www.cdc.gov/foodnet/**.

Outbreak surveillance provides insights into the causes of foodborne illness, types of implicated foods, and settings where transmission occurs. The CDC collects data on foodborne disease outbreaks submitted from all states and territories (**www.cdc.gov/foodsafety/fdoss/index.html**). Public health, regulatory, and agricultural professionals can use this information when creating targeted control strategies and to support efforts to promote safe food preparation practices among food industry employees and the public. Data on foodborne disease outbreaks are available online through the Foodborne Outbreak Online Database (**wwwn.cdc.gov/foodborneoutbreaks**).

Four general rules should be followed to maintain safety of foods:

1. **Clean:** Wash hands and surfaces thoroughly and often.
2. **Separate:** Do not cross contaminate.
3. **Chill:** Refrigerate foods promptly.
4. **Cook:** Cook food to the proper temperature.

The following preventive measures can be implemented to decrease the risk of infection and disease from specific foods.

---

[1]Centers for Disease Control and Prevention. Diagnosis and management of foodborne illnesses: a primer for physicians. *MMWR Recomm Rep.* 2004;53(RR–4):1–33

[2]Centers for Disease Control and Prevention. Surveillance for foodborne disease outbreaks—United States, 2008. *MMWR Morb Mortal Wkly Rep.* 2011;60(35):1197–1202

[3]Centers for Disease Control and Prevention. Surveillance for foodborne disease outbreaks—United States, 1998-2008. *MMWR Morb Mortal Wkly Rep.* 2013;62(SS–2):1–34

Unpasteurized Milk and Milk Products

The American Academy of Pediatrics (AAP) endorses the use of pasteurized milk and recommends that parents be fully informed of the important risks associated with consumption of unpasteurized milk.[1] Interstate sale of unpasteurized (raw) milk and products made from unpasteurized milk (with the exception of certain cheeses) is banned by the US Food and Drug Administration (FDA). The most vulnerable populations, such as children, pregnant women, elderly people, and immunocompromised people, should not consume unpasteurized milk or products made from unpasteurized milk, including cheese, butter, yogurt, pudding, or ice cream from any species, including cows, sheep, and goats. Serious infections attributable to *S enterica*, *Campylobacter* species, *Mycobacterium bovis*, *L monocytogenes*, *Brucella* species, *E coli* O157:H7, and *Y enterocolitica* have been linked to consumption of unpasteurized milk. Although some states allow the sale of raw milk that meets specific standards (certified milk), certified raw milk has also been linked to outbreaks. In particular, a number of outbreaks of campylobacteriosis among children have been associated with school field trips to farms that include consumption of raw milk. School officials should take precautions to prevent raw milk from being served to children during educational trips. Cheeses made from unpasteurized milk also have been associated with illnesses attributable to *Brucella* species, *L monocytogenes*, *S enterica*, *Campylobacter* species, *Shigella* species, *M bovis*, and STEC.

Eggs

At-risk populations, including children, should not eat raw or undercooked eggs, unpasteurized powdered eggs, or foods that may contain raw or undercooked eggs. Ingestion of raw or improperly cooked eggs can result in severe illness attributable to *Salmonella* species. Examples of foods that may contain raw or undercooked eggs include some homemade frostings and mayonnaise, ice cream from uncooked custard, tiramisu, eggs prepared "sunny-side up," fresh Caesar salad dressing, Hollandaise sauce, cookie dough, and cake batter.

Raw and Undercooked Meat

Children should not eat raw or undercooked meat or meat products, particularly ground beef. Various raw or undercooked meat products have been associated with harmful bacteria, including with *S enterica* and *Campylobacter* species; ground beef with STEC and *Salmonella* species; hot dogs with *Listeria* species; pork with *Trichinella* species; and wild game with *Brucella* species, *Francisella* species, STEC, and *Trichinella* species. Ground meats should be cooked to an internal temperature of 160°F; roasts and steaks should be cooked to an internal temperature of 145°F, and poultry should be cooked to an internal temperature of 165°F. Use of a food thermometer is the only sure way of knowing that food has reached a high enough temperature to destroy bacteria. Color is not a reliable indicator that ground beef patties have been cooked to a temperature high enough to kill harmful bacteria. Knives, cutting boards, plates, and other utensils used for raw meats should not be used for preparation of fresh fruits or vegetables until they have been cleaned properly (see Web sites at end of this Appendix for details).

---

[1]American Academy of Pediatrics, Committee on Infectious Diseases and Committee on Nutrition. Consumption of raw or unpasteurized milk and milk products by pregnant women and children. *Pediatrics.* 2014;133(1):175–179

Unpasteurized Juices

Children should drink only pasteurized fruit juice or juice that has been otherwise treated to eliminate harmful bacteria. Consumption of packaged fruit juices that have not undergone pasteurization or a comparable treatment have been associated with foodborne illness attributable to *E coli* O157:H7 and *S enterica*. To identify a packaged juice that has not undergone pasteurization or a comparable treatment, consumers should look for a warning statement that the product has not been pasteurized.

Seed Sprouts

The FDA and the CDC have reaffirmed health advisories that people who are at high risk of severe foodborne disease, including children, people with compromised immune systems, and the elderly, should avoid eating raw seed sprouts.[1] Raw seed sprouts have been associated with outbreaks of illness attributable to *S enterica* and STEC.

Fresh Fruits and Vegetables and Raw Nuts

Many fresh fruits and vegetables have been associated with disease attributable to *Cryptosporidium* species, *Cyclospora* species, norovirus, hepatitis A virus, *Giardia* species, STEC, *S enterica*, *L monocytogenes*, and *Shigella* species. Raw shelled nuts, commercially processed vegetable snacks, spinach, lettuce, tomatoes, melons, basil, and alfalfa sprouts all have been associated with outbreaks of salmonellosis. Nuts that have been roasted or otherwise treated can help minimize the risk of foodborne illness. Washing can decrease but not eliminate contamination of fresh fruits and vegetables. Knives, cutting boards, utensils, and plates used for raw meats should not be used for preparation of fresh fruits or vegetables until the utensils have been cleaned properly (see Web sites at end of this Appendix for details).

Raw Shellfish and Fish

Children should not eat raw shellfish. Raw shellfish, including mussels, clams, oysters, scallops, and other mollusks, can carry many pathogens, including norovirus, *Vibrio* species, and hepatitis A virus as well as toxins (see Appendix VII, p 1008). *Vibrio* species contaminating raw shellfish may cause severe disease in people with liver disease or other conditions associated with decreased immune function. Some experts caution against children ingesting raw fish, which has been associated with transmission of parasites (*Anisakis simplex*, *Diphyllobothrium latum*, and others).

Honey

Children younger than 1 year should not be given honey. Honey has been shown to contain spores of *Clostridium botulinum*. Light and dark corn syrups are manufactured under sanitary conditions, and although the manufacturer cannot ensure that any product will be free of *C botulinum* spores, no cases associated with corn syrup have been documented.

---

[1] For additional information, contact the FDA Food Information Line at 1-800-FDA-4010 or the US Department of Agriculture at 1-800-535-4555 or 1-202-720-2791 or visit the following Web sites: **www.usda.gov** and **www.foodsafety.gov.**

Powdered Infant Formula

For many reasons, infants should be fed human milk rather than infant formula whenever possible. Powdered infant formula is not commercially sterile and has been associated with severe illnesses attributable to *Cronobacter* species and *S enterica*. Although such infections are rare, if infant formula must be used, caregivers can reduce the risk of infection by choosing sterile, liquid formula products rather than powdered products. This may be particularly important for those at greatest risk of severe infection, such as neonates and infants with immunocompromising conditions. Additionally, the World Health Organization (WHO) has issued guidance to improve the safety of powdered infant formula.[1] Recommendations include reconstituting powdered infant formula with water at or above 70°C (158°F), which is high enough to inactivate *Cronobacter* and other pathogens. Although some cite concerns about the risk of burns and possible loss of vitamin C associated with this procedure, health authorities in several countries have issued guidance for powdered infant formula preparation based on the WHO recommendations. Additional recommendations include careful bottle cleaning and handling of prepared formula to minimize the risk of cross-contamination.

Food Irradiation[2]

No single process to eliminate all foodborne diseases exists. However, irradiation of food can be an effective tool in helping to control foodborne pathogens. Irradiation involves exposing food briefly to ionizing radiation (eg, gamma rays, x-rays, or high-voltage electrons). More than 40 countries worldwide, including the United States, have approved the use of irradiation for various types of foods. In addition, every governmental and professional organization that has reviewed the efficacy and safety of food irradiation has endorsed its use. Meat, spices, shell eggs, seeds for sprouting, and some produce items may be irradiated for sale in the United States. The risk of foodborne illness in children could be decreased significantly with the routine consumption of irradiated meat, poultry, and produce.

Detailed information on food safety issues and practices, including steps consumers can take to protect themselves, is available on the following Web sites:

* **www.foodsafetyworkinggroup.gov**
* **www.foodsafety.gov**
* **www.fightbac.org**
* **www.cdc.gov/foodsafety**

---

[1] **www.who.int/foodsafety/publications/micro/pif_guidelines.pdf**

[2] **www.fsis.usda.gov/wps/portal/fsis/topics/food-safety-education/get-answers/ food-safety-fact-sheets/production-and-inspection/irradiation-resources/ irradiation-resources**

·····················
APPENDIX VII

Clinical Syndromes Associated With Foodborne Diseases[1,2]

Foodborne disease results from consumption of contaminated foods or beverages and causes morbidity and mortality in children and adults. The epidemiology of foodborne disease is complex and dynamic because of many pathogens, the variety of disease manifestations, the increasing prevalence of immunocompromised children and adults, dietary habits changes, and trends toward centralized food production and widespread distribution.

Consideration of a foodborne etiology is important in any patient with a gastrointestinal tract illness and patients with certain acute neurologic findings. A detailed history is invaluable, with important questions including time of onset and duration of symptoms, history of recent travel or antimicrobial use, and presence of blood or mucus in stool. To aid in diagnosis, foodborne disease syndromes have been categorized by incubation period, duration, predominant symptoms, causative agent, and foods commonly associated with specific etiologic agents (food vehicles) (see Table 1, p 1009). Diagnosis can be confirmed by laboratory testing of stool, vomitus, or blood, depending on the causative agent. Sporadic (ie, non-outbreak associated) cases account for the majority of foodborne illnesses. In localized outbreaks that affect individuals who shared a common meal, the incubation period can be estimated. However, in more widely dispersed outbreaks and in sporadic cases, the incubation period typically is unknown.

An outbreak should be considered when 2 or more people who have ingested the same food develop an acute illness characterized by nausea, vomiting, diarrhea, or neurologic signs or symptoms. If an outbreak is suspected, local or state public health officials should be notified immediately so they can work with local health care professionals, coordinate laboratory testing, and conduct epidemiologic investigations to potentially curtail the outbreak.

---

[1]Centers for Disease Control and Prevention. Surveillance for foodborne-disease outbreaks—United States, 2008. *MMWR Morb Mortal Wkly Rep.* 2011;60(35):1197–1202. Additional information can be found at **www.cdc.gov/foodsafety** and **www.fsis.usda.gov/wps/portal/fsis/home**

[2]Centers for Disease Control and Prevention. Surveillance for foodborne disease outbreaks-United States, 1998–2008. *MMWR Morb Mortal Wkly Rep.* 2013;62(SS-2):1–34

Table 1. Clinical Syndromes Associated With Foodborne Diseases

Clinical Syndrome	Incubation Period	Causative Agents	Commonly Associated Vehicles[a]
Nausea and vomiting	<1–6 h	*Staphylococcus aureus* (preformed enterotoxins, A through V but excluding F)	Ham, poultry, beef, cream-filled pastries, potato and egg salads, mushrooms, unpasteurized cheese
	<1–6 h	Preformed *Bacillus cereus* (emetic toxin cereulide)	Rice
	1h	Heavy metals (copper, tin, cadmium, iron, zinc)	Acidic beverages, metallic container
		Vomitoxin	Foods made from grains such as wheat, corn, barley
Flushing, dizziness, burning of mouth and throat, palpitations, headache, gastrointestinal tract symptoms, urticaria	<1 h	Histamine (scombroid)	Fish (bluefish, bonita, mackerel, mahi-mahi, marlin, tuna, skipjack, and many other fish types)
Diverse array of neurologic, gastrointestinal tract, and cardiovascular symptoms. Facial and extremity paresthesias and hot/cold temperature sensation reversal are characteristic	<1–6 h	Ciguatera toxin	Large reef-dwelling carnivorous fish (eg, amberjack, barracuda, grouper, snapper)
Paresthesias, nausea, vomiting, diarrhea		Carchatoxins	Shark (particularly liver)
Gastrointestinal tract and neurologic symptoms including paresthesia	According to CDC (**www.bt.cdc.gov/agent/brevetoxin/casedef.asp**) can be up to 18 h	Neurotoxic shellfish toxin (brevetoxin)	Shellfish (eg, mussels, oysters, clams)

Table 1. Clinical Syndromes Associated With Foodborne Diseases, continued

Clinical Syndrome	Incubation Period	Causative Agents	Commonly Associated Vehicles[a]
As above, and short-term memory loss	1 day (www.cdc. gov/mmwr/ preview/ mmwrhtml/ rr5304a1. htm and www.cdc. gov/ncidod/ dbmd/ diseaseinfo/ marinetoxins _g.htm)	Domoic acid (amnesiac shellfish toxin)	Mussels, clams
Variable (gastrointestinal tract, neurologic, chest pain, flushing)		Monosodium glutamate (MSG)	Asian food
Neurologic, including confusion, salivation, hallucinations; gastrointestinal tract manifestations	0–2 h	Mycotoxins (early onset)	Mushrooms
Neuromuscular weakness, symmetric descending paralysis, respiratory weakness, neurologic symptoms may be preceded by gastrointestinal tract manifestations	12–48 h	*Clostridium botulinum* (preformed toxin)	Home-canned vegetables, fruits and fish, salted fish, meats, bottled garlic, potatoes baked in aluminum foil, cheese sauce; honey-associated infantile botulism has a longer incubation period[b]
Neurologic, constipation	3–30 days	*Clostridium botulinum*	Honey
Neurologic, gastrointestinal tract	<30 min	Tetrodotoxin (ascending paralysis)	Puffer fish
	0.5–3 h	Paralytic shellfish toxins (saxitoxins, etc)	Shellfish (clams, mussels, oysters, scallops, other mollusks)

Table 1. Clinical Syndromes Associated With Foodborne Diseases, continued

Clinical Syndrome	Incubation Period	Causative Agents	Commonly Associated Vehicles[a]
Abdominal cramps and watery diarrhea, vomiting	8–16 h	B cereus	Meats, stews, gravies, vanilla sauce
	8–16 h	Clostridium perfringens	Meat, poultry, gravy, dried or precooked foods
	16–72 h	Norovirus	Shellfish, salads, ice, cookies, water, sandwiches, fruit, leafy vegetables, ready-to-eat foods handled by infected food worker
	1–3 days	Rotavirus	Salads, fruits, ready-to-eat foods handled by infected food worker
Abdominal cramps, watery diarrhea	1–4 days	Enterotoxigenic Escherichia coli	Seafood, herbs, fruits, vegetables, water, often acquired abroad—"traveler's diarrhea"
	1–5 days	Vibrio cholerae O1 and O139	Shellfish (including crabs and shrimp), fish, water
		V cholerae non-O1	Shellfish, especially oysters
	1–14 days	Cyclospora species	Raspberries, vegetables, water
	2–14 days	Cryptosporidium species	Vegetables, fruits, milk, water
	1–4 wk	Giardia intestinalis	Water, ready-to-eat foods handled by infected food worker
Diarrhea, fever, abdominal cramps, blood and mucus in stools	12–72 h	Salmonella species (non-typhoidal)	Poultry; pork; beef; eggs; dairy products, including ice cream; raw vegetables (eg, alfalfa sprouts); fruit, including unpasteurized juices; peanut butter
	1–3 days	Shigella species	Lettuce-based salads, potato and egg salads, salsas, dips, and oysters, ready-to-eat foods handled by infected food worker
	2–4 wk	Amebiasis (Entameba histolytica)	Fecally contaminated food or water

Table 1. Clinical Syndromes Associated With Foodborne Diseases, continued

Clinical Syndrome	Incubation Period	Causative Agents	Commonly Associated Vehicles[a]
Bloody diarrhea, abdominal cramps, HUS	1–10 days	Shiga toxin-producing *E coli*	Beef (hamburger); raw milk; roast beef; salami; salad dressings; lettuce; game meats, unpasteurized juices, including apple cider; sprouts; water
Febrile diarrhea or, especially in older children, abdominal pain resembling that of appendicitis	1–11 days	*Yersinia enterocolitica*	Pork chitterlings, tofu, milk
Hepatorenal failure, watery diarrhea	6–48 h	Mushroom toxins (late onset)	Mushrooms (especially *Amanita* species)
Chronic, urgent diarrhea	Varied	Brainerd diarrhea (unknown agent)	Unknown vehicle, but may include unpasteurized milk, and contaminated water
Other extraintestinal manifestations	Varied, up to months	*Brucella* species	Goat cheese, queso fresco, raw milk, meats
Fever, chills, headache, pharyngitis, arthralgia		Group A streptococcus	Egg and potato salad
Fever, malaise, anorexia, jaundice	15–50 days	Hepatitis A virus	Shellfish, raw produce (eg, strawberries, lettuce, green onions)
Meningoencephalitis, sepsis	3–70 days	*Listeria monocytogenes*	Soft cheeses, raw milk, hot dogs, cole slaw, ready-to eat delicatessen meats, produce (eg, sprouts, cantaloupe)
Muscle soreness and pain	Varied, up to weeks	*Trichinella spiralis*	Wild game, pork, meat
Fever, lymphadenopathy, neurologic (reactivation)	5–23 days	*Toxoplasma gondii*	Undercooked meat (especially pork, lamb, and game meat), fruits, vegetables, raw shellfish
Sepsis, meningitis		*Cronobacter (Enterobacter) sakazakii*	Powdered infant formula
		Salmonella species	Powdered infant formula

Table 1. Clinical Syndromes Associated With Foodborne Diseases, continued

Clinical Syndrome	Incubation Period	Causative Agents	Commonly Associated Vehicles[a]
Seizures, behavioral disturbances, and other neurologic signs and symptoms		Taenia solium (neurocysticercosis)	Food contaminated with feces from a human carrier of adult pork tapeworm
Epigastric discomfort, abdominal pain, cholangitis, obstructive jaundice, pancreatitis		Clonorchis sinensis (liver fluke) Opisthorchis species (liver fluke)	Fish Fish
Guillain-Barré syndrome (ascending paralysis)	Varied	Campylobacter species Shigella Enteroinvasive E coli Yersinia enterocolitica Vibrio parahaemolyticus	Poultry, raw milk, water Fecally contaminated food or water Vegetables, hamburger, raw milk Pork chitterlings, tofu, raw milk Fish, shellfish
Postdiarrheal hemolytic-uremic syndrome (acute renal failure, hemolytic anemia, thrombocytopenia)	Varied	Shiga toxin-producing E coli (especially serotype O157:H7) Shigella dysenteriae 1 and rarely other Shiga toxin-producing Enterobacteriaceae	Beef (hamburger); raw milk; roast beef; salami; salad dressings; lettuce; unpasteurized juices, including apple cider; alfalfa and radish sprouts; water Water, milk, other contaminated food
Reactive arthritis	Varied	Campylobacter species Salmonella species Shigella species Yersinia enterocolitica	Poultry, raw milk, water Poultry, pork, beef, eggs, dairy products, including ice cream; vegetables (alfalfa sprouts and fresh produce); fruit, including unpasteurized juices; peanut butter Fecally contaminated food or water Pork chitterlings, tofu, raw milk

[a]List of vehicles in several categories is not exhaustive, because any number of foods can be contaminated; current online literature may be helpful to sort through commonly associated vehicles.
[b]Honey has been implicated in infant botulism but follows ingestion of spores with production of toxin in the intestine; longer incubation period.

••••••••••••••••••••••••••
APPENDIX VIII

Diseases Transmitted by Animals (Zoonoses)

Important zoonoses that may be encountered in North America are listed in this Appendix and reviewed in the *Red Book* (see disease-specific chapters in Section 3 for further information). Morbidity resulting from selected zoonotic diseases in the United States is reported annually by the Centers for Disease Control and Prevention (see "Summary of Notifiable Diseases" at **www.cdc.gov/mmwr/mmwr_nd/**). Information also can be obtained via the Web site of the National Center for Emerging and Zoonotic Infectious Diseases (**www.cdc.gov/ncezid/about-ncezid.html**) or through the main Centers for Disease Control and Prevention Web site (**www.cdc.gov**).

Table 1. Diseases Transmitted by Animals

Disease and/or Organism	Common Animal Sources/Reservoirs	Vector or Modes of Transmission
Bacterial Diseases		
Aeromonas species	Aquatic animals, especially shellfish	Wound infection, ingestion of contaminated food or water
Anthrax (*Bacillus anthracis*)	Herbivores (cattle, goats, sheep)	Direct contact with infected animals or their carcasses, or contact with products from infected animals (eg, meat, hides or hair) contaminated with *B anthracis* spores
Bartonellosis (*Bartonella* species, *Bartonella vinsonii, B vinsonii berkhoffi, B vinsonii arupensis, Bartonella koehleri, Bartonella rochalimae, Bartonella quintana*)	Dogs, cattle, cats, body lice	Bites of arthropods suspected, but evidence is lacking in many species
Brucellosis (*Brucella* species)	Cattle, goats, sheep, swine, dogs, elk, bison, deer	Direct contact with birth products, ingestion of contaminated undercooked meat or dairy products, inhalation of aerosols, contact through mucous membranes or skin wounds
Campylobacteriosis (*Campylobacter jejuni*)	Poultry, dogs (especially puppies), kittens, ferrets, hamsters, birds	Ingestion of contaminated food, water, milk, direct contact (particularly with animals with diarrhea), person-to-person (fecal-oral)
Capnocytophaga canimorsus	Dogs, rarely cats	Bites, scratches, and prolonged contact with dogs
Cat-scratch disease (*Bartonella henselae*)	Cats, infrequently other animals (less than 10%)	Scratches, bites; fleas play a role in cat-to-cat transmission (evidence for transmission from cat fleas to humans is lacking)
Erysipelothrix rhusiopathiae	Pigs, sheep, cattle, horses, birds, fish, shellfish	Direct contact with animal or contaminated animal product
Hemolytic-uremic syndrome (eg, Shiga toxin-producing *Escherichia coli*) (STEC)	Cattle, sheep, goats, deer	Ingestion of undercooked contaminated ground beef, unpasteurized milk, or other contaminated foods or water; person-to-person contact (fecal-oral); contact with infected animals or their environments; contact with animals in public settings including petting zoos and agricultural fairs (fecal-oral)

Table 1. Diseases Transmitted by Animals, continued

Disease and/or Organism	Common Animal Sources/Reservoirs	Vector or Modes of Transmission
Leptospirosis (*Leptospira* species)	Dogs, rodents, livestock, other wild animals	Contact with or ingestion of water, food, or soil contaminated with urine or fluids from infected animals, or direct contact with infected animals
Lyme disease (*Borrelia burgdorferi*)	Mice, squirrels, shrews, and other small vertebrates	Black-legged or deer tick bites (*Ixodes scapularis* or *Ixodes pacificus*)
Mycobacteriosis (*Mycobacterium marinum*, others)	Fish (and cleaning aquaria)	Skin injury or contamination of existing wound
Mycobacterium bovis and *Mycobacterium tuberculosis*	Cattle, elephants, giraffes, rhinoceroses, bison, deer, elk	*M bovis* usually is transmitted from cattle through ingestion of contaminated food and unpasteurized milk, although airborne transmission from cattle or other species is possible; *M tuberculosis* is uncommon in most nonhuman species except for elephants and primates, and it is transmitted by the airborne route
Pasteurella multocida	Cats, dogs, other animals	Bites, scratches, licks
Plague (*Yersinia pestis*)	Rodents, cats, ground squirrels, prairie dogs	Bite of rodent fleas, (especially tropical rat fleas, *Xenopsylla cheopis*), direct contact with infected animal tissues, airborne from other human or animal (eg, cat) with pneumonic plague
Q fever (*Coxiella burnetii*)	Sheep, goats, cows, cats, dogs, wild rodents, birds	Contact with excreta (birth products, urine, feces, milk) of infected animals, inhalation of pathogen-contaminated dust, ingestion of unpasteurized milk, and fomite transmission; consumption of unpasteurized milk (possible role of ticks not well defined)
Rat-bite fever (*Streptobacillus moniliformis*, *Spirillum minus*)	Rodents (especially rats, occasionally squirrels), cats, weasels, gerbils	Bites, secretions, and contaminated food, milk, and water
Relapsing fever (tickborne) (*Borrelia* species)	Wild rodents	Soft tick bites (*Ornithodoros* species)

Table 1. Diseases Transmitted by Animals, continued

Disease and/or Organism	Common Animal Sources/Reservoirs	Vector or Modes of Transmission
Salmonellosis (*Salmonella* species)	Many animals, especially poultry, turtles, frogs, lizards, snakes, salamanders, iguanas, dogs, cats, hedgehogs hamsters, mice, rats and other rodents, ferrets, other wild and domestic animals, Komodo dragons	Ingestion of contaminated food (eg meat, poultry, dairy, eggs, produce, processed foods), unpasteurized milk and other raw dairy products,, or contaminated water; contact with infected animals or their environments; animal products including dry dog and cat food and pet treats contact with fecally contaminated surfaces; person-to-person (fecal-oral)
Streptococcus iniae	Fish grown by aquaculture	Skin injury during handling of fish
Tetanus (*Clostridium tetani*)	Any animal, usually indirect via soil containing animal feces	Wound infection, skin injury or soft tissue injury with inoculation of bacteria (as from soil or a contaminated object), contaminated bites
Tularemia (*Francisella tularensis*)	Wild rabbits, hares, voles, sheep, cattle, muskrats, moles, cats, hamsters Wood tick bites (*Dermacentor andersoni*), dog tick bites (*D variabilis*), Lone-star tick bites (*Amblyomma americanum*), deerfly bites, direct contact with infected animal, ingestion of contaminated water, mechanical transmission from claws or teeth (cats), aerosolization of tissues or excreta	Ingestion of contaminated food or water; skin injury or contamination of existing wound

Table 1. Diseases Transmitted by Animals, continued

Disease and/or Organism	Common Animal Sources/Reservoirs	Vector or Modes of Transmission
Yersiniosis (*Yersinia enterocolitica, Yersinia pseudotuberculosis*)	Swine, deer, elk, horses, goats, sheep, cattle, rodents, birds, rabbits	Ingestion of contaminated food, water, or milk; rarely direct contact, person-to-person (fecal-oral)
Fungal Diseases		
Cryptococcosis (*Cryptococcus neoformans*)	Excreta of birds, particularly pigeons	Inhalation of aerosols from accumulations of bird feces
Histoplasmosis (*Histoplasma capsulatum*)	Excreta of bats, birds, particularly starlings	Inhalation of aerosols from accumulations of bat and bird feces
Ringworm/tinea corporis (*Microsporum* and *Trichophyton* species)	Cats, dogs, fowl, pigs, moles, horses, rodents, cattle, monkeys, goats	Direct contact
Parasitic Diseases		
Anisakiasis (*Anisakis* species)	Saltwater and anadromous fish	Ingestion of larvae in raw or undercooked fish (eg, sushi)
Babesiosis (several *Babesia* species)	Mice and various other rodents and small mammals; wildlife	Tick bite (in the United States, *Babesia microti* is transmitted mainly by *Ixodes scapularis*; in Europe, *Babesia divergens* is mainly transmitted by *Ixodes ricinus*); transmission via blood transfusion also can occur (rarely)
Balantidiasis (*Balantidium coli*)	Swine	Ingestion of contaminated food or water
Baylisascariasis (*Baylisascaris procyonis*)	Raccoons	Ingestion of eggs shed in raccoon feces
Cryptosporidiosis (*Cryptosporidium* species)	Domestic animals (including cattle, sheep, goats, horses, pigs, dogs, cats, birds), particularly young animals	Ingestion of contaminated water or foods, person-to-person (fecal-oral)
Cutaneous larva migrans (*Ancylostoma* species)	Dogs, cats	Penetration of skin by larvae, which develop in soil contaminated with animal feces

Table 1. Diseases Transmitted by Animals, continued

Disease and/or Organism	Common Animal Sources/Reservoirs	Vector or Modes of Transmission
Dog tapeworm (*Dipylidium caninum*)	Dogs, cats	Ingestion of fleas infected with larvae
Dwarf tapeworm (*Hymenolepis nana*)	Rodents	Ingestion of eggs from feces (contaminated food, water), person-to-person and animal-to-person (fecal-oral)
Echinococcosis, hydatid disease (*Echinococcus* species)	Dogs, foxes, possibly other carnivores, coyotes, wolves	Ingestion of eggs shed in animal feces
Fish tapeworm (*Diphyllobothrium latum*)	Saltwater and freshwater fish	Ingestion of larvae in raw or undercooked fish
Giardiasis (*Giardia intestinalis*)	Wild and domestic animals, including dogs, cats, cattle, pigs, beavers, muskrats, rats, pet rodents, rabbits, nonhuman primates	Ingestion of contaminated water or foods, person-to-person and animal-to-person (fecal-oral)
Taeniasis, beef (*Taenia saginata*)	Cattle	Ingestion of larvae in raw or undercooked beef
Taeniasis/pork tapeworm (*Taenia solium*)	Swine (intermediate host)	Ingestion of larvae in raw or undercooked meat (adult tapeworm infection)
Toxoplasmosis (*Toxoplasma gondii*)	Cats, livestock	Ingestion of oocysts from cat feces, consumption of cysts in raw or undercooked meat, contact with birth products of cats
Trichinellosis (*Trichinella spiralis* and other *Trichinella* species)	Swine, horses, bears, seals, walruses	Ingestion of larvae in raw or undercooked meat
Ocular or visceral toxocariasis (ocular or visceral larva migrans) Ocular or visceral toxocariasis (*Toxocara canis* and *Toxocara cati*)	Dogs, cats	Ingestion of eggs, usually from soil contaminated by animal feces
Chlamydial and Rickettsial Diseases		
Human ehrlichiosis (*Ehrlichia chaffeensis* and *Ehrlichia ewingii*)	Deer, dogs, gray foxes, goats	Tick bites (lone-star ticks, *Amblyomma americanum*)

Table 1. Diseases Transmitted by Animals, continued

Disease and/or Organism	Common Animal Sources/Reservoirs	Vector or Modes of Transmission
Human anaplasmosis (*Anaplasma phago-cytophilum*)	Deer, dogs, elk, wild rodents, horses, ruminants	Black-legged tick (*I scapularis*) and western black-legged tick (*I pacificus*) bites; rodents, small mammals
Psittacosis (*Chlamydophila psittaci*)	Pet birds (especially psittacine birds) and poultry	Inhalation of aerosols from feces of infected birds
Rickettsialpox (*Rickettsia akari*)	House mice	Mite bites (house mouse mite, *Lipopyssoides sanguineus*)
Rocky Mountain spotted fever (*Rickettsia rickettsii*)	Dogs, wild rodents, rabbits	Tick bites; rarely by direct contamination with infectious material from ticks (American dog tick, *Dermacentor variabilis*; Rocky Mountain wood tick, *Dermacentor andersoni*; and brown dog tick, *Rhipicephalus sanguineus*)
Rickettsia parkeri infection (Maculatum disease, American boutonneuse fever)	Unknown, perhaps small wild rodents	Gulf coast ticks, *Amblyomma maculatum*
Typhus, fleaborne endemic typhus (*Rickettsia typhi*)	Rats, opossums, cats, dogs	Rat flea feces scratched into abrasions; less common, other fleas (Oriental rat flea, *Xenopsylla cheopis*)
Typhus, louseborne epidemic typhus (*Rickettsia prowazekii*)	Flying squirrels	Person-to-person via body louse, contact with flying squirrels, their nests, or ectoparasites (role and species of ectoparasites undefined)
Viral Diseases		
Colorado tick fever	Rodents (squirrels, chipmunks)	Tick bites (Rocky Mountain wood tick, *Dermacentor andersoni*)
La Crosse	Rodents (squirrels, chipmunks)	Mosquito bites (*Ochlerotatus triseriatus*)
Eastern equine encephalitis	Birds	Mosquito bites (*Coquillettidia* species, *Ochlerotatus* species)
Western equine encephalitis	Birds	Mosquito bites (*Culex tarsalis*)
St Louis encephalitis	Birds	Mosquito bites (*Culex* species)
Venezuelan equine encephalitis	Equines	Mosquito bites (*Psorophora* species, *Ochlerotatus* species)
Powassan	Rodents (Groundhogs, squirrels, mice)	Tick bites (*Ixodes cookie, Ixodes scapularis*)
West Nile	Birds	Mosquito bites (*Culex species*)

Table 1. Diseases Transmitted by Animals, continued

Disease and/or Organism	Common Animal Sources/Reservoirs	Vector or Modes of Transmission
Tickborne encephalitis	Rodents	Tick bites (*Ixodes ricinus*, *Ixodes persulcatus*); infected milk products
Yellow fever	Nonhuman primates (Jungle and sylvatic cycles)	Mosquito bites (*Haemagogus* species, *Sabethes* species, *Aedes* species)
Japanese encephalitis	Pigs, birds	Mosquito bites (*Culex tritaeniorhynchus*)
Nipah	Bats; pigs can become infected	Close contact with bats, consumption of bat contaminated fruit/sap
Hendra	Flying foxes; horses become infected	Contact with body fluids of infected horses
Hantaviruses	Wild and peridomestic rodents	Inhalation of aerosols of infected secreta and excreta
Ebola hemorrhagic fever	Bats; primates may become infected	Contact with bats, contact with sick/dead primates
Marburg hemorrhagic fever	Bats	Contact with bats, entering caves or mines inhabited by bats
Rift Valley fever	Cattle, sheep, goats	Animal slaughter; mosquito bites
Crimean Congo hemorrhagic fever	Small rodents, farm animals	Animal slaughter; tick bites
Kyasanur forest disease/Alkhurma hemorrhagic fever	Camels, primates, possibly farm animals	Animal slaughter; tick bites
Omsk hemorrhagic fever	Muskrat	Slaughtering muskrat, tick bites
Lassa fever	Mastomys rodents	Inhalation of aerosols of infected secreta or excreta
South American arenaviruses (Junin, Machupo, Guanarito, Sabia, Chapare)	Rodents	Inhalation of aerosols of infected secreta or excreta
B virus (formerly herpesvirus simiae)	Macaque monkeys	Bite or exposure to secretions

Table 1. Diseases Transmitted by Animals, continued

Disease and/or Organism	Common Animal Sources/Reservoirs	Vector or Modes of Transmission
Lymphocytic choriomeningitis	Rodents, particularly house mice and pet hamsters (includes feeder rodents used as reptile food), guinea pigs	Direct contact, inhalation of aerosols, ingestion of food contaminated with rodent excreta, mother-to-fetus transmission, organ transplant
Rabies (Lyssavirus)	In the United States, primarily wildlife (bats, raccoons, skunks, foxes, coyotes, mongooses) or, less frequently, domestic animals (dogs, cats, cattle, horses, sheep, goats, ferrets)	Bites, rarely contact of open wounds, abrasions (including scratches), or mucous membranes with saliva or other infectious materials (eg, neural tissue)
Monkeypox	Prairie dogs, African rodents	Direct contact, bite, scratch
Influenza (H5N1)	Chickens, birds, swine	Contact with infected animals or aerosols (markets, slaughter house)
Orf (pox virus of sheep)	Sheep, goats	Contact with infected saliva
Severe acute respiratory virus (coronavirus)	Bats, civet cats, potentially other animal species	Unclear; person-to-person (respiratory, contact)

Index

Page numbers followed by "t" indicate a table. Page numbers followed by "f" indicate a figure.